Thompson & Thompson

GENETICS IN MEDICINE

Seventh Edition

Thompson & Thompson

GENETICS IN MEDICINE

Seventh Edition

Robert L. Nussbaum, MD

Holly Smith Distinguished Professor in Science and Medicine
Chief, Division of Medical Genetics
Department of Medicine and The Institute for Human Genetics
University of California, San Francisco
San Francisco, California

Roderick R. McInnes, MD, PhD, FRS(C)

University Professor
Anne and Max Tanenbaum Chair in Molecular Medicine
Professor of Pediatrics and Molecular and Medical Genetics
University of Toronto and The Hospital for Sick Children
Toronto, Ontario, Canada
Scientific Director, Institute of Genetics
Canadian Institutes of Health Research

Huntington F. Willard, PhD

Director
Institute for Genome Sciences and Policy
Vice Chancellor for Genome Sciences
Nanaline H. Duke Professor of Genome Sciences
Duke University
Durham, North Carolina

With Clinical Case Studies updated and new cases prepared by

Ada Hamosh, MD, MPH

Clinical Director
Institute of Genetic Medicine
Scientific Director, OMIM
Associate Professor, Pediatrics
Johns Hopkins University School of Medicine
Baltimore, Maryland

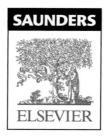

SAUNDERS

ELSEVIER

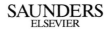

SAUNDERS
ELSEVIER

1600 John F. Kennedy Blvd.
Ste 1800
Philadelphia, PA 19103-2899

THOMPSON & THOMPSON GENETICS IN MEDICINE   ISBN: 9781416030805

Library of Congress Cataloging-in-Publication Data

Nussbaum, Robert L, 1950—
Thompson & Thompson Genetics in Medicine. — 7th ed. / Robert L. Nussbaum, Roderick R.
McInnes, Huntington F. Willard.
     p. ; cm.
     Includes bibliographical references and index.
     ISBN 978-1-4160-3080-5
  1. Medical genetics. I. McInnes, Roderick R. II. Willard, Huntington F. III. Thompson,
Margaret W. (Margaret Wilson), 1920 — Thompson & Thompson Genetics in Medicine.
IV. Title. V. Title: Genetics in medicine. VI. Title: Thompson and Thompson Genetics in
Medicine.
     [DNLM: 1. Genetics, Medical. QZ 50 N975t 2007]
     RB155.T52 2007
     616'.042—dc22   2006033374

ISBN: 978-1-4160-3080-5

Acquisitions Editor: Kate Dimock
Developmental Editor: Marybeth Thiel
Publishing Services Manager: Linda Van Pelt
Design Direction: Karen O'Keefe Owens
Cover Design Direction: Karen O'Keefe Owens

Printed in Canada

Last digit is the print number: 9 8 7 6

Preface

In their preface to the first edition of *Genetics in Medicine*, published over 40 years ago, James and Margaret Thompson wrote:

> *Genetics is fundamental to the basic sciences of preclinical medical education and has important applications to clinical medicine, public health and medical research. With recognition of the role of genetics in medicine has come the problem of providing a place for it in the undergraduate curriculum, a problem which is as yet only partly solved in most medical schools. This book has been written to introduce the medical student to the principles of genetics as they apply to medicine, and to give him (her) a background for his own reading of the extensive and rapidly growing literature in the field. If his (her) senior colleagues also find it useful, we shall be doubly satisfied.*

What was true then is even more so now as our knowledge of genetics and of the human genome is rapidly becoming an integral part of public health and the practice of medicine. This new edition of *Genetics in Medicine*, the seventh, seeks to fulfill the goals of the previous six by providing an accurate exposition of the fundamental principles of human and medical genetics. Using illustrative examples drawn from medicine, we continue to emphasize the genes and molecular mechanisms operating in human diseases.

Much has changed, however, since the last edition of this book. Completion of the Human Genome Project provides us with a catalogue of all human genes, their sequence, and an extensive, and still growing, database of human variation. Genomic information has stimulated the creation of powerful new tools that are changing human genetics research and medical genetics practice. We therefore have expanded the scope of the book to incorporate the concepts of "Personalized Medicine" into *Genetics in Medicine* by providing more examples of how genomics is being used to identify the contributions made by genetic variation to disease susceptibility and treatment outcomes.

The book is not intended to be a compendium of genetic diseases nor is it an encyclopedic treatise on human genetics and genomics in general. Rather, the authors hope that the seventh edition of *Genetics in Medicine* will provide students with a framework for understanding the field of medical genetics while giving them a basis on which to establish a program of continuing education in this area. The clinical cases, first introduced in the last edition to demonstrate and reinforce general principles of disease inheritance, pathogenesis, diagnosis, management, and counseling, continue to be an important feature of the book. We have expanded the set of cases to add more common complex disorders to the original set of cases, which comprised mostly highly informative and important disorders with mendelian inheritance. To enhance further the teaching value of the Clinical Cases, we have added an additional feature to the seventh edition: at specific points throughout the text, we provide a case number (highlighted in blue) to direct readers to the case in the Clinical Case Studies section that is relevant to the concepts being discussed at that point in the text.

Any medical or genetic counseling student, advanced undergraduate, graduate student in genetics, resident in any field of clinical medicine, practicing physician, or allied medical professional in nursing or physical therapy should find this book to be a thorough but not exhaustive (or exhausting!) presentation of the fundamentals of human genetics and genomics as applied to health and disease.

Robert L. Nussbaum, MD
Roderick R. McInnes, MD, PhD
Huntington F. Willard, PhD

Acknowledgments

The authors wish to express their appreciation and gratitude to their many colleagues who, through their ideas, suggestions, and criticisms, improved the seventh edition of *Genetics in Medicine*. In particular, we are grateful to Leslie Biesecker for sharing his knowledge and experience in molecular dysmorphology and genetics in the writing of Chapter 14, "Developmental Genetics and Birth Defects." We also thank Win Arias of the National Institutes of Health; Peter Byers and George Stamatoyannopoulos of the University of Washington; Diane Cox of the University of Alberta; Gary Cutting and David Valle of the Johns Hopkins School of Medicine; Robert Desnick of the Mount Sinai School of Medicine; Curt Harris of the National Cancer Institute; Douglas R. Higgs of the Weatherall Institute of Molecular Medicine; Katherine High of the Children's Hospital of Philadelphia; Jennifer Jennings of the Institute of Genetics of the Canadian Institutes of Health Research; Mark Kay of Stanford University; Muin Khoury of the Centers for Disease Control; Joe Clarke, Don Mahuran, Chris Pearson, Peter Ray, and Steve Scherer of the Hospital for Sick Children, Toronto; Joseph Nevins and Hutton Kearney of Duke University; John Phillips III of the Vanderbilt University School of Medicine; Jennifer Puck and Mel Grumbach of the University of California, San Francisco; Eric Shoubridge of McGill University; Richard Spielman of the University of Pennsylvania; Peter St. George-Hyslop of the University of Toronto; Lyuba Varticovski of the National Cancer Institute; Paula Waters of the University of British Columbia; Huda Zoghbi and Arthur Beaudet of the Baylor College of Medicine; and David Ledbetter and Christa Lees Martin of Emory University. We also thank the many students in the Johns Hopkins/NIH Genetic Counseling Training Program for their constructive criticisms of the previous edition during the gestation of this new edition.

We once again express our deepest gratitude to Dr. Margaret Thompson for providing us the opportunity to carry on the legacy of the textbook she created 40 years ago with her late husband, James S. Thompson. Finally, we again thank our families for their patience and understanding for the many hours we spent creating this, the seventh edition of *Genetics in Medicine*.

Contents

Chapter 1

Introduction, 1

Genetics and Genomics in Medicine, 1
Onward, 2

Chapter 2

The Human Genome and the Chromosomal Basis of Heredity, 5

The Human Genome and Its
  Chromosomes, 6
Cell Division, 13
Human Gametogenesis and Fertilization, 20
Medical Relevance of Mitosis and
  Meiosis, 22

Chapter 3

The Human Genome: Gene Structure and Function, 25

Information Content of the Human
  Genome, 25
The Central Dogma:
  DNA → RNA → Protein, 26
Gene Organization and Structure, 28
Fundamentals of Gene Expression, 30
Gene Expression in Action: The β-Globin
  Gene, 33
Gene Regulation and Changes in Activity of the
  Genome, 36
Variation in Gene Expression and its Relevance
  to Medicine, 38

Chapter 4

Tools of Human Molecular Genetics, 41

Analysis of Individual DNA and RNA
  Sequences, 41
Methods of Nucleic Acid Analysis, 48
The Polymerase Chain Reaction, 50
DNA Sequence Analysis, 53
Advanced Techniques Using Digital Image
  Capture of Fluorescence-Tagged
  Nucleotides, 55
Western Blot Analysis of Proteins, 57

Chapter 5

Principles of Clinical Cytogenetics, 59

Introduction to Cytogenetics, 59
Chromosome Abnormalities, 65
Parent-of-Origin Effects, 77
Studies of Chromosomes in Human Meiosis, 81
Mendelian Disorders with Cytogenetic Effects, 82
Cytogenetic Analysis in Cancer, 82

Chapter 6

Clinical Cytogenetics: Disorders of the Autosomes and the Sex Chromosomes, 89

Autosomal Disorders, 89
The Sex Chromosomes and Their
  Abnormalities, 98
Disorders of Gonadal and Sexual
  Development, 109

Chapter 7

Patterns of Single-Gene Inheritance, 115

Overview and Concepts, 115
Mendelian Inheritance, 118
Factors Affecting Pedigree Patterns, 119
Correlating Genotype and Phenotype, 121
Autosomal Patterns of Mendelian
  Inheritance, 122
X-Linked Inheritance, 129
Pseudoautosomal Inheritance, 135
Mosaicism, 135
Imprinting In Pedigrees, 137
Unstable Repeat Expansions, 139
Conditions that May Mimic Mendelian
  Inheritance of Single-Gene Disorders, 144
Maternal Inheritance of Disorders Caused by
  Mutations in the Mitochondrial Genome, 144
Family History as Personalized Medicine, 146

Chapter 8

Genetics of Common Disorders with Complex Inheritance, 151

Qualitative and Quantitative Traits, 152
Genetic and Environmental Modifiers of
  Single-Gene Disorders, 159

Examples of Multifactorial Traits for which
Genetic and Environmental Factors Are
Known, 160

Chapter 9

Genetic Variation in Individuals and Populations: Mutation and Polymorphism, 175

Mutation, 175
Types of Mutations and Their Consequences, 177
Human Genetic Diversity, 183
Inherited Variation and Polymorphism in
DNA, 184
Inherited Variation and Polymorphism in
Proteins, 186
Genotypes and Phenotypes in Populations, 192
Factors that Disturb Hardy-Weinberg
Equilibrium, 195
Ethnic Differences in the Frequency of Various
Genetic Diseases, 199

Chapter 10

Human Gene Mapping and Disease Gene Identification, 207

The Genetic Landscape of the Human
Genome, 207
Mapping Human Genes by Linkage
Analysis, 217
Mapping of Complex Traits, 222
From Gene Mapping to Gene Identification, 226

Clinical Case Studies Illustrating Genetic Principles, 231

Chapter 11

Principles of Molecular Disease: Lessons from the Hemoglobinopathies, 323

The Effect of Mutation on Protein Function, 323
How Mutations Disrupt the Formation of
Biologically Normal Proteins, 325
The Hemoglobins, 326
The Hemoglobinopathies, 329

Chapter 12

The Molecular, Biochemical, and Cellular Basis of Genetic Disease, 345

Diseases due to Mutations in Different Classes of
Proteins, 345
Diseases Involving Enzymes, 348

Defects in Receptor Proteins, 360
Transport Defects, 364
Disorders of Structural Proteins, 367
Neurodegenerative Disorders, 377

Chapter 13

The Treatment of Genetic Disease, 393

The Current State of Treatment of Genetic
Disease, 393
Special Considerations in Treating Genetic
Disease, 395
Treatment Strategies, 396
The Molecular Treatment of Disease, 399

Chapter 14

Developmental Genetics and Birth Defects, 419

(with the assistance of Leslie G. Biesecker, MD)

Developmental Biology in Medicine, 419
Introduction to Developmental Biology, 422
Genes and Environment in Development, 424
Basic Concepts of Developmental Biology, 426
Cellular and Molecular Mechanisms in
Development, 434
Interaction of Developmental Mechanisms in
Embryogenesis, 440

Chapter 15

Prenatal Diagnosis, 443

Indications for Prenatal Diagnosis by Invasive
Testing, 443
Methods of Prenatal Diagnosis, 444
Laboratory Studies, 453
Emerging Technologies for Prenatal
Diagnosis, 456
Prenatal Prevention and Management of Genetic
Disease, 457
Genetic Counseling for Prenatal Diagnosis, 458

Chapter 16

Cancer Genetics and Genomics, 461

Genetic Basis of Cancer, 461
Oncogenes, 464
Tumor-Suppressor Genes, 467
Tumor Progression, 479
Applying Genomics to Individualize Cancer
Therapy, 479
Cancer and the Environment, 482

Chapter 17

Personalized Genetic Medicine, 485

Family History as Personalized Genetic
  Medicine, 485
Genetic Screening in Populations, 487
Screening for Genetic Susceptibility to
  Disease, 490

Chapter 18

**Pharmacogenetics and
Pharmacogenomics, 497**

Using Risk Information to Improve Care:
  Pharmacogenetics, 497
Pharmacogenomics, 504
Role of Ethnicity and Race in Personalized
  Medicine, 504

Chapter 19

Genetic Counseling and Risk Assessment, 507

The Process of Genetic Counseling, 507
Determining Recurrence Risks, 509

Application of Molecular Genetics to
  Determination of Recurrence Risks, 516
Empirical Recurrence Risks, 519

Chapter 20

Ethical Issues in Medical Genetics, 523

Ethical Dilemmas Arising in Medical
  Genetics, 523
Eugenic and Dysgenic Effects of Medical
  Genetics, 528
Genetics in Medicine, 529

Glossary, 531

Answers to Problems, 551

Index, 567

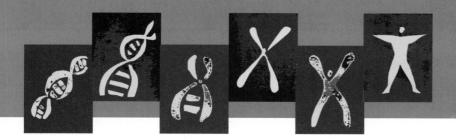

Chapter 1

Introduction

GENETICS AND GENOMICS IN MEDICINE

Genetics in medicine had its start at the beginning of the 20th century, with the recognition by Garrod and others that Mendel's laws of inheritance could explain the recurrence of certain disorders in families. During the ensuing 100 years, medical genetics grew from a small subspecialty concerned with a few rare hereditary disorders to a recognized medical specialty whose concepts and approaches are important components of the diagnosis and management of many disorders, both common and rare. This is even more the case now at the beginning of the 21st century, with the completion of the **Human Genome Project,** an international effort to determine the complete content of the human genome, defined as the sum total of the genetic information of our species (the suffix -ome is from the Greek for "all" or "complete"). We can now study the human genome as an entity, rather than one gene at a time. Medical genetics has become part of the broader field of genomic medicine, which seeks to apply a large-scale analysis of the human genome, including the control of gene expression, human gene variation, and interactions between genes and the environment, to improve medical care.

Medical genetics focuses not only on the patient but also on the entire family. A comprehensive family history is an important first step in the analysis of any disorder, whether or not the disorder is known to be genetic. As pointed out by Childs, "to fail to take a good family history is bad medicine." A family history is important because it can be critical in diagnosis, may show that a disorder is hereditary, can provide information about the natural history of a disease and variation in its expression, and can clarify the pattern of inheritance. Furthermore, recognizing a familial component

to a medical disorder allows the risk in other family members to be estimated so that proper management, prevention, and counseling can be offered to the patient *and* the family.

In the past few years, the Human Genome Project has made available the complete sequence of all human DNA; knowledge of the complete sequence allows the identification of all human genes, a determination of the extent of variation in these genes in different populations, and, ultimately, the delineation of how variation in these genes contributes to health and disease. In partnership with all the other disciplines of modern biology, the Human Genome Project has revolutionized human and medical genetics by providing fundamental insights into many diseases and promoting the development of far better diagnostic tools, preventive measures, and therapeutic methods based on a comprehensive view of the genome.

Genetics is rapidly becoming a central organizing principle in medical practice. Here are just a few examples of the vast array of applications of genetics and genomics to medicine today:

- A child who has multiple congenital malformations and a normal routine chromosome analysis undergoes a high-resolution genomic test for submicroscopic chromosomal deletions or duplications.
- A young woman with a family history of breast cancer receives education, test interpretation, and support from a counselor specializing in hereditary breast cancer.
- An obstetrician sends a chorionic villus sample taken from a 38-year-old pregnant woman to a cytogenetics laboratory for examination for abnormalities in the number or structure of the fetal chromosomes.
- A hematologist combines family and medical history with gene testing of a young adult with deep venous

1

thrombosis to assess the benefits and risks of initiating and maintaining anticoagulant therapy.

- Gene expression array analysis of a tumor sample is used to determine prognosis and to guide therapeutic decision-making.
- An oncologist tests her patients for genetic variations that can predict a good response or an adverse reaction to a chemotherapeutic agent.
- A forensic pathologist uses databases of genetic polymorphisms in his analysis of DNA samples obtained from victims' personal items and surviving relatives to identify remains from the September 11, 2001 World Trade Center attack.
- Discovery of an oncogenic signaling pathway inappropriately reactivated by a somatic mutation in a form of cancer leads to the development of a specific and powerful inhibitor of that pathway that successfully treats the cancer.

Genetic principles and approaches are not restricted to any one medical specialty or subspecialty but are permeating many areas of medicine. To give patients and their families the full benefit of expanding genetic knowledge, all physicians and their colleagues in the health professions need to understand the underlying principles of human genetics. These principles include the existence of alternative forms of a gene (**alleles**) in the population; the occurrence of similar **phenotypes** developing from mutation and variation at different loci; the recognition that familial disorders may arise from gene variants that cause susceptibility to diseases in the setting of gene-gene and gene-environmental interactions; the role of somatic mutation in cancer and aging; the feasibility of prenatal diagnosis, presymptomatic testing, and population screening; and the promise of powerful gene-based therapies. These concepts now influence all medical practice and will only become more important in the future.

Classification of Genetic Disorders

In clinical practice, the chief significance of genetics is in elucidating the role of genetic variation and mutation in predisposing to disease, modifying the course of disease, or causing the disease itself. Virtually any disease is the result of the combined action of genes and environment, but the relative role of the genetic component may be large or small. Among disorders caused wholly or partly by genetic factors, three main types are recognized: chromosome disorders, single-gene disorders, and multifactorial disorders.

In **chromosome disorders,** the defect is due not to a single mistake in the genetic blueprint but to an excess or a deficiency of the genes contained in whole chromosomes or chromosome segments. For example, the presence of an extra copy of one chromosome, chromosome 21, produces a specific disorder, Down syndrome, even though no individual gene on the chromosome is abnormal. As a group, chromosome disorders are common, affecting about 7 per 1000 liveborn infants and accounting for about half of all spontaneous first-trimester abortions. These disorders are discussed in Chapter 6.

Single-gene defects are caused by individual mutant genes. The mutation may be present on only one chromosome of a pair (matched with a normal allele on the homologous chromosome) or on both chromosomes of the pair. In a few cases, the mutation is in the mitochondrial rather than in the nuclear genome. In any case, the cause is a critical error in the genetic information carried by a single gene. Single-gene disorders such as cystic fibrosis, sickle cell anemia, and Marfan syndrome usually exhibit obvious and characteristic pedigree patterns. Most such defects are rare, with a frequency that may be as high as 1 in 500 to 1000 individuals but is usually much less. Although individually rare, single-gene disorders as a group are responsible for a significant proportion of disease and death. Taking the population as a whole, single-gene disorders affect 2% of the population sometime during an entire life span. In a population study of more than 1 million live births, the incidence of serious single-gene disorders in the pediatric population was estimated to be 0.36%; among hospitalized children, 6% to 8% probably have single-gene disorders. These disorders are discussed in Chapter 7.

Multifactorial inheritance is responsible for the majority of diseases, all of which have a genetic contribution, as evidenced by increased risk for recurrence in relatives of affected individuals or by increased frequency in identical twins, and yet show inheritance patterns in families that do not fit the characteristic patterns seen in single-gene defects. Multifactorial diseases include prenatal developmental disorders, resulting in congenital malformations such as Hirschsprung disease, cleft lip and palate, or congenital heart defects, as well as many common disorders of adult life, such as Alzheimer disease, diabetes, and hypertension. There appears to be no single error in the genetic information in many of these conditions. Rather, the disease is the result of one, two, or more different genes that together can produce or predispose to a serious defect, often in concert with environmental factors. Estimates of the impact of multifactorial disease range from 5% in the pediatric population to more than 60% in the entire population. These disorders are the subject of Chapter 8.

● ONWARD

During the 50-year professional life of today's professional and graduate students, extensive changes are likely to take place in the discovery, development, and use of genetic and genomic knowledge and tools in medicine. It is difficult to imagine that any period could encompass changes greater than those seen in the past 50 years, during which the field has gone from first recognizing the identity of DNA as the active agent of inheritance, to uncovering the molecular structure of DNA and chromosomes and determining the complete code of the human genome. And yet, judging from the quickening pace of discovery within only the past decade, it is virtually certain that we are just at the beginning of a revolution in integrating knowledge of genetics and the genome into public health and the practice of medicine. An introduction to the language and concepts of human and medical genetics and an appreciation of the genetic and genomic perspective on health and disease will form a framework for lifelong learning that is part of every health professional's career.

◎ GENERAL REFERENCES

Guttmacher AE, Collins FS: Genomic medicine—a primer. N Engl J Med 347:1512-1520, 2002.

Peltonen L, McKusick VA: Genomics and medicine. Dissecting human disease in the postgenomic era. Science 291:1224-1229, 2001.

Willard HF, Angrist M, Ginsburg GS: Genomic medicine: genetic variation and its impact on the future of health care. Philos Trans R Soc Lond B Biol Sci 360:1543-1550, 2005.

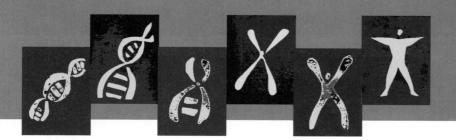

The Human Genome and the Chromosomal Basis of Heredity

Appreciation of the importance of genetics to medicine requires an understanding of the nature of the hereditary material, how it is packaged into the human **genome,** and how it is transmitted from cell to cell during cell division and from generation to generation during reproduction. The human genome consists of large amounts of the chemical deoxyribonucleic acid (**DNA**) that contains within its structure the genetic information needed to specify all aspects of embryogenesis, development, growth, metabolism, and reproduction—essentially all aspects of what makes a human being a functional organism. Every nucleated cell in the body carries its own copy of the human genome, which contains, by current estimates, about 25,000 **genes.** Genes, which at this point we define simply as units of genetic information, are encoded in the DNA of the genome, organized into a number of rod-shaped organelles called **chromosomes** in the nucleus of each cell. The influence of genes and genetics on states of health and disease is profound, and its roots are found in the information encoded in the DNA that makes up the human genome. Our knowledge of the nature and identity of genes and the composition of the human genome has increased exponentially during the past several decades, culminating in the determination of the DNA sequence of virtually the entire human genome in 2003.

Each species has a characteristic chromosome complement (**karyotype**) in terms of the number and the morphology of the chromosomes that make up its genome. The genes are in linear order along the chromosomes, each gene having a precise position or **locus.** A **gene map** is the map of the chromosomal location of the genes and is characteristic of each species and the individuals within a species.

The study of chromosomes, their structure, and their inheritance is called **cytogenetics.** The science of modern human cytogenetics dates from 1956, when it was first established that the normal human chromosome number is 46. Since that time, much has been learned about human chromosomes, their normal structure, their molecular composition, the locations of the genes that they contain, and their numerous and varied abnormalities.

Chromosome and genome analysis has become an important diagnostic procedure in clinical medicine. As described more fully in subsequent chapters, some of these applications include the following:

Clinical Diagnosis Numerous medical disorders, including some that are common, such as Down syndrome, are associated with microscopically visible changes in chromosome number or structure and require chromosome or genome analysis for diagnosis and genetic counseling (see Chapters 5 and 6).

Gene Mapping and Identification A major goal of medical genetics today is the mapping of specific genes to chromosomes and elucidating their roles in health and disease. This topic is referred to repeatedly but is discussed in detail in Chapter 10.

Cancer Cytogenetics Genomic and chromosomal changes in somatic cells are involved in the initiation and progression of many types of cancer (see Chapter 16).

Prenatal Diagnosis Chromosome and genome analysis is an essential procedure in prenatal diagnosis (see Chapter 15).

The ability to interpret a chromosome report and some knowledge of the methodology, the scope, and the limitations of chromosome studies are essential skills for physicians and others working with patients with birth defects, mental retardation, disorders of sexual development, and many types of cancer.

● THE HUMAN GENOME AND ITS CHROMOSOMES

With the exception of cells that develop into gametes (the **germline**), all cells that contribute to one's body are called **somatic cells** (*soma,* body). The genome contained in the nucleus of human somatic cells consists of 46 chromosomes, arranged in 23 pairs (Fig. 2-1). Of those 23 pairs, 22 are alike in males and females and are called **autosomes,** numbered from the largest to the smallest. The remaining pair comprises the **sex chromosomes:** two X chromosomes in females and an X and a Y chromosome in males. Each chromosome carries a different subset of genes that are arranged linearly along its DNA. Members of a pair of chromosomes (referred to as **homologous chromosomes** or **homologues**) carry matching genetic information; that is, they have the same genes in the same sequence. At any specific locus, however, they may have either identical or slightly different forms of the same gene, called

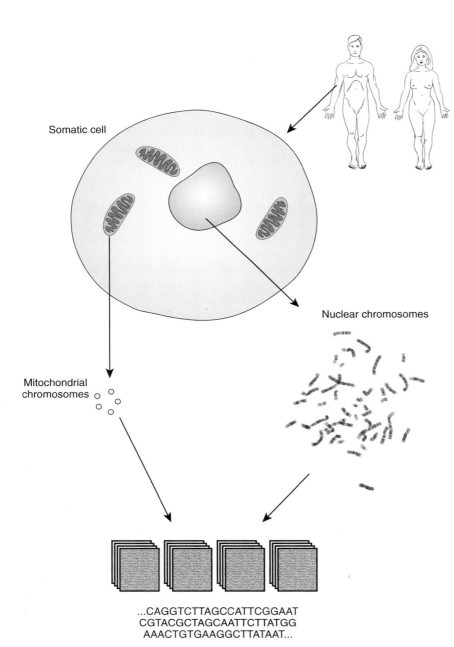

Somatic cell

Nuclear chromosomes

Mitochondrial chromosomes

...CAGGTCTTAGCCATTCGGAAT
CGTACGCTAGCAATTCTTATGG
AAACTGTGAAGGCTTATAAT...

Human Genome Sequence

Figure 2-1 ■ The human genome, encoded on both nuclear and mitochondrial chromosomes. (Modified from Brown TA: Genomes, 2nd ed. New York, Wiley-Liss, 2002.)

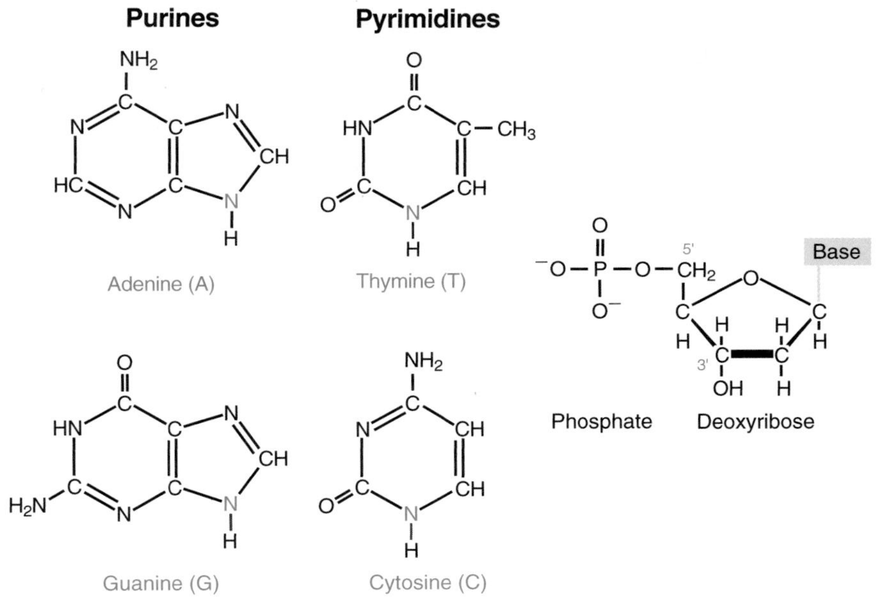

Purines

Pyrimidines

Adenine (A)

Thymine (T)

Figure 2-2 ■ The four bases of DNA and the general structure of a nucleotide in DNA. Each of the four bases bonds with deoxyribose (through the nitrogen shown in blue) and a phosphate group to form the corresponding nucleotides.

Phosphate   Deoxyribose

Base

Guanine (G)

Cytosine (C)

alleles. One member of each pair of chromosomes is inherited from the father, the other from the mother. Normally, the members of a pair of autosomes are microscopically indistinguishable from each other. In females, the sex chromosomes, the two **X chromosomes,** are likewise largely indistinguishable. In males, however, the sex chromosomes differ. One is an X, identical to the X's of the female, inherited by a male from his mother and transmitted to his daughters; the other, the **Y chromosome,** is inherited from his father and transmitted to his sons. In Chapter 6, we look at some exceptions to the simple and almost universal rule that human females are XX and human males are XY.

In addition to the nuclear genome, a small but important part of the human genome resides in mitochondria in the cytoplasm (see Fig. 2-1). The mitochondrial chromosome, to be described later in this chapter, has a number of unusual features that distinguish it from the rest of the human genome.

DNA Structure: A Brief Review

Before the organization of the human genome and its chromosomes is considered in detail, it is necessary to review the nature of the DNA that makes up the genome. DNA is a polymeric nucleic acid macromolecule composed of three types of units: a five-carbon sugar, deoxyribose; a nitrogen-containing base; and a phosphate group (Fig. 2-2). The bases are of two types, **purines** and **pyrimidines.** In DNA, there are two purine bases, **adenine** (A) and **guanine** (G), and two pyrimidine bases, **thymine** (T) and **cytosine** (C). Nucleotides, each composed of a base, a phosphate, and a sugar

moiety, polymerize into long polynucleotide chains by 5'-3' phosphodiester bonds formed between adjacent deoxyribose units (Fig. 2-3). In the human genome, these polynucleotide chains (in the form of a double helix; Fig. 2-4) are hundreds of millions of nucleotides long, ranging in size from approximately 50 million base pairs (for the smallest chromosome, chromosome 21) to 250 million base pairs (for the largest chromosome, chromosome 1).

The anatomical structure of DNA carries the chemical information that allows the exact transmission of genetic information from one cell to its daughter cells and from one generation to the next. At the same time, the primary structure of DNA specifies the amino acid sequences of the polypeptide chains of proteins, as described in the next chapter. DNA has elegant features that give it these properties. The native state of DNA, as elucidated by James Watson and Francis Crick in 1953, is a double helix (see Fig. 2-4). The helical structure resembles a right-handed spiral staircase in which its two polynucleotide chains run in opposite directions, held together by hydrogen bonds between pairs of bases: A of one chain paired with T of the other, and G with C. The specific nature of the genetic information encoded in the human genome lies in the sequence of C's, A's, G's, and T's on the two strands of the double helix along each of the chromosomes, both in the nucleus and in mitochondria (see Fig. 2-1). Because of the complementary nature of the two strands of DNA, knowledge of the sequence of nucleotide bases on one strand automatically allows one to determine the sequence of bases on the other strand. The double-stranded structure of DNA molecules allows them to replicate precisely by separation of the two strands,

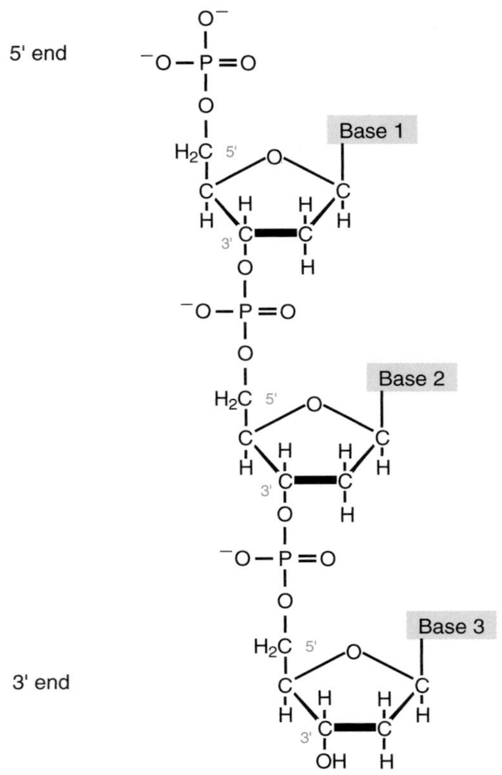

5' end

Base 1

Base 2

Base 3

3' end

Figure 2-3 ■ A portion of a DNA polynucleotide chain, showing the 3'-5' phosphodiester bonds that link adjacent nucleotides.

followed by synthesis of two new complementary strands, in accordance with the sequence of the original template strands (Fig. 2-5). Similarly, when necessary, the base complementarity allows efficient and correct repair of damaged DNA molecules.

Organization of Human Chromosomes

The composition of genes in the human genome, as well as the determinants of their expression, is specified in the DNA of the 46 human chromosomes in the nucleus plus the mitochondrial chromosome. *Each human chromosome consists of a single, continuous DNA double helix;* that is, each chromosome in the nucleus is a long, linear double-stranded DNA molecule, and the nuclear genome consists, therefore, of 46 DNA molecules, totaling more than 6 billion nucleotides (see Fig. 2-1).

Chromosomes are not naked DNA double helices, however. Within each cell, the genome is packaged as **chromatin,** in which genomic DNA is complexed with several classes of chromosomal proteins. Except during cell division, chromatin is distributed throughout the nucleus and is relatively homogeneous in appearance under the microscope. When a cell divides, however, its genome condenses to appear as microscopically visible chromosomes. Chromosomes are thus visible as discrete structures only in dividing cells, although they retain their integrity between cell divisions.

The DNA molecule of a chromosome exists in chromatin as a complex with a family of basic chromosomal proteins called histones and with a heteroge-

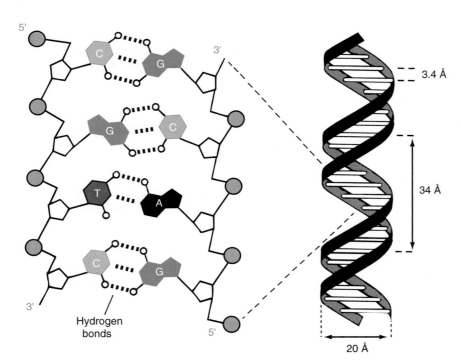

Figure 2-4 ■ The structure of DNA. **Left,** A two-dimensional representation of the two complementary strands of DNA, showing the AT and GC base pairs. Note that the orientation of the two strands is antiparallel. **Right,** The double-helix model of DNA, as proposed by Watson and Crick. The horizontal "rungs" represent the paired bases. The helix is said to be right-handed because the strand going from lower left to upper right crosses over the opposite strand. (Based on Watson JD, Crick FHC: Molecular structure of nucleic acids—a structure for deoxyribose nucleic acid. Nature 171:737-738, 1953.)

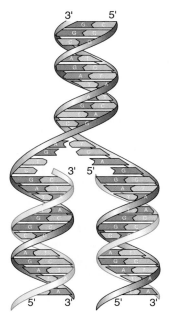

Figure 2-5 ■ Replication of a DNA double helix, resulting in two identical daughter molecules, each composed of one parental strand *(gray)* and one newly synthesized strand *(blue).*

neous group of nonhistone proteins that are much less well characterized but that appear to be critical for establishing a proper environment to ensure normal chromosome behavior and appropriate gene expression.

Five major types of histones play a critical role in the proper packaging of chromatin. Two copies each of the four core histones H2A, H2B, H3, and H4 constitute an octamer, around which a segment of DNA double helix winds, like thread around a spool (Fig. 2-6). Approximately 140 base pairs of DNA are associated with each histone core, making just under two turns around the octamer. After a short (20- to 60–base pair) "spacer" segment of DNA, the next core DNA complex forms, and so on, giving chromatin the appearance of beads on a string. Each complex of DNA with core histones is called a **nucleosome,** which is the basic structural unit of chromatin, and each of the 46 human chromosomes contains several hundred thousand to well over a million nucleosomes. The fifth histone, H1, appears to bind to DNA at the edge of each nucleosome, in the internucleosomal spacer region. The amount of DNA associated with a core nucleosome, together with the spacer region, is about 200 base pairs.

In addition to the major histone types, a number of specialized histones can substitute for H3 and H2A and confer specific characteristics on the genomic DNA at that location. Histones H3 and H4 can also be modified by chemical changes to the encoded proteins. These so-called post-translational modifications (see Chapter 3) can change the properties of nucleosomes that contain them. The pattern of major and specialized histone types and their modifications is often called the **histone code,** which can vary from cell type to cell type and is thought to specify how DNA is packaged and how

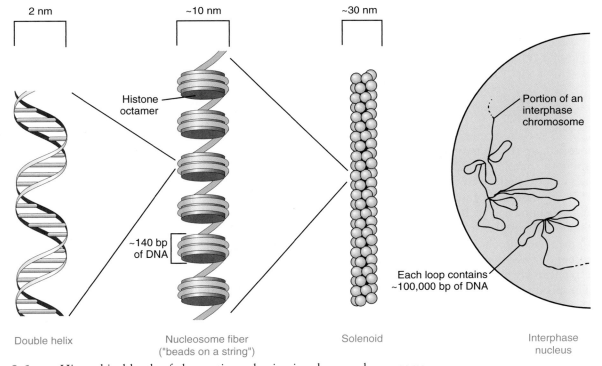

Figure 2-6 ■ Hierarchical levels of chromatin packaging in a human chromosome.

accessible it is to regulatory molecules that determine gene expression or other genome functions.

During the cell cycle, as we will see later in this chapter, chromosomes pass through orderly stages of condensation and decondensation. However, even when chromosomes are in their most decondensed state, in a stage of the cell cycle called **interphase**, DNA packaged in chromatin is substantially more condensed than it would be as a native, protein-free double helix. Further, the long strings of nucleosomes are themselves compacted into a secondary helical chromatin structure that appears under the electron microscope as a thick, 30-nm-diameter fiber (about three times thicker than the nucleosomal fiber; see Fig. 2-6). This cylindrical "solenoid" fiber (from the Greek *solenoeides*, "pipe shaped") appears to be the fundamental unit of chromatin organization. The solenoids are themselves packed into **loops** or domains attached at intervals of about 100,000 base pairs (equivalent to 100 kilobase pairs, or 100 kb, as 1 kb = 1000 base pairs) to a protein **scaffold** or matrix within the nucleus. It has been speculated that these loops are, in fact, functional units of DNA replication or gene transcription, or both, and that the attachment points of each loop are fixed along the chromosomal DNA. Thus, one level of control of gene expression may depend on how DNA and genes are packaged into chromosomes and on their association with chromatin proteins in the packaging process.

The enormous amount of genomic DNA packaged into a chromosome can be appreciated when chromosomes are treated to release the DNA from the underlying protein scaffold (Fig. 2-7). When DNA is released in this manner, long loops of DNA can be visualized, and the residual scaffolding can be seen to reproduce the outline of a typical chromosome.

The Mitochondrial Chromosome

As mentioned earlier, a small but important subset of genes encoded in the human genome resides in the cytoplasm in the mitochondria (see Fig. 2-1). Mitochondrial genes exhibit exclusively maternal inheritance (see Chapter 7). Human cells can have hundreds to thousands of mitochondria, each containing a number of copies of a small circular molecule, the mitochondrial chromosome. The mitochondrial DNA molecule is only 16 kb in length (less than 0.03% of the length of the smallest nuclear chromosome!) and encodes only 37 genes. The products of these genes function in mitochondria, although the majority of proteins within the mitochondria are, in fact, the products of nuclear genes. Mutations in mitochondrial genes have been demonstrated in several maternally inherited as well as sporadic disorders (Case 28) (see Chapters 7 and 12).

Organization of the Human Genome

Regions of the genome with similar characteristics or organization, replication, and expression are not arranged randomly but rather tend to be clustered together. This functional organization of the genome correlates remarkably well with its structural organization as revealed by laboratory methods of chromosome analysis (introduced later in this chapter and discussed in detail in Chapter 5). The overall significance of this functional organization is that chromosomes are not just a random collection of different types of genes and other DNA sequences. Some chromosome regions, or even whole chromosomes, are high in gene content ("gene rich"), whereas others are low ("gene poor") (Fig. 2-8). Certain types of sequence are characteristic of the different structural features of human chromosomes. The clinical consequences of abnormalities of genome structure reflect the specific nature of the genes and sequences involved. Thus, abnormalities of gene-rich chromosomes or chromosomal regions tend to be much more severe clinically than similar-sized defects involving gene-poor parts of the genome.

As a result of knowledge gained from the Human Genome Project, it is apparent that the organization of DNA in the human genome is far more varied than was once widely appreciated. Of the 3 billion base pairs of DNA in the genome, less than 1.5% actually encodes proteins and only about 5% is thought to contain regulatory elements that influence or determine patterns of gene expression during development or in different tissues. Only about half of the total linear length of the genome consists of so-called **single-copy** or **unique DNA**, that is, DNA whose nucleotide sequence is represented only once (or at most a few times). The rest of the genome consists of several classes of **repetitive DNA** and includes DNA whose nucleotide sequence is repeated, either perfectly or with some variation, hundreds to millions of times in the genome. Whereas most (but not all) of the estimated 25,000 genes in the genome are represented in single-copy DNA, sequences in the repetitive DNA fraction contribute to maintaining chromosome structure and are an important source of variation between different individuals; some of this variation can predispose to pathological events in the genome, as we will see in Chapter 6.

Single-Copy DNA Sequences

Although single-copy DNA makes up at least half of the DNA in the genome, much of its function remains a mystery because, as mentioned, sequences actually encoding proteins (i.e., the coding portion of genes) constitute only a small proportion of all the single-copy DNA. Most single-copy DNA is found in short stretches (several kilobase pairs or less), interspersed with

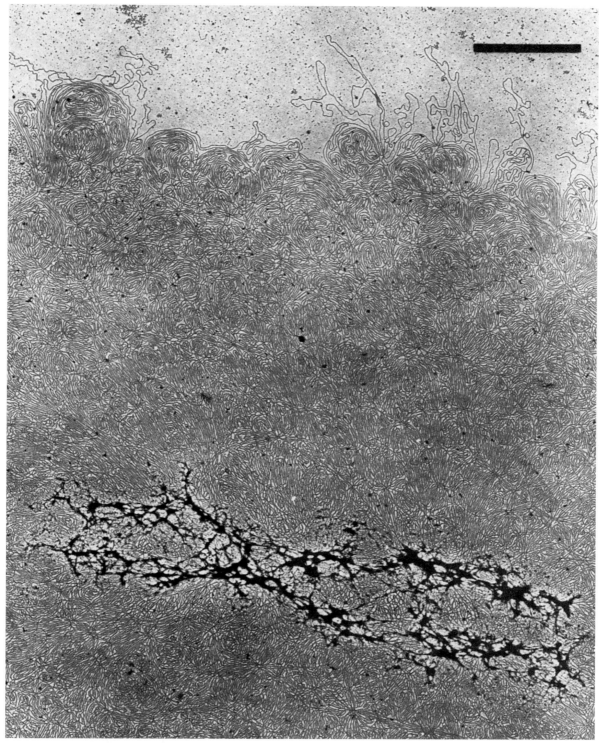

Figure 2-7 ■ Electron micrograph of a protein-depleted human metaphase chromosome, showing the residual chromosome scaffold and loops of DNA. Individual DNA fibers can be best seen at the edge of the DNA loops. Bar = 2 μm. (From Paulson JR, Laemmli UK: The structure of histone-depleted metaphase chromosomes. Cell 12:817-828, 1977. Reprinted by permission of the authors and Cell Press.)

A

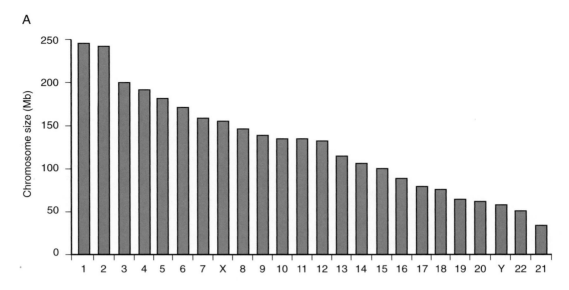

B

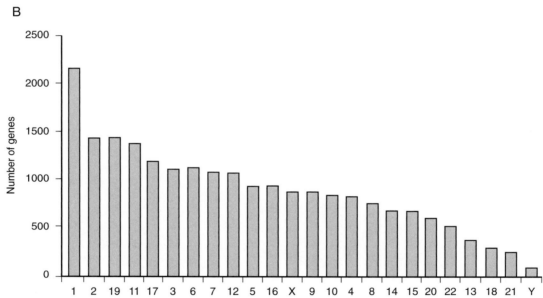

Figure 2-8 ■ Size and gene content of the 24 human chromosomes. **A,** Size of each human chromosome, in millions of base pairs (1 million base pairs = 1 Mb). Chromosomes are ordered left to right by size. **B,** Number of genes identified on each human chromosome. Chromosomes are ordered left to right by gene content. (Based on data from *www.ensembl.org,* v36.)

members of various repetitive DNA families. The organization of genes in single-copy DNA is addressed in depth in Chapter 3.

Repetitive DNA Sequences

Several different categories of repetitive DNA are recognized. A useful distinguishing feature is whether the repeated sequences ("repeats") are clustered in one or a few locations or whether they are interspersed, throughout the genome, with single-copy sequences along the chromosome. Clustered repeated sequences constitute an estimated 10% to 15% of the genome and

consist of arrays of various short repeats organized tandemly in a head-to-tail fashion. The different types of such tandem repeats are collectively called satellite DNAs, so named because many of the original tandem repeat families could be separated by biochemical methods from the bulk of the genome as distinct ("satellite") fractions of DNA.

Tandem repeat families vary with regard to their location in the genome, the total length of the tandem array, and the length of the constituent repeat units that make up the array. In general, such arrays can stretch several million base pairs or more in length and constitute up to several percent of the DNA content of an individual human chromosome. Many tandem repeat sequences are important as molecular tools that have revolutionized clinical cytogenetic analysis because of their relative ease of detection (see Chapter 5). Some human tandem repeats are based on repetitions (with some variation) of a short sequence such as a pentanucleotide. Long arrays of such repeats are found in large genetically inert regions on chromosomes 1, 9, and 16 and make up more than half of the Y chromosome (see Chapter 5). Other tandem repeat families are based on somewhat longer basic repeats. For example, the α-satellite family of DNA is composed of tandem arrays of different copies of an approximately 171–base pair unit, found at the **centromere** of each human chromosome, which is critical for attachment of chromosomes to microtubules of the spindle apparatus during cell division. This repeat family is believed to play a role in centromere function by ensuring proper chromosome segregation in mitosis and meiosis, as is described later in this chapter.

In addition to tandem repeat DNAs, another major class of repetitive DNA in the genome consists of related sequences that are dispersed throughout the genome rather than localized. Although many small DNA families meet this general description, two in particular warrant discussion because together they make up a significant proportion of the genome and because they have been implicated in genetic diseases. Among the best-studied dispersed repetitive elements are those belonging to the so-called *Alu* **family**. The members of this family are about 300 base pairs in length and are recognizably related to each other although not identical in DNA sequence. In total, there are more than a million *Alu* family members in the genome, making up at least 10% of human DNA. In some regions of the genome, however, they make up a much higher percentage of the DNA. A second major dispersed repetitive DNA family is called the long interspersed nuclear element (**LINE**, sometimes called L1) family. LINEs are up to 6 kb in length and are found in about 850,000 copies per genome, accounting for about 20% of the genome. They also are plentiful in some regions of the genome but relatively sparse in others.

Repetitive DNA and Disease   Families of repeats dispersed throughout the genome are clearly of medical importance. Both *Alu* and LINE sequences have been implicated as the cause of mutations in hereditary disease. At least a few copies of the LINE and *Alu* families generate copies of themselves that can integrate elsewhere in the genome, occasionally causing insertional inactivation of a medically important gene. The frequency of such events causing genetic disease in humans is unknown currently, but they may account for as many as 1 in 500 mutations. In addition, aberrant recombination events between different LINE or *Alu*

repeats can also be a cause of mutation in some genetic diseases (see Chapter 9).

An important additional class of repetitive DNA includes sequences that are duplicated, often with extraordinarily high sequence conservation, in many different locations around the genome. Duplications involving substantial segments of a chromosome, called **segmental duplications**, can span hundreds of kilobase pairs and account for at least 5% of the genome. When the duplicated regions contain genes, genomic rearrangements involving the duplicated sequences can result in the deletion of the region (and the genes) between the copies and thus give rise to disease (see Chapter 6). In addition, rearrangements between segments of the genome are a source of significant variation between individuals in the number of copies of these DNA sequences, as is discussed in Chapter 9.

CELL DIVISION

There are two kinds of cell division, mitosis and meiosis. **Mitosis** is ordinary somatic cell division, by which the body grows, differentiates, and effects tissue regeneration. Mitotic division normally results in two daughter cells, each with chromosomes and genes identical to those of the parent cell. There may be dozens or even hundreds of successive mitoses in a lineage of somatic cells. In contrast, **meiosis** occurs only in cells of the germline. Meiosis results in the formation of reproductive cells (**gametes**), each of which has only 23 chromosomes—one of each kind of autosome and either an X or a Y. Thus, whereas somatic cells have the **diploid** (*diploos*, double) or the 2n chromosome complement (i.e., 46 chromosomes), gametes have the **haploid** (*haploos*, single) or the n complement (i.e., 23 chromosomes). Abnormalities of chromosome number or structure, which are usually clinically significant, can arise either in somatic cells or in cells of the germline by errors in cell division.

The Cell Cycle

A human being begins life as a fertilized ovum (**zygote**), a diploid cell from which all the cells of the body (estimated at about 100 trillion in number) are derived by a series of dozens or even hundreds of mitoses. Mitosis is obviously crucial for growth and differentiation, but it takes up only a small part of the life cycle of a cell. The period between two successive mitoses is called **interphase**, the state in which most of the life of a cell is spent.

Immediately after mitosis, the cell enters a phase, called G_1, in which there is no DNA synthesis (Fig. 2-9). Some cells pass through this stage in hours; others

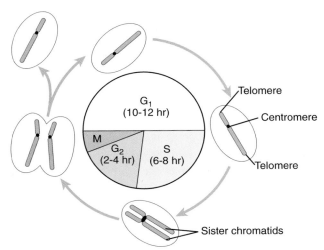

Figure 2-9 ■ A typical mitotic cell cycle, described in the text. The telomeres, the centromere, and sister chromatids are indicated.

spend a long time, days or years, in G_1. In fact, some cell types, such as neurons and red blood cells, do not divide at all once they are fully differentiated; rather, they are permanently arrested during G_1 in a distinct, nondividing phase known as G_0 ("G zero"). Other cells, such as liver cells, may enter G_0 but, after organ damage, eventually return to G_1 and continue through the cell cycle.

Although the molecular mechanisms controlling cell-cycle progression are incompletely understood, the cell cycle is governed by a series of **checkpoints** that determine the timing of each step in mitosis. In addition, checkpoints monitor and control the accuracy of DNA synthesis as well as the assembly and attachment of an elaborate network of microtubules that facilitate chromosome movement. If damage to the genome is detected, these mitotic checkpoints halt cell-cycle progression until repairs are made or, if the damage is excessive, until the cell is instructed to die by programmed cell death (a process called **apoptosis**).

During G_1, each cell contains one diploid copy of the genome. G_1 is followed by the **S phase,** the stage of DNA synthesis. During this stage, each chromosome, which in G_1 has been a single DNA molecule, replicates to become a bipartite chromosome consisting of two **sister chromatids** (see Fig. 2-9), each of which contains an identical copy of the original linear DNA double helix. The ends of each chromosome (or chromatid) are marked by **telomeres,** which consist of specialized repetitive DNA sequences that ensure the integrity of the chromosome during cell division. Correct maintenance of the ends of chromosomes requires a special enzyme called **telomerase,** which ensures that DNA synthesis includes the very ends of each chromosome. In the absence of telomerase, chromosome ends get shorter and shorter, eventually leading to cell death.

The two sister chromatids are held together physically at the **centromere,** a region of DNA that associates with a number of specific proteins to form the **kinetochore.** This complex structure serves to attach each chromosome to the microtubules of the mitotic spindle and to govern chromosome movement during mitosis. DNA synthesis during S phase is not synchronous throughout all chromosomes or even within a single chromosome; rather, along each chromosome, it begins at hundreds to thousands of sites, called **origins of DNA replication.** Individual chromosome segments have their own characteristic time of replication during the 6- to 8-hour S phase.

By the end of S phase, the DNA content of the cell has doubled, and each cell now contains two copies of the diploid genome. After S phase, the cell enters a brief stage called G_2. Throughout the whole cell cycle, ribonucleic acids and proteins are produced and the cell gradually enlarges, eventually doubling its total mass before the next mitosis. G_2 is ended by mitosis, which begins when individual chromosomes begin to condense and become visible under the microscope as thin, extended threads, a process that is considered in greater detail in the following section.

The G_1, S, and G_2 phases together constitute interphase. In typical dividing human cells, the three phases take a total of 16 to 24 hours, whereas mitosis lasts only 1 to 2 hours (see Fig. 2-9). There is great variation, however, in the length of the cell cycle, which ranges from a few hours in rapidly dividing cells, such as those of the dermis of the skin or the intestinal mucosa, to months in other cell types.

Mitosis

During the mitotic phase of the cell cycle, an elaborate apparatus is brought into play to ensure that each of the two daughter cells receives a complete set of genetic information. This result is achieved by a mechanism that distributes one chromatid of each chromosome to each daughter cell (Fig. 2-10). The process of distributing a copy of each chromosome to each daughter cell is called **chromosome segregation.** The importance of this process for normal cell growth is illustrated by the observation that many tumors are invariably characterized by a state of genetic imbalance resulting from mitotic errors in the distribution of chromosomes to daughter cells.

The process of mitosis is continuous, but five stages are distinguished: prophase, prometaphase, metaphase, anaphase, and telophase.

Prophase   This stage initiates mitosis and is marked by gradual condensation of the chromosomes and the beginning of the formation of the **mitotic spindle.** A pair of microtubule organizing centers, also called **centrosomes,** form foci from which microtubules radiate.

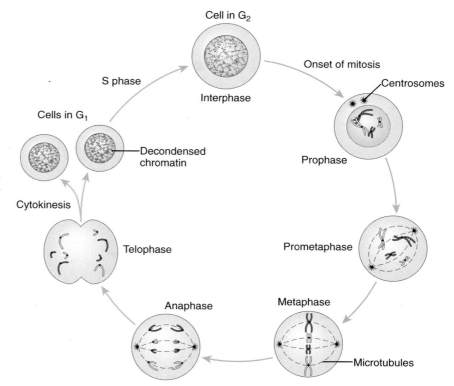

Figure 2-10 ■ Mitosis. Only two chromosome pairs are shown. For further details, see text.

The centrosomes gradually move to take up positions at the poles of the cell.

Prometaphase The cell enters prometaphase when the nuclear membrane breaks up, allowing the chromosomes to disperse within the cell and to attach, by their kinetochores, to microtubules of the mitotic spindle. The chromosomes begin to move toward a point midway between the spindle poles, a process called **congression.** The chromosomes continue to condense throughout this stage.

Metaphase At metaphase, the chromosomes reach maximal condensation. They become arranged at the equatorial plane of the cell, balanced by the equal forces exerted on the kinetochore of each chromosome by microtubules emanating from the two spindle poles. The chromosomes of a dividing human cell are most readily analyzed at the metaphase or the prometaphase stage of mitosis (see later discussion and Chapter 5).

Anaphase Anaphase begins abruptly when the chromosomes separate at the centromere. The sister chromatids of each chromosome now become independent **daughter chromosomes,** which move to opposite poles of the cell (see Fig. 2-10).

Telophase In telophase, the chromosomes begin to decondense from their highly contracted state, a nuclear membrane begins to re-form around each of the two daughter nuclei, and each nucleus gradually resumes its interphase appearance.

To complete the process of cell division, the cytoplasm cleaves by a process known as **cytokinesis,** which begins as the chromosomes approach the spindle poles. Eventually there are two complete daughter cells, each with a nucleus containing all the genetic information of the original cell.

There is an important difference between a cell entering mitosis and one that has just completed the process. The parent cell's chromosomes in G_2 each have a pair of chromatids, but the chromosomes of the daughter cell each consist of only one copy of the genetic material. This copy will not be duplicated until the daughter cell in its turn reaches the S phase of the next cell cycle (see Fig. 2-9). The entire process of mitosis thus ensures the orderly duplication and distribution of the genome through successive cell divisions.

The Human Karyotype

The condensed chromosomes of a dividing human cell are most readily analyzed at metaphase or prometaphase. At these stages, the chromosomes are visible under the microscope as a **chromosome spread;** each chromosome consists of its sister chromatids, although in most chromosome preparations, the two chromatids are held together so tightly that they are rarely visible as separate entities.

Most chromosomes can be distinguished not only by their length but also by the location of the centro-

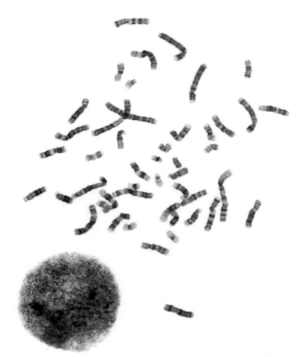

Figure 2-11 ■ A chromosome spread prepared from a lymphocyte culture that has been stained by the Giemsa-banding (G-banding) technique. The darkly stained nucleus adjacent to the chromosomes is from a different cell in interphase, when chromosomal material is diffuse throughout the nucleus. (Courtesy of Stuart Schwartz, University Hospitals of Cleveland, Ohio.)

mere. The centromere is apparent as a **primary constriction,** a narrowing or pinching-in of the sister chromatids due to formation of the kinetochore. This is a recognizable cytogenetic landmark, dividing the chromosome into two **arms**, a short arm designated **p** (for *petit*) and a long arm designated **q**. All 24 types of chromosome (22 autosomes, X, and Y) can be individually identified by a variety of cytogenetic and molecular techniques now in common use.

Figure 2-11 shows a prometaphase cell in which the chromosomes have been stained by the Giemsa-staining (**G-banding**) method, the technique most widely used in clinical cytogenetics laboratories. The chromosomes are treated first with trypsin to digest the chromosomal proteins and then with Giemsa stain. Each chromosome pair stains in a characteristic pattern of alternating light and dark bands (G bands) that correlates roughly with features of the underlying DNA sequence, such as base composition (i.e., the percentage of base pairs that are GC or AT) and the distribution of repetitive DNA elements. With G-banding and other banding techniques, all of the chromosomes can be individually distinguished. Further, the nature of any structural or numerical abnormalities can be readily determined, as we examine in greater detail in Chapters 5 and 6.

Although experts can often analyze metaphase chromosomes directly under the microscope, a common procedure is to cut out the chromosomes from a photomicrograph and arrange them in pairs in a standard classification (Fig. 2-12). The completed picture is called a **karyotype.** The word *karyotype* is also used to refer to the standard chromosome set of an individual ("a normal male karyotype") or of a species ("the human karyotype") and, as a verb, to the process of preparing such a standard figure ("to karyotype").

Unlike the chromosomes seen in stained preparations under the microscope or in photographs, the chromosomes of living cells are fluid and dynamic structures. During mitosis, for example, the chromatin of each interphase chromosome condenses substantially (see Fig. 2-12). At prophase, when chromosomes become visible under the light microscope, chromosome 1 (containing about 250 million base pairs of DNA) has condensed to an overall length of about 50 μm. When maximally condensed at metaphase, DNA in chromosomes is about 1/10,000 of its fully extended state. When chromosomes are prepared to reveal bands (see Figs. 2-11 and 2-12), as many as 1000 or more bands can be recognized in stained preparations of all the chromosomes. Each cytogenetic band therefore contains as many as 50 or more genes, although the density of genes in the genome, as mentioned previously, is variable. After metaphase, as cells complete mitosis, chromosomes decondense and return to their relaxed state as chromatin in the interphase nucleus, ready to begin the cycle again (Fig. 2-13).

Meiosis

Meiosis, the process by which diploid cells give rise to haploid gametes, involves a type of cell division that is unique to germ cells. Meiosis consists of one round of DNA synthesis followed by two rounds of chromosome segregation and cell division (see Fig. 2-12). The cells in the germline that undergo meiosis, primary spermatocytes or primary oocytes, are derived from the zygote by a long series of mitoses before the onset of meiosis.

Male and female gametes have different histories; although the sequence of events is the same, their timing is very different. The two successive meiotic divisions are called meiosis I and meiosis II. Meiosis I is also known as the **reduction division** because it is the division in which the chromosome number is reduced by half through the pairing of homologues in prophase and by their segregation to different cells at anaphase of meiosis I. The X and Y chromosomes are not homologues in a strict sense but do have homologous segments at the ends of their short and long arms (see Chapter 6), and they pair in both regions during meiosis I.

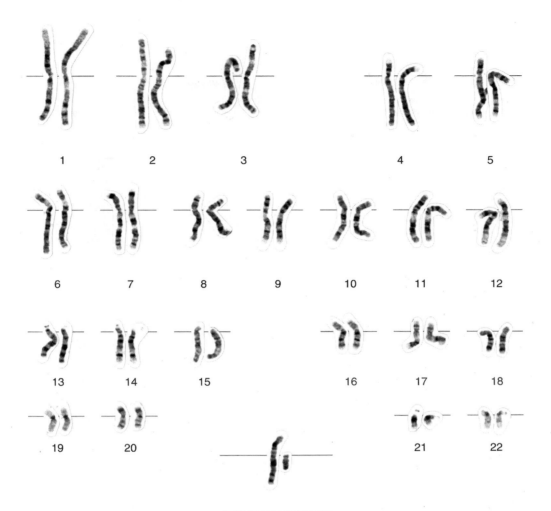

SEX CHROMOSOMES

Figure 2-12 ■ A human male karyotype with Giemsa banding (G-banding). The chromosomes are at the prometaphase stage of mitosis and are arranged in a standard classification, numbered 1 to 22 in order of length, with the X and Y chromosomes shown separately. (Courtesy of Stuart Schwartz, University Hospitals of Cleveland, Ohio.)

Meiosis I is also notable because it is the stage at which genetic **recombination** (also called **meiotic crossing over**) occurs. In this process, homologous segments of DNA are exchanged between non-sister chromatids of a pair of homologous chromosomes, thus ensuring that none of the gametes produced by meiosis is identical to another. The concept of recombination is fundamental to the process of mapping genes responsible for inherited disorders, as we discuss at length in Chapter 10. Because recombination involves the physical intertwining of the two homologues until the appropriate point during meiosis I, it is also critical for ensuring proper chromosome segregation during meiosis. Failure to recombine properly can lead to chromosome missegregation in meiosis I and is a frequent cause of chromosome abnormalities like Down syndrome (see Chapters 5 and 6).

Meiosis II follows meiosis I without an intervening step of DNA replication. As in ordinary mitosis, the chromatids separate, and one chromatid of each chromosome passes to each daughter cell (Fig. 2-14).

The First Meiotic Division (Meiosis I)

Prophase I   The prophase of meiosis I is a complicated process that differs from mitotic prophase in a number of ways, with important genetic consequences. Several stages are defined. Throughout all the stages, the chromosomes continually condense and become shorter and thicker (Fig. 2-15).

Leptotene   The chromosomes, which have already replicated during the preceding S phase, become visible as thin threads that are beginning to condense. At this early stage, the two sister chromatids of each chromosome are so closely aligned that they cannot be distinguished.

Zygotene   At this stage, homologous chromosomes begin to align along their entire length. The process of

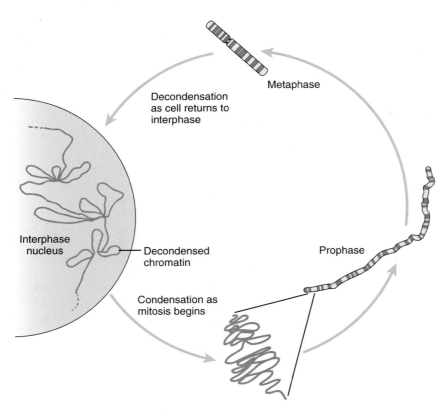

Metaphase

Decondensation
as cell returns to
interphase

Interphase
nucleus

Decondensed
chromatin

Condensation as
mitosis begins

Prophase

Figure 2-13 ■ Cycle of condensation and decondensation as a chromosome proceeds through the cell cycle.

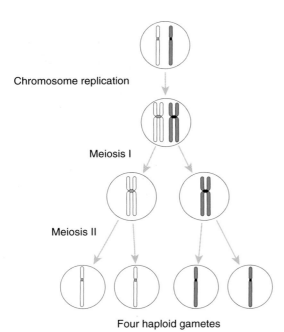

Chromosome replication

Meiosis I

Meiosis II

Four haploid gametes

Figure 2-14 ■ A simplified representation of the essential steps in meiosis, consisting of one round of DNA replication followed by two rounds of chromosome segregation, meiosis I and meiosis II.

pairing or **synapsis** is normally precise, bringing corresponding DNA sequences into alignment along the length of the entire chromosome.

Although the molecular basis of synapsis is not completely understood, electron microscopy reveals that the chromosomes are held together by a **synaptonemal complex,** a ribbon-like protein-containing structure (Fig. 2-16). The synaptonemal complex is essential to the process of recombination.

Pachytene During this stage, the chromosomes become much more tightly coiled. Synapsis is complete, and each pair of homologues appears as a **bivalent** (sometimes called a **tetrad** because it contains four chromatids). Pachytene is the stage at which meiotic crossing over takes place (see Fig. 2-15).

Diplotene After recombination, the synaptonemal complex begins to break down, and the two components of each bivalent now begin to separate from each other. Eventually the two homologues of each bivalent are held together only at points called **chiasmata** (crosses), which are believed to mark the locations of crossovers. The average number of chiasmata seen in human spermatocytes is about 50, that is, several per bivalent.

Diakinesis In this stage, the chromosomes reach maximal condensation.

Metaphase I Metaphase I begins, as in mitosis, when the nuclear membrane disappears. A spindle forms, and the paired chromosomes align themselves on the equatorial plane with their centromeres oriented toward different poles.

Anaphase I   The two members of each bivalent move apart, and their respective centromeres with the attached sister chromatids are drawn to opposite poles of the cell, a process termed **disjunction** (see Fig. 2-15). Thus, the chromosome number is halved, and each cellular product of meiosis I has the haploid chromosome number. The different bivalents assort independently of one another, and as a result, the original paternal and maternal chromosome sets are sorted into random combinations. The possible number of combinations of the 23 chromosome pairs that can be present in the gametes is 2^{23} (more than 8 million). In fact, the variation in the genetic material that is transmitted from parent to child is actually much greater than this because of the process of crossing over. As a result of this process, each chromatid typically contains segments derived from each member of the parental chromosome pair; for example, at this stage, a typical chromosome 1 is composed of three to five segments, alternately paternal and maternal in origin. (See additional discussion in Chapter 10.)

Many errors can occur in cell division. Some result in meiotic arrest and the death of the cell, whereas others lead to missegregation of chromosomes at anaphase. For example, both homologues of a chromosome pair may travel to the same rather than opposite poles during anaphase I. This pathogenic process is termed **nondisjunction.** Some of the consequences of meiotic irregularities are discussed in Chapters 5 and 6.

Telophase I   By telophase, the two haploid sets of chromosomes have normally grouped at opposite poles of the cell.

Cytokinesis

After telophase I, the cell divides into two haploid daughter cells and enters meiotic interphase. In spermatogenesis, the cytoplasm is more or less equally

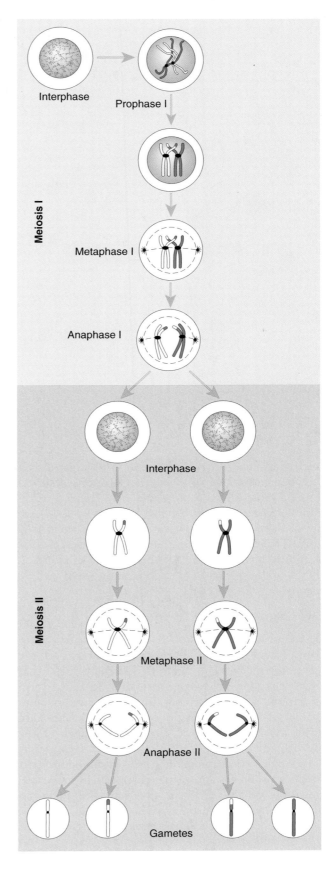

Figure 2-15   ■   Meiosis and its consequences. A single chromosome pair and a single crossover are shown, leading to formation of four distinct gametes. The chromosomes replicate during interphase and begin to condense as the cell enters prophase of meiosis I. In meiosis I, the chromosomes synapse and recombine. Chiasmata are visible as the homologues align at metaphase I, with the centromeres oriented toward opposite poles. In anaphase I, the exchange of DNA between the homologues is apparent as the chromosomes are pulled to opposite poles. After completion of meiosis I and cytokinesis, meiosis II proceeds with a mitosis-like division. The sister kinetochores separate and move to opposite poles in anaphase II, yielding four haploid products.

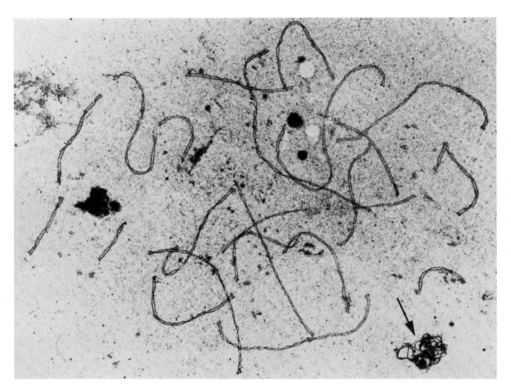

Figure 2-16 ■ Electron micrograph of a human primary spermatocyte in meiosis, showing the 22 autosomal synaptonemal complexes and the XY pair *(arrow)*. The DNA of each bivalent is not visible but extends laterally on each side of the synaptonemal complexes. (Courtesy of A. C. Chandley, Western General Hospital, Edinburgh, Scotland.)

divided between the two daughter cells (Fig. 2-17); but in oogenesis, one product (the secondary oocyte) receives almost all the cytoplasm, and the reciprocal product becomes the first polar body (Fig. 2-18). In contrast to mitosis, interphase is brief, and meiosis II begins. The notable point that distinguishes meiotic and mitotic interphase is that there is no S phase (i.e., no DNA synthesis) between the first and second meiotic divisions.

The Second Meiotic Division (Meiosis II)

The second meiotic division is similar to an ordinary mitosis except that the chromosome number of the cell entering meiosis II is haploid. The end result is that the two daughter cells from meiosis I divide to form four haploid cells, each containing 23 chromosomes (see Fig. 2-15). As mentioned earlier, because of crossing over in meiosis I, the chromosomes of the resulting gametes are not identical. Just as each maternal and paternal chromosome in a homologous pair segregates randomly into a daughter cell in meiosis I, segregation of the different paternal and maternal alleles of each gene also takes place during meiosis. However, whether the alleles segregate during the first or the second meiotic division (see Box) depends on whether they have been involved in a crossover event in meiosis I.

● ● ● Genetic Consequences of Meiosis

- **Reduction of the chromosome number** from diploid to haploid, the essential step in the formation of gametes.
- **Segregation of alleles**, at either meiosis I or meiosis II, in accordance with Mendel's first law.
- Shuffling of the genetic material by **random assortment of the homologues**, in accordance with Mendel's second law.
- Additional shuffling of the genetic material by **crossing over**, which is thought to have evolved as a mechanism for substantially increasing genetic variation but is, in addition, critical to ensure normal chromosome disjunction.

● HUMAN GAMETOGENESIS AND FERTILIZATION

The human primordial germ cells are recognizable by the fourth week of development outside the embryo proper, in the endoderm of the yolk sac. From there, they migrate during the sixth week to the genital ridges and associate with somatic cells to form the primitive gonads, which soon differentiate into testes or ovaries, depending on the cells' sex chromosome constitution (XY or XX), as we examine in greater detail in Chapter 6. Both spermatogenesis and oogenesis require meiosis but have important differences in detail and timing that may have clinical and genetic consequences for the offspring. Female meiosis is initiated once, early during fetal life, in a limited number of cells. In contrast, male meiosis is initiated continuously in many cells from a dividing cell population throughout the adult life of a male.

It is difficult to study human meiosis directly. In the female, successive stages of meiosis take place in the fetal ovary, in the oocyte near the time of ovulation, and after fertilization. Although postfertilization stages can be studied in vitro, access to the earlier stages is limited. Testicular material for the study of male meiosis is less difficult to obtain, inasmuch as testicular biopsy is included in the assessment of many men attending infertility clinics. Much remains to be learned about the cytogenetic, biochemical, and molecular mechanisms involved in normal meiosis and about the causes and consequences of meiotic irregularities.

Spermatogenesis

The stages of spermatogenesis are shown in Figure 2-17. **Sperm** (spermatozoa) are formed in the seminiferous tubules of the testes after sexual maturity is reached. The tubules are lined with **spermatogonia**, which are in different stages of differentiation. These cells have developed from the primordial germ cells by a long series of mitoses. The last cell type in the developmental sequence is the **primary spermatocyte,** which undergoes meiosis I to form two haploid **secondary spermatocytes.** Secondary spermatocytes rapidly undergo meiosis II, each forming two **spermatids,** which differentiate without further division into sperm. In humans, the entire process takes about 64 days. The enormous number of sperm produced, typically about 200 million per ejaculate and an estimated 10^{12} in a lifetime, requires several hundred successive mitoses.

Oogenesis

In contrast to spermatogenesis, which is initiated at puberty and continues throughout adult life, oogenesis begins during prenatal development (see Fig. 2-18). The ova develop from **oogonia,** cells in the ovarian cortex that have descended from the primordial germ cells by a series of about 20 mitoses. Each oogonium is the central cell in a developing follicle. By about the third month of prenatal development, the oogonia of the embryo have begun to develop into **primary oocytes,** most of which have already entered prophase of meiosis I. The process of oogenesis is not synchronized, and both early and late stages coexist in the fetal ovary.

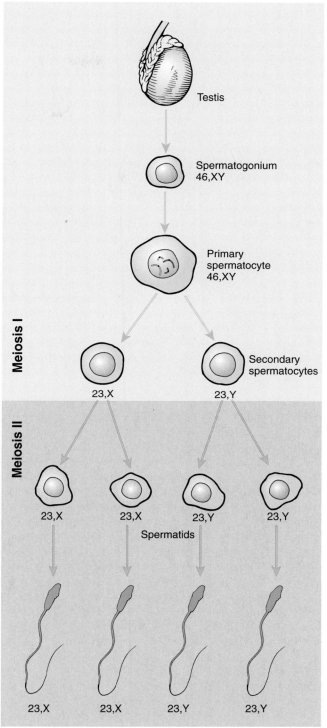

Figure 2-17 ■ Human spermatogenesis in relation to the two meiotic divisions. The sequence of events begins at puberty and takes about 64 days to be completed. The chromosome number (46 or 23) and the sex chromosome constitution (X or Y) of each cell are shown. (Modified from Moore KL, Persaud TVN: The Developing Human: Clinically Oriented Embryology, 6th ed. Philadelphia, WB Saunders, 1998.)

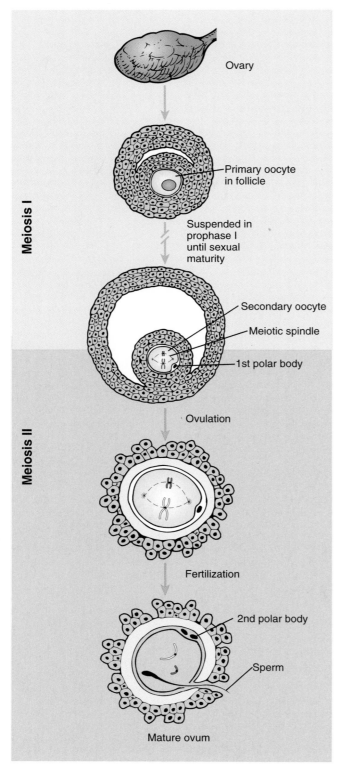

Meiosis I

Ovary

Primary oocyte
in follicle

Suspended in
prophase I
until sexual
maturity

Secondary oocyte

Meiotic spindle

1st polar body

Ovulation

Meiosis II

Fertilization

2nd polar body

Sperm

Mature ovum

Figure 2-18 ■ Human oogenesis and fertilization in relation to the two meiotic divisions. The primary oocytes are formed prenatally and remain suspended in prophase of meiosis I for years until the onset of puberty. An oocyte completes meiosis I as its follicle matures, resulting in a secondary oocyte and the first polar body. After ovulation, each oocyte continues to metaphase of meiosis II. Meiosis II is completed only if fertilization occurs, resulting in a fertilized mature ovum and the second polar body.

There are several million oocytes at the time of birth, but most of these degenerate, and only about 400 eventually mature and are ovulated. The primary oocytes have all nearly completed prophase I by the time of birth, and those that do not degenerate remain arrested in that stage for years, until ovulation as part of a woman's menstrual cycle.

After a woman has reached sexual maturity, individual follicles begin to grow and mature, and a few (on average one per month) are ovulated. Just before ovulation, the oocyte rapidly completes meiosis I, dividing in such a way that one cell becomes the secondary oocyte (an egg or **ovum**), containing most of the cytoplasm with its organelles, and the other becomes the first polar body (see Fig. 2-18). Meiosis II begins promptly and proceeds to the metaphase stage during ovulation, where it halts, only to be completed if fertilization occurs.

Fertilization

Fertilization of the egg usually takes place in the fallopian tube within a day or so of ovulation. Although multiple sperm may be present, the penetration of a single sperm into the ovum sets up a series of biochemical events that helps prevent the entry of other sperm.

Fertilization is followed by the completion of meiosis II, with the formation of the second polar body (see Fig. 2-18). The chromosomes of the fertilized egg and sperm become **pronuclei,** each surrounded by a nuclear membrane. The chromosomes of the diploid **zygote** replicate soon after fertilization, and the zygote divides by mitosis to form two diploid daughter cells. This mitosis is the first of the series of cleavage divisions that initiate the process of embryonic development (see Chapter 14).

Although development begins with the formation of the zygote (conception), in clinical medicine, the stage and duration of pregnancy are usually measured as the "menstrual age," dating from the beginning of the mother's last menstrual period, about 14 days before conception.

◉ MEDICAL RELEVANCE OF MITOSIS AND MEIOSIS

The biological significance of mitosis and meiosis lies in ensuring the constancy of chromosome number—and thus the integrity of the genome—from one cell to its progeny and from one generation to the next. The medical relevance of these processes lies in errors of one or the other mechanism of cell division, leading to formation of an individual or of a cell lineage with an abnormal number of chromosomes and thus abnormal dosage of genomic material.

As we see in detail in Chapter 5, meiotic nondisjunction, particularly in oogenesis, is the most common mutational mechanism in our species, responsible for chromosomally abnormal fetuses in at least several percent of all recognized pregnancies. Among pregnancies that survive to term, chromosome abnormalities are a leading cause of developmental defects, failure to thrive in the newborn period, and mental retardation.

Mitotic nondisjunction also contributes to genetic disease. Nondisjunction soon after fertilization, either in the developing embryo or in extraembryonic tissues like the placenta, leads to chromosomal mosaicism that can underlie some medical conditions, such as a proportion of patients with Down syndrome. Further, abnormal chromosome segregation in rapidly dividing tissues, such as in cells of the colon, is frequently a step in the development of chromosomally abnormal tumors, and thus evaluation of chromosome and genome balance is an important diagnostic and prognostic test in many cancers.

● GENERAL REFERENCES

Brown TA: Genomes, 3rd ed. New York, Garland, 2007.

Miller OJ, Therman E: Human Chromosomes, 4th ed. New York, Springer-Verlag, 2001.

Moore KL, Persaud TVN: Developing Human: Clinically Oriented Embryology, 7th ed. Philadelphia, WB Saunders, 2003.

● REFERENCES FOR SPECIFIC TOPICS

Deininger PL, Batzer MA: Alu repeats and human disease. Mol Genet Metab 67:183-193, 1999.

International Human Genome Sequencing Consortium: Initial sequencing and analysis of the human genome. Nature 409:860-921, 2001.

International Human Genome Sequencing Consortium: Finishing the euchromatic sequence of the human genome. Nature 431:931-945, 2004.

Kazazian HH, Moran JV: The impact of L1 retrotransposons on the human genome. Nat Genet 19:19-24, 1998.

Trask BJ: Human cytogenetics: 46 chromosomes, 46 years and counting. Nat Rev Genet 3:769-778, 2002.

Venter JC, Adams MD, Myers EW, et al: The sequence of the human genome. Science 291:1304-1351, 2001.

● USEFUL WEBSITES

Human Genome Resources: A compilation of useful websites for the study of genes, genomes and medicine. *http://www.ncbi.nlm.nih.gov/genome/guide/human/*

University of California, Santa Cruz: Genome Bioinformatics. *http://genome.ucsc.edu/*

Ensembl genome browser: European Bioinformatics Institute/Wellcome Trust Sanger Institute, Hinxton, Cambridge, United Kingdom. *http://www.ensembl.org/Homo_sapiens/index.html*

PROBLEMS

1. At a certain locus, a person has two alleles *A* and *a*.
   a. What are the genotypes of this person's gametes?
   b. When do *A* and *a* segregate (i) if there is no crossing over between the locus and the centromere of the chromosome? (ii) if there is a single crossover between the locus and the centromere?

2. What is the main cause of numerical chromosome abnormalities in humans?

3. Disregarding crossing over, which increases the amount of genetic variability, estimate the probability that all your chromosomes have come to you from your father's mother and your mother's mother. Would you be male or female?

4. A chromosome entering meiosis is composed of two chromatids, each of which is a single DNA molecule.
   a. In our species, at the end of meiosis I, how many chromosomes are there per cell? How many chromatids?
   b. At the end of meiosis II, how many chromosomes are there per cell? How many chromatids?
   c. When is the diploid chromosome number restored? When is the two-chromatid structure of a typical metaphase chromosome restored?

5. From Figure 2-8, estimate the number of genes per million base pairs on chromosomes 1, 13, 18, 19, 21, and 22. Would a chromosome abnormality of equal size on chromosome 18 or 19 be expected to have greater clinical impact? on chromosome 21 or 22?

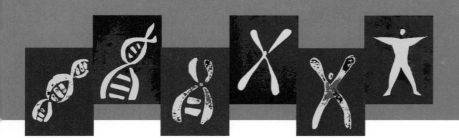

Chapter 3

The Human Genome:
Gene Structure and Function

During the past 20 years, remarkable progress has been made in our understanding of the structure and function of genes and chromosomes at the molecular level. More recently, as a direct result of the Human Genome Project, this knowledge has been supplemented by an in-depth understanding of the organization of the human genome at the level of its DNA sequence. These advances have been aided in large measure by the applications of molecular genetics and genomics to many clinical problems, thereby providing the tools for a distinctive new approach to medical genetics. In this chapter, we present an overview of gene structure and function and the aspects of molecular genetics that are required for an understanding of the genetic approach to medicine. To supplement the information discussed here, Chapter 4 describes many experimental approaches of modern molecular genetics and genomics that are becoming critical to the practice and understanding of human and medical genetics.

The increased knowledge of genes and of their organization in the genome has had an enormous impact on medicine and on our perception of human physiology. As 1980 Nobel laureate Paul Berg stated presciently at the dawn of this new era:

> *Just as our present knowledge and practice of medicine relies on a sophisticated knowledge of human anatomy, physiology, and biochemistry, so will dealing with disease in the future demand a detailed understanding of the molecular anatomy, physiology, and biochemistry of the human genome.... We shall need a more detailed knowledge of how human genes are organized and how they function and are regulated. We shall also have to have physicians who are as conversant with the molecular anatomy and physiology of chromosomes and genes as the cardiac surgeon is with the structure and workings of the heart.*

● INFORMATION CONTENT OF THE HUMAN GENOME

How does the 3-billion-letter digital code of the human genome guide the intricacies of human anatomy, physiology, and biochemistry to which Berg refers? The answer lies in the enormous expansion of information content that occurs as one moves from genes in the genome to proteins of the **proteome** that orchestrate the many functions of cells, organs, and the entire organism, as well as their interactions with the environment. Even with the essentially complete sequence of the human genome in hand, we still do not know the precise number of genes in the genome. Current estimates are that the genome contains about 25,000 genes, but this figure only begins to hint at the levels of complexity that emerge from the decoding of this digital information (Fig. 3-1).

As we discussed in Chapter 2, the product of most genes is a protein whose structure ultimately determines its particular functions in the cell. But if there were a simple one-to-one correspondence between genes and proteins, we could have at most 25,000 different proteins. This number seems insufficient to account for the vast array of functions that occur in human cells. The answer to this dilemma is found in two features of gene structure and function. First, many genes are capable of generating multiple different proteins, not just one (see Fig. 3-1). This process, discussed later in this chapter, is accomplished through the use of

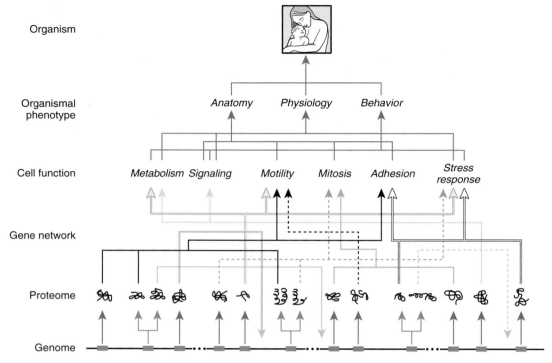

Organism

Organismal phenotype   *Anatomy*   *Physiology*   *Behavior*

Cell function   *Metabolism* *Signaling*   *Motility*   *Mitosis*   *Adhesion*   *Stress response*

Gene network

Proteome

Genome

Figure 3-1 ■ The amplification of genetic information from genome to proteome to gene networks and ultimately to cellular function and phenotype. Many genes in the genome use alternative coding information to generate multiple different proteins. Many proteins participate in multigene networks that respond to cellular signals in a coordinated and combinatorial manner, thus further expanding the range of cellular functions that underlie organismal phenotypes. (Based on an original figure courtesy of Greg Wray, Duke University, Durham, North Carolina.)

alternative coding segments in genes and through the subsequent biochemical modification of the encoded protein; these two features of complex genomes result in a substantial amplification of information content. Indeed, it has been estimated that in this way, the 25,000 human genes can encode as many as a million different proteins. Second, individual proteins do not function by themselves. They form elaborate networks of functions, involving many different proteins and responding in a coordinated fashion to many different genetic, developmental, or environmental signals. The combinatorial nature of gene networks results in an even greater diversity of possible cellular functions.

The genes are located throughout the genome but tend to cluster in some regions and on some chromosomes and to be relatively sparse in other regions or on other chromosomes. To illustrate this point, we use as an example chromosome 11, which, as we saw in Chapter 2, is a relatively gene-rich chromosome with about 1300 protein-coding genes (see Fig. 2-8). These genes are not distributed randomly along the chromosome, and their localization is particularly enriched in two chromosomal regions with gene density as high as one gene every 10 kb (Fig. 3-2). Some of the genes are organized into families of related genes, as we will describe more fully later in this chapter. Other regions are gene poor, and there are several so-called gene

deserts of a million base pairs or more without any known genes.

For genes located on the autosomes, there are two copies of each gene, one on the chromosome inherited from the mother and one on the chromosome inherited from the father. For most autosomal genes, both copies are expressed and generate a product. There are, however, a small number of genes in the genome that are exceptions to this general rule and are expressed only from one of the two copies. Examples of this unusual form of genetic regulation, called genomic imprinting, and its medical significance are discussed in greater detail both later in this chapter and in Chapters 5 and 7.

● THE CENTRAL DOGMA: DNA → RNA → PROTEIN

How does the genome specify the functional diversity evident in Figure 3-1? As we saw in the previous chapter, genetic information is contained in DNA in the chromosomes within the cell nucleus. However, protein synthesis, the process through which the information encoded in the genome is actually used to specify cellular functions, takes place in the cytoplasm. This compartmentalization reflects the fact that the human organism is a **eukaryote.** This means that human cells have a genuine

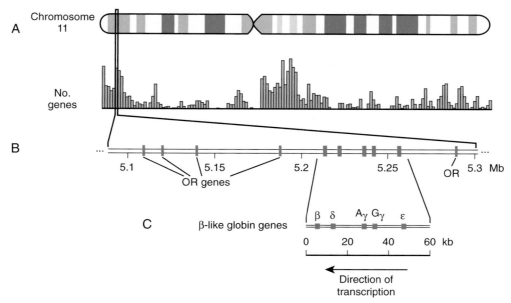

Figure 3-2 ■ Gene content on chromosome 11, which consists of 134.45 Mb of DNA. **A,** The distribution of genes is indicated along the chromosome and is high in two regions of the chromosome and low in other regions. **B,** An expanded region from 5.1 to 5.3 Mb (measured from the short-arm telomere), which contains 10 genes, five belonging to the olfactory receptor (OR) gene family and five belonging to the globin gene family. **C,** The five β-like globin genes expanded further. (Data from European Bioinformatics Institute and Wellcome Trust Sanger Institute: Ensembl v37, February 2006, *http://www.ensembl.org/Homo_sapiens/mapview?chr = 11.*)

nucleus containing the genome, which is separated by a nuclear membrane from the cytoplasm. In contrast, in prokaryotes like the intestinal bacterium *Escherichia coli,* DNA is not enclosed within a nucleus. Because of the compartmentalization of eukaryotic cells, information transfer from the nucleus to the cytoplasm is a complex process that has been a focus of much attention among molecular and cellular biologists.

The molecular link between these two related types of information (the DNA code of genes and the amino acid code of proteins) is **ribonucleic acid (RNA).** The chemical structure of RNA is similar to that of DNA, except that each nucleotide in RNA has a ribose sugar component instead of a deoxyribose; in addition, uracil (U) replaces thymine as one of the pyrimidines of RNA (Fig. 3-3). An additional difference between RNA and DNA is that RNA in most organisms exists as a single-stranded molecule, whereas DNA, as we saw in Chapter 2, exists as a double helix.

The informational relationships among DNA, RNA, and protein are intertwined: genomic DNA directs the synthesis and sequence of RNA, RNA directs the synthesis and sequence of polypeptides, and specific proteins are involved in the synthesis and metabolism of DNA and RNA. This flow of information is referred to as the central dogma of molecular biology.

Genetic information is stored in the DNA of the genome by means of a code (the **genetic code,** discussed later) in which the sequence of adjacent bases ultimately determines the sequence of amino acids in the encoded

polypeptide. First, RNA is synthesized from the DNA template through a process known as **transcription.** The RNA, carrying the coded information in a form called **messenger RNA (mRNA),** is then transported from the nucleus to the cytoplasm, where the RNA sequence is decoded, or translated, to determine the sequence of amino acids in the protein being synthesized. The process of **translation** occurs on **ribosomes,** which are cytoplasmic organelles with binding sites for all of the interacting molecules, including the mRNA, involved in protein synthesis. Ribosomes are themselves made up of many different structural proteins in association with specialized types of RNA known as **ribosomal RNA (rRNA).** Translation involves yet a third type of RNA, **transfer RNA (tRNA),** which provides the molecular link between the code contained in the base sequence of each mRNA and the amino acid sequence of the protein encoded by that mRNA.

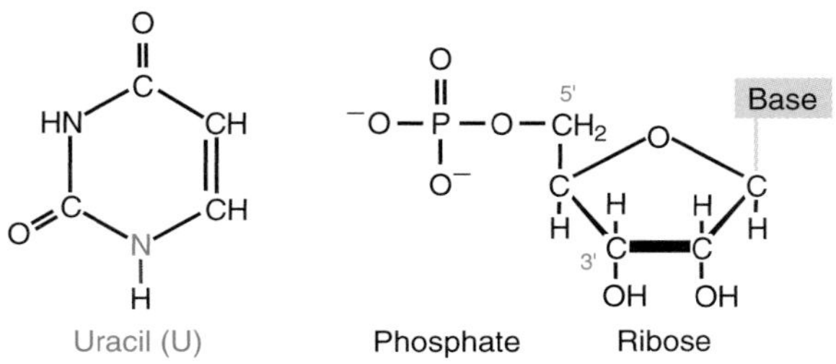

Figure 3-3 ■ The pyrimidine uracil and the structure of a nucleotide in RNA. Note that the sugar ribose replaces the sugar deoxyribose of DNA. Compare with Figure 2-2.

Because of the interdependent flow of information represented by the central dogma, one can begin discussion of the molecular genetics of gene expression at any of its three informational levels: DNA, RNA, or protein. We begin by examining the structure of genes in the genome as a foundation for discussion of the genetic code, transcription, and translation.

GENE ORGANIZATION AND STRUCTURE

In its simplest form, a gene can be visualized as a segment of a DNA molecule containing the code for the amino acid sequence of a polypeptide chain and the regulatory sequences necessary for its expression. This description, however, is inadequate for genes in the human genome (and indeed in most eukaryotic genomes) because few genes exist as continuous coding sequences. Rather, the majority of genes are interrupted by one or more noncoding regions. These intervening sequences, called **introns,** are initially transcribed into RNA in the nucleus but are not present in the mature mRNA in the cytoplasm. Thus, information from the intronic sequences is not normally represented in the final protein product. Introns alternate with **exons,** the segments of genes that ultimately determine the amino acid sequence of the protein, as well as certain flanking sequences that contain the 5' and 3' untranslated regions (Fig. 3-4). Although a few genes in the human genome have no introns, most genes contain at least one and usually several introns. Surprisingly, in many genes, the cumulative length of the introns makes up a far greater proportion of a gene's total length than do the exons. Whereas some genes are only a few kilobase pairs in length, others stretch on for hundreds of kilobase pairs. There are a few exceptionally large genes, such as the dystrophin gene on the X chromosome (mutations in which lead to Duchenne muscular dystrophy [Case 12]), which spans more than 2 million base pairs (2000 kb), of which, remarkably, less than 1% consists of coding exons.

Structural Features of a Typical Human Gene

A range of features characterize human genes (see Fig. 3-4). In Chapters 1 and 2, we briefly defined "gene" in general terms. At this point, we can provide a molecular definition of a gene. In typical circumstances, we define a gene as *a sequence of DNA in the genome that is required for production of a functional product,* be it a polypeptide or a functional RNA molecule. A gene includes not only the actual coding sequences but also adjacent nucleotide sequences required for the proper expression of the gene—that is, for the production of a

normal mRNA molecule, in the correct amount, in the correct place, and at the correct time during development or during the cell cycle.

The adjacent nucleotide sequences provide the molecular "start" and "stop" signals for the synthesis of mRNA transcribed from the gene. At the 5' end of each gene lies a **promoter** region that includes sequences responsible for the proper initiation of transcription. Within the 5' region are several DNA elements whose sequence is conserved among many different genes. This conservation, together with functional studies of gene expression, indicates that these particular sequences play an important role in gene regulation. Only a subset of genes in the genome is expressed in any given tissue. There are several different types of promoter found in the human genome, with different regulatory properties that specify the developmental patterns as well as the levels of expression of a particular gene in different tissues and cell types. The roles of individual conserved promoter elements are discussed in greater detail in the section "Fundamentals of Gene Expression." Both promoters and other **regulatory elements** (located either 5' or 3' of a gene or in its introns) can be sites of mutation in genetic disease that can interfere with the normal expression of a gene. These regulatory elements, including **enhancers, silencers, and locus control regions,** are discussed more fully later in this chapter. Some of these elements lie a significant distance away from the coding portion of a gene, thus reinforcing the concept that the genomic environment in which a gene resides is an important feature of its evolution and regulation as well as accounting for, in some cases, the type of mutations that can interfere with its normal expression and function. By comparative analysis of many thousands of genes now being analyzed as a result of the Human Genome Project, additional important genomic elements are being identified and their role in human disease clarified.

At the 3' end of the gene lies an untranslated region of importance that contains a signal for the addition of a sequence of adenosine residues (the so-called polyA tail) to the end of the mature mRNA. Although it is generally accepted that such closely neighboring regulatory sequences are part of what is called a gene, the precise dimensions of any particular gene will remain somewhat uncertain until the potential functions of more distant sequences are fully characterized.

Gene Families

Many genes belong to gene families, which share closely related DNA sequences and encode polypeptides with closely related amino acid sequences.

Members of two such gene families are located within a small region on chromosome 11 (see Fig. 3-2)

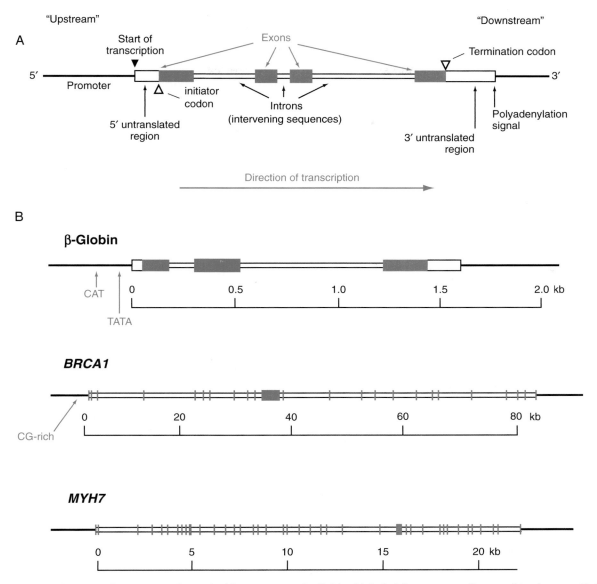

Figure 3-4 ■ **A,** General structure of a typical human gene. Individual labeled features are discussed in the text. **B,** Examples of three medically important human genes. Different mutations in the β-globin gene, with three exons, cause a variety of important disorders of hemoglobin (Cases 37 and 39). Mutations in the *BRCA1* gene (24 exons) are responsible for many cases of inherited breast or breast and ovarian cancer (Case 5). Mutations in the β-myosin heavy chain (*MYH7*) gene (40 exons) lead to inherited hypertrophic cardiomyopathy.

and illustrate a number of features that characterize gene families in general. One small and medically important gene family is composed of genes that encode the protein chains found in hemoglobins. The β-globin gene cluster on chromosome 11 and the related α-globin gene cluster on chromosome 16 are believed to have arisen by duplication of a primitive precursor gene about 500 million years ago. These two clusters contain multiple genes coding for closely related globin chains expressed at different developmental stages, from embryo to adult. Each cluster is believed to have evolved by a series of sequential gene duplication events within the past 100 million years. The exon-intron patterns of

the functional globin genes appear to have been remarkably conserved during evolution; each of the functional globin genes has two introns at similar locations (see the β-globin gene in Fig. 3-4), although the sequences contained within the introns have accumulated far more nucleotide base changes over time than have the coding sequences of each gene. The control of expression of the various globin genes, in the normal state as well as in the many inherited disorders of hemoglobin, is considered in more detail both later in this chapter and in Chapter 11.

The second gene family shown in Figure 3-2 is the family of olfactory receptor (OR) genes. There are estimated to be at least 350 functional OR genes in the genome, which are responsible for our acute sense of smell that can recognize and distinguish thousands of structurally diverse chemicals. The OR genes are located throughout the genome on nearly every chromosome, although more than half are found on chromosome 11, including those family members near the β-globin cluster. The OR gene family is actually part of a much larger **gene superfamily** encoding a large variety of what are called G protein–coupled receptors, which are characterized by a conserved membrane-spanning protein motif that is critical for the function of a diverse repertoire of receptors. Members of this class of proteins are mutated in a wide range of inherited diseases, some of which are described in Chapter 12.

Pseudogenes

Within both the β-globin and OR gene families are sequences that are related to the functional globin and OR genes but that do not produce any RNA or protein product. DNA sequences that closely resemble known genes but are nonfunctional are called **pseudogenes**, and there are many thousands of pseudogenes related to many different genes and gene families. Pseudogenes are widespread in the genome and are of two general types, processed and nonprocessed. **Nonprocessed pseudogenes** are thought to be byproducts of evolution, representing "dead" genes that were once functional but are now vestigial, having been inactivated by mutations in coding or regulatory sequences. In some cases, as in the pseudo–α-globin and pseudo–β-globin genes, the pseudogenes presumably arose through gene duplication, followed by the accumulation of numerous mutations in the extra copies of the once-functional gene. In contrast to nonprocessed pseudogenes, **processed pseudogenes** are pseudogenes that have been formed, not by mutation, but by a process called **retrotransposition,** which involves transcription, generation of a DNA copy of the mRNA (reverse transcription), and finally integration of such DNA copies back into the genome. Because such pseudogenes are created by retrotransposition of a DNA copy of processed mRNA, they lack introns and are not necessarily or usually on the same chromosome (or chromosomal region) as their progenitor gene. In many gene families, there are as many pseudogenes as there are functional gene members, or more. In the OR gene family, for example, there are an estimated 600 or more OR pseudogenes spread throughout the human genome.

Noncoding RNA Genes

Not all genes in the human genome encode proteins. Chromosome 11, for example, in addition to its 1300 protein-coding genes, has an estimated 200 **noncoding RNA genes,** whose final product is an RNA, not a protein. Although the functions of these genes are incompletely understood, some are involved in the regulation of other genes, whereas others may play structural roles in various nuclear or cytoplasmic processes. An important class of noncoding RNA genes are known as **microRNA** (miRNA) genes, of which there are at least 250 in the human genome; miRNAs are short 22-nucleotide-long noncoding RNAs, at least some of which control the expression or repression of other genes during development.

FUNDAMENTALS OF GENE EXPRESSION

As introduced earlier, for genes that encode proteins, the flow of information from gene to polypeptide involves several steps (Fig. 3-5). Initiation of transcription of a gene is under the influence of promoters and other regulatory elements as well as specific proteins known as **transcription factors,** which interact with specific sequences within these regions and determine the spatial and temporal pattern of expression of a gene. Transcription of a gene is initiated at the transcriptional "start site" on chromosomal DNA at the beginning of a 5′ transcribed but *un*translated *r*egion (called the 5′ UTR), just upstream from the coding sequences, and continues along the chromosome for anywhere from several hundred base pairs to more than a million base pairs, through both introns and exons and past the end of the coding sequences. After modification at both the 5′ and 3′ ends of the primary RNA transcript, the portions corresponding to introns are removed, and the segments corresponding to exons are spliced together. After **RNA splicing,** the resulting mRNA (containing a central segment that is co-linear with the coding portions of the gene) is transported from the nucleus to the cytoplasm, where the mRNA is finally translated into the amino acid sequence of the encoded polypeptide. Each of the steps in this complex pathway is subject to error, and mutations that interfere with the individual steps have been implicated in a number of inherited genetic disorders (see Chapters 7, 8, 11, and 12).

Transcription

Transcription of protein-coding genes by RNA polymerase II (one of several classes of RNA polymerases) is initiated at the transcriptional start site, the point in the 5′ UTR that corresponds to the 5′ end of the final RNA product (see Figs. 3-4 and 3-5). Synthesis of the primary RNA transcript proceeds in a 5′ to 3′ direction, whereas the strand of the gene that is transcribed and that serves as the template for RNA synthesis is actually read in a 3′ to 5′ direction with respect to the

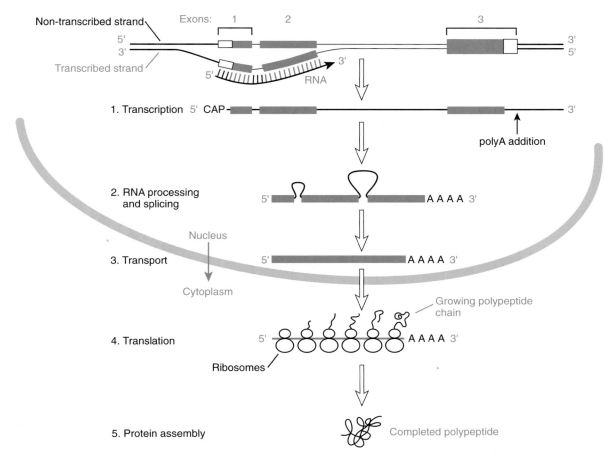

Figure 3-5 ■ Flow of information from DNA to RNA to protein for a hypothetical gene with three exons and two introns. Within the exons, blue indicates the coding sequences. Steps include transcription, RNA processing and splicing, RNA transport from the nucleus to the cytoplasm, and translation.

direction of the deoxyribose phosphodiester backbone (see Fig. 2-3). Because the RNA synthesized corresponds both in polarity and in base sequence (substituting U for T) to the 5′ to 3′ strand of DNA, the 5′ to 3′ strand of nontranscribed DNA is sometimes called the *coding,* or **sense,** DNA strand. The 3′ to 5′ transcribed template strand of DNA is then referred to as the *noncoding,* or **antisense,** strand. Transcription continues through both intronic and exonic portions of the gene, beyond the position on the chromosome that eventually corresponds to the 3′ end of the mature mRNA. Whether transcription ends at a predetermined 3′ termination point is unknown.

The primary RNA transcript is processed by addition of a chemical "cap" structure to the 5′ end of the RNA and cleavage of the 3′ end at a specific point downstream from the end of the coding information. This cleavage is followed by addition of a polyA tail to the 3′ end of the RNA; the polyA tail appears to increase the stability of the resulting polyadenylated RNA. The location of the polyadenylation point is specified in part by the sequence AAUAAA (or a variant of this), usually found in the 3′ untranslated portion of the RNA tran-

script. All of these post-transcriptional modifications take place in the nucleus, as does the process of RNA splicing. The fully processed RNA, now called mRNA, is then transported to the cytoplasm, where translation takes place (see Fig. 3-5).

Translation and the Genetic Code

In the cytoplasm, mRNA is translated into protein by the action of a variety of tRNA molecules, each specific for a particular amino acid. These remarkable molecules, each only 70 to 100 nucleotides long, have the job of bringing the correct amino acids into position along the mRNA template, to be added to the growing polypeptide chain. Protein synthesis occurs on ribosomes, macromolecular complexes made up of rRNA (encoded by the 18S and 28S rRNA genes), and several dozen ribosomal proteins (see Fig. 3-5).

The key to translation is a code that relates specific amino acids to combinations of three adjacent bases along the mRNA. Each set of three bases constitutes a **codon,** specific for a particular amino acid (Table 3-1). In theory, almost infinite variations are possible in the

Table 3-1

The Genetic Code

First Base	Second Base								Third Base
	U		C		A		G		
U	UUU	phe	UCU	ser	UAU	tyr	UGU	cys	U
	UUC	phe	UCC	ser	UAC	tyr	UGC	cys	C
	UUA	leu	UCA	ser	UAA	stop	UGA	stop	A
	UUG	leu	UCG	ser	UAG	stop	UGG	trp	G
C	CUU	leu	CCU	pro	CAU	his	CGU	arg	U
	CUC	leu	CCC	pro	CAC	his	CGC	arg	C
	CUA	leu	CCA	pro	CAA	gln	CGA	arg	A
	CUG	leu	CCG	pro	CAG	gln	CGG	arg	G
A	AUU	ile	ACU	thr	AAU	asn	AGU	ser	U
	AUC	ile	ACC	thr	AAC	asn	AGC	ser	C
	AUA	ile	ACA	thr	AAA	lys	AGA	arg	A
	AUG	met	ACG	thr	AAG	lys	AGG	arg	G
G	GUU	val	GCU	ala	GAU	asp	GGU	gly	U
	GUC	val	GCC	ala	GAC	asp	GGC	gly	C
	GUA	val	GCA	ala	GAA	glu	GGA	gly	A
	GUG	val	GCG	ala	GAG	glu	GGG	gly	G

ABBREVIATIONS FOR AMINO ACIDS

ala (A)	alanine	leu (L)	leucine
arg (R)	arginine	lys (K)	lysine
asn (N)	asparagine	met (M)	methionine
asp (D)	aspartic acid	phe (F)	phenylalanine
cys (C)	cysteine	pro (P)	proline
gln (Q)	glutamine	ser (S)	serine
glu (E)	glutamic acid	thr (T)	threonine
gly (G)	glycine	trp (W)	tryptophan
his (H)	histidine	tyr (Y)	tyrosine
ile (I)	isoleucine	val (V)	valine

Stop = termination codon.
Codons are shown in terms of messenger RNA, which are complementary to the corresponding DNA codons.

arrangement of the bases along a polynucleotide chain. At any one position, there are four possibilities (A, T, C, or G); thus, for three bases, there are 4^3, or 64, possible triplet combinations. These 64 codons constitute the **genetic code.**

Because there are only 20 amino acids and 64 possible codons, most amino acids are specified by more than one codon; hence the code is said to be **degenerate.** For instance, the base in the third position of the triplet can often be either purine (A or G) or either pyrimidine (T or C) or, in some cases, any one of the four bases, without altering the coded message (see Table 3-1). Leucine and arginine are each specified by six codons. Only methionine and tryptophan are each specified by a single, unique codon. Three of the codons are called **stop** (or **nonsense**) **codons** because they designate termination of translation of the mRNA at that point.

Translation of a processed mRNA is always initiated at a codon specifying methionine. Methionine is therefore the first encoded (amino-terminal) amino acid of each polypeptide chain, although it is usually removed before protein synthesis is completed. The codon for methionine (the initiator codon, AUG) establishes the **reading frame** of the mRNA; each subsequent codon is

read in turn to predict the amino acid sequence of the protein.

The molecular links between codons and amino acids are the specific tRNA molecules. A particular site on each tRNA forms a three-base **anticodon** that is complementary to a specific codon on the mRNA. Bonding between the codon and anticodon brings the appropriate amino acid into the next position on the ribosome for attachment, by formation of a peptide bond, to the carboxyl end of the growing polypeptide chain. The ribosome then slides along the mRNA exactly three bases, bringing the next codon into line for recognition by another tRNA with the next amino acid. Thus, proteins are synthesized from the amino terminus to the carboxyl terminus, which corresponds to translation of the mRNA in a 5′ to 3′ direction.

As mentioned earlier, translation ends when a stop codon (UGA, UAA, or UAG) is encountered in the same reading frame as the initiator codon. (Stop codons in either of the other unused reading frames are not read and therefore have no effect on translation.) The completed polypeptide is then released from the ribosome, which becomes available to begin synthesis of another protein.

Post-translational Processing

Many proteins undergo extensive post-translational modifications. The polypeptide chain that is the primary translation product is folded and bonded into a specific three-dimensional structure that is determined by the amino acid sequence itself. Two or more polypeptide chains, products of the same gene or of different genes, may combine to form a single mature protein complex. For example, two α-globin chains and two β-globin chains associate noncovalently to form a tetrameric hemoglobin molecule (see Chapter 11). The protein products may also be modified chemically by, for example, addition of methyl groups, phosphates, or carbohydrates at specific sites. These modifications can have significant influence on the function or abundance of the modified protein. Other modifications may involve cleavage of the protein, either to remove specific amino-terminal sequences after they have functioned to direct a protein to its correct location within the cell (e.g., proteins that function within the nucleus or mitochondria) or to split the molecule into smaller polypeptide chains. For example, the two chains that make up mature insulin, one 21 and the other 30 amino acids long, are originally part of an 82–amino acid primary translation product called proinsulin.

Transcription of the Mitochondrial Genome

The previous sections described fundamentals of gene expression for genes contained in the nuclear genome. The mitochondrial genome has a distinct transcription and protein-synthesis system. A specialized RNA polymerase, encoded in the nuclear genome, is used to transcribe the mitochondrial genome, which contains two related promoter sequences, one for each strand of the circular genome. Each strand is transcribed in its entirety, and the mitochondrial transcripts are then processed to generate the various individual mitochondrial mRNAs, tRNAs, and rRNAs.

● GENE EXPRESSION IN ACTION: THE β-GLOBIN GENE

The flow of information outlined in the preceding sections can best be appreciated by reference to a particular well-studied gene, the β-globin gene. The β-globin chain is a 146–amino acid polypeptide, encoded by a gene that occupies approximately 1.6 kb on the short arm of chromosome 11. The gene has three exons and two introns (see Fig. 3-4). The β-globin gene, as well as the other genes in the β-globin cluster (see Fig. 3-2), is transcribed in a centromere-to-telomere direction. The orientation, however, is different for other genes in the genome and depends on which strand of the chromosomal double helix is the coding strand for a particular gene.

DNA sequences required for accurate initiation of transcription of the β-globin gene are located in the promoter within approximately 200 base pairs upstream from the transcription start site. The double-stranded DNA sequence of this region of the β-globin gene, the corresponding RNA sequence, and the translated sequence of the first 10 amino acids are depicted in Figure 3-6 to illustrate the relationships among these three information levels. As mentioned previously, it is the 3′ to 5′ strand of the DNA that serves as template and is actually transcribed, but it is the 5′ to 3′ strand of DNA that directly corresponds to the 5′ to 3′ sequence of the mRNA (and, in fact, is identical to it except that U is substituted for T). Because of this correspondence, the 5′ to 3′ DNA strand of a gene (i.e., the strand that is *not* transcribed) is the strand generally reported in the scientific literature or in databases.

In accordance with this convention, the complete sequence of approximately 2.0 kb of chromosome 11 that includes the β-globin gene is shown in Figure 3-7. (It is sobering to reflect that this page of nucleotides represents only 0.000067% of the sequence of the entire human genome!) Within these 2.0 kb are contained most but not all of the sequence elements required to encode and regulate the expression of this gene.

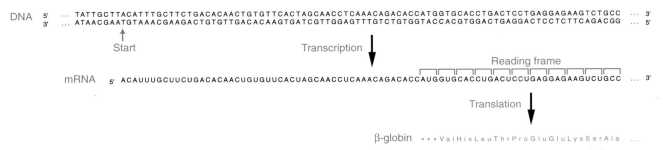

Figure 3-6 ■ Structure and nucleotide sequence of the 5′ end of the human β-globin gene on the short arm of chromosome 11. Transcription of the 3′ to 5′ *(lower)* strand begins at the indicated start site to produce β-globin mRNA. The translational reading frame is determined by the AUG initiator codon (***); subsequent codons specifying amino acids are indicated in blue. The other two potential frames are not used.

5'....agccacaccctagggttggccaatctactcccaggagcagggagggcaggagccagggctgggcataaaa

gtcagggcagagccatctattgcttACATTTGCTTCTGACACAACTGTGTTCACTAGCAACCTCAAACAGACACCATG

Exon 1

ValHisLeuThrProGluGluLysSerAlaValThrAlaLeuTrpGlyLysValAsnValAspGluValGlyGlyGlu
GTGCACCTGACTCCTGAGGAGAAGTCTGCCGTTACTGCCCTGTGGGGCAAGGTGAACGTGGATGAAGTTGGTGGTGAG

AlaLeuGlyAr-
GCCCTGGGCAGgttggtatcaaggttacaagacaggtttaaggagaccaatagaaactgggcatgtggagacagagaag

Intron 1

-gLeuLeuValValTyr
actcttgggtttctgataggcactgactctctctgcctattggtctattttcccacccttagGCTGCTGGTGGTCTAC

Exon 2

ProTrpThrGlnArgPhePheGluSerPheGlyAspLeuSerThrProAspAlaValMetGlyAsnProLysValLys
CCTTGGACCCAGAGGTTCTTTGAGTCCTTTGGGGATCTGTCCACTCCTGATGCTGTTATGGGCAACCCTAAGGTGAAG

AlaHisGlyLysLysValLeuGlyAlaPheSerAspGlyLeuAlaHisLeuAspAsnLeuLysGlyThrPheAlaThr
GCTCATGGCAAGAAAGTGCTCGGTGCCTTTAGTGATGGCCTGGCTCACCTGGACAACCTCAAGGGCACCTTTGCCACA

LeuSerGluLeuHisCysAspLysLeuHisValAspProGluAsnPheArg
CTGAGTGAGCTGCACTGTGACAAGCTGCACGTGGATCCTGAGAACTTCAGGgtgagtctatgggacccttgatgtttt

ctttccccttctttttctatggttaagttcatgtcataggaaggggagaagtaacagggtacagtttagaatgggaaac

agacgaatgattgcatcagtgtggaagtctcaggatcgttttagtttcttttatttgctgttcataacaattgttttc

ttttgtttaattcttgctttctttttttttttcttctccgcaatttttactattatacttaatgccttaacattgtgtat

Intron 2

aacaaaaggaaatatctctgagatacattaagtaacttaaaaaaaaaactttacacagtctgcctagtacattactatt

tggaatatatgtgtgcttatttgcatattcataatgtccctactttattttctttttatttttaattgatacataatca

ttatacatatttatgggttaaagtgtaatgtttttaatatgtgtacacatattgaccaaatcagggtaattttgcatt

tgtaattttaaaaaatgctttcttcttttaatatactttttttgtttatcttatttctaatactttccctaatctcttt

ctttcagggcaataatgatacaatgtatcatgcctctttgcaccattctaaagaataacagtgataatttctgggtta

aggcaatagcaatatttctgcatataaatatttctgcatataaattgtaactgatgtaagaggtttcatattgctaa

tagcagctacaatccagctaccattctgcttttatttttatggttggggataaggctggattattctgagtccaagctag

LeuLeuGlyAsnValLeuValCysValLeuAla
gccctttttgctaatcatgttcatacctcttatcttcctcccacagCTCCTGGGCAACGTGCTGGTCTGTGTGCTGGCC

Exon 3

HisHisPheGlyLysGluPheThrProProValGlnAlaAlaTryGlnLysValValAlaGlyValAlaAsnAlaLeu
CATCACTTTGGCAAAGAATTCACCCCACCAGTGCAGGCTGCCTATCAGAAAGTGGTGGCTGGTGTGGCTAATGCCCTG

AlaHisLysTyrHisTer
GCCCACAAGTATCACTAAGCTCGCTTTCTTGCTGTCCAATTTCTATTAAAGGTTCCTTTGTTCCCTAAGTCCAACTAC

TAAACTGGGGGGATATTATGAAGGGCCTTGAGCATCTGGATTCTGCCTAATAAAAAACATTTATTTTCATTGCaatgat

gtatttaaattatttctgaatattttactaaaaagggaatgtgggaggtcagtgcatttaaaacataaagaaatgatg

agctgttcaaaccttgggaaaatacactatatcttaaactccatgaaagaaggtgaggctgcaaccagctaatgcaca

ttggcaacagcccctgatgcctatgccttattcatccctcagaaaaggattcttgtagaggcttga.... 3'

Figure 3-7 ■ Nucleotide sequence of the complete human β-globin gene. The sequence of the 5' to 3' strand of the gene is shown. Light blue areas with capital letters represent exonic sequences corresponding to mature mRNA. Lowercase letters indicate introns and flanking sequences. The CAT and TATA box sequences in the 5' flanking region are indicated in dark blue. The GT and AG dinucleotides important for RNA splicing at the intron-exon junctions and the AATAAA signal important for addition of a poly-A tail also are highlighted. The ATG initiator codon (AUG in mRNA) and the TAA stop codon (UAA in mRNA) are shown in blue letters. The amino acid sequence of β-globin is shown above the coding sequence; the three-letter abbreviations in Table 3-1 are used here. (Modified from Lawn RM, Efstratiadis A, O'Connell C, et al: The nucleotide sequence of the human β-globin gene. Cell 21:647-651, 1980.)

Indicated in Figure 3-7 are many of the important structural features of the β-globin gene, including conserved promoter sequence elements, intron and exon boundaries, 5' and 3' untranslated regions, RNA splice sites, the initiator and termination codons, and the polyadenylation signal, all of which are known to be mutated in various inherited defects of the β-globin gene (see Chapter 11).

Initiation of Transcription

The β-globin promoter, like many other gene promoters, consists of a series of relatively short functional elements that interact with specific proteins (generically called **transcription factors**) that regulate transcription, including, in the case of the globin genes, those proteins that restrict expression of these genes to erythroid cells, the cells in which hemoglobin is produced. One important promoter sequence is the **TATA box,** a conserved region rich in adenines and thymines that is approximately 25 to 30 base pairs upstream of the start site of transcription (see Figs. 3-4 and 3-7). The TATA box appears to be important for determining the position of the start of transcription, which in the β-globin gene is approximately 50 base pairs upstream from the translation initiation site (see Fig. 3-6). Thus, in this gene there are about 50 base pairs of sequence that are transcribed but are not translated. In other genes, this 5' UTR can be much longer and can even be interrupted by one or more introns. A second conserved region, the so-called CAT box (actually CCAAT), is a few dozen base pairs farther upstream (see Fig. 3-7). Both experimentally induced and naturally occurring mutations in either of these sequence elements, as well as in other regulatory sequences even farther upstream, lead to a sharp reduction in the level of transcription, thereby demonstrating the importance of these elements for normal gene expression. Many mutations in these regulatory elements have been identified in patients with the hemoglobin disorder β-thalassemia (see Chapter 11).

Not all gene promoters contain the two specific elements described. In particular, genes that are constitutively expressed in most or all tissues (called housekeeping genes) often lack the CAT and TATA boxes that are more typical of tissue-specific genes. Promoters of many housekeeping genes often contain a high proportion of cytosines and guanines in relation to the surrounding DNA (see the promoter of the *BRCA1* breast cancer gene in Fig. 3-4). Such CG-rich promoters are often located in regions of the genome called **CpG islands,** so named because of the unusually high concentration of the dinucleotide 5'-CG-3' that stands out from the more general AT-rich genomic landscape. Some of the CG-rich sequence elements found in these promoters are thought to serve as binding sites for specific transcription factors. CpG islands are also important because they are targets for DNA modification by the addition of a methyl group to one of the available carbons in cytosine (see Fig. 2-2). Extensive DNA methylation at CpG islands is usually associated with repression of gene transcription. This type of gene inactivation is seen in many cancers (see Chapter 16) and is a hallmark of several important developmental regulatory events, such as genomic imprinting and X chromosome inactivation (see Chapters 5 and 6).

In addition to the sequences that constitute a promoter itself, there are other sequence elements that can markedly alter the efficiency of transcription. The best characterized of these "activating" sequences are called **enhancers.** Enhancers are sequence elements that can act at a distance (often several kilobases or more) from a gene to stimulate transcription. Unlike promoters, enhancers are both position and orientation independent and can be located either 5' or 3' of the transcription start site. Enhancer elements function only in certain cell types and thus appear to be involved in establishing the tissue specificity or level of expression of many genes, in concert with one or more transcription factors. In the case of the β-globin gene, several tissue-specific enhancers are present both within the gene itself and in its flanking regions. The interaction of enhancers with particular proteins leads to increased levels of transcription.

Normal expression of the β-globin gene during development also requires more distant sequences called the **locus control region (LCR),** located upstream of the ε-globin gene (see Fig. 3-2), which is required for establishing the proper chromatin context needed for appropriate high-level expression. As expected, mutations that disrupt or delete either enhancer or LCR sequences interfere with or prevent β-globin gene expression (see Chapter 11).

RNA Splicing

The primary RNA transcript of the β-globin gene contains two introns, approximately 100 and 850 base pairs in length, that need to be spliced out. The process of RNA splicing is exact and highly efficient; 95% of β-globin transcripts are thought to be accurately spliced to yield functional globin mRNA. The splicing reactions are guided by specific sequences in the primary RNA transcript at both the 5' and the 3' ends of introns. The 5' sequence consists of nine nucleotides, of which two (the dinucleotide GT [GU in the RNA transcript] located in the intron immediately adjacent to the splice site) are virtually invariant among splice sites in different genes (see Fig. 3-7). The 3' sequence consists of about a dozen nucleotides, of which, again, two, the AG located immediately 5' to the intron-exon boundary, are obligatory for normal splicing. The splice sites themselves are unrelated to the reading frame of the particular mRNA. In some instances, as in the case of intron 1 of the β-globin gene, the intron actually splits a specific codon (see Fig. 3-7).

The medical significance of RNA splicing is illustrated by the fact that mutations within the conserved sequences at the intron-exon boundaries commonly impair RNA splicing, with a concomitant reduction in the amount of normal, mature β-globin mRNA; mutations in the GT or AG dinucleotides mentioned earlier invariably eliminate normal splicing of the intron containing the mutation. Representative splice site mutations identified in patients with β-thalassemia are discussed in detail in Chapter 11.

Alternative Splicing

As just discussed, when introns are removed from the primary RNA transcript by RNA splicing, the remaining exons are spliced together to generate the final, mature mRNA. However, for many genes, the primary transcript can follow multiple alternative splicing pathways, leading to the synthesis of multiple related but different mRNAs, each of which can be subsequently translated to generate different protein products (see Fig. 3-1). At least one third of all human genes undergo alternative splicing, and it has been estimated that there are an average of two or three alternative transcripts per gene in the human genome, thus greatly expanding the information content of the human genome beyond the estimated 25,000 genes. A particularly impressive example of this involves the gene for a potassium channel that is mutated in an inherited form of epilepsy. The gene has 35 exons, and eight of these are subject to alternative splicing. More than 500 different mRNAs can be generated from this one gene, each encoding a channel with different functional properties.

Polyadenylation

The mature β-globin mRNA contains approximately 130 base pairs of 3′ untranslated material (the 3′ UTR) between the stop codon and the location of the polyA tail (see Fig. 3-7). As in other genes, cleavage of the 3′ end of the mRNA and addition of the polyA tail is controlled, at least in part, by an AAUAAA sequence approximately 20 base pairs before the polyadenylation site. Mutations in this polyadenylation signal in patients with β-thalassemia document the importance of this signal for proper 3′ cleavage and polyadenylation (see Chapter 11). The 3′ UTR of some genes can be quite long, up to several kilobase pairs. Other genes have a number of alternative polyadenylation sites, selection among which may influence the stability of the resulting mRNA and thus the steady-state level of each mRNA.

GENE REGULATION AND CHANGES IN ACTIVITY OF THE GENOME

Most examples of changes in gene expression are accomplished by alterations in the level of transcription, alternative splicing, or post-translational modification. The activation or repression of a given gene in a given tissue or at a given time during development usually involves changes in transcriptional control, carried out by combinations of specific transcription factors and other proteins interacting with the gene regulatory machinery in response to developmental, spatial, or environmental cues or stimuli. In such examples, the genome itself is unchanged, and it is the regulation, not the structure, of genes that changes dynamically.

There are, however, several important examples of changes in activity of the genome where the genes themselves do change as a result of physical rearrangement of the genome and elevated rates of somatic mutation in specific cell lineages.

Immunoglobulin and T-Cell Receptor Diversity

Antibodies are immunoglobulins that are elicited in response to a stimulus by a foreign antigen and can recognize and bind that antigen and facilitate its elimination. A number of genetic diseases are due to deficiencies of immunoglobulins. However, the primary significance of immunoglobulins from the perspective of the genome is that they exhibit a unique property, **somatic rearrangement**, by which cutting and pasting of DNA sequences in lymphocyte precursor cells is used to rearrange genes in somatic cells to generate diversity.

It is estimated that each human being can generate a repertoire of about 10^{11} different antibodies, yet the genome is composed of only 6 billion base pairs of DNA. This seeming disparity has been reconciled by the demonstration that antibodies are encoded in the germline by a relatively small number of genes that, during B-cell development, undergo a unique process of somatic rearrangement and somatic mutation that allows the generation of enormous diversity.

Immunoglobulin molecules are composed of four polypeptide chains, two identical heavy (H) chains and two identical light (L) chains. Each H and L chain of an immunoglobulin protein consists of two segments, the constant (C) and the variable (V) regions. The constant region determines the class of the immunoglobulin molecule (M, G, A, E, or D), and its amino acid sequence is relatively conserved among immunoglobulins of the same class. In contrast, the amino acid sequence of the V region shows wide variation among different antibodies. The V regions of the H and L chains form the antigen-binding site and determine antibody specificity.

Remarkably, there are no complete genes in the human genome for the immunoglobulin H and L chains. Instead, each H and L chain is encoded by multiple genes that are widely separated by hundreds of kilobases in germline DNA. For example, the H-chain V region is made up of three domains, the V, D, and J segments (Fig. 3-8). More than 200 different V-segment genes are present in the H-chain locus (although some of these are likely to be pseudogenes); farther down the chromosome are approximately 30 D-segment genes and 9 J-segment genes, followed by the various constant segment genes for each of the immunoglobulin types. In total, the H-chain cluster of immunoglobulin genes as well as the similarly arranged L-chain clusters span many millions of base pairs in the genome.

During the differentiation of antibody-producing cells (but *not* in any other cell lineages), DNA at the immunoglobulin loci needs to be rearranged to produce the functional H and L chains. For the H-chain locus, a complete variable region gene is created by generating double-stranded DNA breaks and connecting the free DNA ends, resulting in the juxtaposition of one of the V segments to one of the D segments, which in turn is joined to one of the J regions with deletion of the intervening genomic DNA (see Fig. 3-8). This rearranged segment is then transcribed, and the intronic sequences between the newly formed VDJ fusion exon and C segments are removed, as usual, by RNA splicing to generate a mature mRNA for translation into a specific H-chain. The L-chain loci

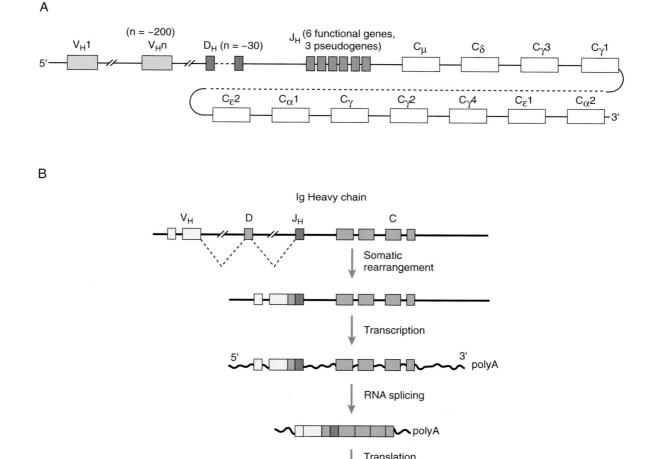

Figure 3-8 ■ Immunoglobulin gene organization and somatic rearrangement to generate a functional gene. **A,** Organization of the heavy chain locus on chromosome 14 in germline genomic DNA, in which many V, D, and J segments are distributed across an extensive region, together with different constant (C) genes. **B,** Rearrangement of the heavy chain genes during antibody formation. Not drawn to scale. (Modified from Abbas AK, Lichtman AH, Pober JS: Cellular and Molecular Immunology, 5th ed. Philadelphia, WB Saunders, 2003.)

undergo a similar process of DNA rearrangement before transcription.

Additional antibody diversity is generated by deletions caused by imprecise joining of gene segments during the somatic rearrangement process. Insertions at the site of joining can also occur when nucleotides (so-called N sequences that are not present in the original germline DNA) are inserted at the site of religation. Loss or gain of a few nucleotides produces frameshifts that encode different amino acids in the final rearranged gene.

Finally, once antigen stimulation occurs, B cells that produce antibodies with some affinity for the particular antigen are stimulated to proliferate and undergo frequent point mutations within the rearranged coding sequences. This rate of spontaneous mutation (one mutation per 10^3 DNA base pairs per cell division) is strikingly high, 100 to 1000 times greater than the average mutation rate elsewhere in the genome (see Chapters 2 and 9). These spontaneous mutations can change the amino acid sequence within the variable (antigen recognition) domain of antibody molecules and are a "fine-tuning" mechanism for improving the affinity of an antibody. The diversity provided by pairing different H and L chains, the DNA rearrangements that join together different germline V, D, and J gene segments, the imprecise VDJ joining, and finally somatic mutation of the variable region are all important mechanisms for expanding the potential repertoire of antibody specificities.

The mechanism of somatic rearrangement is shared by another member of the immunoglobulin gene superfamily, the **T-cell receptor** (TCR). The TCR is a highly variable transmembrane glycoprotein that plays a key role in antigen recognition and T-cell function. The TCR resembles the immunoglobulin molecule structurally; all chains have both constant and variable sections, the variable sections being generated by an assortment of V, D, and J segments. Just as for the immunoglobulin genes, the recombination of multiple germline elements, the imprecision of joining, and the possibility of various chain combinations create extensive diversity in TCR gene expression. However, the genesis of TCRs, unlike that of immunoglobulins, does not involve somatic mutation.

Somatic rearrangement occurs only in the immunoglobulin and TCR gene clusters in the B- and T-cell lineages, respectively. Such behavior is unique to these gene families and cell lineages; the rest of the genome remains highly stable throughout development and differentiation.

Allelic Exclusion

The somatic rearrangements just described occur on only one of the two copies of the immunoglobulin and TCR loci in a given B or T cell. This is an example of **allelic exclusion,** in which the two alleles of autosomal loci are treated differently, and its basis is still poorly understood. Whereas the majority of autosomal loci are expressed from both copies, there are several other examples of monoallelic expression. An extreme form of allelic exclusion is seen in the OR gene family described earlier (see Fig. 3-2). In this case, only a single allele of one OR gene is expressed in each olfactory sensory neuron; the several hundred other copies of the OR family remain repressed in that cell.

For allelic exclusion at the immunoglobulin, TCR, and OR loci, the choice of which allele is expressed is not dependent on parental origin; as with genes that undergo X chromosome inactivation in the female (see Chapters 6 and 7), either the maternal or paternal copy can be expressed in different cells. This distinguishes allelic exclusion from **genomic imprinting,** in which the choice of the allele to be expressed is determined solely by parental origin (see Chapter 5).

⦿ VARIATION IN GENE EXPRESSION AND ITS RELEVANCE TO MEDICINE

The regulated expression of the estimated 25,000 genes encoded in the human genome involves a set of complex interrelationships among different levels of control, including proper gene dosage (controlled by mechanisms of chromosome replication and segregation), gene structure, and, finally, transcription, RNA splicing, mRNA stability, translation, protein processing, and protein degradation. For some genes, fluctuations in the level of functional gene product, due either to inherited variation in the structure of a particular gene or to changes induced by nongenetic factors such as diet or the environment, are of relatively little importance. For other genes, changes in the level of expression can have dire clinical consequences, reflecting the importance of those gene products in particular biological pathways. The nature of inherited variation in the structure and function of chromosomes and genes, and the influence of this variation on the expression of specific traits, is the very essence of medical and molecular genetics and is dealt with in subsequent chapters.

⦿ GENERAL REFERENCES

Alberts B, Bray D, Lewis J, et al: Molecular Biology of the Cell, 4th ed. New York, Garland Publishing, 2002.
Brown TA: Genomes, 3rd ed. New York, Garland, 2007.
Lewin B: Genes VIII. New York, Prentice Hall, 2003.
Strachan T, Read A: Human Molecular Genetics, 3rd ed. New York, Garland Publishing, 2003.

REFERENCES FOR SPECIFIC TOPICS

Abbas AK, Lichtman AH, Pober JS: Cellular and Molecular Immunology, 5th ed. Philadelphia, WB Saunders, 2003.

Bartel DP: MicroRNAs: genomics, biogenesis, mechanism, and function. Cell 116:281-297, 2004.

Berg P: Dissections and reconstructions of genes and chromosomes [Nobel Prize lecture]. Science 213:296-303, 1981.

International Human Genome Sequencing Consortium: The human genome: sequencing and initial analysis. Nature 409:860-921, 2001.

International Human Genome Sequencing Consortium: Finishing the euchromatic sequence of the human genome. Nature 431:931-945, 2004.

Matlin AJ, Clark F, Smith CW: Understanding alternative splicing: towards a cellular code. Nat Rev Mol Cell Biol 6:386-398, 2005.

Mostoslavsky R, Alt FW, Rajewsky K: The lingering enigma of the allelic exclusion mechanism. Cell 118:539-544, 2004.

Proudfoot NJ, Furger A, Dye MJ: Integrating mRNA processing with transcription. Cell 108:501-512, 2002.

Shykind BM: Regulation of odorant receptors: one allele at a time. Hum Mol Genet 14:R33-R39, 2005.

Stamatoyannopoulos G: Control of globin gene expression during development and erythroid differentiation. Exp Hematol 33:259-271, 2005.

Venter JC, Adams MD, Myers EW, et al: The sequence of the human genome. Science 291:1304-1351, 2001.

Xie X, Lu J, Kulbokas EJ, et al: Systematic discovery of regulatory motifs in human promoters and 3′ UTRs by comparison of several mammals. Nature 434:338-345, 2005.

Young JM, Trask BJ: The sense of smell: genomics of vertebrate odorant receptors. Hum Mol Genet 11:1153-1160, 2002.

 PROBLEMS

1. The following amino acid sequence represents part of a protein. The normal sequence and four mutant forms are shown. By consulting Table 3-1, determine the double-stranded sequence of the corresponding section of the normal gene. Which strand is the strand that RNA polymerase "reads"? What would the sequence of the resulting mRNA be? What kind of mutation is each mutant protein most likely to represent?

Normal	-lys-arg-his-his-tyr-leu-
Mutant 1	-lys-arg-his-his-cys-leu-
Mutant 2	-lys-arg-ile-ile-ile-
Mutant 3	-lys-glu-thr-ser-leu-ser-
Mutant 4	-asn-tyr-leu-

2. The following items are related to each other in a hierarchical fashion: chromosome, base pair, nucleosome, kilobase pair, intron, gene, exon, chromatin, codon, nucleotide, promoter. What are these relationships?

3. Describe how mutation in each of the following might be expected to alter or interfere with normal gene function and thus cause human disease: promoter, initiator codon, splice sites at intron-exon junctions, one base pair deletion in the coding sequence, stop codon.

4. Most of the human genome consists of sequences that are not transcribed and do not directly encode gene products. For each of the following, consider ways in which these genome elements might contribute to human disease: introns, *Alu* or LINE repetitive sequences, locus control regions, pseudogenes.

5. Contrast the mechanisms and consequences of RNA splicing and somatic rearrangement.

Chapter 4

Tools of Human Molecular Genetics

One of the principal aims of modern medical genetics is to characterize mutations that lead to genetic disease, to understand how these mutations affect health, and to use that information to improve diagnosis and management. Advances in our understanding of molecular genetics have been driven by the development of technologies that permit the detailed analysis of both normal and abnormal genes and the expression of thousands of genes in normal and disease states. The application of these techniques has increased the understanding of molecular processes at all levels, from the gene to the whole organism.

This chapter is not intended to be a "cookbook" of recipes for genetic experiments or laboratory diagnostic methods. Rather, it serves as an introduction to the techniques and concepts that are largely responsible for advances in both basic and applied genetic research. The contents of this chapter supplement the basic material presented in Chapters 2 and 3 and provide a basis for understanding much of the molecular information contained in the chapters that follow. Readers who have had a course or laboratory experience in human molecular genetics may use this chapter as review or skip over it entirely without interfering with the continuity of the text. For others who find the material in this chapter too brief, far more detailed accounts of modern techniques, along with complete references, can be found in the general references listed at the end of this chapter.

● ANALYSIS OF INDIVIDUAL DNA AND RNA SEQUENCES

Molecular geneticists face two fundamental obstacles to their investigations of the molecular basis of hereditary disease. The first obstacle is that of obtaining a sufficient quantity of a DNA or RNA sequence of inter-est to allow it to be analyzed. Each cell generally has only two copies of a gene and some genes may be transcribed only in a subset of tissues or only at low levels, or both, providing only a small number of messenger RNA (mRNA) molecules. The second obstacle is that of purifying the sequence of interest from all the other segments of DNA or mRNA molecules present in the cell. **Molecular cloning** and the **polymerase chain reaction (PCR)** are technological revolutions that solved the problem of obtaining DNA or RNA in sufficient quantity and purity for detailed analysis (Fig. 4-1). These technological advances come with their own jargon (see Box, "The Language of Genomics and Molecular Genetics").

Molecular Cloning

The purpose of molecular cloning is to isolate a particular gene or other DNA sequence in large quantities for further study. Molecular cloning requires the transfer of a DNA sequence of interest into a single cell of a microorganism. The microorganism is subsequently grown in culture so that it reproduces the DNA sequence along with its own DNA. Because every individual microorganism in the colony is derived from that original single cell and contains the same identical transferred segment of DNA, it is referred to as a **clone,** and the entire process of growing large quantities of the sequence of interest is called molecular cloning (see Fig. 4-1). Large quantities of the sequence of interest can then be isolated in pure form from an individual clone for detailed molecular analysis.

Restriction Enzymes

One of the key advances in the development of molecular cloning was the discovery in the early 1970s of bacterial **restriction endonucleases** (often referred to as

••• The Language Of Genomics And Molecular Genetics

Clone: a recombinant DNA molecule containing a gene or other DNA sequence of interest; also, the act of generating such a molecule. Usage: "to isolate a clone" or "to clone a gene."

Complementary DNA (cDNA): a synthetic DNA made by reverse transcriptase, a special DNA polymerase enzyme that uses messenger RNA (mRNA) as a template; used to refer to either a single-stranded copy or its double-stranded derivative. Usage: "a cDNA clone," "a cDNA library," or "to isolate a cDNA."

Host: the organism used to isolate and propagate a recombinant DNA molecule, usually a strain of the bacterium *Escherichia coli* or the yeast *Saccharomyces cerevisiae*. Usage: "What host did they clone the cDNA in?"

Hybridization: the act of two complementary single-stranded nucleic acid molecules forming bonds according to the rules of base pairing (A with T or U, G with C) and becoming a double-stranded molecule. Usage: "The probe hybridized to a gene sequence."

Insert: a fragment of foreign DNA cloned into a particular vector. Usage: "They purified the insert."

Library: a collection of recombinant clones from a source known to contain the gene, cDNA, or other DNA sequences of interest. In principle, a library may contain all the DNA or cDNA sequences represented in the original cell, tissue, or chromosome. Usage: "a muscle cDNA library" or "a human genomic library."

Ligation: the act of forming phosphodiester bonds to join two double-stranded DNA molecules with the enzyme DNA ligase. Usage: "The fragments were ligated together."

Microarray: a wafer made of glass, plastic, or silicon onto which a large number of different nucleic acids have been spotted individually in a matrix pattern; often referred to as a "chip." The array is used as a target for hybridization with probes consisting of complex mixtures of cDNA or genomic DNA, in order to measure differential gene expression or DNA copy number.

Northern blot: a filter to which RNA has been transferred after gel electrophoresis to separate the RNA molecules by size, named for the compass point, as a pun on Southern blot (see later); also, the act of generating such a filter and hybridizing it to a specific probe. Usage: "to probe a Northern blot" or "they did a Northern."

Oligonucleotide: a short strand of nucleic acid, ranging in length from a few base pairs to a few dozen base pairs, often synthesized chemically; often referred to as an oligo or oligomer. The number of bases is often written with the -mer as a suffix: a 20-mer.

Polymerase chain reaction (PCR): enzymatic amplification of a fragment of DNA located between a pair of primers. Usage: "I PCR'd the fragment" or "I isolated the fragment using PCR."

Primers (for PCR): two oligonucleotides, one on each side of a target sequence, designed so that one of the primers is complementary to a segment of DNA on one strand of a double-stranded DNA molecule and the other is complementary to a segment of DNA on the other strand. A specific pair of primers serves to prime synthesis of DNA in a PCR reaction. Usage: "I designed primers for PCR."

Probe: a cloned DNA or RNA molecule, labeled with radioactivity or another detectable tracer, used to identify its complementary sequences by molecular hybridization; also, the act of using such a molecule. Usage: "the β-globin probe" or "to probe a patient's DNA."

Quantitative PCR: a technique that measures in real time the increase in the amount of PCR product being made during the PCR reaction. The rate of increase can be used as a measure of the amount of template present at the start of the PCR; often referred to as qPCR.

Restriction endonucleases (restriction enzymes): enzymes that recognize specific double-stranded DNA sequences and cleave the DNA at or near the recognition site. Usage: "a restriction enzyme digest" (or just "a restriction digest") or "the restriction enzyme *EcoRI*."

Southern blot: a filter to which DNA has been transferred, usually after restriction enzyme digestion and gel electrophoresis to separate DNA molecules by size (named after the developer of the technique, Ed Southern); also, the act of generating such a filter and hybridizing it to a specific probe. Usage: "to probe a Southern blot" or "they did a Southern."

Vector: the DNA molecule into which the gene or other DNA fragment of interest is cloned; the resulting recombinant molecule is capable of replicating in a particular host. Examples include plasmids, bacteriophage lambda, and bacterial artificial chromosomes (BACs). Usage: "a cloning vector."

Western blot: a filter to which protein molecules have been transferred after gel electrophoresis to separate the protein molecules by size (named, tongue in cheek, for a direction on a compass other than Southern or Northern); also, the act of generating such a filter and exposing it to a specific antibody. Usage: "to probe a Western blot" or "they did a Western."

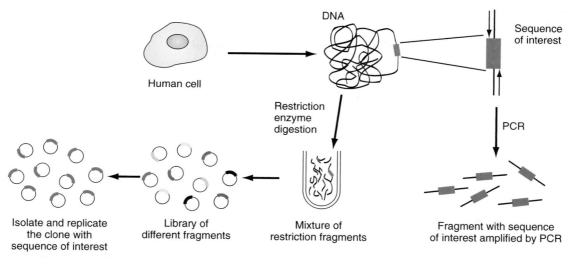

Figure 4-1 ■ Two approaches to isolating arbitrarily large quantities of a particular DNA sequence in pure form: molecular cloning and amplification by the polymerase chain reaction (PCR).

restriction enzymes), enzymes that recognize specific double-stranded sequences in DNA and cleave both phosphodiester backbones of the DNA double helix at or near the recognition site (see Chapter 3). These cleavages can be immediately opposite each other, in which case they will leave blunt-ended DNA strands, or the nicks can be offset by a few bases in either direction, producing single-stranded overhangs on either the 5′ or 3′ end of the DNA strands.

More than 3500 restriction enzymes are now known, each with its own recognition site that consists of four or six base pairs, although a few have longer sites. The sequences are usually **palindromes**; that is, the sequence of bases in the recognition site, when read 5′ to 3′, is the same on both strands. For example, the restriction enzyme *Eco*RI recognizes the specific palindromic six–base pair sequence 5′-GAATTC-3′ wherever it occurs in a double-stranded DNA molecule (Fig. 4-2). The enzyme cleaves the DNA at that site by introducing two nicks offset by four bases, one on each strand between the G and the adjacent A of the GAATTC recognition sequence. Cleavage generates two fragments, each with a four-base, single-stranded overhang 5′-AATT-3′ at the end.

Cleavage of a DNA molecule with a particular restriction enzyme digests the DNA into a characteristic and reproducible collection of fragments whose length distribution reflects the frequency and the location of the enzyme's specific cleavage sites. For example, *Eco*RI cleaves double-stranded DNA specifically at the six-base sequence 5′-GAATTC-3′. *Eco*RI digestion of DNA from the entire human genome generates a collection of approximately 1 million *Eco*RI fragments of varying lengths, each from a particular location in the genome. On average, an enzyme with a six–base pair recognition site like *Eco*RI should cleave human DNA every 4^6 base pairs, or once every 4096 base pairs. In reality, however, such sites are not uniformly distributed because of the differing base composition and sequence along the genome. Thus, *Eco*RI fragments ranging in size from a dozen base pairs to many hundreds of thousands of base pairs are observed; the length of each fragment is determined by how much DNA sits between two consecutive *Eco*RI sites.

Because all DNA molecules digested with *Eco*RI, regardless of their origin, have identical single-stranded sticky ends, *any* two DNA molecules that have been generated by *Eco*RI digestion can be joined together in vitro by pairing of their complementary four-base overhangs followed by rejoining of the phosphodiester backbones on each strand by an enzyme called **DNA ligase**. This ligation step creates a **recombinant** DNA molecule, one end derived from one DNA source and the other end derived from a different source (see Fig. 4-2). When a restriction enzyme cuts both strands at the same location, leaving blunt ends, DNA ligase can also join them together without any need for compatibility of single-stranded overhangs.

Vectors

A vector is a DNA molecule that can replicate autonomously in a host such as bacterial or yeast cells, from which it can be subsequently isolated in pure form for analysis. If a human DNA fragment is inserted into a vector by means of DNA ligase, the novel DNA molecule that results can be introduced into a bacterial host for the propagation of the inserted fragment along with the vector molecule. Replicating vectors can often achieve a high number of copies per cell and the bacte-

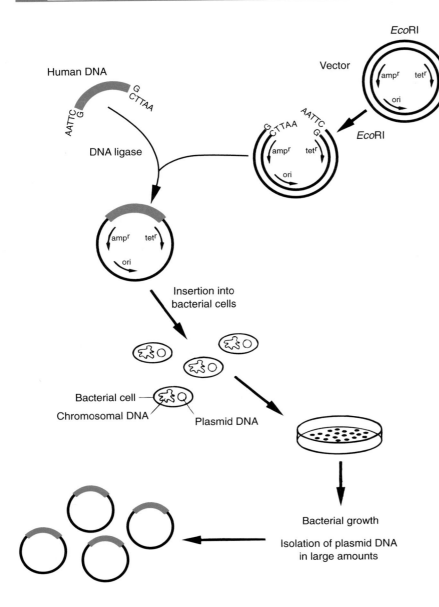

Figure 4-2 ■ The process of cloning a segment of human DNA into an *Eco*RI site in a plasmid cloning vector; *ori* denotes an origin of DNA replication for replicating the plasmid in bacterial cells, *amp^r* and *tet^r* denote bacterial genes conferring resistance to ampicillin and tetracycline. Growth of bacteria on plates containing antibiotics selects for those cells that contain copies of the plasmid, with its cloned human insert. (Modified from Fritsch EF, Wozney JM: Methods of molecular genetics. In Stamatoyannopoulos G, Nienhuis AW, Majerus PW, Varmus H [eds]: The Molecular Basis of Blood Diseases, 2nd ed. Philadelphia, WB Saunders, 1994.)

rial hosts can be grown indefinitely in the laboratory, making vast quantities of the inserted DNA sequence of interest readily available. The ligation of DNA molecules from different sources, such as a fragment of human DNA and a vector, is referred to as **recombinant DNA technology**. A number of vectors are commonly used for this purpose, each with its own set of advantages and limitations, but we will restrict our attention to the most commonly used vector, the plasmid.

Plasmids

Plasmids used as vectors are circular double-stranded DNA molecules that exist separately from the bacterial or yeast chromosome and are replicated independently from the microorganism's own chromosomes. Vector plasmids are derived from naturally occurring mole-

cules that were first discovered in bacteria because they carried antibiotic resistance genes and could be passed easily from one bacterium to another, thereby spreading antibiotic resistance rapidly throughout the microbial population. Plasmids specifically designed for molecular cloning are usually small (several kilobase pairs in size) and contain three critical components: an origin of replication (for replication either in *Escherichia coli* or in yeast), one or more selectable markers (such as a gene that confers resistance to antibiotics), and one or more restriction sites that can be cut and used for the ligation of foreign DNA molecules. The important steps involved in cloning of foreign DNA into the *Eco*RI site of a plasmid are shown in Figure 4-2. Identification of colonies that contain the desired recombinant plasmid, followed by mass growth and isolation of pure plasmid DNA, allows the isolation of large amounts of the cloned insert.

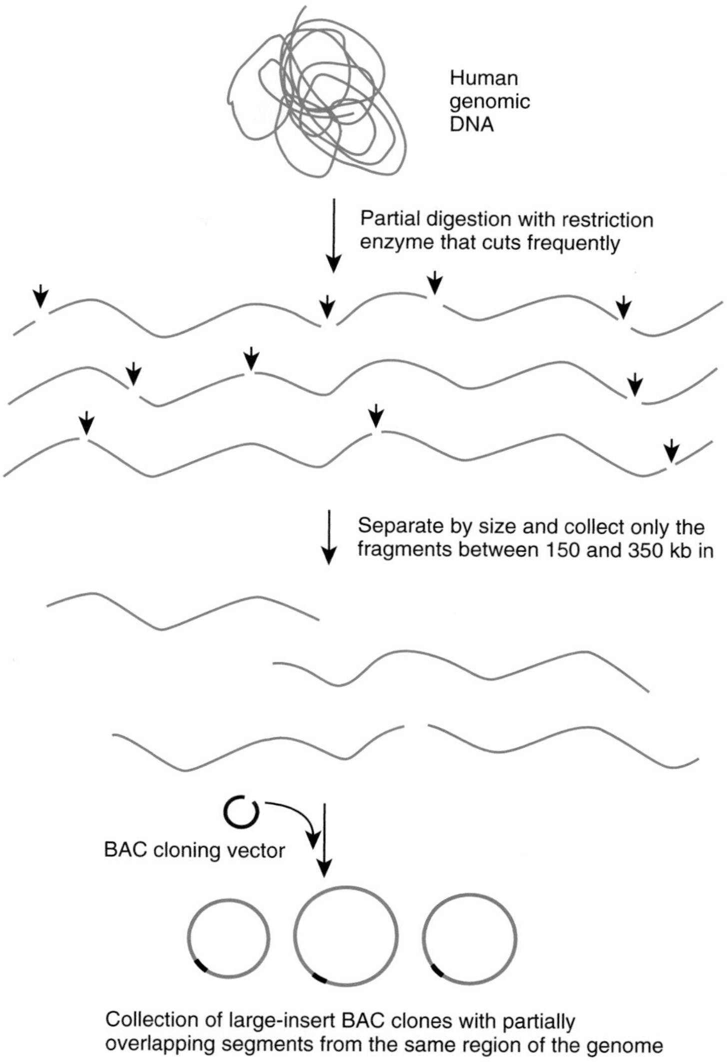

Human genomic DNA

Partial digestion with restriction enzyme that cuts frequently

Separate by size and collect only the fragments between 150 and 350 kb in

BAC cloning vector

Collection of large-insert BAC clones with partially overlapping segments from the same region of the genome

Figure 4-3 ■ Construction of a "library" of DNA from the human genome in a bacterial artificial chromosome (BAC) vector. Shown here are three DNA molecules from the same segment of the genome, cut by chance (*arrows*) at different sites in a partial digest, thereby generating a series of overlapping fragments. Each of the resulting BAC clones at the bottom contains a different but partly overlapping fragment of human DNA. A collection of several tens of thousands of such BACs would represent all of the DNA from the human genome. In the final collection of BAC clones, the vector is shown in black while the genomic DNA inserts are in blue.

Certain plasmids that are especially useful for molecular cloning are those used as bacterial artificial chromosome (BAC) vectors. BACs are specially designed plasmids containing large inserts of DNA, 100 to 350 kb. The development of BAC technology required numerous modifications in the genes of the plasmids and the host bacteria to ensure that the large inserts they carry remained stable and are replicated faithfully when propagated in the bacterial host. BACs played a critical role in the Human Genome Project by allowing the partitioning of the total human genome into fragments of a manageable size, suitable for sequencing.

Libraries

A library is a collection of clones, each of which carries vector molecules into which a different fragment of DNA derived from the total DNA or RNA of a cell or tissue has been inserted. If the collection of clones is large enough, it should theoretically contain all of the sequences found in the original DNA source. One can

then identify a clone carrying a DNA fragment of interest in the library by using sensitive screening methods that are capable of finding it in a collection of millions of different cloned fragments, called a "library".

Genomic Libraries

One useful type of library contains fragments of genomic DNA generated by deliberately using limiting amounts of a restriction enzyme that cuts at sites present at high frequency in the genome. The consequence of using limiting amounts of enzyme is a partial digestion of the DNA so that only a few of the enzyme's recognition sites are cleaved, at random, while most others are not (Fig. 4-3). This approach generates a collection of overlapping fragments of length suitable for cloning into a cloning vector. For example, a plasmid specially designed to create bacterial artificial chromosomes is prepared so that human DNA fragments from 100 to 350 kb in length, generated from a partial restriction enzyme digestion, can be ligated into the vector

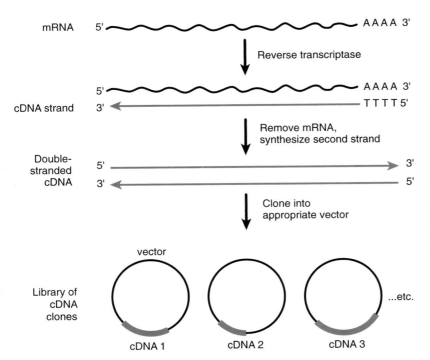

mRNA   5' ~~~~~~~~~~~~~~~~~~~~~~~~ AAAA 3'

↓ Reverse transcriptase

5' ~~~~~~~~~~~~~~~~~~~~~~~~ AAAA 3'
cDNA strand   3' ←———————————————————— T T T T 5'

↓ Remove mRNA, synthesize second strand

Double-
stranded   5' ——————————————————————→ 3'
cDNA   3' ←—————————————————————— 5'

↓ Clone into appropriate vector

vector

Library of
cDNA
clones

cDNA 1   cDNA 2   cDNA 3   ...etc.

Figure 4-4 ■ Construction of a cDNA library in a plasmid vector. RNA from a particular tissue source is copied into DNA by the enzyme reverse transcriptase. Reverse transcriptase requires a primer to initiate DNA synthesis, such as an oligonucleotide consisting of thymidines (oligo-dT); this short homopolymer binds to the polyA tail at the 3′ end of mRNA molecules (see Chapter 3) and provides a primer that reverse transcriptase extends to synthesize a complementary copy. After synthesis of the complementary second strand, the double-stranded cDNA is then cloned.

(Fig. 4-3). After the recombinant plasmids containing large fragments of human DNA are introduced into bacteria, the library, containing many thousands of clones, each containing a different fragment of partially overlapping genomic DNA, can be stored for the future isolation of many genes. If the library is large enough, every segment of the genome will be represented on at least one of these partially overlapping fragments.

Complementary DNA (cDNA) Libraries

Another common type of library used to isolate sequences from a gene is a complementary DNA library, which contains complementary DNA (cDNA) copies of the mRNA population present within a particular tissue. Complementary DNA sequences are preferable to genomic libraries as a source of cloned genes for some applications because (1) cDNA contains only the exons of a gene and is therefore a direct representation of the coding sequence of a gene without the introns or promoter sequences, (2) sets of cDNAs representing transcripts from a single gene may differ, which indicates that alternative promoters or sites of polyadenylation are being used, or differential splice site usage is occurring, so that some exons may be either included or excluded from some of the transcripts, and (3) the use of a particular mRNA source enriches substantially for sequences of a gene known to be expressed selectively in that tissue. For example, the few kilobase pairs of DNA containing the β-globin gene are represented at only one part per million in a human genomic library, but it is a major mRNA transcript in red blood cells. Thus, a cDNA library prepared from red blood cell precursors is the optimal source for isolating cDNA corresponding to β-globin mRNA. Similarly, a liver or muscle cDNA library is a preferred source of cDNA clones for genes known to be expressed preferentially or exclusively in those tissues. A cDNA does not, however, provide any indication of the size or number of exons or the sequence of the 5′ and 3′ splice sites (see Chapter 3).

Cloning of cDNAs relies on the enzyme **reverse transcriptase,** an RNA-dependent DNA polymerase derived from retroviruses that can synthesize a single-stranded cDNA fragment complementary to an RNA template (Fig. 4-4). This single-stranded cDNA is then used as the template for DNA polymerase, which converts the single-stranded molecule to a double-stranded molecule, which can then be ligated into a suitable vector to create a cDNA library representing all of the original mRNA transcripts found in the starting cell type or tissue (see Fig. 4-4). A cDNA representing an individual mRNA in its entirety is particularly useful as it provides the full length of the coding sequence of a gene. Some cleverly engineered vectors, called **expression vectors,** contain transcription and translation signals adjacent to the site of insertion of the cDNA so that a full-length cDNA can be transcribed and translated in bacteria, yeast, or cultured cells to produce the protein it encodes.

Thousands of cDNA libraries from many different tissues or different stages of development from many different organisms have been constructed and have proved to be an invaluable source of cDNAs for a vast array of mRNA transcripts. Making a large library increases the chances that any mRNA of interest, no matter how rare, will be represented at least once in the library.

Screening Libraries with Nucleic Acid Hybridization Probes

Once a library is made, the next step is to identify the clone carrying a sequence of interest among the millions of other clones carrying other fragments. Identifying the clone carrying the DNA insert of interest is called **library screening.** Library screening is often performed by **nucleic acid hybridization.** In its most general form, a hybridization reaction proceeds by mixing single-stranded nucleic acids under conditions of temperature and salt concentration that permit only correct base pairing (A with T, G with C) between DNA strands (see Chapter 3). Only those strands that are correctly base paired can form a stable *double-stranded* nucleic acid; no stable double-stranded molecules will form between noncomplementary sequences in the mixture (Fig. 4-5). Nucleic acid hybridization is a fundamental concept in molecular biology. The technique is used not only for screening libraries of cloned DNA but also more generally for the analysis of DNA or RNA in cells and tissues, as described in later sections of this chapter.

The usefulness of nucleic acid probes resides in the specificity of nucleic acid hybridization between complementary strands. One sequence (the "target") in a mixture of nucleic acids is tested for its ability to form stable base pairing with a DNA or RNA fragment of known sequence (the "probe"), which has been tagged with either a radioactive tracer, a histochemical compound, or a fluorescent dye, to allow the probe to be subsequently detected. If the probe is complementary to the target, it will form a stable double-stranded molecule. The target sequence in the original DNA or RNA sample is now identified by the tag on the probe, thus facilitating its subsequent detection and analysis or isolation.

To tag a probe with a radioactive tracer, one can label it with phosphorus-32 (^{32}P), whose high energy exposes x-ray film. One introduces ^{32}P into a probe by a variety of methods that substitute ^{32}P into the phosphodiester backbone of a strand of DNA. Probes can also be tagged with fluorescent dyes. The probe is made by synthesizing it with nucleotides to which a fluorescent dye tag either has been or can be attached. Many different fluorescent dyes are commercially available. Each dye is excited by a specific wavelength of light and subsequently emits light at a wavelength characteristic of that particular dye. The fluorescence emitted by the probe is captured by digital photography and is therefore available for digital signal processing by computer.

Probes can be obtained from a number of different sources. They can be cloned genomic or cDNA molecules, DNA fragments generated enzymatically by PCR (see later discussion), or chemically synthesized nucleic acid (DNA or RNA) molecules. Probes derived from cloned DNA or generated by PCR are usually several hundred to several thousand nucleotides in length. Chemically synthesized single-stranded DNA probes, typically 18 to 60 nucleotides in length, are known as **oligonucleotide probes** or, simply, **oligonucleotides.**

Genome Database Resources

Although library construction and screening remain important tools for gene discovery and characterization, the Human Genome Project and its many applications (see Chapter 10) are having a profound impact on the study of human genetics. For example, the rapid expansion of vast databases of sequence information accessible through the Internet is making the construction and screening of libraries increasingly unnecessary.

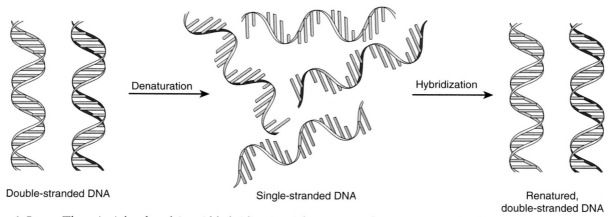

Double-stranded DNA   Single-stranded DNA   Renatured, double-stranded DNA

Figure 4-5 ■ The principle of nucleic acid hybridization. The two complementary strands of a Watson-Crick double helix can be "denatured" by a variety of treatments (such as high temperature, high pH, or very low salt conditions) to yield a collection of single-stranded DNA molecules. Under conditions that favor formation of double-stranded DNA, complementary strands will anneal (or "hybridize") to each other but not to other fragments of DNA that have a different nucleotide sequence.

Large numbers of BAC and full-length cDNA libraries from humans and other species are now in common use, and the complete sequence of many individual BAC and cDNA clones from these libraries are already deposited in searchable public databases (the URLs for a number of such comprehensive genomic databases are provided at the end of this chapter). A BAC or cDNA clone with a particular sequence of interest can be identified electronically by use of software that matches the sequence to all the sequences stored in sequence databases. Many of the actual libraries in which extensive sequencing of individual clones has been done are stored in centralized commercial clone repositories from which any clone found by database searching to carry a sequence of interest can be easily obtained.

METHODS OF NUCLEIC ACID ANALYSIS

Examination of the RNA or DNA from a particular gene requires that we be able to distinguish the specific DNA segments or RNA molecules corresponding to that gene from among all the many other DNA segments or RNA molecules present in a sample of cells or tissue. When genomic DNA is analyzed, the problem is to find and examine the specific DNA fragment in which one is interested from within a complex mixture of genomic DNA containing several million DNA fragments generated by restriction enzyme digestion of total human genomic DNA. With RNA samples, the problem is to detect and measure the amount and the quality of a particular mRNA transcript in an RNA sample from a tissue in which the desired mRNA might account for only 1/1000 or less of the total RNA transcripts. The solution to the problem of detecting one rare sequence among many involves use of gel electrophoresis to separate the molecules of DNA or RNA by size, then carrying out nucleic acid hybridization with a probe to identify the molecule of interest.

Southern Blotting

The Southern blotting technique allows one to find and examine, at a gross level, a number of DNA fragments of interest in a seemingly uninformative collection of a million or so restriction enzyme fragments. Thus, Southern blotting, developed in the mid-1970s, is the standard method for examining particular fragments of DNA cleaved by restriction enzymes. In this procedure, DNA is first isolated from an accessible source (Fig. 4-6). Any cell in the body can be used as the source of DNA, except for mature red blood cells, which have no nuclei. For the analysis of patient DNA samples, one typically prepares genomic DNA from lymphocytes obtained by routine venipuncture. A 10-mL (10 cc) sample of peripheral blood contains approximately 10^8 white blood cells and provides more than 100 µg of DNA, enough for dozens of restriction enzyme digestions. Genomic DNA can also be prepared from other tissues, however, including cultured skin fibroblasts, amniotic fluid or chorionic villus cells for prenatal diagnosis (see Chapter 15), or any organ biopsy specimen (e.g., liver, kidney, placenta). The millions of distinct DNA fragments generated by restriction enzyme cleavage of a genomic DNA sample are first put in a well cut into the agarose at the top of the gel. They are then separated on the basis of size by agarose gel electrophoresis, in which small fragments move through an electric field more rapidly than do larger ones. When digested DNA separated in this way is stained with a fluorescent DNA dye such as ethidium bromide, the genomic DNA fragments appear as a smear of fluorescing material distributed along a lane in the gel, with the smaller fragments at the bottom and the larger fragments at the top. The DNA appears as a smear instead of discrete bands on the gel because there are usually far too many DNA fragments for any fragment of a particular size to stand out from the others (Fig. 4-7, *left*). The smear of double-stranded DNA fragments is first denatured with a strong base to separate the two complementary DNA strands (see Fig. 4-5). The now single-stranded DNA molecules are then transferred from the gel to a piece of filter paper by blotting and capillarity (hence, the name "Southern blot" or "Southern transfer").

To identify the one or more fragments of interest among the millions of fragments on the filter, a single-stranded labeled probe is incubated with the filter under conditions that favor formation of pairing of complementary double-stranded DNA molecules (as in Fig. 4-5). After being washed to remove unbound probe, the filter (with its bound radioactive probe) is exposed to x-ray film to reveal the position of the one or more fragments to which the probe hybridized. Thus, specific radioactive bands are detectable on the x-ray film for each lane of human DNA on the original agarose gel (Fig. 4-7, *right*).

The ability of Southern blotting to identify mutations is limited because a probe can detect only mutations that have an appreciable effect on the size of a fragment, such as a large deletion or insertion. A mutation that changes a single base or inserts or deletes a small number of bases will escape detection, unless the mutation happens to destroy or create a restriction enzyme cleavage site so that the size of the fragment detected by the probe is substantially altered. There are, however, many techniques other than Southern blotting for finding mutations affecting one or just a few base pairs in a gene; some of these are discussed here and in Chapter 19.

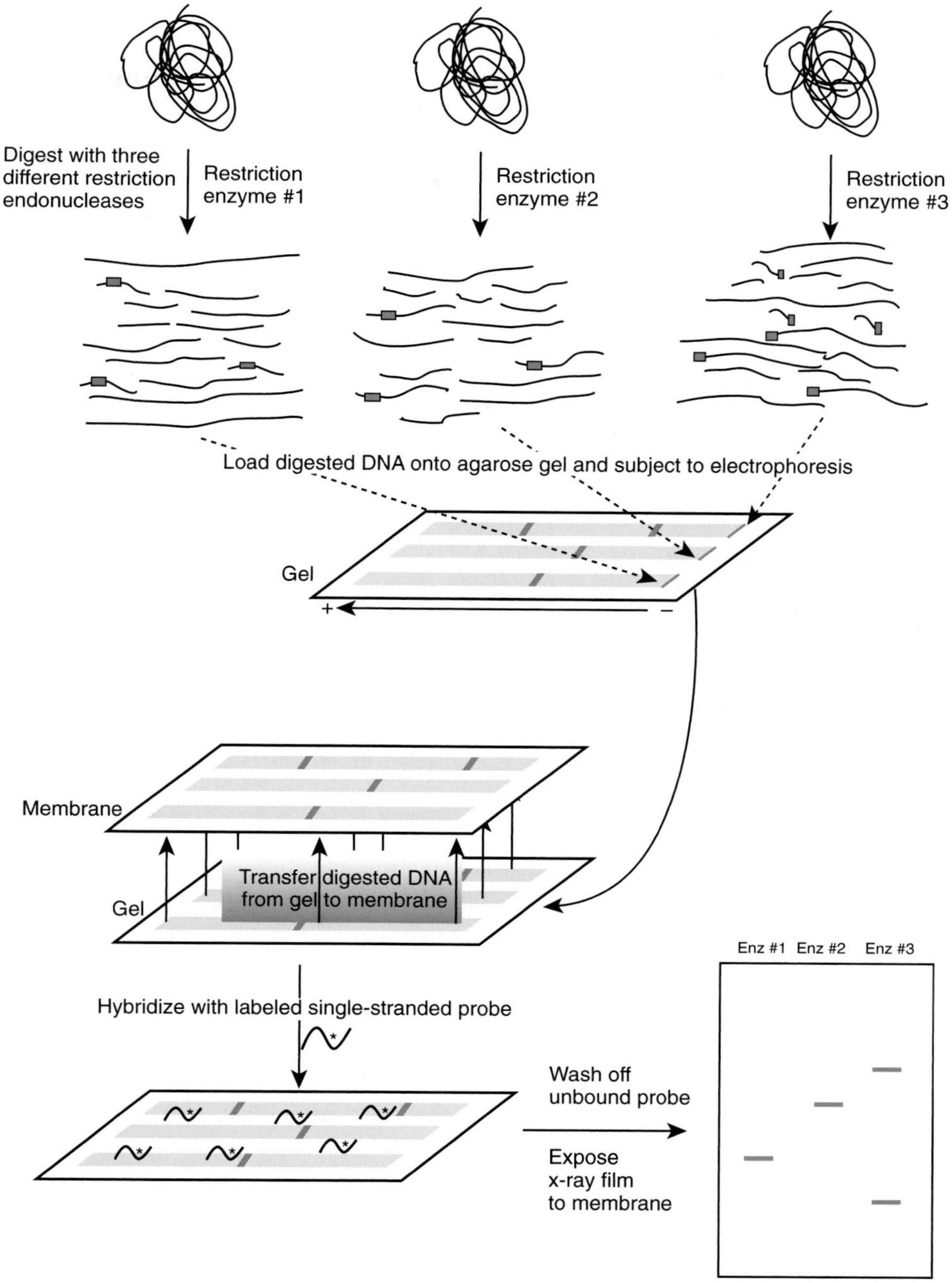

Figure 4-6 ■ The Southern blotting procedure for analyzing specific DNA sequences in a complex mixture of different sequences, such as genomic DNA. In this example, a sample of DNA is digested with three different restriction enzymes. The fragments are separated according to size within an agarose gel under an electric field (the fragments containing a sequence of interest are shown for illustrative purposes only as blue bands in each lane of DNA). After electrophoresis, the fragments are rendered single stranded and transferred to a membrane by capillary action. The labeled single-stranded probe is applied to the membrane, and the probe is allowed to anneal to its complementary DNA sequences. After unannealed probe is washed off, the membrane is placed against an x-ray film. The pattern of fragments containing sequences complementary to the probe generated with each restriction enzyme is revealed.

Analysis with Allele-Specific Oligonucleotide Probes

In certain genetic diseases, the same mutation affecting one or a small number of bases is known to be responsible for a significant fraction of cases of the disease. Examples include the mutation that causes **sickle cell anemia**, a single base change that converts a glutamate to valine in β-globin (see Chapter 11) **(Case 37)**, and the three-base in-frame deletion in the gene encoding the cystic fibrosis transmembrane conductance regulator that comprises approximately 60% of all mutations causing severe **cystic fibrosis** in white individuals (see Chapter 12) **(Case 10)**. In other situations, one is testing for a less common mutation in the family member of someone in whom a mutation has already been defined. In these cases, one can target the analysis of DNA to ask whether a particular mutation is present or absent in an individual patient. The best probe to use for detection of a single base mutation or a small insertion or deletion

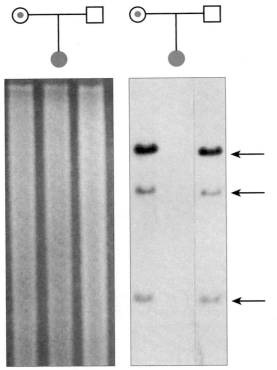

Figure 4-7 ■ Detection of a deletion of the X-linked androgen receptor gene by Southern blotting. *Left,* When genomic DNA from family members is digested with a restriction enzyme and the DNA stained with a fluorescent DNA dye (such as ethidium bromide) after electrophoresis, all samples appear the same. *Right,* After Southern blotting and hybridization to a cDNA probe for the human androgen receptor gene, the individual with androgen insensitivity syndrome (see Chapter 6) is deleted for this gene *(middle lane).* The individual with androgen insensitivity has a 46,XY karyotype but is phenotypically female and therefore depicted by a circle in the pedigree. (Courtesy of R. Lafreniere, Stanford University, Stanford, California.)

mutation is a synthetic oligonucleotide, because its shorter length makes it much more sensitive to even single–base pair mismatches between the probe and the sample to be analyzed. Thus, an oligonucleotide probe synthesized to match precisely the normal DNA sequence in a gene (an **allele-specific oligonucleotide [ASO]**) hybridizes only to the normal complementary sequence but not to an imperfect complementary sequence in which there are one or more mismatches between target and probe (Fig. 4-8). Similarly, an ASO made to the sequence corresponding to a mutant gene hybridizes only to the mutant complementary sequence but not to the sequence in a normal gene.

It is important to recognize the distinction between ASO analysis and conventional Southern blot analysis with DNA probes. In most cases, mutant genes due to single base changes or small changes in the DNA (small deletions or insertions, for example) are indistinguishable from normal genes by Southern blot analysis done with use of standard, cloned DNA probes. Only short

ASO probes have the ability to reliably detect single nucleotide changes.

ASO analysis permits precise identification of a particular DNA sequence and can distinguish among individuals who carry the normal DNA sequence on both homologous chromosomes, individuals with the mutant sequence on both homologous chromosomes, and individuals with the normal sequence on one chromosome and the mutant sequence on the other (see Fig. 4-8). Care must be taken, however, in interpreting results from ASO analysis because not all mutant genes at a given locus share exactly the same DNA sequence alteration. Thus, failure to hybridize to a specific mutant gene ASO does not necessarily mean that the patient's gene is normal throughout its entire sequence; there may be a mutation elsewhere in the gene at a location other than that examined by a particular ASO.

Northern or RNA Blotting

For the analysis of RNA, the counterpart of the Southern blotting technique is called Northern or RNA blotting. Northern blotting is a standard approach for determining the size and abundance of the mRNA from a specific gene in a sample of RNA. RNA cannot be cleaved by the restriction enzymes used for DNA analysis. Different RNA transcripts are naturally of different lengths, however, depending on the size and number of exons within a transcribed gene (see Chapter 3). Thus, total cellular RNA (or purified mRNA) obtained from a particular cell type can be separated according to size by agarose gel electrophoresis. Although RNA is naturally single stranded, it may need to be denatured before gel electrophoresis to prevent base-pairing between short stretches of complementary bases within the same molecule; such intramolecular base-pairing produces secondary structure that causes the molecules to migrate aberrantly in the gel. After electrophoresis, the RNA is transferred to a filter. As in the Southern blotting procedure, the filter is then incubated with a denatured, labeled probe that hybridizes to one or more specific RNA transcripts. After exposure of the washed filter to x-ray film, one or more bands may be apparent, revealing the position and abundance of the specific transcript of interest. Although Northern blotting still has a role in the analysis of mRNA transcripts, it has been replaced in some of its applications by techniques that are based on the polymerase chain reaction, described next.

● THE POLYMERASE CHAIN REACTION

The polymerase chain reaction (PCR) is an alternative to cloning for generating essentially unlimited amounts of a sequence of interest (see Fig. 4-1). PCR can selec-

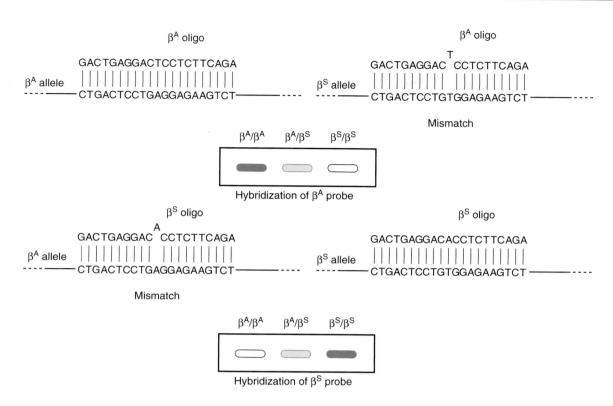

Figure 4-8 ■ Detection of the single–base pair mutation in the β-globin gene that causes sickle cell disease by allele-specific oligonucleotide (ASO) probes. *Top left,* The "normal" β^A probe will base pair only to DNA sequences that are identical to the probe. *Bottom right,* The "mutant" β^S probe will pair only to DNA sequences carrying the sickle cell hemoglobin mutation that differ from the normal sequence by a specific single–base pair mutation. The β^A probe will mismatch with a β^S globin sequence and vice versa. Beneath each sequence is a diagram of the hybridization of each labeled probe with samples of DNA obtained from individuals of all three genotypes. The intensity of hybridization distinguishes each of the three genotypes.

tively amplify a single molecule of DNA several billion–fold in a few hours and has revolutionized both molecular diagnosis and the molecular analysis of genetic disease. PCR is an enzymatic amplification of a fragment of DNA (the target) located between two oligonucleotide "primers" (Fig. 4-9). These primers are designed so that one is complementary to one strand of a DNA molecule on one side of the target sequence and the other primer is complementary to the other strand of the DNA molecule on the opposite side of the target sequence. The oligonucleotide primers therefore flank the target sequence, and their 3′ ends are directed toward the target sequence to be amplified. DNA polymerase is then used to synthesize two new strands of DNA with the sequence located between the primers as the template. The newly synthesized strands of DNA are themselves complementary and can form a second copy of the original target sequence (Fig. 4-9). Repeated cycles of heat denaturation, hybridization of the primers, and enzymatic DNA synthesis result in the exponential amplification (2, 4, 8, 16, 32,…copies) of the target DNA sequence (see Fig. 4-9). As a result, a staggering number of copies of the segment of DNA

between the primers are generated until the substrates (primer, deoxynucleotides) are used up. With the use of specifically designed PCR machines, a round of amplification takes only a few minutes. Thus, in only a few hours, many billions of copies of a starting DNA molecule can be created.

PCR amplification can generate sufficient quantities of specific genes from DNA samples for the analysis of mutations (see Fig. 4-1). Particular portions of a gene (usually the exons) are rapidly amplified with use of primers known to be specific to the gene. The amplified segment can then either be easily sequenced (see later discussion) or tested by ASO hybridization methods to detect a mutation. The analysis of DNA generated by PCR can be carried out in less than a day, thereby greatly facilitating the development and clinical application of many DNA diagnostic tests.

PCR can be applied to the analysis of small samples of RNA as well, a procedure referred to as **reverse transcriptase PCR (RT-PCR)**. A single-stranded cDNA is first synthesized from the mRNA of interest with the same reverse transcriptase enzyme that is used to prepare cDNA clone libraries (see Fig. 4-5). PCR primers

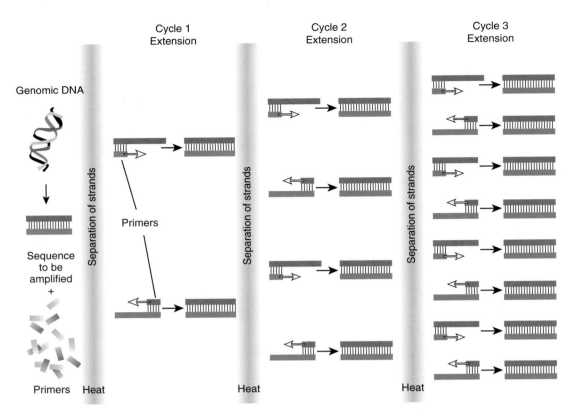

Figure 4-9 ■ The polymerase chain reaction. By repeated synthesis of the DNA between two primers, this DNA segment is specifically and selectively amplified in an exponential fashion. Three successive rounds of amplification are shown, resulting in a total of eight copies of the targeted sequence. After 30 rounds of amplification, more than a billion copies of the sequence are created. (From Eisenstein BI: The polymerase chain reaction. A new method of using molecular genetics for medical diagnosis. N Engl J Med 322[3]:178-183, 1990.)

are then added, along with DNA polymerase, as in the case of DNA PCR. One of the oligonucleotides primes synthesis of the second strand of the cDNA, which in its double-stranded form then serves as a target for PCR amplification.

PCR is an extremely sensitive technique that is faster, less expensive, more sensitive, and less demanding of patients' samples than any other method for nucleic acid analysis. It allows the detection, analysis, and quantification of specific gene sequences in a patient's sample without cloning and without the need for Southern or Northern blotting. Analyses can even be performed on the few buccal cells present in mouth rinses, from a single cell removed from a 3-day-old embryo containing four to eight cells, from the sperm in a vaginal swab obtained from a rape victim, or from a drop of dried blood at a crime scene. PCR thus eliminates the need to prepare large amounts of DNA or RNA from tissue samples. PCR is rapidly becoming a standard method for analysis of DNA and RNA samples for research, for clinical diagnosis, and for forensic and law enforcement laboratories. Specific examples of its use for the detection of mutations in genetic disorders are presented in Chapter 19.

Quantitative PCR

PCR can also be used as a quantitative technique to measure the amount of a particular DNA sequence in a sample. Early in a PCR reaction, the number of molecules of the region of DNA being amplified doubles with each cycle of denaturation, hybridization of the primers, and DNA synthesis. If we plot the amount of material synthesized early in the PCR reaction, we get a straight line on a semilogarithmic plot when the amount of product is doubling with each cycle (Fig. 4-10). The number of cycles required to reach an arbitrary threshold is a measure of how much template was initially present at the start of the PCR: the fewer cycles to reach a given threshold, the more template must have been present at the beginning. This technique, known as real-time PCR, is most frequently used to measure small amounts of one particular DNA or RNA in one sample (sample A) relative to the amount of a control RNA or DNA in another sample (sample B). It is important that the efficiency of the amplification of sample A and sample B be comparable; i.e., the two straight line segments should be parallel.

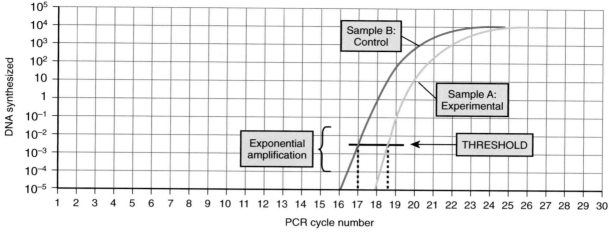

Figure 4-10 ■ Quantitative PCR. The number of PCR cycles required to reach an arbitrary threshold chosen within the exponential portion of PCR amplification is a measure of how much template was initially present when the PCR reaction was initiated. In this example, the experimental sample reaches the threshold 1.5 cycles later than the control, which means there was $1/(2^{1.5})$ or 29% the amount of experimental versus control sample at the start of the PCR reaction.

▪▪▪ The Molecular Analysis of a Human Mutation

How does one proceed to identify a mutation in a gene in a patient with a genetic disorder known to be or suspected of being due to defects in that gene?

Consider a patient with a diagnosis of **β-thalassemia**, an autosomal recessive defect in the β-globin gene (see Chapter 11) (Case 39). The initial diagnosis is generally made on the basis of clinical and hematological findings alone. It is important to examine the gene itself, however, first to confirm the clinical diagnosis and, second, to identify the specific mutation in the β-globin locus for future use in carrier testing and possible prenatal diagnosis in the patient's family. In addition, identification of the mutation increases our understanding of the relationship between specific mutations in a gene and the resulting pathophysiological changes.

Several tests can be used initially to examine the gross integrity of the β-globin gene itself and its mRNA. Are both copies of the gene present in the patient, and is their structure normal? Or is one or both copies of the gene deleted, as has been described in some cases of β-thalassemia? **Southern blotting** of the β-globin gene can address the question of whether the gene is present and whether it is grossly normal in structure. By this method, one can detect large molecular defects (e.g., deletions, rearrangements) that are well below the level of sensitivity of chromosome analysis. Southern blotting cannot reveal the presence of most single nucleotide mutations, or very small deletions of only a few base pairs, unless they disrupt a restriction endonuclease site.

If the mutated gene is present, is it transcribed? To determine whether a specific transcript is present, **Northern blotting** is used. This approach also enables one to detect major changes in mRNA levels or in the structure of a specific gene, but not to detect minor alterations (e.g., a mutation that changes a codon in an exon).

Having asked whether there are gross changes in the gene or in its mRNA, one can proceed to examine gene structure and expression at increasingly finer levels of analysis. In β-thalassemia, as in many other genetic disorders, many mutations are already known that are responsible for the disease (see Fig. 11-11). To determine whether one of the known mutations is responsible for a particular case of β-thalassemia, one can use **allele-specific oligonucleotides (ASOs)** that enable one to detect specific single–base pair mutations (see Fig. 4-8). If ASO analysis fails to reveal a known mutation, it may be necessary to compare the sequence of the mutant β-globin gene (or cDNA) from the patient with a normal β-globin gene by use of the **polymerase chain reaction (PCR)** to specifically generate many copies of a particular gene fragment in order to sequence it. In this way, the specific mutation responsible for the genetic disorder in the patient can be identified and used to develop direct screening tests for that mutation in the patient's family.

● DNA SEQUENCE ANALYSIS

The most widely used approach for DNA sequence analysis is **Sanger sequencing** (named after Fred Sanger, who, with Walter Gilbert, received the Nobel Prize in 1980 for developing DNA sequencing). The sequence of virtually any purified DNA segment can now be determined, whether it is a cloned fragment or a target sequence amplified by PCR. The Sanger sequencing method takes advantage of certain chemical analogues of the four nucleotides known as dideoxy nucleotides (ddA, ddC, ddG and ddT) because they lack a 3'-

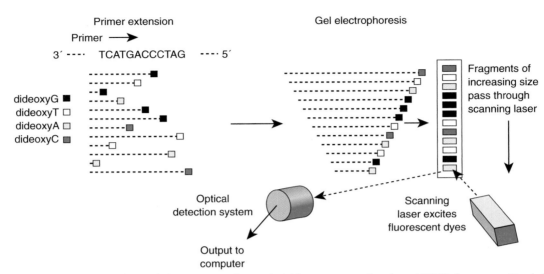

Figure 4-11 ■ The Sanger method of determining the nucleotide sequence of a cloned DNA fragment. To define the location of C residues, for example, in a segment of DNA, a dideoxyG analogue is included in the reaction, so that a proportion of individual molecules will not be extended when DNA polymerase incorporates the analogue. The relative amounts of the normal G nucleotide and the G analogue in this reaction are adjusted so that the polymerase incorporates the analogue of G in some newly synthesized strands the very first time it incorporates a G, whereas in other strands, a G analogue is incorporated at the second G, or at the third, or at the fourth, and so on. When the different-sized fragments are separated by electrophoresis, many fragments are observed, each of which corresponds to the location of each G residue at which a dideoxyG was incorporated, thereby causing a chain termination. Similar reactions for the A, T, and G residues provide corresponding series of fragments. The fragments generated in all four reactions constitute a series of fragments differing by one base. The fragments are separated on the basis of size by electrophoresis, and the particular dideoxy nucleotide responsible for terminating each fragment is identified by the emission wavelength of the fluorescent dye corresponding to that dideoxy nucleotide. The sequence is read as a series of fragments, each one terminated by a dideoxy base at its 3' end. (Modified from an original figure by Eric D. Green, National Human Genome Research Institute.)

hydroxyl group on their deoxyribose (in addition to the 2'-hydroxyl normally missing in DNA). If incorporated into a growing strand of DNA, dideoxy nucleotides do not allow the enzyme DNA polymerase to attach the next base complementary to the original template being sequenced, and therefore terminate the growing DNA chain (Fig. 4-11).

In Sanger sequencing, a fragment of DNA to be sequenced is used as a template for DNA synthesis primed by a short oligonucleotide, and the DNA polymerase proceeds along the template sequence, extending the primer and incorporating nucleotides. To obtain sequence information, one first adds the dideoxy analogues along with all four normal nucleotides into the sequencing reactions. Each analogue is labeled with a different fluorescent dye with its own distinctive emission. The polymerase will incorporate either a normal nucleotide and continue to extend the strand, or it will incorporate a dideoxy base, thereby terminating synthesis. These terminated strands are separated by electrophoresis, and the particular dideoxy nucleotide responsible for the termination is identified by the particular fluorescent dye molecule that is incorporated.

Machines have been designed that automate the procedure of DNA sequencing.

DNA sequence information is critical for predicting the amino acid sequence encoded by a gene, for detecting individual mutations in genetic disease, and for designing either ASO probes or PCR primers used in molecular diagnostic procedures. Automated sequencing was massively applied in the Human Genome Project to obtain the nucleotide sequence of all 3 billion base pairs of the entire human genome (see Chapter 10) as well as the complete sequence of other organisms of medical and scientific importance, including *E. coli* and other pathogenic bacteria, the yeast *Saccharomyces cerevisiae*, the malaria parasite and the *Anopheles* mosquito that carries the parasite, the worm *Caenorhabditis elegans*, the fruit fly *Drosophila melanogaster*, various fish species, the chicken, the rat and mouse, the chimpanzee, and a host of other organisms occupying the many twigs and branches of the evolutionary tree. Catalogues of similarities in the protein-coding and noncoding sequences of these organisms are being compiled at a rapid rate. The sequence of an entire genome, with the comprehensive catalogue of the genes in that organism that such sequence data provide, is a critical source of information for understanding the complete metabolic systems of cells and for finding vulnerabilities in pathogenic organisms that may be suitable for attack by vaccines and antibiotics. Furthermore, comparing the 99% of human genomic sequence that is not coding sequence with the sequences of other species to find similarities in DNA segments conserved during hundreds of millions of years of evolution, is an important tool for identifying important functional elements within the human genome.

ADVANCED TECHNIQUES USING DIGITAL IMAGE CAPTURE OF FLUORESCENCE-TAGGED NUCLEOTIDES

Southern and Northern hybridization are useful techniques for studying a small number of genes or gene transcripts at a time. However, new and more powerful methods using nucleic acid hybridization have now been developed to allow entire genomes or large collections of mRNA transcripts to be examined in a single experiment. These newer methods rely on developments in two areas of technology. The first is in the detection and processing of high-resolution fluorescent signals and images. With this technology, the levels of fluorescence emitted from every portion of an image can measured, pixel by pixel, over an entire microscopic field. The second rapidly developing area is **microarray** technology. Borrowing techniques from the semiconductor industry, researchers have designed and produced miniature wafers or "chips" on which small amounts of nucleic acid are fixed in a dense two-dimensional microarray of hundreds of thousands of spots over an area of, at most, a few square centimeters. The nucleic acid in each spot can range from oligonucleotides as short as 25 bases to BAC clones with inserts as large as 350 kb. After sequence-specific hybridization of probes labeled with fluorescent dyes to these dense arrays, each spot is examined under a fluorescence microscope, and the light emitted by the probe bound to each spot is quantified. If the probe contains a mixture of two fluorescent dyes that emit light at different wavelengths, the brightness of each wavelength can be analyzed and the relative contributions of each dye to the total emitted light determined, thus allowing researchers to determine the relative contributions of each of the fluorescent dyes in the probe to the overall emission spectrum.

Fluorescence In Situ Hybridization to Chromosomes

Just as nucleic acid hybridization probes are used to identify fragments of DNA in Southern blot analysis, cytogeneticists can hybridize probes labeled with fluo-

rescent dyes to DNA contained within chromosomes immobilized on microscope slides to visualize chromosomal aberrations (see Chapters 5 and 6). This technique is called **fluorescence in situ hybridization (FISH)** because the DNA, either in interphase chromatin or in metaphase chromosomes, is fixed on a slide and denatured in place (hence "in situ") to expose the two strands of DNA and allow a denatured labeled probe to hybridize to the chromosomal DNA. The hybridized probe fluoresces when the chromosomes are viewed with a wavelength of light that excites the fluorescent dye. The location of the hybridization signal, and thus the location of the DNA segment to which the probe hybridizes, is then determined under a microscope.

One commonly used class of probe for FISH is a fragment of DNA derived from a unique location on a chromosome. Such probes hybridize and label the site on each homologous chromosome corresponding to the normal location of the probe sequence. A FISH probe can also be a complex mixture of DNA obtained from all or part of a chromosome arm or even from an entire chromosome. Depending on how the probe is constituted, some or all of a chromosome will stain with the fluorescent hybridized probe. Such probe mixtures are known as **chromosome "painting" probes** (see Chapters 5 and 6 for examples). Finally, one can combine 24 different chromosome painting probes, one for each of the 24 human chromosomes, each labeled with a different combination of fluorescent dyes that emit at different wavelengths. Every human chromosome will be labeled by a probe that fluoresces with its own characteristic combination of wavelengths of light. All 24 probes for the human chromosomes are then combined and used for FISH of metaphase chromosomes, a technique known as **spectral karyotyping** (SKY; see Fig. 5-B, *color insert*). Because each chromosome-specific probe emits its own signature combination of wavelengths of fluorescence, abnormal chromosomes consisting of pieces of different chromosomes are easily seen with SKY, and the chromosomes involved in the rearrangement can be readily identified. FISH using a single contiguous genomic sequence, a chromosome-specific painting probe, or SKY using painting probes for all the chromosomes combined, is used widely in diagnostic clinical cytogenetics to detect chromosomal aberrations such as deletions, duplications, and translocations (see Chapters 5 and 6).

Comparative Genome Hybridization

Deletions and duplications of individual DNA segments too small (less than approximately 1 to 2 Mb) to be seen in routine metaphase chromosome preparations are important aberrations that can occur in birth defect syndromes and in cancer. Such small changes in the number of copies of a DNA segment can be identified and characterized by another fluorescent imaging tech-

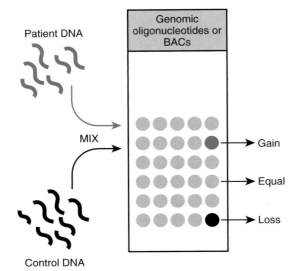

Patient DNA

MIX

Control DNA

Genomic
oligonucleotides or
BACs

→ Gain

→ Equal

→ Loss

Figure 4-12 ■ Comparative genome hybridization. Patient DNA, labeled with a green dye (shown here in blue), and control DNA, labeled with a red dye (shown here in black), are mixed in equal proportions and hybridized to an array of unique genomic DNA sequences spotted individually on a surface. Spots containing a sequence that is present in equal amounts in the patient and control will give a yellow signal (gray) indicating that equal amounts of patient DNA and control DNA were hybridizing to those spots (see *Equal*). Any spots corresponding to sequences that are increased in the patient relative to the control will hybridize disproportionately more patient DNA in the probe than control DNA, giving a spot that is more green (here, blue) (see *Gain*). In contrast, any spots corresponding to sequences that are decreased in the patient relative to the control will hybridize disproportionately less patient DNA than control DNA, giving a spot that is more red (here, black) (see *Loss*).

nique, **comparative genome hybridization (CGH;** Fig. 4-12). CGH is used to measure the difference between two different DNA samples in copy number, or dosage, of a particular DNA segment.

One rapidly emerging technique for high-resolution CGH is called **array CGH.** In this method, total DNA from one sample (test) is labeled with a red fluorescent dye, and the other (control) sample is labeled with a green dye. The two labeled DNA samples are mixed in equal amounts and hybridized to a microarray chip containing approximately 100,000 or more short single-stranded oligonucleotides, each corresponding to a different unique sequence from the human genome. These unique sequences are chosen so that they are uniformly distributed, less than 30 kb apart, throughout the genome. The ratio of red-to-green fluorescence emitted by the probe at each spotted oligonucleotide location is a measure of how much of the particular segment of DNA represented by that oligonucleotide is present in the test sample versus the control sample.

When the DNA from a particular region of a chromosome is represented equally in the two samples that make up the CGH probe, the ratio of red-to-green fluo-

rescence in the fluorescent signal will be 1:1. But if, for example, the DNA labeled with green is from a normal cell line and the DNA labeled with red comes from cells with only a single copy or three copies of a genomic region, the ratio of red-to-green fluorescence at all the oligonucleotide spots corresponding to sequences from within the region of abnormal dosage will shift from 1:1 to 0.5:1, in the case of one copy, and from 1:1 to 1.5:1, when there are three copies of that region (see Fig. 4-12).

CGH is particularly useful for finding changes in gene dosage in cancer tissues versus noncancerous tissue from the same individual (see Chapter 16). The array CGH is also being used successfully to find cytogenetically undetected deletions and duplications in some of the patients seen in genetics clinics with unexplained malformations or mental retardation but with apparently normal chromosome analysis by routine cytogenetic analysis (see Chapter 5). It has also revealed previously unappreciated normal variation in the number of copies of certain segments of DNA, known as copy number polymorphisms, in human populations (see Chapter 9).

RNA Expression Arrays

As described earlier, Northern blot analysis allows researchers to examine the size and abundance of one or a small set of transcripts detected by a probe specific for those RNAs. Diseases such as cancer or systemic autoimmune disorders, however, may have alterations in the abundance of hundreds of mRNAs or of regulatory microRNAs, yet Northern analysis of a small number of genes cannot provide sufficiently comprehensive information in such situations. In contrast, RNA expression microarrays do provide such information and are a powerful method of analyzing, in one experiment, the abundance of a large number, perhaps all, of the transcripts made in a particular cell type, tissue, or disease state relative to those made in another cell type, tissue, or disease state. The RNA samples to be analyzed could be from patients and controls, from samples of different histological types of cancer, or from cell lines treated or untreated with a drug.

For RNA expression analysis using arrays, RNA is first obtained from the cells or tissue to be tested and from a standard RNA source. Each RNA is reverse transcribed into cDNA. The test and standard cDNA samples are labeled separately with a red or green fluorescent dye, mixed in equal proportions, and hybridized to a chip by the same comparative hybridization approach just illustrated for genomic DNA samples. In this case, however, the expression array contains nucleotide sequences uniquely corresponding to each RNA. The sequence unique to a particular RNA can be a 25-mer oligonucleotide or a partial or complete cDNA clone. The ratio of the intensity of fluorescence of the two different dyes at each spot in the array is a measure of the relative abundance in the two samples of the RNA transcript represented by the sequence at that spot in the array (Fig. 4-A; *see color insert*).

Clinical Applications of Expression Arrays for Molecular Phenotyping and Functional Pathway Analysis

The simplest application of expression array data is to treat the pattern of changes in a test sample of RNA versus a standard sample as if it were a fingerprint that is characteristic of the source of the test RNA, without paying much attention to the identity or function of the particular genes whose transcripts are increased, decreased, or remain the same compared with the standard RNA sample. Such patterns of gene expression are **molecular phenotypes** that can characterize various disease states. Molecular phenotyping of mRNAs and microRNAs (see Chapter 3) is currently being used in oncology to differentiate histologically similar tumors and to provide a more accurate prediction of clinically relevant features, such as the tendency to metastasize or response to treatment (Chapter 16). More sophisticated expression array analysis is also being attempted in which the proteins encoded by the specific transcripts that show changes in a disease state are placed, first theoretically and then with actual experimentation, into **functional pathways**. In this way, researchers can begin to make inferences as to the molecular pathogenesis of disease on the basis of the knowledge of how the transcripts of genes of known or suspected function are perturbed by the disease process. The use of RNA expression arrays is revolutionizing the study of cancer and is now being widely applied to all areas of human disease.

◉ WESTERN BLOT ANALYSIS OF PROTEINS

The analysis of both normal and abnormal gene function often requires an examination of the protein encoded by a normal or mutant gene of interest. In most instances, one wants to know not only the molecular defect in the DNA but also how that defect alters the encoded protein to produce the clinical phenotype. The most commonly used technique for examining one or more proteins in a sample of cells or tissues is Western blotting.

For Western blot analysis, proteins isolated from a cell extract are separated according to size or charge by polyacrylamide gel electrophoresis and then transferred to a membrane. The membrane containing the separated proteins is then incubated with antibodies that

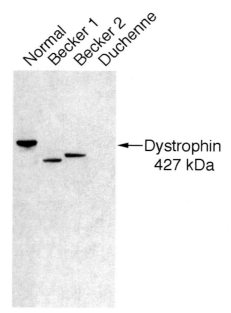

Figure 4-13 ■ A Western blot demonstrating the presence or absence of the muscle protein dystrophin *(arrow)* in protein extracts from patients with the severe Duchenne or mild Becker form of X-linked muscular dystrophy. See Chapter 12 for additional information. (Courtesy of P. Ray, Hospital for Sick Children, Toronto, Ontario, Canada.)

specifically recognize the protein to be analyzed. A second antibody against the first, tagged with a detectable histochemical, fluorescent, or radioactive substance, can then detect the specific interaction between the first antibody and its protein target. For example, a Western blot can be used to detect the presence and size of the muscle protein dystrophin in patients with X-linked **Duchenne or Becker muscular dystrophy** (Fig. 4-13).

◉ GENERAL REFERENCES

Dieffenbach C, Dveksler G: PCR Primer: A Laboratory Manual. Cold Spring Harbor, NY, Cold Spring Harbor Laboratory, 2003.

Elles R, Mountford R: Molecular Diagnosis of Genetic Diseases, 2nd ed. Totowa, NJ, Humana Press, 2003.

Gibson G, Muse SV: A Primer of Genome Science, 2nd ed. Sunderland, Mass, Sinauer Publishers, 2004.

Sambrook J, Russell DW, Sambrook J: Molecular Cloning: A Laboratory Manual, 3rd ed. Cold Spring Harbor, NY, Cold Spring Harbor Laboratory, 2001.

◉ REFERENCES FOR SPECIFIC TOPICS

Choi S, Kim UJ: Construction of a bacterial artificial chromosome library. Methods Mol Biol 175:57-68, 2001.

Fan Y-S: Molecular Cytogenetics: Protocols and Applications. Methods in Cell Biology, vol 204. Totowa, NJ, Humana Press, 2002.

Freeman WM, Robertson DJ, Vrana KE: Fundamentals of DNA hybridization arrays for gene expression analysis. Biotechniques 29:1042-1055, 2000.

Handyside AH: Clinical evaluation of preimplantation genetic diagnosis. Prenat Diagn 18:1345-1348, 1998.

Jobanputra V, Sebat J, Troge J, et al: Application of ROMA (representational oligonucleotide microarray analysis) to patients with cytogenetic rearrangements. Genet Med 7:111-118, 2005.

Lockhart DJ, Winzeler EA: Genomics, gene expression and DNA arrays. Nature 405:827-836, 2000.

Lucito R, Healy J, Alexander J, et al: Representational oligonucleotide microarray analysis: a high-resolution method to detect genome copy number variation. Genome Res 13:2291-2305, 2003.

Pagon RA: Molecular genetic testing for inherited disorders. Expert Rev Mol Diagn 4:135-140, 2004.

Sebat J, Lakshmi B, Troge J: Large scale copy number polymorphism in the human genome. Science 305:525-528, 2004.

Slater HR, Bailey DK, Ren H, et al: High-resolution identification of chromosomal abnormalities using oligonucleotide arrays containing 116,204 SNPs. Am J Hum Genet 77:709-726, 2005.

Weedn VW: Forensic DNA tests. Clin Lab Med 16:187-196, 1996.

● USEFUL WEBSITES

Children's Hospital Oakland Research Institute, Oakland, California: Bacterial Artificial Chromosome (BAC) Resource Database. *http://bacpac.chori.org/*

European Bioinformatics Institute/Wellcome Trust Sanger Institute, Hinxton, Cambridge, United Kingdom: Ensembl (genome browser). *http://www.ensembl.org/index.html*

National Center for Biotechnology Information/National Library of Medicine, Bethesda, Maryland: Entrez, The Life Sciences Search Engine. *http://www.ncbi.nlm.nih.gov/gquery/gquery.fcgi*

University of California, Santa Cruz: Genome Bioinformatics. *http://genome.ucsc.edu/*

PROBLEMS

1. Consider the following diagnostic situations. What laboratory method or methods would be most appropriate?

    a. Prenatal diagnosis of a male fetus at risk for Duchenne muscular dystrophy (DMD). Previous studies in this family have already documented a complete gene deletion.

    b. You want to estimate the amount of dystrophin mRNA present in a muscle specimen from a mildly affected obligate carrier of DMD.

    c. Prenatal diagnosis of a male fetus at risk for DMD. Previous studies have already documented a particular nucleotide base change that is responsible for the defect in this family.

2. What are some of the advantages or disadvantages of PCR for the diagnosis of genetic defects in comparison with Southern blotting? with biochemical assays of enzyme levels to diagnose enzyme deficiencies?

3. From which of the following tissues can DNA be obtained for diagnostic procedures: tissue biopsy specimens, white blood cells, cultured amniotic fluid cells, red blood cells?

4. Why is cloning of a gene considered such a significant advance for the field of medical genetics? What does the availability of a cloned gene allow one to do that one could not do before?

5. A patient with a genetic disease has a mutation (**C** to **T**, underlined) in exon 18 of a gene. The normal sequence is:

    CTGTGCCGTATGAAAAGACCAATC**C**GAGAAGT
    TCCTGTTACCAAACTCATAGAC

    The sequence in the patient is:

    CTGTGCCGTATGAAAAGACCAATC**T**GAGAAGT
    TCCTGTTACCAAACTCATAGAC

    a. What is the consequence of this mutation on gene function? (The first three nucleotides in each sequence constitute a codon of the gene.)

    b. You need to develop an ASO assay for the mutation in genomic DNA. Which of the following oligonucleotides would be useful in an ASO for the normal sequence? for the mutant sequence? Give your reasons for selecting or rejecting each oligonucleotide.

       1. 5′ GCCGTATGAAAAGACCAATCTG
       2. 5′ GACCAATCCGAGAAGTTCC
       3. 5′ GACCAATCTGAGAAGTTCC
       4. 5′ GGAACTTCTCAGATTGGTC
       5. 5′ ATCTGAG

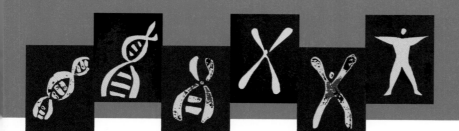

Chapter 5

Principles of Clinical Cytogenetics

Clinical cytogenetics is the study of chromosomes, their structure and their inheritance, as applied to the practice of medical genetics. It has been apparent for nearly 50 years that chromosome abnormalities—microscopically visible changes in the number or structure of chromosomes—could account for a number of clinical conditions that are thus referred to as **chromosome disorders.** Directing their focus to the complete set of chromosome material, cytogeneticists were the first to bring a genome-wide perspective to medical genetics. Today, chromosome analysis—now with dramatically improved resolution and precision at both the cytological and genomic levels—is an increasingly important diagnostic procedure in numerous areas of clinical medicine.

Chromosome disorders form a major category of genetic disease. They account for a large proportion of all reproductive wastage, congenital malformations, and mental retardation and play an important role in the pathogenesis of malignant disease. Specific chromosome abnormalities are responsible for hundreds of identifiable syndromes that are collectively more common than all the mendelian single-gene disorders together. Cytogenetic disorders are present in nearly 1% of live births, in about 2% of pregnancies in women older than 35 years who undergo prenatal diagnosis, and in fully half of all spontaneous first-trimester abortions.

In this chapter, we discuss the general principles of clinical cytogenetics and the various types of numerical and structural abnormalities observed in human karyotypes. Some of the most common and best-known abnormalities of the autosomes and the sex chromosomes are described in the next chapter.

● INTRODUCTION TO CYTOGENETICS

The general morphology and organization of human chromosomes as well as their molecular and genomic composition were introduced in Chapters 2 and 3. To be examined by chromosome analysis for routine clinical purposes, cells must be capable of growth and rapid division in culture. The most readily accessible cells that meet this requirement are white blood cells, specifically T lymphocytes. To prepare a short-term culture that is suitable for cytogenetic analysis of these cells, a sample of peripheral blood is obtained, usually by venipuncture, and mixed with heparin to prevent clotting. The white blood cells are collected, placed in tissue culture medium, and stimulated to divide. After a few days, the dividing cells are arrested in **metaphase** with chemicals that inhibit the mitotic spindle, collected, and treated with a hypotonic solution to release the chromosomes. Chromosomes are then fixed, spread on slides, and stained by one of several techniques, depending on the particular diagnostic procedure being performed. They are then ready for analysis.

Increasingly, routine karyotype analysis at the cytological level is being complemented by what might be called molecular karyotyping, the application of genomic techniques to assess the integrity and dosage of the karyotype genome-wide. The determination of what approaches are most appropriate for particular diagnostic or research purposes is a rapidly evolving area, as the resolution, sensitivity, and ease of chromosome and genome analysis increase.

Clinical Indications for Chromosome Analysis

Chromosome analysis is indicated as a routine diagnostic procedure for a number of specific phenotypes encountered in clinical medicine, as described in this chapter and in Chapter 6. In addition, there are also some nonspecific general clinical situations and findings that indicate a need for cytogenetic analysis:

- **Problems of early growth and development.** Failure to thrive, developmental delay, dysmorphic facies, multiple malformations, short stature, ambiguous genitalia, and mental retardation are frequent findings in children with chromosome abnormalities, although they are not restricted to that group. Unless there is a definite non-chromosomal diagnosis, chromosome analysis should be performed for patients presenting with a combination of such problems.
- **Stillbirth and neonatal death.** The incidence of chromosome abnormalities is much higher among stillbirths (up to approximately 10%) than among live births (about 0.7%). It is also elevated among infants who die in the neonatal period (about 10%). Chromosome analysis should be performed for all stillbirths and neonatal deaths that might have a cytogenetic basis to identify a possible specific cause or, alternatively, to rule out a chromosome abnormality as the reason for the loss. In such cases, karyotyping (or other comprehensive ways of scanning the genome) is essential for accurate genetic counseling and may provide important information for prenatal diagnosis in future pregnancies.
- **Fertility problems.** Chromosome studies are indicated for women presenting with amenorrhea and for couples with a history of infertility or recurrent miscarriage. A chromosome abnormality is seen in one or the other parent in a significant proportion (3% to 6%) of cases in which there is infertility or two or more miscarriages.
- **Family history.** A known or suspected chromosome abnormality in a first-degree relative is an indication for chromosome analysis under some circumstances.
- **Neoplasia.** Virtually all cancers are associated with one or more chromosome abnormalities (see Chapter 16). Chromosome and genome evaluation in the appropriate tissue sample (the tumor itself, or bone marrow in the case of hematological malignant neoplasms) can provide useful diagnostic or prognostic information.
- **Pregnancy in a woman of advanced age.** There is an increased risk of chromosome abnormality in fetuses conceived by women older than about 35 years (see Chapter 15). Fetal chromosome analysis should be offered as a routine part of prenatal care in such pregnancies.

Although ideal for rapid clinical analysis, cell cultures prepared from peripheral blood have the disadvantage of being short-lived (3 to 4 days). Long-term cultures suitable for permanent storage or molecular studies can be derived from a variety of other tissues. Skin biopsy, a minor surgical procedure, can provide samples of tissue that in culture produce **fibroblasts**, which can be used for a variety of biochemical and molecular studies as well as for chromosome and genome analysis. White blood cells can also be transformed in culture to form **lymphoblastoid** cell lines that are potentially immortal. **Bone marrow** can be obtained only by the relatively invasive procedure of marrow biopsy, but it has the advantage of containing a high proportion of dividing cells, so that little if any culturing is required. Its main use is in the diagnosis of suspected hematological malignant neoplasms. Its disadvantage is that the chromosome preparations obtained from marrow are relatively poor, with short, poorly resolved chromosomes that are more difficult to analyze than are those from peripheral blood. **Fetal cells** derived from amniotic fluid (amniocytes) or obtained by chorionic villus biopsy can also be cultured successfully for cytogenetic, genomic, biochemical, or molecular analysis. Chorionic villus cells can also be analyzed directly, without the need for culturing (see Chapter 15 for further discussion).

Molecular analysis of the genome can be carried out on any appropriate clinical material, provided that good-quality DNA can be obtained. Cells do not have to be dividing for this purpose, and thus it is possible to perform tests on tissue and tumor samples, for example, as well as on peripheral blood.

Chromosome Identification

The 24 types of chromosome found in the human genome can be readily identified at the cytological level by a number of specific staining procedures. There are three commonly used staining methods that can distinguish among human chromosomes. In Chapter 2, we examined chromosomes stained by Giemsa banding (**G banding**), the most common method used in clinical laboratories. Other procedures used in some laboratories or for specific purposes include the following:

Q Banding This method requires staining with quinacrine mustard or related compounds and examination by fluorescence microscopy. The chromosomes stain in a specific pattern of bright and dim bands (Q bands), the bright Q bands corresponding almost exactly to the dark bands seen after G banding. Q banding, as well

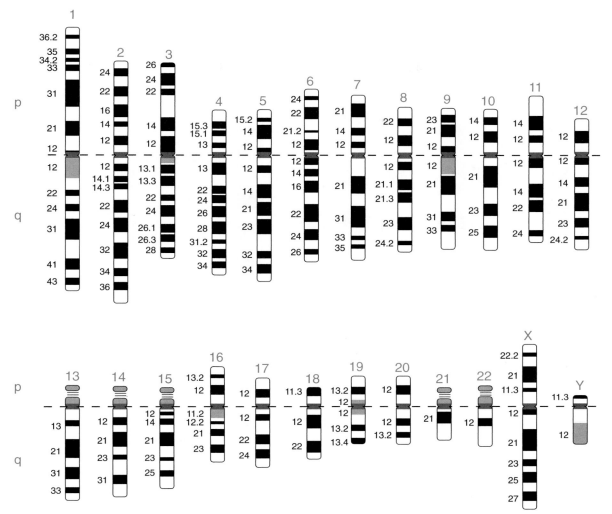

Figure 5-1 ■ Ideogram showing G-banding patterns for human chromosomes at metaphase, with about 400 bands per haploid karyotype. As drawn, chromosomes are typically represented with the sister chromatids so closely aligned that they are not recognized as distinct structures. Centromeres are indicated by the narrow dark gray regions separating the p and q arms. For convenience and clarity, only the G-positive bands are numbered. For examples of full numbering scheme, see Figure 5-2. (Redrawn from ISCN 2005.)

as C banding (see next section), is particularly useful for detecting occasional variants in chromosome morphology or staining, called **heteromorphisms.** These variants are generally benign and reflect differences in the amount or type of satellite DNA sequences (see Chapter 2) at a particular location along a chromosome.

R Banding If the chromosomes receive special treatment (such as heating) before staining, the resulting dark and light bands are the reverse of those produced by G or Q banding and are accordingly referred to as R bands. Especially when regions that stain poorly by G or Q banding are examined, R banding gives a pattern that is easier to analyze than that given by G or Q banding. It is the standard method in some laboratories, particularly in Europe.

A uniform system of chromosome classification is internationally accepted for the identification of human chromosomes stained by any of the three staining procedures mentioned. Figure 5-1 is an ideogram of the banding pattern of a set of normal human chromosomes at metaphase, illustrating the alternating pattern of dark and light bands used for chromosome identification. The pattern of bands on each chromosome is numbered on each arm from the centromere to the telomere, as shown in detail in Figure 5-2 for several chromosomes. By use of this numbering system, the location of any particular band as well as the DNA sequences and genes within it and its involvement in a chromosomal abnormality can be described precisely and unambiguously.

Human chromosomes are often classified by the position of the **centromere** into three types that can

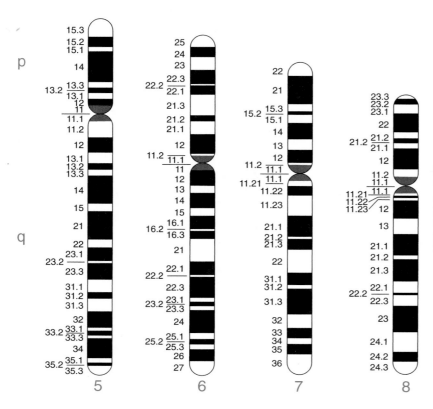

Figure 5-2 ■ Examples of G-banding patterns for chromosomes 5, 6, 7, and 8 at the 550-band stage of condensation. Band numbers permit unambiguous identification of each G-dark or G-light band, for example, chromosome 5p15.2 or chromosome 8q24.1. (Redrawn from ISCN 2005.)

be easily distinguished at metaphase (see Fig. 5-1): **metacentric** chromosomes, with a more or less central centromere and arms of approximately equal length; **submetacentric** chromosomes, with an off-center centromere and arms of clearly different lengths; and **acrocentric** chromosomes, with the centromere near one end. A potential fourth type of chromosome, **telocentric,** with the centromere at one end and only a single arm, does not occur in the normal human karyotype, but it is occasionally observed in chromosome rearrangements and is a common type in some other species. The human acrocentric chromosomes (chromosomes 13, 14, 15, 21, and 22) have small, distinctive masses of chromatin known as **satellites** attached to their short arms by narrow stalks (secondary constrictions). The stalks of these five chromosome pairs contain hundreds of copies of genes encoding ribosomal RNA (the major component of ribosomes; see Chapter 3) as well as a variety of repetitive sequences.

Special Cytological Procedures

For particular situations, a number of specialized techniques can be used.

C Banding   This method specifically involves staining the centromeric region of each chromosome and other regions containing **constitutive heterochromatin,** namely, sections of chromosomes 1q, 9q, and 16q adjacent to the centromere and the distal part of Yq. Heterochromatin is the type of chromatin defined by its

property of remaining in the condensed state and staining darkly in nondividing (interphase) cells.

High-Resolution Banding   This type of banding (also called **prometaphase banding**) is achieved through G-banding or R-banding techniques to stain chromosomes that have been obtained at an early stage of mitosis (prophase or prometaphase), when they are still in a relatively uncondensed state (see Chapter 2). High-resolution banding is especially useful when a subtle structural abnormality of a chromosome is suspected; some laboratories, however, routinely use prometaphase banding, as shown in Figures 2-11 and 2-12. Prometaphase chromosomes reveal 550 to 850 bands or even more in a haploid set, whereas standard metaphase preparations show only about 450. A comparison of the banding patterns of the X chromosome at three different stages of resolution is shown in Figure 5-3. The increase in diagnostic precision obtained with these longer chromosomes is evident.

Fragile Sites   Fragile sites are non-staining gaps that are occasionally observed at characteristic sites on several chromosomes. To demonstrate fragile sites, it is usually necessary to expose the cells to growth conditions or chemicals that alter or inhibit DNA synthesis. Many fragile sites are known to be heritable variants. The fragile site most clearly shown to be clinically significant is seen near the end of Xq in males with a specific and common form of X-linked mental retardation (see discussion of the **fragile X syndrome** in Chapter 7

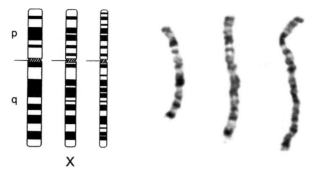

p

q

X

Figure 5-3 ■ The X chromosome: ideograms and photomicrographs at metaphase, prometaphase, and prophase *(left to right)*. (Ideograms redrawn from ISCN 2005; photomicrographs courtesy of Yim Kwan Ng, The Hospital for Sick Children, Toronto.)

and Case 15), as well as in some female carriers of the same genetic defect. Detection of the fragile site on the X chromosome is a diagnostic procedure specific for the fragile X syndrome (see Fig. 7-30), although in most laboratories this has been replaced by (or is complemented by) molecular testing to detect expansion of

the CGG repeat in the *FMR1* gene characteristic of this disorder (see Chapter 7).

Fluorescence In Situ Hybridization

As introduced in Chapter 4, both research and clinical cytogenetics have been revolutionized by the development of fluorescence in situ hybridization (**FISH**) techniques to examine the presence or absence of a particular DNA sequence or to evaluate the number or organization of a chromosome or chromosomal region. This confluence of genomic and cytogenetic approaches—**molecular cytogenetics**—has dramatically expanded both the range and precision of routine chromosome analysis.

In FISH, DNA probes specific for individual chromosomes, chromosomal regions, or genes can be used to identify particular chromosomal rearrangements or to rapidly diagnose the existence of an abnormal chromosome number in clinical material (Fig. 5-4). Suitable probes can be prepared by any number of techniques introduced in Chapter 4. Gene-specific or locus-specific probes can be used to detect the presence, absence, or

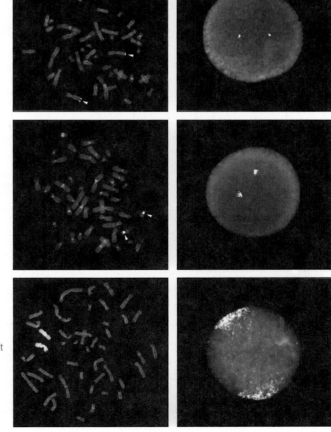

Metaphase   Interphase

Locus-specific probe

Satellite DNA probe

Chromosome paint probe

Figure 5-4 ■ Fluorescence in situ hybridization to human chromosomes at metaphase and interphase, with three different types of DNA probe. *Top,* A single-copy DNA probe specific for the factor VIII gene on the X chromosome. *Middle,* A repetitive α-satellite DNA probe specific for the centromere of chromosome 17. *Bottom,* A whole-chromosome "paint" probe specific for the X chromosome. (Images courtesy of Karen Gustashaw, Case Western Reserve University.)

location of a particular gene, both in metaphase chromosomes and in interphase cells. Repetitive DNA probes allow detection of satellite DNA or other localized repeated DNA elements at specific chromosomal loci including centromeres (see Fig. 5-4), telomeres, and regions of heterochromatin. Satellite DNA probes, especially those belonging to the α-satellite family of centromere repeats (see Chapter 2), are widely used for determining the number of copies of a particular chromosome (Fig. 5-A; *see color insert*). Lastly, probes for entire chromosomes or chromosome arms contain a mixture of single-copy DNA sequences that are located along the length of an entire chromosome (or arm). These probes "paint" the target chromosome; a comparison of cells in metaphase and interphase, as in Figure 5-4, visually documents the dynamic nature of chromosome condensation and decondensation throughout the cell cycle, as introduced in Chapter 2 (compare with Fig. 2-13).

One of the more important applications of FISH technology in clinical cytogenetics involves the use of different fluorochromes to detect multiple probes simultaneously. Two-, three-, and even four-color applications are routinely used to diagnose specific deletions, duplications, or rearrangements, both in prometaphase or metaphase preparations and in interphase. With highly specialized imaging procedures, it is even possible to detect and distinguish 24 different colors simultaneously by spectral karyotyping (SKY; see Chapter 4), allowing dramatic evaluation of the karyotype in a single experiment (Figs. 5-B and 5-C; *see color insert*).

Chromosome and Genome Analysis by Use of Microarrays

With the availability of resources from the Human Genome Project, chromosome analysis can also be carried out at a genomic level by a variety of array-based methods that use **comparative genome hybridization** (**CGH;** see Chapter 4). To assess the relative copy number of genomic DNA sequences in a comprehensive, genome-wide manner, microarrays containing either a complete representation of the genome or a series of cloned fragments, spaced at various intervals, from throughout the genome can be hybridized to control and patient samples (Fig. 5-5). This approach, which is being used in an increasing number of clinical laboratories, complements conventional karyotyping and has the potential to provide a much more sensitive, high-resolution assessment of the genome. However, array-based CGH methods measure the relative copy number of DNA sequences but not whether they have been translocated or rearranged from their normal position in the genome. Thus, confirmation of suspected chromosome abnormalities by karyotyping or FISH is important to determine the nature of the abnormality and its risk of recurrence, either for the individual or for other family members.

High-resolution genome and chromosome analysis can reveal variants, in particular small changes in copy number between samples, that are of uncertain clinical significance. An increasing number of such variants are being documented and catalogued even within the phe-

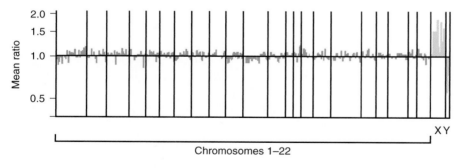

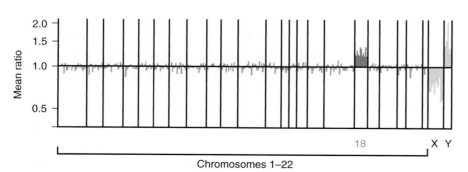

Figure 5-5 ■ Array CGH analysis from two individuals with use of BAC arrays. Intensities of hybridization signals are typically presented as ratios on a log$_2$ scale, where a ratio of 1.0 indicates signal equivalent to a control sample. Trisomy for an autosome is expected to give a mean signal intensity of 1.5 (i.e., case-to-control ratio of 3:2); monosomy should give a mean ratio of 0.5 (i.e., case-to-control ratio of 1:2). Samples are routinely hybridized with a control of the opposite sex, so a male sample shows a reduced ratio for X chromosome BACs and a high ratio for Y chromosome BACs (relative to a 46,XX control). A female sample shows an increased ratio for X BACs and a low ratio for Y BACs (relative to a 46,XY control). *Top,* Sample from a normal female. *Bottom,* Sample from a male with trisomy 18, showing increased ratios for chromosome 18 BACs. (Original data courtesy of Emory Genetics Laboratory.)

Table 5-1

Incidence of Chromosome Abnormalities at Different Stages of Fetal or Postnatal Life

Abnormal Karyotype	First-Trimester Abortuses	Fetuses of Mothers > 35 Years*	Live Births
Total incidence	1/2	1/50	1/160
Percentage of abnormalities			
Numerical abnormalities	96%	85%	60%
Structural abnormalities			
Balanced	0%	10%	30%
Unbalanced	4%	5%	10%

*Studied at amniocentesis; data summarized from Hsu LYF: Prenatal diagnosis of chromosomal abnormalities through amniocentesis. In Milunsky A (ed): Genetic Disorders and the Fetus, 4th ed. Baltimore, Johns Hopkins University Press, 1998, pp 179-248.

notypically normal population. These genomic variants can range from a few kilobase pairs to several million base pairs in size, and although they are found throughout the karyotype, they are particularly common in the subtelomeric and centromeric regions of chromosomes. Many are likely to be benign **copy number polymorphisms** or **variants,** which collectively underscore the unique nature of each individual's genome (see Chapter 9) and emphasize the diagnostic challenge of assessing what is considered a "normal" karyotype and what is likely to be pathogenic.

⊙ CHROMOSOME ABNORMALITIES

Abnormalities of chromosomes may be either numerical or structural and may involve one or more autosomes, sex chromosomes, or both simultaneously. The clinical and social impact of chromosome abnormalities is enormous. By far the most common type of clinically significant chromosome abnormality is **aneuploidy,** an abnormal chromosome number due to an extra or missing chromosome, which is always associated with physical or mental maldevelopment or both. **Reciprocal translocations** (an exchange of segments between nonhomologous chromosomes) are also relatively common but usually have no phenotypic effect, although, as explained later, there may be an associated increased risk of abnormal offspring. The relative frequencies of numerical and structural abnormalities observed in spontaneous abortions, in fetuses of mothers older than 35 years that are analyzed in amniocentesis, and in live births are presented in Table 5-1.

Chromosome abnormalities are described by a standard set of abbreviations and nomenclature that indicate the nature of the abnormality and (in the case of analyses performed by FISH or microarrays) the technology used. Some of the more common abbreviations and examples of abnormal karyotypes and abnormalities are listed in Table 5-2.

The phenotypic consequences of a chromosome abnormality depend on its specific nature, the resulting imbalance of involved parts of the genome, the specific genes contained in or affected by the abnormality, and the likelihood of its transmission to the next generation. Predicting such outcomes can be an enormous challenge for genetic counseling, particularly in the prenatal setting. Many such diagnostic dilemmas will be presented later in this chapter and in Chapters 6 and 15, but there are a number of general principles that should be kept in mind as we explore specific types of chromosome abnormality (see Box).

▪▪▪ Unbalanced Karyotypes in Liveborns: General Guidelines for Counseling

Monosomies are more deleterious than trisomies.
• Complete monosomies are generally not viable except for monosomy X.
• Complete trisomies are viable for chromosomes 13, 18, 21, X, and Y.

Phenotype in partial aneusomies depends on:
• the size of the unbalanced segment;
• whether the imbalance is monosomic or trisomic; and
• which regions of the genome are affected and which genes are involved.

In a mosaic karyotype, "all bets are off."

Rings give a phenotype specific to the genomic region involved, but are commonly mosaic.

Inversions
• Pericentric: risk of birth defects in offspring increases with size of inversion.
• Paracentric: very low risk of abnormal phenotype.

Abnormalities of Chromosome Number

A chromosome complement with any chromosome number other than 46 is said to be **heteroploid.** An exact multiple of the haploid chromosome number (n) is called **euploid,** and any other chromosome number is **aneuploid.**

Triploidy and Tetraploidy

In addition to the diploid (2n) number characteristic of normal somatic cells, two other euploid chromosome

Table 5-2

Some Abbreviations Used for Description of Chromosomes and Their Abnormalities, with Representative Examples

Abbreviation	Meaning	Example	Condition
		46,XX	Normal female karyotype
		46,XY	Normal male karyotype
cen	centromere		
del	deletion	46,XX,del(5p)	Female with cri du chat syndrome (see Chapter 6), due to deletion of part of short arm of one chromosome 5
der	derivative chromosome	der(1)	Translocation chromosome derived from chromosome 1 and containing the centromere of chromosome 1
dic	dicentric chromosome	dic(X;Y)	Translocation chromosome containing the centromeres of both the X and Y chromosomes
dup	duplication		
fra	fragile site	46,Y,fra(X)(q27.3)	Male with fragile X chromosome
i	isochromosome	46,X,i(X)(q10)	Female with isochromosome for the long arm of the X chromosome
ins	insertion		
inv	inversion	inv(3)(p25q21)	Pericentric inversion of chromosome 3
mar	marker chromosome	47,XX,+mar	Female with an extra, unidentified chromosome
mat	maternal origin	47,XY,+der(1)mat	Male with an extra der(1) chromosome inherited from his mother
p	short arm of chromosome		
pat	paternal origin		
q	long arm of chromosome		
r	ring chromosome	46,X,r(X)	Female with ring X chromosome
rcp	reciprocal translocation		
rob	Robertsonian translocation	rob(13;21)(q10;q10)	Breakage and reunion have occurred at band 13q10 and band 21q10 in the centromeric regions of chromosomes 13 and 21
t	translocation	46,XX,t(2;8)(q22;p21)	Female with balanced translocation between chromosome 2 and chromosome 8, with breaks in 2q22 and 8p21
ter	terminal or telomere	46,X,del(X)(pter → q21:)	Female with partial deletion of the X chromosome, distal to band Xq21 (nomenclature shows the portion of the chromosome that is present)
+	gain of	47,XX,+21	Female with trisomy 21
−	loss of	45,XX,−22	Female with monosomy 22
:	break	5qter → 5p15:	Deleted chromosome 5, with deletion breakpoint in 5p15
::	break and join	2pter → 2q22::8p21 → 8pter	Description of der(2) portion of t(2;8)
/	mosaicism	46,XX/47,XX,+8	Female with two populations of cells, one with a normal karyotype and one with trisomy 8
ish	in situ hybridization	ish 22q11.2(D22S75 × 2)	FISH with a probe from the DiGeorge syndrome (see Chapter 6) region of chromosome 22 (for locus D22S75 in 22q11.2) showed a normal hybridization pattern (two signals = ×2) on metaphase chromosomes
		46,XX.ish del(22)(q11.2q11.2)(D22S75−)	A female with a normal karyotype by G-banding analysis, with a deletion of proximal region on chromosome 22q (within band 22q11.2) identified by FISH with a probe for locus D22S75
arr	array		
cgh	comparative genome hybridization	arr cgh 1-22(#BACs tested) × 2, X(#BACs) × 2, Y(#BACs) × 0	Normal female array CGH pattern, detected by use of the indicated number of BAC clones from the autosomes, X, and Y; pattern showed level of hybridization expected for two copies (×2) of autosomes and the X, but zero copies (×0) of the Y
		arr cgh 1-22(#BACs) × 2, X(#BACs) × 1, Y(#BACs) × 1	Normal male array CGH pattern by use of the indicated number of BAC clones
		arr cgh 22q11.2(BAC name) × 1 *or* arr cgh 22q11.2(D22S75) × 1	Loss of the DiGeorge syndrome critical region on chromosome 22q11.1 identified by array CGH

Abbreviations from ISCN 2005: An International System for Human Cytogenetic Nomenclature. Basel, Karger, 2005.

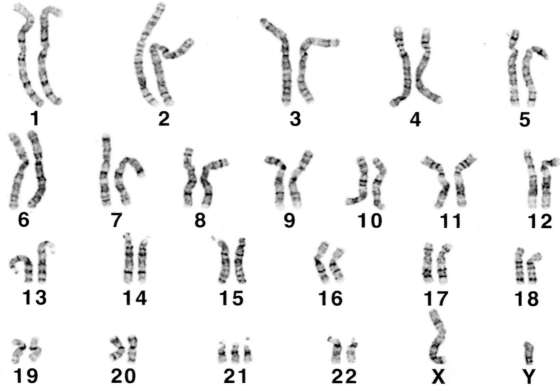

Figure 5-6 ■ Karyotype from a male patient with Down syndrome, showing three copies of chromosome 21. (Courtesy of Center for Human Genetics Laboratory, University Hospitals of Cleveland.)

complements, **triploid** (3n) and **tetraploid** (4n), are occasionally observed in clinical material. Both triploidy and tetraploidy have been seen in fetuses, and although triploid infants can be liveborn, they do not survive long. Triploidy is observed in 1% to 3% of recognized conceptions, and among those that survive to the end of the first trimester, most result from fertilization by two sperm (dispermy). Failure of one of the meiotic divisions, resulting in a diploid egg or sperm, can also account for a proportion of cases. The phenotypic manifestation of a triploid karyotype depends on the source of the extra chromosome set; triploids with an extra set of paternal chromosomes typically have an abnormal placenta and are classified as **partial hydatidiform moles** (see later section), but those with an additional set of maternal chromosomes are spontaneously aborted earlier in pregnancy. Tetraploids are always 92,XXXX or 92,XXYY; the absence of XXXY or XYYY sex chromosome constitutions suggests that tetraploidy results from failure of completion of an early cleavage division of the zygote.

Aneuploidy

Aneuploidy is the most common and clinically significant type of human chromosome disorder, occurring in at least 5% of all clinically recognized pregnancies.

Most aneuploid patients have either **trisomy** (three instead of the normal pair of a particular chromosome) or, less often, **monosomy** (only one representative of a particular chromosome). Either trisomy or monosomy can have severe phenotypic consequences.

Trisomy can exist for any part of the genome, but trisomy for a whole chromosome is rarely compatible with life. By far the most common type of trisomy in liveborn infants is **trisomy 21** (karyotype 47,XX or XY,+21), the chromosome constitution seen in 95% of patients with Down syndrome (Fig. 5-6). Other trisomies observed in liveborns include trisomy 18 (see Fig. 5-5) and trisomy 13. It is notable that these autosomes (13, 18, and 21) are the three with the lowest number of genes located on them (see Fig. 2-8); presumably, trisomy for autosomes with a greater number of genes is lethal in most instances. Monosomy for an entire chromosome is almost always lethal; an important exception is monosomy for the X chromosome, as seen in Turner syndrome. These conditions are described in greater detail in Chapter 6.

Although the causes of aneuploidy are not well understood, it is known that the most common chromosomal mechanism is meiotic **nondisjunction**. This refers to the failure of a pair of chromosomes to disjoin properly during one of the two meiotic divisions, usually during meiosis I. The consequences of nondisjunction

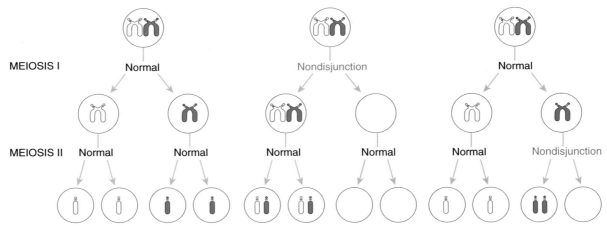

MEIOSIS I

MEIOSIS II

Figure 5-7 ■   The different consequences of nondisjunction at meiosis I *(center)* and meiosis II *(right)*, compared with normal disjunction *(left)*. If the error occurs at meiosis I, the gametes either contain a representative of both members of the chromosome 21 pair or lack a chromosome 21 altogether. If nondisjunction occurs at meiosis II, the abnormal gametes contain two copies of one parental chromosome 21 (and no copy of the other) or lack a chromosome 21.

during meiosis I and meiosis II are different (Fig. 5-7). If the error occurs during meiosis I, the gamete with 24 chromosomes contains both the paternal and the maternal members of the pair. If it occurs during meiosis II, the gamete with the extra chromosome contains both copies of either the paternal or the maternal chromosome. (Strictly speaking, the statements mentioned refer only to the paternal or maternal centromere, because recombination between homologous chromosomes has usually taken place in the preceding meiosis I, resulting in some genetic differences between the chromatids and thus between the corresponding daughter chromosomes; see Chapter 2.) The propensity of a chromosome pair to nondisjoin has been strongly associated with aberrations in the frequency or placement, or both, of recombination events in meiosis I. A chromosome pair with too few (or even no) recombinations, or with recombination too close to the centromere or telomere, may be more susceptible to nondisjunction than a chromosome pair with a more typical number and distribution of recombination events.

In addition to classic nondisjunction, in which improper chromosome segregation is the result of the failure of chromosomes either to pair or to recombine properly, or both, another mechanism underlying aneuploidy involves premature separation of sister chromatids in meiosis I instead of meiosis II. If this happens, the separated chromatids may by chance segregate to the oocyte or to the polar body, leading to an unbalanced gamete.

More complicated forms of multiple aneuploidy have also been reported. A gamete occasionally has an extra representative of more than one chromosome. Nondisjunction can take place at two successive meiotic divisions or by chance in both male and female gametes simultaneously, resulting in zygotes with unusual chromosome numbers, which are extremely rare except for the sex chromosomes (Fig. 5-D; *see color insert*). Nondisjunction can also occur in a mitotic division after formation of the zygote. If this happens at an early cleavage division, clinically significant **mosaicism** may result (see later section). In some malignant cell lines and some cell cultures, mitotic nondisjunction can lead to highly abnormal karyotypes.

An important development in the diagnosis of aneuploidy, especially prenatally, is the application of multicolor FISH to interphase cells (Fig. 5-E; *see color insert*). This approach allows rapid diagnosis without the need to culture cells. A large number of prenatal cytogenetics laboratories are now performing prenatal interphase analysis to evaluate aneuploidy for chromosomes 13, 18, 21, X, and Y, the five chromosomes that account for the vast majority of aneuploidy in liveborn individuals (see Chapters 6 and 15).

Abnormalities of Chromosome Structure

Structural rearrangements result from chromosome breakage, followed by reconstitution in an abnormal combination. Whereas rearrangements can take place in many ways, they are together less common than aneuploidy; overall, structural abnormalities are present in about 1 in 375 newborns. Chromosome rearrangement occurs spontaneously at a low frequency and may also be induced by breaking agents (clastogens), such as ionizing radiation, some viral infections, and many chemicals. Like numerical abnormalities, structural rearrangements may be present in all cells of a person or in mosaic form.

Structural rearrangements are defined as **balanced,** if the chromosome set has the normal complement of chromosomal material, or **unbalanced,** if there is addi-

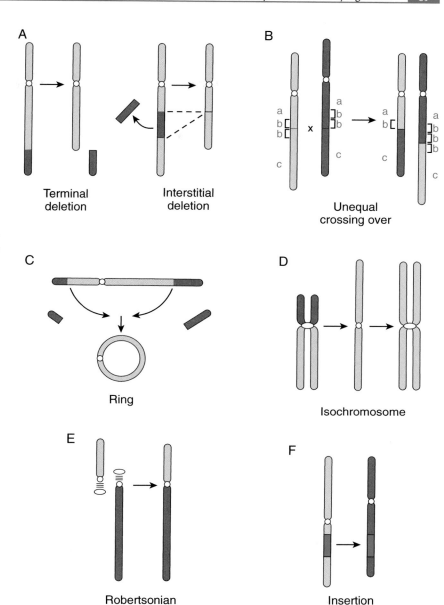

Figure 5-8 ■ Structural rearrangements of chromosomes, described in the text. **A,** Terminal and interstitial deletions, each generating an acentric fragment. **B,** Unequal crossing over between segments of homologous chromosomes or between sister chromatids (duplicated or deleted segment indicated by the brackets). **C,** Ring chromosome with two acentric fragments. **D,** Generation of an isochromosome for the long arm of a chromosome. **E,** Robertsonian translocation between two acrocentric chromosomes. **F,** Insertion of a segment of one chromosome into a nonhomologous chromosome.

tional or missing material. Some rearrangements are stable, capable of passing through mitotic and meiotic cell divisions unaltered, whereas others are unstable. To be completely stable, a rearranged chromosome must have a functional centromere and two telomeres. Some of the types of structural rearrangements observed in human chromosomes are illustrated in Figure 5-8.

Unbalanced Rearrangements

In unbalanced rearrangements, the phenotype is likely to be abnormal because of deletion, duplication, or (in some cases) both. Duplication of part of a chromosome leads to partial trisomy; deletion leads to partial monosomy. Any change that disturbs the normal balance of

functional genes can result in abnormal development. Large deletions or duplications involving imbalance of at least a few million base pairs can be detected at the level of routine chromosome banding, including high-resolution karyotyping. Detection of smaller deletions or duplications generally requires more sophisticated analysis, involving FISH (Fig. 5-F; *see color insert*) or microarray analysis (Fig. 5-9).

An important class of unbalanced rearrangement involves submicroscopic changes of a telomere region in patients with idiopathic mental retardation. Small deletions, duplications, and translocations have been detected in several percent of such patients. Targeted cytogenetic or genomic analysis of telomeric and subtelomeric regions by FISH (Fig. 5-G; *see color insert*)

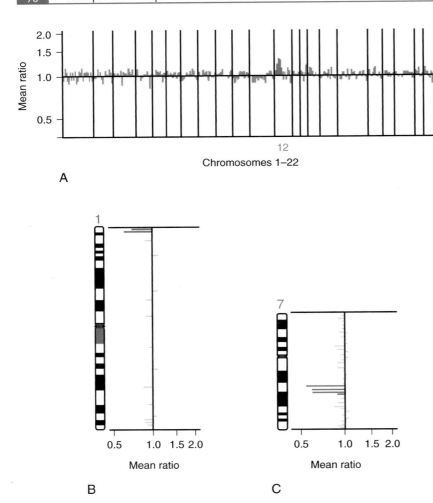

Figure 5-9 ■ Array CGH analysis of chromosome abnormalities. **A,** Detection of a partial duplication of chromosome 12p in a patient with an apparently normal routine karyotype and symptoms of Pallister-Killian syndrome. (Sex chromosome data are not shown.) **B,** Detection of terminal deletion of chromosome 1p by array CGH in a patient with mental retardation. **C,** Detection of an approximately 5 Mb de novo deletion of chromosome 7q22 by array CGH in a patient with a complex abnormal phenotype; this deletion was originally undetected by routine karyotyping. (Original data courtesy of Arthur Beaudet, Baylor College of Medicine; Hutton Kearney, Duke University Medical Center; Stephen Scherer, The Hospital for Sick Children, Toronto; and Charles Lee, Brigham and Women's Hospital, Boston.)

or by array CGH (see Fig. 5-9B) may be indicated in unexplained mental retardation because of the profound implications of a positive result for genetic counseling.

Deletions Deletions involve loss of a chromosome segment, resulting in chromosome imbalance (see Fig. 5-8A). A carrier of a chromosomal deletion (with one normal homologue and one deleted homologue) is monosomic for the genetic information on the corresponding segment of the normal homologue. The clinical consequences generally reflect **haploinsufficiency** (literally, the inability of a single copy of the genetic material to carry out the functions normally performed by two copies) and, where examined, appear to depend on the size of the deleted segment and the number and function of the genes that it contains. Cytogenetically visible autosomal deletions have an incidence of approximately 1 in 7000 live births. Smaller, submicroscopic deletions detected by microarray analysis are much more common, but as mentioned earlier, the clinical significance of many such variants has yet to be fully determined.

A deletion may occur at the end of a chromosome (**terminal**) or along a chromosome arm (**interstitial**). Deletions may originate simply by chromosome breakage and loss of the acentric segment. Alternatively, unequal crossing over between misaligned homologous chromosomes or sister chromatids may account for deletion in some cases (see Fig. 5-8B). Deletions can also be generated by abnormal segregation of a balanced translocation or inversion, as described later. Numerous deletions have been identified in the investigation of dysmorphic patients and in prenatal diagnosis, and knowledge of the functional genes lost in the deleted segments and their relation to the phenotypic consequences has increased markedly from the Human Genome Project. Specific examples of these syndromes are discussed in Chapter 6.

Both high-resolution banding techniques and FISH can reveal deletions that are too small to be seen in ordinary metaphase spreads. To be identifiable cytogenetically by high-resolution banding, a deletion must typically span at least several million base pairs, but karyotypically undetectable deletions or uncertain deletions with phenotypic consequences can be detected routinely by FISH (Figs. 5-F and 5-H; *see color insert*) or microarray analysis (see Fig. 5-9B and C) with the use of probes specific for the region of interest.

Duplications Duplications, like deletions, can originate by unequal crossing over (see Fig. 5-8B) or by abnormal segregation from meiosis in a carrier of a translocation or inversion. In general, duplication appears to be less harmful than deletion. Because duplication in a gamete results in chromosomal imbalance (i.e., partial trisomy), however, and because the chromosome breaks that generate it may disrupt genes, duplication often leads to some phenotypic abnormality.

Although many duplications have been reported, few of any one kind have been studied thus far. Nonetheless, certain phenotypes appear to be associated with duplications of particular chromosomal regions. For example, duplication of all or a portion of chromosome 12p (see Fig. 5-9A) leads to Pallister-Killian syndrome, in which patients show characteristic craniofacial features, mental retardation, and a range of other birth defects likely to be related to trisomy or tetrasomy for specific genes present in the duplicated region.

Marker and Ring Chromosomes Very small, unidentified chromosomes, called marker chromosomes, are occasionally seen in chromosome preparations, frequently in a mosaic state. They are usually in addition to the normal chromosome complement and are thus also referred to as **supernumerary chromosomes** or **extra structurally abnormal chromosomes.** Cytogeneticists find it difficult to characterize marker chromosomes specifically by banding, even by high-resolution techniques, because they are usually so small that the banding pattern is ambiguous or not apparent. FISH with various probes is usually required for precise identification; tiny marker chromosomes often consist of little more than centromeric heterochromatin that can be identified with a variety of chromosome-specific satellite or "paint" FISH probes.

Larger marker chromosomes invariably contain some material from one or both chromosome arms, creating an imbalance for whatever genes are present. The prenatal frequency of de novo supernumerary marker chromosomes has been estimated to be approximately 1 in 2500. Because of the problem of identification, the clinical significance of a marker chromosome is difficult to assess, and the finding of a marker in a fetal karyotype can present a serious problem in assessment and genetic counseling. Depending on the origin of the marker chromosome, the risk of a fetal abnormality can range from very low to as high as 100%. A relatively high proportion of such markers derive from chromosome 15 and from the sex chromosomes. Specific syndromes are associated with bisatellited chromosome 15–derived markers and with markers derived

from the centric portion of the X chromosome (see Chapter 6).

An intriguing subclass of marker chromosomes lacks identifiable centromeric DNA sequences, despite being mitotically stable. These markers represent small fragments of chromosome arms (usually some distance from the normal centromere) that have somehow acquired centromere activity. Such markers are said to contain **neocentromeres.**

Many marker chromosomes lack identifiable telomeric sequences and are thus likely to be small ring chromosomes that are formed when a chromosome undergoes two breaks and the broken ends of the chromosome reunite in a ring structure (see Fig. 5-8C). **Ring chromosomes** are quite rare but have been detected for every human chromosome. When the centromere is within the ring, a ring chromosome is expected to be mitotically stable. However, some rings experience difficulties at mitosis, when the two sister chromatids of the ring chromosome become tangled in their attempt to disjoin at anaphase. There may be breakage of the ring followed by fusion, and larger and smaller rings may thus be generated. Because of this mitotic instability, it is not uncommon for ring chromosomes to be found in only a proportion of cells.

Isochromosomes An isochromosome (see Fig. 5-8D) is a chromosome in which one arm is missing and the other duplicated in a mirror-image fashion. A person with 46 chromosomes carrying an isochromosome, therefore, has a single copy of the genetic material of one arm (partial monosomy) and three copies of the genetic material of the other arm (partial trisomy). A person with two normal homologues in addition to the isochromosome is tetrasomic for the chromosome arm involved in the isochromosome. Although the basis for isochromosome formation is not precisely known, at least two mechanisms have been documented: (1) misdivision through the centromere in meiosis II and, more commonly, (2) exchange involving one arm of a chromosome and its homologue (or sister chromatid) in the region of the arm immediately adjacent to the centromere. (Formally, these latter isochromosomes are termed isodicentric chromosomes because they have two centromeres, although the two centromeres are usually not distinguishable cytogenetically because they are so close together.)

The most common isochromosome is an isochromosome of the long arm of the X chromosome, i(Xq), in some individuals with Turner syndrome (see Chapter 6). Isochromosomes for a number of autosomes have also been described, however, including isochromosomes for the short arm of chromosome 18, i(18p), and for the short arm of chromosome 12, i(12p). Isochromosomes are also frequently seen in karyotypes of both solid tumors and hematological malignant neoplasms (see Chapter 16).

Dicentric Chromosomes   A dicentric is a rare type of abnormal chromosome in which two chromosome segments (from different chromosomes or from the two chromatids of a single one), each with a centromere, fuse end to end, with loss of their acentric fragments. Dicentric chromosomes, despite their two centromeres, may be mitotically stable if one of the two centromeres is inactivated or if the two centromeres always coordinate their movement to one or the other pole during anaphase. Such chromosomes are formally called **pseudodicentric**. The most common pseudodicentrics involve the sex chromosomes or the acrocentric chromosomes (Robertsonian translocations; see later).

Balanced Rearrangements

Chromosomal rearrangements do not usually have a phenotypic effect if they are balanced because all the chromosomal material is present even though it is packaged differently. It is important to distinguish here between truly balanced rearrangements and those that appear balanced cytogenetically but are really unbalanced at the molecular level. Further, because of the high frequency of copy number polymorphisms around the genome (see Chapter 9), collectively adding up to differences of many million base pairs between genomes of unrelated individuals, the concept of what is balanced or unbalanced is somewhat arbitrary and subject to ongoing investigation and refinement.

Even when structural rearrangements are truly balanced, they can pose a threat to the subsequent generation because carriers are likely to produce a high frequency of unbalanced gametes and therefore have an increased risk of having abnormal offspring with unbalanced karyotypes; depending on the specific rearrangement, the risk can range from 1% to as high as 20%. There is also a possibility that one of the chromosome breaks will disrupt a gene, leading to mutation. This is a well-documented cause of X-linked diseases in female carriers of balanced X;autosome translocations (see Chapter 6), and such translocations can be a useful clue to the location of the gene responsible for a genetic disease.

Inversions   An inversion occurs when a single chromosome undergoes two breaks and is reconstituted with the segment between the breaks inverted. Inversions are of two types (Fig. 5-10): **paracentric** (not including the

A Paracentric

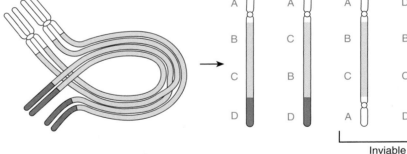

B Pericentric

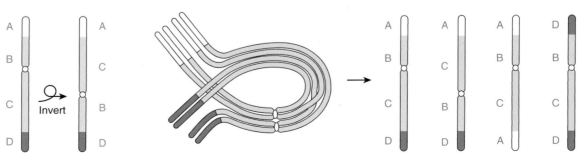

Figure 5-10 ■ Crossing over within inversion loops formed at meiosis I in carriers of a chromosome with segment B-C inverted (order A-C-B-D, instead of A-B-C-D). **A,** Paracentric inversion. Gametes formed after the second meiosis usually contain either a normal (A-B-C-D) or a balanced (A-C-B-D) copy of the chromosome because the acentric and dicentric products of the crossover are inviable. **B,** Pericentric inversion. Gametes formed after the second meiosis may be normal, balanced, or unbalanced. Unbalanced gametes contain a copy of the chromosome with a duplication or a deficiency of the material flanking the inverted segment (A-B-C-A or D-B-C-D).

centromere), in which both breaks occur in one arm; and **pericentric** (including the centromere), in which there is a break in each arm. Because paracentric inversions do not change the arm ratio of the chromosome, they can be identified only by banding or FISH with locus-specific probes, if at all. Pericentric inversions are easier to identify cytogenetically because they may change the proportion of the chromosome arms as well as the banding pattern.

An inversion does not usually cause an abnormal phenotype in carriers because it is a balanced rearrangement. Its medical significance is for the progeny; a carrier of either type of inversion is at risk of producing abnormal gametes that may lead to unbalanced offspring because, when an inversion is present, a loop is formed when the chromosomes pair in meiosis I (see Fig. 5-10). Although recombination is somewhat suppressed within inversion loops, when it occurs it can lead to the production of unbalanced gametes. Both gametes with balanced chromosome complements (either normal or possessing the inversion) and gametes with unbalanced complements are formed, depending on the location of recombination events. When the inversion is paracentric, the unbalanced recombinant chromosomes are typically acentric or dicentric and may not lead to viable offspring (see Fig. 5-10A), although there have been rare exceptions. Thus, the risk that a carrier of a paracentric inversion will have a liveborn child with an abnormal karyotype is very low indeed.

A pericentric inversion, on the other hand, can lead to the production of unbalanced gametes with both **duplication** and **deficiency** of chromosome segments (see Fig. 5-10B). The duplicated and deficient segments are the segments that are distal to the inversion. Overall, the apparent risk of a carrier of a pericentric inversion producing a child with an unbalanced karyotype is estimated to be 5% to 10%. Each pericentric inversion, however, is associated with a particular risk. Large pericentric inversions are more likely than are smaller ones to lead to viable recombinant offspring because the unbalanced segments in the recombinant progeny are smaller in the case of large inversions. Three well-described inversions illustrate this point.

A pericentric inversion of chromosome 3, originating in a couple from Newfoundland married in the early 1800s, is one of the few for which sufficient data have been obtained to allow an estimate of the segregation of the inversion chromosome in the offspring of carriers. The inv(3)(p25q21) has since been reported from a number of North American centers, in families whose ancestors have been traced to the maritime provinces of Canada. Carriers of the inv(3) chromosome are normal, but some of their offspring have a characteristic abnormal phenotype (Fig. 5-11) associated with a recombinant chromosome 3, in which there is duplication of the segment distal to 3q21 and deficiency of the

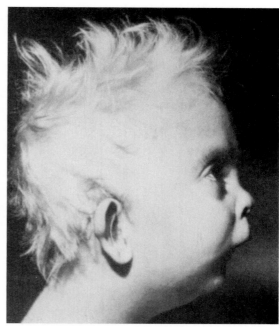

Figure 5-11 ■ A child with an abnormal karyotype, the offspring of a carrier of a pericentric inversion. See text for discussion. (From Allderdice PW, Browne N, Murphy DP: Chromosome 3 duplication q21-qter, deletion p25-pter syndrome in children of carriers of a pericentric inversion inv(3)(p25q21). Am J Hum Genet 27:699-718, 1975.)

segment distal to 3p25. Nine individuals who were carriers of the inversion have had 53 recorded pregnancies. The high empirical risk of an abnormal pregnancy outcome in this group (22/53, or >40%) indicates the importance of family chromosome studies to identify carriers and to offer genetic counseling and prenatal diagnosis.

Another pericentric inversion associated with a severe duplication or deficiency syndrome in recombinant offspring involves chromosome 8, inv(8) (p23.1q22.1), and is found primarily among Hispanics from the southwestern United States. Empirical studies have shown that carriers of the inv(8) have a 6% chance of having a child with the recombinant 8 syndrome, a lethal disorder with severe cardiac abnormalities and mental retardation. The recombinant chromosome is duplicated for sequences distal to 8q22.1 and deleted for sequences distal to 8p23.1.

The most common inversion seen in human chromosomes is a small pericentric inversion of chromosome 9, which is present in up to 1% of all individuals tested by cytogenetics laboratories. The inv(9)(p11q12) has no known deleterious effect on carriers and does not appear to be associated with a significant risk of miscarriage or unbalanced offspring; it is therefore generally considered a normal variant.

In addition to cytogenetically visible inversions, an increasing number of smaller inversions are being detected by genomic approaches. Many of these are

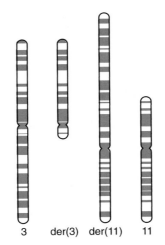

3   der(3)   der(11)   11

A

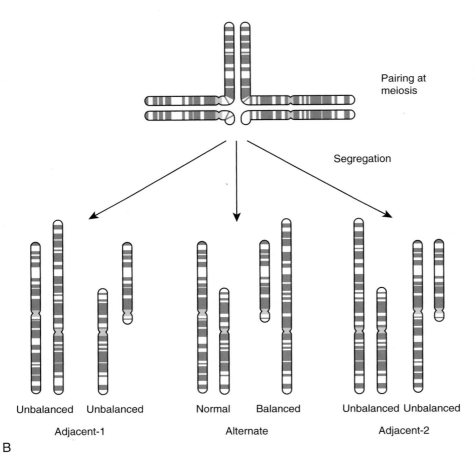

Pairing at
meiosis

Segregation

Unbalanced   Unbalanced   Normal   Balanced   Unbalanced Unbalanced

Adjacent-1   Alternate   Adjacent-2

B

Figure 5-12 ■ **A,** Diagram of a balanced translocation between chromosome 3 and chromosome 11, t(3;11)(q12;p15.5). **B,** Quadrivalent formation in meiosis and 2:2 segregation in a carrier of the t(3;11) translocation, leading to either balanced or unbalanced gametes. See text for discussion.

believed to be clinically benign, with no negative effect on reproduction.

Translocations   Translocation involves the exchange of chromosome segments between two, usually nonhomologous, chromosomes. There are two main types: reciprocal and Robertsonian.
Reciprocal Translocations   This type of rearrangement results from breakage of nonhomologous chromo-

somes, with reciprocal exchange of the broken-off segments. Usually only two chromosomes are involved, and because the exchange is reciprocal, the total chromosome number is unchanged (Fig. 5-12A). (Complex translocations involving three or more chromosomes have been described but are rare.) Reciprocal translocations are relatively common and are found in approximately 1 in 600 newborns. Such translocations are usually harmless, although they are more common in institutionalized mentally retarded individuals than in the general population. Like other balanced structural rearrangements, they are associated with a high risk of unbalanced gametes and abnormal progeny. They come to attention either during prenatal diagnosis or when the parents of an abnormal child with an unbalanced translocation are karyotyped. Balanced translocations are more commonly found in couples that have had two or more spontaneous abortions and in infertile males than in the general population.

When the chromosomes of a carrier of a balanced reciprocal translocation pair at meiosis, a **quadrivalent** (cross-shaped) figure is formed, as shown in Figure 5-12B. At anaphase, the chromosomes usually segregate from this configuration in one of three ways, described as **alternate, adjacent-1,** and **adjacent-2 segregation.** Alternate segregation, the usual type of meiotic segregation, produces gametes that have either a normal chromosome complement or the two reciprocal chromosomes; both types of gamete are balanced. In adjacent-1 segregation, homologous centromeres go to separate daughter cells (as is normally the case in meiosis I), whereas in adjacent-2 segregation (which is rare), homologous centromeres pass to the same daughter cell. Both adjacent-1 and adjacent-2 segregation yield unbalanced gametes (see Fig. 5-12B).

In addition to the examples mentioned of 2:2 segregation (i.e., two chromosomes going to each pole), balanced translocation chromosomes can also segregate 3:1, leading to gametes with 22 or 24 chromosomes. Although monosomy in a resulting fetus is rare, trisomy can result. Such 3:1 segregation is observed in 5% to 20% of sperm from balanced translocation carriers, depending on the specific translocation.

Robertsonian Translocations This type of rearrangement involves two acrocentric chromosomes that fuse near the centromere region with loss of the short arms (see Fig. 5-8E). The resulting balanced karyotype has only 45 chromosomes, including the translocation chromosome, which in effect is made up of the long arms of two chromosomes. Because the short arms of all five pairs of acrocentric chromosomes have multiple copies of genes for ribosomal RNA, loss of the short arms of two acrocentric chromosomes is not deleterious. Robertsonian translocations can be either monocentric or pseudodicentric, depending on the location of the breakpoint on each acrocentric chromosome.

Although Robertsonian translocations involving all combinations of the acrocentric chromosomes have been detected, two (13q14q and 14q21q) are relatively common. The translocation involving 13q and 14q is found in about 1 person in 1300 and is thus by far the single most common chromosome rearrangement in our species. Rare homozygotes for the 13q14q Robertsonian translocation have been described; these phenotypically normal individuals have only 44 chromosomes and lack any normal 13's or 14's, replaced by two copies of the translocation.

Although a carrier of a Robertsonian translocation is phenotypically normal, there is a risk of unbalanced gametes and therefore of unbalanced offspring. The risk of unbalanced offspring varies according to the particular Robertsonian translocation and the sex of the carrier parent; carrier females in general have a higher risk of transmitting the translocation to an affected child. The chief clinical importance of this type of translocation is that carriers of a Robertsonian translocation involving chromosome 21 are at risk of producing a child with translocation Down syndrome, as will be explored further in Chapter 6.

Insertions An insertion is a nonreciprocal type of translocation that occurs when a segment removed from one chromosome is inserted into a different chromosome, either in its usual orientation or inverted (see Fig. 5-8F). Because they require three chromosome breaks, insertions are relatively rare. Abnormal segregation in an insertion carrier can produce offspring with duplication or deletion of the inserted segment as well as normal offspring and balanced carriers. The average risk of producing an abnormal child is high, up to 50%, and prenatal diagnosis is indicated.

Mosaicism

When a person has a chromosome abnormality, the abnormality is usually present in all of his or her cells. Sometimes, however, two or more different chromosome complements are present in an individual; this situation is called **mosaicism.** Mosaicism may be either numerical or, less commonly, structural. Mosaicism is typically detected by conventional karyotyping but can also be suspected on the basis of interphase FISH analysis or array CGH.

A common cause of mosaicism is nondisjunction in an early postzygotic mitotic division. For example, a zygote with an additional chromosome 21 might lose the extra chromosome in a mitotic division and continue to develop as a 46/47,+21 mosaic. The significance of a finding of mosaicism is often difficult to assess, especially if it is identified prenatally. The effects of mosaicism on development vary with the timing of the nondisjunction event, the nature of the chromosome abnormality, the proportions of the different chromosome complements present, and the tissues affected. An additional problem is that the proportions of the different chromosome complements seen in the tissue being analyzed (e.g., cultured amniocytes or lymphocytes) may not necessarily reflect the proportions present in other tissues or in the embryo during its early developmental stages. In laboratory studies, cytogeneticists attempt to differentiate between true mosaicism, present in the individual, and **pseudomosaicism,** in

Table 5-3

Incidence of Chromosomal Abnormalities in Newborn Surveys

Type of Abnormality	Number	Approximate Incidence
SEX CHROMOSOME ANEUPLOIDY		
Males (43,612 newborns)		
47,XXY	45	1/1,000
47,XYY	45	1/1,000
Other X or Y aneuploidy	32	1/1,350
Total	122	1/360 male births
Females (24,547 newborns)		
45,X	6	1/4,000
47,XXX	27	1/900
Other X aneuploidy	9	1/2,700
Total	42	1/580 female births
AUTOSOMAL ANEUPLOIDY (68,159 NEWBORNS)		
Trisomy 21	82	1/830
Trisomy 18	9	1/7,500
Trisomy 13	3	1/22,700
Other aneuploidy	2	1/34,000
Total	96	1/700 live births
STRUCTURAL ABNORMALITIES (68,159 NEWBORNS)		
Balanced rearrangements		
Robertsonian	62	1/1,100
Other	77	1/885
Unbalanced rearrangements		
Robertsonian	5	1/13,600
Other	38	1/1,800
Total	182	1/375 live births
All Chromosome Abnormalities	442	1/154 live births

Data from Hsu LYF: Prenatal diagnosis of chromosomal abnormalities through amniocentesis. In Milunsky A (ed): Genetic Disorders and the Fetus, 4th ed. Baltimore, Johns Hopkins University Press, 1998, pp 179-248.

which the mosaicism probably arose in cells in culture after they were taken from the individual. The distinction between these types is not always easy or certain. In particular, mosaicism is relatively common in cytogenetic studies of chorionic villus cultures and can lead to major interpretive difficulties in prenatal diagnosis (see Chapter 15).

Clinical studies of the phenotypic effects of mosaicism have two main weaknesses. First, because people are hardly ever karyotyped without some clinical indications, clinically normal mosaic persons are rarely ascertained; second, there have been few follow-up studies of prenatally diagnosed mosaic fetuses. Nonetheless, it is often believed that individuals who are mosaic for a given trisomy, such as mosaic Down syndrome or mosaic Turner syndrome, are less severely affected than nonmosaic individuals.

Incidence of Chromosome Anomalies

The incidence of different types of chromosomal aberration has been measured in a number of large surveys (Tables 5-3 and 5-4). The major numerical disorders of chromosomes are three autosomal trisomies (trisomy 21, trisomy 18, and trisomy 13) and four types of sex chromosomal aneuploidy: Turner syndrome (usually 45,X), Klinefelter syndrome (47,XXY), 47,XYY, and 47,XXX (see Chapter 6). Triploidy and tetraploidy account for a small percentage of cases, particularly in spontaneous abortions. The classification and incidence of chromosomal defects measured in these surveys can be used to summarize the fate of 10,000 conceptuses, as presented in Table 5-5.

Live Births

The overall incidence of chromosome abnormalities in newborns has been found to be about 1 in 160 births (0.7%). The findings are summarized in Table 5-3, classified separately for specific numerical abnormalities of sex chromosomes and autosomes and for balanced and unbalanced structural rearrangements. Most of the autosomal abnormalities can be diagnosed at birth, but most sex chromosome abnormalities, with the exception of Turner syndrome, are not recognized clinically until puberty (see Chapter 6). Balanced rearrangements are rarely identified clinically unless a carrier of a rearrangement gives birth to a child with an unbalanced chromosome complement and family studies are initiated; unbalanced rearrangements are likely to come to clinical attention because of abnormal appearance and delayed physical and mental development in the chromosomally abnormal individual.

Spontaneous Abortions

The overall frequency of chromosome abnormalities in spontaneous abortions is at least 40% to 50%, and the

Table 5-4

Frequency of Chromosome Abnormalities in Spontaneous Abortions with Abnormal Karyotypes

Type	Approximate Proportion of Abnormal Karyotypes
Aneuploidy	
Autosomal trisomy	0.52
Autosomal monosomy	<0.01
45,X	0.19
Triploidy	0.16
Tetraploidy	0.06
Other	0.07

Based on analysis of 8841 unselected spontaneous abortions, as summarized by Hsu LYF: Prenatal diagnosis of chromosomal abnormalities through amniocentesis. In Milunsky A (ed): Genetic Disorders and the Fetus, 4th ed. Baltimore, Johns Hopkins University Press, 1998, pp 179-248.

Table 5-5

Outcome of 10,000 Pregnancies*

Outcome	Pregnancies	Spontaneous Abortions (%)	Live Births
Total	10,000	1500 (15)	8500
Normal chromosomes	9,200	750 (8)	8450
Abnormal chromosomes	800	750 (94)	50
Triploid or tetraploid	170	170 (100)	0
45,X	140	139 (99)	1
Trisomy 16	112	112 (100)	0
Trisomy 18	20	19 (95)	1
Trisomy 21	45	35 (78)	10
Trisomy, other	209	208 (99.5)	1
47,XXY, 47,XXX, 47,XYY	19	4 (21)	15
Unbalanced rearrangements	27	23 (85)	4
Balanced rearrangements	19	3 (16)	16
Other	39	37 (95)	2

*These estimates are based on observed frequencies of chromosome abnormalities in spontaneous abortuses and in liveborn infants. It is likely that the frequency of chromosome abnormalities in all conceptuses is much higher than this, as many spontaneously abort before they are recognized clinically.

kinds of abnormalities differ in a number of ways from those seen in liveborns (see Table 5-4). The single most common abnormality in abortuses is 45,X (Turner syndrome), which accounts for nearly 20% of chromosomally abnormal spontaneous abortuses but less than 1% of chromosomally abnormal live births. The other sex chromosome abnormalities, which are common in live births, are rare in abortuses. Another difference is the distribution of kinds of trisomy; for example, trisomy 16 accounts for about one third of trisomies in abortuses but is not seen at all in live births.

Because the overall spontaneous abortion rate (about 15%) is known, as is the overall incidence of specific chromosome defects in both abortuses and live births, one can estimate the proportion of all clinically recognized pregnancies of a given karyotype that is lost by spontaneous abortion (see Table 5-5).

● PARENT-OF-ORIGIN EFFECTS

Genomic Imprinting

For some disorders, the expression of the disease phenotype depends on whether the mutant allele or abnormal chromosome has been inherited from the father or from the mother. Differences in gene expression between the allele inherited from the mother and the allele inherited from the father are the result of **genomic imprinting**. Imprinting is a normal process caused by alterations in chromatin that occur in the germline of one parent, but not the other, at characteristic locations in the genome. These alterations include the covalent modification of DNA, such as methylation of cytosine to form **5-methylcytosine,** or the modification or substitution in chromatin of specific histone types (see **histone code,** in Chapter 2), which can influence gene expression within a chromosomal region. Notably, imprinting affects the expression of a gene but not its primary DNA sequence. It is a reversible form of gene inactivation but not a mutation, and thus it is an example of what is called an *epi*genetic effect. **Epigenetics** is an area of increasing importance in human and medical genetics, with significant influences on gene expression and phenotype, both in normal individuals and in a variety of disorders, including cytogenetic abnormalities (as discussed here and in Chapter 6), inherited single-gene conditions (see Chapter 7), and cancer (see Chapter 16).

Imprinting takes place during gametogenesis, before fertilization, and marks certain genes as having come from the mother or father. After conception, the imprint controls gene expression within the imprinted region in some or all of the somatic tissues of the embryo. The imprinted state persists postnatally into adulthood through hundreds of cell divisions so that only the maternal or paternal copy of the gene is expressed. Yet, imprinting must be reversible: a paternally derived allele, when it is inherited by a female, must be converted in her germline so that she can then pass it on with a maternal imprint to her offspring. Likewise, an imprinted maternally derived allele, when it is inherited by a male, must be converted in his germline so that he can pass it on as a paternally imprinted allele to his offspring (Fig. 5-13). Control over this conversion process appears to be governed by DNA elements called **imprinting centers** that are located within imprinted regions throughout the genome; whereas their precise mechanism of action is not known, they must initiate the epigenetic change in chromatin, which then spreads outward along the chromosome over the imprinted region.

The effect of genomic imprinting on inheritance patterns in pedigrees is discussed in Chapter 7. Here, we focus on the relevance of imprinting to clinical cytogenetics, as many imprinting effects come to light because of chromosome abnormalities. Evidence of

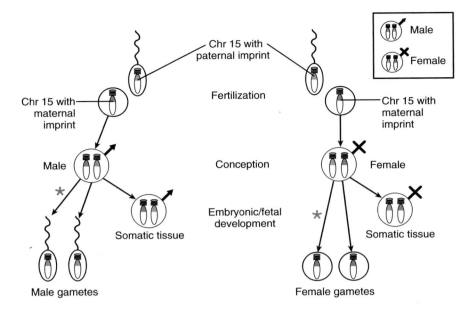

Figure 5-13 ■ Diagram of conversion of maternal and paternal imprinting during passage through the germline to make male or female gametes. Erasure of uniparental imprint on one chromosome and conversion to imprint of the other sex is marked by the asterisk.

genomic imprinting has been obtained for a number of chromosomes or chromosomal regions throughout the genome, as revealed by comparing phenotypes of individuals carrying the same cytogenetic abnormality affecting either the maternal or paternal homologue. Although estimates vary, it is likely that at least several dozen and perhaps as many as a hundred genes in the human genome show imprinting effects (Fig. 5-14). Some regions contain a single imprinted gene; others contain clusters, spanning in some cases well over 1 Mb along a chromosome, of multiple imprinted genes.

The hallmark of imprinted genes that distinguishes them from other autosomal loci is that only one allele, either maternal or paternal, is expressed in the relevant tissue. In contrast, nonimprinted loci (i.e., the overwhelming majority of loci in the genome) are expressed from both maternal and paternal alleles in each cell.

Prader-Willi and Angelman Syndromes

Perhaps the best-studied examples of the role of genomic imprinting in human disease are **Prader-Willi syndrome** (Case 33) and **Angelman syndrome.** Prader-Willi syndrome is a relatively common dysmorphic syndrome characterized by obesity, excessive and indiscriminate eating habits, small hands and feet, short stature, hypogonadism, and mental retardation (Fig. 5-15). In approximately 70% of cases of the syndrome, there is a cytogenetic deletion (Fig. 5-I; *see color insert*) involving the proximal long arm of chromosome 15 (15q11-q13), occurring only on the chromosome 15 inherited from the patient's father (Table 5-6). Thus, the genomes of these patients have genetic information in 15q11-q13 that derives only from their mothers. In contrast, in approximately 70% of patients with the rare Angelman syndrome, characterized by unusual

facial appearance, short stature, severe mental retardation, spasticity, and seizures (Fig. 5-16), there is a deletion of approximately the same chromosomal region but now on the chromosome 15 inherited from the mother. Patients with Angelman syndrome, therefore, have genetic information in 15q11-q13 derived only from their fathers. This unusual circumstance demonstrates strikingly that the parental origin of genetic material (in this case, on chromosome 15) can have a profound effect on the clinical expression of a defect.

Approximately 30% of patients with Prader-Willi syndrome do not have cytogenetically detectable deletions; instead, they have two cytogenetically normal chromosome 15's, both of which were inherited from the mother (see Table 5-6). This situation illustrates **uniparental disomy,** defined as the presence of a disomic cell line containing two chromosomes, or portions thereof, inherited from only one parent. If the identical chromosome is present in duplicate, the situation is described as **isodisomy;** if both homologues from one parent are present, the situation is **heterodisomy.** Approximately 3% to 5% of patients with Angelman syndrome also have uniparental disomy, in their case with two intact chromosome 15's of paternal origin (see Table 5-6). These patients add additional confirmation that Prader-Willi syndrome and Angelman syndrome result from loss of the paternal and maternal contribution of genes in 15q11-q13, respectively.

In addition to chromosomal deletion and uniparental disomy, a few patients with Prader-Willi syndrome and Angelman syndrome appear to have a defect in the imprinting center itself (see Table 5-6). As a result, the switch from female to male imprinting during spermatogenesis or from male to female imprinting during oogenesis (see Fig. 5-13) fails to occur. Fertilization by a sperm carrying an abnormally persistent female

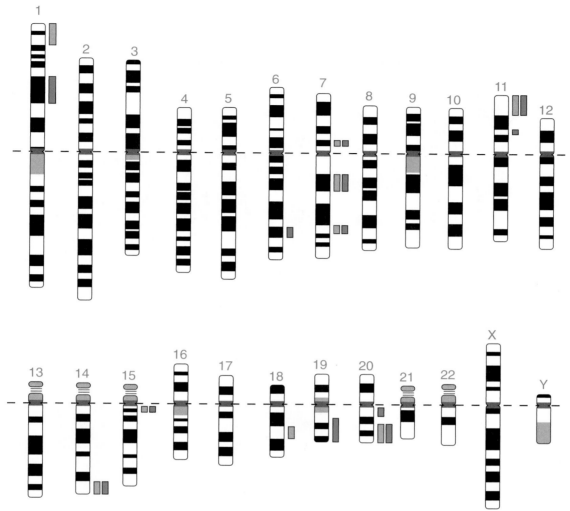

Figure 5-14 ■ Map of imprinted regions in the human genome. Chromosomal regions containing one or more genes expressed only from the maternally inherited copy are indicated in gray; regions containing one or more genes expressed only from the paternally inherited copy are indicated in blue. Some regions contain clusters of imprinted genes, some of which are maternally imprinted (i.e., expressed only from the paternal allele) and some of which are paternally imprinted (i.e., expressed only from the maternal allele). (Based on Morison IA, Ramsay JP, Spencer HG: A census of mammalian imprinting. Trends Genet 21:457-465, 2005.)

imprint would produce a child with Prader-Willi syndrome; fertilization of an egg that bears an inappropriately persistent male imprint would result in Angelman syndrome.

Finally, mutations in the maternal copy of a single gene, the E6-AP ubiquitin-protein ligase gene, have been found to cause Angelman syndrome (see Table 5-6). The E6-AP ubiquitin-protein ligase gene is located in 15q11-q13 and is normally imprinted (expressed only from the maternal allele) in the central nervous system. It is likely that the large maternal 15q11-q13 deletions and the uniparental disomy of paternal 15 seen in Angelman syndrome cause the disorder because they result in loss of the maternal copy of this critically important, imprinted gene. Mutations in a single imprinted gene have not yet been found in Prader-Willi syndrome.

Other Disorders due to Uniparental Disomy of Imprinted Regions

Uniparental disomy has been documented for most chromosomes in the karyotype, although clinical abnormalities have been demonstrated for only some of these, presumably reflecting the location of one or more imprinted genes. Uniparental disomy for a portion of chromosome 11 (11p15) is implicated in **Beckwith-Wiedemann syndrome** (Case 4). Affected children are very large at birth and have an enlarged tongue and frequent protrusion of the umbilicus. Severe hypoglycemia is a life-threatening complication, as are the development of malignant neoplasms of kidney, adrenal, and liver. The condition results from an excess of paternal or a loss of maternal contribution of genes, or both, on

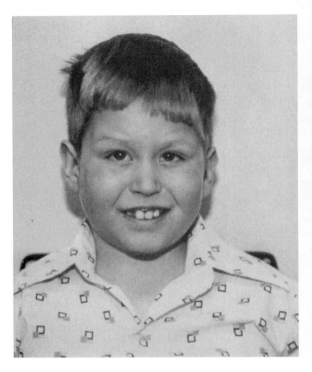

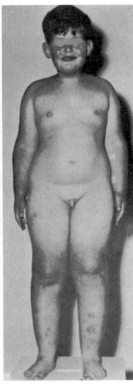

Figure 5-15 ■ Prader-Willi syndrome. *Left,* Typical facies in a 9-year-old affected boy. (From Pettigrew AL, Gollin SM, Greenberg F, et al: Duplication of proximal 15q as a cause of Prader-Willi syndrome. Am J Med Genet 28:791-802, 1987. Copyright © 1990, Wiley-Liss, Inc. Reprinted by permission of John Wiley and Sons, Inc.) *Right,* Obesity, hypogonadism, and small hands and feet in a 9.5-year-old affected boy who also has short stature and developmental delay. (From Jones KL: Smith's Recognizable Patterns of Human Malformation, 4th ed. Philadelphia, WB Saunders, 1988, p 173.)

Figure 5-16 ■ Angelman syndrome in a 4-year-old affected girl. Note wide stance and position of arms. Compare with phenotype of Prader-Willi syndrome in Figure 5-15. See text for discussion. (Photographs courtesy of Jan M. Friedman. From Magenis RE, Toth-Fejel S, Allen LJ, et al: Comparison of the 15q deletions in Prader-Willi and Angelman syndromes: specific regions, extent of deletions, parental origin, and clinical consequences. Am J Med Genet 35:333-349, 1990. Copyright © 1990, Wiley-Liss, Inc. Reprinted by permission of John Wiley and Sons, Inc.)

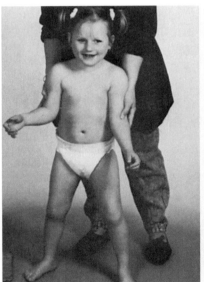

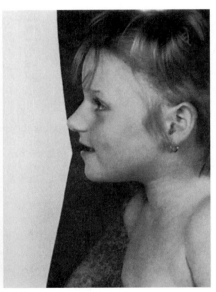

Table 5-6

Molecular Mechanisms Causing Prader-Willi and Angelman Syndromes

	Prader-Willi Syndrome	Angelman Syndrome
15q11-q13 deletion	~70% (paternal)	~70% (maternal)
Uniparental disomy	~30% (maternal)	~5% (paternal)
Single-gene mutation	None detected	E6-AP ubiquitin-protein ligase (10% of total but seen only in familial cases)
Imprinting center mutation	5%	5%
Unidentified	<1%	10%-15%

Data from Nicholls RD, Knepper JL: Genome organization, function and imprinting in Prader-Willi and Angelman syndromes. Annu Rev Genomics Hum Genet 2:153-175, 2001; and Horsthemke B, Buiting K: Imprinting defects on human chromosome 15. Cytogenet Genome Res 113:292-299, 2006.

chromosome 11p15, including the insulin-like growth factor 2 gene. In addition, a few rare patients with **cystic fibrosis** and short stature have been described with two identical copies of most or all of their maternal chromosome 7. In both cases, the mother happened to be a carrier for cystic fibrosis, and because the child received two maternal copies of the mutant cystic fibrosis gene and no paternal copy of a normal cystic fibrosis gene, the child developed the disease. The growth failure was unexplained but might be related to loss of unidentified paternally imprinted genes on chromosome 7.

Although it is unclear how common uniparental disomy is, it may provide an explanation for a disease when an imprinted region is present in two copies from one parent (see Fig. 5-14). Thus, physicians and genetic counselors must keep imprinting in mind as a possible cause of genetic disorders, especially in cases of autosomal recessive disorders in patients who have only one documented carrier parent or in cases of X-linked disorders transmitted from father to son or expressed in homozygous form in females.

Cytogenetics of Hydatidiform Moles and Ovarian Teratomas

On occasion, in an abnormal pregnancy, the placenta is converted into a mass of tissue resembling a bunch of grapes, called a hydatid cyst. This is due to abnormal growth of the chorionic villi, in which the epithelium proliferates and the stroma undergoes cystic cavitation. Such an abnormality is called a **mole**. A mole may be complete, with no fetus or normal placenta present, or partial, with remnants of placenta and perhaps a small atrophic fetus.

Most **complete moles** are diploid, with a 46,XX karyotype. The chromosomes are all paternal in origin, however, and with rare exceptions, all genetic loci are homozygous. Complete moles originate when a single 23,X sperm fertilizes an ovum that lacks a nucleus, and its chromosomes then double. The absence of any maternal contribution is thought to be responsible for the very abnormal development, with hyperplasia of the trophoblast and grossly disorganized or absent fetal tissue. About half of all cases of choriocarcinoma (a malignant neoplasm of fetal, not maternal, tissue) develop from hydatidiform moles. The reciprocal genetic condition is apparent in **ovarian teratomas**, benign tumors that arise from 46,XX cells containing only maternal chromosomes; no paternal contribution is evident. Thus, normal fetal development requires both maternal and paternal genetic contributions. It appears that the paternal genome is especially important for extraembryonic development, whereas the maternal genome is critical for fetal development.

In contrast to complete moles, **partial moles** are triploid; in about two thirds of cases, the extra chromosome set is of paternal origin. Comparing cases of maternal or paternal origin, fetal development is severely abnormal in both, but the defects are different. An extra paternal set results in abundant trophoblast but poor embryonic development, whereas an extra maternal set results in severe retardation of embryonic growth with a small, fibrotic placenta. The specificity of the effect is another example of genomic imprinting.

Confined Placental Mosaicism

One specific type of chromosomal mosaicism occurs when the karyotype of the placenta is mosaic for an abnormality, usually a trisomy, that is not apparent in the fetus. For example, the placenta may be 46,XX/47,XX,+15, whereas the fetus may be 46,XX. This situation, called **confined placental mosaicism,** may lead to a phenotypically abnormal fetus or liveborn, despite the apparently euploid karyotype. In one mechanism, both copies of the relevant chromosome (e.g., chromosome 15) in the fetus may originate from the same parent. The interpretation is that a trisomic state, not normally consistent with survival, may be "rescued" by loss of one of the copies of the chromosome involved in the trisomy. By chance, the chromosome lost may be the only copy that originated from one of the parents, leading to **uniparental disomy** in the remaining cells.

The possibility of confined placental mosaicism is a frequent diagnostic dilemma in prenatal cytogenetics laboratories (see Chapter 15).

● STUDIES OF CHROMOSOMES IN HUMAN MEIOSIS

Two general approaches have been used to study the chromosome constitution of sperm or ova in human males and females, respectively. In the first approach, one can analyze abnormal meioses retrospectively, using DNA polymorphisms (see Chapter 9) or cytogenetic heteromorphisms to study the parental origin of aneuploid fetuses or liveborns. Extensive analysis of more than 1000 conceptuses has indicated a significantly different contribution of either maternal or paternal nondisjunction to different cytogenetic abnormalities; for example, maternal nondisjunction accounts for more than 90% of cases of trisomy 21 and fully 100% of trisomy 16 but only about half of cases of Klinefelter syndrome (47,XXY) and only 20% to 30% of Turner syndrome (45,X).

A second approach involves direct analysis of chromosomes in human germ cells. By use of FISH with chromosome-specific probes, a large number of sperm can be scored quickly to evaluate aneuploidy levels for individual human chromosomes (Fig. 5-D; *see color insert*). A number of large studies have indicated chromosome-specific rates of disomy of about 1 in 1000 to 2000 sperm, with some variation between chromosomes. Nondisjunction of the sex chromosomes appears to be several-fold more frequent than nondisjunction of the autosomes.

A number of studies have suggested that the frequency of chromosomally abnormal sperm is elevated in males who exhibit infertility. This is an important area of investigation because of the increasing use of intracytoplasmic sperm injection (ICSI) in human in vitro fertilization (IVF) procedures; in many IVF centers, ICSI is the procedure of choice in male infertility cases. There are a number of indications that suggest a sharp increase in chromosomal abnormalities (particularly involving the sex chromosomes) as well as imprinting defects in ICSI pregnancies.

Sperm FISH can also be used to evaluate the proportion of normal, balanced, or unbalanced sperm in male carriers of reciprocal translocations or inversions. Results of such studies can be useful for genetic counseling, although comparison of the findings in sperm, fetuses, and liveborns must be made with caution. For example, half the sperm in carriers of reciprocal translocations have unbalanced karyotypes; this is in contrast to the observations in liveborn offspring of male translocation carriers, very few of whom have unbalanced chromosome sets.

Direct visualization of chromosomes during oogenesis is more difficult than during spermatogenesis. As a result of improvements in IVF technology, however, oocytes can be obtained at the time of ovulation, matured in vitro, and examined by FISH (Fig. 5-J; *see color insert*), SKY, or array CGH during meiosis. Such studies provide estimates of the frequency of nondisjunction in oogenesis as well as insights into mechanisms of maternal nondisjunction and the relationship between advancing maternal age, the frequency and placement of recombination events, and the increasing incidence of aneuploidy.

● MENDELIAN DISORDERS WITH CYTOGENETIC EFFECTS

There are several rare single-gene syndromes, in addition to the relatively common fragile X syndrome (see Chapter 7), in which there is a characteristic cytogenetic abnormality. Collectively, these autosomal recessive disorders are referred to as **chromosome instability syndromes.** In each disorder, a detailed chromosome study can be an important element of diagnosis. The nature of the chromosome defect and the underlying molecular defect in chromosome replication or repair is different in each of these disorders. For example, Bloom syndrome is caused by a defect in a DNA heli-

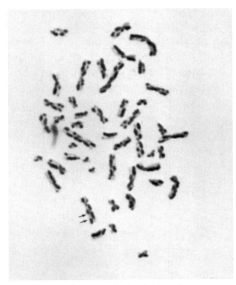

Figure 5-17 ■ Characteristic high frequency of sister chromatid exchanges in chromosomes from a patient with Bloom syndrome. Two exchanges are indicated by the arrows. (Photomicrograph courtesy of Chin Ho, Cytogenetics Laboratory, The Hospital for Sick Children, Toronto.)

case that leads to a striking increase in somatic recombination and **sister chromatid exchange** (Fig. 5-17). ICF syndrome (characterized by *i*mmunodeficiency, *c*entromeric instability, and *f*acial anomalies) is caused by a deficiency in one of the DNA methyltransferases that are required for establishing and maintaining normal patterns of DNA methylation (at 5-methylcytosine residues) in the genome. Chromosomes from patients with ICF syndrome show a characteristic abnormal association of pericentromeric heterochromatin involving chromosomes 1, 9, and 16.

Several chromosome instability syndromes are associated with an increased risk of malignant transformation. Further analysis of the correlation between decreased ability to replicate or repair DNA and increased risk of malignant neoplasms might be expected to provide insight into the relationship between mutagenesis and carcinogenesis (see Chapter 16).

● CYTOGENETIC ANALYSIS IN CANCER

An important area in cancer research is the delineation of cytogenetic changes in specific forms of cancer and the relation of the breakpoints of the various structural rearrangements to oncogenes. The cytogenetic changes seen in cancer cells are numerous and diverse. Many are repeatedly seen in the same type of tumor. Several hundred nonrandom chromosome changes involving all chromosomes except the Y chromosome have been identified in various neoplasias. The association of cytogenetic and genome analysis with tumor type and with the effectiveness of therapy is already an important part of the management of patients with cancer. The types of chromosome changes seen in cancer and the role of chromosome abnormalities in the etiology or progression, or both, of different malignant neoplasms are discussed further in Chapter 16. Their detection in clinical cytogenetics laboratories, by use of FISH, SKY (Fig. 5-C; *see color insert*), and array CGH, can have important diagnostic and prognostic value for oncologists.

● GENERAL REFERENCES

Epstein CJ: The Consequences of Chromosome Imbalance: Principles, Mechanisms, and Models. New York, Cambridge University Press, 1986.

Gardner RJM, Sutherland GR: Chromosome Abnormalities and Genetic Counseling, 3rd ed. Oxford, England, Oxford University Press, 2004.

Hsu LYF: Prenatal diagnosis of chromosomal abnormalities through amniocentesis. In Milunsky A (ed): Genetic Disorders and the Fetus, 4th ed. Baltimore, Johns Hopkins University Press, 1998, pp 179-248.

Miller OJ, Therman E: Human Chromosomes, 4th ed. New York, Springer-Verlag, 2001.

Shaffer LG, Tommerup N (eds): ISCN 2005: An International System for Human Cytogenetic Nomenclature. Basel, Karger, 2005.

Speicher MR, Carter NP: The new cytogenetics: blurring the boundaries with molecular biology. Nat Rev Genet 6:782-792, 2005.

Trask B: Human cytogenetics: 46 chromosomes, 46 years and counting. Nat Rev Genet 3:769-778, 2002.

● REFERENCES FOR SPECIFIC TOPICS

Allderdice PW, Browne N, Murphy DP: Chromosome 3 duplication q21-qter, deletion p25-pter syndrome in children of carriers of a pericentric inversion inv(3)(p25q21). Am J Hum Genet 27:699-718, 1975.

BAC Resource Consortium: Integration of cytogenetic landmarks into the draft sequence of the human genome. Nature 409:953-958, 2001.

Callinan PA, Feinberg AP: The emerging science of epigenomics. Hum Mol Genet 15:R95-R101, 2006.

de Vries BB, Pfundt R, Leisink M, et al: Diagnostic genome profiling in mental retardation. Am J Hum Genet 77:606-616, 2005.

Feuk L, Marshall CR, Wintle RF, Scherer SW: Structural variants: changing the landscape of chromosomes and design of disease studies. Hum Mol Genet 15:R57-R66, 2006.

Hassold T, Hunt P: To err (meiotically) is human: the genesis of human aneuploidy. Nat Rev Genet 2:280-291, 2001.

Jacobs PA, Browne C, Gregson N, et al: Estimates of the frequency of chromosome abnormalities detectable in unselected newborns using moderate levels of banding. J Med Genet 29:103-108, 1992.

Jiang YH, Bressler J, Beaudet AL: Epigenetics and human disease. Annu Rev Genomics Hum Genet 5:479-510, 2004.

Linardopoulou EV, Williams EM, Fan Y, et al: Human subtelomeres are hot spots of interchromosomal recombination and segmental duplication. Nature 437:94-100, 2005.

Morison IA, Ramsay JP, Spencer HG: A census of mammalian imprinting. Trends Genet 21:457-465, 2005.

Pellestor F, Andreo B, Anahory T, Hamamah S: The occurrence of aneuploidy in human: lessons from the cytogenetic studies of human oocytes. Eur J Med Genet 49:103-116, 2006.

Redon R, Ishikawa S, Fitch KR, et al: Global variation in copy number in the human genome. Nature 444:444–454, 2006.

Reid T: Cytogenetics—in color and digitized. N Engl J Med 350:1597-1600, 2004.

Sharp AJ, Locke DP, McGrath SD, et al: Segmental duplications and copy-number variation in the human genome. Am J Hum Genet 77:78-88, 2005.

Shianna KV, Willard HF: Human genomics: in search of normality. Nature 444:428-429, 2006.

Slater HR, Bailey DK, Ren H, et al: High-resolution identification of chromosome abnormalities using oligonucleotide arrays containing 116,204 SNPs. Am J Hum Genet 77:709-726, 2005.

Warburton D: De novo balanced chromosome rearrangements and extra marker chromosomes identified at prenatal diagnosis: clinical significance and distribution of breakpoints. Am J Hum Genet 49:995-1013, 1991.

Warburton PE: Chromosomal dynamics of human neocentromere formation. Chromosome Res 12:617-626, 2004.

● USEFUL WEBSITES

Chromosome Abnormality Database (CAD). *www.ukcad.org.uk/ cocoon/ukcad* A collection of constitutional and acquired abnormal karyotypes reported by UK Regional Cytogenetics Centers.

Database of Chromosomal Imbalance and Phenotype in Humans using Ensembl Resources (DECIPHER). *www.sanger.ac.uk/ PostGenomics/decipher/* A database of submicroscopic chromosomal variants with links to phenotypes.

Developmental Genome Anatomy Project (DGAP). *www. bwhpathology.org/dgap/* A database of balanced chromosome rearrangements critical to development.

Imprinted Gene Catalogue. *www.otago.ac.nz/IGC* A catalogue of imprinted genes and parent-of-origin effects in humans and animals.

Mitelman Database of Chromosome Aberrations in Cancer. *cgap. nci.nih.gov/chromosomes/mitelman* A database relating chromosomal aberrations to tumor characteristics.

PROBLEMS

1. You send a blood sample from a dysmorphic infant to the chromosome laboratory for analysis. The laboratory's report states that the child's karyotype is 46,XY,del(18)(q12).
   a. What does this karyotype mean?
   b. The laboratory asks for blood samples from the clinically normal parents for analysis. Why?
   c. The laboratory reports the mother's karyotype as 46,XX and the father's karyotype as 46,XY,t(7;18)(q35;q12). What does the latter karyotype mean? Referring to the normal chromosome ideograms in Figure 5-1, sketch the translocation chromosome or chromosomes in the father and in his son. Sketch these chromosomes in meiosis in the father. What kinds of gametes can he produce?
   d. In light of this new information, what does the child's karyotype mean now? What regions are monosomic? trisomic? Given information from Chapters 2 and 3, estimate the number of genes present in the trisomic or monosomic regions.

2. A spontaneously aborted fetus is found to have trisomy 18.
   a. What proportion of fetuses with trisomy 18 are lost by spontaneous abortion?
   b. What is the risk that the parents will have a liveborn child with trisomy 18 in a future pregnancy?

3. A newborn child with Down syndrome, when karyotyped, is found to have two cell lines: 70% of her cells have the typical 47,XX,+21 karyotype, and 30% are normal 46,XX. When did the nondisjunctional event probably occur? What is the prognosis for this child?

4. Which of the following persons is or is expected to be phenotypically normal?
   a. a female with 47 chromosomes, including a small supernumerary chromosome derived from the centromeric region of chromosome 15

   b. a female with the karyotype 47,XX,+13
   c. a male with deletion of a band on chromosome 4
   d. a person with a balanced reciprocal translocation
   e. a person with a pericentric inversion of chromosome 6

   What kinds of gametes can each of these individuals produce? What kinds of offspring might result, assuming that the other parent is chromosomally normal?

5. For each of the following, state whether chromosome analysis is indicated or not. For which family members, if any? For what kind of chromosome abnormality might the family in each case be at risk?
   a. a pregnant 29-year-old woman and her 41-year-old husband, with no history of genetic defects
   b. a pregnant 41-year-old woman and her 29-year-old husband, with no history of genetic defects
   c. a couple whose only child has Down syndrome
   d. a couple whose only child has cystic fibrosis
   e. a couple who have two severely retarded boys

6. Explain the nature of the chromosome abnormality and the method of detection indicated by the following nomenclature.
   a. inv(X)(q21q26)
   b. 46,XX,del(1)(1qter → p36.2:)
   c. 46,XX.ish del(15)(q11.2q11.2)(SNRPN–,D15S10–)
   d. 46,XX,del(15)(q11q13).ish del(15)(q11.2q11.2) (SNRPN–,D15S10–)
   e. 46,XX.arr cgh 1p36.3(RP11-319A11,RP11-58A11, RP11-92O17) × 1
   f. 46,XY.ish dup(X)(q28q28)(MECP2++)
   g. 47,XY,+mar.ish r(8)(D8Z1+)
   h. 46,XX,rob(13;21)(q10;q10),+21
   i. 45,XY,rob(13;21)(q10;q10)

7. Using the nomenclature system in Table 5-2, describe the "molecular karyotypes" that correspond to the array CGH data in Figures 5-5 and 5-9.

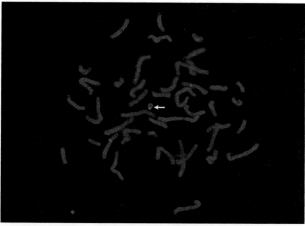

Figure 5-A ■ Identification of a ring chromosome derived from chromosome 8 by fluorescence in situ hybridization with use of a centromeric α-satellite probe specific for chromosome 8 (D8Z1). Two normal 8's and the r(8) *(arrow)* are evident by the red hybridization signals. (Courtesy of Barbara Goodman, Duke University Medical Center.)

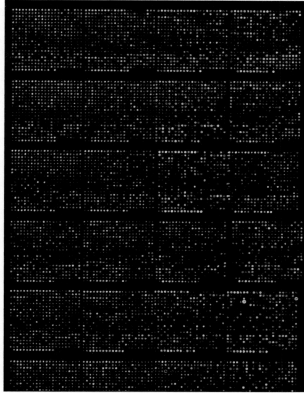

Figure 4-A ■ A microarray of oligonucleotides corresponding to cDNA sequences. The basic principle is similar to comparative genome hybridization (see Fig. 4-12), except the red- and green-labeled probes are made by reverse transcription of RNA from test and control, respectively. Spots in red are individual mRNA sequences that are enriched in test versus control; spots in green are those mRNA sequences enriched in control versus test. The majority of spots are yellow and represent mRNAs present in equal amounts in the two different RNA samples.

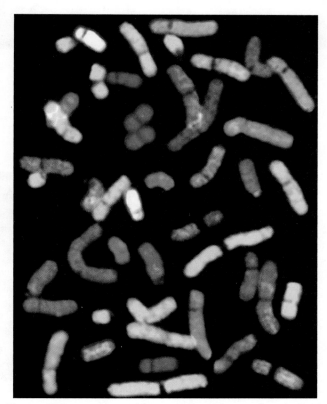

Figure 5-B ■ Spectral karyotyping. Twenty-four individual chromosome painting probes are labeled with different fluorescent dyes and used as a total genome chromosome paint. The fluorescent signals are analyzed by sophisticated imaging software and stored in a computer. To generate the photograph, the computer assigns a different color to each of the 24 different fluorescence spectra generated by the individual chromosome painting probes. In this metaphase from a 46,XX female, only 23 colors are present; the unique color generated by the Y chromosome painting probe is not seen. (Courtesy of Amalia Dutra, National Human Genome Research Institute.)

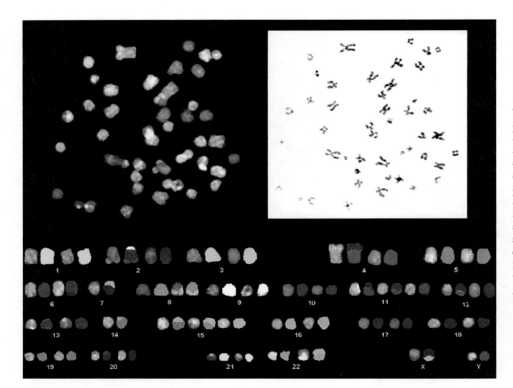

Figure 5-C ■ Spectral karyotyping analysis of chromosomes from a medulloblastoma cell line. Numerous structural and numerical abnormalities are evident and can be identified by image analysis of the 24 different chromosome paint probes used. Karyotype shows both original image *(left member of each pair)* and false-colored image *(right member of each pair)* in which each of the 24 chromosome types is assigned a different color to aid visual scoring. (Courtesy of Amalia Dutra, National Human Genome Research Institute.)

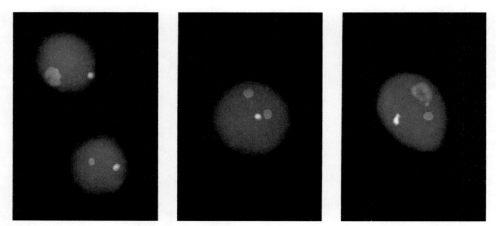

Figure 5-D ■ Three-color fluorescence in situ hybridization analysis of human sperm with repetitive probes for chromosome 18 *(yellow-white)*, the Y chromosome *(green)*, and the X chromosome *(red)*. The two haploid sperm on the left are monosomic for these chromosomes (one 23,X and one 23,Y sperm). The abnormal sperm in the middle panel is disomic for the X chromosome (24,XX karyotype), whereas the abnormal sperm on the right is disomic for the sex chromosomes (24, XY karyotype). (Courtesy of Terry Hassold, Washington State University.)

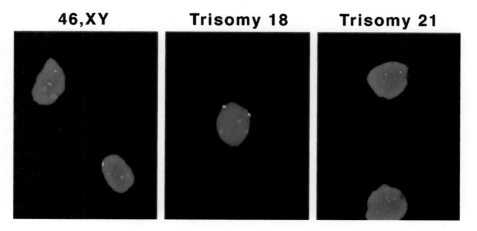

46,XY   **Trisomy 18**   **Trisomy 21**

Figure 5-E ■ Multicolor fluorescence in situ hybridization analysis of interphase amniotic fluid cells. *Left panel*, 46,XY cells (chromosome 18, *aqua*; X chromosome, *green*; Y chromosome, *red*). *Middle panel*, 47,XX, +18 cell (chromosome 18, *aqua*; X chromosome, *green*). *Right panel*, trisomy 21 cells (chromosome 13, *green*; chromosome 21, *red*). (Courtesy of Stuart Schwartz, University of Chicago.)

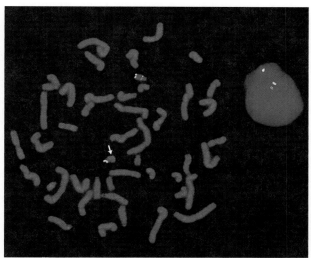

Figure 5-F ■ Two-color fluorescence in situ hybridization analysis of proband with DiGeorge syndrome (see Chapter 6), demonstrating deletion of 22q11.2 on one homologue. Green signal is hybridization to a control probe in distal chromosome 22q. Red signal on proximal 22q is a single-copy probe for a region that is present on one chromosome 22 but deleted from the other *(arrow)*. (Courtesy of Hutton Kearney, Duke University Medical Center.)

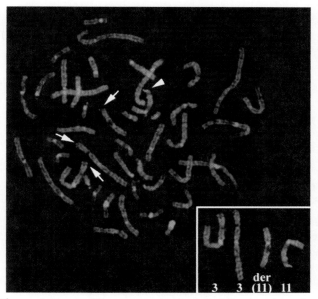

Figure 5-G ■ Fluorescence in situ hybridization detection of a cryptic translocation in a developmentally delayed proband by use of specific probes for the telomere of chromosome 3p *(red)* and chromosome 11q *(green)*. An unbalanced translocation between 3p and 11q was not evident by standard G-band analysis but was revealed by FISH. The arrows show three chromosome 3p hybridization signals, indicative of partial trisomy for 3p, whereas the arrowhead shows only a single hybridization signal for 11q, indicating partial monosomy for 11q. (Courtesy of Christa Lese Martin and David Ledbetter, Emory University.)

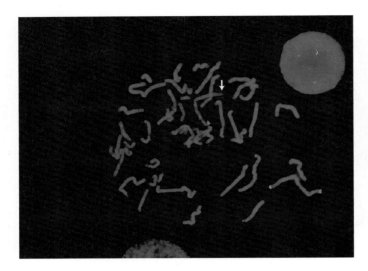

Figure 5-H ■ Fluorescence in situ hybridization detection of a terminal deletion of chromosome 1p by use of subtelomeric probes for 1p *(green)* and 1q *(red)*. Arrow indicates the 1p deletion. (Courtesy of Leah Stansberry and Hutton Kearney, Duke University Medical Center.)

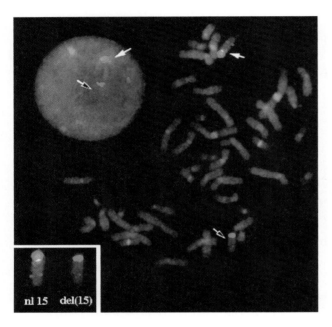

Figure 5-I ■ Two-color fluorescence in situ hybridization analysis of proband with Prader-Willi syndrome, demonstrating deletion of 15q11-q13 on one homologue. Green signal is hybridization to α-satellite DNA at the centromere of chromosome 15. Red signal on distal 15q is a control single-copy probe. Red signal on proximal 15q is a probe for the *SNRPN* gene, which is present on one chromosome 15 *(white arrow)* but deleted from the other *(dark arrow)*. (Courtesy of Christa Lese Martin and David Ledbetter, Emory University.)

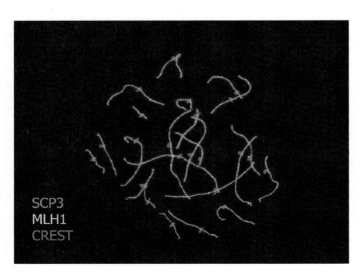

Figure 5-J ■ Combined immunohistochemical analysis of human oocyte chromosome bivalents. Each of the 23 bivalents is detected by an antibody to the synaptonemal complex (SCP3, *in red*). The location of the centromere in each bivalent is shown in blue with an antibody to centromere proteins (CREST). The position of recombination events (0 to 7 per bivalent in this cell) is indicated by presence of recombination protein *(yellow)*. (Courtesy of Rhea Vallente, Washington State University.)

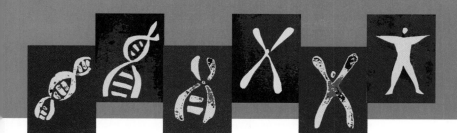

Chapter **6**

Clinical Cytogenetics: Disorders of the Autosomes and the Sex Chromosomes

In Chapter 5, we introduced general principles of clinical cytogenetics and the different types of abnormalities detected in clinical practice. In this chapter, we present more detailed accounts of several specific chromosomal disorders and their causes and consequences. We first discuss the most common autosomal abnormalities, including Down syndrome, followed by consideration of the X and Y chromosomes, their unique biology, and their abnormalities. Because sex determination is chromosomally based, we include in this chapter disorders of gonadal development and sexual differentiation. Even though many such disorders are determined by single genes, a clinical approach to evaluation of ambiguous genitalia usually includes a detailed cytogenetic analysis.

● AUTOSOMAL DISORDERS

In this section, the major autosomal disorders of clinical significance are described. Although there are numerous rare chromosome disorders in which gain or loss of an entire chromosome or a chromosome segment has been reported, many of these either have been seen only in fetuses that were aborted spontaneously or involve relatively short chromosome segments. There are only three well-defined non-mosaic chromosome disorders compatible with postnatal survival in which there is trisomy for an entire autosome: **trisomy 21** (Down syndrome), **trisomy 18**, and **trisomy 13**.

Each of these autosomal trisomies is associated with growth retardation, mental retardation, and multiple congenital anomalies. Nevertheless, each has a fairly distinctive phenotype. The developmental abnormalities characteristic of any one trisomic state are

determined by the extra dosage of the particular genes on the additional chromosome. Knowledge of the specific relationship between the extra chromosome and the consequent developmental abnormality has been limited to date. Current research, however, is beginning to show that specific genes on the extra chromosome are responsible, through direct and indirect modulation of developmental pathways, for specific aspects of the abnormal phenotype. More generally, any chromosomal imbalance, whether it involves addition or loss of genes, is expected to have a specific phenotypic effect determined by the dosage of the specific genes on the extra or missing chromosome segment.

Down Syndrome

Down syndrome, or trisomy 21, is by far the most common and best known of the chromosome disorders and is the single most common genetic cause of moderate mental retardation. About 1 child in 800 is born with Down syndrome (see Table 5-3), and among liveborn children or fetuses of mothers 35 years of age or older, the incidence rate is far higher (Fig. 6-1).

The syndrome was first described clinically by Langdon Down in 1866, but its cause remained a deep mystery for almost a century. Two noteworthy features of its population distribution drew attention: increased maternal age and a peculiar distribution within families—concordance in monozygotic twins but almost complete discordance in dizygotic twins and other family members. Although it was recognized as early as the 1930s that a chromosome abnormality might explain these observations, at that time no one was prepared to believe that humans are really likely to

89

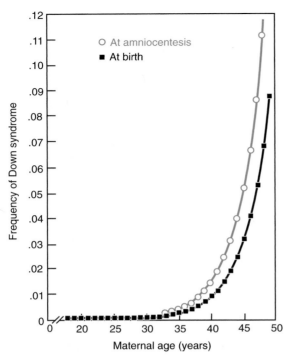

Figure 6-1 ■ Maternal age dependence on incidence of trisomy 21 at birth and at time of amniocentesis. See also Chapter 15. (Data from Hook EB, Cross PK, Schreinemachers DM: Chromosomal abnormality rates at amniocentesis and in live-born infants. JAMA 249:2034-2038, 1983.)

have chromosome abnormalities. However, when techniques for detailed analysis of human chromosomes became available, Down syndrome was one of the first conditions to be examined chromosomally. In 1959, it was established that most children with Down syndrome have 47 chromosomes, the extra member being a small acrocentric chromosome that has since been designated chromosome 21 (see Fig. 5-6).

Phenotype

Down syndrome can usually be diagnosed at birth or shortly thereafter by its dysmorphic features, which vary among patients but nevertheless produce a distinctive phenotype (Fig. 6-2). Hypotonia may be the first abnormality noticed in the newborn. In addition to characteristic dysmorphic facial features evident to even the untrained observer, the patients are short in stature and have brachycephaly with a flat occiput. The neck is short, with loose skin on the nape. The nasal bridge is flat; the ears are low-set and have a characteristic folded appearance; the eyes have Brushfield spots around the margin of the iris; and the mouth is open, often showing a furrowed, protruding tongue. Characteristic epicanthal folds and upslanting palpebral fissures gave rise to the term *mongolism*, once used to refer to this condition but now considered inappropriate. The hands are short and broad, often with a single

transverse palmar crease ("simian crease") and incurved fifth digits, or clinodactyly. The dermatoglyphics (patterns of the ridged skin) are highly characteristic. The feet show a wide gap between the first and second toes, with a furrow extending proximally on the plantar surface.

The major cause for concern in Down syndrome is mental retardation. Even though in early infancy the child may not seem delayed in development, the delay is usually obvious by the end of the first year. The intelligence quotient (IQ) is usually 30 to 60 when the child is old enough to be tested. Nevertheless, many children with Down syndrome develop into happy, responsive, and even self-reliant persons in spite of these limitations (see Fig. 6-2).

Congenital heart disease is present in at least one third of all liveborn Down syndrome infants and in a somewhat higher proportion of abortuses with the syndrome. Certain malformations, such as duodenal atresia and tracheoesophageal fistula, are much more common in Down syndrome than in other disorders. There is a high degree of variability in the phenotype of Down syndrome individuals; specific abnormalities are detected in almost all patients, but others are seen only in a subset of cases.

Each of these birth defects must reflect to some degree the direct or indirect effects of overexpression of one or more genes on chromosome 21 on patterning events during early development (see Chapter 14). Large-scale gene expression studies have shown that a significant proportion of genes encoded on chromosome 21 are expressed at higher levels in Down syndrome brain and heart samples than in corresponding samples from euploid individuals. As the complete catalogue of chromosome 21 genes is known, current efforts are directed toward determining which genes are responsible for particular phenotypes.

Prenatal and Postnatal Survival

Because trisomy 21 accounts for about half of all abnormalities identified prenatally, the incidence of Down syndrome seen in live births, in amniocentesis, and in chorionic villus sampling at different maternal ages can provide a basis for estimating the amount of fetal loss between the 11th and 16th weeks and between the 16th week and birth (see Table 15-1). At all maternal ages, there is some loss between the 11th and 16th weeks (as would be expected from the high rate of chromosome abnormality seen in spontaneous abortions) and an additional loss later in pregnancy. In fact, probably only 20% to 25% of trisomy 21 conceptuses survive to birth (see Table 5-5).

Among Down syndrome conceptuses, those least likely to survive are those with congenital heart disease; about one fourth of the liveborn infants with heart

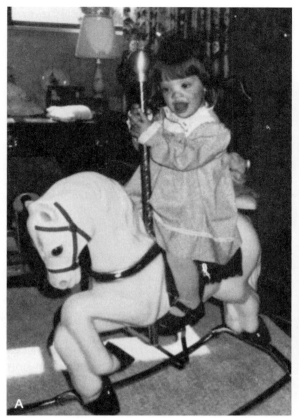 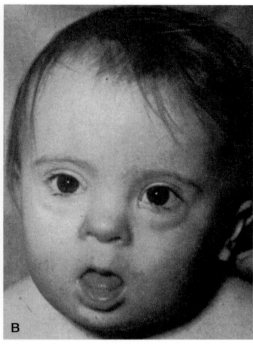

Figure 6-2 ■ Two children with Down syndrome. (**A** courtesy of David Patterson, Eleanor Roosevelt Institute, Denver. **B** from Jones KL: Smith's Recognizable Patterns of Human Malformation, 4th ed. Philadelphia, WB Saunders, 1988.)

defects die before their first birthday. There is a 15-fold increase in the risk of leukemia among Down syndrome patients who survive the neonatal period. Premature dementia, associated with the neuropathological findings characteristic of Alzheimer disease (cortical atrophy, ventricular dilatation, and neurofibrillar tangles), affects nearly all Down syndrome patients, several decades earlier than the typical age at onset of Alzheimer disease in the general population.

The Chromosomes in Down Syndrome

The clinical diagnosis of Down syndrome usually presents no particular difficulty. Nevertheless, karyotyping is necessary for confirmation and to provide a basis for genetic counseling. Although the specific abnormal karyotype responsible for Down syndrome usually has little effect on the phenotype of the patient, it is essential for determining the recurrence risk.

Trisomy 21   In about 95% of all patients, Down syndrome involves trisomy for chromosome 21 (see Fig. 5-6), resulting from meiotic nondisjunction of the chromosome 21 pair, as discussed in the preceding chapter. As noted earlier, the risk of having a child with trisomy 21 increases with maternal age, especially after the age

of 30 years (see Fig. 6-1). The meiotic error responsible for the trisomy usually occurs during maternal meiosis (about 90% of cases), predominantly in meiosis I, but about 10% of cases occur in paternal meiosis, usually in meiosis II.

Robertsonian Translocation   About 4% of Down syndrome patients have 46 chromosomes, one of which is a Robertsonian translocation between chromosome 21q and the long arm of one of the other acrocentric chromosomes (usually chromosome 14 or 22). The translocation chromosome replaces one of the normal acrocentric chromosomes, and the karyotype of a Down syndrome patient with a Robertsonian translocation between chromosomes 14 and 21 is therefore 46,XX or XY,rob(14;21)(q10;q10),+21 (see Table 5-2 for nomenclature). Such a chromosome can also be designated der(14;21), and both nomenclatures are used in practice. In effect, patients with a Robertsonian translocation involving chromosome 21 are trisomic for genes on 21q.

Unlike standard trisomy 21, translocation Down syndrome shows no relation to maternal age but has a relatively high recurrence risk in families when a parent, especially the mother, is a carrier of the translocation. For this reason, karyotyping of the parents and possibly

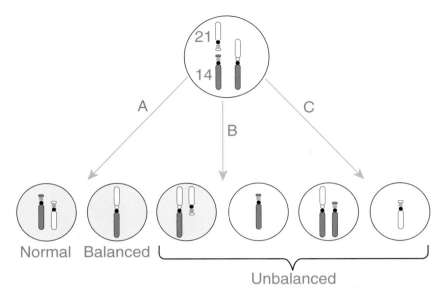

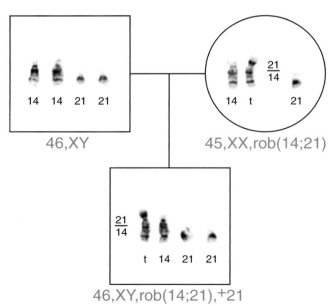

Figure 6-3 ■ Chromosomes of gametes that theoretically can be produced by a carrier of a Robertsonian translocation, rob(14;21). **A,** Normal and balanced complements. **B,** Unbalanced, one product with both the translocation chromosome and the normal chromosome 21, and the reciprocal product with chromosome 14 only. **C,** Unbalanced, one product with both the translocation chromosome and chromosome 14, and the reciprocal product with chromosome 21 only. Only the three shaded gametes at the left can lead to viable offspring; see text for a description of the eventual fate of these gametes.

other relatives is essential before accurate genetic counseling can be provided.

A carrier of a Robertsonian translocation involving chromosomes 14 and 21 has only 45 chromosomes; one chromosome 14 and one chromosome 21 are missing and are replaced by the translocation chromosome. The gametes that can be formed by such a carrier are shown in Figure 6-3. Theoretically, there are six possible types of gamete, but three of these appear unable to lead to viable offspring. Of the three viable types, one is normal, one is balanced, and one is unbalanced, having both the translocation chromosome and the normal chromosome 21. In combination with a normal gamete, this could produce a child with translocation Down syndrome (Fig. 6-4). Theoretically, the three types of gametes are produced in equal numbers, and thus the theoretical risk of a Down syndrome child should be 1 in 3. However, extensive population studies have shown that unbalanced chromosome complements appear in only about 10% to 15% of the progeny of carrier mothers and in only a few percent of the progeny of carrier fathers who have translocations involving chromosome 21.

21q21q Translocation   A 21q21q translocation chromosome is a chromosome composed of two chromosome 21 long arms; it is seen in a few percent of Down syndrome patients. It is thought to originate as an isochromosome rather than by Robertsonian translocation. Many such cases appear to arise postzygotically, and accordingly, the recurrence risk is low. Nonetheless, it is particularly important to evaluate if a parent is a carrier (or a mosaic) because all gametes of a carrier of such a chromosome must either contain the 21q21q chromosome, with its double dose of chromosome 21 genetic material, or lack it and have no chromosome 21 representative at all. The potential progeny, therefore, inevitably have either Down syndrome or monosomy 21, which is rarely viable. Mosaic carriers are at an increased risk of recurrence, and thus prenatal diagnosis should be considered in any subsequent pregnancy.

Mosaic Down Syndrome   About 2% of Down syndrome patients are mosaic, usually for cell populations with either a normal or a trisomy 21 karyotype. The phenotype may be milder than that of typical trisomy 21, but there is wide variability in phenotypes among

Figure 6-4 ■ Robertsonian translocation 14q21q transmitted by a carrier mother to her child, who has Down syndrome. The father's chromosomes are normal. Only chromosomes 14, 21, and rob(14;21) are shown. t, translocation. (Original karyotype courtesy of R. G. Worton, The Hospital for Sick Children, Toronto.)

mosaic patients, possibly reflecting the variable proportion of trisomy 21 cells in the embryo during early development. Those patients ascertained with mosaic Down syndrome probably represent the more clinically severe cases because mildly affected persons are less likely to be karyotyped.

Partial Trisomy 21   Very rarely, Down syndrome is diagnosed in a patient in whom only a part of the long arm of chromosome 21 is present in triplicate, and a Down syndrome patient with no cytogenetically visible chromosome abnormality is even more rarely identified. These patients are of particular interest because they can show what region of chromosome 21 is likely to be responsible for specific components of the Down syndrome phenotype and what regions can be triplicated *without* causing that aspect of the phenotype.

Although chromosome 21 contains only a few hundred genes (see Fig. 2-8B), attempts to correlate triple dosage of specific genes with specific aspects of the Down syndrome phenotype have had limited success so far. The most notable success has been identification of a region that is critical for the heart defects seen in about 40% of Down syndrome patients. Sorting out the specific genes crucial to the expression of the Down syndrome phenotype from those that merely happen to be syntenic with them on chromosome 21 is a focus of current investigation, especially with the mouse as a surrogate model. Mice engineered to contain extra dosage of genes from human chromosome 21 (or even a nearly complete copy of human chromosome 21) can show phenotypic abnormalities in behavior, brain function, and cardiac development, and this is a potentially promising avenue of research.

Etiology of Trisomy 21

Although the chromosomal basis of Down syndrome is clear, the cause of the chromosome abnormality is still poorly understood. The high percentage of all cases of trisomy 21 in which the abnormal gamete originated during maternal meiosis I suggests that something about maternal meiosis I is the underlying cause. Because of the increased risk of Down syndrome to older mothers (see next section), one obvious possibility is the "older egg" model; it has been suggested that the older the oocyte, the greater the chance that the chromosomes will fail to disjoin correctly. As mentioned in Chapter 5, analyses of trisomy 21 (as well as of other autosomal trisomies) have implicated the number or placement of recombination events as a determinant of whether the chromosome pair will disjoin properly during the two meiotic divisions. Older eggs may be less able to overcome a susceptibility to nondisjunction established by the recombination machinery. A remarkable feature of this model (and one that greatly complicates its investigation) is that the etiological event leading to the birth

of a Down syndrome infant today may have taken place 35 to 40 years ago, when the child's mother was herself a fetus whose primary oocytes were in prophase of the first meiotic division. Despite recognition of the important association between recombination patterns and chromosome segregation, a full understanding of chromosome 21 nondisjunction and the maternal age effect continues to be elusive.

Risk of Down Syndrome

A frequent problem in genetic counseling, especially in prenatal genetics, is how to assess the risk of the birth of a Down syndrome child. Down syndrome can be detected prenatally by cytogenetic or array comparative genome hybridization (CGH) analysis of chorionic villus or amniotic fluid cells. In fact about 80% of prenatal diagnoses are performed because increased maternal age or prenatal biochemical screening (see Chapter 15) gives rise to concern about the risk of Down syndrome in the fetus. A commonly accepted guideline is that a woman is eligible for prenatal diagnosis if the risk that her fetus has Down syndrome outweighs the risk that the procedure of amniocentesis or chorionic villus sampling used to obtain fetal tissue for chromosome analysis will lead to fetal loss (see Chapter 15). The risk depends chiefly on the mother's age but also on both parents' karyotypes.

The population incidence of Down syndrome in live births is currently estimated to be about 1 in 800, reflecting the maternal age distribution for all births and the proportion of older mothers who make use of prenatal diagnosis and selective termination. At about the age of 30 years, the risk begins to rise sharply, reaching 1 in 25 births in the oldest maternal age group (see Fig. 6-1). Even though younger mothers have a much lower risk, their birth rate is much higher, and therefore more than half of the mothers of all Down syndrome babies are younger than 35 years. The risk of Down syndrome due to translocation or partial trisomy is unrelated to maternal age. The paternal age appears to have no influence on the risk.

In the United States and Canada, 50% or more of pregnant women 35 years old and older undergo prenatal diagnosis for fetal chromosome analysis, but only about 1% of the fetuses tested are found to have trisomy 21. Current approaches to more precise or efficient identification of fetuses at risk, by means of biochemical screening assays and ultrasonography, are discussed in Chapter 15. Methods to examine rare fetal cells found in the maternal circulation are also being developed.

Recurrence Risk

The recurrence risk of trisomy 21 or some other autosomal trisomy, after one such child has been born in a family, is about 1% overall. The risk is about 1.4% for mothers younger than 30 years, and it is the same as the age-related risk for older mothers; that is, there is a significant increase in risk for the younger mothers but not for the older mothers, whose risk is already elevated. The reason for the increased risk for the younger mothers is not known. One possibility is that unrecognized germline mosaicism in one parent, with a trisomic cell line as well as a normal cell line, may be a factor. A history of trisomy 21 elsewhere in the family, although often a cause of maternal anxiety, does not appear to significantly increase the risk of having a Down syndrome child.

The recurrence risk for Down syndrome due to a translocation is much higher, as described previously.

Trisomy 18

The phenotype of an infant with trisomy 18 is shown in Figure 6-5. The features of trisomy 18 always include mental retardation and failure to thrive and often include severe malformation of the heart. Hypertonia is a typical finding. The head has a prominent occiput, and the jaw recedes. The ears are low-set and malformed. The sternum is short. The fists clench in a characteristic way, the second and fifth digits overlapping the third and fourth (see Fig. 6-5). The feet have a "rocker-bottom" appearance, with prominent calcanei. The dermal patterns are distinctive, with single creases on the palms and arch patterns on most or all digits. The nails are usually hypoplastic.

The incidence of this condition in liveborn infants is about 1 in 7500 births (see Table 5-3). The incidence

at conception is much higher, but about 95% of trisomy 18 conceptuses are aborted spontaneously. Postnatal survival is also poor, and survival for more than a few months is rare. At least 60% of the patients are female, perhaps because of their preferential survival. As in most other trisomies, increased maternal age is a factor, and the risk of a trisomy 18 infant is substantially greater for women older than 35 years.

The trisomy 18 phenotype, like that of trisomy 21, can result from a variety of rare karyotypes other than complete trisomy, and karyotyping of affected infants or fetuses is essential for genetic counseling. In about 20% of cases, there is a translocation involving all or most of chromosome 18, which may be either de novo or inherited from a balanced carrier parent. The trisomy may also be present in mosaic form, with variable but usually somewhat milder expression.

Trisomy 13

The striking phenotype of trisomy 13 is shown in Figure 6-6. Growth retardation and severe mental retardation are present, accompanied by severe central nervous system malformations such as arhinencephaly and holoprosencephaly. The forehead is sloping; there is microcephaly and wide open sutures; and there may be microphthalmia, iris coloboma, or even absence of the eyes. The ears are malformed. Cleft lip and cleft palate are often present. The hands and feet may show postaxial polydactyly, and the hands clench with the second and fifth digits overlapping the third and fourth, as in trisomy 18. The feet, again as in trisomy 18, have a rocker-bottom appearance. The palms often have

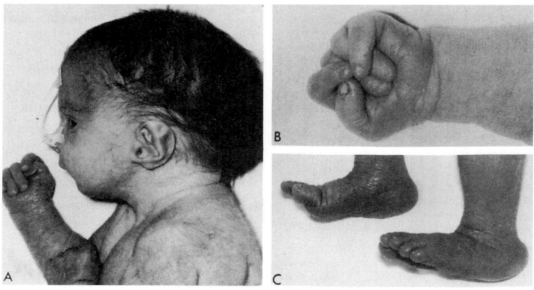

Figure 6-5 ■ An infant with trisomy 18. Note the clenched fist with the second and fifth digits overlapping the third and fourth; rocker-bottom feet with prominent calcanei; and large, malformed, and low-set ears. (Courtesy of H. Medovy, Children's Centre, Winnipeg, Canada.)

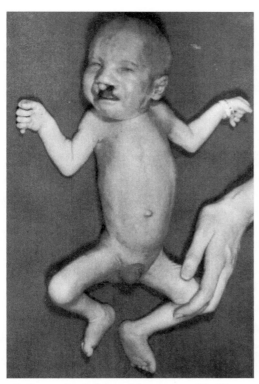

Figure 6-6 ■ An infant with trisomy 13. Note particularly the bilateral cleft lip and polydactyly. (Courtesy of P. E. Conen, The Hospital for Sick Children, Toronto.)

simian creases. Internally, there are usually congenital heart defects (in particular, ventricular septal defect and patent ductus arteriosus) and urogenital defects, including cryptorchidism in males, bicornuate uterus and hypoplastic ovaries in females, and polycystic kidneys. Of this constellation of defects, the most distinctive are the general facial appearance with cleft lip and palate and ocular abnormalities, polydactyly, the clenched fists, and rocker-bottom feet.

The incidence of trisomy 13 is about 1 in 15,000 to 25,000 births. Trisomy 13 is clinically severe, and about half of such individuals die within the first month. Like most other trisomies, it is associated with increased maternal age, and the extra chromosome usually arises from nondisjunction in maternal meiosis I. Karyotyping of affected infants or fetuses is indicated to confirm the clinical diagnosis; about 20% of the cases are caused by an unbalanced translocation. The recurrence risk is low; even when one parent of a translocation patient is a carrier of the translocation, the empirical risk that a subsequent liveborn child will have the syndrome is less than 2%.

Autosomal Deletion Syndromes

There are many reports of cytogenetically detectable deletions in dysmorphic patients, but most of these deletions have been seen in only a few patients and are not associated with recognized syndromes. However, there are a number of well-delineated autosomal deletion syndromes in which a series of patients have the same or similar deletion, resulting in a clearly recognizable syndrome. Overall, cytogenetically visible autosomal deletions occur with an estimated incidence of 1 in 7000 live births.

Cri du Chat Syndrome

One such syndrome is the cri du chat syndrome, in which there is either a terminal or interstitial deletion of part of the short arm of chromosome 5. This deletion syndrome was given its common name because crying infants with this disorder sound like a mewing cat. The syndrome accounts for about 1% of all institutionalized mentally retarded patients. The facial appearance, shown in Figure 6-7A, is distinctive, with microcephaly, hypertelorism, epicanthal folds, low-set ears sometimes with preauricular tags, and micrognathia. Other features include moderate to severe mental retardation and heart defects.

Most cases of cri du chat syndrome are sporadic; 10% to 15% of the patients are the offspring of translocation carriers. The breakpoints and extent of the deleted segment of chromosome 5p vary in different patients, but the critical region, missing in all patients with the phenotype, has been identified as band 5p15. By use of fluorescence in situ hybridization (FISH) and array CGH (see Chapters 4 and 5), a number of genes have been demonstrated to be deleted from del(5p) chromosomes, and the basis for the relationship between monosomy for such genes and the clinical phenotype is beginning to be elucidated. Many of the clinical findings appear to be due to haploinsufficiency for a gene or genes within band 5p15.2, and the distinctive cat cry appears to result from deletion of a gene or genes within a small region in band 5p15.3. The degree of mental retardation usually correlates with the size of the deletion, although array CGH analysis suggests that haploinsufficiency for particular regions within 5p14-p15 may contribute disproportionately to severe mental retardation. The phenotypic map shown in Figure 6-7B illustrates the increasing precision and refinement that genomic approaches can bring to the general concept of karyotype-phenotype correlations in clinical cytogenetics. This is an important goal of research in many recurring chromosome abnormalities, both for understanding pathophysiological changes and for genetic counseling.

Genomic Disorders: Microdeletion and Duplication Syndromes

Several dysmorphic syndromes are associated with small but sometimes cytogenetically visible deletions that lead

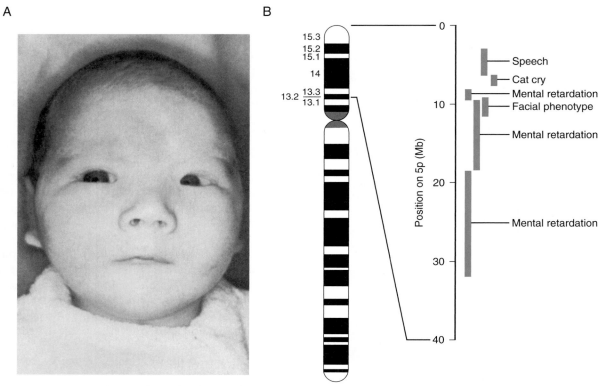

Figure 6-7 ■ A, An infant with cri du chat syndrome, which results from deletion of part of chromosome 5p. Note characteristic facies with hypertelorism, epicanthus, and retrognathia. B, Phenotype-karyotype map, based on array CGH analysis of del(5p) chromosomes. (Based on data from Zhang X, Snijders A, Segraves R, et al: High-resolution mapping of genotype-phenotype relationships in cri du chat syndrome using array comparative genome hybridization. Am J Hum Genet 76:312-326, 2005.)

to a form of genetic imbalance referred to as **segmental aneusomy** (Table 6-1). These deletions produce syndromes that are usually clinically recognizable and that can be detected by high-resolution chromosome analysis, by FISH (Figs. 5-F and 5-I; *see color insert*), or by array CGH. The term **contiguous gene syndrome** has

been applied to many of these conditions, as the phenotype is attributable to haploinsufficiency for multiple, contiguous genes within the deleted region. For other such disorders, the phenotype is apparently due to deletion of only a single gene, despite the typical association of a chromosomal deletion with the condition.

Table 6-1

Examples of Genomic Disorders Involving Recombination Between Low-Copy Repeat Sequences

Disorder	Location	REARRANGEMENT		
		Type	Size (kb)	Repeat Length (kb)
Smith-Magenis syndrome	17p11.2	Deletion ⎤	4000	175-250
dup(17)(p11.2p11.2)		Duplication ⎦		
Charcot-Marie-Tooth (*CMT1A*)/HNLPP	17p12	Duplication ⎤	1400	24
		Deletion ⎦		
DiGeorge syndrome/velocardiofacial syndrome	22q11.2	Deletion ⎤	3000, 1500	225-400
Cat-eye syndrome/22q11.2 duplication syndrome		Duplication ⎦		
Prader-Willi/Angelman syndromes	15q11-q13	Deletion	3500	400
Williams syndrome	7q11.23	Deletion	1600	300-400
Neurofibromatosis	17q11.2	Deletion	1400	85
Sotos syndrome	5q35	Deletion	2000	400
Azoospermia (AZFc)	Yq11.2	Deletion	3500	230

HNLPP, hereditary neuropathy with liability to pressure palsies.
Based on Lupski JR, Stankiewicz P: Genomic Disorders: The Genomic Basis of Disease. Totowa, NJ, Humana Press, 2006.

For each syndrome, the extent of the deletions in different patients is similar. Indeed, for the syndromes listed in Table 6-1, molecular and FISH studies have demonstrated that the centromeric and telomeric breakpoints cluster among different patients, suggesting the existence of deletion-prone sequences. Fine mapping in a number of these disorders has shown that the breakpoints localize to low-copy repeated sequences and that aberrant recombination between nearby copies of the repeats causes the deletions, which span several hundred to several thousand kilobase pairs. This general sequence-dependent mechanism has been implicated in several syndromes involving contiguous gene rearrangements, which have therefore been termed **genomic disorders** (see Table 6-1).

Several deletions and duplications mediated by unequal recombination have been documented within the proximal short arm of chromosome 17 and illustrate the general concept of genomic disorders (Fig. 6-8). For example, a cytogenetically visible segment of 17p11.2 of approximately 4 Mb is deleted de novo in about 70% to 80% of patients with **Smith-Magenis syndrome** (SMS), a usually sporadic condition characterized by multiple congenital anomalies and mental retardation. Unequal recombination between large blocks of flanking repeated sequences that are nearly 99% identical in sequence results in the SMS deletion, del(17)(p11.2p11.2), as well as the reciprocal duplication, dup(17)(p11.2p11.2), which is seen in patients with a milder, neurobehavioral phenotype. Slightly

more distally on the chromosome, duplication or deletion of a 1400-kb region in chromosome 17p11.2-p12, mediated by recombination between a different set of nearly identical repeated sequences, leads to another pair of inherited genomic disorders. Duplication of the region between the repeats leads to a form of **Charcot-Marie-Tooth disease (Case 6)**; deletion leads to a different condition, hereditary neuropathy with liability to pressure palsies (HNLPP) (see Table 6-1). These two distinct peripheral neuropathies result from different dosages of the gene for peripheral myelin protein that is encoded within the deleted or duplicated segment.

A particularly common microdeletion that is frequently evaluated in clinical cytogenetics laboratories involves chromosome 22q11.2 and is associated with diagnoses of **DiGeorge syndrome, velocardiofacial syndrome,** or **conotruncal anomaly face syndrome.** All three clinical syndromes are autosomal dominant conditions with variable expressivity, caused by a deletion within 22q11.2, spanning about 3 Mb. This microdeletion, also mediated by homologous recombination between low-copy repeated sequences, is one of the most common cytogenetic deletions associated with an important clinical phenotype and is detected in 1 in 2000 to 4000 live births (Fig. 6-9). Patients show characteristic craniofacial anomalies, mental retardation, and heart defects. The deletion in the 22q11.2 deletion syndromes is thought to play a role in as many as 5% of all congenital heart defects and is a particularly frequent cause of certain defects. For example, more than

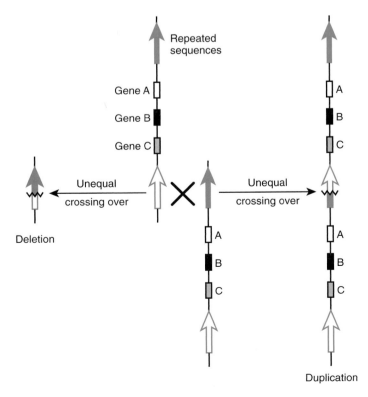

Figure 6-8 ■ Model of rearrangements underlying genomic disorders. Unequal crossing over between misaligned sister chromatids or homologous chromosomes containing highly homologous copies of a long repeated DNA sequence can lead to deletion or duplication products, which differ in the number of copies of the sequence. The copy number of any gene or genes (such as A, B, and C) that lie between the copies of the repeat will change as a result of these genome rearrangements. For examples of genomic disorders, the size of the repeated sequences, and the size of the deleted or duplicated region, see Table 6-1.

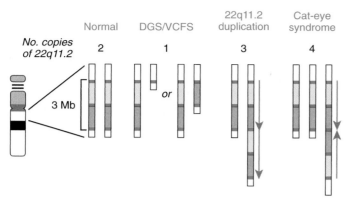

No. copies
of 22q11.2

Normal   DGS/VCFS   22q11.2
duplication   Cat-eye
syndrome

2   1   3   4

3 Mb

or

Figure 6-9 ■ Chromosomal deletions, duplications, and rearrangements in 22q11.2 mediated by homologous recombination. Normal karyotypes show two copies of 22q11.2, each containing three copies of an approximately 200-kb repeated segment (dark blue) within a 3-Mb genomic region, which is composed of two duplicated segments (light blue and grey). In DiGeorge syndrome (DGS) or velocardiofacial syndrome (VCFS), the full 3-Mb region (or, less frequently, the proximal 1.5 Mb within it) is deleted from one homologue. The reciprocal duplication is seen in patients with dup(22)(q11.2q11.2). Tetrasomy for 22q11.2 is seen in patients with cat-eye syndrome. Note that the duplicated region in the cat-eye syndrome chromosome is in an inverted orientation relative to the duplication seen in dup(22) patients.

40% of patients with tetralogy of Fallot and pulmonary atresia and more than 60% of patients with tetralogy of Fallot and absent pulmonary valve have this microdeletion. The typical deletion removes approximately 30 genes, although a related, smaller deletion is seen in approximately 10% of cases. Haploinsufficiency for at least one of these genes, *TBX1*, which encodes a transcription factor involved in development of the pharyngeal system, has been implicated in the phenotype; it is contained within the deleted region and is mutated in patients with a similar phenotype but without the chromosomal deletion.

In contrast to the relatively common deletion of 22q11.2, the reciprocal duplication of 22q11.2 is much rarer and leads to a series of dysmorphic malformations and birth defects called the 22q11.2 duplication syndrome. Diagnosis of this duplication generally requires analysis by FISH on interphase cells or array CGH. Some patients have a quadruple complement of this segment of chromosome 22 and are said to have **cat-eye syndrome,** which is characterized clinically by ocular coloboma, congenital heart defects, craniofacial anomalies, and moderate mental retardation. The karyotype in cat-eye syndrome is 47,XX or XY,+inv dup(22)(pter→q11.2).

The constellation of different disorders associated with varying dosage of genes in this segment of chromosome 22 (see Fig. 6-9) reflects two major principles in clinical cytogenetics. First, with few exceptions, altered gene dosage for any extensive chromosomal or genomic region is likely to result in a clinical abnormality, the phenotype of which will, in principle, depend on haploinsufficiency for or overexpression of one or more genes encoded within the region. Second, even patients carrying what appears to be the same chromosomal deletion or duplication can present with a range of variable phenotypes. Although the precise basis for this variability is unknown, it could be due to nongenetic causes or to differences in the genome sequence among unrelated individuals.

● THE SEX CHROMOSOMES AND THEIR ABNORMALITIES

The X and Y chromosomes have long attracted interest because they differ between the sexes, because they have their own specific patterns of inheritance, and because they are involved in primary sex determination. They are structurally distinct and subject to different forms of genetic regulation, yet they pair in male meiosis. For all these reasons, they require special attention. In this section, we review the common sex chromosome abnormalities and their clinical consequences, the current state of knowledge concerning the control of sex determination, and mendelian abnormalities of sexual differentiation.

The Chromosomal Basis of Sex Determination

The different sex chromosome constitution of normal human male and female cells has been appreciated for more than 50 years. Soon after cytogenetic analysis became feasible, the fundamental basis of the XX/XY system of sex determination became apparent. Males with Klinefelter syndrome were found to have 47 chromosomes with two X chromosomes as well as a Y chromosome (karyotype 47,XXY), whereas most Turner syndrome females were found to have only 45 chromosomes with a single X chromosome (karyotype 45,X). These findings promptly and unambiguously established the crucial role of the Y chromosome in normal male development. Furthermore, compared with the dramatic consequences of autosomal aneuploidy, these karyotypes underscored the relatively modest effect of varying the number of X chromosomes in either males or females. The basis for both observations is now understood in terms of the unique biology of the Y and X chromosomes.

Whereas the sex chromosomes play a determining role in specifying primary (gonadal) sex, a number of genes located on both the sex chromosomes and the autosomes are involved in sex determination and subsequent sexual differentiation. In most instances, the role of these genes has come to light as a result of patients with abnormalities in sexual development, whether cytogenetic, mendelian, or sporadic, and many of these are discussed in a section later in this chapter.

The Y Chromosome

The structure of the Y chromosome and its role in sexual development have been determined at both the molecular and genomic levels (Fig. 6-10). In male meiosis, the X and Y chromosomes normally pair by segments at the ends of their short arms (see Chapter 2) and undergo recombination in that region. The pairing segment includes the **pseudoautosomal region** of the X and Y chromosomes, so called because the X- and Y-linked copies of this region are essentially identical to one another and undergo homologous recombination in meiosis I, like pairs of autosomes (see Chapter 7). (A second, smaller pseudoautosomal segment is located at the distal ends of Xq and Yq.) By comparison with autosomes and the X chromosome, the Y chromosome is relatively gene poor and contains only about 50 genes (see Fig. 2-8). Notably, however, the functions of a high proportion of these genes are related to gonadal and genital development.

Embryology of the Reproductive System

The effect of the Y chromosome on the embryological development of the male and female reproductive systems is summarized in Figure 6-11. By the sixth week of development in both sexes, the primordial germ cells have migrated from their earlier extraembry-

onic location to the gonadal ridges, where they are surrounded by the sex cords to form a pair of primitive gonads. Up to this time, the developing gonad, whether chromosomally XX or XY, is bipotential and is often referred to as indifferent.

The current concept is that development into an ovary or a testis is determined by the coordinated action of a sequence of genes that leads normally to ovarian development when no Y chromosome is present or to testicular development when a Y is present. The ovarian pathway is followed unless a Y-linked gene, designated testis-determining factor (*TDF*), acts as a switch, diverting development into the male pathway.

In the presence of a Y chromosome (with the *TDF* gene), the medullary tissue forms typical testes with seminiferous tubules and Leydig cells that, under the stimulation of chorionic gonadotropin from the placenta, become capable of androgen secretion (see Fig. 6-11). The spermatogonia, derived from the primordial germ cells by successive mitoses, line the walls of the seminiferous tubules, where they reside together with supporting Sertoli cells.

If no Y chromosome is present, the gonad begins to differentiate to form an ovary, beginning as early as the eighth week of gestation and continuing for several weeks; the cortex develops, the medulla regresses, and oogonia begin to develop within follicles (see Fig. 6-11). Beginning at about the third month, the oogonia enter meiosis I, but (as described in Chapter 2) this process is arrested at dictyotene until ovulation occurs many years later.

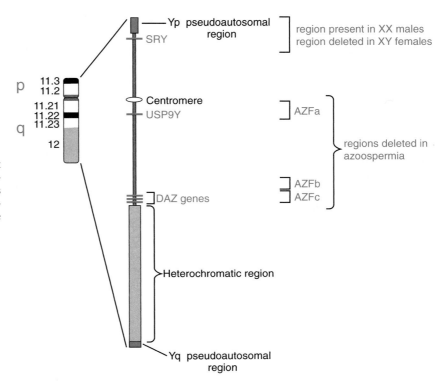

Figure 6-10 ■ The Y chromosome in sex determination and in disorders of sexual differentiation. Individual genes and regions implicated in sex determination, sex reversal, and defects of spermatogenesis are indicated.

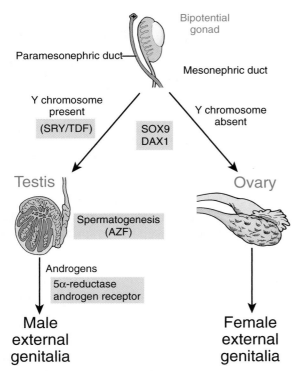

Figure 6-11 ■ Scheme of developmental events in sex determination and differentiation of the male and female gonads. Involvement of individual genes in key developmental steps or in genetic disorders is indicated in blue boxes. See text for discussion.

While the primordial germ cells are migrating to the genital ridges, thickenings in the ridges indicate the developing genital ducts, the **mesonephric** (formerly called wolffian) and **paramesonephric** (formerly called müllerian) ducts. In the male, the Leydig cells of the fetal testes produce androgen, which stimulates the mesonephric ducts to form the male genital ducts. The Sertoli cells produce a hormone (müllerian inhibitory substance) that suppresses formation of the paramesonephric ducts. In the female (or in an embryo with no gonads), the mesonephric ducts regress, and the paramesonephric ducts develop into the female duct system. Duct formation is usually completed by the third month of gestation.

In the early embryo, the external genitalia consist of a genital tubercle, paired labioscrotal swellings, and paired urethral folds. From this undifferentiated state, male external genitalia develop under the influence of androgens. In the absence of a testis, female external genitalia are formed regardless of whether an ovary is present.

The Testis-Determining Gene, SRY

The earliest cytogenetic studies established the testis-determining function of the Y chromosome. In the ensuing three decades, different deletions of the pseu-

doautosomal region and of the sex-specific region of the Y chromosome in sex-reversed individuals were used to map the precise location of the primary testis-determining region on Yp (Case 36).

Whereas the X and Y chromosomes normally exchange in meiosis I within the Xp/Yp pseudoautosomal region, in rare instances, genetic recombination occurs outside of the pseudoautosomal region (Fig. 6-12), leading to two rare but highly informative abnormalities: **XX males** and **XY females**. Each of these sex-reversal disorders occurs with an incidence of approximately 1 in 20,000 births. XX males are phenotypic males with a 46,XX karyotype who usually possess some Y chromosomal sequences translocated to the short arm of the X. Similarly, a proportion of phenotypic females with a 46,XY karyotype have lost the testis-determining region of the Y chromosome.

The *SRY* gene (*sex-determining region on the Y*) lies near the pseudoautosomal boundary on the Y chromosome, is present in many 46,XX males, and is deleted or mutated in a proportion of female 46,XY patients, thus strongly implicating *SRY* in male sex determination. *SRY* is expressed only briefly early in development in cells of the germinal ridge just before differentiation of the testis. *SRY* encodes a DNA-binding protein that is likely to be a transcription factor, although the specific genes that it regulates are unknown. Thus, by all available genetic and developmental criteria, *SRY* is equivalent to the *TDF* gene on the Y chromosome.

However, the presence or absence of *SRY* does not explain all cases of abnormal sex determination. *SRY* is not present in about 10% of unambiguous XX males and in most cases of XX true hermaphrodites (see later) or XX males with ambiguous genitalia. Further, mutations in the *SRY* gene account for only about 15% of 46,XY females. Thus, other genes are implicated in the sex-determination pathway and are discussed in later sections in this chapter.

Y-Linked Genes in Spermatogenesis

Interstitial deletions in Yq have been associated with at least 10% of cases of nonobstructive azoospermia (no sperm detectable in semen) and with approximately 6% of cases of severe oligospermia (low sperm count). These findings suggest that one or more genes, termed azoospermia factors (*AZF*), are located on the Y chromosome, and three nonoverlapping regions on Yq (AZFa, AZFb, and AZFc) have been defined (see Fig. 6-10). Molecular analysis of these deletions has led to identification of a series of genes that may be important in spermatogenesis. For example, the AZFc deletion region contains several families of genes expressed in the testis, including the *DAZ* genes (*deleted in azoospermia*) that encode RNA-binding proteins expressed only in the premeiotic germ cells of the testis. De novo

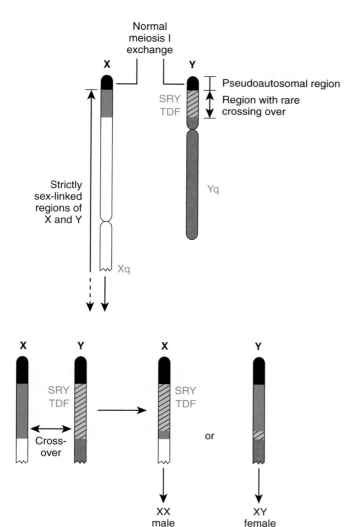

Figure 6-12 ■ Etiological factors of XX male or XY female phenotypes by aberrant exchange between X- and Y-linked sequences. X and Y chromosomes normally recombine within the Xp/Yp pseudoautosomal segment in male meiosis. If recombination occurs below the pseudoautosomal boundary, between the X-specific and Y-specific portions of the chromosomes, sequences responsible for male sexual differentiation (including the *SRY* gene) may be translocated from the Y to the X. Fertilization by a sperm containing such an X chromosome leads to an XX male. In contrast, fertilization by a sperm containing a Y chromosome that has lost *SRY* will lead to an XY female.

deletions of AZFc arise in about 1 in 4000 males and are mediated by recombination between long repeated sequences (see Table 6-1). AZFa and AZFb deletions, although less common, also involve recombination.

The prevalence of AZF mutations, deletions, and sequence variants in the general male population as well as their contribution to spermatogenic failure remain to be fully elucidated. Approximately 2% of otherwise healthy males are infertile because of severe defects in sperm production, and it appears likely that de novo deletions or mutations account for at least a

proportion of these. Thus, men with idiopathic infertility should be karyotyped, and Y chromosome molecular testing and genetic counseling may be appropriate before the initiation of assisted reproduction for such couples.

Not all cases of male infertility are due to chromosomal deletions. For example, a de novo point mutation has been described in one Y-linked gene, *USP9Y*, the function of which is unknown but which must be required for normal spermatogenesis (see Fig. 6-10).

The X Chromosome

As pointed out in Chapter 5, aneuploidy for the X chromosome is among the most common of cytogenetic abnormalities. The relative tolerance of the human karyotype for X chromosome abnormalities can be explained in terms of **X chromosome inactivation**, the process by which most genes on one of the two X chromosomes in females are silenced epigenetically and fail to produce any product. X inactivation and its consequences in relation to X-linked disorders are discussed in Chapter 7. Here we discuss the chromosomal and molecular mechanisms of X inactivation.

X Chromosome Inactivation

As will be discussed at greater length in Chapter 7, the theory of X inactivation is that in somatic cells in normal females (but not in normal males), one X chromosome is inactivated early in development, thus equalizing the expression of X-linked genes in the two sexes. In normal female cells, the choice of which X chromosome is to be inactivated is a random one that is then maintained in each clonal lineage. Thus, females are mosaic with respect to X-linked gene expression; some cells express alleles on the paternally inherited X but not the maternally inherited X, whereas other cells do the opposite (Fig. 6-13). This pattern of gene expression distinguishes most X-linked genes from imprinted genes (which are also expressed from only one allele but determined by parental origin, not randomly) as well as from the majority of autosomal genes that are expressed from both alleles.

Although the inactive X chromosome was first identified cytologically by the presence of a heterochromatic mass (called the Barr body) in interphase cells, there are many epigenetic features that distinguish the active and inactive X chromosomes (Table 6-2). As well as providing insight into the mechanisms of X inactivation, these features can be useful diagnostically for identifying the inactive X chromosome in clinical material (Fig. 6-14).

The promoter region of many genes on the inactive X chromosome is extensively modified by addition of a methyl group to cytosine (see Fig. 2-2) by the enzyme DNA methyltransferase. As introduced in the context

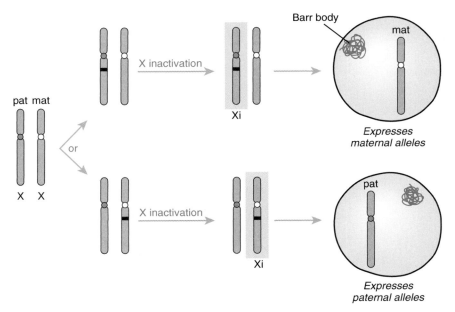

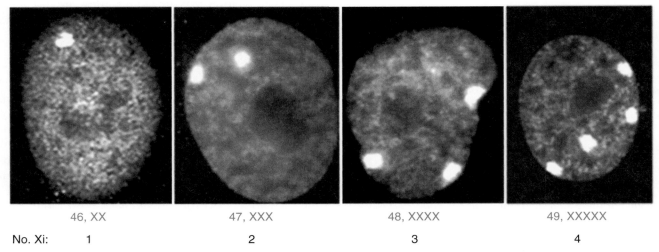

Figure 6-13 ■ Random X chromosome inactivation early in female development. Shortly after conception of a female embryo, both the paternally and maternally inherited X chromosomes (pat and mat, respectively) are active. Within the first week of embryogenesis, one or the other X is chosen at random to become the future inactive X, through a series of events involving the X inactivation center in Xq13.2 (black box). That X then becomes the inactive X (Xi, indicated by the blue shading) in that cell and its progeny and forms the Barr body in interphase nuclei.

Figure 6-14 ■ Detection of the histone variant macroH2A in interphase nuclei from females with 46,XX, 47,XXX, 48,XXXX, and 49,XXXXX karyotypes. Regions of bright fluorescence indicate presence of macroH2A associated with inactive X chromosomes and illustrate that the number of inactive X chromosomes (Xi) is always one less than the total number of X chromosomes. (Courtesy of Brian Chadwick, Duke University Medical Center.)

Table 6-2

Chromosomal Features of X Inactivation

- Inactivation of most X-linked genes on the inactive X
- Random choice of one of two X chromosomes in female cells
- Inactive X:
  Heterochromatic (Barr body)
  Late-replicating in S phase
  Expresses XIST RNA
  Associated with macroH2A histone modifications in chromatin

---

of genomic imprinting in Chapter 5, such **DNA methylation** is restricted to CpG dinucleotides (see Chapter 2) and contributes to formation of an inactive chromatin state. Additional differences between the active and inactive X chromosomes involve the histone code and appear to be an essential part of the X inactivation mechanism. For example, the histone variant macroH2A is highly enriched in inactive X chromatin and distinguishes the two X's in female cells (see Fig. 6-14).

In patients with extra X chromosomes, any X chromosome in excess of one is inactivated (see Fig. 6-14 and Box). Thus, all diploid somatic cells in both males

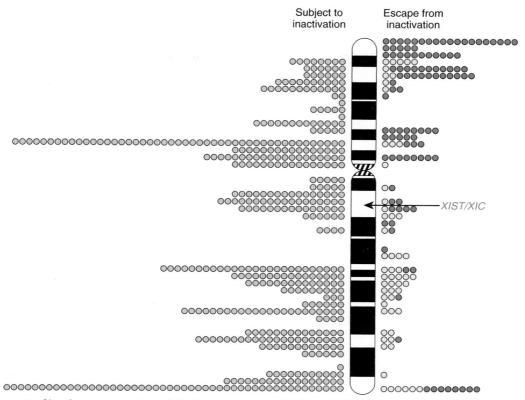

Figure 6-15 ■ Profile of gene expression of the X chromosome. Each symbol indicates X inactivation status of an X-linked gene. Location of each symbol indicates its approximate map position on the X chromosome. Genes not expressed from the inactive X (subject to inactivation) are on the left. Genes expressed from the inactive X (escape from inactivation) are on the right; genes represented in light blue are those that escape inactivation in only a subset of females tested. The location of the *XIST* gene and the X inactivation center (XIC) are indicated in Xq13.2. (Data based on Carrel L, Willard HF: X inactivation profile reveals extensive variability in X-linked gene expression in females. Nature 434:400-404, 2005.)

and females have a single active X chromosome, regardless of the total number of X or Y chromosomes present.

Although X chromosome inactivation is clearly a chromosomal phenomenon, not all genes on the X chromosome are subject to inactivation (Fig. 6-15). Extensive analysis of expression of nearly all X-linked genes has demonstrated that at least 15% of the genes escape inactivation and are expressed from both active and inactive X chromosomes. In addition, another 10% show variable X inactivation; that is, they escape inactivation in some females but not in others. Notably, these genes are not distributed randomly along the X; many more genes escape inactivation on distal Xp (as many as 50%) than on Xq (just a few percent) (see Fig. 6-15). This finding has important implications for genetic counseling in cases of partial X chromosome aneuploidy, as imbalance for genes on Xp may have greater clinical significance than imbalance of Xq.

The X Inactivation Center and the *XIST* Gene   From the study of structurally abnormal, inactivated X chromosomes, the **X inactivation center** has been mapped

to proximal Xq, in band Xq13 (see Figs. 6-13 and 6-15). The X inactivation center contains an unusual gene, ***XIST,*** that appears to be a key master regulatory locus for X inactivation. *XIST,* an acronym for inactive X (X*i*)–specific *t*ranscripts, has the novel feature that it is expressed only from the allele on the inactive X; it is transcriptionally silent on the active X in both male and female cells. Although the exact mode of action of

•••	**Sex Chromosomes and X Inactivation**		
Sexual Phenotype	Karyotype	No. of Active X's	No. of Inactive X's
Male	46,XY; 47,XYY	1	0
	47,XXY; 48,XXYY	1	1
	48,XXXY; 49,XXXYY	1	2
	49,XXXXY	1	3
Female	45,X	1	0
	46,XX	1	1
	47,XXX	1	2
	48,XXXX	1	3
	49,XXXXX	1	4

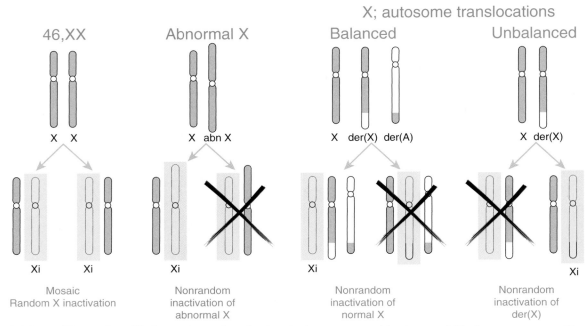

Figure 6-16 ■ Nonrandom X chromosome inactivation in karyotypes with abnormal X chromosomes or X;autosome translocations. Normal female cells (46,XX) undergo random X inactivation; resulting tissues are a mosaic of two cell populations in which either the paternal or maternal X is the inactive X (Xi, indicated by blue box). Individuals carrying a structurally abnormal X (abn X) or X;autosome translocation in a balanced or unbalanced state show nonrandom X inactivation in which virtually all cells have the same X inactive. The other cell population is inviable or at a growth disadvantage because of genetic imbalance and is thus underrepresented or absent. See text for further discussion. der(X) and der(A) represent the two derivatives of the X;autosome translocation.

XIST is unknown, X inactivation cannot occur in its absence. The product of *XIST* is a noncoding RNA that stays in the nucleus in close association with the inactive X chromosome and the Barr body.

Nonrandom X Chromosome Inactivation As shown in Figure 6-13, X inactivation is normally random in female somatic cells and leads to mosaicism for two cell populations expressing alleles from one or the other X. However, there are exceptions to this when the karyotype involves a structurally abnormal X. For example, in almost all patients with unbalanced structural abnormalities of an X chromosome (including deletions, duplications, and isochromosomes), the structurally abnormal chromosome is always the inactive X, probably reflecting secondary selection against genetically unbalanced cells that could lead to significant clinical abnormalities (Fig. 6-16). Because of this preferential inactivation of the abnormal X, such X chromosome anomalies have less of an impact on phenotype than similar abnormalities of autosomes and consequently are more frequently observed.

Nonrandom inactivation is also observed in most cases of X;autosome translocations (see Fig. 6-16). If such a translocation is balanced, the normal X chromosome is preferentially inactivated, and the two parts of the translocated chromosome remain active, again

probably reflecting selection against cells in which autosomal genes have been inactivated. In the unbalanced offspring of a balanced carrier, however, only the translocation product carrying the X inactivation center is present, and this chromosome is invariably inactivated; the normal X is always active. These nonrandom patterns of inactivation have the general effect of minimizing, but not always eliminating, the clinical consequences of the particular chromosomal defect. Because patterns of X inactivation are strongly correlated with clinical outcome, determination of an individual's X inactivation pattern by cytogenetic or molecular analysis is indicated in all cases involving X;autosome translocations.

One consequence sometimes observed in balanced carriers of X;autosome translocations is that the break itself may cause a mutation by disrupting a gene on the X chromosome at the site of the translocation. The only normal copy of the particular gene is inactivated in most or all cells because of nonrandom X inactivation of the normal X, thus allowing expression in a female of an X-linked trait normally observed only in hemizygous males (see Chapter 7). Several X-linked genes have been identified when a typical X-linked phenotype has been found in a female who then proved to have an X;autosome translocation. The general clinical message of these findings is that if a female patient manifests an

X-linked phenotype normally seen only in males, high-resolution chromosome analysis is indicated. The finding of a balanced translocation can explain the phenotypic expression and show the gene's probable map position on the X chromosome.

X-Linked Mental Retardation

An additional feature of the X chromosome is the high frequency of mutations, microdeletions, or duplications that cause X-linked mental retardation. The collective incidence of X-linked mental retardation has been estimated to be 1 in 500 to 1000 live births. In many instances, mental retardation is but one of several abnormal phenotypic features that together define an X-linked syndrome, and more than 50 X-linked genes have been identified in families with such disorders. However, there are many other genes at which mutations lead to isolated or nonsyndromic X-linked mental retardation, often of the severe to profound kind. The number of such genes is consistent with the finding in many large-scale surveys that there is a 20% to 40% excess of males among persons with mental retardation. Detailed chromosome analysis is indicated as an initial evaluation to rule out an obvious cytogenetic abnormality, such as a deletion.

Cytogenetic Abnormalities of the Sex Chromosomes

Sex chromosome abnormalities, like abnormalities of the autosomes, can be either numerical or structural and can be present in all cells or in mosaic form. As a group, disorders of the sex chromosomes tend to occur as isolated events without apparent predisposing factors, except for an effect of late maternal age in the cases that

originate from errors of maternal meiosis I. Their incidence in liveborn children, in fetuses examined prenatally, and in spontaneous abortions was compared in Chapter 5 with the incidence of similar abnormalities of the autosomes and is summarized in Table 6-3. There are a number of clinical indications that raise the possibility of a sex chromosome abnormality and thus the need for cytogenetic or molecular studies. These especially include delay in onset of puberty, primary or secondary amenorrhea, infertility, and ambiguous genitalia.

X and Y chromosome aneuploidy is relatively common, and sex chromosome abnormalities are among the most common of all human genetic disorders, with an overall incidence of about 1 in 400 to 500 births. The phenotypes associated with these chromosomal defects are, in general, less severe than those associated with comparable autosomal disorders because X chromosome inactivation, as well as the low gene content of the Y, minimizes the clinical consequences of sex chromosome imbalance. By far the most common sex chromosome defects in liveborn infants and in fetuses are the trisomic types (XXY, XXX, and XYY), but all three are rare in spontaneous abortions. In contrast, monosomy for the X (Turner syndrome) is less frequent in liveborn infants but is the most common chromosome anomaly reported in spontaneous abortions (see Table 5-4).

Structural abnormalities of the sex chromosomes are less common; the defect most frequently observed is an isochromosome of the long arm of the X, i(Xq), seen in complete or mosaic form in at least 15% of females with Turner syndrome. Mosaicism is more common for sex chromosome abnormalities than for autosomal abnormalities, and in some patients it is associated with relatively mild expression of the associated phenotype.

Table 6-3

Incidence of Sex Chromosome Abnormalities

Sex	Disorder	Karyotype	Approximate Incidence
Male	Klinefelter syndrome	47,XXY	1/1000 males
		48,XXXY	1/25,000 males
		Others (48,XXYY; 49,XXXYY; mosaics)	1/10,000 males
	47,XYY syndrome	47,XYY	1/1000 males
	Other X or Y chromosome abnormalities		1/1500 males
	XX males	46,XX	1/20,000 males
			Overall incidence: 1/400 males
Female	Turner syndrome	45,X	1/5000 females
		46,X,i(Xq)	1/50,000 females
		Others (deletions, mosaics)	1/15,000 females
	Trisomy X	47,XXX	1/1000 females
	Other X chromosome abnormalities		1/3000 females
	XY females	46,XY	1/20,000 females
	Androgen insensitivity syndrome	46,XY	1/20,000 females
			Overall incidence: 1/650 females

Data adapted from Table 5-3 and Robinson A, Linden MG, Bender BG: Prenatal diagnosis of sex chromosome abnormalities. In Milunsky A (ed): Genetic Disorders of the Fetus, 4th ed. Baltimore, Johns Hopkins University Press, 1998, pp 249-285.

Table 6-4

Follow-up Observations on Patients with Sex Chromosome Aneuploidy

Disorder	Karyotype	Phenotype	Sexual Development	Intelligence	Behavioral Problem
Klinefelter syndrome	47,XXY	Tall male (see text)	Infertile; hypogonadism	Learning difficulties (some patients)	May have poor psychosocial adjustment
XYY syndrome	47,XYY	Tall male	Normal	Normal	Frequent
Trisomy X	47,XXX	Female, usually tall	Usually normal	Learning difficulties (some patients)	Occasional
Turner syndrome	45,X	Short female, distinctive features (see text)	Infertile; streak gonads	Slightly reduced	Rare (but see text)

Data from Ratcliffe SG, Paul N (eds): Prospective studies on children with sex chromosome aneuploidy. March of Dimes Birth Defects Foundation, Birth Defects Original Article Series, vol 22. New York, Alan R. Liss, 1986; and Rovert J, Netley C, Bailey J, et al: Intelligence and achievement in children with extra X aneuploidy: a longitudinal perspective. Am J Med Genet 60:356-363, 1995.

The four well-defined syndromes associated with sex chromosome aneuploidy are important causes of infertility or abnormal development, or both, and thus warrant a more detailed description. The effects of these chromosome abnormalities on development have been studied in long-term multicenter studies of more than 300 affected individuals, some of whom have been monitored for more than 35 years. To avoid the bias inherent in studying cases unusual enough to be referred to a medical center for assessment, only cases ascertained by screening of newborns or by prenatal diagnosis have been used. The major conclusions of this important clinical study are summarized in Table 6-4. As a group, those with sex chromosome aneuploidy show reduced levels of psychological adaptation, educational achievement, occupational performance, and economic independence, and on average, they scored slightly lower on intelligence (IQ) tests. However, each group showed high variability, making it impossible to generalize to specific cases. In fact, the overall impression is a high degree of normalcy, particularly in adulthood, which is remarkable among those with chromosomal anomalies. Because almost all patients with sex chromosome abnormalities have only mild developmental abnormalities, a parental decision regarding potential termination of a pregnancy in which the fetus is found to have this type of defect can be a very difficult one.

Klinefelter Syndrome (47,XXY)

The phenotype of Klinefelter syndrome, the first human sex chromosome abnormality to be reported, is shown in Figure 6-17. The patients are tall and thin and have relatively long legs. They appear physically normal until puberty, when signs of hypogonadism become obvious. Puberty occurs at a normal age, but the testes remain small, and secondary sexual characteristics remain underdeveloped. Gynecomastia is a feature of some patients; because of this, the risk of breast cancer is 20 to 50 times that of 46,XY males. Klinefelter

patients are almost always infertile because of the failure of germ cell development, and patients are often identified clinically for the first time because of infertility. Klinefelter syndrome is relatively common among infertile males (about 3%) or males with oligospermia

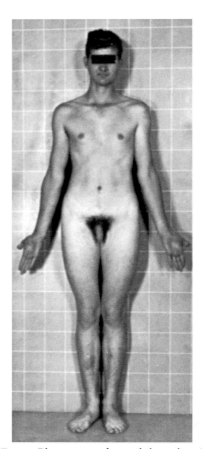

Figure 6-17 ■ Phenotype of an adult male with 47,XXY Klinefelter syndrome. Note long limbs, narrow shoulders and chest, and relatively small genitalia. Gynecomastia, not present in this patient, is a feature of some Klinefelter males. (From Grumbach MM, Hughes IA, Conte FA: Disorders of sex differentiation. In Larsen PR, Kronenberg HM, Melmed S, Polonsky KS [eds]: Williams Textbook of Endocrinology, 10th ed. Philadelphia, WB Saunders, 2003.)

or azoospermia (5% to 10%). In adulthood, persistent androgen deficiency may result in decreased muscle tone, a loss of libido, and decreased bone mineral density.

The incidence is at least 1 in 1000 male live births (1 in 2000 total births). As discussed earlier, one of the two X chromosomes is inactivated. Because of the relatively mild yet variable phenotype, many cases are presumed to go undetected.

About half the cases of Klinefelter syndrome result from errors in paternal meiosis I because of a failure of normal Xp/Yp recombination in the pseudoautosomal region. Among cases of maternal origin, most result from errors in maternal meiosis I and the remainder from errors in meiosis II or from a postzygotic mitotic error leading to mosaicism. Maternal age is increased in the cases associated with maternal meiosis I errors.

About 15% of Klinefelter patients have mosaic karyotypes. As a group, such mosaic patients have variable phenotypes; some may have normal testicular development. The most common mosaic karyotype is 46,XY/47,XXY, probably as a consequence of loss of one X chromosome in an XXY conceptus during an early postzygotic division.

There are several variants of Klinefelter syndrome, with karyotypes other than 47,XXY, including 48,XXYY, 48,XXXY, and 49,XXXXY. As a rule, the additional X chromosomes (even though they are mostly inactive) cause a correspondingly more severe phenotype, with a greater degree of dysmorphism, more defective sexual development, and more severe mental impairment.

Although there is wide phenotypic variation among patients with this and other sex chromosome aneuploidies, some consistent phenotypic differences have been identified between patients with Klinefelter syndrome and chromosomally normal males. Verbal comprehension and ability are below those of normal males, and 47,XXY males score slightly lower on certain intelligence performance tests. Patients with Klinefelter syndrome have a several-fold increased risk of learning difficulties, especially in reading, that may require educational intervention. Klinefelter syndrome is overrepresented among boys requiring special education. Many of the affected boys have relatively poor psychosocial adjustment, in part related to poor body image. Language difficulties may lead to shyness, unassertiveness, and immaturity.

47,XYY Syndrome

Among all male live births, the incidence of the 47,XYY karyotype is about 1 in 1000. The 47,XYY chromosome constitution is not associated with an obviously abnormal phenotype, and males with this karyotype cannot be distinguished from normal 46,XY males by any marked physical or behavioral features.

The origin of the error that leads to the XYY karyotype must be paternal nondisjunction at meiosis II, producing YY sperm. The less common XXYY and XXXYY variants, which share the features of the XYY and Klinefelter syndromes, probably also originate in the father as a result of sequential nondisjunction in meiosis I and meiosis II.

XYY males identified in newborn screening programs without ascertainment bias are tall and have an increased risk of educational or behavioral problems in comparison with chromosomally normal males. They have normal intelligence and are not dysmorphic. Fertility is usually normal, and there appears to be no particularly increased risk that a 47,XYY male will have a chromosomally abnormal child. About half of 47,XYY boys require educational intervention as a result of language delays and reading and spelling difficulties. Their IQ scores are about 10 to 15 points below average.

Parents whose child is found, prenatally or postnatally, to be XYY are often extremely concerned about the behavioral implications. Attention deficits, hyperactivity, and impulsiveness have been well documented in XYY males, but marked aggression or psychopathological behavior is not a common feature of the syndrome. This is an important point to emphasize because of reports in the 1960s and 1970s that the proportion of XYY males was elevated in prisons and mental hospitals, especially among the tallest inmates. This stereotypic impression is now known to be incorrect.

Nonetheless, inability to predict the outcome in individual cases makes identification of an XYY fetus one of the more difficult genetic counseling problems in prenatal diagnosis programs.

Trisomy X (47,XXX)

Trisomy X occurs with an incidence of 1 in 1000 female births. Trisomy X females, although somewhat above average in stature, are not abnormal phenotypically. Some are first identified in infertility clinics, but probably most remain undiagnosed. Follow-up studies have shown that XXX females develop pubertal changes at an appropriate age, and they are usually fertile although with a somewhat increased risk of chromosomally abnormal offspring. There is a significant deficit in performance on IQ tests, and about 70% of the patients have some learning problems. Severe psychopathological and antisocial behaviors appear to be rare; however, abnormal behavior is apparent, especially during the transition from adolescence to early adulthood.

In 47,XXX cells, two of the X chromosomes are inactivated. Almost all cases result from errors in maternal meiosis, and of these, the majority are in meiosis I. There is an effect of increased maternal age, restricted to those patients in whom the error was in maternal meiosis I.

The tetrasomy X syndrome (48,XXXX) is associated with more serious retardation in both physical and mental development. The pentasomy X syndrome (49,XXXXX), despite the presence of four inactive X chromosomes (see Fig. 6-14), usually includes severe developmental retardation with multiple physical defects.

Turner Syndrome (45,X and Variants)

Unlike patients with other sex chromosome aneuploidies, females with Turner syndrome can often be identified at birth or before puberty by their distinctive phenotypic features (Fig. 6-18). Turner syndrome is much less common than other sex chromosome aneuploidies. The incidence of the Turner syndrome phenotype is approximately 1 in 4000 female live births, although much higher numbers have been reported in some surveys (Case 42).

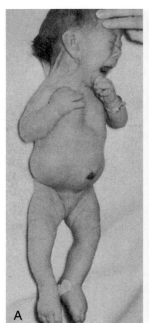
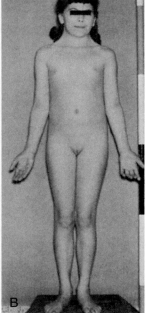

Figure 6-18 ■ Phenotype of females with 45,X Turner syndrome. **A,** Newborn infant. Note the webbed neck and lymphedema of the hands and feet. **B,** A 13-year-old girl showing classic Turner syndrome features, including short stature, webbed neck, delayed sexual maturation, and broad, shieldlike chest with widely spaced nipples. (From Moore KL: The Sex Chromatin. Philadelphia, WB Saunders, 1966.)

The most frequent chromosome constitution in Turner syndrome is 45,X (sometimes written incorrectly as 45,XO), with no second sex chromosome. However, about 50% of cases have other karyotypes. About one quarter of Turner syndrome cases involve mosaic karyotypes, in which only a proportion of cells are 45,X. The most common karyotypes and their approximate relative prevalences are as follows:

45,X	50%
46,X,i(Xq)	15%
45,X/46,XX mosaics	15%
45,X/46,X,i(Xq) mosaics	about 5%
45,X, other X abnormality	about 5%
Other 45,X/? mosaics	about 5%

The chromosome constitution is clinically significant. For example, patients with i(Xq) are similar to classic 45,X patients, whereas patients with a deletion of Xp have short stature and congenital malformations, and those with a deletion of Xq often have only gonadal dysfunction.

Typical abnormalities in Turner syndrome include short stature, gonadal dysgenesis (usually streak gonads reflecting a failure of ovarian maintenance), characteristic unusual facies, webbed neck, low posterior hairline, broad chest with widely spaced nipples, and elevated frequency of renal and cardiovascular anomalies. At birth, infants with this syndrome often have edema of the dorsum of the foot, a useful diagnostic sign (see Fig. 6-18A). Many patients have coarctation of the aorta, and Turner syndrome females are at particular risk for cardiovascular abnormalities. Lymphedema may be present in fetal life, causing cystic hygroma (visible by ultrasonography), which is the cause of the neck webbing seen postnatally. Turner syndrome should be suspected in any newborn female with edema of the hands and feet or with hypoplastic left-sided heart or coarctation of the aorta. The diagnosis should also be considered in the teenage years for girls with primary or secondary amenorrhea, especially if they are of short stature. Growth hormone therapy should be considered for all girls with Turner syndrome and can result in gains of 6 to 12 cm to the final height.

Intelligence in Turner syndrome females is usually considered to be normal, although approximately 10% of patients will show significant developmental delay requiring special education. Even among those with normal intelligence, however, patients often display a deficiency in spatial perception, perceptual motor organization, or fine motor execution. As a consequence, the nonverbal IQ score is significantly lower than the verbal IQ score, and many patients require educational intervention, especially in mathematics. Turner syndrome females have an elevated risk of impaired social adjustment. A comparison of 45,X girls with a maternal X and those with a paternal X provided evidence of significantly worse social cognition skills in those with

Table 6-5

Examples of Genes Involved in Abnormalities of Sex Determination and Differentiation

Gene	Cytogenetic Locus	Abnormal Sexual Phenotype
SRY	Yp11.3	XY female (mutation)
		XX male (gene translocated to X)
SOX9	17q24	XY female (with camptomelic dysplasia)
		XX male (gene duplication)
SF1	9q33	XY sex reversal and adrenal insufficiency
WT1	11p13	XY female (Frasier syndrome) or male pseudohermaphrodite (Denys-Drash syndrome)
DAX1	Xp21.3	XY female (gene duplication)
ATRX	Xq13.3	XY sex reversal (variable)
WNT4	1p35	XY female, cryptorchidism (gene duplication)
FOXL2	3q23	Premature ovarian failure

Updated from Fleming A, Vilain E: The endless quest for sex determination genes. Clin Genet 67:15-25, 2004; and Grumbach MM, Hughes IA, Conte FA: Disorders of sex differentiation. In Larsen PR, Kronenberg HM, Melmed S, Polonsky KS (eds): Williams Textbook of Endocrinology, 10th ed. Philadelphia, WB Saunders, 2003.

a maternally-derived X. Because imprinting could explain this parent-of-origin effect, the possibility of an imprinted X-linked gene that influences phenotype is under investigation.

The high incidence of a 45,X karyotype in spontaneous abortions has already been mentioned. This single abnormality is present in an estimated 1% to 2% of all conceptuses; survival to term is a rare outcome, and more than 99% of such fetuses abort spontaneously. The single X is maternal in origin in about 70% of cases; in other words, the chromosome error leading to loss of a sex chromosome is usually paternal. The basis for the unusually high frequency of X or Y chromosome loss is unknown. Furthermore, it is not clear why the 45,X karyotype is usually lethal in utero but is apparently fully compatible with postnatal survival. The "missing" genes responsible for the Turner syndrome phenotype must reside on both the X and Y chromosomes. It has been suggested that the responsible genes are among those that escape X chromosome inactivation, particularly on Xp, including those in the pseudoautosomal region.

Small ring X chromosomes are occasionally observed in patients with short stature, gonadal dysgenesis, and mental retardation. Because mental retardation is not a typical feature of Turner syndrome, the presence of mental retardation with or without other associated physical anomalies in individuals with a 46,X,r(X) karyotype has been attributed to the fact that small ring X chromosomes lack the X inactivation center. The failure to inactivate the ring X in these patients leads to overexpression of X-linked genes that are normally subject to inactivation. The discovery of a ring X in a prenatal diagnosis can lead to great uncertainty, and studies of *XIST* expression are indicated. Large rings containing the X inactivation center and expressing *XIST* predict a Turner syndrome phenotype; a small ring lacking or not expressing *XIST* predicts a much more severe phenotype.

DISORDERS OF GONADAL AND SEXUAL DEVELOPMENT

The genetic sex of an embryo is established at the time of fertilization. Earlier in this chapter, we discussed the primary sex-determining role of the Y chromosome and the *SRY* gene. Here we examine the role of various X-linked and autosomal genes in ovarian and testicular development and in the development of male and female external genitalia (Table 6-5).

For some newborn infants, determination of sex is difficult or impossible because the genitalia are ambiguous, with anomalies that tend to make them resemble those of the opposite chromosomal sex (Case 36). Such anomalies may vary from mild hypospadias in males (a developmental anomaly in which the urethra opens on the underside of the penis or on the perineum) to an enlarged clitoris in females. In some patients, both ovarian and testicular tissue is present, a condition known as **hermaphroditism.** Abnormalities of either external or internal genitalia do not necessarily indicate a cytogenetic abnormality of the sex chromosomes but may be due to chromosomal changes elsewhere in the karyotype, to single-gene defects, or to nongenetic causes. Nonetheless, determination of the child's karyotype is an essential part of the investigation of such patients and can help guide both surgical and psychosocial management as well as genetic counseling. The detection of cytogenetic abnormalities, especially when seen in multiple patients, can also provide important clues about the location and nature of genes involved in sex determination and sex differentiation (Table 6-6).

Gonadal Dysgenesis

A number of autosomal and X-linked genes have been implicated in conversion of the bipotential gonad to either a testis or ovary (see Fig. 6-11). Detailed analysis

Table 6-6

Cytogenetic Abnormalities Associated with Cases of Sex Reversal or Ambiguous Genitalia

Cytogenetic Abnormality	Phenotype
dup 1p31-p35	XY female (*WNT4* gene duplication)
del 2q31	XY female, mental retardation
del 9p24.3	XY female, ambiguous genitalia
del 10q26-qter	XY female
del 12q24.3	XY ambiguous genitalia, mental retardation
dup 22q	XY true hermaphroditism
dup Xp21.3	XY female (*DAX1* gene duplication)

Updated from Fleming A, Vilain E: The endless quest for sex determination genes. Clin Genet 67:15-25, 2004; and Pinsky L, Erickson RP, Schimke RN: Genetic Disorders of Human Sexual Development. Oxford, England, Oxford University Press, 1999.

of a subset of **sex-reversed 46,XY females** in whom the *SRY* gene was not deleted or mutated revealed a duplication of a portion of the short arm of the X chromosome. The *DAX1* gene in Xp21.3 encodes a transcription factor that plays a dosage-sensitive role in determination of gonadal sex, implying a tightly regulated interaction between *DAX1* and *SRY*. An excess of *SRY* at a critical point in development leads to testis formation; an excess of *DAX1* resulting from duplication of the gene can suppress the normal male-determining function of *SRY*, and ovarian development results.

Camptomelic dysplasia, due to mutations in the *SOX9* gene on chromosome 17q, is an autosomal dominant disorder with usually lethal skeletal malformations. However, about 75% of 46,XY patients with this disorder are sex reversed and are phenotypic females (see Table 6-5). *SOX9* is normally expressed early in development in the genital ridge and thus appears to be required for normal testis formation (in addition to its role in other aspects of development). In the absence of one copy of the *SOX9* gene, testes fail to form, and the default ovarian pathway is followed. Interestingly, duplication of *SOX9* has been reported to lead to XX sex reversal, suggesting that overproduction of *SOX9*, even in the absence of *SRY*, can initiate testis formation.

Other autosomal loci have also been implicated in gonadal development. Chromosomally male patients with **Denys-Drash syndrome** have ambiguous external genitalia; patients with the more severe **Frasier syndrome** show XY complete gonadal dysgenesis. The *WT1* gene in 11p13 (also implicated in Wilms tumor, a childhood kidney neoplasia) encodes a transcription factor that is involved in interactions between Sertoli and Leydig cells in the developing gonad. Dominant *WT1* mutations apparently disrupt normal testicular development.

The X-linked *ATRX* gene is responsible for an X-linked mental retardation syndrome with α-thalassemia (see also Chapter 11) and, in many patients, genital anomalies ranging from undescended testes to micropenis to varying degrees of XY sex reversal.

Ovarian Development and Maintenance

In contrast to testis determination, much less is known about development of the ovary, although a number of genes have been implicated in normal ovarian maintenance. It has long been thought that two X chromosomes are necessary for ovarian maintenance, as 45,X females, despite normal initiation of ovarian development in utero, are characterized by germ cell loss, oocyte degeneration, and ovarian dysgenesis. Patients with cytogenetic abnormalities involving Xq frequently show **premature ovarian failure.** Because many nonoverlapping deletions on Xq show the same effect, this finding may reflect a need for two structurally normal X chromosomes in oogenesis or simply a requirement for multiple X-linked genes.

Specific genes have been implicated in familial cases of premature ovarian failure and in mendelian forms of 46,XX gonadal dysgenesis. For example, mutations in the *FOXL2* gene (see Table 6-5) are seen in patients with blepharophimosis/ptosis/epicanthus inversus (BPES) syndrome, and the phenotype in affected females ranges from ovarian dysgenesis to premature ovarian failure.

Female Pseudohermaphroditism

Pseudohermaphrodites are "pseudo" because, unlike true hermaphrodites, they have gonadal tissue of only one sex that matches their chromosomal constitution. Female pseudohermaphrodites have 46,XX karyotypes with normal ovarian tissue but with ambiguous or male external genitalia. Male pseudohermaphrodites, as we will see in the next section, are 46,XY with incompletely masculinized or female external genitalia. In general, ambiguous development of the genital ducts and external genitalia should always be evaluated cytogenetically, both to determine the sex chromosome constitution of the patient and to identify potential chromosome abnormalities frequently associated with dysgenetic gonads (see Table 6-6).

Female pseudohermaphroditism is usually due to **congenital adrenal hyperplasia** (CAH), an inherited disorder arising from specific defects in enzymes of the adrenal cortex required for cortisol biosynthesis and resulting in virilization of female infants. In addition to being a frequent cause of female pseudohermaphroditism, CAH accounts for approximately half of all cases presenting with ambiguous external

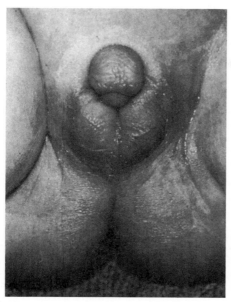

Figure 6-19 ■ Masculinized external genitalia of a 46,XX infant caused by congenital adrenal hyperplasia (virilizing form). See text for discussion. (From Moore KL, Persaud TVN: The Developing Human: Clinically Oriented Embryology, 5th ed. Philadelphia, WB Saunders, 1993.)

genitalia. Ovarian development is normal, but excessive production of androgens causes masculinization of the external genitalia, with clitoral enlargement and labial fusion to form a scrotum-like structure (Fig. 6-19).

Although any one of several enzymatic steps may be defective in CAH, by far the most common defect is deficiency of 21-hydroxylase, which has an incidence of about 1 in 12,500 births. Deficiency of 21-hydroxylase blocks the normal biosynthetic pathway of glucocorticoids and mineralocorticoids. This leads to overproduction of the precursors, which are then shunted into the pathway of androgen biosynthesis, causing abnormally high androgen levels in both XX and XY embryos. Whereas female infants with 21-hydroxylase deficiency are born with ambiguous genitalia, affected male infants have normal external genitalia and may go unrecognized in early infancy. Of patients with classic 21-hydroxylase deficiency, 25% have the simple virilizing type, and 75% have a salt-losing type due to mineralocorticoid deficiency that is clinically more severe and may lead to neonatal death. A screening test developed to identify the condition in newborns, in which heel-prick blood specimens are blotted onto filter paper, is now in use in many countries (see Chapter 15). It is valuable in preventing the serious consequences of the salt-losing defect in early infancy and in prompt diagnosis of and hormone replacement therapy for affected males and females.

Prompt medical, surgical, and psychosocial management of 46,XX CAH patients is associated with improved fertility rates and normal female gender identity.

Male Pseudohermaphroditism

In addition to disorders of testis formation during embryological development, causes of pseudohermaphroditism in 46,XY individuals include abnormalities of gonadotropins, inherited disorders of testosterone biosynthesis and metabolism, and abnormalities of androgen target cells. These disorders are heterogeneous both genetically and clinically, and in some cases they may correspond to milder manifestations of the same cause underlying true hermaphroditism. Whereas the gonads are exclusively testes in male pseudohermaphroditism, the genital ducts or external genitalia are incompletely masculinized.

In addition to mutation or deletion of any of the genes involved in testes determination and differentiation and presented earlier (see Table 6-5), there are several forms of androgen insensitivity that result in male pseudohermaphroditism. One example is deficiency of the steroid **5α-reductase,** the enzyme responsible for converting the male hormone testosterone to its active form dihydrotestosterone. This inherited condition results in feminization of external genitalia in affected males. Although testicular development is normal, the penis is small, and there is a blind vaginal pouch. Gender assignment can be difficult.

Another well-studied disorder is an X-linked syndrome known as **androgen insensitivity syndrome** (formerly known as **testicular feminization**). In this disorder, affected persons are chromosomal males (karyotype 46,XY), with apparently normal female external genitalia, who have a blind vagina and no uterus or uterine tubes (Fig. 6-20). The incidence of androgen insensitivity is about 1 in 20,000 live births. Axillary and pubic hair is sparse or absent. As the original name "testicular feminization" indicates, testes are present either within the abdomen or in the inguinal canal, where they are sometimes mistaken for hernias in infants who otherwise appear to be normal females. Thus, gender assignment is not an issue, and psychosexual development and sexual function are that of a normal female (except for fertility).

Although the testes secrete androgen normally, end-organ unresponsiveness to androgens results from absence of androgen receptors in the appropriate target cells. The receptor protein, specified by the normal allele at the X-linked androgen receptor locus, has the role of forming a complex with testosterone and dihydrotestosterone. If the complex fails to form, the

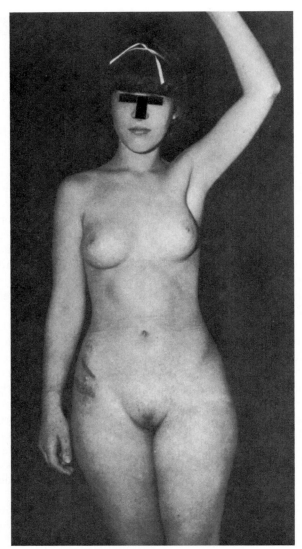

Figure 6-20 ■ Complete androgen insensitivity syndrome (testicular feminization) in a 46,XY individual. Note female body contours, absence of axillary hair, sparse pubic hair, and breast development. (Courtesy of L. Pinsky, McGill University, Montreal.)

hormone fails to stimulate the transcription of target genes required for differentiation in the male direction. The molecular defect has been determined in hundreds of cases and ranges from a complete deletion of the androgen receptor gene (see Fig. 4-7) to point mutations in the androgen-binding or DNA-binding domains of the androgen receptor protein.

● GENERAL REFERENCES

Gardner RJM, Sutherland GR: Chromosome Abnormalities and Genetic Counseling, 3rd ed. Oxford, England, Oxford University Press, 2004.

Grumbach MM, Hughes IA, Conte FA: Disorders of sex differentiation. In Larsen PR, Kronenberg HM, Melmed S, Polonsky KS (eds): Williams Textbook of Endocrinology, 10th ed. Philadelphia, WB Saunders, 2003, pp 842-1002.

Lupski JR, Stankiewicz P (eds): Genomic Disorders: The Genomic Basis of Disease. Totowa, NJ, Humana Press, 2006.

Moore KL, Persaud TVN: The Developing Human: Clinically Oriented Embryology, 7th ed. Philadelphia, WB Saunders, 2003.

Pinsky L, Erickson RP, Schimke RN: Genetic Disorders of Human Sexual Development. Oxford, England, Oxford University Press, 1999.

● REFERENCES FOR SPECIFIC TOPICS

Antonarakis SE, Lyle R, Dermitzakis ET, et al: Chromosome 21 and Down syndrome: from genomics to pathophysiology. Nat Rev Genet 5:725-738, 2004.

Carrel L, Willard HF: X inactivation profile reveals extensive variability in X-linked gene expression in females. Nature 434:400-404, 2005.

Fleming A, Vilain E: The endless quest for sex determination genes. Clin Genet 67:15-25, 2004.

Lamb NE, Yu K, Shaffer J, et al: Association between maternal age and meiotic recombination for trisomy 21. Am J Hum Genet 76:91-99, 2005.

Lupski JR, Stankiewicz P: Genomic disorders: molecular mechanisms for rearrangements and conveyed phenotypes. PLoS Genet 1:627-633, 2005.

McDermid HE, Morrow BE: Genomic disorders on 22q11. Am J Hum Genet 70:1077-1088, 2002.

McElreavey K, Ravel C, Chantot-Bastaraud S, Siffroi J-P: Y chromosome variants and male reproductive failure. Int J Androl 29:298-303, 2006.

O'Doherty A, Ruf S, Mulligan C, et al: An aneuploid mouse strain carrying human chromosome 21 with Down syndrome phenotypes. Science 309:2033-2037, 2005.

Pont SJ, Robbins JM, Bird TM, et al: Congenital malformations among liveborn infants with trisomies 18 and 13. Am J Med Genet 140:1749-1756, 2006.

Ratcliffe SG, Paul N (eds): Prospective studies on children with sex chromosome aneuploidy. March of Dimes Birth Defects Foundation, Birth Defects Original Article Series, vol 22. New York, Alan R. Liss, 1986.

Ropers H-H: X-linked mental retardation: many genes for a complex disorder. Curr Opin Genet Dev 16:260-269, 2006.

Rovert J, Netley C, Bailey J, et al: Intelligence and achievement in children with extra X aneuploidy: a longitudinal perspective. Am J Med Genet 60:356-363, 1995.

Sybert VP, McCauley E: Turner's syndrome. N Engl J Med 351:1227-1238, 2004.

Toniolo D: X-linked premature ovarian failure: a complex disease. Curr Opin Genet Dev 16:293-300, 2006.

Zhang X, Snijders A, Segraves R, et al: High-resolution mapping of genotype-phenotype relationships in cri du chat syndrome using array comparative genome hybridization. Am J Hum Genet 76:312-326, 2005.

PROBLEMS

1. In a woman with a 47,XXX karyotype, what types of gametes would theoretically be formed and in what proportions? What are the *theoretical* karyotypes and phenotypes of her progeny? What are the *actual* karyotypes and phenotypes of her progeny?

2. One of your patients is a girl with severe hemophilia A, an X-linked inherited disorder typically seen only in males.
   a. You are advised to arrange for chromosome analysis of this child. Why? What mechanisms can allow the occurrence of an X-linked phenotype in a female?
   b. The laboratory reports that the child has an X;autosome translocation, with a breakpoint in the X chromosome at Xq28. How could this explain her phenotype?

3. The birth incidence rates of 47,XXY and 47,XYY males are approximately equal. Is this what you would expect on the basis of the possible origins of the two abnormal karyotypes? Explain.

4. How can a person with an XX karyotype differentiate as a phenotypically normal male?

5. A baby girl presents with bilateral inguinal masses that are thought to be hernias but are found to be testes in the inguinal canals. What karyotype would you expect to find in the child? What is her disorder? What genetic counseling would you offer to the parents?

6. A baby girl with ambiguous genitalia is found to have 21-hydroxylase deficiency of the salt-wasting type. What karyotype would you expect to find? What is

the disorder? What genetic counseling would you offer to the parents?

7. What are the expected clinical consequences of the following deletions? If the same amount of DNA is deleted in each case, why might the severity of each be different?
   a. 46,XX,del(13)(pter→p11.1:)
   b. 46,XY,del(Y)(pter→q12:)
   c. 46,XX,del(5)(p15)
   d. 46,XX,del(X)(q23q26)

8. Discuss the clinical consequences of X chromosome inactivation. Provide possible explanations for the fact that persons with X chromosome aneuploidy are clinically not completely normal.

9. In genetics clinic, you are counseling five pregnant women who inquire about their risk of having a Down syndrome fetus. What are their risks and why?
   a. a 23-year-old mother of a previous trisomy 21 child
   b. a 41-year-old mother of a previous trisomy 21 child
   c. a 27-year-old woman whose niece has Down syndrome
   d. a carrier of a 14;21 Robertsonian translocation
   e. a woman whose husband is a carrier of a 14;21 Robertsonian translocation

10. A young girl with Down syndrome is karyotyped and found to carry a 21q21q translocation. With use of standard cytogenetic nomenclature, what is her karyotype?

Chapter 7

Patterns of Single-Gene Inheritance

In Chapter 1, the three main categories of genetic disorders—single-gene, chromosomal, and complex—were briefly characterized. In this chapter, the typical patterns of transmission of single-gene disorders are discussed in further detail; the emphasis is on the molecular and genetic mechanisms by which mutations in genes result in recessive, dominant, X-linked, and mitochondrial inheritance patterns. In the next chapter, we go on to describe more complex patterns of inheritance, including multifactorial disorders that result from the interaction between variants at multiple loci and environmental factors to cause disease.

Single-gene traits caused by mutations in genes in the nuclear genome are often called **mendelian** because, like the characteristics of garden peas studied by Gregor Mendel, they occur on average in fixed proportions among the offspring of specific types of matings. The single-gene diseases known so far are listed in Victor A. McKusick's classic reference, *Mendelian Inheritance in Man,* which has been indispensable to medical geneticists for decades. The online version of *Mendelian Inheritance in Man* (OMIM), available on the Internet through the National Library of Medicine, currently lists more than 3917 diseases with mendelian patterns of inheritance. Of these, 3310, or about 84%, are known to be caused by mutations in 1990 genes. The number of diseases with known genetic causes and the number of genes in which mutations can cause disease are not the same because different mutations in the same gene can cause different diseases, and mutations in different genes can cause similar or indistinguishable diseases. The remaining 16% of diseases in OMIM are diseases with clear mendelian inheritance patterns, but the mutant genes responsible are still unknown. Thus, of the approximately 25,000 human genes, about 8% have already been directly implicated in human genetic disease. This is probably a great underestimate. The pace at which geneticists are identifying genes with disease-causing alleles is high, and it appears certain to accelerate because of the powerful new tools made available through the Human Genome Project.

As a whole, single-gene disorders are often considered to be primarily but by no means exclusively disorders of the pediatric age range; less than 10% manifest after puberty, and only 1% occur after the end of the reproductive period. Although individually rare, as a group they are responsible for a significant proportion of childhood diseases and deaths. In a population study of more than 1 million live births, the incidence of serious single-gene disorders was estimated to be 0.36%; among hospitalized children, 6% to 8% are thought to have single-gene disorders. Mendelian disorders are important to consider in adult medicine as well. A survey of OMIM for mendelian forms of 17 of the most common adult diseases, such as heart disease, stroke, cancer, and diabetes, revealed nearly 200 mendelian disorders whose phenotypes included these common adult illnesses. Although by no means the major contributory factor in causing these common diseases in the population at large, the mendelian forms are important in individual patients because of their significance for the health of other family members and because of the availability of genetic testing and detailed management options for many of them.

● OVERVIEW AND CONCEPTS

Even though the principles of medical genetics are easy to understand, the unfamiliar terminology may make the subject seem inaccessible at first. To help address the language problem, we review some terms and introduce others that have not been defined previously.

Variation in Genes

Inherited variation in the genome is the cornerstone of human and medical genetics. As described in Chapter 2, a segment of DNA occupying a particular position or location on a chromosome is a **locus.** If the segment contains a gene, that DNA segment is the locus for that gene. Alternative variants of a gene are called **alleles.** For many genes, there is a single prevailing allele, present in the majority of individuals, that geneticists call the **wild-type** or common allele. The other versions of the gene are **variant** or **mutant** alleles that differ from the wild-type allele because of the presence of a **mutation,** a permanent change in the nucleotide sequence or arrangement of DNA. A given set of alleles at a locus or cluster of loci on a chromosome is referred to as a **haplotype.**

Variant alleles arose by mutation at some time in the recent or remote past. If there are at least two relatively common alleles at the locus in the population, the locus is said to exhibit **polymorphism** (literally "many forms"), as is discussed in detail in subsequent chapters. In addition to a normal allele or to common polymorphic alleles, loci may also have one or more rare, variant alleles. Some of these rare alleles were originally identified because they cause genetic disease; others may increase susceptibility to disease, and yet others are of no known significance to health.

The term **mutation** is used in medical genetics in two senses: sometimes to indicate a new genetic change that has not been previously known in a family, and sometimes merely to indicate a disease-causing mutant allele. Mutation and mutant, however, are never used to refer to the human beings who carry mutant alleles.

Genotype and Phenotype

The **genotype** of a person is the set of alleles that make up his or her genetic constitution, either collectively at all loci or, more typically, at a single locus. In contrast, the **phenotype** is the observable expression of a genotype as a morphological, clinical, cellular, or biochemical trait. The phenotype is usually thought of as the presence or absence of a disease, but phenotype can refer to any manifestation, including characteristics that can be detected only by blood or tissue testing. A phenotype may, of course, be either normal or abnormal in a given individual, but in this book, which emphasizes disorders of medical significance, the focus is on abnormal phenotypes—that is, genetic disorders. Although each gene usually encodes a polypeptide chain or RNA molecule, a single abnormal gene or gene pair often produces multiple diverse phenotypic effects and determines which organ systems are involved, which particular signs and symptoms occur, and when

they occur. Under these circumstances, the expression of the gene defect is said to be **pleiotropic.** At present, for many pleiotropic disorders, the connection between the gene defect and the various manifestations is neither obvious nor well understood.

A **single-gene disorder** is one that is determined primarily by the alleles at a single locus. When a person has a pair of identical alleles at a locus encoded in nuclear DNA, he or she is said to be **homozygous** (a **homozygote**); when the alleles are different, he or she is **heterozygous** (a **heterozygote** or **carrier**). The term **compound heterozygote** is used to describe a genotype in which two different mutant alleles of the same gene are present, rather than one normal and one mutant. These terms (homozygous, heterozygous, and compound heterozygous) can be applied either to a person or to a genotype. In the special case in which a male has an abnormal allele for a gene located on the X chromosome and there is no other copy of the gene, he is neither homozygous nor heterozygous and is referred to as **hemizygous.** Mitochondrial DNA is still another special case. In contrast to the two copies of each gene per diploid cell, mitochondrial DNA molecules, and the genes encoded by the mitochondrial genome, are present in tens to thousands of copies per cell (see Chapter 2). For this reason, the terms homozygous, heterozygous, and hemizygous are not used to describe genotypes at mitochondrial loci.

Pedigrees

Single-gene disorders are characterized by their patterns of transmission in families. To establish the pattern of transmission, a usual first step is to obtain information about the family history of the patient and to summarize the details in the form of a **pedigree,** a graphical representation of the family tree, with use of standard symbols (Fig. 7-1). The extended family depicted in such pedigrees is a **kindred** (Fig. 7-2). The member through whom a family with a genetic disorder is first brought to the attention of the geneticist (i.e., is ascertained) is the **proband** (synonyms: **propositus** or **index case**) if he or she is affected. The person who brings the family to attention by consulting a geneticist is referred to as the **consultand;** the consultand may be an affected individual or an unaffected relative of a proband. A family may have more than one proband, if they are ascertained through more than one source. Brothers and sisters are called **sibs,** and a family of sibs forms a **sibship.** Relatives are classified as **first degree** (parents, sibs, and offspring of the proband), **second degree** (grandparents and grandchildren, uncles and aunts, nephews and nieces, and half-sibs), **third degree** (e.g., first cousins), and so forth, depending on the number of steps in the pedigree between the two relatives. The offspring of first cousins are second cousins,

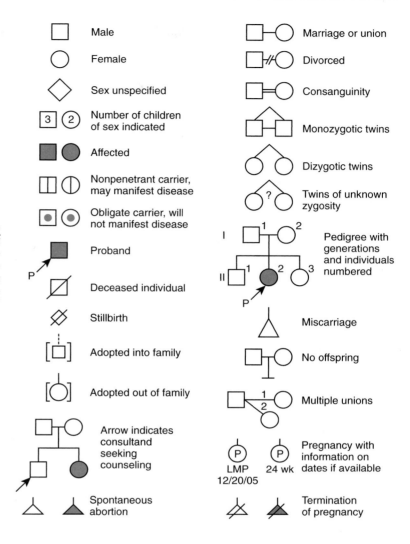

Figure 7-1 ■ Symbols commonly used in pedigree charts. Although there is no uniform system of pedigree notation, the symbols used here are according to recent recommendations made by professionals in the field of genetic counseling. (From Bennett RL, Steinhaus KA, Uhrich SB, et al: Recommendations for standardized pedigree nomenclature. J Genet Counsel 4:267-279, 1995.)

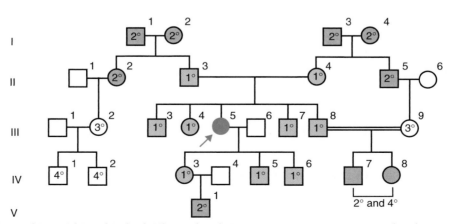

Figure 7-2 ■ Relationships within a kindred. The proband, III-5 *(arrow),* represents an isolated case of a genetic disorder. She has four siblings, III-3, III-4, III-7, and III-8. Her partner/spouse is III-6, and they have three children (their F1 progeny). The proband has nine first-degree relatives (her parents, siblings, and offspring), nine second-degree relatives (grandparents, uncles and aunts, nieces and nephews, and grandchildren), two third-degree relatives (first cousins), and four fourth-degree relatives (first cousins once removed). IV-3, IV-5, and IV-6 are second cousins of IV-1 and IV-2. IV-7 and IV-8, whose parents are consanguineous, are doubly related to the proband: second-degree relatives through their father and fourth-degree relatives through their mother.

and a child is a "first cousin once removed" of his or her parents' first cousins. Couples who have one or more ancestors in common are **consanguineous.** If there is only one affected member in a family, he or she is an **isolated** case or, if the disorder is determined to be due to new mutation in the propositus, a **sporadic** case (see Fig. 7-2). When there is a strong similarity of phenotype among different families with the same defect, well-established patterns of inheritance in other families with the same disorder can often be used as a basis for diagnosis and counseling even if the patient is an isolated case in the family. Thus, many patients with genetic disorders have no similarly affected relatives, but it may still be possible to recognize that the disorder is genetic.

In many disorders, whether or not a condition will demonstrate an obvious familial pattern of transmission in families depends on whether individuals affected by the disorder can reproduce. Geneticists coined the term **fitness** as a measure of the impact of a condition on reproduction. Fitness is defined as the number of offspring individuals affected with the condition can have who survive to reproductive age, in comparison with an appropriate control group. Fitness is *not* a measure of physical or mental disability. For example, in some disorders, an affected individual can have normal mental capacities and health but yet have a fitness of 0 because the condition interferes with normal reproduction. In other cases, a severe, debilitating genetic disorder may have normal fitness because the onset of the disease is well past the usual reproductive age.

● MENDELIAN INHERITANCE

The patterns shown by single-gene disorders in pedigrees depend chiefly on two factors:

1. whether the phenotype is **dominant** (expressed when only one chromosome of a pair carries the mutant allele and the other chromosome has a wild-type allele at that locus) or **recessive** (expressed only when both chromosomes of a pair carry mutant alleles at a locus); and
2. the chromosomal location of the gene locus, which may be on an **autosome** (chromosomes 1 to 22) or on a sex chromosome (chromosomes X and Y).

It is necessary, however, to distinguish between genes that are physically located on the sex chromosomes (X or Y **synteny**) and genes that show **X-linked** (or **Y-linked**) inheritance. The majority of loci on the X show X-linked inheritance because they participate in meiotic recombination only during female gametogenesis, when there are two X chromosomes, but cannot recombine with the Y during male gametogenesis. There are,

however, a small number of genes (referred to as **pseudoautosomal** loci, discussed subsequently in this chapter) located on the X chromosome that do not show X-linked inheritance because they *can* recombine with counterparts on the Y chromosome. Thus, there are four basic patterns of single-gene inheritance (if we group autosomal and pseudoautosomal patterns together):

	Dominant	Recessive
Autosomal	Autosomal dominant	Autosomal recessive
X-linked	X-linked dominant	X-linked recessive

In addition to these classic pedigree patterns seen with disease-causing alleles at loci on the chromosomes located in the nucleus, another class of disorders with a distinctive maternal pattern of inheritance can be due to mutations in the mitochondrial genome (described later in this chapter).

Autosomal and X-Linked Inheritance

Whether an abnormal gene is on an autosome or is X-linked has a profound effect on the clinical expression of the disease. First, autosomal disorders, in general, affect males and females equally. (The only exceptions are referred to as sex-limited disorders, discussed later in the chapter.) For X-linked disorders, the situation is quite different. Males have only a single X and are therefore hemizygous with respect to X-linked genes; 46,XY males are never heterozygous for alleles at X-linked loci, whereas females can be heterozygous or homozygous at X-linked loci. Second, to compensate for the double complement of X-linked genes in females, alleles for most X-linked genes are expressed from only one of the two X chromosomes in any given cell of a female (as described in Chapter 6).

Dominant and Recessive Inheritance

Recessive Inheritance

As classically defined, a phenotype expressed only in homozygotes (or, for X-linked traits, male hemizygotes) and not in heterozygotes is recessive. Most of the recessive disorders described to date are due to mutations that reduce or eliminate the function of the gene product, so-called **loss-of-function** mutations. For example, many recessive diseases are caused by mutations that impair or eliminate the function of an enzyme. These are usually inherited as recessive diseases because heterozygotes, with only one of a pair of alleles functioning and the other (abnormal) allele not, can typically make sufficient product (~50% of the amount made by wild-type homozygotes) to carry out the enzymatic reaction required for normal physiological function, thereby preventing disease (see Chapter 12).

Dominant Inheritance

In contrast, a phenotype expressed in both homozygotes and heterozygotes for a mutant allele is inherited as a dominant. Dominant disorders occur whether or not there is normal gene product made from the remaining normal allele. In a **pure dominant** disease, homozygotes and heterozygotes for the mutant allele are both affected equally. Pure dominant disorders rarely if ever exist in medical genetics. On occasion, phenotypic expression of two different alleles for a locus occurs, in which case the two alleles are termed **codominant.** One well-known example of codominant expression is the ABO blood group system (see Chapter 9). Most commonly, dominant disorders are more severe in homozygotes than in heterozygotes, in which case the disease is called **incompletely dominant** (or **semidominant**). The different molecular mechanisms to explain why certain mutations produce a dominantly rather than recessively inherited disease are discussed in Chapter 12.

Strictly speaking, it is the inheritance of a phenotype rather than the allele that is dominant or recessive. However, mutant alleles are often referred to as dominant or recessive on the basis of whether they can cause a change in phenotype in the heterozygous or homozygous state, respectively. Consequently, the terms *dominant allele or gene* and *recessive allele or gene* are widely, albeit loosely, used.

● FACTORS AFFECTING PEDIGREE PATTERNS

Penetrance and Expressivity

Many genetic conditions segregate sharply within families; that is, the abnormal phenotype can be readily distinguished from the normal one. In clinical experience, however, some disorders are not expressed at all in an individual despite his having the same genotype that causes the disorder in others in his family. In others, the same disorder may have extremely variable expression in terms of clinical severity, the range of symptoms, or age at onset. Phenotypic expression of an abnormal genotype may be modified by the effects of aging, other genetic loci, or the effects of environment. These differences in expression can often lead to difficulties in diagnosis and pedigree interpretation. There are two distinct ways in which such differences in expression can occur: reduced penetrance and variable expressivity.

Penetrance is the probability that a gene will have any phenotypic expression at all. When the frequency of expression of a phenotype is less than 100%—that is, when some of those who have the appropriate genotype completely fail to express it—the gene is said to show **reduced penetrance.** Penetrance is an all-or-none concept. It is the percentage of people with a predisposing genotype who are actually affected, at least to some degree.

Expressivity is the severity of expression of the phenotype among individuals with the same disease-causing genotype. When the severity of disease differs in people who have the same genotype, the phenotype is said to have **variable expressivity.** Even in the same kindred, two individuals carrying the same mutant genes may have some signs and symptoms in common, whereas their other disease manifestations may be quite different, depending on which tissues or organs happen to be affected.

Some of the difficulties raised by age-dependent penetrance and variable expressivity in understanding the inheritance of a disease phenotype are demonstrated by the autosomal dominant disease **neurofibromatosis** (NF1) (Case 29). NF1 is a common disorder of the nervous system, the eye, and the skin that occurs in approximately 1 in 3500 births. There is no significant variation in disease frequency among different ethnic groups. A typical clinical presentation is shown in Figure 7-3. NF1 is characterized by growth of multiple benign fleshy tumors, neurofibromas, in the skin; presence of multiple flat, irregular pigmented skin lesions known as café au lait spots; growth of small benign tumors (hamartomas) called Lisch nodules on the iris of the eye; and less frequently, mental retardation, central nervous system tumors, diffuse plexiform

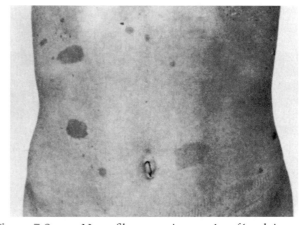

Figure 7-3 ■ Neurofibromatosis, type 1: café au lait spots, hyperpigmented spots on the skin, are a useful diagnostic sign in family members who otherwise may appear unaffected. Most patients have six or more spots at least 15 mm in diameter, usually on the trunk. (Courtesy of Rosanna Weksberg, The Hospital for Sick Children, Toronto, Canada.)

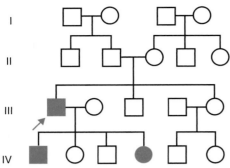

Figure 7-4 ■ Pedigree of family with neurofibromatosis, type 1, apparently originating as a new mutation in the proband of generation III *(arrow)*. This individual appears to have a new mutant allele of *NF1* because his parents and their parents are all unaffected.

neurofibromas, and the development of cancer of the nervous system or muscle. Thus, the condition has a pleiotropic phenotype.

NF1 was first fully described by the physician von Recklinghausen in 1882, but the disease has probably been known since ancient times. Although adult heterozygotes almost always demonstrate some sign of the disease (penetrance is therefore said to be 100% in adults), some may have only café au lait spots, freckles on the axillary skin, and Lisch nodules, whereas others may have life-threatening benign tumors involving the spinal cord or malignant sarcomas of an extremity. Thus, there is variable expressivity; even within a kindred, some individuals are severely affected and others only mildly so. Diagnosis is further complicated in children because the signs develop gradually during childhood. For example, in the newborn period, less than half of all affected newborns show even the most subtle sign of the disease, an increased incidence of café au lait spots. Penetrance, therefore, is age dependent.

Many different mutations have been found in the *NF1* gene, all of which appear to cause loss of function of its gene product, neurofibromin. Approximately half the cases of NF1 result from a new rather than an inherited mutation (Fig. 7-4).

The chief genetic problem in counseling families of patients with NF1 is to decide between two equally likely possibilities: Is the disease in the proband sporadic, that is, due to new mutation, or has the patient inherited a clinically significant form of the disorder from a parent in whom the gene is present but only mildly expressed? If the proband has inherited the defect, the risk that any of his or her sibs will also inherit it is 50%; but if the proband has a new mutant gene, there is very little risk that any sib will be affected. Significantly, in either case, the risk that the patient will pass the gene on to any one of his or her offspring is 50%. In view of these uncertainties, it is reassuring to families of patients with NF1 to know that the disorder

can be detected presymptomatically and even prenatally by molecular genetic analysis (see Chapter 17). Unfortunately, molecular testing can generally only answer whether the condition will occur and not how severe it will be. Except for the association of complete gene deletions with dysmorphic features, mental retardation, and increased number of neurofibromas at an early age, there is no correlation between severity of the phenotype and particular mutant *NF1* alleles.

Another example of an autosomal dominant malformation with reduced penetrance is the **split-hand deformity,** a type of ectrodactyly (Fig. 7-5). The malformation originates in the sixth or seventh week of development, when the hands and feet are forming. The disorder demonstrates locus heterogeneity, with at least five loci recognized, although the actual gene responsible has been identified in only a few. Failure of penetrance in pedigrees of split-hand malformation can lead to apparent skipping of generations, and this complicates genetic counseling because an at-risk person with normal hands may nevertheless carry the gene for the condition and thus be capable of having children who are affected.

Figure 7-6 is a pedigree of split-hand deformity in which the unaffected person is the **consultand** (the person who asks for genetic counseling). Her mother is a nonpenetrant carrier of the split-hand mutation. Review of the literature on split-hand deformity suggests that there is reduced penetrance of about 70% (i.e., only 70% of the people who have the gene exhibit the defect). Using this information in Bayesian analysis, a mathematical method for determining conditional probabilities in pedigrees (see further discussion in Chapter 19), one can calculate the risk that the consultand might have a child with the abnormality.

Age at Onset

Genetic disorders can appear at any time in the lifetime of an individual, ranging from early in intrauterine development all the way to the postreproductive years, and all ages in between. Some may be lethal prenatally, whereas others may interfere with normal fetal development and can be recognized prenatally (e.g., by ultrasonography; see Chapter 15) but are consistent with a full-liveborn infant; still others may be recognized only at birth (**congenital**). (The terms *genetic* and *congenital* are frequently confused. Keep in mind that a genetic disorder is one that is determined by genes, whereas a congenital disorder is merely one that is present at birth and may or may not have a genetic basis.) Thus, in a pedigree of a family with a lethal disorder affecting a fetus early in pregnancy, the pattern of disease occurrence may be obscure because all that one observes are multiple miscarriages and fetal losses or apparently reduced fertility, rather than recurrence of the prenatal

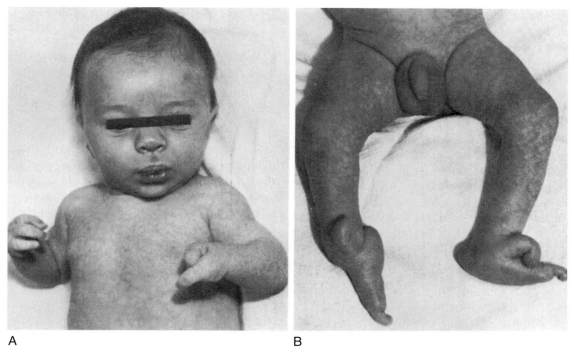

A   B

Figure 7-5 ■ Split-hand deformity, an autosomal dominant trait involving the hands and feet, in a 3-month-old boy. **A,** Upper part of body. **B,** Lower part of body. (From Kelikian H: Congenital Deformities of the Hand and Forearm. Philadelphia, WB Saunders, 1974.)

disease itself. Conversely, in a family with a late-onset dominant disorder, an affected individual may have parents and children reportedly free of disease because the carrier parent died of unrelated causes before the disease could develop, and the children at risk have not reached the age at which the mutant gene reveals itself in a disease phenotype.

Other Factors Affecting Pedigree Patterns

Although as a general rule pedigrees of single-gene disorders can be readily classified as autosomal or X-linked and as dominant or recessive, the inheritance pattern of an individual pedigree may be obscured by

a number of other factors that may make the mode of inheritance difficult to interpret. Diagnostic difficulties may be due to reduced penetrance or variable expressivity of the disease; other genes and environmental factors may affect gene expression; persons of some genotypes may fail to survive to the time of birth; accurate information about the presence of the disorder in relatives or about family relationships may be lacking; the occurrence of new mutations can contribute to the occurrence of dominant and X-linked disease; and finally, with the small family size typical of most developed countries today, the patient may by chance alone be the only affected family member, making determination of any inheritance pattern very difficult.

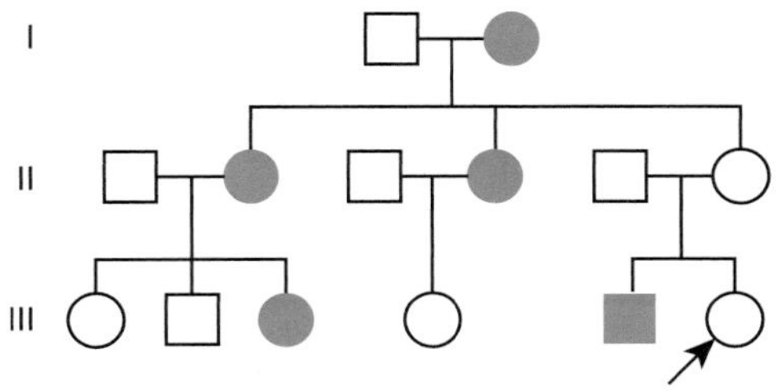

○ CORRELATING GENOTYPE AND PHENOTYPE

An important component of medical genetics is identifying and characterizing the genotypes responsible for particular disease phenotypes. It is important not to adhere to an overly simplistic view of the relationship between single-gene mutations and disease phenotypes. When a genetic disorder that appears to be inherited as a single-gene disorder is thoroughly analyzed, it is frequently found to be genetically heterogeneous; that is, it includes a number of phenotypes that are similar but

Figure 7-6 ■ Pedigree of split-hand deformity demonstrating failure of penetrance in the mother of the consultand *(arrow).* Reduced penetrance must be taken into account in genetic counseling.

are actually determined by different genotypes at different loci. **Genetic heterogeneity** may be the result of different mutations at the same locus (**allelic heterogeneity**), mutations at different loci (**locus heterogeneity**), or both (see Chapter 12). Recognition of genetic heterogeneity is an important aspect of clinical diagnosis and genetic counseling. On the other hand, distinct phenotypes inherited in different families can result from different mutant alleles in the same gene. This phenomenon, known as **clinical** or **phenotypic heterogeneity,** is well known and must be taken into account in correlating genotype and phenotype.

Allelic Heterogeneity

Allelic heterogeneity is an important cause of clinical variation. Many loci possess more than one mutant allele; in fact, at a given locus, there may be several or many mutations. As one example, nearly 1400 different mutations have been found worldwide in the **cystic fibrosis** transmembrane conductance regulator (CFTR) among patients with cystic fibrosis (see Chapter 12) (Case 10). Sometimes, these different mutations result in clinically indistinguishable disorders. In other cases, different mutant alleles at the same locus produce a similar phenotype but along a continuum of severity; for example, some CFTR mutations cause patients to have classic cystic fibrosis with pancreatic insufficiency, severe progressive lung disease, and congenital absence of the vas deferens in males, whereas patients carrying other mutant alleles have lung disease but normal pancreatic function, and still others have only the abnormality of the male reproductive tract.

Since any particular mutant allele is generally uncommon in the population, most people with rare autosomal recessive disorders are compound heterozygotes rather than true homozygotes. Because different allelic combinations may have somewhat different clinical consequences, clinicians must be aware of allelic heterogeneity as one possible explanation for variability among patients considered to have the same disease. There are, however, some well-recognized exceptions to the observation that compound heterozygotes are more common than true homozygotes. The first is when the affected individuals inherited the same mutant allele from consanguineous parents, who both carry the same mutant allele they inherited from a common ancestor. Second, one mutant allele may be responsible for a large proportion of the cases of an autosomal recessive condition in a particular ethnic group, and so many patients from that group will be homozygous for this allele. The third is when the disorder normally has little if any allelic heterogeneity because the disease phenotype caused by a particular mutation is specific to that mutation (e.g., **sickle cell disease;** see Chapter 11) (Case 37).

Locus Heterogeneity

For many phenotypes, pedigree analysis alone has been sufficient to demonstrate locus heterogeneity. For example, **retinitis pigmentosa,** a common cause of visual impairment due to photoreceptor degeneration, has long been known to occur in autosomal dominant, autosomal recessive, and X-linked forms. In recent years, the heterogeneity has been shown to be even more extensive; pedigree analysis combined with gene mapping has demonstrated that there are at least 43 loci responsible for 5 X-linked forms, 14 autosomal dominant forms, and 24 autosomal recessive forms of retinitis pigmentosa that are not associated with other phenotypic abnormalities. If one includes disorders in which retinitis pigmentosa is found in conjunction with other defects such as mental retardation or deafness, there are nearly 70 different genetic diseases manifesting retinitis pigmentosa.

Phenotypic Heterogeneity

Different mutations in the same gene can sometimes give rise to strikingly different phenotypes. For example, certain loss-of-function mutations in the *RET* gene, which encodes a receptor tyrosine kinase, can cause dominantly inherited failure of development of colonic ganglia, leading to defective colonic motility and severe chronic constipation (**Hirschsprung disease;** see Chapter 8) (Case 20). Other mutations in the same gene result in unregulated hyperfunction of the kinase, leading to dominantly inherited cancer of the thyroid and adrenal glands (**multiple endocrine neoplasia type 2A and 2B;** see Chapter 16). A third group of mutations in *RET* causes both Hirschsprung disease and multiple endocrine neoplasia in the same individuals. A comparable situation occurs with the *LMNA* gene, which encodes lamin A/C, a nuclear membrane protein. Different *LMNA* mutations have been associated with half a dozen phenotypically distinct disorders, including Emery-Dreifuss muscular dystrophy, one form of hereditary dilated cardiomyopathy, one form of the Charcot-Marie-Tooth peripheral neuropathy, a disorder of normal adipose tissue called lipodystrophy, and the premature aging syndrome known as Hutchinson-Gifford progeria.

⊙ AUTOSOMAL PATTERNS OF MENDELIAN INHERITANCE

Autosomal Recessive Inheritance

Autosomal recessive disease occurs only in homozygotes or compound heterozygotes, individuals with two mutant alleles and no normal allele, because in these diseases, one normal gene copy is able to compensate for the mutant allele and prevent the disease from occurring. Because an individual inherits only one of the two alleles at any locus from one parent, homozygotes must have inherited a mutant allele from each parent (barring uniparental disomy or new mutation, which is rare in autosomal recessive disorders).

Three types of matings can lead to homozygous offspring affected with an autosomal recessive disease. The mutant recessive allele is symbolized as *r* and its normal dominant allele as *R*. Although any mating in which each parent has at least one recessive allele can produce homozygous affected offspring, the most common mating by far is between two unaffected heterozygotes.

Parental Mating	Offspring	Risk of Disease
Carrier by carrier $R/r \times R/r$	1/4 R/R, 1/2 R/r, 1/4 r/r	3/4 unaffected, 1/4 affected
Carrier by affected $R/r \times r/r$	1/2 R/r, 1/2 r/r	1/2 unaffected, 1/2 affected
Affected by affected $r/r \times r/r$	r/r only	All affected

When both parents of an affected person are heterozygotes (**carriers**), their children's risk of receiving a recessive allele is one half from each parent, and so the chance of inheriting two recessive alleles and therefore being affected is $1/2 \times 1/2$ or 1 in 4. The proband may be the only affected family member, but if any others are affected, they are usually in the same sibship and not elsewhere in the kindred (Fig. 7-7).

Sex-Influenced Disorders

Since males and females both have the same complement of autosomes, autosomal recessive disorders generally show the same frequency and severity in males and females. There are, however, exceptions. Some autosomal recessive phenotypes are sex-influenced, that is, expressed in both sexes but with different frequen-

cies or severity. Among autosomal disorders, **hemochromatosis** is an example of a phenotype more common in males (Case 17). This autosomal recessive disorder of iron metabolism occurs most commonly in the approximately 0.5% of individuals of northern European extraction that are homozygous for a missense mutation replacing cysteine at position 282 with a tyrosine (Cys282Tyr) in the *HFE* gene. Cys282Tyr homozygotes have enhanced absorption of dietary iron and often demonstrate laboratory abnormalities suggestive of excessive body stores of iron, although the condition only rarely leads to iron overload and serious damage to the heart, liver, and pancreas. The lower incidence of the clinical disorder in females (one fifth to one tenth that of males) is believed to be related, among other factors, to lower dietary intake of iron, lower alcohol usage, and increased iron loss through menstruation among females.

Gene Frequency and Carrier Frequency

The mutant alleles responsible for a recessive disorder are generally rare, and so most people will not have even one copy of the mutant allele. Among individuals with at least one copy of the mutant allele, however, the frequency of clinically unaffected heterozygotes with one normal allele and one mutant allele is always much greater than the frequency of affected individuals with two rare mutant alleles. (We discuss how to calculate actual carrier and disease frequencies in Chapter 9.) Because an autosomal recessive disorder must be inherited through *both* parents, the risk that any carrier will have an affected child depends partly on the chance that his or her mate is also a carrier of a mutant allele for the condition. Thus, knowledge of the carrier frequency of a disease is clinically important for genetic counseling.

The most common autosomal recessive disorder in white children is **cystic fibrosis** (CF), caused by mutations in the *CFTR* gene (see Chapter 12) (Case 10). CF is virtually unknown in Asian populations and is relatively rare in African American populations, but in white populations, about 1 child in 2000 has two

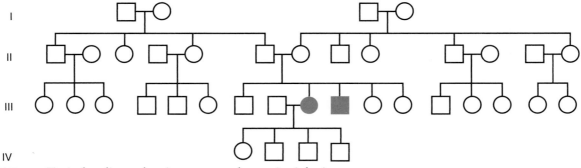

Figure 7-7 ■ Typical pedigree showing autosomal recessive inheritance.

mutant *CFTR* alleles and has the disease. The frequency of carriers for one of the hundreds of possible mutant *CFTR* alleles can be calculated to be approximately 1/29 (see Chapter 9). In a population of 3247 white individuals, therefore, you can expect 1 CF patient, 112 unaffected carriers of a *CFTR* mutation, and 3134 normal homozygotes. Because a patient has two mutant *CFTR* alleles and a carrier has only one, $(112 \times 1)/(112 \times 1 + 1 \times 2) = 112/114$ (about 98%) of all mutant *CFTR* alleles in this population of 3247 individuals are hidden in carriers (who usually are unaware that they are carriers), and only 2% are in patients.

Consanguinity

Because the majority of the mutant alleles responsible for autosomal recessive disorders are in carriers rather than in homozygotes, mutant alleles can be handed down in families for numerous generations without ever appearing in the homozygous state and causing overt disease. The presence of such hidden recessive genes is not revealed unless the carrier happens to mate with someone who also carries a mutant allele at the same locus and the two deleterious alleles are both inherited by a child. It is believed that everyone carries at least 8 to 10 mutant alleles, of which perhaps half are lethal in homozygotes before birth. The remainder cause well-known, easily recognizable autosomal recessive disorders in homozygotes. This is, however, a minimal estimate that does not take into account mutant alleles that exert their effect by interacting with mutant alleles at other loci (**multifactorial inheritance;** see Chapter 8).

The chance that both parents are carriers of a mutant allele at the same locus is increased substantially if the parents are related and could each have inherited the mutant allele from a single common ancestor, a situation called **consanguinity.** Consanguinity is defined arbitrarily as a union of individuals related to each other as close as or closer than second cousins. Consanguinity of the parents of a patient with a genetic disorder is strong evidence (although not proof) for the autosomal recessive inheritance of that condition. For example, the disorder in the pedigree in Figure 7-8 is likely to be an autosomal recessive trait, even though other information in the pedigree may seem insufficient to establish this inheritance pattern.

The genetic risk to the offspring of marriages between related people is not as great as is sometimes imagined. For marriages between first cousins, the absolute risks of abnormal offspring, including not only known autosomal recessive diseases but also stillbirth, neonatal death, and congenital malformations, is 3% to 5%, about double the overall background risk of 2% to 3% for offspring born to any unrelated couple (see Chapter 19). Consanguinity at the level of third cousins or more remote relationships is not considered to be genetically significant, and the increased risk of abnormal offspring is negligible in such cases.

Although the incidence of cousin marriage is low (~1 to 10 per 1000) in many populations in Western societies today, it remains relatively common in some ethnic groups, for example, in families from rural areas of the Indian subcontinent, in other parts of Asia, and in the Middle East, where between 20% and 60% of all marriages are between cousins. In general, however, the frequency of first-cousin marriages, and consanguinity in general, is declining in many traditional societies.

Consanguinity is not the most common explanation for an autosomal recessive trait. The mating of unrelated persons, each of whom happens by chance to be a carrier, accounts for most cases of autosomal recessive disease, particularly if a recessive trait has a high frequency in the population. Thus, most affected persons with a relatively common disorder, such as CF, are *not* the result of consanguinity, because the mutant allele is so common in the general population. However, consanguinity is more frequently found in the background of patients with very rare conditions. For example, in **xeroderma pigmentosum** (Case 43), a very rare autosomal recessive condition of DNA repair (see Chapter 16), more than 20% of cases occur among the offspring of marriages between first cousins.

The Measurement of Consanguinity

The measurement of consanguinity is relevant in medical genetics because the risk of a child's being homozygous for a rare recessive allele is proportional to how related the parents are. Some types of consanguineous mating carry an increased risk (Fig. 7-9).

Consanguinity is measured by the **coefficient of inbreeding** (F), the probability that a homozygote has received both alleles at a locus from the same ancestral

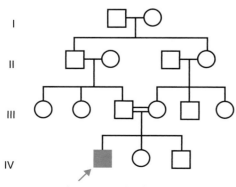

Figure 7-8 ■ Pedigree in which parental consanguinity suggests autosomal recessive inheritance.

Table 7-1

Consanguineous Matings

Type	Degree of Relationship	Proportion of Genes in Common	Coefficient of Inbreeding of Child (F)
Monozygotic twins	NA	1	NA
Parent-child	1st	1/2	1/4
Brother-sister (including dizygotic twins)	1st	1/2	1/4
Brother–half sister	2nd	1/4	1/8
Uncle-niece or aunt-nephew	2nd	1/4	1/8
Half uncle–niece	3rd	1/8	1/16
First cousins	3rd	1/8	1/16
Double first cousins	2nd	1/4	1/8
Half first cousins	4th	1/16	1/32
First cousins once removed	4th	1/16	1/32
Second cousins	5th	1/32	1/64

Coefficients of inbreeding for the offspring of a number of consanguineous matings. If a person is inbred through more than one line of descent, the separate coefficients are summed to find his or her total coefficient of inbreeding. NA, not applicable

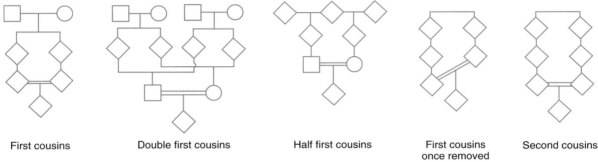

First cousins   Double first cousins   Half first cousins   First cousins once removed   Second cousins

Figure 7-9 ■ Types of consanguineous mating. The probability that the offspring in each of these matings is homozygous by descent at any one locus is equal to the coefficient of inbreeding, F.

source; it is also the proportion of loci at which a person is homozygous for an allele from the same ancestral source, a situation referred to as **identity by descent.** In Figure 7-10, individual IV-1 is the offspring of a first-cousin mating. Each of the four alleles at locus A (A^1, A^2, A^3, and A^4) in generation I has a $1/8 \times 1/8 = 1/64$ chance of being homozygous in IV-1; thus, the

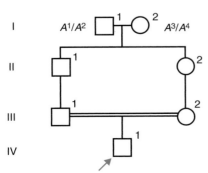

Figure 7-10 ■ A cousin marriage, used in the text to demonstrate how to calculate the coefficient of inbreeding, F, of the child IV-1.

probability that IV-1 is homozygous for *any* one of the four alleles is $4 \times 1/64 = 1/16$. Table 7-1 shows the coefficients of inbreeding for the offspring of a number of consanguineous matings. If a person is inbred through more than one line of descent, the separate coefficients are summed to find his or her total coefficient of inbreeding. (See Problem 7 at the end of the chapter.)

Genetic counseling for the risk of birth defects and genetic disease in the children of consanguineous matings is discussed in Chapter 19.

Inbreeding

Inbreeding is closely related to consanguinity. Inbreeding describes the situation in which individuals from a small population tend to choose their mates from within the same population for cultural, geographical, or religious reasons. In this situation, the parents may consider themselves unrelated but still may have common ancestry within the past few generations. Just as with consanguinity, inbreeding increases the chance that individuals will be homozygous for an allele inherited from a common ancestor. Thus, in taking a family history, it is important to ask not only about consanguinity but also about the geographical origins of ancestors, especially if a couple seeking counseling is of similar ethnic or geographical origin. As with consanguineous matings, it is possible to estimate a coefficient of inbreeding for individuals in a population even if they are not known to be related to each other.

Although we make a distinction between consanguinity occurring within a family and inbreeding, which occurs between unrelated individuals from the same small ethnic group, an increased risk for mating between heterozygous carriers of autosomal recessive disorders exists in both situations.

Rare Recessive Disorders in Genetic Isolates

There are many small groups in which the frequency of certain rare recessive genes is greater than that in the general population. Such groups, genetic **isolates,** may have become separated from their neighbors by geographical, religious, or linguistic barriers. Although such populations are not consanguineous, the chance of mating with another carrier of a particular recessive condition may be as high as that observed in cousin marriages.

Tay-Sachs disease (GM_2 gangliosidosis) is an example of an autosomal recessive disease with increased frequency in certain genetic isolates (Case 38). The disease is a neurological degenerative disorder that develops when a child is about 6 months old. Affected children become blind and regress mentally and physically (see Chapter 12). The disease is fatal in early childhood. Among Ashkenazi Jews in North America, for example, Tay-Sachs disease is 100 times more frequent (1 in 3600) than in other groups of European ancestry. This increased disease frequency is because the Tay-Sachs carrier frequency among Ashkenazi Jews, approximately 1 in 30, is 10-fold higher than in similar non-Ashkenazi European populations (calculated as described in Chapter 9).

When the mutant alleles causing a recessive disease are relatively frequent in a particular population, unrelated spouses have a reasonable chance of both being heterozygous, and therefore consanguinity is generally not a striking feature in the families with affected children. For example, among Ashkenazi Jews, the parents of children with Tay-Sachs disease are usually not closely related. When the mutant allele is rare, however, the frequency of carriers is very low and consanguinity is often the explanation for how both members of a couple came to be heterozygotes. For example, consanguinity is often present in the parents of Tay-Sachs patients in the population of French ancestry in Quebec, Canada, where mutant alleles for Tay-Sachs disease are rare.

••• Characteristics of Autosomal Recessive Inheritance

- An autosomal recessive phenotype, if it appears in more than one member of a kindred, typically is seen only in the sibship of the proband, not in parents, offspring, or other relatives.
- For most autosomal recessive diseases, males and females are equally likely to be affected.
- Parents of an affected child are asymptomatic carriers of mutant alleles.
- The parents of the affected person may in some cases be consanguineous. This is especially likely if the gene responsible for the condition is rare in the population.
- The recurrence risk for each sib of the proband is 1 in 4.

New Mutation in Autosomal Recessive Disorders

When a child is affected with an autosomal recessive condition, the assumption is generally made that both parents are heterozygous carriers for the condition (see Box). Yet, new mutations occur all the time during the generation of gametes (see Chapter 9). Might not an individual have two mutant alleles for an autosomal recessive condition by virtue of inheriting one mutant allele from a carrier parent while the other mutant allele arose de novo in a gamete that came from a parent who was not a carrier? Such a situation is, of course, not impossible but is relatively unlikely compared with the situation in which both parents are heterozygous carriers. This is because the chance that the gamete from a noncarrier parent had acquired a mutant allele by spontaneous mutation ranges from 1 in 10^5 to 1 in 10^6 (see Chapter 9), which is thousands of times less likely than the typical 1 in 20 to 1 in 1000 chance that the gamete contained the mutant allele because the parent is a heterozygous carrier. The relative unimportance of new mutations in autosomal recessive disease is in stark contrast to the situation with dominant and X-linked disorders, as will be discussed later in this chapter.

Autosomal Dominant Inheritance

More than half of all mendelian disorders are inherited as autosomal dominant traits. The incidence of some autosomal dominant disorders is high, at least in specific geographical areas: for example, 1 in 500 for **familial hypercholesterolemia** (Case 14) in populations of European or Japanese descent; 1 in 550 for myotonic dystrophy in the Charlevoix and Saguenay–Lac Saint Jean regions in northeastern Quebec; and about 1 in 2500 to 3000 for several conditions, such as Hunting-

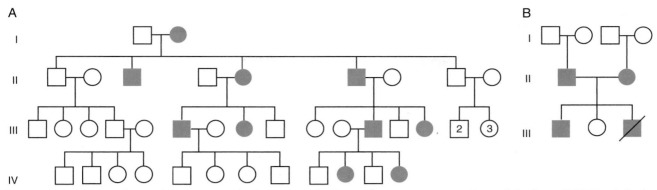

Figure 7-11 ■ **A,** Pedigree showing typical inheritance of a form of progressive sensorineural deafness (DFNA1) inherited as an autosomal dominant trait. **B,** Pedigree showing inheritance of achondroplasia, an incompletely dominant (or semidominant) trait.

ton disease (Case 22) in populations of northern European origin, neurofibromatosis (Case 29), and polycystic kidney disease (Case 32). Although many autosomal dominant disorders are individually much less common, they are so numerous in the aggregate that their total incidence is appreciable. The burden of autosomal dominant disorders is further increased because of their hereditary nature; when they are transmitted through families, they become problems not only for individuals but also for whole kindreds, often through many generations. In some cases, the burden is compounded by social difficulties resulting from physical or mental disability.

The risk and severity of dominantly inherited disease in the offspring depend on whether one or both parents are affected and whether the trait is strictly dominant or incompletely dominant. Denoting D as the mutant allele and d as the normal allele, matings that produce children with an autosomal dominant disease can be between two heterozygotes (D/d) for the mutation or, more frequently, between a heterozygote for the mutation (D/d) and a homozygote for a normal allele (d/d):

Parental Mating	Offspring	Risk to Offspring
Affected by unaffected $D/d \times d/d$	1/2 D/d, 1/2 d/d	1/2 affected 1/2 unaffected
Affected by affected $D/d \times D/d$	1/4 D/D, 1/2 D/d, 1/4 d/d	If strictly dominant: 3/4 affected 1/4 unaffected
		If incompletely dominant: 1/2 affected similarly to the parents 1/4 affected more severely than the parents 1/4 unaffected

Each child of a D/d by d/d mating has a 50% chance of receiving the affected parent's abnormal allele D and a 50% chance of receiving the normal allele d. In the population as a whole, the offspring of D/d by d/d parents are approximately 50% D/d and 50% d/d. Of course, each pregnancy is an independent event, not governed by the outcome of previous pregnancies. Thus, within a family, the distribution of affected and unaffected children may be quite different from the theoretical expected ratio of 1:1, especially if the sibship is small. Typical autosomal dominant inheritance can be seen in the pedigree of a family with a dominantly inherited form of hereditary deafness (Fig. 7-11A).

In medical practice, homozygotes for dominant phenotypes are not often seen because matings that could produce homozygous offspring are rare. Again denoting the mutant allele as D and the normal allele as d, the matings that can produce a D/D homozygote might theoretically be D/d by D/d, D/D by D/d, or D/D by D/D, or the patient might, in exceedingly rare instances, have received a new mutation from a genetically unaffected parent. Practically speaking, however, only the mating of two heterozygotes need be considered because D/D homozygotes are very rare and generally too severely affected to reproduce (fitness = 0). In the case of two heterozygotes mating, 3/4 of the offspring of a D/d by D/d mating will be affected to some extent and 1/4 unaffected. In theory, the 3/4 affected could all have the same condition if it is a pure dominant, or 1/3 of the affected would be homozygotes and much more severely affected than the D/d heterozygotes if it is an incompletely dominant condition. In fact, as mentioned earlier, no dominant human disorders have been clearly proved to be pure dominants. Even **Huntington disease**, which is the disorder most frequently claimed to be a pure dominant because the disease is generally similar in the nature and severity of symptoms in heterozygotes and homozygotes, appears to have a somewhat accelerated time course from the onset

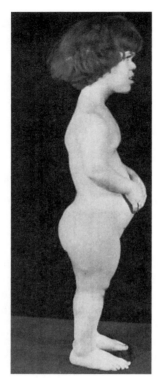

Figure 7-12 ■ Achondroplasia, an autosomal dominant disorder that often occurs as a new mutation. Note small stature with short limbs, large head, low nasal bridge, prominent forehead, and lumbar lordosis in this typical presentation. (From Tachdjian MO: Pediatric Orthopedics, vol 1. Philadelphia, WB Saunders, 1972, p 284.)

coronary heart disease (Case 14). In this disorder, the rare homozygous patients have a more severe disease, with an earlier age at onset and much shorter life expectancy, than do the relatively more common heterozygotes (Fig. 7-13).

New Mutation in Autosomal Dominant Inheritance

In typical autosomal dominant inheritance, every affected person in a pedigree has an affected parent, who also has an affected parent, and so on as far back as the disorder can be traced or until the occurrence of an original mutation. This is also true, as discussed later, of X-linked dominant pedigrees. In fact, most dominant conditions of any medical importance come about not only through transmission of the mutant allele from a carrier parent but also through inheritance of a spontaneous, new mutation in a gamete inherited from a nonheterozygous parent. This is because dominant disorders can occur when only one of the pair of

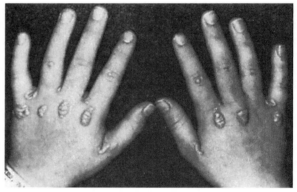

A

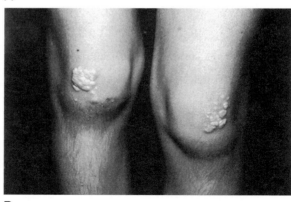

B

Figure 7-13 ■ Cutaneous xanthomas in a familial hypercholesterolemia homozygote. (**A** courtesy of J. L. Goldstein, University of Texas Southwestern Medical Center, Dallas. **B** from Teruel JL, Lasunción MA: Cutaneous xanthomas in homozygous familial hypercholesterolemia. N Engl J Med 332:1137, 1995. Copyright © 1995 Massachusetts Medical Society. All rights reserved.)

of disease to death in homozygous individuals compared with heterozygotes.

Incompletely Dominant Inheritance

Achondroplasia is a well known, incompletely dominant skeletal disorder of short-limbed dwarfism and large head (Fig. 7-12) (Case 1). Most achondroplastic individuals have normal intelligence and lead normal lives within their physical capabilities. Marriages between two achondroplastic individuals are not uncommon. A homozygous child of two heterozygotes is often recognizable on clinical grounds alone; individuals homozygous for achondroplasia are much more severely affected than are heterozygotes and commonly do not survive the immediate postnatal period. A pedigree of a mating between two individuals heterozygous for the mutation that causes achondroplasia is shown in Figure 7-11B. The deceased child, individual III-3, was a homozygote for the condition and had a disorder far more severe than in either parent, resulting in death soon after birth.

Another example of an incompletely dominant disorder is **familial hypercholesterolemia** (see Chapter 12), an autosomal dominant disorder leading to premature alleles at a locus is defective, whether it is inherited from a heterozygous parent or arises through a new, spontaneous mutation in the gamete transmitted from a nonheterozygous parent (see Fig. 7-11B).

Relationship Between New Mutation and Fitness in Autosomal Dominant Disorders

Once a new mutation has arisen, its survival in the population depends on the fitness of persons carrying it, that is, the ability of a heterozygote for the new mutant allele to reproduce. There is an inverse relation between the fitness of a given autosomal dominant disorder and the proportion of all patients with the disorder who received the defective gene as a new muta-tion rather than inheriting it from a heterozygous parent. At one extreme are disorders that have a fitness of zero; in other words, patients with such disorders never reproduce, and the disorder is referred to as a **genetic lethal.** All autosomal dominant genetic lethal diseases must be due to new mutations because these mutations cannot be inherited. The affected individual will appear as an isolated case in the pedigree. At the other extreme are disorders that have virtually normal reproductive fitness because of a late age at onset or a mild phenotype that does not interfere with reproduc-tion. If the fitness is normal, the disorder is rarely the result of fresh mutation; a patient is much more likely to have inherited the disorder than to have a new mutant gene, and the pedigree is likely to show multiple affected individuals with clear-cut autosomal dominant inheri-tance. The measurement of mutation frequency and the relation of mutation frequency to fitness are discussed further in Chapter 9.

Sex-Limited Phenotype in Autosomal Dominant Disease

As discussed earlier for the autosomal recessive condi-tion hemochromatosis, autosomal dominant pheno-types may also demonstrate a sex ratio that differs significantly from 1:1. Extreme divergence of the sex ratio is seen in sex-limited phenotypes, in which the defect is autosomally transmitted but expressed in only one sex. An example is **male-limited precocious puberty** (familial testotoxicosis), an autosomal dominant disor-der in which affected boys develop secondary sexual characteristics and undergo an adolescent growth spurt at about 4 years of age (Fig. 7-14). In some families, the defect has been traced to mutations in the gene that encodes the receptor for luteinizing hormone (*LCGR*); these mutations constitutively activate the receptor's signaling action even in the absence of its hormone. The defect is not manifested in heterozygous females. The pedigree in Figure 7-15 shows that although the disease can be transmitted by unaffected females, it can also

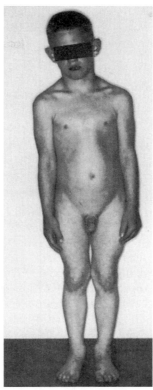

Figure 7-14 ■ Male-limited precocious puberty (familial testotoxicosis), an autosomal dominant disorder expressed exclusively in males. This child, at 4.75 years, is 120 cm in height (above the 97th percentile for his age). Note the muscle bulk and precocious development of the external genitalia. Epiphyseal fusion occurs at an early age, and affected persons are relatively short as adults.

be transmitted directly from father to son, showing that it is autosomal, not X-linked.

Males with precocious puberty due to activating *LCGR* mutations have normal fertility, and numerous multigeneration pedigrees are known. For disorders in which affected males do not reproduce, however, it is not always easy to distinguish sex-limited autosomal inheritance from X-linkage because the critical evi-dence, absence of male-to-male transmission, cannot be provided. In that case, other lines of evidence, espe-cially gene mapping to learn whether the responsible gene maps to the X chromosome or to an autosome (see Chapter 10), can determine the pattern of inheritance and the consequent recurrence risk (see Box).

● X-LINKED INHERITANCE

The X and Y chromosomes, which are responsible for sex determination (see Chapter 6), are distributed unequally to males and females in families. For this reason, phenotypes determined by genes on the X have a characteristic sex distribution and a pattern of inheri-

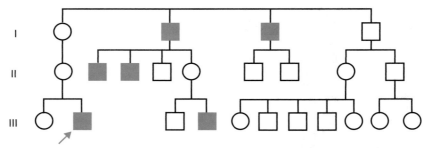

Figure 7-15 ■ Pedigree pattern (part of a much larger pedigree) of male-limited precocious puberty in the family of the child shown in Figure 7-14. This autosomal dominant disorder can be transmitted by affected males or by unaffected carrier females. Male-to-male transmission shows that the inheritance is autosomal, not X-linked. Because the trait is transmitted through unaffected carrier females, it cannot be Y-linked.

tance that is usually easy to identify. Approximately 1100 genes are thought to be located on the X chromosome, of which approximately 40% are presently known to be associated with disease phenotypes.

Because males have one X chromosome but females have two, there are only two possible genotypes in males and three in females with respect to a mutant

allele at an X-linked locus. A male with a mutant allele at an X-linked locus is **hemizygous** for that allele, whereas females may be homozygous for either the wild-type or mutant allele or may be heterozygous. For example, if X_H is the wild-type allele for the gene for coagulation factor VIII and a mutant allele, X_h, causes hemophilia A, the genotypes expected in males and females would be as follows:

	Genotypes	Phenotypes
Males	Hemizygous X_H	Unaffected
	Hemizygous X_h	Affected
Females	Homozygous X_H/X_H	Unaffected
	Heterozygous X_H/X_h	Unaffected (usually)
	Homozygous X_h/X_h	Affected

● ■ ■ Characteristics of Autosomal Dominant Inheritance

- The phenotype usually appears in every generation, each affected person having an affected parent.

  Exceptions or apparent exceptions to this rule in clinical genetics are (1) cases originating from fresh mutations in a gamete of a phenotypically normal parent and (2) cases in which the disorder is not expressed (nonpenetrant) or is expressed only subtly in a person who has inherited the responsible mutant allele.

- Any child of an affected parent has a 50% risk of inheriting the trait.

  This is true for most families, in which the other parent is phenotypically normal. Because statistically each family member is the result of an "independent event," wide deviation from the expected 1:1 ratio may occur by chance in a single family.

- Phenotypically normal family members do not transmit the phenotype to their children.

  Failure of penetrance or subtle expression of a condition may lead to apparent exceptions to this rule.

- Males and females are equally likely to transmit the phenotype, to children of either sex. In particular, male-to-male transmission can occur, and males can have unaffected daughters.

- A significant proportion of isolated cases are due to new mutation. The less the fitness, the greater is the proportion due to new mutation.

X Inactivation, Dosage Compensation, and the Expression of X-Linked Genes

As introduced in Chapter 6, X inactivation is a normal physiological process in which one X chromosome is largely inactivated in somatic cells in normal females (but not in normal males), thus equalizing the expression of most X-linked genes in the two sexes.

The clinical relevance of X inactivation is profound. It leads to females having two cell populations, one in which one of the X chromosomes is active, the other in which the other X chromosome is active (see Chapter 6). Both cell populations in human females are readily detected for some disorders. For example, in **Duchenne muscular dystrophy**, female carriers exhibit typical mosaic expression, allowing carriers to be identified by dystrophin immunostaining (Fig. 7-16) (Case 12). Depending on the pattern of random X inactivation of the two X chromosomes, two female heterozygotes for an X-linked disease may have very different clinical presentations because they differ in the proportion of cells that have the mutant allele on the active X in a relevant tissue (as seen in **manifesting heterozygotes** described later).

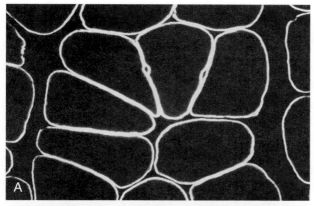

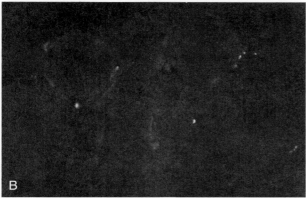

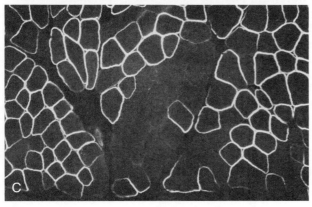

Figure 7-16 ■ Immunostaining for dystrophin in muscle specimens. **A,** A normal female (magnification ×480). **B,** A male with Duchenne muscular dystrophy (×480). **C,** A carrier female (×240). Staining creates the bright lines seen here encircling individual muscle fibers. Muscle from DMD patients lacks dystrophin staining. Muscle from DMD carriers exhibits both positive and negative patches of dystrophin immunostaining, reflecting X inactivation. (Courtesy of K. Arahata, National Institute of Neuroscience, Tokyo.)

Recessive and Dominant Inheritance of X-Linked Disorders

X-linked "dominant" and "recessive" patterns of inheritance are distinguished on the basis of the phenotype in heterozygous females. Some X-linked phenotypes are consistently expressed in carriers (dominant), whereas

others usually are not (recessive). The difficulty in classifying an X-linked disorder as dominant or recessive arises because females who are heterozygous for the same mutant allele in the same family may or may not demonstrate the disease, depending on the pattern of random X inactivation and the proportion of the cells in pertinent tissues that have the mutant allele on the active versus inactive chromosome. Some geneticists have recommended dispensing altogether with the terms recessive and dominant for X-linked disorders. This recommendation is based on the observation that dominance and recessiveness for X-linked disorders is not absolute. Nearly 40% of commonly known X-linked disorders might be classified as recessive because they show little or no penetrance (less than a few percent of female heterozygotes), and 30% would be considered dominant because they are penetrant in most (>85%) female heterozygotes; the remaining 30% are penetrant in some (15% to 85%) but not all female heterozygotes and cannot be classified as either dominant or recessive. Be that as it may, the terms recessive and dominant are widely applied to X-linked disorders and we will continue to use them, recognizing that they describe extremes of a continuum of penetrance and expressivity in female carriers of X-linked diseases.

X-Linked Recessive Inheritance

The inheritance of X-linked recessive phenotypes follows a well-defined and easily recognized pattern (Fig. 7-17 and Box). An X-linked recessive mutation is typically expressed phenotypically in all males who receive it but only in those females who are homozygous for the mutation. Consequently, X-linked recessive disorders are generally restricted to males and rarely seen among females (see section on manifesting heterozygotes later in this chapter).

Hemophilia A is a classic X-linked recessive disorder in which the blood fails to clot normally because of a deficiency of factor VIII, a protein in the clotting cascade (Case 18). The hereditary nature of hemophilia and even its pattern of transmission have been recognized since ancient times, and the condition became known as the "royal hemophilia" because of its occurrence among descendants of Britain's Queen Victoria, who was a carrier.

As in the earlier discussion, X_h represents the mutant factor VIII allele causing hemophilia A, and X_H represents the normal allele. If a hemophiliac mates with a normal female, all the sons receive their father's Y chromosome and a maternal X and are unaffected, but all the daughters receive the paternal X chromosome with its hemophilia allele and are obligate carriers:

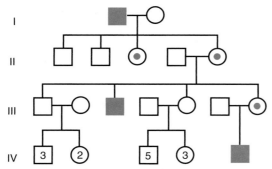

Figure 7-17 ■ Pedigree pattern demonstrating an X-linked recessive disorder such as hemophilia A, transmitted from an affected male through females to an affected grandson and great-grandson.

AFFECTED MALE BY NORMAL FEMALE: $X_h/Y \times X_H/X_H$

	X_H	X_H	
X_h	X_H/X_h	X_H/X_h	Daughters: *all* carriers
Y	X_H/Y	X_H/Y	Sons: *all* unaffected

Now assume that a daughter of the affected male mates with an unaffected male. Four genotypes are possible in the progeny, with equal probabilities:

NORMAL MALE BY CARRIER FEMALE: $X_H/Y \times X_H/X_h$

	X_H	X_h	
X_H	X_H/X_H	X_H/X_h	Daughters: 1/2 normal, 1/2 carriers
Y	X_H/Y	X_h/Y	Sons: 1/2 normal, 1/2 affected

> **••• Characteristics of X-Linked Recessive Inheritance**
>
> - The incidence of the trait is much higher in males than in females.
> - Heterozygous females are usually unaffected, but some may express the condition with variable severity as determined by the pattern of X inactivation.
> - The gene responsible for the condition is transmitted from an affected man through all his daughters. Any of his daughters' sons has a 50% chance of inheriting it.
> - The mutant allele is ordinarily never transmitted directly from father to son, but it is transmitted by an affected male to all his daughters.
> - The mutant allele may be transmitted through a series of carrier females; if so, the affected males in a kindred are related through females.
> - A significant proportion of isolated cases are due to new mutation.

The hemophilia of an affected grandfather, which did not appear in any of his own children, has a 50% chance of appearing in the son of each of his daughters. It will not reappear among the descendants of his sons, however. A daughter of a carrier has a 50% chance of being a carrier herself (see Fig. 7-17). By chance, an X-linked recessive allele may be transmitted undetected through a series of female carriers before it is expressed in a male descendant.

Homozygous Affected Females   A gene for an X-linked disorder is occasionally present in both a father and a carrier mother, and female offspring can then be homozygous affected, as shown in the pedigree of X-linked **color blindness**, a relatively common X-linked disorder (Fig. 7-18). Most X-linked diseases are so rare, however, that it is unusual for a female to be homozygous unless her parents are consanguineous:

AFFECTED MALE BY CARRIER FEMALE: $X_h/Y \times X_H/X_h$

	X_H	X_h	
X_h	X_H/X_h	X_h/X_h	Daughters: 1/2 carriers, 1/2 affected
Y	X_H/Y	X_h/Y	Sons: 1/2 normal, 1/2 affected

Manifesting Heterozygotes and Unbalanced Inactivation for X-Linked Disease   In those rare instances in which a female carrier of a recessive X-linked allele has phenotypic expression of the disease, she is referred to as a **manifesting heterozygote**. Manifesting heterozygotes have been described for many X-linked recessive disorders, including color blindness, hemophilia A (classic hemophilia, factor VIII deficiency), hemophilia B (Christmas disease, factor IX deficiency), Duchenne muscular dystrophy, Wiskott-Aldrich syndrome (an X-linked immunodeficiency), and several X-linked eye disorders.

Whether a female heterozygote will be a manifesting heterozygote depends on a number of factors. First,

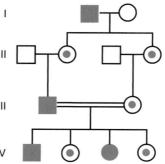

Figure 7-18 ■ Consanguinity in an X-linked recessive pedigree for red-green color blindness, resulting in a homozygous affected female.

because X inactivation is random but established at a stage of embryonic development when the embryo has fewer than 100 cells (see Chapter 6), the fraction of cells in various tissues of carrier females in which the normal or mutant allele happens to remain active can be quite variable. If it happens that the deleterious allele finds itself located on the active X while the normal allele happens to be located on the inactive X, **unbalanced** or "skewed" X inactivation results. If such skewed inactivation is present in pertinent tissues, it can cause a female carrier to have signs and symptoms of the disorder. Second, depending on the disorder in question, female heterozygotes can have very different degrees of disease penetrance and expression, even if their degree of skewed inactivation is the same, because of the underlying physiological functioning of the genes. For example, in the lysosomal storage disease (see Chapter 12) caused by iduronate sulfatase deficiency (**Hunter syndrome**), those cells in which the X carrying the normal gene is active can export the enzyme to the extracellular space, where it is picked up by cells in which the X carrying the mutant allele is active, and correct the defect in those cells. As a result, the penetrance for Hunter syndrome in female heterozygotes is extremely low even when X inactivation diverges significantly from the expected random 50%-50% pattern. On the other hand, nearly half of all female heterozygotes for the **fragile X syndrome** (see Chapter 12) show developmental abnormalities, although generally to a lesser extent than in males with the disorder (Case 15).

In addition to manifesting heterozygotes, the opposite pattern of unbalanced or skewed inactivation (i.e., with the mutant allele found preferentially on the inactive X in some or all tissues of the heterozygous female) can also occur and is characteristic of several X-linked disorders. In general, such skewed inactivation is seen in asymptomatic heterozygotes and is believed to reflect a cell survival or proliferative disadvantage for those cells that originally had the mutant allele on the active X (see Chapter 6). A pattern of skewed inactivation in relevant tissues has been used to diagnose the carrier state for some X-linked conditions, including certain X-linked immunodeficiencies, dyskeratosis congenita (an X-linked form of skin disease and bone marrow failure), and incontinentia pigmenti (an X-linked condition affecting skin and teeth).

X-Linked Dominant Inheritance

As discussed earlier, an X-linked phenotype is described as dominant if it is regularly expressed in heterozygotes. X-linked dominant inheritance can readily be distinguished from autosomal dominant inheritance by the lack of **male-to-male transmission,** which is obviously impossible for X-linked inheritance because males

transmit the Y chromosome, not the X, to their sons. Thus, the distinguishing feature of a fully penetrant X-linked dominant pedigree (Fig. 7-19) is that *all* the daughters and *none* of the sons of affected males are affected; if any daughter is unaffected or any son is affected, the inheritance must be autosomal, not X-linked. The pattern of inheritance through females is no different from the autosomal dominant pattern; because females have a pair of X chromosomes just as they have pairs of autosomes, each child of an affected female has a 50% chance of inheriting the trait, regardless of sex. Across multiple families with an X-linked dominant disease, the expression is usually milder in females, who are almost always heterozygotes, because the mutant allele is located on the inactive X chromosome in a proportion of their cells. Thus, most X-linked dominant disorders are incompletely dominant, as is the case with most autosomal dominant disorders (see Box).

> **••• Characteristics of X-Linked Dominant Inheritance**
>
> - Affected males with normal mates have no affected sons and no normal daughters.
> - Both male and female offspring of female carriers have a 50% risk of inheriting the phenotype. The pedigree pattern is similar to that seen with autosomal dominant inheritance.
> - Affected females are about twice as common as affected males, but affected females typically have milder (although variable) expression of the phenotype.

Only a few genetic disorders are classified as X-linked dominant. One example is X-linked **hypophosphatemic rickets** (also called vitamin D–resistant rickets), in which the ability of the kidney tubules to reabsorb filtered phosphate is impaired. The defective gene product appears to be a member of a family of

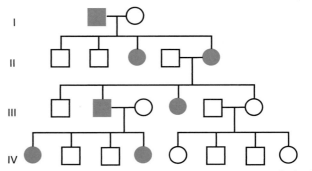

Figure 7-19 ■ Pedigree pattern demonstrating X-linked dominant inheritance.

endopeptidases that activate or degrade a variety of peptide hormones. The pathogenic mechanism by which a deficiency of this endopeptidase results in a disorder of phosphate metabolism and rickets is not known. This disorder fits the criterion of an X-linked dominant disorder in that although both sexes are affected, the serum phosphate level is less depressed and the rickets less severe in heterozygous females than in affected males.

X-Linked Dominant Disorders with Male Lethality

Some of the rare genetic defects expressed exclusively or almost exclusively in females appear to be X-linked dominant conditions that are lethal in males before birth (Fig. 7-20). Typical pedigrees of these conditions show transmission by affected females, who produce affected daughters, normal daughters, and normal sons in equal proportions (1:1:1).

Rett syndrome is a striking disorder that occurs nearly exclusively in females and meets all criteria for being an X-linked dominant disorder that is usually lethal in hemizygous males (Case 35). The syndrome is characterized by normal prenatal and neonatal growth and development, followed by the rapid onset of neurological symptoms and loss of milestones between 6 and 18 months of age. The children become spastic and ataxic, develop autistic features and irritable behavior

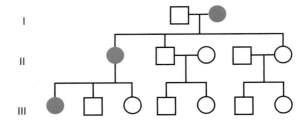

Figure 7-20 ■ Pedigree pattern demonstrating an X-linked dominant disorder, lethal in males during the prenatal period.

with outbursts of crying, and demonstrate characteristic purposeless wringing or flapping movements of the hands and arms (Fig. 7-21). Head growth slows and microcephaly develops. Seizures are common (~50%). Surprisingly, the mental deterioration stops after a few years and the patients can then survive for many decades with a stable but severe neurological disability.

Most cases of Rett syndrome are caused by spontaneous mutations in an X-linked gene, *MECP2*, encoding a DNA-binding protein known as methyl-CpG–binding protein 2. The disease mechanism is unknown but is thought to reflect abnormalities in the regulation of a set of genes in the developing brain. Most female heterozygotes have full-blown Rett syndrome. Males who survive with the syndrome usually have two X chromosomes (as in a 47,XXY Klinefelter

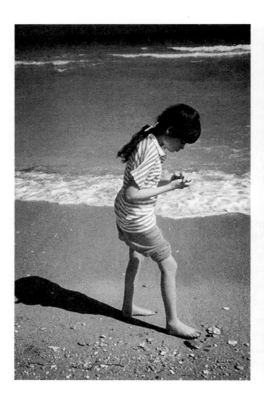

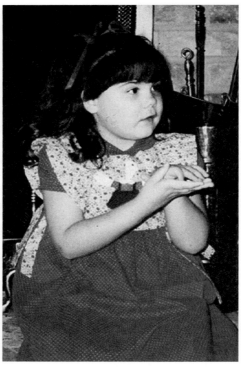

Figure 7-21 ■ Typical appearance and hand posture of girls with Rett syndrome. (Courtesy of Dr. Huda Zoghbi, Baylor College of Medicine and Howard Hughes Medical Institute.)

individual or in a 46,X,der(X) male with the male-determining *SRY* gene translocated from the Y to an X) or are mosaic for a mutation that is absent in most of their cells. There are a few apparently unaffected women who have given birth to more than one child with Rett syndrome. In these cases, the mother may be heterozygous for an *MECP2* mutation but was protected from the effects of the mutant allele because her X inactivation pattern was highly skewed and the chromosome bearing the mutant gene was inactive in most of her cells. Alternatively, the phenotypically normal mother of more than one child affected with Rett syndrome can be a germline mosaic who does not have the mutant gene in her own somatic tissues (mosaicism is discussed subsequently in this chapter).

New Mutation in X-Linked Disorders

In males, genes for X-linked disorders are exposed to selection that is complete for some disorders, partial for others, and absent for still others, depending on the fitness of the genotype. Patients with **hemophilia** (Case 18) have only about 70% as many offspring as unaffected males do; that is, the fitness of affected males is about 0.70. Selection against mutant alleles is more dramatic for X-linked disorders such as **Duchenne muscular dystrophy** (DMD) (Case 12), a disease of muscle that affects young boys (see Chapter 12). The disorder is usually apparent by the time the child begins to walk and progresses inexorably, so that the child is confined to a wheelchair by about the age of 10 years and usually does not survive his teens. Although the situation may change as a result of advances in research aimed at therapy for affected boys, DMD is currently a genetic lethal because affected males usually fail to reproduce. It may, of course, be transmitted by carrier females, who themselves rarely show any clinical manifestation of the disease.

New mutations constitute a significant fraction of isolated cases of many X-linked diseases. When patients are affected with a severe X-linked recessive disease, such as DMD, they cannot reproduce (i.e., selection is complete), and therefore the mutant alleles they carry are lost from the population. Because the incidence of DMD is not changing, mutant alleles lost through failure of the affected males to reproduce are continually replaced by new mutations. For hemophilia, in which reproduction is reduced but not eliminated, a proportionately smaller fraction of cases will be due to new mutation. The balance between new mutation and selection is discussed more fully in Chapter 9.

PSEUDOAUTOSOMAL INHERITANCE

Pseudoautosomal inheritance describes the inheritance pattern seen with genes in the pseudoautosomal region

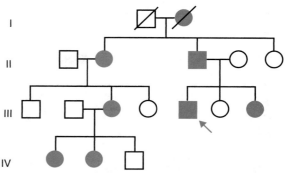

Figure 7-22 ■ Pedigree showing inheritance of dyschondrosteosis due to mutations in a pseudoautosomal gene on the X and Y chromosomes. The arrow shows a male who inherited the trait on his Y chromosome from his father. His father, however, inherited the trait on his X chromosome from his mother. (From Shears DJ, et al: Mutation and deletion of the pseudoautosomal gene SHOX cause Leri-Weill dyschondrosteosis. Nat Genet 19:70-73, 1998.)

of the X and Y chromosome that can exchange regularly between the two sex chromosomes. Alleles for genes in the pseudoautosomal region can show male-to-male transmission, and therefore mimic autosomal inheritance, because they can cross over from the X to the Y during male gametogenesis and be passed on from a father to his male offspring. **Dyschondrosteosis,** a dominantly inherited skeletal dysplasia with disproportionate short stature and deformity of the forearm, is an example of a pseudoautosomal condition inherited in a dominant manner. A greater prevalence of the disease was seen in females as compared with males, suggesting an X-linked dominant disorder, but the presence of male-to-male transmission clearly ruled out strict X-linked inheritance (Fig. 7-22). Mutations in the *SHOX* gene encoding a homeodomain-containing transcription factor have been found responsible for this condition. *SHOX* is located in the pseudoautosomal region on Xp and Yp and escapes X inactivation.

MOSAICISM

Mosaicism is the presence in an individual or a tissue of at least two cell lines that differ genetically but are derived from a single zygote. Although we are used to thinking of ourselves as being composed of cells that all carry exactly the same complement of genes and chromosomes, this is in reality an oversimplified view. We already introduced the concept of mosaicism due to X inactivation that generates two different populations of somatic cells in females, those in which the paternal X is the active chromosome and those in which the maternal X is the active chromosome. More generally, mutations arising in a single cell in either prenatal or postnatal life can give rise to clones of cells genetically

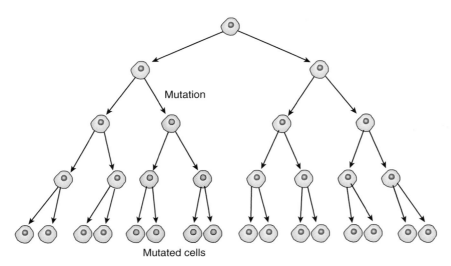

Mutation

Mutated cells

Figure 7-23 ■ Schematic presentation of mitotic cell divisions. A mutation occurring during cell proliferation, in somatic cells or during gametogenesis, leads to a proportion of cells carrying the mutation—that is, to either somatic or germline mosaicism.

different from the original zygote because once the mutation occurs, it could persist in all the clonal descendants of that cell (Fig. 7-23). Mosaicism for numerical or structural abnormalities of chromosomes is a clinically important phenomenon (see Chapter 5), and somatic mutation is recognized as a major contributor to many types of cancer (see Chapter 16). Mosaicism for mutations in single genes, in either somatic or germline cells, explains a number of unusual clinical observations, such as **segmental neurofibromatosis,** in which skin manifestations are not uniform and occur in a patchy distribution, and the recurrence of **osteogenesis imperfecta,** a highly penetrant autosomal dominant disease, in two or more children born to unaffected parents.

The population of cells that carry a mutation in a mosaic individual could theoretically be present in some tissues of the body but not in the gametes (pure **somatic mosaicism**), be restricted to the gamete lineage only and nowhere else (pure **germline mosaicism**), or be present in both somatic lineages and the germline, depending on when the mutation occurred in embryological development. Whether mosaicism for a mutation involves only somatic tissues, the germline, or both depends on whether during embryogenesis the mutation occurred before or after the separation of germline cells from somatic cells. If before, both somatic and germline cell lines would be mosaic and the mutation could be transmitted to the offspring as well as being expressed somatically in mosaic form. A mutation occurring later would be found only in the germline or only in a subset of somatic tissues. Thus, for example, if a mutation were to occur in a germline precursor cell, a proportion of the gametes would carry the mutation (see Fig. 7-23). There are about 30 mitotic divisions in the cells of the germline before meiosis in the female and several hundred in the male (see Chapter 2), allow-

ing ample opportunity for mutations to occur during the mitotic stages of gamete development.

Determining whether mosaicism for a mutation is present only in the germline or only in somatic tissues may be difficult because failure to find a mutation in a subset of cells from a readily accessible somatic tissue (such as peripheral white blood cells, skin, or buccal cells) does not ensure that the mutation is not present elsewhere in the body, including the germline. Characterizing the extent of somatic mosaicism is made more difficult when the mutant allele in a mosaic fetus occurs exclusively in the extraembryonic tissues (i.e., the placenta) and is not present in the fetus itself.

Somatic Mosaicism

A mutation affecting morphogenesis and occurring during embryonic development might be manifested as a segmental or patchy abnormality, depending on the stage at which the mutation occurred and the lineage of the somatic cell in which it originated. For example, NF1 is sometimes segmental, affecting only one part of the body. Segmental NF1 is caused by mosaicism for a mutation that occurred after conception. In such cases, the patient has normal parents, but if he or she has an affected child, the child's phenotype is typical for NF1, that is, not segmental. In such cases, the mutation has to be in the patient's gametes and therefore must have occurred before separation of germline cells from the somatic cell line that carries the mutation.

Germline Mosaicism

As discussed earlier in this chapter, the chance that an autosomal or X-linked disorder caused by a new mutation could occur more than once in a sibship is low because spontaneous mutations are generally rare (on

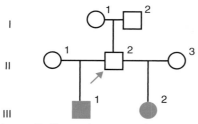

Figure 7-24 ■ Pedigree demonstrating recurrence of the autosomal dominant disorder osteogenesis imperfecta. Both affected children have the same point mutation in a collagen gene. Their father *(arrow)* is unaffected and has no such mutation in DNA from examined somatic tissues. He must have been a mosaic for the mutation in his germline.

the order of 1 chance in 10^4 to 10^6; see Chapter 9), and having two occur independently in the same gene in the same family is thus very unlikely (less than 1 in 10^8 to 10^{12}). After even subtle evidence of the disease had been ruled out in the unaffected parents of a child with an autosomal dominant or X-linked disorder and with negative results of molecular testing for the carrier state, it therefore used to be customary to advise the parents that the disease in their child was the result of a new mutation and that the chance of the same defect in a subsequent child was negligible, equivalent to the population risk. There are, however, well-documented examples where parents who are phenotypically normal and test negative for being carriers have more than one child affected with a highly penetrant autosomal dominant or X-linked disorder. Such unusual pedigrees can be explained by germline mosaicism. Germline mosaicism is well documented in as many as 6% of severe, lethal forms of the autosomal dominant disorder **osteogenesis imperfecta** (Fig. 7-24) (see Chapter 12), in which mutations in type I collagen genes lead to abnormal collagen, brittle bones, and frequent fractures. Pedigrees that could be explained by germline mosaicism have also been reported for several other well-known disorders, such as **hemophilia A** (Case 18), **hemophilia B**, and **DMD** (Case 12), but have only very rarely been seen in other dominant diseases, such as **achondroplasia** (Case 1). Accurate measurement of the frequency of germline mosaicism is difficult, but estimates suggest that the highest incidence is in DMD, in which up to 15% of the mothers of isolated cases show no evidence of the mutation in their somatic tissues and yet carry the mutation in their germline.

Now that the phenomenon of germline mosaicism has been recognized, geneticists and genetic counselors are aware of the potential inaccuracy of predicting that a specific autosomal dominant or X-linked phenotype that appears by every test to be a new mutation must have a negligible recurrence risk in future offspring. Obviously, in diseases known to show germline mosa-

icism, phenotypically normal parents of a child whose disease is believed to be due to a new mutation should be informed that the recurrence risk is not negligible. Furthermore, apparently noncarrier parents of a child with any autosomal dominant or X-linked disorder in which mosaicism is possible but unproven may have a recurrence risk that may be as high as 3% to 4%; these couples should be offered whatever prenatal diagnostic tests are appropriate. The exact recurrence risk is difficult to assess, however, because it depends on what proportion of gametes contains the mutation.

● IMPRINTING IN PEDIGREES

Unusual Inheritance Patterns due to Genomic Imprinting

According to Mendel's laws of heredity, a mutant allele of an autosomal gene is equally likely to be transmitted from a parent, of either sex, to an offspring of either sex; similarly, a female is equally likely to transmit a mutated X-linked gene to a child of either sex. Originally, little attention was paid to whether the sex of the parent had any effect on the *expression* of the genes each parent transmits. As discussed in Chapter 5, we now know, however, that in some genetic disorders such as **Prader-Willi syndrome** (Case 33) and **Angelman syndrome**, the expression of the disease phenotype depends on whether the mutant allele has been inherited from the father or from the mother, a phenomenon known as **genomic imprinting**.

Imprinting can cause unusual inheritance patterns in pedigrees, as clearly demonstrated by a rare condition known as **Albright hereditary osteodystrophy (AHO)**. AHO is characterized by obesity, short stature, subcutaneous calcifications, and brachydactyly, particularly of the fourth and fifth metacarpal bones (Fig. 7-25). AHO is inherited as a fully penetrant autosomal dominant trait. What is unusual, however, is that in families of individuals affected by AHO, some but not all of the affected patients have an additional clinical disorder known as **pseudohypoparathyroidism** (PHP; Table 7-2). In PHP, an abnormality of calcium metabolism typically seen with a *deficiency* of parathyroid hormone occurs but with *elevated* levels of parathyroid hormone (hence the use of the prefix *pseudo*) that is secondary to renal tubular resistance to the effects of parathyroid hormone. PHP in an individual with the AHO phenotype is known as **pseudohypoparathyroidism type 1a (PHP1a)**. AHO with or without PHP is caused by a defect in the *GNAS* gene. GNAS is involved in transmitting the parathyroid hormone signal from the surface of renal cells to inside the cell.

A careful examination of PHP1a pedigrees shows that some individuals have AHO only, without the

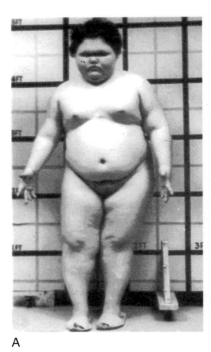

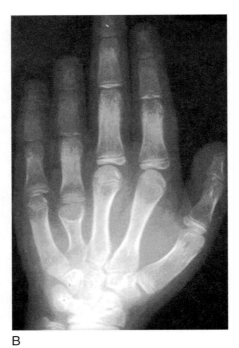

A   B

Figure 7-25 ■ A, Characteristic appearance of a patient with Albright hereditary osteodystrophy. B, Hand radiograph showing shortened metacarpals and distal phalanges, especially and characteristically the fourth metacarpal. (Courtesy of L. S. Weinstein, National Institute of Diabetes and Digestive and Kidney Diseases, National Institutes of Health, Bethesda, Maryland.)

calcium and renal problems, whereas others have the physical characteristics as a component of PHP1a (Fig. 7-26A). When AHO occurs *without* the renal tubular dysfunction in families in which other relatives have PHP1a, it is often referred to (perhaps inelegantly) as **pseudopseudohypoparathyroidism (PPHP)**. Interestingly, when PPHP and PHP1a occur within the same family, affected brothers and sisters in any one sibship either *all* have PPHP or *all* have PHP1a; what does not happen is that one sib will have one condition while another has the other.

Why is it that in any one family, there are some individuals affected with AHO and others with pseudohypoparathyroidism, while *within any one* sibship, brothers and sisters either all have PHP1a or all have PPHP? This unusual pattern of inheritance can be explained by the fact that the defective gene (*GNAS*)

in PHP1a and PPHP is imprinted only in certain tissues, including renal tubular cells, so that only the *GNAS* allele inherited from the mother is expressed in these cells while the father's allele is normally silent. PHP1a therefore occurs only when an individual inherits an inactivating mutation in *GNAS* from his or her mother; since the paternal copy is not expressed anyway, these tissues have no normal, functioning copy of *GNAS*, and resistance to the effects of parathyroid hormone ensues. There is no imprinting, however, in most of the tissues of the body. In the tissues without *GNAS* imprinting, heterozygotes for one mutant *GNAS* allele all develop AHO, which is passed on as a simple autosomal dominant trait.

The effect of imprinting for understanding certain unusual patterns of disease inheritance is also seen in another form of autosomal dominant pseudohypopara-

Table 7-2

Pseudohypoparathyroidism and Related Disorders

Disorder	Phenotype	Molecular Basis
AHO	Obesity, short stature, subcutaneous calcifications, brachydactyly	Constitutional haploinsufficiency for *GNAS*
PHP1a	AHO with pseudohypoparathyroidism, hypothyroidism, growth hormone deficiency	Constitutional haploinsufficiency for *GNAS* inherited from a female parent, which also causes complete loss of expression in critical renal and endocrine tissues
PPHP	AHO alone in a member of a family in which PHP1a is also occurring	Constitutional haploinsufficiency for *GNAS* inherited from a male parent, which leaves intact expression of the maternal copy in critical renal and endocrine tissues
PHP1b	Only the endocrine defects of PHP1a without the features of AHO	Mutation in the imprinting center whose normal function is required for expression of the maternal copy of *GNAS* in critical renal and endocrine tissues; no loss of constitutional *GNAS* expression

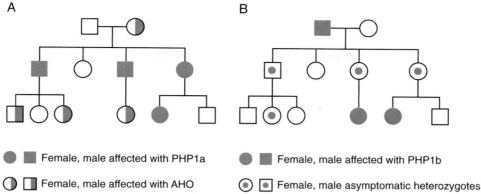

Figure 7-26 ■ Pedigrees of pseudohypoparathyroidism. **A,** Family with pseudohypoparathyroidism 1a (PHP1a, *solid-blue symbols*) and pseudopseudohypoparathyroidism (PPHP, *half-blue symbols*), showing that all PHP1a patients inherit the mutant *GNAS* gene from their mothers, whereas all PPHP patients have a paternally derived mutant allele. **B,** Pedigree of family with PHP1b *(solid-blue symbols)* due to a deletion in the imprinting control region. All affected patients inherit the deletion allele from their mothers; heterozygotes with a paternal allele are unaffected. Heterozygotes for a deletion mutation in the imprinting regulatory region of the *GNAS* gene are indicated by the blue dots.

thyroidism, known as PHP type 1b (Fig. 7-26B). PHP1b has the calcium abnormalities seen in PHP1a but without the physical signs of AHO. PHP1b is caused by a mutation in upstream regulatory elements (the "imprinting center") that control the imprinting of the *GNAS* gene; the normal function of these regulatory elements is to specify that the maternally inherited GNAS allele, and only that allele, will be expressed in renal tubules. When a mutation of the imprinting control region is inherited from the mother, both the paternal allele, which is normally silent in kidney tubules, and the maternal allele, which is silenced in these tissues because of the deletion, fail to be expressed, and PHP1b ensues. Individuals who inherit the mutation from their fathers, however, are asymptomatic heterozygotes because their maternal copy of *GNAS,* with its imprinting control region intact, is expressed normally in these tissues. Outside of the kidney and a few other tissues, both maternal and paternal *GNAS* alleles are expressed independently of any imprinting, and AHO therefore does not occur.

● UNSTABLE REPEAT EXPANSIONS

In all of the types of inheritance presented earlier in this chapter, the responsible mutation, once it occurs, is *stable* from generation to generation; that is, all affected members of a family share the identical inherited mutation. In contrast, an entirely new class of genetic disease has been recognized, diseases due to *unstable repeat expansions.* By definition, these conditions are characterized by an expansion within the affected gene of a segment of DNA consisting of repeating units of three or more nucleotides in tandem (i.e., adjacent to each other). For example, the repeat unit

often consists of three nucleotides, such as CAG or CCG, and the repeat will be CAGCAGCAG...CAG or CCGCCGCCG...CCG. In general, the genes associated with these diseases all have wild-type alleles that are polymorphic; that is, there is a variable but relatively low number of repeat units in the normal population. As the gene is passed from generation to generation, however, the number of repeats can increase (undergoes **expansion**), far beyond the normal polymorphic range, leading to abnormalities in gene expression and function. The molecular mechanisms by which such expansions occur are not clearly understood but are likely to be due to a type of DNA replication error known as **slipped mispairing** (see Chapter 12, Fig. 12-32). The discovery of this unusual group of conditions has dispelled the orthodox notions of germline stability and provided a biological basis for such eccentric genetic phenomena as **anticipation** and **parental transmission bias**, discussed later in this section, that previously had no known mechanistic explanation.

More than a dozen diseases are known to result from unstable repeat expansions. All of these conditions are primarily neurological. A dominant inheritance pattern occurs in some, X-linked in others, and recessive inheritance in still others. The degree of expansion of the repeat unit that causes disease is sometimes subtle (as in the rare disorder **oculopharyngeal muscular dystrophy**) and sometimes explosive (as in **congenital myotonic dystrophy** or severe **fragile X syndrome**). Other differences between the various unstable repeat expansion diseases include the length and base sequence of the repeated unit; the number of repeated units in normal, presymptomatic and fully affected individuals; the location of the repeated unit within genes; the pathogenesis of the disease; the degree to which the repeated units are unstable during meiosis

Table 7-3

Four Representative Examples of Unstable Repeat Expansion Diseases

Disease	Inheritance Pattern	Repeat	Gene Affected	Location in Gene	Repeat Number		
					Normals	*Intermediate*	*Affected*
Huntington disease	Autosomal dominant	CAG	*HD*	coding region	<36	36-39 usually affected	>40
Fragile X	X-linked	CGG	*FMR1*	5′ untranslated	<60	60-200 usually unaffected*	>200
Myotonic dystrophy	Autosomal dominant	CTG	*DMPK*	3′ untranslated	<30	50-80 may be mildly affected	80-2000
Friedreich ataxia	Autosomal recessive	AAG	*FRDA*	intron	<34	36-100	>100

*May have tremor-ataxia syndrome or premature ovarian failure.

or mitosis; and parental bias in when expansion occurs.

We review the inheritance patterns of four different diseases to illustrate the major similarities and differences among the most common unstable repeat expansion diseases (Table 7-3). These disorders are Huntington disease and other progressive neurodegenerative diseases, such as spinobulbar muscular atrophy and autosomal dominant spinocerebellar ataxias (referred to as **polyglutamine disorders** because they result from expansions of the triplet CAG encoding glutamine residues); fragile X syndrome; myotonic dystrophy; and Friedreich ataxia. The mechanisms by which repeat expansion occurs and causes these diseases will be discussed in more detail in Chapter 12.

Polyglutamine Disorders

Huntington Disease

Huntington disease (HD) is a well-known disorder that illustrates many of the common genetic features of the polyglutamine disorders caused by expansion of an unstable repeat (Case 22). HD was first described by the physician George Huntington in 1872 in an American kindred of English descent. The neuropathology is dominated by degeneration of the striatum and the cortex. Patients first present clinically in midlife and manifest a characteristic phenotype of motor abnormalities (chorea, dystonia), personality changes, a gradual loss of cognition, and ultimately death.

For a long time, HD was thought to be a typical, autosomal dominant condition. The disease is passed from generation to generation with a 50% risk to each offspring, and heterozygous and homozygous patients carrying the mutation have very similar phenotypes, although homozygotes may have a more rapid course of their disease. There are, however, obvious peculiarities in its inheritance that could not be explained by simple autosomal dominant inheritance. First, the age at onset of HD is variable; only about half the

individuals who carry a mutant *HD* allele show symptoms by the age of 40 years. Second, the disease appears to develop at an earlier and earlier age when it is transmitted through the pedigree, a phenomenon referred to as **anticipation,** but only when it is transmitted by an affected father and not by an affected mother.

The peculiarities of inheritance of HD are now readily explained by the discovery that the mutation is composed of an abnormally long expansion of a stretch of the nucleotides CAG, the codon specifying the amino acid glutamine, in the coding region of a gene for a protein of unknown function called huntingtin. Normal individuals carry between 9 and 35 CAG repeats in their *HD* gene, with the average being 18 or 19. Individuals affected with HD have 40 or more repeats, with the average being around 46. A borderline repeat number of 36 to 39, although usually associated with HD, can be found in a few individuals who show no signs of the disease even at a fairly advanced age. Once an expansion increases to greater than 39, however, disease always occurs, and the larger the expansion, the earlier the onset of the disease (Fig. 7-27).

How, then, does an individual come to have an expanded CAG repeat in his or her *HD* gene (Fig. 7-28)? Most commonly, he or she inherits it as a straightforward autosomal dominant trait from an affected parent who already has an expanded repeat (>36). In contrast to stable mutations, however, the size of the repeat may expand on transmission, resulting in earlier onset disease in later generations (thus explaining anticipation); on the other hand, repeat numbers in the range of 40 to 50 may not result in disease until later in life, thereby explaining the age-dependent penetrance. In the pedigree shown in Figure 7-28, individual I-1, now deceased, was diagnosed with HD at the age of 64 years and had an expansion of 37 CAG repeats. Four of his children inherited the expanded allele, and in all four of them, the expansion increased over that found in individual I-1. Individual II-5, in particular, has the largest number of repeats and became symptomatic during adolescence. Individual II-1, in

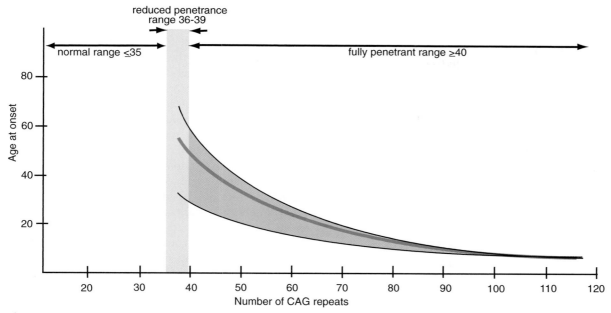

Figure 7-27 ■ Graph correlating approximate age at onset of Huntington disease with the number of CAG repeats found in the *HD* gene. The solid line is the average age at onset, and the shaded area shows the range of age at onset for any given number of repeats. (Data courtesy of Dr. M. Macdonald, Massachusetts General Hospital, Boston, Massachusetts.)

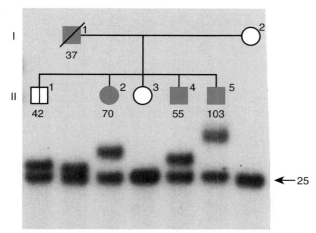

Figure 7-28 ■ Pedigree of family with Huntington disease. Shown beneath the pedigree is a Southern blot analysis for CAG repeat expansions in the huntingtin gene. In addition to a normal allele containing 25 CAG repeats, individual I-1 and his children II-1, II-2, II-4, and II-5 are all heterozygous for expanded alleles, each containing a different number of CAG repeats. I-1, who developed HD at the age of 64 years and is now deceased, had an abnormal repeat length of 37. He has three affected children, two of whom have repeat lengths of 55 and 70 and developed disease in their 40s, and a son with juvenile HD and 103 CAG repeats in his huntingtin gene. Individual II-1 is unaffected at the age of 50 years but will develop the disease later in life. Individuals I-2 and II-3 have two alleles of normal length (25). Repeat lengths were confirmed by PCR analysis. (Data courtesy of Dr. Ben Roa, Baylor College of Medicine, Houston, Texas.)

contrast, inherited an expanded allele but remains asymptomatic and will likely develop the disease sometime later in life.

On occasion, unaffected individuals carry alleles with repeat lengths at the upper limit of the normal range (29 to 35 CAG repeats) that, however, can expand during meiosis to 40 or more repeats. CAG repeat alleles at the upper limits of normal that do not cause disease but are capable of expanding into the disease-causing range are known as **premutations**. Expansion in HD shows a paternal transmission bias and occurs most frequently during male gametogenesis, which is why the severe early-onset juvenile form of the disease, seen with the largest expansions (70 to 121 repeats), is always paternally inherited. Expanded repeats may continue to be unstable during mitosis in somatic cells, resulting in some degree of somatic mosaicism (see later) for the number of repeats in different tissues from the same patient.

The largest known group of HD patients lives in the region of Lake Maracaibo, Venezuela; these patients are descendants of a single individual who introduced the gene into the population early in the 19th century. About 100 living affected persons and another 900, each at 50% risk, are currently known in the Lake Maracaibo community. High frequency of a disease in a local population descended from a small number of individuals, one of whom carried the gene responsible for the disease, is an example of **founder effect** (see Chapter 9).

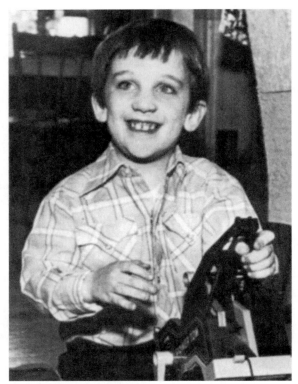

Figure 7-29 ■ Characteristic facial appearance of a patient with the fragile X syndrome. (Photograph courtesy of Michael Partington, Queen's University, Kingston, Ontario, Canada.)

Spinobulbar Muscular Atrophy and Other Polyglutamine Disorders

In addition to HD, other neurological diseases are caused by CAG expansions encoding polyglutamine, such as X-linked recessive spinobulbar muscular atrophy and the various autosomal dominant spinocerebellar ataxias. These conditions differ in the gene involved, the normal range of the repeat, the threshold for clinical disease caused by expansion, and the regions of the brain affected; they all share with HD the fundamental characteristic that results from instability of a stretch of repeated CAG nucleotides leading to expansion of a glutamine tract in a protein.

Fragile X Syndrome

The **fragile X syndrome** (Fig. 7-29) is the most common heritable form of moderate mental retardation and is second only to Down syndrome among all causes of mental retardation in males (Case 15). The name refers to a cytogenetic marker on the X chromosome at Xq27.3, a "fragile site" in which the chromatin fails to condense properly during mitosis (Fig. 7-30). The syndrome is inherited as an X-linked disorder with penetrance in females in the 50% to 60% range. The fragile X syndrome has a frequency of at least 1 in 4000

male births and is so common that it requires consideration in the differential diagnosis of mental retardation in both males and females. Testing for the fragile X syndrome is among the most frequent indications for DNA analysis, genetic counseling, and prenatal diagnosis.

Genetic analysis of the syndrome revealed some unexpected findings that were initially puzzling but can now be explained by the discovery that the disorder is caused by another unstable repeat expansion, a massive expansion of another triplet repeat, CGG, located in the 5′ untranslated region of the first exon of a gene called *FMR1* (fragile X mental retardation 1). The normal number of repeats is up to 60, whereas as many as several thousand repeats are found in patients with the "full" fragile X syndrome mutation. More than 200 copies of the repeat lead to excessive methylation of cytosines in the promoter of *FMR1*; this interferes with replication or chromatin condensation or both, producing the characteristic chromosomal fragile site, a form of DNA modification that prevents normal promoter function or blocks translation.

Triplet repeat numbers between 60 and 200 constitute a special intermediate premutation stage of the fragile X syndrome. Expansions in this range are unstable when they are transmitted from mother to child and have an increasing tendency to undergo full expansion to more than 200 copies of the repeat during gametogenesis in the female (but almost never in the male), with the risk of expansion increasing dramatically with increasing premutation size (Fig. 7-31). In addition to the risk of expansion to a full mutation and the development of fragile X syndrome in offspring, carriers of premutations can develop an adult-onset neurological disorder of cerebellar dysfunction and neurological deterioration, known as the **fragile X–associated tremor/ataxia syndrome**. In addition, approximately one quarter of female carriers of premutations will experience **premature ovarian failure** by the age of 40 years.

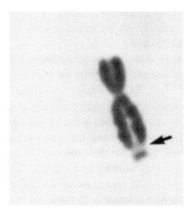

Figure 7-30 ■ The fragile site at Xq27.3 associated with X-linked mental retardation.

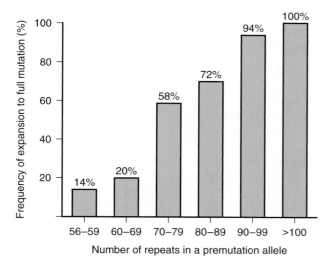

Figure 7-31 ■ Frequency of expansion of a premutation triplet repeat in *FMR1* to a full mutation in oogenesis as a function of the length of the premutation allele carried by a heterozygous female. The risk of fragile X syndrome to her sons is approximately half this frequency, since there is a 50% chance a son will inherit the expanded allele. The risk of fragile X syndrome to her daughters is approximately one-fourth this frequency, since there is a 50% chance a daughter would inherit the full mutation, and penetrance of the full mutation in a female is approximately 50%. (From Nolin SL: Familial transmission of the *FMR1* CGG repeat. Am J Hum Genet 59:1252-1261, 1996. The University of Chicago Press.)

Myotonic Dystrophy

A third unstable repeat expansion disease is **myotonic dystrophy** (dystrophia myotonica, or DM), inherited as an autosomal dominant myopathy characterized by myotonia, muscular dystrophy, cataracts, hypogonadism, diabetes, frontal balding, and changes in the electroencephalogram. The disease is notorious for lack of penetrance, pleiotropy, and its variable expression in both clinical severity and age at onset (Fig. 7-32). One form of DM, the congenital form, is particularly severe and may be life-threatening as well as a cause of mental retardation. Virtually every child with the congenital form is the offspring of an affected mother, who herself may have only a mild expression of the disease and may not even know that she is affected. Thus, pedigrees of DM, like those of HD and fragile X syndrome, show clear evidence of anticipation.

Some of the puzzling features of the inheritance of DM, such as incomplete penetrance and anticipation, can be explained by the discovery that this disease is also associated with amplification of a triplet repeat, in this case a CTG triplet located in the 3′ untranslated region of a protein kinase gene (*DMPK*). The normal range for repeats in *DMPK* is 5 to 30; carriers of repeats in the range of 38 to 54 (premutations) are usually asymptomatic but have an increased risk of passing on fully expanded repeats. Mildly affected individuals have about 50 to 80 copies; the severity increases and age at onset decreases the longer the expansion. Severely affected individuals can have more than 2000 copies. Either parent can transmit an amplified copy, but males can pass on up to 1000 copies of repeat, whereas really massive expansions containing many thousands of repeats occur only in female gametogenesis. Because congenital DM is due to huge expansions in the many thousands, this form of myotonic dystrophy is therefore almost always inherited from an affected mother.

Friedreich Ataxia

Friedreich ataxia (FRDA), a spinocerebellar ataxia, constitutes a fourth category of triplet repeat disease.

Figure 7-32 ■ Myotonic dystrophy, an autosomal dominant condition with variable expression in clinical severity and age at onset. The grandmother in this family *(left)* had bilateral cataracts but has no facial weakness or muscle symptoms; her daughter was thought to be unaffected until after the birth of her severely affected child, but she now has moderate facial weakness and ptosis, with myotonia, and has had cataract extraction. The child has congenital myotonic dystrophy. (From Harper PS: Myotonic Dystrophy, 2nd ed. Philadelphia, WB Saunders, 1989, p 18.)

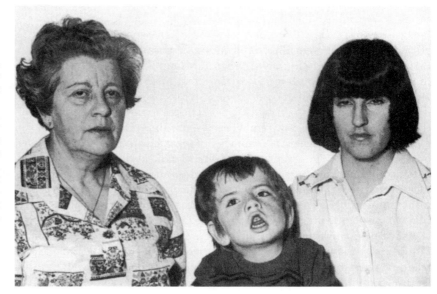

The disease is inherited in an autosomal recessive pattern, in contrast to HD, DM, and fragile X syndrome. The disorder is usually manifested before adolescence and is generally characterized by incoordination of limb movements, difficulty with speech, diminished or absent tendon reflexes, impairment of position and vibratory senses, cardiomyopathy, scoliosis, and foot deformities. In most cases, Friedreich ataxia is caused by amplification of still another triplet repeat, AAG, located this time in an intron of a gene that encodes a mitochondrial protein called frataxin, which is involved in iron metabolism. How a repeat expansion in a frataxin intron can lead to FRDA will be discussed in Chapter 12. In normal individuals, the repeat length varies from 7 to 34 copies, whereas repeat expansions in the patients are typically between 100 and 1200 copies. Expansion within the intron interferes with normal expression of the frataxin gene; because Friedreich ataxia is recessive, loss of expression from both alleles is required to produce the disease. In fact, 1% to 2% of FRDA patients are known to be compound heterozygotes in whom one allele is the common amplified intronic AAG repeat mutation and the other a nucleotide mutation.

Similarities and Differences Among Unstable Repeat Expansion Disorders

A comparison of HD (and the other polyglutamine neurodegeneration diseases) with the fragile X syndrome, DM, and FRDA reveals some similarities but also many differences (see Table 7-3). Although unstable repeat expansions of a trinucleotide are involved in all four types of disease, the expansion in the polyglutamine diseases is in the coding region and ranges from 40 to 120 copies of the CAG, whereas the repeat expansions in fragile X syndrome, DM, and FRDA involve different triplet nucleotides, contain hundreds to thousands of repeated triplets, and are located in untranslated portions of the *FMR1*, *DMPK*, and *FRDA* genes, respectively. Premutation expansions causing an increased risk for passing on full mutations are the rule in all four of these disorders, and anticipation is commonly seen in pedigrees of the dominant and X-linked diseases (HD, fragile X syndrome, and DM). However, the number of repeats in premutation alleles in HD is 29 to 35, similar to what is seen in DM but far less than in fragile X syndrome. Premutation carriers can develop significant disease in fragile X syndrome but are, by definition, disease-free in HD and DM. The expansion of premutation alleles occurs in the female primarily in FRDA, DM, and fragile X syndrome; the largest expansions causing juvenile onset HD occur in the male germline. Finally, the degree of mitotic instability in fragile X syndrome, DM, and FRDA is far greater than that seen in HD and results in much greater variability in the numbers of repeats found among cells of the same tissue and between different somatic tissues in a single individual.

CONDITIONS THAT MAY MIMIC MENDELIAN INHERITANCE OF SINGLE-GENE DISORDERS

A pedigree pattern sometimes simulates a single-gene pattern even though the disorder does not have a single-gene basis. It is easy to be misled in this way by teratogenic effects; by certain types of inherited chromosome disorders, such as balanced translocations; or by environmental exposures shared among family members. Inherited single-gene disorders can usually be distinguished from these other types of familial disorders by their typical mendelian segregation ratios within kindreds. Confirmation that a familial disease is due to mutations in a single gene eventually requires demonstration of defects at the level of the gene product, or the gene itself.

There is also a class of disorders called **segmental aneusomies,** in which there is a deficiency or excess of two or more genes at neighboring loci on a chromosome, due to a deletion or a duplication or triplication of an entire segment of DNA (see Chapter 5). Here the phenotype, referred to as a **contiguous gene syndrome,** results from alterations in the copy number of more than one gene and yet shows typical mendelian segregation ratios, with a usually dominant inheritance pattern, because the segmental aneusomy is passed on as if it were a single mutant allele. Examples include autosomal dominant Parkinson disease due to a triplication of an approximately 2-Mb region of chromosome 4q; autosomal dominant velocardiofacial syndrome, where the phenotype is caused by deletions of millions of base pairs of DNA encoding multiple genes at 22q11.2; and the X-linked syndrome of choroideremia (a retinal degeneration), deafness, and mental retardation, caused by a deletion of at least three loci in band Xq21.

MATERNAL INHERITANCE OF DISORDERS CAUSED BY MUTATIONS IN THE MITOCHONDRIAL GENOME

Some pedigrees of inherited diseases that could not be explained by typical mendelian inheritance of nuclear genes are now known to be caused by mutations of the mitochondrial genome and to manifest maternal inheritance. Disorders caused by mutations in mitochondrial DNA demonstrate a number of unusual features that result from the unique characteristics of mitochondrial biology and function.

The Mitochondrial Genome

As described in Chapter 2, not all the RNA and protein synthesized in a cell are encoded in the DNA of the nucleus; a small but important fraction is encoded by genes within the mitochondrial genome. This genome consists of a circular chromosome, 16.5 kb in size, that is located inside the mitochondrial organelle, not in the nucleus (see Fig. 12-28). Most cells contain at least 1000 mtDNA molecules, distributed among hundreds of individual mitochondria. A remarkable exception is the mature oocyte, which has more than 100,000 copies of mtDNA, composing about one third of the total DNA content of these cells.

Mitochondrial DNA (mtDNA) contains 37 genes. The genes encode 13 polypeptides that are subunits of enzymes of oxidative phosphorylation, two types of ribosomal RNA, and 22 transfer RNAs required for translating the transcripts of the mitochondria-encoded polypeptides. The remaining polypeptides of the oxidative phosphorylation complex are encoded by the nuclear genome.

More than 100 different rearrangements and 100 different point mutations have been identified in mtDNA that can cause human disease, often involving the central nervous and musculoskeletal systems (e.g., myoclonic epilepsy with ragged-red fibers) (Case 28). The diseases that result from these mutations show a distinctive pattern of inheritance because of three unusual features of mitochondria: **replicative segregation, homoplasmy** and **heteroplasmy,** and **maternal inheritance.**

Replicative Segregation

The first unique feature of the mitochondrial chromosome is the absence of the tightly controlled segregation seen during mitosis and meiosis of the 46 nuclear chromosomes. At cell division, the multiple copies of mtDNA in each of the mitochondria in a cell replicate and sort randomly among newly synthesized mitochondria. The mitochondria, in turn, are distributed randomly between the two daughter cells. This process is known as **replicative segregation.**

Homoplasmy and Heteroplasmy

The second unique feature of the genetics of mtDNA arises from the fact that most cells contain many copies of mtDNA molecules. When a mutation arises in the mtDNA, it is at first present in only one of the mtDNA molecules in a mitochondrion. With replicative segregation, however, a mitochondrion containing a mutant mtDNA will acquire multiple copies of the mutant molecule. With cell division, a cell containing a mixture of normal and mutant mtDNAs can distribute very different proportions of mutant and wild-type mitochondrial DNA to its daughter cells. One daughter cell may, by chance, receive mitochondria that contain only a pure population of normal mtDNA or a pure population of mutant mtDNA (a situation known as **homoplasmy**). Alternatively, the daughter cell may receive a mixture of mitochondria, some with and some without mutation (**heteroplasmy**; Fig. 7-33). Because the phenotypic expression of a mutation in mtDNA depends on the

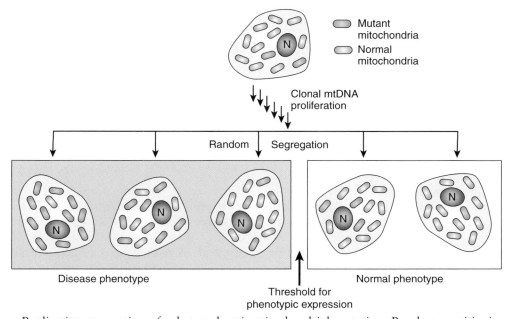

Figure 7-33 ■ Replicative segregation of a heteroplasmic mitochondrial mutation. Random partitioning of mutant and wild-type mitochondria through multiple rounds of mitosis produces a collection of daughter cells with wide variation in the proportion of mutant and wild-type mitochondria carried by each cell. Cell and tissue dysfunction results when the fraction of mitochondria that are carrying a mutation exceeds a threshold level. N, nucleus.

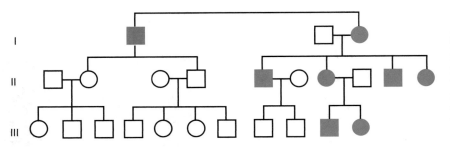

Figure 7-34 ■ Pedigree of Leber hereditary optic neuropathy, a form of spontaneous blindness caused by a defect in mitochondrial DNA. Inheritance is only through the maternal lineage, in agreement with the known maternal inheritance of mitochondrial DNA. No affected male transmits the disease.

relative proportions of normal and mutant mtDNA in the cells making up different tissues, reduced penetrance, variable expression, and pleiotropy are all typical features of mitochondrial disorders.

Maternal Inheritance of mtDNA

The final defining characteristic of the genetics of mtDNA is its **maternal inheritance.** Sperm mitochondria are generally eliminated from the embryo, so that mtDNA is inherited from the mother. Thus, all the children of a *female* who is homoplasmic for a mtDNA mutation will inherit the mutation, whereas none of the offspring of a *male* carrying the same mutation will inherit the defective DNA. The maternal inheritance of a homoplasmic mtDNA mutation causing **Leber hereditary optic neuropathy** is shown in Figure 7-34.

Maternal inheritance in the presence of heteroplasmy in the mother is associated with additional features of mtDNA genetics that are of medical significance. First, the number of mtDNA molecules within developing oocytes is reduced before being subsequently amplified to the huge total seen in mature oocytes. This restriction and subsequent amplification of mtDNA during oogenesis is termed the **mitochondrial genetic bottleneck.** Consequently, the variability in the percentage of mutant mtDNA molecules seen in the offspring of a mother with heteroplasmy for a mtDNA mutation arises, at least in part, from the sampling of only a subset of the mtDNAs during oogenesis. As might be expected, mothers with a high proportion of mutant mtDNA molecules are more likely to produce eggs with a higher proportion of mutant mtDNA and therefore are more likely to have clinically affected offspring than are mothers with a lower proportion. One exception to maternal inheritance occurs when the mother is heteroplasmic for deletion mutation in her mtDNA; for unknown reasons, deleted mtDNA molecules are generally not transmitted from clinically affected mothers to their children (see Table 12-11).

Although mitochondria are almost always inherited exclusively through the mother, at least one instance of paternal inheritance of mtDNA has occurred in a

patient with a mitochondrial myopathy. Consequently, in patients with apparently sporadic mtDNA mutations, the rare occurrence of paternal mtDNA inheritance must be considered (see Box).

••• Characteristics of Mitochondrial Inheritance

- All children of females *homoplasmic* for a mutation will inherit the mutation; the children of males carrying a similar mutation will not.
- Females *heteroplasmic* for *point mutations* and *duplications* will pass them on to all of their children. However, the fraction of mutant mitochondria in the offspring, and therefore the risk and severity of disease, can vary considerably, depending on the fraction of mutant mitochondria in their mother as well as on random chance operating on small numbers of mitochondria per cell at the oocyte bottleneck. Heteroplasmic *deletions* are generally not heritable.
- The fraction of mutant mitochondria in different tissues of an individual heteroplasmic for a mutation can vary tremendously, thereby causing a spectrum of disease among the members of a family in which there is heteroplasmy for a mitochondrial mutation. Pleiotropy and variable expressivity in different affected family members are frequent.

⊙ FAMILY HISTORY AS PERSONALIZED MEDICINE

An accurate determination of the family pedigree is an important part of the work-up of every patient. Pedigrees may demonstrate a straightforward, typical mendelian inheritance pattern; one that is more atypical, as is seen with mitochondrial mutations and germline mosaicism; or a complex pattern of familial occurrence that matches no obvious inheritance pattern (see Chapter 8). Not only is a determination of the inheritance pattern important for making a diagnosis in the proband, but it also identifies other individuals in the family who may be at risk and in need of evaluation and counseling. Despite the sophisticated cytogenetic and molecular testing available to geneticists, an accurate family history, including the family pedigree, remains a fundamental tool for all physicians and genetic counselors to use in designing an individualized management and treatment plan for their patients.

◉ GENERAL REFERENCES

Rimoin DL, Connor JM, Pyeritz RE: Emery and Rimoin's Principles and Practice of Medical Genetics, 4th ed. Philadelphia, WB Saunders, 2001.

Scriver CR, Beaudet AL, Sly WS, Valle D (eds): The Metabolic and Molecular Bases of Inherited Disease, 8th ed. New York, McGraw-Hill, 2000. Updated in an online version at *http://genetics. accessmedicine.com/.*

◉ REFERENCES FOR SPECIFIC TOPICS

Baird PA, Anderson TW, Newcombe HB, Lowry RB: Genetic disorders in children and young adults: a population study. Am J Hum Genet 42:677-693, 1998.

Bastepe M, Juppner H: *GNAS* locus and pseudohypoparathyroidism. Horm Res 63:65-74, 2005.

Bennett RL, Motulsky AG, Bittles A, et al: Genetic counseling and screening of consanguineous couples and their offspring: recommendations of the National Society of Genetic Counselors. J Genet Counsel 11:97-119, 2002.

Bennett RL, Steinhaus KA, Uhrich SB, et al: Recommendations for standardized pedigree nomenclature. J Genet Counsel 4:267-279, 1995.

Costa T, Scriver CR, Childs B: The effect of mendelian disease on human health: a measurement. Am J Med Genet 21:231-242, 1985.

Dobyns WB, Filauro A, Tomson BN, et al: Inheritance of most X-linked traits is not dominant or recessive, just X-linked. Am J Med Genet A 129:136-143, 2004.

Jacquemont S, Hagerman RJ, Leehey M, et al: Fragile X premutation tremor/ataxia syndrome: molecular, clinical, and neuroimaging correlates. Am J Hum Genet 72:869-878, 2003.

Johns DR: Mitochondrial DNA and disease. N Engl J Med 333:638-644, 1995.

Lightowlers RN, Chinnery PF, Turnbull DM, Howell N: Mammalian mitochondrial genetics: heredity, heteroplasmy and disease. Trends Genet 13:450-454, 1997.

Lyon MF: X-chromosome inactivation and human genetic disease. Acta Paediatr Suppl 91:107-112, 2002.

Nolin SL, Lewis FA 3rd, Ye LL, et al: Familial transmission of the FMR1 CGG repeat. Am J Hum Genet 59:1252-1261, 1996.

Pearson CE, Edamura KN, Cleary JD: Repeat instability: mechanisms of dynamic mutations. Nat Rev Genet 6:729-742, 2005.

Scheuner MT, Yoon PW, Khoury MJ: Contribution of mendelian disorders to common chronic disease: opportunities for recognition, intervention, and prevention. Am J Med Genet C Semin Med Genet 125:50-65, 2004.

Squiteri F, Gellera C, Cannella M, et al: Homozygosity for CAG mutation in Huntington disease is associated with a more severe clinical course. Brain 126:946-955, 2003.

Waalen J, Nordestgaard BG, Beutler E: The penetrance of hereditary hemochromatosis. Best Pract Res Clin Haematol 18:203-220, 2005.

Walter J, Paulsen M: Imprinting and disease. Semin Cell Dev Biol 14:101-110, 2003.

Wattendorf DJ, Hadley DW: Family history: the three-generation pedigree. Am Fam Physician 72:441-448, 2005.

Willemsen R, Mientjes E, Oostra BA: FXTAS: a progressive neurologic syndrome associated with fragile X premutation. Curr Neurol Neurosci Rep 5:405-410, 2005.

Zlotogora J: Germ line mosaicism. Hum Genet 102:381-386, 1998.

◉ USEFUL WEBSITE

McKusick VA: Online Mendelian Inheritance in Man. *http://www3. ncbi.nlm.nih.gov* Catalogues of autosomal dominant, autosomal recessive, and X-linked phenotypes.

PROBLEMS

1. Cathy is pregnant for the second time. Her first child, Donald, has CF. Cathy has two brothers, Charles and Colin, and a sister, Cindy. Colin and Cindy are unmarried. Charles is married to an unrelated woman, Carolyn, and has a 2-year-old daughter, Debbie. Cathy's parents are Bob and Betty. Betty's sister Barbara is the mother of Cathy's husband, Calvin, who is 25. There is no previous family history of CF.
   a. Sketch the pedigree, using standard symbols.
   b. What is the pattern of transmission of CF, and what is the risk of CF for Cathy's next child?
   c. Which people in this pedigree are obligate heterozygotes?

2. George and Grace, who have normal hearing, have 8 children; 2 of their 5 daughters and 2 of their 3 sons are congenitally deaf. Another couple, Harry and Helen, both with normal hearing, also have 8 children; 2 of their 6 daughters and one of their 2 sons is deaf. A third couple, Gilbert and Gisele, who are congenitally deaf, have 4 children, also deaf. Their daughter Hedy marries Horace, a deaf son of George and Grace, and Hedy and Horace in turn have 4 deaf children. Their eldest son Isaac marries Ingrid, a daughter of Harry and Helen; although both Isaac and Ingrid are deaf, their 6 sons all have *normal* hearing. Sketch the pedigree and answer the following questions. (Hint: how many different types of

congenital deafness are segregating in this pedigree?)
a. State the probable genotypes of the children in the last generation.
b. Why are all the children of Gilbert and Gisele and of Hedy and Horace deaf?

3. Consider the following situations:
   a. Retinitis pigmentosa occurs in X-linked and autosomal forms.
   b. Two parents each have a typical case of familial hypercholesterolemia diagnosed on the basis of hypercholesterolemia, arcus corneae, tendinous xanthomas, and demonstrated deficiency of LDL receptors, together with a family history of the disorder; they have a child who has a very high plasma cholesterol level at birth and within a few years develops xanthomas and generalized atherosclerosis.
   c. A couple with normal vision, from an isolated community, have a child with autosomal recessive gyrate atrophy of the retina. The child grows up, marries another member (with normal vision) of the same community, and has a child with the same eye disorder.
   d. A child has severe neurofibromatosis (NF1). Her father is phenotypically normal; her mother seems clinically normal but has several large café au lait spots and areas of hypopigmentation, and slit-lamp examination shows that she has a few Lisch nodules (hamartomatous growths on the iris).
   e. Parents of normal stature have a child with achondroplasia.
   f. An adult male with myotonic dystrophy has cataracts, frontal balding, and hypogonadism, in addition to myotonia.
   g. A man with vitamin D–resistant rickets transmits the condition to all his daughters, who have a milder form of the disease than their father has; none of his sons is affected. The daughters have approximately equal numbers of unaffected sons, affected sons, unaffected daughters, and affected daughters, the affected sons being more severely affected than their affected sisters.
   h. A boy has progressive muscular dystrophy with onset in early childhood and is wheelchair bound by the age of 12 years. An unrelated man also has progressive muscular dystrophy but is still ambulant at the age of 30 years. Molecular analysis shows that both patients have large deletions in the dystrophin gene, which encodes the protein that is deficient or defective in the Duchenne and Becker types of muscular dystrophy.
   i. A patient with a recessive disorder is found to have inherited both copies of one chromosome from the same parent and no representative of that chromosome from the other parent.
   j. A child with maple syrup urine disease is born to parents who are first cousins.
   Which of the concepts listed here are illustrated by the situations a-j?
   Variable expressivity
   Uniparental disomy
   Consanguinity
   Inbreeding
   X-linked dominant inheritance
   New mutation
   Allelic heterogeneity
   Locus heterogeneity
   Autosomal incompletely dominant trait
   Pleiotropy

4. Don and his maternal grandfather Barry both have hemophilia A. Don's partner Diane is his maternal aunt's daughter. Don and Diane have one son, Edward, and two daughters, Elise and Emily, all of whom have hemophilia A. They also have an unaffected daughter, Enid.
   a. Draw the pedigree.
   b. Why are Elise and Emily affected?
   c. What is the probability that a son of Elise would be hemophilic? What is the probability that her daughter would be hemophilic?
   d. What is the probability that a son of Enid would be hemophilic? a daughter?

5. A boy is born with a number of malformations but does not have a recognized syndrome. The parents are unrelated, and there is no family history of a similar condition. Which of the following conditions could explain this situation? Which are unlikely? Why?
   a. autosomal dominant inheritance with new mutation
   b. autosomal dominant inheritance with reduced penetrance
   c. autosomal dominant inheritance with variable expressivity
   d. autosomal recessive inheritance
   e. X-linked recessive inheritance
   f. autosomal dominant inheritance, misattributed paternity
   g. maternal ingestion of a teratogenic drug at a sensitive stage of embryonic development

6. A couple has a child with NF1. Both parents are clinically normal, and neither of their families shows a positive family history.
   a. What is the probable explanation for NF1 in their child?
   b. What is the risk of recurrence in other children of this couple?
   c. If the husband has another child by a different mother, what would the risk of NF1 be?
   d. What is the risk that any offspring of the affected child will also have NF1?

7. The consultand (*arrow*) wants to know her risk for having a child with a birth defect before starting her family because she and her husband are related (see pedigree). The family history reveals no known recessive disease. What is the coefficient of inbreeding of the offspring of this couple?

8. Given the pedigree below, what is/are: the *most likely* inheritance pattern(s); *possible* but less likely inheritance pattern(s); *incompatible* inheritance pattern(s)? Patterns are autosomal recessive, autosomal dominant, X-linked recessive, X-linked dominant, mitochondrial. Justify your choices.

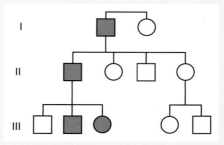

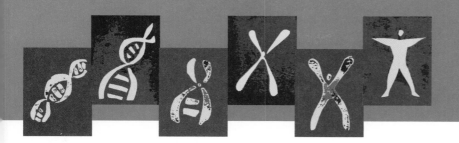

Chapter 8

Genetics of Common Disorders with Complex Inheritance

Diseases such as congenital birth defects, myocardial infarction, cancer, mental illness, diabetes, and Alzheimer disease cause morbidity and premature mortality in nearly two of every three individuals during their lifetimes (Table 8-1). Many of these diseases "run in families"—they seem to recur in the relatives of affected individuals more frequently than in the general population. And yet their inheritance generally does not follow one of the mendelian patterns seen in the single-gene disorders (described in Chapter 7). Instead, they are thought to result from complex *interactions* between a number of genetic and environmental factors and therefore are said to follow a **multifactorial** (or **complex**) inheritance pattern. The familial clustering can be explained by recognizing that family members share a greater proportion of their genetic information and environmental exposures than do individuals chosen at random in the population. Thus, the relatives of an affected individual are more likely to experience the same **gene-gene** and **gene-environment interactions** that led to disease in the proband in the first place than are individuals who are unrelated to the proband. The multifactorial inheritance pattern that results represents an interaction between the collective effect of the genotype at one or, more commonly, multiple loci (**polygenic** or **multigenic** effects) either to raise or to lower susceptibility to disease, combined with a variety of environmental exposures that may trigger, accelerate, exacerbate, or protect against the disease process. The gene-gene interactions in polygenic inheritance may be simply additive or much more complicated. For example, there may be synergistic amplification of sus-

ceptibility by the genotypes at multiple loci or dampening of the effect of genotype at one locus by the genotypes at other loci. Gene-environment interactions, including systematic exposures or chance encounters with environmental factors in one's surroundings, add even more complexity to individual disease risk and the pattern of disease inheritance.

In this chapter, we first address the question of how we determine that genes predispose to common diseases and, therefore, that these diseases are, at least in part, "genetic." We describe how studies of familial aggregation, twin studies, and estimates of heritability are used by geneticists to quantify the relative contributions of genes and environment to diseases and clinically important physiological measures with complex inheritance. Second, we illustrate the general concept of gene-gene interaction, starting with one of the simplest examples, one in which **modifier genes** affect the occurrence or severity of a mendelian disorder. We then give a few examples of more complicated multifactorial diseases in which knowledge of the alleles and loci that confer disease susceptibility is leading to an increased understanding of the mechanisms by which these alleles interact with each other or the environment to cause disease. Unfortunately, we do not understand the underlying mechanisms of the gene-gene and gene-environment interactions for the majority of complex disorders. Geneticists must therefore continue to rely on **empirically derived risk figures** to give our patients and their relatives some answers to basic questions about disease risk and approaches to reducing that risk. We provide such risk figures here but expect that, with

Table 8-1

Frequency of Different Types of Genetic Disease

Type	Incidence at Birth (per 1000)	Prevalence at Age 25 Years (per 1000)	Population Prevalence (per 1000)
Disorders due to genome and chromosome mutations	6	1.8	3.8
Disorders due to single-gene mutations	10	3.6	20
Disorders with multifactorial inheritance	~50	~50	~600

Data from Rimoin DL, Connor JM, Pyeritz RE: Emery and Rimoin's Principles and Practice of Medical Genetics, 3rd ed. Edinburgh, Churchill Livingstone, 1997.

time, research will make them obsolete, replaced by more robust measures of individual risk. As the information gained through the Human Genome Project is applied to the problem of diseases with complex inheritance, physicians and genetic counselors in the years ahead will have the information they need to provide accurate molecular diagnosis and risk assessment and to develop rational preventive and therapeutic measures.

● QUALITATIVE AND QUANTITATIVE TRAITS

We can divide the complex phenotypes of multifactorial disorders into two major categories: **qualitative** and **quantitative** traits. A genetic disease that is either present or absent is referred to as a discrete or qualitative trait; one has the disease or not. In contrast are quantitative traits, which are measurable physiological or biochemical quantities such as height, blood pressure, serum cholesterol concentration, and body mass index (a measure of obesity) that underlie many common and devastating illnesses in the population.

Genetic Analysis of Qualitative Disease Traits

Familial Aggregation of Disease

A primary characteristic of diseases with complex inheritance is that affected individuals may cluster in families (**familial aggregation**). The converse, however, is not necessarily true: familial aggregation of a disease does not mean that a disease must have a genetic contribution. Family members may develop the same disease or trait by chance alone, particularly if it is a common one in the population. Even if familial aggregation is not due to chance, families share more than their genes; for example, they often have cultural attitudes and behaviors, socioeconomic status, diet, and environmental exposures in common. It is the task of the genetic epidemiologist to determine whether familial aggregation is coincidental or the result of factors common to members of the family and to assess the extent to which those common factors are genetic or

environmental. Ultimately, gene mapping studies to locate and identify the particular loci and alleles involved provide the definitive proof of a genetic contribution to multifactorial disease (see Chapter 10).

Concordance and Discordance

When two related individuals in a family have the same disease, they are said to be **concordant** for the disorder. Conversely, when only one member of the pair of relatives is affected and the other is not, the relatives are **discordant** for the disease. Diseases with complex inheritance result from the impact of environmental factors on individuals with certain genotypes. Discordance for phenotype between relatives who share a genotype at loci that predispose to disease can be explained if the unaffected individual has not experienced the other factors (environmental or chance occurrences) necessary to trigger the disease process and make it manifest. Conversely, concordance for a phenotype may occur even when the two affected relatives have different predisposing genotypes, if the disease in one relative is a **genocopy** or **phenocopy** of the disease in the other relative. Lack of penetrance and frequent genocopies and phenocopies contribute to obscuring the inheritance pattern in multifactorial genetic disease.

Measuring Familial Aggregation in Qualitative Traits

Relative Risk λ_r The familial aggregation of a disease can be measured by comparing the frequency of the disease in the relatives of an affected proband with its frequency (prevalence) in the general population. The **relative risk ratio λ_r** is defined as:

$$\lambda_r = \frac{\text{Prevalence of the disease in the relatives of an affected person}}{\text{Prevalence of the disease in the general population}}$$

(The subscript r for λ is used here to refer to relatives; in practice, one measures λ for a particular class of relatives, e.g., r = s for sibs, r = p for parents.) The value of λ_r is a measure of familial aggregation that depends

Table 8-2

Risk Ratios λ_r for Siblings of Probands with Diseases with Familial Aggregation and Complex Inheritance

Disease	Relationship	λ_r
Schizophrenia	Siblings	12
Autism	Siblings	150
Manic-depressive (bipolar) disorder	Siblings	7
Type 1 diabetes mellitus	Siblings	35
Crohn's disease	Siblings	25
Multiple sclerosis	Siblings	24

Data from Rimoin DL, Connor JM, Pyeritz RE: Emery and Rimoin's Principles and Practice of Medical Genetics, 3rd ed. Edinburgh, Churchill Livingstone, 1997; and King RA, Rotter JI, Motulsky AG: The Genetic Basis of Common Diseases, 2nd ed. Oxford, England, Oxford University Press, 2002.

both on the risk of the disease's recurrence in the family and on the population prevalence; the larger λ_r is, the greater is the familial aggregation. The population prevalence enters into the calculation because the more common a disease is, the greater is the likelihood that aggregation may be just a coincidence rather than a result of sharing the alleles that predispose to disease. A value of $\lambda_r = 1$ indicates that a relative is no more likely to develop the disease than is any individual in the population. Examples of approximate λ_r values for various diseases are shown in Table 8-2.

Case-Control Studies Another approach to assessing familial aggregation is the case-control study, in which patients with a disease (the cases) are compared with suitably chosen individuals without the disease (the controls), with respect to family history of disease (as well as other factors, such as environmental exposures, occupation, geographical location, parity, and previous illnesses). To assess a possible genetic contribution to familial aggregation of a disease, the frequency with which the disease is found in the extended families of the cases (**positive family history**) is compared with the frequency of positive family history among suitable controls, matched for age and ethnicity, but who do not have the disease. Spouses are often used as controls in this situation because they usually match the cases in age and ethnicity and share the same household environment. Other frequently used controls are patients with unrelated diseases matched for age, occupation, and ethnicity. Thus, for example, in a study of **multiple sclerosis (MS)**, approximately 3.5% of siblings of patients with MS also had MS, prevalences that were much higher than among the relatives of matched controls without MS (0.2%). One can conclude, therefore, that a family history of MS in a sibling is found more frequently among patients with MS than in controls, indicating that some familial aggregation is occurring in MS.

Case-control studies for familial aggregation are subject to many different kinds of errors or **bias**. One of the most troublesome is **ascertainment bias,** a difference in the likelihood that affected relatives of the cases will be reported to the epidemiologist as compared with the affected relatives of controls. A proband's relatives may be more likely than a control's relatives to know of other family members with the same or similar disease or may be more motivated to respond to questioning because of familiarity with the disease (**recall bias**). Another confounding factor is the choice of controls. Controls should differ from the cases only in their disease status and not in ethnic background, occupation, gender, or socioeconomic status, any of which may distinguish them as being different from the cases in important ways that have little or nothing to do with the fact that they are not affected by the disease. Finally, an association found in a case-control study does not prove causation. If two factors are not independent of each other, such as ethnic background and dietary consumption of certain foods, a case-control study may find a significant association between the disease and ethnic background when it is actually the dietary habits associated with ethnic background that are responsible. For example, the lower frequency of coronary artery disease among Japanese compared with North Americans becomes less pronounced in first-generation Japanese who emigrated to North America and adopted the dietary customs of their new home.

Determining the Relative Contributions of Genes and Environment to Complex Disease

Concordance and Allele Sharing Among Relatives

The more closely related two individuals are in a family, the more alleles they have in common, inherited from their common ancestors. Conversely, the more distantly related the relative is to the proband, the fewer the alleles shared between the proband and the relative. One approach to dissecting the contribution of genetic influences from environmental effects in multifactorial disease is to compare disease concordance in relatives who are more or less closely related to the proband. When genes are important contributors to a disease, the frequency of disease concordance increases as the degree of relatedness increases. The most extreme examples of two individuals having alleles in common are identical (**monozygotic**) twins (see later in this chapter), who have the same alleles at every locus. The next most closely related individuals in a family are first-degree relatives, such as a parent and child or a pair of sibs, including fraternal (**dizygotic**) twins. In a parent-child pair, the child has one allele in common with each parent at every locus, that is, the allele the child inherited from that parent. For a sibpair (including dizygotic twins), the situation is slightly different. A pair of sibs inherits the same two alleles at a locus 25% of the time, no alleles in common 25% of the time, and one allele in common 50% of the time (Fig. 8-1). At any one locus, the average number of alleles one sibling is expected to share with another is given by:

$$0.25 \ (2 \ \text{alleles}) + 0.5 \ (1 \ \text{allele}) + 0.25 \ (0 \ \text{alleles}) = 1 \ \text{allele}$$

For example, if genes predispose to a disease, one would expect λ_r to be greatest for monozygotic twins, then to decrease for first-degree relatives such as sibs or parent-child pairs, and to continue to decrease as allele sharing decreases among the more distant relatives in a family (Table 8-3).

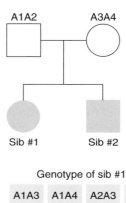

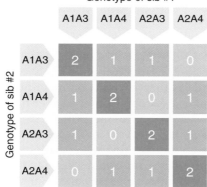

Figure 8-1 ■ Allele sharing at an arbitrary locus between sibs concordant for a disease. The parents' genotypes are shown as *A1A2* for the father and *A3A4* for the mother. All four possible genotypes for sib #1 are given across the top of the table, and all four possible genotypes for sib #2 are given along the left side of the table. The numbers inside the boxes represent the number of alleles both sibs have in common for all 16 different combinations of genotypes for both sibs. For example, the upper left-hand corner has the number 2 because sib #1 and sib #2 both have the genotype *A1A3* and so have both *A1* and *A3* alleles in common. The bottom left-hand corner contains the number 0 because sib #1 has genotype *A1A3* whereas sib #2 has genotype *A2A4*, so there are no alleles in common.

Table 8-3

Degree of Relationship and Alleles in Common

Relationship to Proband	Proportion of Alleles in Common with Proband
Monozygotic twin	1
First-degree relative	1/2
Second-degree relative	1/4
Third-degree relative	1/8

See Chapter 7, Figure 7-2, for description of degrees of relationship.

Unrelated Family Member Controls

The more closely related two individuals are, the more likely they are to share home environment as well as genes. One way to separate family environment from genetic influence is to compare the incidence of disease in unrelated family members (adoptees, spouses) with that in biological relatives. In one study of MS, for example, $\lambda_r = 20$ to 40 in first-degree biological relatives (parents, children, and sibs) but $\lambda_r = 1$ for siblings or children adopted into the family, suggesting that most of the familial aggregation in MS is genetic rather than environmental in origin. These values of λ_r translate into a risk for MS for the monozygotic twin of an affected individual, who shares 100% of his genetic information with his twin, that is 190 times the risk for MS in an adopted child or sibling of an MS proband, who shares with the affected individual much of the same environmental exposures but none of the genetic information.

Twin Studies

Another common method for separating genetic from environmental influences on disease is to study twins, both monozygotic (MZ) and dizygotic (DZ). Twins are "experiments of nature" that come closest to providing an opportunity to assess environmental and genetic influences separately in humans. DZ twins reared together allow geneticists to measure disease concordance in relatives who grow up in similar environments but do not share all their genes, whereas MZ twins provide an opportunity to compare relatives with identical genotypes who may or may not be reared together in the same environment. Studies of twins have played a significant role in helping geneticists to assess the relative contributions of genes and environment to disease causation.

MZ twins arise from the cleavage of a single fertilized zygote into two separate zygotes early in embryogenesis (see Fig. 14-12). As a result, MZ twins have identical genotypes at every locus and are always of the same sex. They occur in approximately 0.3% of all births, without significant differences among different ethnic groups. DZ twins arise from the simultaneous fertilization of two eggs by two sperm; genetically, DZ twins are siblings who share a womb and, like all siblings, share, on average, 50% of the alleles at all loci. DZ twins are of the same sex half the time and of opposite sex the other half. DZ twins occur with a frequency that varies as much as 5-fold in different populations, from a low of 0.2% among Asians to more than 1% of births in parts of Africa and among African Americans.

Disease Concordance in Monozygotic Twins An examination of how frequently MZ twins are concordant for a disease is a powerful method for determining whether genotype alone is sufficient to produce a particular disease. For example, if one MZ twin has sickle cell disease, the other twin will also have sickle cell disease. In contrast, when one MZ twin has type 1 diabetes mellitus (previously known as insulin-dependent or juvenile diabetes), only about 40% of the other twins will also have type 1 diabetes. *Disease concordance less than 100% in MZ twins is strong evidence that nongenetic factors play a role in the disease.* Such factors could include environmental influences, such as exposure to infection or diet, as well as other effects, such as somatic mutation, effects of aging, and differences in X inactivation in one female twin compared with the other.

Concordance of Monozygotic Versus Dizygotic Twins MZ and same-sex DZ twins share a common intrauterine environment and sex and are usually reared together in the same household by the same parents. Thus, a comparison of concordance for a disease between MZ and same-sex DZ twins shows how frequently disease occurs when relatives who experience the same prenatal and possibly postnatal environment have all their genes in common, compared with only 50% of their genes in common. *Greater concordance in MZ versus DZ twins is strong evidence of a genetic component to the disease* (Table 8-4). This conclusion is strongest for conditions with early onset, such as birth defects. For late-onset diseases, such as neurodegenerative disease of late adulthood, the assumption that MZ and DZ twins are exposed to similar environments throughout their adult lives becomes less valid, and thus a difference in concordance provides less strong evidence for genetic factors in disease causation.

Twins Reared Apart If MZ twins are separated at birth and raised apart, geneticists have the opportunity to observe disease concordance in individuals with identical genotypes reared in different environments. Such studies have been used primarily in research in psychiatric disorders, substance abuse, and eating disorders, in which strong environmental influences within the family are believed to play a role in the development of disease. For example, in one study of alcoholism, five

Table 8-4

Concordance Rates in MZ and DZ Twins

Disorder	Concordance (%)	
	MZ	DZ
Nontraumatic epilepsy	70	6
Multiple sclerosis	17.8	2
Type 1 diabetes	40	4.8
Schizophrenia	46	15
Bipolar disease	62	8
Osteoarthritis	32	16
Rheumatoid arthritis	12.3	3.5
Psoriasis	72	15
Cleft lip with or without cleft palate	30	2
Systemic lupus erythematosus	22	0

Data from Rimoin DL, Connor JM, Pyeritz RE: Emery and Rimoin's Principles and Practice of Medical Genetics, 3rd ed. Edinburgh, Churchill Livingstone, 1997; King RA, Rotter JI, Motulsky AG: The Genetic Basis of Common Diseases. Oxford, England, Oxford University Press, 1992; and Tsuang MT: Recent advances in genetic research on schizophrenia. J Biomed Sci 5:28-30, 1998.

of six MZ twin pairs reared apart were concordant for alcoholism, a concordance rate at least as high as that seen among MZ twins reared together, suggesting that shared genetic factors are far more important than shared environment.

Limitations of Twin Studies As useful as twin studies are for dissecting genetic and environmental factors in disease, they must be interpreted with care for several reasons. First, MZ twins do not have precisely identical genes or gene expression despite starting out with identical genotypes at the time the zygote cleaves in two to create the MZ twins. For example, somatic rearrangements in the immunoglobulin and T-cell receptor loci will differ between MZ twins in various lymphocyte subsets (see Chapter 3). In addition, on the X chromosome, random X inactivation after cleavage into two female MZ zygotes produces significant differences in the expression of alleles of X-linked genes in different tissues (see Chapter 6).

Second, environmental exposures may not be the same for twins, especially once the twins reach adulthood and leave their childhood home. Even intrauterine environment may not be the same. For example, MZ twins frequently share a placenta, and there may be a disparity between the twins in blood supply, intrauterine development, and birth weight.

Third, measurements of disease concordance in MZ twins give an average estimate that may not be accurate if the relevant predisposing alleles or environmental factors are different in different twin pairs. Suppose the genotype of one pair of twins generates a greater risk for disease than does the genotype of another pair; the observed concordance will be an average that really applies to neither pair of twins. As

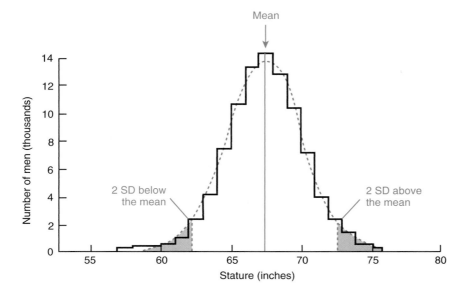

Figure 8-2 ■ Distribution of stature in a sample of 91,163 young English males in 1939 (black line). The blue line is a normal (gaussian) curve with the same mean and standard deviation (SD) as the observed data. The shaded areas indicate persons of unusually tall or short stature (>2 SD above or below the mean). (Modified from Harrison GA, Weiner JS, Tanner JM, et al: Human Biology, 2nd ed. Oxford, England, Oxford University Press, 1977.)

a more extreme example, the disease may not always be genetic in origin, that is, nongenetic phenocopies may exist. If genotype alone causes the disease in some pairs of twins (MZ twin concordance 100%) and a nongenetic phenocopy affects one twin of the pair in another group of twins (MZ twin concordance 0%), twin studies will show an intermediate level of concordance greater than 0% and less than 100% that really applies to neither form of the disease.

Finally, ascertainment bias is a problem, particularly when one twin with a particular disease is asked to recruit the other twin to participate in a study (**volunteer-based ascertainment**), rather than if they are ascertained first as twins and only then is their health status examined (**population-based ascertainment**). Volunteer-based ascertainment can give biased results because twins, particularly MZ twins who may be emotionally close, are more likely to volunteer if they are concordant than if they are not, which inflates the concordance rate. In properly designed studies, however, twins offer an unusual opportunity to study disease occurrence when genetic influences are held constant (measuring disease concordance in MZ twins reared together or apart) or when genetic differences are present but environmental influences are similar (comparing disease concordance in MZ versus DZ twins).

Genetic Analysis of Quantitative Traits

Measurable physiological quantities, such as blood pressure, serum cholesterol concentration, and body mass index, vary among different individuals and are important determinants of health and disease in the population. Such variation is usually due to differences in genotype as well as nongenetic (i.e., environmental) factors. The challenge to geneticists is to determine the extent to which genes contribute to this variability, to identify these genes, and to ascertain the alleles responsible.

The Normal Distribution

As is often the case with physiological quantities measured in a population, a graph of the number of individuals in the population (y-axis) having a particular quantitative value (x-axis) produces the familiar bell-shaped curve known as the **normal (gaussian) distribution** (Fig. 8-2). In a graph of the population frequency of a normally distributed value, the position of the peak of the graph and the shape of the graph are governed by two quantities, the **mean** (μ) and the **variance** (σ^2), respectively. The mean is the arithmetic average of the values, and because more people have values for the trait near the average, the curve has its peak at the mean value. The variance (or its square root, the **standard deviation**, σ), is a measure of the degree of spread of values to either side of the mean and therefore determines the breadth of the curve. Any physiological quantity that can be measured is a **quantitative phenotype**, with a mean and a variance. The variance of a measured quantity in the population is called the **total phenotypic variance**.

The Normal Range

The concept of the normal range of a physiological quantity is fundamental to clinical medicine. For example, extremely tall or short stature, hypertension, hypercholesterolemia, and obesity are all considered abnormal when a value sits clearly outside the normal range. In assessing health and disease in children, height, weight, head circumference, and other measurements are compared with the "normal" expected mea-

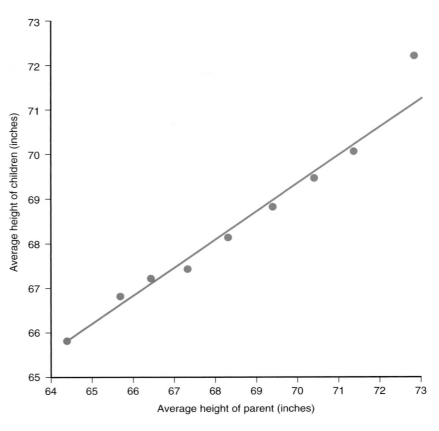

Figure 8-3 ■ Correlation between average parental height and height of children. The average height of parents within intervals of 1 inch (64 to 65 inches, 65 to 66 inches, and so on) is plotted along the abscissa; the average height within a 1-inch interval of their children is plotted on the ordinate. The straight line is a "best fit" through the data points. (The astute observer will note that the slope of the line is not 45 degrees. This reflects the fact that children of tall parents, although still taller than average, tend to be shorter than their parents, whereas the children of short parents, although still shorter than average, tend to be taller than their parents. This phenomenon, known as regression to the mean, was observed more than 100 years ago by Galton.)

surements for a child's sex and age. But how is the "normal" range determined? In many situations in medicine, a particular measured physiological value is "normal" or "abnormal" depending on how far it is above or below the mean. The normal distribution provides guidelines for setting the limits of the normal range. Basic statistical theory states that when a quantitative trait is normally distributed in a population, only 5% of the population will have measurements more than 2 standard deviations above or below the population mean. (Note that the word "normal" is used here in two different ways. Asserting that a physiological quantity has a normal distribution in the population and stating that an individual's value is in the normal range are different uses of the same word.)

Familial Aggregation of Quantitative Traits

Just as familial aggregation, as measured by λ_r and case-control studies, is used to assess the role of heredity in qualitative disease traits, family studies can also be used to determine the role of heredity in quantitative traits. Quantitative traits, however, are not either present or absent; they are measurements. Consequently, one cannot simply compare the prevalence of disease in relatives versus controls or the degree of concordance in twins. Instead, geneticists measure the **correlation** of particular physiological quantities among relatives, that is, the tendency for the actual values of

a physiological measurement to be more similar among relatives than among the general population. The **coefficient of correlation** (symbolized by the letter r) is a statistical measure applied to a pair of measurements, such as, for example, a person's blood pressure and the mean blood pressures of that person's siblings. Accordingly, a **positive correlation** exists between the blood pressure measurements in a group of patients and the blood pressure measurements of their relatives if it is found that the higher a patient's blood pressure, the higher are the blood pressures of the patient's relatives. (A **negative correlation** exists when the greater the increase in the patient's measurement, the lower the measurement is in the patient's relatives. The measurements are still correlated, but in the opposite direction.) The value of r can range from 0 when there is no correlation to +1 for perfect positive correlation and to −1 for perfect negative correlation.

Figure 8-3 shows a graph of the average height of more than 200 parent couples plotted against the average height of their nearly 1000 adult children. There is a positive but not perfect correlation ($r = {\sim}0.6$) between the average parental height and the mean height of their children.

The correlation among relatives can be used to estimate genetic influence on a quantitative trait if you assume that the degree of similarity in the values of the trait measured among relatives is proportional to the number of alleles they share at the relevant loci for that trait. The more closely related the individuals are in a family, the more likely they are to share alleles at loci that determine a quantitative trait and the more strongly correlated will be their values. However, just as with disease traits that are found to aggregate in families because relatives share genes and environmental factors, correlation of a particular physiological value among relatives reflects the influence of both heredity and common environmental factors. A correlation does not indicate that genes are wholly responsible for whatever correlation there is.

Heritability

The concept of **heritability** (symbolized as h^2) was developed to quantify the role of genetic differences in determining variability of quantitative traits. Heritability is defined as the fraction of the total phenotypic variance of a quantitative trait that is caused by genes and is therefore a measure of the extent to which different alleles at various loci are responsible for the variability in a given quantitative trait seen across a population. The higher the heritability, the greater is the contribution of genetic differences among people in causing variability of the trait. The value of h^2 varies from 0, if genes contribute nothing to the total phenotypic variance, to 1, if genes are totally responsible for the phenotypic variance.

Heritability of a trait is a somewhat theoretical concept; it is estimated from the correlation between measurements of that trait among relatives of known degrees of relatedness, such as parents and children, siblings, or, as described next, MZ and DZ twins. There are, however, a number of practical difficulties in measuring and interpreting h^2. One is that relatives share more than their genes; they also share environmental exposures, and so the correlation between relatives may not reflect simply their familial genetic relationship. Second, even when the heritability of a trait is high, it does not reveal the underlying mechanism of inheritance of the trait, such as the number of loci involved or how the various alleles at those loci interact. Finally, as tempting as it is to think of heritability as an intrinsic quality of a particular quantitative trait, it cannot be considered in isolation from the population group and living conditions in which the estimate is being made.

Estimating Heritability from Twin Studies Just as twin data may be used to assess the separate roles of genes and environment in qualitative disease traits, they can also be used to estimate the heritability of a quantitative trait. The variance in the values of a physiological measurement made in a set of MZ twins (who share 100% of their genes) is compared with the variance in the values of that measurement made in a set of DZ twins (who share 50% of their genes, on average). The formula for calculating h^2 is given by

$$h^2 = \frac{\text{Variance in DZ pairs} - \text{Variance in MZ pairs}}{\text{Variance in DZ pairs}}$$

If the variability of the trait is determined chiefly by environment, the variance within pairs of DZ twins will be similar to that seen within pairs of MZ twins, and the numerator, and therefore h^2 itself, will approach 0. If the variability is determined exclusively by genetic makeup, variance of MZ pairs is zero, and h^2 is 1.

Adult stature has been studied by geneticists for decades as a model of how genetic and environmental contributions to a quantitative trait can be apportioned. Large numbers of measurements have been collected (from military recruits, for example). A graph of the frequency of various heights in the population (see Fig. 8-2) demonstrates a bell-shaped curve that fits the normal distribution. By use of the twin method in samples of northern European extraction, h^2 for stature is estimated to be approximately 0.8, indicating that most of the variability in height among individuals is due to genotypic differences between them, not differences in environmental exposures. Thus, genes play a far greater role in determining adult height than does environment.

As another example, a comparison of MZ twins reared together or apart with DZ twins reared together or apart is a classic way of measuring heritability of complex traits. Studies of the body mass index of twins showed a high heritability value ($h^2 = .70$ to $.80$), indicating that there is a strong influence of heredity on this trait.

One has to make a number of simplifying assumptions when using twins to estimate heritability. The first is that MZ and same-sex DZ twins reared together differ only in that they share all (MZ) or, on average, half (DZ) of their genes, although their experiences and environmental exposures are identical. In analyzing the heritability of stature or body mass index, such assumptions may not be too far off the mark, but they are much more difficult to justify in estimating the heritability of more complicated quantitative measurements, such as scores on personality profiles and IQ tests. Another important caveat is that one may not always be able to extrapolate heritability estimated from twins to the population as a whole, to different ethnic groups, or even to the same group if socioeconomic conditions change over time.

Limitations of Studies of Familial Aggregation, Disease Concordance, and Heritability

Familial aggregation studies, the analysis of twin concordance, and estimates of heritability do not specify which loci and alleles are involved, how many loci there are, or how a particular genotype and set of environmental influences interact to cause a disease or to determine the value of a particular physiological parameter. In most cases, all we can show is that there is a genetic contribution but little else.

Historically, geneticists lacked the tools needed to study families and populations directly to identify the factors involved in most multifactorial disease. Instead, they attempted to understand the underlying mechanisms by which complex diseases are inherited by creating theoretical models. In these models, geneticists would specify a set of alleles at various unknown loci, a number of environmental factors, and the nature of the interactions among these factors and then test the models for how well they could predict the inheritance pattern of a disease observed in actual families. A good match between theoretical prediction and observation would suggest that the theoretical model is a good approximation of the true underlying mechanism of disease. Unfortunately, many different models can fit an inheritance pattern to a first approximation, making it difficult to know which model, if any, is closest to the correct underlying mechanism. The powerful genetic analysis tools that have come out of the Human Genome Project now make it possible to analyze families and populations directly to find specific genes and alleles that contribute to disease susceptibility. Empirical studies designed to identify how particular alleles at specific loci interact with relevant environmental factors to alter susceptibility to complex disease are a central

focus of the field of **genetic epidemiology** (to be discussed more fully in Chapter 10). The field is developing rapidly, and it is clear that the genetic basis of many more complex diseases in humans will be elucidated in the coming years.

GENETIC AND ENVIRONMENTAL MODIFIERS OF SINGLE-GENE DISORDERS

As discussed in Chapter 7, differences in one's genotype can explain variation in the phenotype in many single-gene disorders. In **cystic fibrosis (CF)**, for example, whether or not a patient has pancreatic insufficiency requiring enzyme replacement can be largely explained by which mutant alleles are present in the *CFTR* gene. The correlation may be imperfect, however, for other alleles, loci, and phenotypes. With CF again as an example, the variation in the degree of pulmonary disease remains unexplained even after correction for allelic heterogeneity. It has been proposed that the genotypes at other genetic loci could act as genetic modifiers, that is, genes whose alleles have an effect on the severity of pulmonary disease seen in CF patients. For example, reduction in FEV_1 (forced expiratory volume after 1 second) is a commonly used measure of deterioration in pulmonary function in CF patients. FEV_1, calculated as percentage of the value expected for CF patients (a CF-specific FEV_1 percent), can be considered a quantitative trait and compared in MZ versus DZ twins to get an estimate of the heritability of the severity of lung disease in CF patients independent of the *CFTR* genotype (since twins have the same CF mutations). The decrease in CF-specific FEV_1 percent was found to correlate better in MZ versus DZ twins, with a heritability of 0.5, suggesting that modifier genes play a role in determining this measure of lung disease. On the other hand, since the heritability was not 1, the analysis also shows that environmental factors are likely to be important in influencing lung disease severity in CF patients with identical genotypes at the *CFTR* locus.

The specific loci harboring alleles responsible for modifying the severity of pulmonary disease in CF are currently not completely known. Two candidates are *MBL2*, a gene that encodes a serum protein called mannose-binding lectin, and the *TGFB1* locus encoding the cytokine transforming growth factor β (TGFβ). Mannose-binding lectin is a plasma protein in the innate immune system that binds to carbohydrates on the surface of many pathogenic organisms and aids in their destruction by phagocytosis and complement activation. A number of common alleles that result in reduced blood levels of the lectin exist at the *MBL2* locus in European populations. Lower levels of

---

■ ■ ■ Characteristics of Inheritance of Complex Diseases

- Genes contribute to diseases with complex inheritance, but these diseases are not single-gene disorders and do not demonstrate a simple mendelian pattern of inheritance.
- Diseases with complex inheritance often demonstrate familial aggregation because relatives of an affected individual are more likely to have disease-predisposing alleles in common with the affected person than are unrelated individuals.
- Pairs of relatives who share disease-predisposing genotypes at relevant loci may still be discordant for phenotype (show lack of penetrance) because of the crucial role of nongenetic factors in disease causation. The most extreme examples of lack of penetrance despite identical genotypes are discordant monozygotic twins.
- The disease is more common among the close relatives of the proband and becomes less common in relatives who are less closely related and therefore share fewer predisposing alleles. Greater concordance for disease is expected among monozygotic versus dizygotic twins.

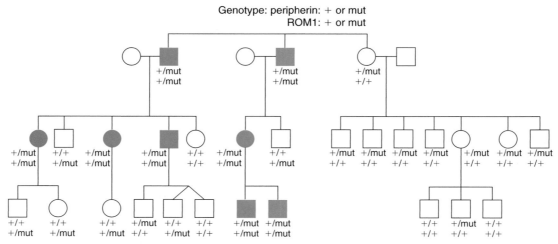

Figure 8-4 ■ Pedigree of a family with retinitis pigmentosa due to digenic inheritance. Filled symbols are affected individuals. Each individual's genotypes at the peripherin locus (*first line*) and *ROM1* locus (*second line*) are written below each symbol. The normal allele is +; the mutant allele is mut. (From Kajiwara K, Berson EL, Dryja TP: Digenic retinitis pigmentosa due to mutations at the unlinked peripherin/RDS and ROM1 loci. Science 264:1604-1608, 1994.)

mannose-binding lectin appear associated with worse outcomes, perhaps because of difficulties with containing respiratory tract infection and inflammation. Alleles at the *TGFB1* locus that result in higher TGFβ production are also associated with worse outcome, perhaps because TGFβ promotes lung scarring and fibrosis after inflammation.

● EXAMPLES OF MULTIFACTORIAL TRAITS FOR WHICH GENETIC AND ENVIRONMENTAL FACTORS ARE KNOWN

Digenic Retinitis Pigmentosa

The simplest example of a multigenic trait (i.e., one determined by the additive effect of the genotypes at multiple loci) has been found in a few families of patients with a form of retinal degeneration called **retinitis pigmentosa** (Fig. 8-4). Two rare mutations in two different unlinked genes encoding proteins found in the photoreceptor are present in these families. Patients heterozygous either for a particular missense mutation in one gene, encoding the photoreceptor membrane protein peripherin, or for a null allele in the other gene, encoding a related photoreceptor membrane protein called Rom1, do *not* develop the disease. However, patients heterozygous for *both* mutations *do* develop the disease. Thus, this disease is caused by the simplest form of multigenic inheritance, inheritance due to the effect of mutant alleles at two loci without any known environmental factors that influence disease occurrence or severity. These two photoreceptor proteins are associated noncovalently in the stacks of membranous disks

found in photoreceptors in the retina. Thus, in patients with digenic retinitis pigmentosa, the deleterious effect of each mutation alone is insufficient to cause disease, but their joint presence is sufficient to cross a threshold of cell damage, photoreceptor death, and loss of vision.

Venous Thrombosis

Another example of gene-gene interaction predisposing to disease is found in the group of conditions referred to as hypercoagulability states, in which venous or arterial clots form inappropriately and cause life-threatening complications (Case 41). With hypercoagulability, however, there is a third factor, an environmental influence that, in the presence of the predisposing genetic factors, increases the risk of disease even more. One such disorder is **idiopathic cerebral vein thrombosis**, a disease in which clots form in the venous system of the brain, causing catastrophic occlusion of cerebral veins in the absence of an inciting event such as infection or tumor. It affects young adults, and although quite rare (<1 per 100,000 in the population), it carries with it a high mortality rate (5% to 30%). Three relatively common factors (two genetic and one environmental) that lead to abnormal coagulability of the clotting system are each known to individually increase the risk for cerebral vein thrombosis: a common missense mutation in a clotting factor, factor V; another common variant in the 3′ untranslated region of the gene for the clotting factor prothrombin; and the use of oral contraceptives (Fig. 8-5).

A mutant allele of factor V (**factor V Leiden, FVL**), in which arginine is replaced by glutamine at position 506 (Arg506Gly), has an allele frequency of approxi-

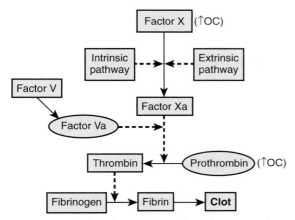

Figure 8-5 ■ The clotting cascade relevant to factor V Leiden and prothrombin mutations. Once factor X is activated, through either the intrinsic or extrinsic pathway, activated factor V promotes the production of the coagulant protein thrombin from prothrombin, which in turn cleaves fibrinogen to generate fibrin required for clot formation. Oral contraceptives (OC) increase blood levels of prothrombin and factor X as well as a number of other coagulation factors. The hypercoagulable state can be explained as a synergistic interaction of genetic and environmental factors that increase the levels of factor V, prothrombin, factor X and others to promote clotting. Activated forms of coagulation proteins are indicated by the letter *a*. Solid arrows are pathways; dashed arrows are stimulators.

mately 2.5% in white people but is rarer in other population groups. This alteration affects a cleavage site used to degrade factor V, thereby making the protein more stable and able to exert its procoagulant effect for a longer duration. Heterozygous carriers of FVL, approximately 5% of the white population, have a risk of cerebral vein thrombosis that, although still quite low, is seven times higher than that in the general population; homozygotes have a risk that is 80 times higher. The second genetic risk factor, a mutation in the **prothrombin** gene, changes a G to an A at position 20210 in the 3′ untranslated region of the gene (prothrombin g.20210G>A). Approximately 2.4% of white individuals are heterozygotes, but it is rare in other ethnic groups. This change appears to increase the level of prothrombin mRNA, resulting in increased translation and elevated levels of the protein. Being heterozygous for the prothrombin 20210G>A allele raises the risk of cerebral vein thrombosis 3-fold to 6-fold. Finally, the use of oral contraceptives containing synthetic estrogen increases the risk of thrombosis 14- to 22-fold, independent of genotype at the factor V and prothrombin loci, probably by increasing the levels of many clotting factors in the blood. Although using oral contraceptives and being heterozygous for FVL cause only a modest increase in risk compared with either factor alone, oral contraceptive use in a heterozygote for prothrombin 20210G>A has an increased relative risk for cerebral vein thrombosis between 30 and 150! Thus, each of

these three factors, two genetic and one environmental, on its own increases the risk for an abnormal hypercoagulable state; having two of these factors at the same time raises the risk for a rare, devastating illness of the cerebral vascular system even more.

These FVL and prothrombin 20210G>A alleles, as well as an allele for a heat-sensitive methylene tetrahydrofolate reductase (see later discussion), have also been implicated as serious predisposing genetic risk factors for **placental artery thrombosis.** Carrying one of these mutations raises the risk an average of 5-fold above the general population risk for this rare but severe obstetrical complication. The resulting placental dysfunction is associated with severe preeclampsia, premature separation of the placenta from the uterine wall, intrauterine growth retardation, and stillbirth.

There is much interest in the role of FVL and prothrombin 20210G>A alleles in **deep venous thrombosis** (DVT) of the lower extremities, a condition that is far more common than idiopathic cerebral venous or placental artery thrombosis. Lower extremity DVT occurs in approximately 1 in 1000 individuals per year, with mortality, primarily due to pulmonary embolus, of up to 10%, depending on age and the presence of other medical conditions. Many environmental factors are known to increase the risk for DVT and include trauma, surgery (particularly orthopedic surgery), malignant disease, prolonged periods of immobility, oral contraceptive use, and advanced age. FVL increases the relative risk of a first episode of DVT 7-fold in heterozygotes and 80-fold in homozygotes; heterozygotes who use oral contraceptives see their risk increased to 30-fold compared with controls. Heterozygotes for prothrombin 20210G>A also have an increase in their relative risk for DVT of 2-fold to 3-fold; double heterozygotes for FVL and prothrombin 20210G>A have a relative increased risk 20-fold above that of the general population. Interestingly, heterozygosity for either FVL or prothrombin 20210G>A alone has little effect on the risk of a recurrence of DVT after the first episode, but together they act synergistically and increase the risk of recurrence 2-fold to 3-fold.

The interaction of these genetic factors with the use of oral contraceptives has led to a proposal that physicians screen all women for the predisposing factor V and prothrombin gene mutations before prescribing birth control pills. Although carriers of the FVL and prothrombin 20210G>A alleles have an increased risk for thrombotic events above that of noncarriers, a risk that increases even more if oral contraceptives are used, these alleles are frequent in the population, as is oral contraceptive use, while the incidence of thrombotic events is small. One can only conclude, therefore, that these factors must not cause significant disease in everyone who uses birth control pills or is heterozygous for one of these alleles. If that were the case, thrombosis would be far more frequent than it is. For example, nearly 1 in 40 white women is heterozygous for prothrombin 20210G>A, yet fewer than 1 in 1000 of these heterozygotes will develop cerebral venous thrombosis when using oral contraception.

The effect of FVL and prothrombin 20210G>A provides a clear example of the difference between increasing susceptibility to an illness and actually causing the illness, and between relative risk and absolute risk conferred by a particular genotype. *A risk factor can increase risk, but still not be a good predictor in any one individual of whether one will develop the complication* (see Chapter 17). As a result, there is significant controversy as to whether being a woman of childbearing age contemplating oral contraceptive use is enough to justify the expense and potential for complications for employment or insurance (in societies that lack genetic discrimination protection) of testing for FVL or prothrombin 20210G>A, unless an additional warning sign is present, such as a personal or family history of unexplained or recurrent venous thrombosis. Thus, consensus recommendations for testing for FVL or prothrombin 20210G>A (see Box) do *not* include screening all young women contemplating starting oral contraceptives in the absence of personal or family history of thrombosis.

••• Consensus Recommendations for Testing for Factor V Leiden or Prothrombin 20210G>A

- Any venous thrombosis in an individual younger than 50 years
- Venous thrombosis in unusual sites (such as hepatic, mesenteric, and cerebral veins)
- Recurrent venous thrombosis
- Venous thrombosis and a strong family history of thrombotic disease
- Venous thrombosis in pregnant women or women taking oral contraceptives
- Relatives of individuals with venous thrombosis younger than 50 years
- Myocardial infarction in female smokers younger than 50 years

---

Hirschsprung Disease

A more complicated set of interacting genetic factors has been described in the pathogenesis of a developmental abnormality of the parasympathetic nervous system in the gut known as **Hirschsprung disease** (HSCR) (Case 20). In HSCR, there is complete absence of some or all of the intrinsic ganglion cells in the myenteric and submucosal plexuses of the colon. An aganglionic colon is incapable of peristalsis, resulting in severe constipation, symptoms of intestinal obstruction, and massive dilatation of the colon (megacolon) proximal to the aganglionic segment. The disorder affects approximately 1 in 5000 newborns. HSCR occurs most commonly as an isolated defect involving a single, short segment of colon, but it can also involve long, continuous colonic segments and can also occur as one element of a broader constellation of congenital abnormalities including deafness and pigmentary abnormalities of hair and eyes (the **Waardenburg-Shah** syndrome).

The hereditary pattern of HSCR has many of the characteristics of a disorder with complex genetics. The relative risk ratio for sibs, λ_s, is very high (approximately 200), but MZ twins do not show perfect concordance. HSCR can occur through multiple generations or can affect multiple siblings in a family, or both, suggesting an autosomal dominant or recessive disorder, but recurrence risks are not strictly 50% or 25% as one might expect for autosomal dominant or autosomal recessive disease traits. Finally, males have a 2-fold higher risk for developing HSCR compared with females within the same family.

Mutations in many different genes may cause the disease. In some families, HSCR affecting long colonic segments is inherited in a mendelian manner. Under these circumstances, the birth defects are most commonly due to mutations in the *RET* gene located at 10q11.2, encoding RET, a tyrosine kinase receptor. A small minority of families with mendelian inheritance of HSCR has mutations in the gene encoding one of the ligands that binds to RET, such as the glial cell line–derived neurotrophic factor (GDNF). Other individuals have been described with mutations in either one of another pair of genes, the *EDNRB* gene at 13q22 encoding the G protein–coupled endothelin receptor B, and the *EDN3* gene encoding its ligand, endothelin 3, at 20q13. Endothelin receptor B and RET can signal independently along parallel pathways, as well as interact with each other to promote development of colonic ganglion cells.

Although a variety of different mutations in the coding exons of *RET* can cause HSCR affecting multiple individuals in a family, the penetrance of these *RET* alleles is far from complete. In some families, penetrance requires that an individual have both a *RET* mutation and a mutation in *GDNF*. The most likely explanation for these observations is that some mutant alleles of *RET* still provide residual function sufficient to prevent development of the disease unless additional dysfunction in another component of the relevant signaling pathways also occurs.

The multifactorial nature of HSCR was brought into even sharper focus when the genetic basis of the most common form of HSCR, involving only a short

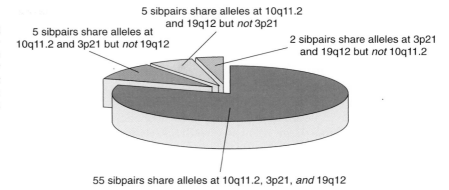

Loci showing allele sharing in 67 sibpairs
concordant for Hirschsprung disease

5 sibpairs share alleles at 10q11.2
and 19q12 but *not* 3p21

5 sibpairs share alleles at
10q11.2 and 3p21 but *not* 19q12

2 sibpairs share alleles at 3p21
and 19q12 but *not* 10q11.2

55 sibpairs share alleles at 10q11.2, 3p21, *and* 19q12

Figure 8-6 ■ Patterns of allele sharing among 67 sibpairs concordant for Hirschsprung disease, divided according to the number of loci for which the sibs show allele sharing. The three loci are located at 10q11.2 (*RET*), 3p21, and 19q12. (Data provided by A. Chakravarti, Johns Hopkins University, Baltimore, Maryland.)

segment of colon, was analyzed in families that did not show any obvious mendelian inheritance pattern for the disorder. When a set of 67 pairs of siblings concordant for HSCR were analyzed to see which loci and which sets of alleles at these loci each sib had in common with an affected brother or sister, alleles at three loci were found to be significantly shared—the 10q11.2 region, where *RET* is located, and two other regions, located at 3p21 and 19q12—although the particular genes responsible in these two regions are not currently known (Fig. 8-6). Most of the concordant sibpairs (55 of 67) were found to share alleles at all three loci. In particular, all of these 55 pairs of siblings had a common DNA variant in the first intron of the *RET* gene that reduced the function of a regulatory element. This variant is common in certain populations, with a frequency of approximately 25% of whites and approximately 40% of Asians. Because most people with the variant do not have HSCR, it must have very low penetrance and must interact with the other genetic loci to cause disease. A minority of concordant sibpairs (12 of 67) was found to share alleles at only two of the three loci, whereas none of the concordant affected sibpairs shared alleles at only one or none of the loci. Thus, HSCR is a multifactorial disease that results from the additive effects of susceptibility alleles at *RET, EDNRB*, and a number of other loci. The identification of a common, low-penetrant DNA variation in a noncoding enhancer within an intron of *RET* serves to illustrate that the gene variants responsible for modifying expression of a multifactorial trait may be subtle in how they exert their effects on gene expression and, as a consequence, on disease penetrance and expressivity. It is also sobering to realize that the underlying genetic mechanisms for this relatively well defined congenital malformation have turned out to be so surprisingly complex; still, they are likely to be far simpler than are the mechanisms involved in the more common complex diseases, such as diabetes.

Type 1 Diabetes Mellitus

There are two major types of diabetes mellitus, **type 1 (insulin dependent; IDDM)** (Case 23) and **type 2 (non–insulin dependent; NIDDM)** (Case 30), representing about 10% and 88% of all cases, respectively. They differ in typical onset age, MZ twin concordance, and association with particular alleles at the major histocompatibility complex (MHC; see Chapter 9). Familial aggregation is seen in both types of diabetes, but in any given family, usually only type 1 or type 2 is present.

Type 1 diabetes has an incidence in the white population of about 1 in 500 (0.2%) but is lower in African and Asian populations. It usually manifests in childhood or adolescence. It results from autoimmune destruction of the β cells of the pancreas, which normally produce insulin. A large majority of children who will go on to have type 1 diabetes develop multiple autoantibodies early in childhood against a variety of endogenous proteins, including insulin, well before they develop overt disease.

MHC Association in Type 1 Diabetes

There is strong evidence for genetic factors in type 1 diabetes: concordance among MZ twins is approximately 40%, which far exceeds the 5% concordance in DZ twins. The risk for type 1 diabetes in siblings of an affected proband is approximately 7%, resulting in an estimated $\lambda_s = 7\%/0.2\% = \sim35$. It has been known for a long time that the MHC locus (see Chapter 9) is a major genetic factor in type 1 diabetes, as suggested by the finding that about 95% of all patients with type 1 diabetes (in comparison with about half the normal population) are heterozygous for certain alleles, *HLA-DR3* or *HLA-DR4*, at the HLA class II locus in the MHC.

The original studies showing an association between *HLA-DR3* and *HLA-DR4* with IDDM relied on the standard method in use at that time for distinguishing between different HLA alleles, one that was based on immunological reactions in a test tube. This method has now been superseded by direct determination of the DNA sequence of different alleles. Sequencing of the MHC in a large number of individuals has revealed that the *DR3* and *DR4* "alleles" are not single alleles at all. Both *DR3* and *DR4* can be subdivided into a dozen or more alleles located at a locus now termed *DRB1*, defined at the level of DNA sequence. Furthermore, it has also become clear that the association between certain *DRB1* alleles and IDDM was due, in part, to alleles at another class II locus, *DQB1*, located about 80 kb away from *DRB1*, that formed a common haplotype (due to linkage disequilibrium; see Chapter 10) with each other. *DQB1* encodes the β chain, one of the chains that forms a dimer to make up the class II DQ protein. It appears that the presence of aspartic acid (Asp) at position 57 of the DQ β chain (see Fig. 9-7) is closely associated with *resistance* to type 1 diabetes, whereas other amino acids at this position (alanine, valine, or serine) confer susceptibility. About 90% of patients with type 1 diabetes are homozygous for *DQB1* alleles that do not encode Asp at position 57. Given that the DQ molecule, and position 57 of the β chain in particular, is critical in peptide antigen binding and presentation to the T cell for response, it is likely that differences in antigen binding, determined by which amino acid is at position 57 of the β chain of DQ, contribute directly to the autoimmune response that destroys the insulin-producing cells of the pancreas. Other loci and alleles in the MHC, however, are also important, as can be seen from the fact that some patients with type 1 diabetes do have an aspartic acid at this position in the DQ β chain.

Genes Other than Class II MHC Loci in Type 1 Diabetes

The MHC haplotype alone accounts for only a portion of the genetic contribution to the risk for type 1 diabetes in siblings of a proband. Family studies in type 1 diabetes (Table 8-5) suggest that even when siblings share the same MHC class II haplotypes, the risk of disease is approximately 17%, still well below the MZ twin concordance rate of approximately 40%. Thus, there must be other genes, elsewhere in the genome, that also predispose to the development of type 1 diabetes, assuming MZ twins and sibs have similar environmental exposures. Besides the MHC, variation at

Table 8-5

Empirical Risks for Counseling in Type 1 Diabetes

Relationship to Affected Individual	Risk for Development of Type 1 Diabetes
MZ twin	40%
Sibling	7%
Sibling with no DR haplotypes in common	1%
Sibling with 1 DR haplotype in common	5%
Sibling with 2 DR haplotypes in common	17% (20%-25% if shared haplotype is *DR3/DR4*)
Child	4%
Child of affected mother	3%
Child of affected father	5%

more than a dozen loci has been proposed to increase susceptibility to type 1 diabetes, but substantial evidence is available for only three. These include a variable number tandem repeat polymorphism in the promoter of the insulin gene itself and single nucleotide polymorphisms in the immune regulatory gene *CTLA4* and in the *PTPN22* gene encoding a protein phosphatase (see Chapter 9). Identification of other susceptibility genes for type 1 diabetes, both within and outside the MHC, remains the target of intensive investigation. At present, the nature of the nongenetic risk factors in type 1 diabetes is largely unknown.

Genetic factors alone, however, do not cause type 1 diabetes, because the MZ twin concordance rate for type 1 diabetes is only approximately 40%, not 100%. Until a more complete picture develops of the genetic and nongenetic factors that cause type 1 diabetes, risk counseling must remain empirical (see Table 8-5).

Alzheimer Disease

Alzheimer disease (AD) (Case 3) is a fatal neurodegenerative disease that affects 1% to 2% of the United States population. It is the most common cause of dementia in the elderly and is responsible for more than half of all cases of dementia. As with other dementias, patients experience a chronic, progressive loss of memory and other intellectual functions, associated with death of cortical neurons. Age, gender, and family history are the most significant risk factors for AD. Once a person reaches 65 years of age, the risk for any dementia, and AD in particular, increases substantially with age and female sex (Table 8-6).

AD can be diagnosed definitively only postmortem, on the basis of neuropathological findings of characteristic protein aggregates (β-amyloid plaques and neurofibrillary tangles; see Chapter 12). The most important constituent of these plaques is a small (39 to 42–amino

Table 8-6

Cumulative Age- and Sex-Specific Risks for Alzheimer Disease and Dementia

Time Interval Past 65 Years of Age	Risk for Development of AD (%)	Risk for Development of Any Dementia (%)
65 to 80 years		
Male	6.3	10.9
Female	12	19
65 to 100 years		
Male	25	32.8
Female	28.1	45

Data from Seshadri S, Wolf PA, Beiser A, et al: Lifetime risk of dementia and Alzheimer's disease. The impact of mortality on risk estimates in the Framingham Study. Neurology 49:1498-1504, 1997.

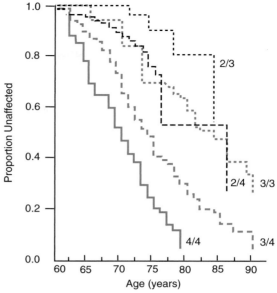

Figure 8-7 ■ Chance of remaining unaffected by Alzheimer disease as a function of age for different *APOE* genotypes. At one extreme is the ε4/ε4 homozygote who has a less than 10% chance of remaining free of the disease by the age of 80 years, whereas an ε2/ε3 heterozygote has a more than 80% chance of remaining disease free at the age of 80 years. (Modified from Strittmatter WJ, Roses AD: Apolipoprotein E and Alzheimer's disease. Annu Rev Neurosci 19: 53-77, 1996.)

acid) peptide, Aβ, derived from cleavage of a normal neuronal protein, the amyloid protein precursor. The secondary structure of Aβ gives the plaques the staining characteristics of amyloid proteins.

In addition to three rare autosomal dominant forms of the disease (see Table 12-9), in which disease onset is in the third to fifth decade, there is a common form of AD with onset after the age of 60 years (late onset). This form has no obvious mendelian inheritance pattern but does show familial aggregation and an elevated relative risk ratio ($\lambda_s = 4$-5) typical of disorders with complex inheritance. Individuals with a first-degree relative with AD have an approximately 3-fold to 4-fold increased risk of developing AD as well. Twin studies have been inconsistent but suggest MZ concordance of about 50% and DZ concordance of about 18%.

The ε4 Allele of Apolipoprotein E

The first significant genetic factor associated with common late-onset AD was the apolipoprotein E (*APOE*) locus. Apolipoprotein E is a protein component of the low-density lipoprotein (LDL) particle and is involved in clearing LDL through an interaction with high-affinity receptors in the liver. Apolipoprotein E is also a constituent of amyloid plaques in AD and is known to bind the Aβ peptide. The *APOE* gene maps to chromosome 19 and has three alleles, ε2, ε3, and ε4, due to substitutions of arginine for two different cysteine residues in the protein (see Table 12-10).

When the genotypes at the *APOE* locus were analyzed in AD patients and controls, a genotype with at least one ε4 allele was found two to three times more frequently among the patients compared with controls (Table 8-7) in both the general United States and Japanese populations, with much less of an association in the Hispanic and African American populations. Even more striking is that the risk for AD appears to increase

further if both *APOE* alleles are ε4, through an effect on the age at onset of AD; patients with two ε4 alleles have an earlier onset of disease than do those with only one. In a study of patients with AD and unaffected controls (Fig. 8-7), the age at which AD developed in the affected patients was earliest for ε4/ε4 homozygotes, next for ε4/ε3 heterozygotes, and significantly less for the other genotypes.

In the population in general, the ε4 allele is clearly a predisposing factor that increases the risk for development of AD by shifting the age at onset to an earlier age. AD develops before most patients die of other life-threatening illnesses of the elderly. Despite this

Table 8-7

Association of Apolipoprotein E ε4 Allele with Alzheimer Disease*

Genotype	Frequency			
	United States		Japan	
	AD	Control	AD	Control
ε4/ε4; ε4/ε3; or ε4/ε2	0.64	0.31	0.47	0.17
ε3/ε3; ε2/ε3; or ε2/ε2	0.36	0.69	0.53	0.83

*Frequency of genotypes with and without the ε4 allele among Alzheimer disease (AD) patients and controls from the United States and Japan.

Table 8-8

Some Common Congenital Malformations with Multifactorial Inheritance

Malformation	Population Incidence (per 1000)
Cleft lip with or without cleft palate	0.4-1.7
Cleft palate	0.4
Congenital dislocation of hip	2*
Congenital heart defects	4-8
Ventricular septal defect	1.7
Patent ductus arteriosus	0.5
Atrial septal defect	1.0
Aortic stenosis	0.5
Neural tube defects	2-10
Spina bifida and anencephaly	Variable
Pyloric stenosis	1†, 5*

*Per 1000 males.
†Per 1000 females.
Note: Population incidence is approximate. Many of these disorders are heterogeneous and are usually but not invariably multifactorial.
Data from Carter CO: Genetics of common single malformations. Br Med Bull 32:21-26, 1976; Nora JJ: Multifactorial inheritance hypothesis for the etiology of congenital heart diseases: the genetic environmental interaction. Circulation 38:604-617, 1968; and Lin AE, Garver KL: Genetic counseling for congenital heart defects. J Pediatr 113:1105-1109, 1988.

Table 8-9

Recurrence Risks (%) for Cleft Lip with or without Cleft Palate and for Neural Tube Malformations*

Affected Relatives	Cleft Lip with or without Cleft Palate	Anencephaly and Spina Bifida
No sibs		
Neither parent	0.1	0.3
One parent	3	4.5
Both parents	34	30
One sib		
Neither parent	3	4
One parent	11	12
Both parents	40	38
Two sibs		
Neither parent	8	10
One parent	19	20
Both parents	45	43
One sib and one second-degree relative		
Neither parent	6	7
One parent	16	18
Both parents	43	42
One sib and one third-degree relative		
Neither parent	4	5.5
One parent	14	16
Both parents	44	42

*These recurrence risks within families were calculated before the widespread introduction of maternal folic acid supplementation during pregnancy (see later).
From Bonaiti-Pellié C, Smith C: Risk tables for genetic counselling in some common congenital malformations. J Med Genet 11:374-377, 1974.

increased risk, other genetic and environmental factors must be important because many ε4/ε4 homozygotes live to extreme old age with no evidence for AD, and 50% to 75% of all heterozygotes carrying one ε4 allele never develop AD. There is also an association between the presence of the ε4 allele and neurodegenerative disease after head injury (as seen in professional boxers), indicating that at least one environmental factor, brain trauma, interacts with the ε4 allele in the pathogenesis of AD. Thus, the ε4 variant of *APOE* represents a prime example of a predisposing allele: *it predisposes to a complex trait in a powerful way but does not predestine any individual carrying the allele to develop the disease.* Additional genes as well as environmental effects are also clearly involved but remain to be identified. Testing of asymptomatic people for the ε4 allele remains inadvisable because knowing that one is a heterozygote or homozygote for the ε4 allele does not mean one will develop AD, nor is there any intervention currently known that can affect the chance one will or will not develop AD (see Chapter 17).

Multifactorial Congenital Malformations

Several common congenital malformations, occurring as isolated defects and not as part of a syndrome, seem to recur in families. The familial aggregation and elevated risk of recurrence in relatives of an affected individual are all characteristic of a complex trait (Tables 8-8 to 8-10). Some of the more important congenital malformations with complex inheritance are **neural tube defects, cleft lip** with or without **cleft palate,** and **congenital heart malformations.**

Neural Tube Defects

Anencephaly and **spina bifida** are neural tube defects (NTDs) that frequently occur together in families and are considered to have a common pathogenesis (Fig. 8-8; also see Table 8-9). In anencephaly, the forebrain, overlying meninges, vault of the skull, and skin are all absent. Many infants with anencephaly are stillborn, and those born alive survive a few hours at most. About two thirds of affected infants are female. In spina bifida, there is failure of fusion of the arches of the

Table 8-10

Empirical Risks for Cleft Lip with or without Cleft Palate in Relatives of Affected Probands

Population Affected	Incidence of Cleft Lip with or without Cleft Palate (%)	$\lambda_{relative}$
General population	0.1	—
First-degree relatives	4.0	40
Second-degree relatives	0.7	7
Third-degree relatives	0.3	3

DEFECTS IN CLOSURE OF NEURAL TUBE

Dorsal view of normal embryo of 23 days

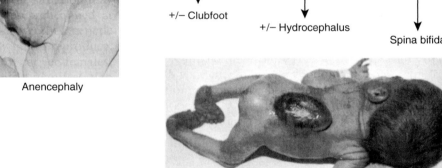

Cephalad neural groove

Caudad neural groove

Somite

Neural tube (normally completely closed by 28 days)

DEFECT IN CLOSURE OF ANTERIOR NEURAL TUBE

DEFECT IN CLOSURE

Figure 8-8 ■ The origin of the neural tube defects anencephaly and spina bifida. (From Jones KL: Smith's Recognizable Patterns of Human Malformation, 4th ed. Philadelphia, WB Saunders, 1988.)

1. Incomplete development of brain, with degeneration
2. Incomplete development of calvaria
3. Alteration in facies +/− auricle

Neural tube

Somite

Neural deficit caudal to lesion

Meningomyelocele

Defect in spinous process

+/− Clubfoot

+/− Hydrocephalus

Spina bifida

Anencephaly

Meningomyelocele with partially epithelialized sac

vertebrae, typically in the lumbar region. There are varying degrees of severity, ranging from spina bifida occulta, in which the defect is in the bony arch only, to spina bifida aperta, in which a bone defect is also associated with meningocele (protrusion of meninges) or meningomyelocele (protrusion of neural elements as well as meninges through the defect; see Fig. 8-8).

As a group, NTDs are a leading cause of stillbirth, death in early infancy, and handicap in surviving children. Their incidence at birth is variable, ranging from almost 1% in Ireland to 0.2% or less in the United States. The frequency also appears to vary with social factors and season of birth and oscillates widely over time (with a marked decrease in recent years; see later discussion).

A small proportion of NTDs have known specific causes, for example, amniotic bands (fibrous connections between the amnion and fetus caused by early rupture of the amnion, which may disrupt structures during their embryological development), some single-gene defects with pleiotropic expression, some chromosome disorders, and some teratogens. Most NTDs, however, are isolated defects of unknown cause.

Maternal Folic Acid Deficiency and Neural Tube Defects   NTDs were long believed to follow a multifactorial inheritance pattern determined by multiple genetic and environmental factors. It was therefore a stunning discovery to find that the single greatest factor in causing NTDs is a vitamin deficiency. The risk of NTDs was found to be inversely correlated with maternal serum folic acid levels during pregnancy, with a threshold of 200 µg/L, below which the risk of NTD becomes significant. Along with reduced blood folate levels, elevated homocysteine levels were also seen in the mothers of children with NTDs, suggesting that a biochemical abnormality was present at the step of recycling of tetrahydrofolate to methylate homocysteine to methionine (see Fig. 12-7). Folic acid levels are strongly influenced by dietary intake and can become depressed during pregnancy even with a typical intake of approximately 230 µg/day. The impact of folic acid deficiency is exacerbated by a genetic variant of the enzyme 5,10-methylenetetrahydrofolate reductase (MTHFR), caused by a common missense mutation that makes the enzyme less stable than normal. Instability of this enzyme hinders the recycling of tetrahydrofolate and interferes with the methylation of homocysteine to methionine. The mutant allele is so common in many populations that between 5% and 15% of the population is homozygous for the mutation. In studies of infants with NTDs and their mothers, it was found that mothers of infants with NTDs were twice as likely as controls to be homozygous for the mutant allele encoding the unstable enzyme. Not all mothers of NTD infants with low folic acid levels are homozygous for the mutant allele of MTHFR, however, indicating that low folic acid levels may be caused by other unknown genetic factors or by simple dietary deficiency alone. How this enzyme defect contributes to NTDs and whether the abnormality is a direct result of elevated homocysteine levels, depressed methionine levels, or some other metabolic derangement remains undefined.

Prevention of Neural Tube Defects   The discovery of folic acid deficiency in NTDs has led to a remarkable public health initiative to educate women to supplement their diets with folic acid 1 month before conception and continuing for 2 months after conception during the period when the neural tube forms. Dietary supplementation with 400 to 800 µg of folic acid per day for women who plan their pregnancies has been shown to reduce the incidence of NTDs by more than 75%. Much active discussion is ongoing as to whether the entire food supply should be supplemented with folic acid as a public health measure to avoid the problem of women failing to supplement their diets individually during pregnancy.

Parents of children with an NTD potentially are at increased risk for a recurrence in future pregnancies (see Table 8-9). These risks are now more potential than real since they can be substantially modified by dietary folic acid supplementation.

NTDs also rank high among the conditions for which prenatal diagnosis is possible; anencephaly and most cases of open spina bifida can be identified prenatally by detection of excessive levels of **alpha-fetoprotein** (AFP) and other fetal substances in the amniotic fluid and by **ultrasonographic scanning** (see Chapter 15 for further discussion). However, less than 5% of all patients with NTDs are born to women with previous affected children. For this reason, screening of all pregnant women for NTDs by measurements of AFP and other fetal substances in maternal serum is becoming more widespread. Thus, we can anticipate that a combination of preventive folic acid therapy and maternal AFP screening will provide major public health benefits by drastically reducing the incidence of NTDs.

Cleft Lip and Cleft Palate

Cleft lip with or without cleft palate, or CL(P), is one of the most common congenital malformations, affecting 1.4 per thousand newborns worldwide. There is considerable variation in frequency in different ethnic groups: about 1.7 per 1000 in Japanese, 1.0 per 1000 in whites, and 0.4 per 1000 in African Americans. Relatively high rates are also seen in some North American populations of Asian descent, for example, in Indians of the southwest United States and the west coast of Canada. The concordance rate is approximately 30% in MZ twins and approximately 2% (the same as the risk for non-twin sibs) in DZ twins (see Table 8-4). CL(P), which is usually etiologically distinct from isolated cleft palate without cleft lip, originates as a failure of fusion of the frontal process with the maxillary process at about the 35th day of gestation. About 60% to 80% of those affected with CL(P) are males.

CL(P) is heterogeneous and includes forms in which the clefting is only one feature of a syndrome that includes other anomalies—**syndromic CL(P)**—as well as forms that are not associated with other birth defects—**nonsyndromic CL(P)**. Syndromic CL(P) can be inherited as a mendelian single-gene disorder or can be caused by chromosome disorders (especially trisomy 13 and 4p−) (see Chapter 6) or teratogenic exposure

Table 8-11

Risk for Cleft Lip with or without Cleft Palate in Siblings of Probands Affected with Clefts of Increasing Severity

Phenotype of Proband	Incidence in Sibs of Cleft Lip with or without Cleft Palate (%)
Unilateral cleft lip without cleft palate	4.0
Unilateral cleft lip and palate	4.9
Bilateral cleft lip without cleft palate	6.7
Bilateral cleft lip and palate	8.0

(rubella embryopathy, thalidomide, or anticonvulsants) (see Chapter 14). Nonsyndromic CL(P) can also be inherited as a single-gene disorder but more commonly is a sporadic occurrence in some families and demonstrates some degree of familial aggregation without an obvious mendelian inheritance pattern in others (see Table 8-9). One of the predictions of multifactorial inheritance is that the recurrence risk increases the more affected relatives an individual has in the family (see Tables 8-9 and 8-10). Another prediction of multifactorial inheritance is that the risk for CL(P) in relatives of probands that are severely affected will be greater than the risk to relatives of mildly affected probands. Indeed, in families with a proband with an isolated case of CL(P), there is an increase in recurrence risk with increasing severity in the proband, from unilateral to bilateral, and from cleft lip alone to CL(P) (Table 8-11). The explanation for all of these observations is that more severe disease and more affected relatives of the proband indicate a greater load of alleles predisposing to disease in the family.

Progress in identifying genes responsible for multifactorial nonsyndromic CL(P) has come from the study of rare single-gene forms of syndromic CL(P). These include X-linked clefting with ankyloglossia (tethering of tongue by short or anterior frenulum) and two forms of autosomal dominant clefting, one associated with missing teeth and the other with infertility and anosmia (inability to smell). These three mendelian forms of syndromic clefting result from mutations in two transcription factor genes, *TBX1* and *MSX1,* and in the gene *FGFR1,* which encodes a cell signaling molecule. The most striking finding, however, is that a variety of rare mutations have now been found in all three of these genes in patients from a variety of different ethnic backgrounds who appear to have *nonsyndromic* CL(P). The frequency of mutation in CL(P) patients is approximately 5% for *TBX1,* approximately 2% for *MSX1,* and 1% for *FGFR1.* In all cases, investigation of additional family members may disclose affected individuals with more typical features of the syndromes associated

with mutations in that gene. Another transcription factor gene, *IRF6,* in which mutations cause the syndromic form of CL(P) known as **Van der Woude syndrome,** is also involved in nonsyndromic clefting. Van der Woude syndrome has pits in the lower lip in 85% of patients, but 15% may present only with cleft lip or palate. What is very likely, however, is that these genes represent only a fraction of the total genetic contribution to this birth defect and that marked locus and allelic heterogeneity will be the rule. It is unknown to what extent the majority of CL(P) patients will turn out to have the defect because of rare alleles at additional single loci, or because of multifactorial interactions between more common alleles at many loci. Finally, maternal smoking is a well recognized risk factor for CL(P). The degree of risk associated with this environmental factor may itself have a genetic basis due to genetic variation in the mother or the fetus that alters how contaminants produced by tobacco smoke are metabolized.

Sequencing of the genes implicated in CL(P) may provide useful information in families seeking genetic counseling, particularly when there is a family history suggestive of some of the anomalies involving tongue, teeth, ability to smell, or infertility. However, the utility of mutation detection is limited by our lack of knowledge of the penetrance of the spectrum of mutant alleles that may be present at all four of these loci. In the absence of any specific information as to the involvement of a particular locus or mutation, the empirical risk figures (see Tables 8-9 to 8-11) are the only guidelines available for genetic counseling.

Congenital Heart Defects

Congenital heart defects (CHDs) are common, with a frequency of about 4 to 8 per 1000 births. They are a heterogeneous group, caused in some cases by single-gene or chromosomal mechanisms and in others by exposure to teratogens, such as rubella infection or maternal diabetes. The cause is usually unknown, and the majority of cases are believed to be multifactorial in origin.

There are many types of CHDs, with different population incidences and empirical risks. It is known that when heart defects recur in a family, however, the affected children do not necessarily have exactly the same anatomical defect but instead show recurrence of lesions that are similar with regard to developmental mechanisms. With use of developmental mechanism as a classification scheme, five main groups of CHDs can be distinguished: flow lesions, defects in cell migration or in cell death, abnormalities in extracellular matrix, and defects in targeted growth. A familial pattern is found primarily in the group with flow lesions, a large category constituting about 50% of all CHDs. Flow

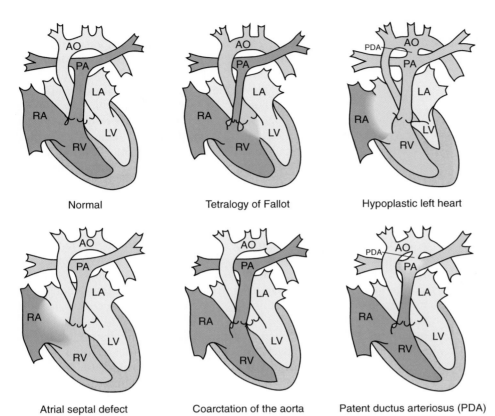

Normal

Tetralogy of Fallot

Hypoplastic left heart

Atrial septal defect

Coarctation of the aorta

Patent ductus arteriosus (PDA)

Figure 8-9 ■ Diagram of various flow lesions seen in congenital heart disease. RA, right atrium; RV, right ventricle; LA, left atrium; LV, left ventricle; PA, pulmonary artery; AO, aorta. Blood on the left side of the circulation is shown in pale blue, on the right side in dark blue. Abnormal admixture of oxygenated and deoxygenated blood is an intermediate blue.

lesions include hypoplastic left heart syndrome, coarctation of the aorta, atrial septal defect of the secundum type, pulmonary valve stenosis, a common type of ventricular septal defect, and other forms (Fig. 8-9). Up to 25% of patients with all flow lesions, particularly tetralogy of Fallot, may have the deletion of chromosome region 22q11 seen in the **velocardiofacial syndrome** (see Chapter 6).

Are isolated CHDs inherited as multifactorial traits? For flow lesions, the relative risk ratios for sibs, λ_s, support familial aggregation for this class of CHD (Table 8-12). Until more is known, the figures given can be used as estimates of the recurrence risk for flow lesions in first-degree relatives. There is, however, a

Table 8-12

Population Incidence and Recurrence Risks for Various Flow Lesions

Defect	Population Incidence (%)	Frequency in Sibs (%)	λ_{sib}
Ventricular septal defect	0.17	4.3	25
Patent ductus arteriosus	0.083	3.2	38
Atrial septal defect	0.066	3.2	48
Aortic stenosis	0.044	2.6	59

rapid fall-off in risk (to levels not much higher than the population risk) in second- and third-degree relatives of index patients with flow lesions. Similarly, relatives of index patients with types of CHDs other than flow lesions can be offered reassurance that their risk is no greater than that of the general population. For further reassurance, many CHDs can now be assessed prenatally by ultrasonography (see Chapter 15).

Mental Illness

Mental illnesses are some of the most common and perplexing of human diseases, affecting 4% of the human population worldwide. The annual cost in medical care and social services exceeds $150 billion in the United States alone. Among the most severe of the mental illnesses are **schizophrenia** and **bipolar disease** (manic-depressive illness).

Schizophrenia affects 1% of the world's population. It is a devastating psychiatric illness, with onset commonly in late adolescence or young adulthood, and is characterized by abnormalities in thought, emotion, and social relationships, often associated with delusional thinking and disordered mood. A genetic contribution to schizophrenia is supported by both twin and

Table 8-13

Recurrence Risks and Relative Risk Ratios in Schizophrenia Families

Relation to Individual Affected by Schizophrenia	Recurrence Risk (%)	λ_r
Child of two schizophrenic parents	46	23
Child	9-16	11.5
Sibling	8-14	11
Nephew or niece	1-4	2.5
Uncle or aunt	2	2
First cousin	2-6	4
Grandchild	2-8	5

From *www.nchpeg.org/cdrom/empiric.html.*

Table 8-14

Recurrence Risks and Relative Risk Ratios in Bipolar Disorder Families

Relation to Individual Affected with Bipolar Disease	Recurrence Risk (%)*	λ_r
Child of two parents with bipolar disease	50-70	75
Child	27	34
Sibling	20-30	31
Second-degree relative	5	6

*Recurrence of bipolar, unipolar, or schizoaffective disorder.
From *www.nchpeg.org/cdrom/empiric.html.*

family aggregation studies. MZ concordance in schizophrenia is estimated to be 40% to 60%; DZ concordance is 10% to 16%. The recurrence risk ratio is elevated in first- and second-degree relatives of schizophrenic patients (Table 8-13).

Although there is considerable evidence of a genetic contribution to schizophrenia, little certainty exists as to the genes and alleles that predispose to the disease. Counseling, therefore, relies on empirical risk figures (see Table 8-13). One exception is the high prevalence of schizophrenia in carriers of the 22q11 deletion responsible for the **velocardiofacial syndrome** (also referred to as the DiGeorge syndrome) (see Chapter 6). It is estimated that 25% of patients with 22q11 deletions develop schizophrenia, even in the absence of many or most of the other physical signs of the syndrome. The mechanism by which a deletion of 3 Mb of DNA on 22q11 causes mental illness in patients with the velocardiofacial syndrome is unknown.

Bipolar disease is predominantly a mood disorder in which episodes of mood elevation, grandiosity, high-risk dangerous behavior, and inflated self-esteem (mania) alternate with periods of depression, decreased interest in what are normally pleasurable activities, feelings of worthlessness, and suicidal thinking. The prevalence of bipolar disease is 0.8%, approximately equal to that of schizophrenia, with a similar age at onset. The seriousness of this condition is underscored by the high (10% to 15%) rate of suicide in affected patients.

A genetic contribution to bipolar disease is strongly supported by twin and family aggregation studies. MZ twin concordance is 62%; DZ twin concordance is 8%. Disease risk is also elevated in relatives of affected individuals (Table 8-14). One striking aspect of bipolar disease in families is that the condition has variable expressivity; some members of the same family demonstrate classic bipolar illness, others have depression alone (unipolar disorder), and others carry a diagnosis of a psychiatric syndrome that involves both thought and mood (**schizoaffective disorder**). As with schizo-

phrenia, the genes and alleles that predispose to bipolar disease are largely unknown. Counseling, therefore, relies on empirical risk figures (see Table 8-14).

Coronary Artery Disease

Coronary artery disease (CAD) kills about 450,000 individuals in the United States yearly and is the number one cause of morbidity and mortality in the developed world. CAD due to atherosclerosis is the major cause of the nearly 1,500,000 cases of myocardial infarction (MI) and the more than 200,000 deaths from acute MI occurring annually. In the aggregate, CAD costs more than $100 billion in health care expenses and lost productivity each year in the United States. For unknown reasons, males are at higher risk for CAD both in the population and within affected families.

Family and twin studies have repeatedly supported a role for heredity in CAD, particularly when it occurs in relatively young individuals. The recurrence risk in male first-degree relatives is greater than that in the general population when the proband is female (7-fold increased) compared with the 2.5-fold increased risk in female relatives of a male index case. When the proband is young (<55 years), the risk for CAD is 11.4-fold that of the general population. Twin studies show similar trends. A study of 21,004 twins in Sweden revealed that after controlling for risk factors such as diabetes, smoking, and hypertension, if one male twin experienced an MI before the age of 65 years, the other twin's risk for MI was increased 6-fold to 8-fold if he was an MZ twin and 3-fold if a DZ twin. Among female twins, the increase in risk for MI in MZ twins was even greater: 15-fold for an MZ twin and only 2.6-fold for a DZ twin when one twin experienced an MI before the age of 65 years. The older the first twin was at time of MI, the less increased was the risk to the other twin. This pattern of increased risk suggests that when the index case is female or young, there is likely to be a greater genetic contribution to MI in the family, thereby increasing the risk for disease in the proband's relatives.

There are many stages in the evolution of athero-sclerotic lesions in the coronary artery at which genetic differences may predispose or protect from CAD (Fig. 8-10; also see Box). What begins as a fatty streak in the intima of the artery evolves into a fibrous plaque containing smooth muscle, lipid, and fibrous tissue. These intimal plaques become vascular and may bleed, ulcerate, and calcify, thereby causing severe vessel narrowing as well as providing fertile ground for thrombosis resulting in sudden, complete occlusion and MI.

A few mendelian disorders with CAD are known. Familial hypercholesterolemia (Case 14), an autosomal dominant defect of the LDL receptor discussed in Chapter 12, is the most common of these but accounts for only about 5% of survivors of MI. Most cases of CAD show multifactorial inheritance, with both non-genetic and genetic predisposing factors. The risk factors for CAD include several other multifactorial disorders with genetic components: hypertension, obesity, and diabetes mellitus. In this context, the metabolic and physiological derangements represented by these disorders also contribute to enhancing the risk of CAD. Diet, physical activity, and smoking are environmental factors that also play a major role in influencing the risk for CAD. Given all the different proteins and environmental factors that contribute to the development of CAD, it is easy to imagine that genetic susceptibility to CAD could be a complex multifactorial condition (see Box).

CAD is often an incidental finding in family histories of patients with other genetic diseases. In view of the high recurrence risk, physicians and genetic coun-selors may need to consider whether first-degree relatives of patients with CAD should be evaluated further and offered counseling and therapy, even when CAD is not the primary genetic problem for which the patient or relative has been referred. Such an evaluation is clearly indicated when the proband is young.

● ■ ■ Genes and Gene Products Involved in the Stepwise Process of Coronary Artery Disease

A large number of genes and gene products have been suggested and, in some cases, implicated in promoting one or more of the developmental stages of coronary artery disease. These include genes encoding proteins involved in the following:

- Serum lipid transport and metabolism—cholesterol, apolipoprotein E, C-III, the LDL receptor, and lipoprotein(a)—as well as total cholesterol level. Elevated low-density lipoprotein (LDL) cholesterol and decreased high-density lipoprotein (HDL) cholesterol, both of which elevate the risk for coronary artery disease, are themselves quantitative traits with significant heritabilities of 40% to 60% and 45% to 75% respectively.
- Vasoactivity, such as angiotensin-converting enzyme
- Blood coagulation, platelet adhesion, and fibrinolysis, such as plasminogen activator inhibitor 1, and the platelet surface glycoproteins Ib and IIIa
- Inflammatory and immune pathways
- Arterial wall components

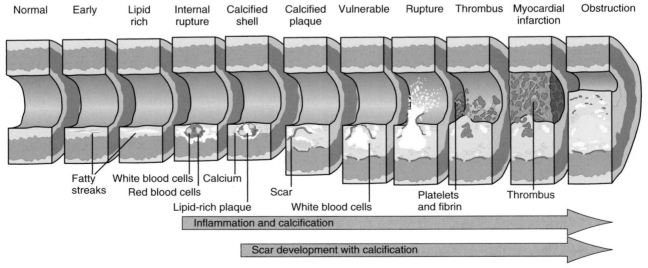

Figure 8-10 ■ Sections of coronary artery demonstrating the steps leading to coronary artery disease. Genetic and environmental factors operating at any or all of the steps in this pathway can contribute to the development of this complex, common disease. (Modified from an original figure by Larry Almonte, with permission.)

••• Genetic Counseling of Families of Patients with Multifactorial Traits

The underlying mechanisms by which genes and environment interact to cause diseases with complex inheritance are largely unknown. For genetic counseling, we are dependent on measuring actual recurrence risks in collections of families to generate average **empirical estimates** of the recurrence risks. Of course, the actual risk for an individual family may be larger or smaller than the average. For now, these population-based empirical risks, although often inadequate, are the only source available for genetic prediction. Certain general principles must be considered, however, in providing genetic counseling for multifactorial disorders:

- The recurrence risk is much higher for first-degree relatives of affected family members than for more distant relatives.
- The best estimate of the recurrence risk is the empirical risk, which is simply the recurrence risk, observed in similar families, for a relative with the same degree of relationship. It is often useful to state the empirical risk as a multiple of the population risk of the defect. The empirical risk is based entirely on past experience and does not imply that the genetic and environmental factors in the pathogenesis of the malformation are understood. An empirical risk is an average for the population and is not necessarily accurate for a specific family.
- In general, the recurrence risk is increased by the presence of more than one affected relative; a severe form or an early onset of the disorder; an affected person of the sex less likely to be affected; and consanguineous parentage.

- Two common errors in risk calculation should be avoided:

  If the parent of a child with a multifactorial birth defect has another child by a different partner, the children are second-degree, not first-degree, relatives, and the empirical risk for the second child is much lower than if the children had both parents in common (usually, the risk is approximately 1% instead of approximately 5%).

  When an unaffected uncle or aunt of a child with a multifactorial defect inquires about the risk of the same defect in his or her offspring, the relevant risk is not the risk to the aunt or uncle (a second-degree relative to the proband) but the risk to the offspring of the aunt or uncle (a third-degree relative).

- For many common disorders with familial aggregation, a minority of cases will be due to single-gene disorders with mendelian inheritance that is masked by small family sizes and incomplete penetrance. Because the recurrence risk is much higher in mendelian forms, the geneticist needs to maintain a high index of suspicion that there may be a single-gene disorder when there is anything unusual about the disease presentation, particularly if there is an unusually early age of onset or if there are associated clinical features not typically found in the disorder. Mendelian forms of the disorder may have characteristic clinical or laboratory features that need to be specifically investigated.

◉ GENERAL REFERENCES

King RA, Rotter JI, Motulsky AG: The Genetic Basis of Common Diseases, 2nd ed. Oxford, England, Oxford University Press, 2002.

Rimoin DL, Connor JM, Pyeritz RE: Emery and Rimoin's Principles and Practice of Medical Genetics, 4th ed. Philadelphia, WB Saunders, 2001.

◉ REFERENCES FOR SPECIFIC TOPICS

Aznar J, Vayá A, Estellés A, et al: Risk of venous thrombosis in carriers of the prothrombin G20210A variant and factor V Leiden and their interaction with oral contraceptives. Haematologica 85:1271-1276, 2000.

Bolk Gabriel S, Salomon R, Pelet A, et al: Segregation at three loci explains familial and population risk in Hirschsprung disease. Nat Genet 31:89-93, 2002.

Concannon P, Erlich HA, Julier C, et al: Type 1 diabetes: evidence for susceptibility loci from four genome-wide linkage scans in 1,435 multiplex families. Diabetes 54:2995-3001, 2005.

Ebers GC, Sadovnick AD, Risch NJ, et al: A genetic basis for familial aggregation in multiple sclerosis. Nature 377:150-151, 1995.

Emison ES, McCallion AS, Kashuk CS, et al: A common sex-dependent mutation in a *RET* enhancer underlies Hirschsprung disease risk. Nature 434:857-863, 2005.

Emmerich J, Rosendaal FR, Cattaneo M, et al: Combined effect of factor V Leiden and prothrombin 20210A on the risk of venous thromboembolism. Thromb Haemost 86:809-816, 2001.

Foy CA, Grant PJ: Genes and the development of vascular disease. Postgrad Med J 73:271-278, 1997.

Grody WW, Griffin JH, Taylor AK, et al: American College of Medical Genetics Consensus Statement on Factor V Leiden Mutation Testing, 2005. *www.acmg.net/resources/policies/pol-009.asp*

Hawkes CH: Twin studies in medicine—what do they tell us? Q J Med 90:311-321, 1997.

Kajiwara K, Berson EL, Dryja TP: Digenic retinitis pigmentosa due to mutations at the unlinked peripherin/*RDS* and *ROM1* loci. Science 264:1604-1608, 1994.

Lin AE, Garver KL: Genetic counseling for congenital heart defects. J Pediatr 113:1105-1109, 1988.

Marenberg ME, Risch N, Berkman LF, et al: Genetic susceptibility to death from coronary heart disease in a study of twins. N Engl J Med 330:1041-1046, 1994.

Martinelli I, Sacchi E, Landi G, et al: High risk of cerebral-vein thrombosis in carriers of a prothrombin-gene mutation and in users of oral contraceptives. N Engl J Med 38:1793-1797, 1998.

Mein CA, Esposito L, Dunn MG, et al: A search for type 1 diabetes susceptibility genes in families from the United Kingdom. Nat Genet 19:297-300, 1998.

Mitchell LE: Epidemiology of neural tube defects. Am J Med Genet C Semin Med Genet 135:88-94, 2005.

Peyser PA: Genetic epidemiology of coronary artery disease. Epidemiol Rev 19:80-90, 1997.

Potter JD: Epidemiology informing clinical practice: from bills of mortality to population laboratories. Nat Clin Pract Oncol 2: 625-634, 2005.

Risch N: Linkage strategies for genetically complex traits. I. Multilocus models. Am J Hum Genet 46:222-228, 1990.

Rosendaal FR: Hematology, the American Society of Hematology Education Program Book. Washington, DC, American Society of Hematology, 2005, pp 1-12.

Sadovnick AD, Dircks A, Ebers GC: Genetic counseling in multiple sclerosis: risks to sibs and children of affected individuals. Clin Genet 56:118-122, 1999.

Strittmatter WJ, Roses AD: Apolipoprotein E and Alzheimer's disease. Annu Rev Neurosci 19:53-77, 1996.

Tsuang MT: Recent advances in genetic research on schizophrenia. J Biomed Sci 5:28-30, 1998.

● USEFUL WEBSITE

National Coalition for Health Professional Education in Genetics (NCHPEG): Mental disorders. *http://www.nchpeg.org/cdrom/empiric.html*

PROBLEMS

1. For a certain malformation, the recurrence risk in sibs and offspring of affected persons is 10%, the risk in nieces and nephews is 5%, and the risk in first cousins is 2.5%.
   a. Is this more likely to be an autosomal dominant trait with reduced penetrance or a multifactorial trait? Explain.
   b. What other information might support your conclusion?

2. A large sex difference in affected persons is often a clue to X-linked inheritance. How would you establish that pyloric stenosis is multifactorial rather than X-linked?

3. A series of children with a particular congenital malformation includes both boys and girls. In all cases, the parents are normal. How would you determine whether the malformation is more likely to be multifactorial than autosomal recessive?

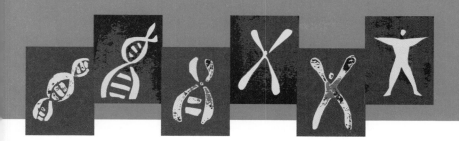

Chapter 9

Genetic Variation in Individuals and Populations: Mutation and Polymorphism

This chapter is one of several in which we explore the nature of genetically determined differences among individuals. The sequence of nuclear DNA is nearly 99.9% identical between any two humans. Yet it is precisely the small fraction of DNA sequence different among individuals that is responsible for the genetically determined variability among humans. Some DNA sequence differences have little or no effect on phenotype, whereas other differences are directly responsible for causing disease. Between these two extremes is the variation responsible for genetically determined phenotypic variability in anatomy, physiology, dietary intolerances, therapeutic responses or adverse reactions to medications, susceptibility to infection, predisposition to cancer, and perhaps even variability in various personality traits, athletic aptitude, and artistic talent. One of the important concepts of human and medical genetics is that genetic disease is only the most obvious and often the most extreme manifestation of genetic differences, one end of a continuum of variation that extends from rare variants that cause illness, through more common variants that can increase susceptibility to disease, to the most common variation in the population that is of no known disease relevance.

◉ MUTATION

Categories of Human Mutation

A mutation is defined as any change in the nucleotide sequence or arrangement of DNA. Mutations can be classified into three categories (Table 9-1): mutations that affect the number of chromosomes in the cell (**genome mutations**), mutations that alter the structure of individual chromosomes (**chromosome mutations**), and mutations that alter individual genes (**gene mutations**). Genome mutations are alterations in the number of intact chromosomes (called **aneuploidy**) arising from errors in chromosome segregation during meiosis or mitosis (see Chapters 5 and 6). Chromosome mutations are changes involving only a part of a chromosome, such as partial duplications or triplications, deletions, inversions, and translocations, which can occur spontaneously or may result from abnormal segregation of translocated chromosomes during meiosis. Gene mutations are changes in DNA sequence of the nuclear or mitochondrial genomes, ranging from a change in as little as a single nucleotide to changes that may affect many millions of base pairs. Many types of mutation are represented among the diverse alleles at individual loci in more than a thousand different genetic disorders as well as among the millions of DNA variants found throughout the genome in the normal population. The description of different mutations not only increases awareness of human genetic diversity and of the fragility of human genetic heritage but also, more significantly, contributes information needed for the detection and screening of genetic disease in particular families at risk as well as for some diseases in the population at large.

A genome mutation that deletes or duplicates an entire chromosome alters the dosage and thus the expression levels of hundreds or thousands of genes. Similarly, a chromosome mutation that deletes or duplicates large portions of one or more chromosomes may also affect the expression of hundreds of genes. Even a

Table 9-1

Types of Mutation and Their Estimated Frequencies

Class of Mutation	Mechanism	Frequency (Approximate)	Examples
Genome mutation	Chromosome missegregation	$2\text{-}4 \times 10^{-2}$/cell division	Aneuploidy
Chromosome mutation	Chromosome rearrangement	6×10^{-4}/cell division	Translocations
Gene mutation	Base pair mutation	10^{-10}/base pair/cell division	Point mutations
		$10^{-5}\text{-}10^{-6}$/locus/generation	

Based on Vogel F, Motulsky AG: Human Genetics, 3rd ed. Berlin, Springer-Verlag, 1997; and Crow JF: The origins, patterns and implications of human spontaneous mutation. Nat Rev Genet 1:40-47, 2000.

small gene mutation can have large effects, depending on which gene has been altered and what effect the alteration has on expression of the gene. A gene mutation consisting of a change in a single nucleotide in the coding sequence may lead to complete loss of expression of the gene or to the formation of a variant protein with altered properties. The phenotypic changes produced by gene mutations are considered in detail in Chapters 11 and 12.

Some DNA changes, however, have no phenotypic effect. A chromosome translocation or inversion may not affect a critical portion of the genome and may have no phenotypic effect whatsoever. A mutation within a gene may have no effect either because the change does not alter the primary amino acid sequence of a polypeptide or because, even if it does, the resulting change in the encoded amino acid sequence does not alter the functional properties of the protein. Not all mutations, therefore, have clinical consequences.

All three types of mutation occur at appreciable frequencies in many different cells. If a mutation occurs in the DNA of cells that will populate the germline, the mutation may be passed on to future generations. In contrast, **somatic mutations** occur by chance in only a subset of cells in certain tissues and result in somatic mosaicism as seen, for example, in many instances of cancer. Somatic mutations cannot be transmitted to the next generation.

The Origin of Mutations

Genome Mutations

As we discussed at length in Chapter 5, missegregation of a chromosome pair during meiosis causes genome mutations responsible for conditions such as trisomy 21 (Down syndrome). Genome mutations produce chromosomal aneuploidy and are the most common mutations seen in humans (see Table 9-1), with a rate of one missegregation event per 25 to 50 meiotic cell divisions (see Chapter 5). This estimate is clearly a minimal one because the developmental consequences of many such events may be so severe that the resulting aneuploid fetuses are spontaneously aborted shortly after conception without being detected. Genome mutations are also common in cancer cells (see Chapter 16).

Chromosome Mutations

Chromosome mutations, occurring at a rate of approximately one rearrangement per 1700 cell divisions, happen much less frequently than genome mutations. Although the frequencies of genome and chromosome mutations may seem high, these mutations are rarely perpetuated from one generation to the next because they are usually incompatible with survival or normal reproduction. Chromosome mutations are also frequently seen in cancer cells (see Chapter 16).

Gene Mutations

Gene mutations, including base pair substitutions, insertions, and deletions (Fig. 9-1), can originate by either of two basic mechanisms: errors introduced during the normal process of DNA replication, or mutations arising from a failure to repair DNA after damage and to return its sequence to what it was before the damage. Some mutations are spontaneous, whereas others are induced by physical or chemical agents called **mutagens**, because they greatly enhance the frequency of mutations.

DNA Replication Errors   The majority of replication errors are rapidly removed from the DNA and corrected by a series of DNA repair enzymes that first recognize which strand in the newly synthesized double helix contains the incorrect base and then replace it with the proper complementary base, a process termed proofreading. DNA replication (see Fig. 2-5) needs to be a remarkably accurate process; otherwise, the burden of mutation on the organism would be intolerable, and our species would cease to exist. The enzyme DNA polymerase faithfully duplicates the double helix, through a combination of strict base pairing rules (A pairs with T, C with G) and molecular proofreading. An incorrect nucleotide is introduced into one of the growing daughter strands only once every 10 million base pairs (all this while moving along a human chromosome at a rate of about 50 base pairs per second!). Additional replication error checking then corrects more than 99.9% of errors of DNA replication. Thus, the overall mutation rate as a

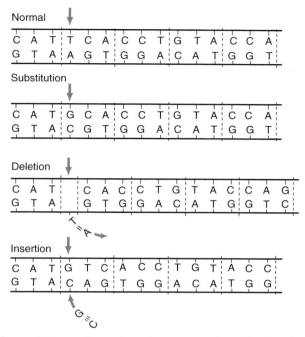

Figure 9-1 ■ Examples of gene mutation. The first base of the second codon is mutated by a base substitution, deletion, or insertion. Both the single–base pair deletion and insertion lead to a frameshift mutation in which the translational reading frame is altered. See text for discussion.

result of replication errors is a remarkably low 10^{-10} per base pair per cell division. Because the human diploid genome contains approximately 6×10^9 base pairs of DNA, replication errors introduce less than one new base pair mutation per cell division.

Repair of DNA Damage In addition to replication errors, it is estimated that between 10,000 and 1,000,000 nucleotides are damaged per human cell per day by spontaneous chemical processes such as depurination, demethylation, or deamination; by reaction with chemical mutagens (natural or otherwise) in the environment; and by exposure to ultraviolet or ionizing radiation. Some but not all of this damage is repaired. Even if the damage is recognized and excised, the repair machinery may not read the complementary strand accurately and, as a consequence, will create mutations by introducing incorrect bases. Thus, in contrast to replication-related DNA changes, which are usually corrected through proofreading mechanisms, nucleotide changes introduced by DNA damage and repair often result in permanent mutations.

⦿ TYPES OF MUTATIONS AND THEIR CONSEQUENCES

Here we consider the nature of different mutations, their underlying mechanisms, and their effect on the

••• Types of Mutation in Human Genetic Disease

Nucleotide Substitutions (Point Mutations)	Percentage of Disease-Causing Mutations	Deletions and Insertions	Percentage of Disease-Causing Mutations
Missense mutations (amino acid substitutions)	50%	Addition or deletion of a small number of bases	25%
Nonsense mutations (premature stop codons)	10%	If the number of bases involved is not a multiple of 3, a frameshift results with likely premature termination downstream.	
RNA processing mutations (destroy consensus splice sites, cap sites, and polyadenylation sites or create cryptic sites).	10%	If the number of bases involved is a multiple of 3, amino acids in the translated product are either lost or gained.	
Splice-site mutations leading to frameshift mutations and premature stop codons	10%	Larger gene deletions, inversions, fusions, and duplications (may be mediated by DNA sequence homology either within or between DNA strands)	5%
Regulatory mutations affecting transcription factor binding, transcriptional control, or other aspects of gene expression	rare	Insertion of a LINE or *Alu* element (disrupting transcription or interrupting the coding sequence)	rare
		Expansion of trinucleotide repeat sequences	rare

genes involved. In Chapters 11 and 12, we turn to the ways in which mutations in specific disease genes cause these diseases. Each type of mutation discussed here is illustrated by one or more disease examples. However, the mutations that underlie a single genetic disease are often heterogeneous. Different cases of a particular disorder will therefore usually be caused by different underlying mutations (see Box on previous page).

Nucleotide Substitutions

Missense Mutations

A single nucleotide substitution (or **point mutation**) in a DNA sequence can alter the code in a triplet of bases and cause the replacement of one amino acid by another in the gene product. Such mutations are called **missense mutations** because they alter the "sense" of the coding strand of the gene by specifying a different amino acid. In many disorders, such as the hemoglobinopathies described in Chapter 11, most of the detected mutations are missense mutations (see Table 11-2).

Other base substitutions occurring either within or outside the coding sequences of a gene can also have extensive effects on the gene product or interfere directly with the transcription process itself. As discussed in detail in Chapter 11, a number of mutations in the 5′ promoter region or the 3′ untranslated region of the β-globin gene lead to a sharp decrease in the amount of mature, processed β-globin mRNA produced. Indeed, such mutations have been critical for elucidating the importance for gene expression of particular nucleotides in these regions.

Chain Termination Mutations

Point mutations in a DNA sequence that cause the replacement of the normal codon for an amino acid by one of the three termination codons are called **nonsense mutations.** Since translation of mRNA ceases when a termination codon is reached (see Chapter 3), a mutation that converts a coding exon into a termination codon causes translation to stop partway through the coding sequence of the mRNA. The consequences of premature termination mutations are 2-fold. First, the mRNA carrying a premature mutation is often unstable (**nonsense-mediated mRNA decay**), and no translation is possible. Even if the mRNA is stable enough to be translated, the truncated protein is usually so unstable that it is rapidly degraded within the cell (see Table 11-4).

A point mutation not only may create a premature termination codon, it also may destroy a termination codon and allow translation to continue until the next termination codon is reached. Such a mutation will create a protein with additional amino acids at its carboxyl terminus and may disrupt any regulatory function provided by the 3′ untranslated region just downstream from the normal stop codon.

RNA Processing Mutations

As described in Chapter 3, the normal mechanism by which initial RNA transcripts are converted into mature mRNAs requires a series of modifications including 5′ capping, polyadenylation, and splicing. All of these steps in RNA maturation depend on specific sequences within the mRNA. In the case of splicing, two general classes of splicing mutations have been described. For introns to be excised from unprocessed RNA and the exons spliced together to form a mature mRNA requires particular nucleotide sequences located at or near the exon-intron (5′ donor site) or the intron-exon (3′ acceptor site) junctions. Mutations that affect these required bases at either the splice donor or acceptor site interfere with (and in some cases abolish) normal RNA splicing at that site (see Fig. 11-12). A second class of splicing mutations involves intron base substitutions that do not affect the donor or acceptor site sequences themselves. This class of mutations creates alternative donor or acceptor sites that compete with the normal sites during RNA processing. Thus, at least a proportion of the mature mRNA in such cases may contain improperly spliced intron sequences. Examples of this mechanism of mutation also are presented in Chapter 11.

"Hotspots" of Mutation

Nucleotide changes that involve the substitution of one purine for the other (A for G or G for A) or one pyrimidine for the other (C for T or T for C) are called **transitions.** In contrast, the replacement of a purine for a pyrimidine (or vice versa) is called a **transversion.** If nucleotide substitutions were random, there should be twice as many transversions as transitions because every base can undergo two transversions but only one transition. Different mutagenic processes preferentially cause one or the other type of substitution.

For example, transitions are overrepresented among single base pair substitutions causing genetic disease. The explanation for this observation is likely to be that the major form of DNA modification in the human genome involves **methylation** of cytosine residues (to form 5-methylcytosine), specifically when they are located immediately 5′ to a guanine (i.e., as the dinucleotide 5′-CG-3′). Spontaneous deamination of 5-methylcytosine to thymidine (compare the structures of cytosine and thymine in Fig. 2-2) in the CG doublet gives rise to C > T or G > A transitions (depending on the strand of DNA in which the 5-methylcytosine is mutated). More than 30% of all single nucleotide substitutions are of this type, and they occur at a rate 25 times greater than does any other single nucleotide mutation. Thus, the CG doublet represents a true "hotspot" for mutation in the human genome.

Deletions and Insertions

Mutations can also be caused by the insertion, inversion, fusion, or deletion of DNA sequences. Some deletions and insertions involve only a few nucleotides and are generally most easily detected by nucleotide sequencing. In other cases, a substantial segment of a gene or an entire gene is deleted, inverted, duplicated, or translocated to create a novel arrangement of gene sequences. As discussed in Chapter 4, such mutations are usually detected at the level of Southern blotting of a patient's DNA, or by polymerase chain reaction (PCR) analysis of the novel junction formed by the translocated segment. In rare instances, deletions are large enough to be visible at the cytogenetic level. To be detected even with high-resolution prometaphase banding, these mutations generally must delete at least 2 to 4 million base pairs of DNA. In many instances, such deletions remove more than a single gene and are associated with a **contiguous gene syndrome** (see Chapter 6). Interchromosomal translocations are most easily detected by spectral karyotyping.

Small Deletions and Insertions

Some deletions and insertions affect only a small number of base pairs. When the number of bases involved is not a multiple of three (i.e., is not an integral number of codons), and when it occurs in a coding sequence, the reading frame is altered beginning at the point of the insertion or deletion. The resulting mutations are called **frameshift mutations**. At the point of the insertion or deletion, a different sequence of codons is thereby generated that encodes a few abnormal amino acids followed by a termination codon in the shifted frame. In contrast, if the number of base pairs inserted or deleted is a multiple of three, no frameshift occurs and there will be an insertion or deletion of the corresponding amino acids in the translated gene product.

Large Deletions and Insertions

Alterations of gene structure large enough to be detected by Southern blotting are relatively uncommon but have been described in many inherited disorders. The frequency of such mutations differs markedly among different genetic diseases; some disorders are characterized by a high frequency of detectable deletions, whereas in others, deletion is a very rare cause of mutation. For example, deletions within the large dystrophin gene on the X chromosome in **Duchenne muscular dystrophy** (Case 12) (see Chapter 12) or the large neurofibromin gene in **neurofibromatosis type 1** (Case 29) are present in more than 60% of cases. Many cases of **α-thalassemia**

are due to deletion of one of the two α-globin genes on chromosome 16, whereas **β-thalassemia** is only rarely due to deletion of the β-globin gene (Case 39) (see Chapter 11). In some cases, the basis for gene deletion is well understood and is probably mediated by aberrant recombination between multiple copies of similar or identical DNA sequences. In other cases, the basis for deletion is unknown.

Insertion of large amounts of DNA is a cause of mutation that is much rarer than deletion. However, a novel mechanism of mutation, the insertion of LINE sequences, has been described in a few unrelated, sporadic patients with hemophilia A (Case 18). As discussed in Chapter 3, the LINE family of interspersed repetitive sequences represents a class of repeated DNA that may be transcribed into an RNA that, when it is reverse transcribed, generates a DNA sequence that can insert itself into different sites in the genome. In a few patients with hemophilia A, LINE sequences several kilobase pairs long were found to be inserted into an exon in the factor VIII gene, interrupting the coding sequence and inactivating the gene. This finding suggests that at least some of the estimated 850,000 copies of the LINE family in the human genome are capable of causing disease by insertional mutagenesis.

Effects of Recombination

An important cause of mutation in some disorders involves deletion or duplication mediated by recombination among highly similar or identical DNA sequences. For example, recombination between different members of the *Alu* family class of interspersed repeated DNA (see Chapter 3) located in introns of the low-density lipoprotein receptor gene has been documented as the cause of a duplication of several exons, resulting in **familial hypercholesterolemia** (Case 14) (see Chapter 12). In other cases, a gene may belong to a gene family represented by similar copies of the gene located in tandem on a chromosome (see Chapter 3). When the members of such a gene family are located in a head-to-tail tandem fashion in the same chromosomal region, they sometimes misalign and pair out of register either in meiosis (when two homologues pair) or in mitosis after replication (when the two sister chromatids often exchange DNA).

Recombination occurring between mispaired chromosomes or sister chromatids can lead to gene deletion or duplication. The mechanism of **unequal crossing over** is believed to be responsible for deletion of one of the α-globin genes in α-thalassemia (see Chapter 11) and for variation in the copy number of green visual pigment genes in the red and green visual pigment gene cluster on the X chromosome, both in persons with normal color vision and in males with X-linked defects in green or red color perception (Fig. 9-2A). Abnormal pairing and recombination between two similar

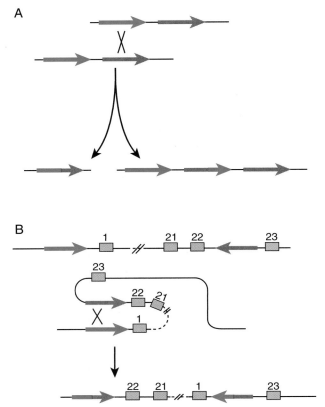

Figure 9-2 ■ **A,** Unequal but homologous recombination between misaligned sister chromatids or homologous chromosomes containing highly homologous sequences *(gray and blue arrows)* leads to two products, one with only a single copy and one with three copies of the sequence. **B,** Recombination between inverted homologous sequences located 500 kb apart on the same strand (one upstream of the factor VIII gene, the other in intron 22 of the gene) results in inversion of exons 1 through 22 of the gene, thereby disrupting the gene and causing hemophilia.

sequences repeated on a single strand of DNA may also occur; depending on the orientation of these sequences, such recombination may lead to deletion or inversion. For example, nearly half of all severe hemophilia A is due to recombination that inverts a number of exons, thereby disrupting gene structure (Fig. 9-2B).

Dynamic Mutations

The mutations in disorders such as **Huntington disease** (Case 22) and **fragile X syndrome** (Case 15) involve amplification of trinucleotide repeat sequences (see Chapters 7 and 12). In these diseases, a simple trinucleotide repeat, located either in the coding region (in the case of Huntington disease) or in a transcribed but untranslated region of a gene (in the case of fragile X syndrome), may expand during gametogenesis, in what is referred to as a **dynamic mutation,** and interfere with normal gene expression. A repeat in the coding region will generate an abnormal protein product, whereas

repeat expansion in transcribed but untranslated parts of a gene may interfere with transcription, mRNA processing, or translation. How dynamic mutations occur is not completely understood. It is thought that during replication, errors can occur when the growing strand slips while the polymerase is attempting to extend the strand and subsequently sits back down on the template strand out of register with where it was when it lost contact with the template strand.

Uniform Nomenclature for Mutations

As researchers identify and catalogue many thousands of mutations in genes causing disease and clinical laboratories report mutations for clinical use in diagnosis and counseling, there is an obvious need for uniform nomenclature to describe these mutations unambiguously, both for research and for clinical purposes (see Box on next page).

Estimates of Germline Mutation Rates in Humans

The mutation rate of a gene is usually expressed as the number of new mutations per locus per generation. The most direct way of estimating the rate is to measure the incidence of new, sporadic cases of an autosomal dominant or X-linked genetic disease that is fully penetrant with a clearly recognizable phenotype at birth or shortly thereafter. **Achondroplasia** (Case 1) is one such disease that meets the requirements for directly estimating a mutation rate. In one study, seven achondroplastic children were born in a series of 242,257 consecutive births. All seven were born to parents of normal stature, and because achondroplasia is fully penetrant, all were considered to represent new mutations. Assuming accurate diagnoses, the new mutation rate can be calculated as seven new mutations in a total of $2 \times 242,257$ alleles, or approximately $1.4 \pm 0.5 \times 10^{-5}$ mutations per locus per generation.

The mutation rate has been estimated for a number of inherited disorders in which the occurrence of a new mutation was determined by the appearance of a detectable disease phenotype (Table 9-2). The median gene mutation rate is approximately 1×10^{-6} mutations per locus per generation, but the rates vary over a 1000-fold range, from 10^{-4} to 10^{-7} mutations per locus per generation. The basis for these differences may be related to some or all of the following: gene size; the fraction of mutant alleles that give a particular observable phenotype; the age and gender of the parent in whom the mutation occurred; the mutational mechanism; and the presence or absence of mutational hotspots, such as methylated CG dinucleotides, in the gene. The Duchenne muscular dystrophy *(DMD)* and the neurofibromatosis *(NF1)* genes are both very large;

▪■▪ Mutation Nomenclature

The position of a mutation is designated as being in genomic (i.e., nuclear) DNA, in a cDNA sequence, in mitochondrial DNA, or in a protein by the prefix g., c., m., or p., respectively.

A nucleotide change is denoted first by the nucleotide number of that base, the original nucleotide, a greater than symbol (>) and the new nucleotide at that position. In genomic DNA, the nucleotide symbols are capitalized; in mRNA, they are lowercase.

If the full genomic sequence is not known, the nucleotides in an intron (referred to by the expression "intervening sequence," or IVS) are counted as +1, +2, and so on, in which +1 is the invariant G of the GT in the 5' splice donor site, or as −1, −2, and so on, counting back from the highly invariant G of the AG 3' splice acceptor site.

Small deletions are indicated by the numbers of the nucleotides deleted, separated by underscore (___), followed by the term *del*, and then the actual nucleotides that have been deleted.

Small insertions are designated by *ins* after the two nucleotides between which the insertion occurred, followed by the actual nucleotides inserted.

A missense or nonsense mutation can be described at the level of the protein by giving the correct amino acid, the position of that residue, and the amino acid that replaced the normal one.

In cDNA, the A of the translational start ATG is designated +1. The next base upstream is −1; there is no 0. The amino-terminal methionine is numbered +1 in the protein.

Examples

c.1444g>a: a mutation at position 1444 in the hexosaminidase A cDNA causing Tay-Sachs disease

g.IVS33+2T>A: a mutation substituting an A for T in a splice donor site GT of intron 33 of a gene

g.IVS33−2A>T: a mutation substituting a T for an A in the highly conserved AG splice acceptor site in the same intron

c.1524_1527delCGTA: a deletion of four nucleotides, numbers 1524 through 1527 in cDNA

c.1277_1278insTATC: a four-base insertion between nucleotides 1277 and 1278 in the hexosaminidase A cDNA, a common mutation causing Tay-Sachs disease

Glu6Val: a missense mutation, glutamic acid to valine at residue 6 in β-globin, that causes sickle cell disease

Gln39X: a nonsense mutation, glutamine to stop codon (X) at position 39 in β-globin, that causes β^0-thalassemia

---

thus, it is not surprising that the mutation rates are high at these loci. The differences in mutation rates between loci cannot be entirely explained by these factors, however. For example, achondroplasia, with a relatively high mutation rate of 1.4×10^{-5}, results almost exclusively from mutation at one particular nucleotide that changes a glycine codon to an arginine at position 380 (Gly380Arg) in a fibroblast growth factor receptor. Why this one nucleotide appears to be so easily mutated

is unknown. The estimates in Table 9-2 reflect measurements made of very visible and deleterious mutations; less severe or obvious mutations would have escaped detection, as would have more severe, lethal mutations. Thus, the overall new mutation rate may be considerably higher.

Despite the limitations of these and other approaches for determining the average gene mutation rate, all methods yield essentially the same range of values for

---

Table 9-2

Estimates of Mutation Rates for Selected Human Genes

Disease	Inheritance	Locus (Protein)	Mutation Rate*
Achondroplasia	AD	*FGFR3* (fibroblast growth factor receptor 3)	1.4×10^{-5}
Aniridia	AD	*AN2* (Pax6)	$2.9\text{-}5 \times 10^{-6}$
Duchenne muscular dystrophy	X-linked	*DMD* (dystrophin)	$3.5\text{-}10.5 \times 10^{-5}$
Hemophilia A	X-linked	*F8* (factor VIII)	$3.2\text{-}5.7 \times 10^{-5}$
Hemophilia B	X-linked	*F9* (factor IX)	$2\text{-}3 \times 10^{-6}$
Neurofibromatosis, type 1	AD	*NF1* (neurofibromin)	$4\text{-}10 \times 10^{-5}$
Polycystic kidney disease, type 1	AD	*PKD1* (polycystin)	$6.5\text{-}12 \times 10^{-5}$
Retinoblastoma	AD	*RB* (Rb)	$5\text{-}12 \times 10^{-6}$

*Expressed as mutations per locus per generation.
AD, autosomal dominant.
Based on data in Vogel F, Motulsky AG: Human Genetics, 3rd ed. Berlin, Springer-Verlag, 1997.

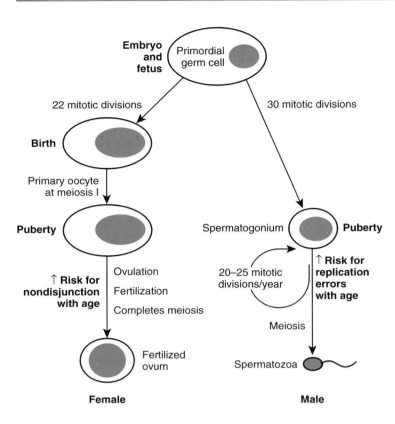

Figure 9-3 ■ Gametogenesis and mutagenesis. The diagram demonstrates the difference in the risk of genome and gene mutations during various stages of female and male gametogenesis.

germline mutation rates: approximately 10^{-4} to 10^{-6} per locus per generation, with the median much closer to 10^{-6}. Taking 10^{-6} per locus per generation as the average and given that there are about 25,000 genes in the human genome, there is a 2.6% risk of a new mutation at one locus per generation. Thus, at a minimum, *1 in 40 persons is likely to have received a newly mutated gene somewhere in the genome from one or the other parent.*

Sex Differences in Mutation Rates

New mutations can occur in the germline during any of the mitotic divisions or during the meiotic division in spermatogenesis or oogenesis. There are, however, marked differences between the sexes in both the number and timing of the mitotic and meiotic divisions, differences that can affect the frequency and types of mutation in paternal versus maternal gametes.

In oogenesis, as we saw in Chapter 2, each haploid ovum is the product of an estimated 22 mitotic divisions in fetal life, after which it becomes a primary oocyte, enters meiosis I, and remains suspended there until ovulation, years or even decades later, when meiosis I is finally completed (Fig. 9-3). No DNA replication occurs once the primary oocyte is formed. There is speculation that the longer oocytes remain in meiosis I, the greater the chance for a nondisjunction error to occur when the cells finally do complete meiosis.

These characteristics of oogenesis may help explain why autosomal trisomies of chromosomes 13, 18, and 21 and the sex chromosome aneuploidy 47,XXX occur between 80% and 100% of the time in the maternal rather than in the paternal germline, and why their frequency increases with increasing age of the mother but not of the father (see Chapter 6).

Spermatogenesis, on the other hand, involves a continuous series of cell divisions throughout life, resulting in a total of approximately 1 trillion sperm. These cells are the result of about 30 mitotic divisions during intrauterine development and childhood up to the time of puberty, and about 20 to 25 replication cycles per year thereafter (see Fig. 9-3). Given a frequency of 10^{-10} replication errors per base of DNA per cell division, each diploid spermatogonium, which contains 6×10^9 base pairs of DNA, will accumulate $10^{-10} \times 6 \times 10^9 =$ ~0.6 new mutation each time it replicates before meiosis. As an example, each sperm in a 25-year-old man is the product of about 30 prepubertal and 270 postpubertal rounds of replication, and so each sperm will contain an estimated $300 \times 0.6 =$ ~180 new mutations somewhere in the DNA as a result of replication errors. In a 55-year-old man, the number of errors per sperm would increase to approximately 600. Of course, most of these mutations will not be deleterious (or will be recessive or lethal to the sperm and thus not phenotypically apparent in a resulting conception and birth). It is estimated that the fraction of random point mutations that is deleterious is about 1/2000, and so we can estimate that depending on the age of the man, *approximately 1 in 10 to 1 in 3 sperm carries a new deleterious mutation* somewhere in the genome.

Because the DNA in sperm has undergone far more replication cycles than has the DNA in ova, one might expect that point mutations are more often paternal rather than maternal in origin. In highly penetrant, dominant diseases such as achondroplasia, certain of the **craniosynostoses (Apert, Pfeiffer,** or **Crouzon syndromes),** and the **multiple endocrine neoplasias** type 2 (MEN2A and 2B), the new mutations responsible are usually missense mutations that arise nearly always in the paternal germline. Furthermore, the older a man is, the more rounds of replication have preceded the meiotic divisions, and thus the frequency of paternal new mutations might be expected to increase with the age of the father. In fact, an increase of gene mutations of paternal origin with increasing age has been observed for some disorders, notably achondroplasia, Apert syndrome, and X-linked **hemophilia B** (where the maternal grandfather is the source of a new mutation in the mother of the proband). In contrast, new mutations in Duchenne muscular dystrophy show little bias overall in parent of origin or age of the parent. However, if the new mutations in this disorder are partitioned into the rarer point mutations and more common intragenic deletions, approximately 90% of all new point mutations are paternal in origin, whereas seven of eight new *DMD* deletion mutations are maternal. In other diseases, however, the parent of origin and age effect on mutational spectrum are, for unknown reasons, not so striking.

In trinucleotide repeat disorders (see Chapter 12), a marked parent-of-origin effect is well known. For example, the very large expansions of the CAG repeat that cause juvenile **Huntington disease** are generally of paternal origin. On the other hand, the massive expansions of the CGG repeat in fragile X syndrome nearly always occur during female gametogenesis. Such differences may be due to fundamental biological differences between oogenesis and spermatogenesis but may also result from selection against gametes carrying repeat expansions, as has been shown for sperm carrying extremely large CGG repeat expansions associated with the fragile X syndrome.

◉ HUMAN GENETIC DIVERSITY

Most of the estimates of mutation rates described involve detection of deleterious mutations with an obvious effect on phenotype. Many mutations, however, are not deleterious but are thought to be selectively neutral; some may even be beneficial. During the course of evolution, the steady influx of new nucleotide varia-

tion has ensured a high degree of genetic diversity and individuality. This theme extends through all fields in human and medical genetics; genetic diversity may manifest as changes in the staining pattern of chromosomes (see Chapter 5), as variation in the copy number of megabase segments of DNA, as nucleotide changes in DNA, as alterations in proteins, or as disease.

The Concept of Genetic Polymorphism

The DNA sequence of exactly the same region of a chromosome is remarkably similar among chromosomes carried by many different individuals from around the world. In fact, a randomly chosen segment of human DNA about 1000 base pairs in length contains, on average, only one base pair that varies between the two homologous chromosomes inherited from the parents (assuming the parents are unrelated). This figure is about 2.5 times higher than the proportion of heterozygous nucleotides estimated for protein-coding regions of the genome (about 1 in 2500 base pairs). The difference is not altogether surprising because it seems intuitively likely that protein-coding regions are under more rigid selective pressure, and thus the incidence of mutations in those regions throughout evolution should be lower.

When a variant is so common that it is found in more than 1% of chromosomes in the general population, the variant constitutes what is known as a **genetic polymorphism.** In contrast, alleles with frequencies of less than 1% are, by convention, called **rare variants.** Although many deleterious mutations that lead to genetic disease are rare variants, there is not a simple correlation between allele frequency and the effect of the allele on health. Many rare variants appear to have no deleterious effect, whereas some variants common enough to be polymorphisms are known to predispose to serious illness.

There are many types of polymorphism. Some polymorphisms are due to variants that consist of deletions, duplications, triplications, and so on, of hundreds to millions of base pairs of DNA and are not associated with any known disease phenotype; other similarly sized alterations are rare variants that clearly cause serious illness. Polymorphisms can also be changes in one or a few bases in the DNA located between genes or within introns, can be inconsequential to the functioning of any gene, and can be detected only by direct DNA analysis. Sequence changes may also be located in the coding sequence of genes themselves and result in different protein variants that may lead in turn to sharply distinct phenotypes. Still others are in regulatory regions and may also be important in determining phenotype by affecting transcription or mRNA stability.

Table 9-3

Types of DNA Polymorphism

Polymorphism	Basis for the Polymorphism	Number of Alleles
SNP	Substitution of one or the other of two bases at one location	2
Indel		
Simple	Presence or absence of a short segment of DNA	2
STRP	~5-25 copies, in tandem, of a repeated 2-, 3-, or 4-nucleotide repeat unit	Typically 5 or more
VNTR	Hundreds to thousands of copies, in tandem, of a 10- to 100-nucleotide repeat unit	Typically 5 or more
CNP	Typically the presence or absence of 200-bp to 1.5-Mb segments of DNA, although tandem duplication of 2, 3, 4, or more copies can also occur	2 up to a few

CNP, copy number polymorphism; SNP, single nucleotide polymorphism; STRP, short tandem repeat polymorphism; VNTR, variable number tandem repeat.

Polymorphisms are key elements in human genetics research and practice. The ability to distinguish different inherited forms of a gene or different segments of the genome provides tools that are crucial for a wide array of applications. As illustrated in this chapter and other chapters to follow, genetic markers are enormously powerful as research tools for mapping a gene to a particular region of a chromosome by linkage analysis or by allelic association (see Chapter 10). They are already commonly in use in medicine for prenatal diagnosis of genetic disease and heterozygote detection (see Chapter 15), as well as in blood banking and tissue typing for transfusions and organ transplantation (see later in this chapter). Polymorphisms are the basis for ongoing efforts to provide genomic-based **personalized medicine** (see Chapter 17) in which one tailors an individual's medical care on the basis of whether he or she carries polymorphic variants that increase or decrease the risk for common adult disorders (such as coronary heart disease, cancer, and diabetes; see Chapter 8), make complications after surgery more likely, or influence the efficacy or safety of particular medications. Finally, polymorphisms have become a powerful new tool in forensic applications such as identity testing for determining paternity, for identifying remains of crime victims, or for matching a suspect's DNA to the perpetrator's.

INHERITED VARIATION AND POLYMORPHISM IN DNA

The vast amount of DNA sequence information obtained as a result of the Human Genome Project from many hundreds of individuals worldwide has provided the information necessary to begin to characterize the types and frequencies of polymorphic variation in human DNA sequence. As a result, we have begun to generate catalogues of human DNA sequence diversity. DNA polymorphisms can be classified according to how the DNA sequence varies between the different alleles (Table 9-3).

Single Nucleotide Polymorphisms

The simplest and most common of all polymorphisms are **single nucleotide polymorphisms (SNPs)**. SNPs usually have only two alleles corresponding to the two different bases occupying a particular location in the genome. SNPs are common and occur on average once every 1000 base pairs, which means that there is an average of 3,000,000 differences between any two human genomes. The total number of variant positions among all humans is far greater and is estimated to be more than 10,000,000, although this estimate is likely to be too low since we certainly do not yet have a complete catalogue of all variants, particularly the rare ones, in every ethnic group across the globe. Many millions of SNPs have been identified and catalogued in populations worldwide. A subset of approximately 10% of the most frequent SNPs were chosen to serve as the markers for a high-density map of the human genome known as the haplotype map (HapMap; see Chapter 10).

The significance for health of the vast majority of polymorphic SNPs is the subject of active research. The fact that SNPs are common does not mean that they must be neutral and without effect on health or longevity. What it does mean is that any effect of common SNPs must be a subtle altering of disease susceptibility rather than a direct cause of serious illness.

Insertion-Deletion Polymorphisms

The next class of polymorphism is the result of variations caused by **insertion or deletion (indels)** of between 2 and 100 nucleotides. Indels number in the hundreds of thousands in the genome. Approximately half of all indels are referred to as **simple** because they have only two alleles, that is, the presence or absence of the inserted or deleted segment; the other half are **multiallelic** due to variable numbers of a segment of DNA that is repeated in tandem at a particular location. Multiallelic indels are further subdivided into **microsatellite** and **minisatellite** polymorphisms.

Microsatellites

Microsatellites are stretches of DNA consisting of units of two, three, or four nucleotides, such as TGTG...TG, CAACAA...CAA, or AAATAAAT...AAAT, repeated between one and a few dozen times. The different alleles in a microsatellite polymorphism are the result of differing numbers of repeated nucleotide units

contained within any one microsatellite and are therefore often referred to as **short tandem repeat polymorphisms** or **STRPs**. A microsatellite locus often has many alleles (repeat lengths) present in the population and can be readily genotyped by determining the size of the PCR fragment generated by primers that flank the microsatellite repeat (Fig. 9-4). Many tens of thousands of microsatellite polymorphic loci are known throughout the human genome.

Minisatellites

Another class of indel polymorphisms results from the insertion, in tandem, of varying numbers (usually in the hundreds to thousands) of copies of a DNA sequence 10 to 100 base pairs in length, known as a **minisatellite**. This class of polymorphism has many alleles (Fig. 9-5) due to variation in the number of copies of the minisatellite that are repeated in tandem, referred to as **variable number tandem repeats (VNTRs)**. The most informative markers have several dozen or more alleles, so no two unrelated individuals are likely to share the same alleles. Although the majority of

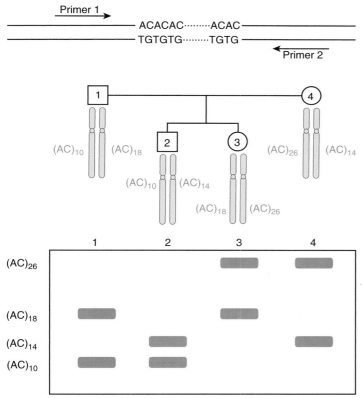

Figure 9-4 ■ Microsatellite markers in human DNA. At top is the DNA containing an $(AC)_n$ microsatellite marker on one chromosome; primers 1 and 2 are PCR primers complementary to unique sequences that flank the dinucleotide repeat. Below is a pedigree demonstrating codominant inheritance of a microsatellite polymorphism due to variable numbers of the dinucleotide AC. The genotype of each individual is shown below his or her symbol in the pedigree. The different-sized fragments are amplified by PCR with primers 1 and 2 flanking the stretch of AC dinucleotides, and their relative lengths are determined by separating them by gel electrophoresis (bottom).

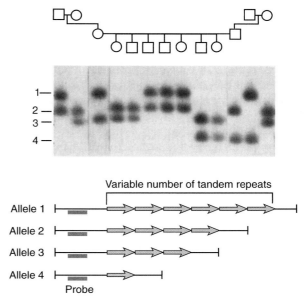

Figure 9-5 ■ Codominant inheritance of an autosomal DNA polymorphism caused by a variable number of tandem repeats. Alleles 1 to 4 are related to one other by a variable number of identical (or nearly so) short DNA sequences (arrows). Size variation can be detected after restriction enzyme digestion and hybridization with a unique probe that lies outside the VNTR sequences themselves but inside the restriction sites used to define the allelic fragments. (Courtesy of A. Bowcock, Washington University, St. Louis, Missouri.)

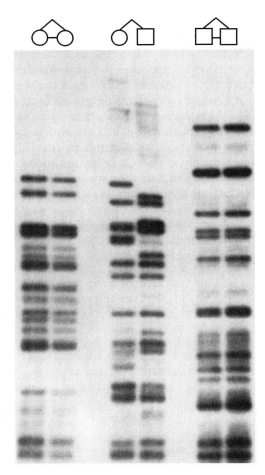

Figure 9-6 ■ DNA fingerprinting of twins by means of a probe that detects VNTR polymorphisms at many loci around the genome. Each pair of lanes contains DNA from a set of twins. The twins of the first set (as well as the twins of the third set) have identical DNA fingerprints, indicating that they are identical (monozygotic) twins. The set in the middle have clearly distinguishable DNA fingerprints, indicating that they are fraternal twins. (Courtesy of Alec Jeffreys, University of Leicester, United Kingdom.)

indels, whether they are simple, STRP, or VNTR polymorphisms, are considered to be of no significance for human health, some VNTRs have been implicated in disease.

The minisatellite repeat sequences found in many different VNTR-type polymorphisms are sufficiently similar to one another to make possible the detection of many different loci simultaneously by use of one minisatellite fragment as a probe in a single Southern blot hybridization. Only identical twins show an indistinguishable pattern (Fig. 9-6), and therefore the simultaneous detection of a number of minisatellite polymorphisms was one of the first methods of **DNA fingerprinting** to be used for identity testing. Detection of minisatellite polymorphisms by Southern blotting

has been largely superseded by typing of microsatellites by PCR. For example, the Federal Bureau of Investigation in the United States currently uses 13 STRP markers for its DNA fingerprinting panel. Two individuals (other than monozygotic twins) are so unlikely to have identical genotypes at all 13 loci that the panel will allow definitive determination of whether two samples came from the same individual.

Copy Number Polymorphisms

The last and most recently discovered form of human polymorphism are **copy number polymorphisms (CNPs)**. CNPs consist of variation in the number of copies of larger segments of the genome, ranging from 200 bp to nearly 2 Mb. CNPs may have only two alleles (i.e., the presence or absence of a segment) or multiple alleles due to the presence of 0, 1, 2, or 3 or more copies of a segment of DNA in tandem. CNPs have only recently been identified and studied because the deleted or repeated regions are usually too small to be seen by cytogenetic examination but too large to be detected by DNA sequencing. Instead, CNPs are most readily discovered by the application of a new technology, **array comparative genome hybridization,** as discussed in Chapter 4. As with all DNA polymorphism, the significance of different CNP alleles in health and disease susceptibility is largely unknown but is the subject of intensive investigation. CNPs constitute a background of common variation that must be understood if alterations in copy number observed in patients are to be interpreted properly.

● INHERITED VARIATION AND POLYMORPHISM IN PROTEINS

Although all polymorphism is ultimately the result of differences in DNA sequence, some polymorphic loci have been studied by examining the variation in the proteins encoded by the alleles rather than by examining the differences in DNA sequence of the alleles themselves. It is estimated that any one individual is likely to be heterozygous for alleles determining structurally different polypeptides at approximately 20% of all loci; when individuals from different ethnic groups are compared, an even greater fraction of proteins has been found to exhibit detectable polymorphism. Thus, a striking degree of biochemical individuality exists within the human species in its makeup of enzymes and other gene products. Furthermore, because the products of many of the encoded biochemical pathways interact, one may plausibly conclude that each individual, regardless of his or her state of health, has a unique, genetically determined chemical makeup and thus responds in a unique manner to environmental, dietary, and pharmacological influences. This concept of **chemi-**

cal individuality, first put forward a century ago by the remarkably foresighted British physician Archibald Garrod, remains true today.

Here we discuss a few polymorphisms of medical significance: the ABO and Rh blood groups important in determining compatibility for blood transfusions, the major histocompatibility complex (MHC) that plays an important role in transplantation medicine. Studying variation in proteins rather than studying the DNA that encodes them has real utility; after all, the variant protein products of various polymorphic alleles are often what is responsible for different phenotypes and therefore are likely to dictate how genetic variation at a locus affects the interaction between an individual and the environment.

Blood Groups and Their Polymorphisms

The first instances of genetically determined protein variation were detected in antigens found in blood, the so-called **blood group antigens.** Numerous polymorphisms are known to exist in the components of human blood, especially in the ABO and Rh antigens of red blood cells. In particular, the ABO and Rh systems are important in blood transfusion, tissue and organ transplantation, and hemolytic disease of the newborn.

The ABO System

Human blood can be assigned to one of four types according to the presence on the surface of red blood cells of two antigens, A and B, and the presence in the plasma of the two corresponding antibodies, anti-A and anti-B. There are four major phenotypes: O, A, B, and AB. Type A persons have antigen A on their red blood cells, type B persons have antigen B, type AB persons have both antigens A and B, and type O persons have neither. The reaction of the red blood cells of each type with anti-A and anti-B antisera is shown in Table 9-4.

One feature of the ABO groups not shared by other blood group systems is the reciprocal relationship, in an individual, between the antigens present on the red blood cells and the antibodies in the serum (see Table

9-4). When the red blood cells lack antigen A, the serum contains anti-A; when the cells lack antigen B, the serum contains anti-B. The reason for this reciprocal relationship is uncertain, but formation of anti-A and anti-B is believed to be a response to the natural occurrence of A-like and B-like antigens in the environment (e.g., in bacteria).

The ABO blood groups are determined by a locus on chromosome 9. The *A, B,* and *O* alleles at this locus are a classic example of multiallelism in which three alleles, two of which (*A* and *B*) are inherited as a codominant trait and the third of which (*O*) is inherited as a recessive trait, determine four phenotypes. The A and B antigens are made by the action of the *A* and *B* alleles on a red blood cell surface glycoprotein called H antigen. The antigenic specificity is conferred by the specific terminal sugars, if any, that are added to the H substance. The *B* allele codes for a glycosyltransferase that preferentially recognizes the sugar D-galactose and adds it to the end of an oligosaccharide chain contained in the H antigen, thereby creating the B antigen. The *A* allele codes for a slightly different form of the enzyme that preferentially recognizes *N*-acetylgalactosamine instead of D-galactose and adds *N*-acetylgalactosamine to the precursor, thereby creating the A antigen. A third allele, *O,* codes for a mutant version of the transferase that lacks transferase activity and does not detectably affect H substance at all.

The molecular differences in the glycosyltransferase gene that are responsible for the *A, B,* and *O* alleles have been determined. Four nucleotide sequence differences between the *A* and *B* alleles result in amino acid changes that alter the specificity of the glycosyltransferase. The *O* allele has a single–base pair deletion in the *ABO* gene coding region, which causes a frameshift mutation that eliminates the transferase activity in type O individuals. Now that the DNA sequences are available, ABO blood group typing is being performed directly at the genotype rather than at the phenotype level, especially when there are technical difficulties in serological analysis, as is often the case in forensic investigations or paternity testing.

The primary medical importance of the ABO blood group is in blood transfusion and tissue or organ transplantation. In the ABO blood group system, there are compatible and incompatible combinations. A compatible combination is one in which the red blood cells of a donor do not carry an A or a B antigen that corresponds to the antibodies in the recipient's serum. Although theoretically there are universal donors (group O) and universal recipients (group AB), a patient is given blood of his or her own ABO group, except in emergencies. The regular presence of anti-A and anti-B explains the failure of many of the early attempts to transfuse blood, because these antibodies can cause immediate destruction of ABO-incompatible cells. In

Table 9-4

ABO Genotypes and Serum Reactivity

RBC Phenotype	Reaction with Anti-A	Reaction with Anti-B	Antibodies in Serum
O	–	–	Anti-A, anti-B
A	+	–	Anti-B
B	–	+	Anti-A
AB	+	+	Neither

– represents no reaction; + represents reaction. RBC, red blood cell.

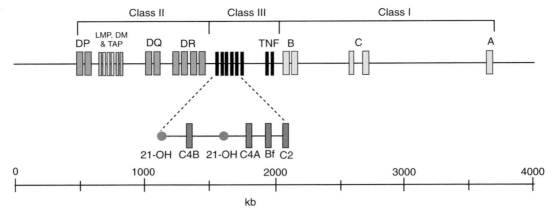

Figure 9-7 ■ A schematic of the major histocompatibility complex on chromosome 6p. *DP, DQ,* and *DR,* class II antigen genes; *B, C,* and *A,* class I antigen genes; *LMP,* genes encoding components of large multifunctional protease; DM, heterodimer of *DMA* and *DMB* genes encoding the antigen-processing molecule required for binding peptide to MHC class II antigens; other genes encode TAP, transporter associated with antigen processing; TNF, tumor necrosis factor; Bf, properdin factor B; C2, C4A, C4B, complement components; 21-OH, 21-hydroxylase. (One of the 21-OH loci is a pseudogene.) For discussion, see text.

tissue and organ transplantation, ABO compatibility of donor and recipient, as well as human leukocyte antigen (HLA) compatibility (described later), is essential to graft survival.

The Rh System

The Rh system ranks with the ABO system in clinical importance because of its role in hemolytic disease of the newborn and in transfusion incompatibilities. The name Rh comes from Rhesus monkeys that were used in the experiments that led to the discovery of the system. In simplest terms, the population is separated into Rh-positive individuals, who express, on their red blood cells, the antigen Rh D, a polypeptide encoded by a gene (*RHD*) on chromosome 1, and Rh-negative individuals, who do not express this antigen. The Rh-negative phenotype usually originates from homozygosity for a nonfunctional allele of the *RHD* gene. The frequency of Rh-negative individuals varies enormously in different ethnic groups. For example, 17% of whites and 7% of African Americans are Rh-negative, whereas the frequency among Japanese is 0.5%.

Hemolytic Disease of the Newborn

Clinically, the chief significance of the Rh system is that Rh-negative persons can readily form anti-Rh antibodies after exposure to Rh-positive red blood cells. This is especially a problem when an Rh-negative pregnant woman is carrying an Rh-positive fetus. Normally during pregnancy, small amounts of fetal blood cross the placental barrier and reach the maternal blood stream. If the mother is Rh-negative and the fetus Rh-positive, the mother will form antibodies that return to the fetal circulation and damage the fetal red blood cells, causing hemolytic disease of the newborn with consequences that can be severe if not treated.

In pregnant Rh-negative women, the risk of immunization by Rh-positive fetal red blood cells can be minimized with an injection of Rh immune globulin at 28 to 32 weeks of gestation and again after pregnancy. Rh immune globulin serves to clear any Rh-positive fetal cells from the mother's circulation before she is sensitized. Rh immune globulin is also given after miscarriage, termination of pregnancy, or invasive procedures such as chorionic villus sampling or amniocentesis, in case any Rh-positive cells gained access to the mother's circulation. The discovery of the Rh system and its role in hemolytic disease of the newborn has been a major contribution of genetics to medicine. At one time ranking as the most common human genetic disease, hemolytic disease of the newborn is now relatively rare because of preventive measures that have become routine practice in obstetrical medicine.

The Major Histocompatibility Complex

The MHC is composed of a large cluster of genes located on the short arm of chromosome 6 (Fig. 9-7). On the basis of structural and functional differences, these genes are categorized into three classes, two of which, the class I and class II genes, correspond to the human leukocyte antigen (HLA) genes, originally discovered by virtue of their importance in tissue transplantation between unrelated individuals. The HLA class I and class II genes encode cell surface proteins that play a critical role in the initiation of an immune response and specifically in the "presentation" of antigen to lymphocytes, which cannot recognize and respond to an antigen unless it is complexed with an HLA molecule on the surface of an antigen-presenting cell. Many hundreds of different alleles of the HLA class I and class II genes are known and more are being

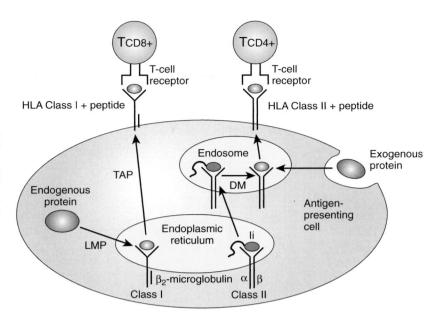

Figure 9-8 ■ The interaction between MHC class I and class II molecules, foreign proteins, and T-cell receptors. LMP, large multifunctional protease; TAP, transporter associated with antigen processing; Ii, invariant chain; DM, heterodimer encoded by the *DMA* and *DMB* genes; CD8+, cytotoxic T cells; CD4+, helper T cells. (Modified from Thorsby E: HLA-associated diseases. Hum Immunol 53:1-11, 1997.)

discovered daily, making them by far the most highly polymorphic loci in the human genome.

The class I genes (*HLA-A, HLA-B,* and *HLA-C*) encode proteins that are an integral part of the plasma membrane of all nucleated cells (Fig. 9-8). A class I protein consists of two polypeptide subunits, a variable heavy chain encoded within the MHC and a nonpolymorphic polypeptide, β_2-microglobulin, that is encoded by a gene outside the MHC, mapping to chromosome 15. Peptides derived from intracellular proteins are generated by proteolytic degradation by a large multifunctional protease; the peptides are then transported to the cell surface and held in a cleft formed in the class I molecule to display the peptide antigen to cytotoxic T cells (see Fig. 9-8).

The class II region is composed of several loci, such as *HLA-DP, HLA-DQ,* and *HLA-DR,* that encode integral membrane cell surface proteins. Each class II molecule is a heterodimer, composed of α and β subunits, both of which are encoded by the MHC. Class II molecules present peptides derived from extracellular proteins that had been taken up into lysosomes and processed into peptides for presentation to T cells (see Fig. 9-8).

Other gene loci are present within the MHC (see Fig. 9-7) but are functionally unrelated to the HLA class I and class II genes and do not function to determine histocompatibility or immune responsiveness. Some of these genes are, however, associated with diseases, such as **congenital adrenal hyperplasia** (see Chapter 6), caused by deficiency of 21-hydroxylase, and **hemochromatosis,** a liver disease caused by iron overload (Case 17).

HLA Alleles and Haplotypes

The HLA system can be confusing at first because the nomenclature used to define and describe different HLA alleles has undergone a fundamental change with the advent of widespread DNA sequencing of the MHC. According to the older, traditional system of HLA nomenclature, the different alleles were distinguished from one another serologically. An individual's HLA type was determined by seeing how a panel of different antisera or reactive lymphocytes reacted to his or her cells. These antisera and cells were obtained from hundreds of multiparous women who developed immune reactivity against the paternal type I and type II antigens expressed by their fetuses during the course of their pregnancies. If cells from two unrelated individuals evoked the same pattern of reaction in a typing panel of antibodies and cells, they would be considered to have the same HLA types and the allele they represented would be given a number, such as *B27* in the class I *HLA-B* locus or *DR3* in the class II *DR* locus. However, as the genes responsible for encoding the class I and class II MHC chains were identified and sequenced, single HLA alleles initially defined serologically were shown to consist of multiple alleles defined by different DNA sequence variants even within the same serological allele. The 100 serological specificities at *HLA-A, B, C, DR, DQ,* and *DP* now comprise more than 1300 alleles defined at the DNA sequence level. For example, more than 24 different nucleic acid sequence variants of the *HLA-B* gene exist in what was previously defined as "the" *B27* allele by serological testing. Most but not all of the DNA variants change a triplet codon and therefore an amino acid in the peptide encoded by that allele. Each allele that changes an amino acid in the HLA-B peptide is given its own number, so allele number 1, number 2, and so on in the group of alleles corresponding to what used to be a single *B27* allele defined serologically, is now referred to as *HLA-B*2701, HLA-B*2702,* and so on.

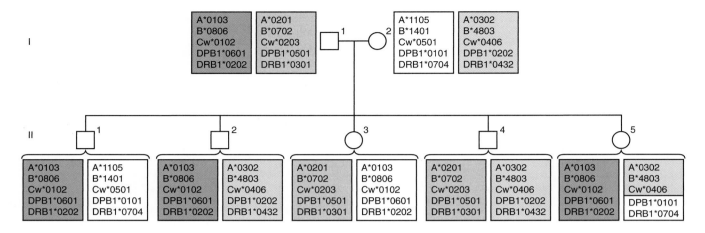

Figure 9-9 ■ The inheritance of HLA haplotypes. A haplotype is usually transmitted, as shown in this figure, as a unit. In extremely rare instances, a parent will transmit a recombinant haplotype to the child, as seen in individual II-5, who received a haplotype that is recombinant between the class I and class II loci.

The set of HLA alleles at the different class I and class II loci on a given chromosome together form a **haplotype.** The alleles are codominant; each parent has two haplotypes and expresses both. These loci are located close enough to each other that, in an individual family, the entire haplotype can be transmitted as a single block to a child (Fig. 9-9). As a result, parent and child share only one haplotype, and there is a 25% chance that two sibs inherit matching HLA haplotypes. Because acceptance of transplanted tissues largely correlates with the degree of similarity between donor and recipient HLA haplotypes (and ABO blood groups), the favored donor for bone marrow or organ transplantation is an ABO-compatible and HLA-identical sibling of the recipient.

Within any one ethnic group, some HLA alleles are found commonly; others are rare or never seen. Similarly, some haplotypes are much more frequent than expected, whereas others are exceptionally rare or nonexistent. For example, most of the 3×10^7 allelic combinations that could theoretically occur to make a haplotype among white individuals have never been observed. This restriction in the diversity of haplotypes possible in a population results from a situation referred to as **linkage disequilibrium** (see Chapter 10) and may be explained by a complex interaction between a number of factors. These factors include low rates of meiotic recombination in the small physical distance between HLA loci; environmental influences that provide positive selection for particular combinations of HLA alleles forming a haplotype; and historical factors, such as how long ago the population was founded, how many founders there were, and how much immigration has occurred (see later in this chapter).

Major differences in allele and haplotype frequencies exist between populations as well. What may be a common allele or haplotype in one population may be very rare in another. Once again, the differences in the distribution and frequency of the alleles and haplotypes within the MHC are the result of complex genetic, environmental, and historical factors at play in each of the different populations.

HLA and Disease Association

Ankylosing Spondylitis   With the increasing delineation of HLA alleles has come an appreciation of the association between certain diseases and specific HLA alleles and haplotypes. The etiological basis for most of the HLA-disease associations remains obscure. Most but not all of these disorders are **autoimmune,** that is, associated with an abnormal immune response apparently directed against one or more self antigens that is thought to be related to variation in the immune response resulting from polymorphism in immune response genes (Table 9-5). **Ankylosing spondylitis,** a chronic inflammatory disease of the spine and sacroiliac joints, is one example. In older studies that relied on serologically defined *B27* alleles, only 9% of Norwegians, for example, are *B27*-positive, whereas more than 95% of those with ankylosing spondylitis are *B27*-positive. Thus, the risk of developing ankylosing spondylitis is at least 150 times higher for people who have *HLA-B27* than for those who do not. Although less than 5% of *B27*-positive individuals develop the disease, as many as 20% of *B27*-positive individuals may have subtle, subclinical manifestations of the disease without any symptoms or disability. One explanation for why some *B27*-positive individuals do not develop disease

Table 9-5

HLA Alleles with Strong Disease Association

Disease	HLA Allele (Serological)	Frequency (%)*		Odds Ratio†
		Patients	*Controls*	
Ankylosing spondylitis	B27	>95	9	>150
Reiter syndrome	B27	>80	9	>40
Acute anterior uveitis	B27	68	9	>20
Subacute thyroiditis	B35	70	14	14
Psoriasis vulgaris	Cw6	87	33	7
Narcolepsy	DQ6	>95	33	>38
Graves disease	DR3	65	27	4
Rheumatoid arthritis	DR4	81	33	9
Juvenile rheumatoid arthritis	DR8	38	7	8
Celiac disease	DQ2	99	28	>250
Multiple sclerosis	DR2, DQ6	86	33	12
Type I diabetes	DQ8	81	23	14
Type I diabetes	DQ6	<1	33	0.02
Hemochromatosis	A3	75	13	20
CAH (21-hydroxylase deficiency)	B47	25	0.2	80-150

*Frequency data are for Norwegian populations and are approximate.

†The odds ratio is approximate and is calculated as ad/bc where a = number of patients with the antigen, b = number of controls with the antigen, c = number of patients without the antigen, and d = number of controls without the antigen (see Chapter 10).

CAH, congenital adrenal hyperplasia.

Modified from Fugger L, Tisch R, Libau R, et al: The role of human major histocompatibility complex (HLA) genes in disease. In Scriver CR, Beaudet AL, Sly WS, Valle D (eds): The Metabolic and Molecular Bases of Inherited Disease, 7th ed. New York, McGraw-Hill, 1995, pp 555-585; Bell JI, Todd JA, McDevitt HO: The molecular basis of HLA-disease association. Adv Hum Genet 18:1-41, 1989; and Thorsby E: HLA associated diseases. Hum Immunol 53:1-11, 1997.

rests in part on that fact that DNA sequencing has revealed more than two dozen different alleles within "the" *HLA-B27* allele originally defined serologically. The frequency of each of these different alleles varies within a given ethnic group and between ethnic groups. If only certain of these *B27* alleles predispose to disease, while others may actually be protective, studies in different ethnic groups that lump all the *B27* alleles into a single allele will find quite different rates of disease in *B27*-positive individuals.

In other cases, the association between a particular HLA allele or haplotype and a disease is not due to functional differences in immune response genes encoded by the HLA alleles. Instead, the association is due to a particular MHC allele being present at a very high frequency on chromosomes that also happen to contain disease-causing mutations in another gene within the MHC, because of linkage disequilibrium (see Chapter 10). As mentioned earlier, the autosomal recessive disorders **congenital adrenal hyperplasia** due to 21-hydroxylase deficiency and primary **hemochromatosis** result from mutations in genes that lie within the MHC. Analysis of 21-hydroxylase mutations responsible for adrenal hyperplasia has revealed that certain of the mutations at this locus originally occurred on chromosomes with particular haplotypes and were subsequently inherited through multiple generations along with these specific haplotype markers as a block. Another example is hemochromatosis, a common autosomal recessive disorder of iron overload. More than

80% of patients with hemochromatosis are homozygous for a common mutation, Cys282Tyr, in the hemochromatosis gene *(HFE)* and have *HLA-A*0301* alleles at their *HLA-A* locus. The association is not the result of *HLA-A*0301* somehow causing hemochromatosis. *HFE* is involved with iron transport or metabolism in the intestine; *HLA-A*, as a class I immune response gene, has no effect on iron transport. The association is due to proximity of the two loci and the linkage disequilibrium between the Cys282Tyr mutation in *HFE* and the *A*0301* allele at *HLA-A*.

The functional basis of most HLA-disease associations is unknown. HLA molecules are integral to T-cell recognition of antigens. Perhaps different polymorphic alleles result in structural variation in these cell surface molecules, leading to differences in the capacity of the proteins to interact with antigen and the T-cell receptor in the initiation of an immune response, thereby affecting such critical processes as immunity against infections and self-tolerance to prevent autoimmunity.

HLA and Tissue Transplantation

As the name major histocompatibility complex implies, the HLA loci are the primary determinants of transplant tolerance and graft rejection and therefore play an important role in transplantation medicine. Despite the impressive progress in the design of powerful immunosuppressive drugs to suppress rejection of organ transplants, only an absolutely perfect match for all

HLA and blood group alleles, such as occurs between monozygotic twins, can provide a 100% transplantation success rate without immunosuppressive therapy. For the transplantation of solid organs, such as kidneys, the percentage of grafts surviving after 10 years when the recipient and the donor are HLA-identical siblings is 72% but falls to 56% when the donor is a sibling who has only one HLA haplotype in common with the recipient.

Bone marrow transplantation is a greater challenge than solid organ transplantation; not only can the host reject the graft, but also the graft, which contains immunocompetent lymphocytes, can attack the host in what is known as graft-versus-host disease (GVHD). Survival out to 8 years after bone marrow transplantation for patients with chronic myelogenous leukemia following chemotherapy is 60% if graft and host mismatch at no more than one class I or class II locus but falls to 25% when there are both class I and class II mismatches. GVHD is also less frequent and severe the better the class I match.

Given the obvious improvement in the success of bone marrow transplantation with the greater number of matches, and the tremendous diversity of HLA haplotypes within a population and between different ethnic groups, millions of HLA-typed unrelated bone marrow donors have been registered in databases that can be searched to look for the best possible match for a patient needing a bone marrow transplantation.

GENOTYPES AND PHENOTYPES IN POPULATIONS

Genetic Variation in Populations

Population genetics is the quantitative study of the distribution of genetic variation in populations and of how the frequencies of genes and genotypes are maintained or change. Population genetics is concerned both with genetic factors, such as mutation and reproduction, and with environmental and societal factors, such as selection and migration, which together determine the frequency and distribution of alleles and genotypes in families and communities. A mathematical description of the behavior of genes in populations is an important element of many disciplines, including anthropology, evolutionary biology, and human genetics. At present, human geneticists are using the principles and methods of population genetics to address many unanswered questions concerning the history and genetic structure of human populations, the flow of genes between populations and between generations, and, very importantly, the optimal methods for identifying genetic susceptibilities to common disease. In medical genetic practice, population genetics provides the knowledge about different disease genes that are common in different populations, information that is needed for clinical diagnosis and genetic counseling, including determining the allele frequencies required for risk calculations.

In this section, we describe the central, organizing concept of population genetics, Hardy-Weinberg equilibrium; we consider its assumptions and the factors that may cause true or apparent deviation from equilibrium in real as opposed to idealized populations. Finally, the chapter provides some insight into how differences in disease gene frequencies arise among members of different, more or less genetically isolated groups.

Genetic Factors in Human Immunodeficiency Virus Resistance

An important example of a common autosomal trait governed by a single pair of alleles can be used to illustrate the basic principles that determine allele and genotype frequencies in populations. Consider the gene *CCR5*, which encodes a cell surface cytokine receptor that serves as an entry point for certain strains of the human immunodeficiency virus (HIV) that causes the acquired immunodeficiency syndrome (AIDS). A 32–base pair deletion in this gene results in an allele (*ΔCCR5*) that encodes a nonfunctional protein due to a frameshift and premature termination. Individuals homozygous for the *ΔCCR5* allele do not express the receptor on their cell surface and, as a consequence, are resistant to HIV infection. Loss of function of *CCR5* appears to be a benign trait, and its only known phenotypic consequence is resistance to HIV infection. The normal allele and the 32–base pair deletion allele, *ΔCCR5*, are easily distinguished by PCR analysis of the gene. A sampling of 788 individuals from Europe provides absolute numbers of individuals who were homozygous for either allele or heterozygous (Table 9-6).

On the basis of the observed genotype frequencies, we can directly determine the allele frequencies by simply counting the alleles. In this context, when we refer to the population frequency of an allele, we are considering a hypothetical **gene pool** as a collection of all the alleles at a particular locus for the entire population. For autosomal loci, the size of the gene pool at one locus is twice the number of individuals in the population because each autosomal genotype consists of two alleles, that is, a *ΔCCR5/ΔCCR5* individual has two *ΔCCR5* alleles, and a *CCR5/ΔCCR5* individual has one of each. In this example, then, the observed frequency of the *CCR5* allele is:

$$\frac{(2 \times 647) + (1 \times 134)}{788 \times 2} = 0.906$$

Similarly, one can calculate the frequency of the *ΔCCR5* allele as 0.094, either by adding up the number of

Table 9-6

Genotype Frequencies for Normal *CCR5* Allele and the Deletion *ΔCCR5* Allele

Genotype	Number of People	Observed Relative Genotype Frequency	Allele	Derived Allele Frequencies
CCR5/CCR5	647	0.821		
CCR5/ΔCCR5	134	0.168	*CCR5*	0.906
ΔCCR5/ΔCCR5	7	0.011	*ΔCCR5*	0.094
Total	788	1.000		

Data from Martinson JJ, Chapman NH, Rees DC, et al: Global distribution of the *CCR5* gene 32-basepair deletion. Nat Genet 16:100-103, 1997.

ΔCCR5 alleles directly [(2 × 7) + (1 × 134) = 148 of a total of 1576 alleles] or simply by subtracting the frequency of the normal *CCR5* allele, 0.906, from 1, because the frequencies of the two alleles must add up to 1.

The Hardy-Weinberg Law

As we have shown with the *CCR5* cytokine receptor gene example, we can use a sample of individuals with known genotypes in a population to derive estimates of the allele frequencies by simply counting the alleles in individuals with each genotype. How about the converse? Can we calculate the proportion of the population with various genotypes once we know the allele frequencies? Deriving genotype frequencies from allele frequencies is not as straightforward as counting because we actually do not know in advance how the alleles are distributed among homozygotes and heterozygotes. If a population meets certain assumptions, however, there is a simple mathematical relationship known as the Hardy-Weinberg law for calculating genotype frequencies from allele frequencies. This law, the cornerstone of population genetics, was named for Godfrey Hardy, an English mathematician, and Wilhelm Weinberg, a German physician, who independently formulated it in 1908.

The Hardy-Weinberg law has two critical components. The first is that under certain ideal conditions (see Box), a simple relationship exists between allele frequencies and genotype frequencies in a population. Suppose p is the frequency of allele A and q is the frequency of allele a in the gene pool and alleles combine into genotypes randomly; that is, mating in the population is completely at random with respect to the genotypes at this locus. The chance that two A alleles will pair up to give the AA genotype is p^2; the chance that two a alleles will come together to give the aa genotype is q^2; and the chance of having one A and one a pair, resulting in the Aa genotype, is $2pq$ (the factor 2 comes from the fact that the A allele could be inherited from the mother and the a allele from the father, or vice versa). *The Hardy-Weinberg law states that the frequency of the three genotypes AA, Aa, and aa is given*

••• The Hardy-Weinberg Law

The Hardy-Weinberg law rests on these assumptions:

• The population is large and matings are random with respect to the locus in question.
• Allele frequencies remain constant over time because:
There is no appreciable rate of mutation.
Individuals with all genotypes are equally capable of mating and passing on their genes, that is, there is no selection against any particular genotype.
There has been no significant immigration of individuals from a population with allele frequencies very different from the endogenous population.

by the terms of the binomial expansion of $(p + q)^2 = p^2 + 2pq + q^2$.

A second component of the Hardy-Weinberg law is that if allele frequencies do not change from generation to generation, the relative proportion of the genotypes will not change either; that is, the *population genotype frequencies from generation to generation will remain constant, at equilibrium, if the allele frequencies p and q remain constant.* More specifically, when there is random mating in a population that is at equilibrium and genotypes AA, Aa, and aa are present in the proportions $p^2 : 2pq : q^2$, then genotype frequencies in the next generation will remain in the same relative proportions, $p^2 : 2pq : q^2$. Proof of this equilibrium is shown in Table 9-7. It is important to note that Hardy-Weinberg equilibrium does not specify any particular values for p and q; whatever allele frequencies happen to be present in the population will result in genotype frequencies of $p^2 : 2pq : q^2$, and these relative genotype frequencies will remain constant from generation to generation as long as the allele frequencies remain constant and other conditions are met.

Applying the Hardy-Weinberg formula to the *CCR5* example given earlier, with relative frequencies of the two alleles in the gene pool of 0.906 (for the normal allele *CCR5*) and 0.094 (for *ΔCCR5*), then the Hardy-Weinberg law states that the relative proportions of the

Table 9-7

Frequencies of Mating Types and Offspring for a Population in Hardy-Weinberg Equilibrium with Parental Genotypes in the Proportion $p^2 : 2pq : q^2$

Types of Matings			Offspring		
Mother	Father	Frequency	AA	Aa	aa
AA	AA	$p^2 \times p^2 = p^4$	(p^4)		
AA	Aa	$p^2 \times 2pq = 2p^3q$	$1/2(2p^3q)$	$1/2(2p^3q)$	
Aa	AA	$2pq \times p^2 = 2p^3q$	$1/2(2p^3q)$	$1/2(2p^3q)$	
AA	aa	$p^2 \times q^2 = p^2q^2$		(p^2q^2)	
aa	AA	$q^2 \times p^2 = p^2q^2$		(p^2q^2)	
Aa	Aa	$2pq \times 2pq = 4p^2q^2$	$1/4(4p^2q^2)$	$1/2(4p^2q^2)$	$1/4(4p^2q^2)$
Aa	aa	$2pq \times q^2 = 2pq^3$		$1/2(2pq^3)$	$1/2(2pq^3)$
aa	Aa	$q^2 \times 2pq = 2pq^3$		$1/2(2pq^3)$	$1/2(2pq^3)$
aa	aa	$q^2 \times q^2 = q^4$			(q^4)

Sum of AA offspring $= p^4 + p^3q + p^3q + p^2q^2 = p^2(p^2 + 2pq + q^2) = p^2(p + q)^2 = p^2$. (Remember that $p + q = 1$.)
Sum of Aa offspring $= p^3q + p^3q + p^2q^2 + p^2q^2 + 2\ p^2q^2 + pq^3 + pq^3 = 2pq(p^2 + 2pq + q^2) = 2pq(p + q)^2 = 2pq$.
Sum of aa offspring $= p^2q^2 + pq^3 + pq^3 + q^4 = q^2(p^2 + 2pq + q^2) = q^2(p + q)^2 = q^2$.

three combinations of alleles (genotypes) are $p^2 = 0.906 \times 0.906 = 0.821$ (for drawing two CCR5 alleles from the pool), $q^2 = 0.094 \times 0.094 = 0.009$ (for two $\Delta CCR5$ alleles), and $2pq = (0.906 \times 0.094) + (0.094 \times 0.906) = 0.170$ (for one CCR5 and one $\Delta CCR5$ allele). When these genotype frequencies, which were *calculated* by the Hardy-Weinberg law, are applied to a population of 788 individuals, the derived numbers of people with the three different genotypes $(647 : 134 : 7)$ are, in fact, identical to the actual *observed* numbers in Table 9-6. As long as the assumptions of the Hardy-Weinberg law are met in a population, we would expect these genotype frequencies $(0.821 : 0.170 : 0.009)$ to remain constant generation after generation in that population.

As we have seen, Hardy-Weinberg distributions of genotypes in populations are simply a binomial distribution $(p + q)^n$, where symbols p and q represent the frequencies of two alternative alleles at a locus (where $p + q = 1$), and $n = 2$, representing the pair of alleles at any autosomal locus or any X-linked locus in females. (Because males are unique in having only a single X chromosome, frequencies of X-linked genes in males are considered separately later.) If a locus has three alleles, with frequencies p, q, and r, the genotypic distribution can be determined from $(p + q + r)^2$. In general terms, the genotypic frequencies for any known number of alleles a_n with allele frequencies $p_1, p_2, \ldots p_n$ can be derived from the terms of the expansion of $(p_1 + p_2 + \ldots p_n)^2$.

The Hardy-Weinberg Law in Autosomal Recessive Disease

The major practical application of the Hardy-Weinberg law in medical genetics is in genetic counseling for autosomal recessive disorders. For a disease such as **phenylketonuria** (PKU; see Chapter 12), the frequency

of affected homozygotes in the population can be determined accurately because the disease is identified through newborn screening programs. Heterozygotes, however, are asymptomatic silent carriers, and their population incidence is impossible to measure directly from phenotype. The Hardy-Weinberg law allows an estimate of heterozygote frequency to be made and used subsequently for counseling. For example, the frequency of PKU is approximately 1/4500 in Ireland. Affected individuals are usually compound heterozygotes for different mutant alleles rather than homozygotes for the same mutant allele. In practice, however, we usually lump all disease-causing alleles together and treat them as a single allele, with frequency q, even when there is significant allelic heterogeneity in disease-causing alleles. Then the frequency of affected individuals $= 1/4500 = q^2$, $q = 0.015$, and $2pq = 0.029$ or approximately 3%. The carrier frequency in the Irish population is therefore 3%, and there would be an approximately 3% chance that a parent known to be a carrier of PKU through the birth of an affected child would find that a new mate of Irish ethnicity would also be a carrier. If the new mate were from Finland, however, where the frequency of PKU is much lower (~1/200,000), his or her chance of being a carrier would be only 0.6%.

The Hardy-Weinberg Law in X-Linked Disease

Recall that for X-linked genes, there are only two possible male genotypes but three female genotypes. To illustrate gene frequencies and genotype frequencies when the gene of interest is X-linked, we use the trait known as **red-green color blindness**, which is caused by mutations in the series of red and green visual pigment genes on the X chromosome. We use color blindness as

Table 9-8

X-Linked Genes and Genotype Frequencies (Color Blindness)

Sex	Genotype	Phenotype	Incidence (Approximate)
Male	X^+	Normal color vision	$p = 0.92$
	X^{cb}	Color blind	$q = 0.08$
Female	X^+/X^+	Normal (homozygote)	$p^2 = (0.92)^2 = 0.8464$
	X^+/X^{cb}	Normal (heterozygote)	$2pq = 2(0.92)(0.08) = 0.1472$
		Normal (total)	$p^2 + 2pq = 0.9936$
	X^{cb}/X^{cb}	Color blind	$q^2 = (0.08)^2 = 0.0064$

an example because, as far as we know, it is not a deleterious trait (except for possible difficulties with traffic lights), and color-blind persons are not subject to selection. As discussed later, allowing for the effect of selection complicates estimates of gene frequencies.

We use the symbol *cb* for all the mutant color-blindness alleles and the symbol + for the normal allele, with frequencies *q* and *p,* respectively (Table 9-8). The frequencies of the normal and mutant alleles can be determined directly from the incidence of the corresponding phenotypes in *males* by simply counting the alleles. Because females have two X chromosomes, their genotypes are distributed like autosomal genotypes, but because color-blindness alleles are recessive, the normal homozygotes and heterozygotes are not distinguishable. As shown in Table 9-8, the frequency of color blindness in females is much lower than that in males, even though the allele frequencies are, of course, the same in both sexes. Less than 1% of females are color-blind, but nearly 15% are carriers of a mutant color-blindness allele and have a 50% chance of having a color-blind son with each male pregnancy.

⦿ FACTORS THAT DISTURB HARDY-WEINBERG EQUILIBRIUM

A number of assumptions underlie the Hardy-Weinberg law. First is that the population is large and mating is random. A very small population in which random events can radically alter an allele frequency may not meet this first assumption. This first assumption is also breached when the population contains subgroups whose members choose to marry within their own subgroup rather than the population at large. Second is that allele frequencies are not changing over time. This means that there is no migration in or out of the population by groups whose allele frequencies at a locus of interest are radically different from the allele frequencies in the population as a whole. Similarly, selection for or against particular alleles and new mutations adding alleles to the gene pool break the assumptions of the Hardy-Weinberg law. In practice, some of these violations are more damaging than others to the appli-

cation of the law to human populations. As shown in the sections that follow, violating the assumption of random mating can cause large deviations from the frequency of individuals homozygous for an autosomal recessive condition that we might expect from population allele frequencies. On the other hand, changes in allele frequency due to mutation, selection, or migration usually cause more minor and subtle deviations from Hardy-Weinberg equilibrium. Finally, when Hardy-Weinberg equilibrium does not hold for a particular disease allele at a particular locus, it may be instructive to investigate *why* the allele and its associated genotypes are not in equilibrium.

Exception to Large Population with Random Mating

The principle of random mating is that for any locus, an individual of a given genotype has a purely random probability of mating with an individual of any other genotype, the proportions being determined only by the relative frequencies of the different genotypes in the population. One's choice of mate, however, may not be at random. In human populations, nonrandom mating may occur because of three distinct but related phenomena: **stratification, assortative mating,** and **consanguinity.**

Stratification

Stratification describes a population in which there are a number of subgroups that have remained relatively genetically separate during modern times. Worldwide, there are numerous stratified populations; for example, the U.S. population is stratified into many subgroups including whites, African Americans, and numerous Native American, Asian, and Hispanic groups. Similarly stratified populations exist in other parts of the world as well. When mate selection in a population is restricted to members of one particular subgroup within that population, the result for any locus with more than one allele is an excess of homozygotes in the population as a whole and a corresponding deficiency of heterozygotes compared with what one would predict under random mating from allele frequencies in the population as a whole.

Suppose a population contains a minority group constituting 10% of the population in which a mutant allele for an autosomal recessive disease has a frequency $q_{min} = 0.05$. In the remaining majority 90% of the population, q_{maj} is 0. An example of just such a situation is the African American population of the United States and the mutant allele at the β-globin locus responsible for **sickle cell disease**. The overall frequency of the disease allele in the total population, q_{pop}, is therefore equal to 0.05/10 = 0.005, and, simply applying the Hardy-Weinberg law, the frequency of the disease in the population as a whole would be $q^2_{pop} = 0.000025$ if mating were perfectly random throughout the entire population. If, however, a minority group mates nearly exclusively with other members of the minority group, then the frequency of affected individuals in the minority group would be $(q^2_{min}) = 0.0025$. Because the minority group is one tenth of the entire population, the true frequency of disease in the total population is 0.0025/10 = 0.00025, 10-fold higher than one would expect from applying the Hardy-Weinberg law to the population as a whole without consideration of stratification. By way of comparison, stratification has no effect on the frequency of autosomal dominant disease and would have only a minor effect on the frequency of X-linked disease by increasing the small number of females homozygous for the mutant allele.

Assortative Mating

Assortative mating is the choice of a mate because the mate possesses some particular trait. Assortative mating is usually positive; that is, people tend to choose mates who resemble themselves (e.g., in native language, intelligence, stature, skin color, musical talent, or athletic ability). To the extent that the characteristic shared by the partners is genetically determined, the overall genetic effect of positive assortative mating is an increase in the proportion of the homozygous genotypes at the expense of the heterozygous genotype.

A clinically important aspect of assortative mating is the tendency to choose partners with similar medical problems, such as congenital deafness or blindness or exceptionally short stature (dwarfism). In such a case, the expectations of Hardy-Weinberg equilibrium do not apply because the genotype of the mate at the disease locus is not determined by the allele frequencies found in the general population. For example, in the case of two parents with **achondroplasia** (Case 1), an autosomal dominant disorder, offspring homozygous for the achondroplasia gene have a severe, lethal form of dwarfism that is almost never seen unless both parents are achondroplasia heterozygotes.

When mates have autosomal recessive disorders caused by the same mutation or by allelic mutations in the same gene, all of their offspring will also have the disease. Of course, not all blindness, deafness, or short stature has the same genetic basis; many families have been described, for example, in which two parents with albinism have had children with normal pigmentation or two deaf parents have had hearing children because of locus heterogeneity (discussed in Chapter 7). Even if there is genetic heterogeneity with assortative mating, however, the chance that two individuals are carrying mutations in the same disease locus is increased over what it would be under true random mating, and therefore the risk of the disorder in their offspring is also increased. Although the long-term population effect of this kind of positive assortative mating on disease gene frequencies is insignificant, a specific family may find itself at very high genetic risk.

Consanguinity and Inbreeding

Consanguinity, like stratification and positive assortative mating, brings about an increase in the frequency of autosomal recessive disease by increasing the frequency with which carriers of an autosomal recessive disorder mate (see Chapter 7). Unlike the disorders in stratified populations, in which each subgroup is likely to have a high frequency of a few alleles, the kinds of recessive disorders seen in the offspring of related parents may be very rare and unusual because consanguineous mating allows uncommon alleles to become homozygous. Similarly, in genetic **isolates**, the chance of mating with another carrier of a particular recessive condition may be as high as that observed in cousin marriages, a phenomenon known as **inbreeding** (see Chapter 7).

For example, among Ashkenazi Jews in North America, mutant alleles for **Tay-Sachs disease** (GM_2 gangliosidosis) (see Chapter 12) (Case 38) are relatively more common than in other ethnic groups. The frequency of Tay-Sachs disease is 100 times higher in Ashkenazi Jews (1 in 3600) than in most other populations (1 in 360,000). Thus, the Tay-Sachs carrier frequency among Ashkenazi Jews is approximately one in 30 ($q^2 = 1/3600$, $q = 1/60$, $2pq = \sim1/30$) as compared to a carrier frequency of about one in 300 in non-Ashkenazis.

Exceptions to Constant Allele Frequencies

Genetic Drift in Small Populations

Chance events can have a much greater effect on allele frequencies in a small population than in a large one. If the population is small, random effects, such as increased fertility or survival of the carriers of a mutation, *occurring for reasons unrelated to carrying the mutant allele* (which would be selection, not a random event), may cause the allele frequency to change from one generation to the next. In a large population, such random effects would average out, but in a small population, allele frequencies can fluctuate from generation to generation by chance. This phenomenon, known as **genetic drift,** can explain how allele frequencies can change as a result of chance operating on the small gene pool contained within a small population.

Mutation and Selection

In contrast to nonrandom mating, which can substantially upset the relative frequency of various genotypes predicted by Hardy-Weinberg equilibrium, changes in allele frequency due to selection or mutation usually occur slowly, in small increments, and cause much less deviation from Hardy-Weinberg equilibrium, at least for recessive diseases. Mutation rates are generally well below the frequency of heterozygotes for autosomal recessive diseases, and so new mutation would have little effect in the short term on allele frequencies for such diseases. In addition, most deleterious recessive alleles are hidden in heterozygotes and not subject to selection. As a consequence, selection is not likely to have major short-term effects on the allele frequency of these recessive alleles. Therefore, to a first approximation, Hardy-Weinberg equilibrium may apply even for alleles that cause severe autosomal recessive disease. For dominant or X-linked disease, however, mutation and selection do perturb allele frequencies from what would be expected under Hardy-Weinberg equilibrium by substantially reducing or increasing certain genotypes.

The molecular basis for mutation was considered earlier in this chapter. Here we examine the concept of **fitness,** the chief factor that determines whether a mutation is lost immediately, becomes stable in the population, or even becomes, over time, the predominant allele at the locus concerned. The frequency of an allele in a population represents a balance between the rate at which mutant alleles appear through mutation and the effects of selection. If either the mutation rate or the effectiveness of selection is altered, the allele frequency is expected to change.

Whether an allele is transmitted to the succeeding generation depends on its fitness *(f),* which is a measure of the number of offspring of affected persons who survive to reproductive age, compared with an appropriate control group. If a mutant allele is just as likely as the normal allele to be represented in the next generation, *f* equals 1. If an allele causes death or sterility, selection acts against it completely, and *f* equals 0. A related parameter is the **coefficient of selection,** *s,* which is a measure of the *loss* of fitness and is defined as $1 - f$, that is, the proportion of mutant alleles that are not passed on and are therefore lost as a result of selection. In the genetic sense, a mutation that prevents reproduction by an adult is just as lethal as one that causes a

very early miscarriage of an embryo, because in neither case is the mutation transmitted to the next generation. Fitness is thus the outcome of the joint effects of survival and fertility. In the biological sense, fitness has no connotation of superior endowment except in a single respect: comparative ability to contribute to the gene pool of the next generation.

Selection in Recessive Disease Selection against harmful recessive mutations has far less effect on the population frequency of the mutant allele than does selection against dominant mutations because only a small proportion of the genes are present in homozygotes and are therefore exposed to selective forces. Even if there were complete selection against homozygotes $(f = 0)$, as in many lethal autosomal recessive conditions, it would take many generations to reduce the gene frequency appreciably because most of the mutant alleles are carried by heterozygotes with normal fitness. For example, the frequency of mutant alleles causing **phenylketonuria** (PKU; see Chapter 12), *q,* is approximately 1% in many white populations. Two percent of the population $(2 \times p \times q)$ is heterozygous, with one mutant allele, whereas only 1 individual in 10,000 (q^2) is a homozygote with two mutant alleles. The proportion of mutant alleles in homozygotes is given by:

$$\frac{2 \times 0.0001}{(2 \times 0.0001) + (1 \times 0.02)} = \sim 0.01$$

Thus, only approximately 1% of all the mutant alleles in the population are in affected homozygotes and therefore are exposed to selection if dietary treatment were not available. Removal of selection against an autosomal recessive disorder such as PKU by successful medical treatment would have just as slow an effect on increasing the gene frequency over many generations. *Thus, as long as mating is random, genotypes in autosomal recessive diseases can be considered to be in Hardy-Weinberg equilibrium, despite selection against homozygotes for the recessive allele.* The mathematical relationship between genotype and allele frequencies described in the Hardy-Weinberg law holds for most practical purposes in recessive disease.

Selection in Dominant Disorders Dominant mutant alleles are directly exposed to selection, in contrast to recessive mutant alleles, most of which are "hidden" in heterozygotes. Consequently, the effects of selection and mutation are more obvious and can be more readily measured for dominant traits. A genetic lethal dominant allele, if fully penetrant, is exposed to selection in heterozygotes, removing all alleles responsible for the disorder in a single generation. Several human diseases are thought or known to be autosomal dominant traits with zero or near-zero fitness and thus always result

Table 9-9

Examples of Disorders Occurring as Sporadic Conditions due to New Mutations with Zero Fitness

Acrodysostosis	Multiple congenital abnormalities, especially short hands with peripheral dysostosis, small nose, and mental deficiency
Apert syndrome	Craniosynostosis, broad thumb and great toe, shallow orbits, hypertelorism, frequent but variable mental deficiency; mutation in fibroblast growth factor receptor 2 gene. Very rarely, a person with this dysmorphic syndrome has offspring; if so, 50% of the offspring are affected.
Atelosteogenesis	Early lethal form of short-limbed dwarfism
Cornelia de Lange syndrome	Mental retardation, micromelia, synophrys, and other abnormalities; can be caused by mutation in the NIPBL gene
Lenz-Majewski hyperostosis syndrome	Dense, thick bone; symphalangism; cutis laxa
Osteogenesis imperfecta, type 2	Perinatal lethal type, with a defect in type 1 collagen (see Chapter 12)
Thanatophoric dysplasia	Early lethal form of short-limbed dwarfism due to mutations in fibroblast growth factor receptor 3 gene

from new rather than inherited autosomal dominant mutations (Table 9-9). In some, the genes and specific mutant alleles are known, and family studies show new mutations in the affected individuals that were not inherited from the parents. In other conditions, the genes are not known, but a paternal age effect (discussed earlier in this chapter) has been seen, suggesting (but not proving) a new mutation in the paternal germline as a possible cause of the disorder. The implication for genetic counseling is that the parents of a child with an autosomal dominant, genetic lethal condition have a low risk of recurrence because the condition would generally require another independent mutation to recur (except that the possibility of germline mosaicism must be kept in mind; see Chapter 7).

Mutation and Selection Balance in Dominant Disease   If a dominant disease is deleterious but not lethal, affected persons may reproduce but will nevertheless contribute fewer than the average number of offspring to the next generation; that is, their fitness, f, may be reduced. Such a mutation is lost through selection at a rate proportional to the loss of fitness of heterozygotes. The frequency of the mutant alleles responsible for the disease in the population therefore represents a balance between loss of mutant alleles through the effects of selection and gain of mutant alleles through recurrent mutation. A stable allele frequency is reached at whatever level balances the two opposing forces: one (selec-

tion) that removes mutant alleles from the gene pool and one (new mutation) that adds new ones back. The mutation rate per generation, μ, at a disease locus must be sufficient to account for that fraction of all the mutant alleles (allele frequency q) that are lost by selection from each generation. Thus,

$$\mu = sq$$

When a genetic disorder limits reproduction so severely that the fitness is zero ($s = 1$), it is referred to as a **genetic lethal**. For a dominant genetic lethal disorder, every allele in the population must be a new mutation since none can be inherited (in the absence of gonadal mosaicism). In achondroplasia, the fitness of affected patients is not zero, but they have only about one fifth as many children as people of normal stature in the population. Thus, their average fitness, f, is 0.20, and the coefficient of selection, s, is 0.80. In the subsequent generation, only 20% of current achondroplasia alleles are passed on from the current generation to the next. Because the frequency of achondroplasia is not decreasing, new mutations must be responsible for replacing the 80% of mutant genes in the population lost through selection.

If the fitness of affected persons suddenly improved (because of medical advances, for example), the observed incidence of the disease in the population would increase and reach a new equilibrium. Retinoblastoma and certain other dominant embryonic tumors with childhood onset are examples of conditions that now have a greatly improved prognosis, with a predicted consequence of increased disease frequency in the population. Allele frequency, mutation rate, and fitness are related; thus, if any two of these three characteristics are known, the third can be estimated.

Mutation and Selection Balance in X-Linked Recessive Mutations   For those X-linked phenotypes of medical interest that are recessive, or nearly so, selection occurs in hemizygous males and not in heterozygous females, except for the small proportion of females who are manifesting heterozygotes with low fitness. In this brief discussion, however, we assume that heterozygous females have normal fitness.

Because males have one X chromosome and females two, the pool of X-linked alleles in the entire population's gene pool will be partitioned, with one third of mutant alleles present in males and two thirds in females. As we saw in the case of autosomal dominant mutations, mutant alleles lost through selection must be replaced by recurrent new mutations to maintain the observed disease incidence. If the incidence of a serious X-linked disease is not changing and selection is operating against, and only against, hemizygous males, the mutation rate, μ, must equal the coefficient of selection, s (the proportion of mutant alleles that are not passed on), times q, the allele frequency, times 1/3 since selection is operating on only one third of the mutant alleles in the population, that is, those present in males. Thus,

$$\mu = sq/3$$

For an X-linked genetic lethal disease, $s = 1$ and one third of all copies of the mutant gene responsible is lost from each generation. Therefore, one third of all persons who have such X-linked lethal disorders are predicted to carry a new mutation, and their genetically normal mothers have a low risk of having subsequent children with the same disorder (assuming no mosaicism). In less severe disorders such as hemophilia A, the proportion of affected individuals representing new mutations is less than one third (currently about 15%). Because the treatment of hemophilia is improving rapidly, the total frequency of mutant alleles can be expected to rise relatively rapidly and to reach a new equilibrium, as we saw in the case of autosomal dominant conditions. Assuming that the mutation rate at this locus stays the same, the *proportion* of hemophiliacs who result from a new mutation will decrease, even though the incidence of the disease increases. Such a change would have significant implications for genetic counseling for this disorder (see Chapter 19).

Migration and Gene Flow

Migration can change allele frequency by the process of **gene flow**, defined as the slow diffusion of genes across a barrier. Gene flow usually involves a large population and a gradual change in gene frequencies. The genes of migrant populations with their own characteristic allele frequencies are gradually merged into the gene pool of the population into which they have migrated. (The term *migrant* is used here in the broad sense of crossing a reproductive barrier, which may be racial, ethnic, or cultural and not necessarily geographical and requiring physical movement from one region to another.)

The frequencies of the 32–base pair deletion allele of the *CCR5* cytokine receptor gene, *ΔCCR5*, have been studied in many populations all over the world. The frequency of the *ΔCCR5* allele is highest, approximately 10%, in western Europe and Russia and declines to a few percent in the Middle East and the Indian subcontinent. The *ΔCCR5* allele is virtually absent from Africa and the Far East, suggesting that the mutation originated in whites and diffused into the more easterly populations (Fig. 9-10).

Another example of gene flow between population groups is reflected in the frequency of specific mutant alleles causing PKU. There is strong evidence that the most common mutations were of Celtic origin. These same mutations have now turned up in many populations around the world. The presence of the same PKU alleles in different populations reflects the geographical migration of the Celts. Thus, the frequency of PKU is approximately 1/4500 in Ireland, but the disorder is progressively less prevalent across northern and southern Europe. There has been considerably less gene flow to East Asia; the incidence of PKU in Japan is only about 1/109,000.

ETHNIC DIFFERENCES IN THE FREQUENCY OF VARIOUS GENETIC DISEASES

The previous discussion of the Hardy-Weinberg law explained how, at equilibrium, genotype frequencies are determined by allele frequencies and remain stable from generation to generation, assuming the allele frequencies in a large, isolated, randomly mating population remain constant. However, there is a problem of interest to human geneticists that the Hardy-Weinberg law does not address: Why are allele frequencies different in different populations in the first place? In particular, why are some mutant alleles that are clearly deleterious when present in homozygotes relatively common in certain population groups and not in others? We address these issues in the rest of this chapter.

The human species of more than 6 billion members is separated into many subpopulations, or ethnic groups, distinguishable by appearance, geographical origin, and history. Although the 25,000 genes and their location and order on the chromosomes are nearly identical in all humans, we saw earlier that extensive polymorphism exists between individuals in a population. Most variation is found in all human populations, at similar frequencies. Other alleles, however, although present in all groups, may demonstrate dramatic differences in frequency among population groups; and finally, some allelic variants are restricted to certain populations, although they are not necessarily present in all members of that group. It is likely that because modern humans lived in small isolated settlements until quite recently, as mutations occurred in the various groups, the differences in the frequency of certain alleles persisted and could even become magnified. A number of factors are thought to allow differences in alleles and allele frequencies among ethnic groups to develop. Two such factors are **genetic drift** (discussed earlier), including nonrandom distribution of alleles among the individuals who founded particular subpopulations (**founder effect**), and **heterozygote advantage** under environmental conditions that favor the reproductive fitness of carriers of deleterious mutations. Both are discussed in the next section.

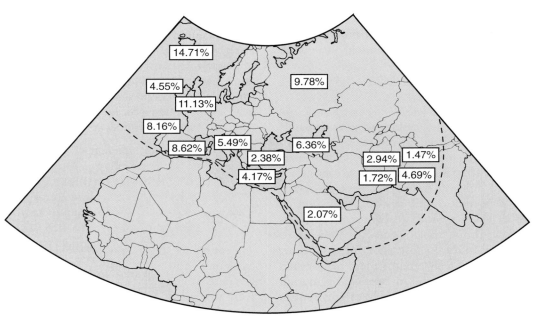

Figure 9-10 ■ Frequency of Δ*CCR5* alleles in populations from Europe, the Middle East, and the Indian subcontinent. (From Martinson JJ, Chapman NH, Rees DC, et al: Global distribution of the *CCR5* gene 32-basepair deletion. Nat Genet 16:100-103, 1997.)

For the population geneticist and anthropologist, selectively neutral genetic markers provide a means of tracing human history by tracking gene flows. For example, some polymorphisms exist only in populations in sub-Saharan Africa, resulting in more polymorphic diversity among sub-Saharan Africans themselves than there is between sub-Saharan Africans and any other ethnic groups. These data support the notion that modern humans in Africa developed substantial genetic diversity over a million years or more, well before the rest of the world's populations were derived 40,000 to 100,000 years ago from smaller subgroups that migrated out of Africa, carrying a more limited genetic diversity.

Differences in frequencies of alleles that cause genetic disease are significant for the medical geneticist and genetic counselor because they cause different disease risks in specific population groups. Well-known examples include Tay-Sachs disease in people of Ashkenazi Jewish ancestry, sickle cell disease in African Americans, and cystic fibrosis and PKU in white populations (Table 9-10).

The inherited disease of hemoglobin, β-thalassemia, is a clear example of ethnic differences both in disease frequency and in which alleles are responsible in populations with a high incidence of disease (see Chapter 11) (Case 39). The disease is common in people of Mediterranean or East Asian descent and very rare in other ethnic groups. Even though dozens of different alleles can cause β-thalassemia, certain alleles tend to be far more common in some populations than in others, so that each population has only a few common alleles. For example, the most common β-thalassemia alleles responsible for more than 90% of the disease in Mediterranean people are very rare in people from Southeast Asia or the Asian subcontinent; similarly, the most common alleles in Southeast Asians and Asian Indians are quite rare in the other two unrelated ethnic groups. This information is of value in genetic counseling and prenatal diagnosis. For example, in North America, when persons of Mediterranean descent are at risk of having a child with β-thalassemia, testing of parental DNA for just seven mutant alleles has a more than 90% probability of providing the information needed for prenatal diagnosis.

Genetic Drift

Genetic drift can explain a high frequency of a deleterious disease allele in a population. For example, when a new mutation occurs in a small population, its frequency is represented by only one copy among all the copies of that gene in the population. Random effects of environment or other chance occurrences that are independent of the genotype and operating in a small population can produce significant changes in the frequency of the disease allele. During the next few generations, although the population size of the new group remains small, there may be considerable fluctuation in gene frequency. These changes are likely to smooth out as the population increases in size. In contrast to gene

Table 9-10

Incidence, Gene Frequency, and Heterozygote Frequency for Selected Autosomal Disorders in Different Populations

Disorder	Population	Incidence	Allele Frequency	Heterozygote Frequency
RECESSIVE		q^2	q	$2pq$
Sickle cell anemia (*S/S* genotype)*	U.S. African American	1 in 400	0.05	1 in 11
	Hispanic American	1 in 40,000	0.005	1 in 101
α_1-Antitrypsin deficiency (*Z/Z* genotype)[†]	Denmark	1 in 2000	0.022	1 in 22
	U.S. African American	1 in 100,000	0.04	1 in 125
Cystic fibrosis (all mutant alleles)[†]	U.S. white	1 in 2000	0.022	1 in 22
	Finland	1 in 25,000	0.0063	1 in 80
	Mexico	1 in 8500	0.011	1 in 47
Phenylketonuria (all mutant alleles)[†]	Scotland	1 in 5300	0.014	1 in 37
	Finland	1 in 200,000	0.002	1 in 250
	Japan	1 in 109,000	0.003	1 in 166
Tay-Sachs disease[†]	U.S. Ashkenazi Jewish	1 in 3900	0.016	1 in 32
	U.S. non-Ashkenazi Jewish	1 in 112,000	0.003	1 in 170
DOMINANT		$2pq + q^2$	q	
Familial hypercholesterolemia[†]	Regions of Quebec, Canada	1 in 122	0.004	—
	Afrikaner, South Africa	1 in 70	0.007	—
Myotonic dystrophy[†]	Europe	1 in 25,000	0.00002	—
	Regions of Quebec, Canada	1 in 475	0.0011	—

*See Chapter 11.
[†]See Chapter 12.

flow, in which allele frequencies change because of admixture, the mechanism of genetic drift is chance.

Founder Effect

When a small subpopulation breaks off from a larger population, the gene frequencies in the small population may be different from those of the population from which it originated because the new group contains a small, random sample of the parent group and, by chance, may not have the same gene frequencies as the parent group. This form of genetic drift is known as the founder effect. If one of the original founders of a new group just happens to carry a relatively rare allele, that allele will have a far higher frequency than it had in the larger group from which the new group was derived. One example is the high incidence of Huntington disease in the region of Lake Maracaibo, Venezuela (see Chapter 12), but there are numerous other examples of founder effect involving other disease alleles in genetic isolates throughout the world.

The founder effect is well illustrated by the Old Order Amish, a religious isolate of European descent that settled in Pennsylvania and gave rise to a number of small, genetically isolated subpopulations throughout the United States and Canada. The Old Order

Amish tend to have large families and a high frequency of consanguineous marriage. The incidence of specific rare autosomal recessive syndromes such as the **Ellis–van Creveld syndrome** of short-limbed dwarfism, polydactyly, abnormal nails and teeth, and high incidence of congenital heart defects (Fig. 9-11) in some Amish communities, but not in others, is an illustration of the founder effect.

The French-Canadian population of Canada also has high frequencies of certain disorders that are rare elsewhere. One disease characteristic of the relatively isolated Lac Saint Jean region of Quebec is hereditary **type I tyrosinemia;** this autosomal recessive condition causes hepatic failure and renal tubular dysfunction due to deficiency of fumarylacetoacetase, an enzyme in the degradative pathway of tyrosine. The disease has an overall frequency of about 1/100,000 in other parts of Quebec and in Norway and Sweden, but its frequency is 1/685 in the Saguenay–Lac Saint Jean region. As expected with a founder effect, 100% of the mutant alleles in the Saguenay–Lac Saint Jean patients are due to the same mutation, a splice donor site mutation in intron 12.

The population of Finland, long isolated genetically by geography, language, and culture, has expanded in the past 300 years from 400,000 to about 5 million.

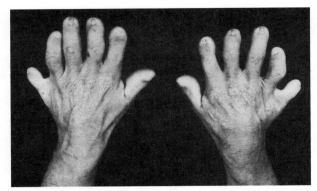

Figure 9-11 ■ The hands of a patient with Ellis–van Creveld syndrome, a very rare disorder seen with increased frequency in some Amish groups. (Courtesy of David Rimoin, Cedars-Sinai Medical Center, Los Angeles, California.)

The isolation and population expansion have allowed the Finnish population to develop a distinctive pattern of single-gene disorders. There is a high frequency of at least 20 diseases that are rare elsewhere. For example, **choroideremia**, an X-linked degenerative eye disease, is very rare worldwide; only about 400 cases have been described. Fully one third of the total number of patients, however, are from a small region in Finland, populated by a large extended family descended from a founding couple born in the 1640s (Fig. 9-12). Another Finnish genetic disease is hyperornithinemia with **gyrate atrophy** of the choroid and retina, an autosomal recessive condition caused by deficiency of ornithine aminotransferase and leading to loss of vision in young adulthood (see Fig. 9-12). As one might expect with a founder effect, one mutation was found in homozygous form in the majority of apparently unrelated cases of gyrate atrophy in Finland, but it was not observed at all in non-Finnish cases. Conversely, disorders that are common in other European populations, such as PKU, are quite rare in Finland.

Thus, one of the outcomes of the founder effect and genetic drift is that each population may be characterized by its own particular mutant alleles as well as by an increase or decrease in specific diseases. As these examples show, genetic drift and founder effect can favor the establishment at high incidence of alleles that are not favorable or even neutral but are actually harmful. The relative mobility of most present-day populations, in comparison with their ancestors of only a few generations ago, may reduce the effect of genetic drift in the future while increasing the effect of gene flow.

Positive Selection for Heterozygotes (Heterozygote Advantage)

Although certain mutant alleles may be deleterious in homozygotes, there may be environmental conditions in which heterozygotes for some diseases have increased fitness not only over homozygotes for the mutant allele

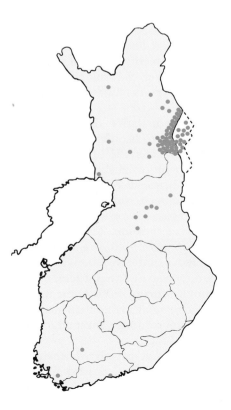

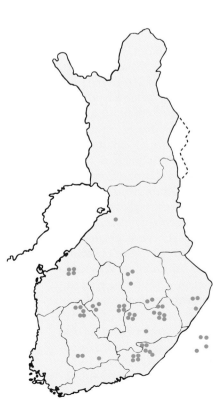

Figure 9-12 ■ The geographical origin of cases of two genetic disorders prevalent in Finland: X-linked choroideremia *(left)* and hyperornithinemia with gyrate atrophy of the choroid and retina *(right)*. Most cases of each disease originate from particular communities in Finland, but the distributions of the diseases differ. (Based on Mitchell GA, Brody LC, Sipila I, et al: At least two mutant alleles of ornithine-δ-aminotransferase cause gyrate atrophy of the choroid and retina in Finns. Proc Natl Acad Sci USA 86:197-201, 1989; and Nario R, Nevanlinna HR, Perheentupa J: Hereditary diseases in Finland: rare flora in rare soil. Ann Clin Res 5:109-141, 1973.)

but also over homozygotes for the normal allele, a situation termed **heterozygote advantage**. Even a slight heterozygote advantage can lead to an increase in frequency of an allele that is severely detrimental in homozygotes, because heterozygotes greatly outnumber homozygotes in the population. A situation in which selective forces operate both to maintain a deleterious allele and to remove it from the gene pool is described as a **balanced polymorphism**.

Malaria and Hemoglobinopathies A well-known example of heterozygote advantage is resistance to malaria in heterozygotes for the sickle cell disease mutation (Case 37) (see Chapter 11). The sickle cell allele has reached its highest frequency in certain regions of West Africa, where heterozygotes are more fit than either type of homozygote because heterozygotes are relatively more resistant to the malarial organism. In regions where malaria is endemic, normal homozygotes are susceptible to malaria; many become infected and are severely, even fatally, affected, leading to reduced fitness. Sickle cell homozygotes are even more seriously disadvantaged, with a fitness approaching zero, because of their severe hematological disease (see Chapter 11). Heterozygotes for sickle cell disease have red cells that are inhospitable to the malaria organism but do not undergo sickling under normal environmental conditions; the heterozygotes are relatively more fit than either homozygote and reproduce at a higher rate. Thus, over time, the sickle cell mutant allele has reached a frequency as high as 0.15 in some areas of West Africa that are endemic for malaria, far higher than could be accounted for by recurrent mutation.

The heterozygote advantage in sickle cell disease demonstrates how violating one of the fundamental assumptions of Hardy-Weinberg equilibrium—that allele frequencies are not significantly altered by selection—causes the mathematical relationship between allele and genotype frequencies to diverge from what is expected under the Hardy-Weinberg law. Consider two alleles, the normal A allele and the mutant S allele, which give rise to three genotypes: A/A (normal), A/S (heterozygous carriers), and S/S (sickle cell disease). In a sample of 12,387 individuals from an adult West African population, the three genotypes were detected in the following proportions: 9365 A/A : 2993 A/S : 29 S/S. By counting the A and S alleles in these three genotypes, one can determine the allele frequencies to be $p = 0.877$ for the A allele and $q = 0.123$ for the S allele. Under Hardy-Weinberg equilibrium, the ratio of genotypes should be $A/A : A/S : S/S = p^2 : 2pq : q^2 = 9527 : 2672 : 188$. The observed ratios, however, $A/A : A/S : S/S = 9365 : 2993 : 29$, differ significantly from expectations. The example of the sickle cell allele illustrates how the forces of selection, operating not only on the relatively rare S/S genotype but also on the other two, much more frequent A/A

and A/S genotypes, distort the transmission of the A and S alleles and cause a deviation from Hardy-Weinberg equilibrium in a population.

Change in the selective pressures would be expected to lead to a rapid change in the relative frequency of the sickle cell allele. Today, many sickle cell heterozygotes live in non-malarial regions, and even in malarial areas, major efforts are being made to eradicate the mosquito responsible for transmitting the disease. There is evidence that in the African American population in the United States, the frequency of the sickle cell gene may already be falling from its high level in the original African population of several generations ago, although other factors, such as the introduction of alleles from non-African populations into the African American gene pool, may also be playing a role.

Some other deleterious alleles, including genes for hemoglobin C, the thalassemias, and glucose-6-phosphate dehydrogenase deficiency (see Chapter 18), as well as the benign FY allele of the Duffy blood group system, are also thought to be maintained at their present high frequencies in certain populations because of the protection that they provide against malaria. Heterozygote advantage has also been proposed to explain the high frequencies of cystic fibrosis in white populations and of Tay-Sachs disease and other disorders affecting sphingolipid metabolism in the Ashkenazi Jewish population.

Drift Versus Heterozygote Advantage Determining whether drift or heterozygote advantage is responsible for the increased frequency of some deleterious alleles in certain populations is not simple to do. The environmental selective pressure responsible for heterozygote advantage may have been operating in the past and not be identifiable in modern times. The northwest to southeast gradient in the frequency of the $\Delta CCR5$ allele, for example, reflects major differences in the frequency of this allele in different ethnic groups. For example, the highest frequency of the $\Delta CCR5$ allele is 21%, seen among Ashkenazi Jews, and it is nearly that high in Iceland and the British Isles. The current AIDS pandemic is too recent to have affected gene frequencies through selection; the variation in allele frequencies in Europe itself is most consistent with genetic drift acting on a neutral polymorphism. It is, however, possible that another selective factor (perhaps another infectious disease such as bubonic plague) may have elevated the frequency of the $\Delta CCR5$ allele in northern European populations during a period of intense selection. Thus, geneticists continue to debate whether genetic drift or heterozygote advantage (or both) adequately accounts for the unusually high frequencies that some deleterious alleles achieve in some populations.

Population genetics uses quantitative methods to explain why and how differences in the frequency of genetic disease and the alleles responsible for them arose among different individuals and ethnic groups. Population genetics is also important to our attempts to identify susceptibility alleles for common, complex disorders by use of population-based association methods, as will be discussed in Chapter 10. Not only can the fascinating history of our species be read in the patterns of genetic variation we now see, but genetic heterogeneity also has important practical implications for professionals seeking to deliver appropriate, personalized health care to the world's populations in ways that are both efficient and sensitive.

● GENERAL REFERENCES

Antonarakis SE: The nature and mechanisms of human gene mutation. In Scriver CR, Beaudet AL, Sly WS, Valle D (eds): The Metabolic and Molecular Bases of Inherited Disease, 8th ed. New York, McGraw-Hill, 2001, pp 343-378.

Cavalli-Sforza LL: The DNA revolution in population genetics. Trends Genet 14:60-65, 1998.

Hartl DL: A Primer of Population Genetics, 3rd ed. Sunderland, Mass, Sinauer Associates, 2000.

Li CC: First Course in Population Genetics. Pacific Grove, Calif, Boxwood Press, 1975.

Peltonen L, Uusitalo A: Rare disease genes—lessons and challenges. Genome Res 7:765-767, 1997.

● REFERENCES FOR SPECIFIC TOPICS

Antonarakis SE: Recommendations for a nomenclature system for human gene mutations. Nomenclature Working Group. Hum Mutat 11:1-3, 1998.

Buckley PG, Mantripragada KK, Piotrowski A, et al: Copy-number polymorphisms: mining the tip of an iceberg. Trends Genet 21:315-317, 2005.

Butler J: Forensic DNA Typing. San Diego, Calif, Academic Press, 2001.

Cox DW: α_1-Antitrypsin deficiency. In Scriver CR, Beaudet AL, Sly WS, Valle D (eds): The Metabolic and Molecular Bases of Inherited Disease, 8th ed. New York, McGraw-Hill, 2000, pp 5559-5586.

Crow JF: The origins, patterns and implications of human spontaneous mutation. Nat Rev Genet 1:40-47, 2000.

Daniels G: The molecular genetics of blood group polymorphism. Transpl Immunol 14:143-153, 2005.

den Dunnen JT, Antonarakis SE: Nomenclature for the description of human sequence variations. Hum Genet 109:121-124, 2001.

den Dunnen JT, Antonarakis SE: Mutation nomenclature extensions and suggestions to describe complex mutations: a discussion. Hum Mutat 15:7-12, 2000.

Erlich HA, Opelz G, Hansen J: HLA DNA typing and transplantation. Immunity 14:347-356, 2001.

Gardner RJ: A new estimate of the achondroplasia mutation rate. Clin Genet 11:31-38, 1977.

Holden AL: The SNP consortium: summary of a private consortium effort to develop an applied map of the human genome. Biotechniques Suppl:22-4, 26, 2002.

Jeffreys AJ: DNA typing: approaches and applications. J Forensic Sci Soc 33:204-211, 1993.

Kunkel TA, Bebenek K: DNA replication fidelity. Annu Rev Biochem 69:497-529, 2000.

Lorey FW, Arnopp J, Cunningham GC: Distribution of hemoglobinopathy variants by ethnicity in a multiethnic state. Genet Epidemiol 13:501-512, 1996.

Lowe JB: Red cell membrane antigens. In Stamatoyannopoulos G, Majerus PW, Perlmutter RM, Varmus H (eds): The Molecular Basis of Blood Diseases, 3rd ed. Philadelphia, WB Saunders, 2001, pp 314-361.

Marth G, Schuler G, Yeh R, et al: Sequence variations in the public human genome data reflect a bottlenecked population history. Proc Natl Acad Sci USA 100:376-381, 2002.

Martinson JJ, Chapman NH, Rees DC, et al: Global distribution of the CCR5 gene 32 basepair deletion. Nat Genet 16:100-103, 1997.

McCluskey J, Au Peh C: The human leucocyte antigens and clinical medicine: an overview. Immunogenetics 1:3-20, 1999.

Nagel RL, Ranney H: Genetic epidemiology of structural mutations of the β-globin gene. Semin Hematol 27:342-359, 1990.

Pearson CE, Edamura KN, Cleary JD: Repeat instability: mechanisms of dynamic mutations. Nat Rev Genet 6:729-742, 2005.

Ramachandran S, Deshpande O, Roseman CC, et al: Support from the relationship of genetic and geographic distance in human populations for a serial founder effect originating in Africa. Proc Natl Acad Sci USA 102:15942-15947, 2005.

Sheffield VC, Weber JL, Buetow KH, et al: A collection of tri- and tetranucleotide repeat markers used to generate high quality, high resolution human genome–wide linkage maps. Hum Mol Genet 4:1837-1844, 1995.

Stephens JC, Reich DE, Goldstein DB, et al: Dating the origin of the CCR5-delta32 AIDS-resistance allele by the coalescence of haplotypes. Am J Hum Genet 62:1507-1515, 1998.

Stockman JA 3rd: Overview of the state of the art of Rh disease: history, current clinical management, and recent progress. J Pediatr Hematol Oncol 23:554-562, 2001.

Wang DG, Fan J, Siao C, et al: Large-scale identification, mapping, and genotyping of single-nucleotide polymorphisms in the human genome. Science 280:1077-1082, 1998.

Watkins WS, Rogers AR, Ostler CT: Genetic variation among world populations: inferences from 100 Alu insertion polymorphisms. Genome Res 13:1607-1618, 2003.

Yamamoto F: Cloning and regulation of the ABO genes. Transfus Med 11:281-294, 2001.

● USEFUL WEBSITES

Human Mutation and Polymorphism Databases

Human Genome Variation Society. http://www.genomic.unimelb.edu.au/mdi/dblist/dblist.html, and Institute of Medical Genetics in Cardiff. http://archive.uwcm.ac.uk/uwcm/mg/hgmd0.html. Comprehensive databases of mutations in hundreds of different human disease genes. Both also include links to locus-specific and disease-specific mutation databases maintained by researchers around the world.

dbSNP at the National Center for Biotechnology Information. http://www.ncbi.nlm.nih.gov/SNP/index.html Central repositories of SNPs.

Human Genome Variation Database. http://hgvbase.cgb.ki.se/cgi-bin/main.pl?page=index_new1.htm. A curated database of human genome variation maintained at the Karolinska Institute in Sweden.

European Bioinformatics Institute HLA Database. http://www.ebi.ac.uk/imgt/hla/ Database of HLA alleles.

PROBLEMS

1. Among 4.5 million births in one population during a period of 40 years, 41 children diagnosed with the autosomal dominant condition aniridia were born to normal parents. Assuming that these cases were due to new mutations, what is the estimated mutation rate at the aniridia locus? On what assumptions is this estimate based, and why might this estimate be either too high or too low?

2. If point mutations are more likely to occur in the paternal germline, what impact would that have on the clinical counseling of a family in which a single affected male child has one of the X-linked recessive diseases most frequently caused by point mutations, such as hemophilia B, Lesch-Nyhan syndrome, or ornithine transcarbamylase deficiency?

3. A VNTR-type DNA polymorphism detects five different alleles, each with a frequency of 0.20. What proportion of individuals would be expected to be heterozygous at this locus?

4. A woman who is Rh-negative marries a man who is Rh-positive. Are the children at risk for hemolytic disease of the newborn? If their children are at risk, is the risk for disease greater or less during the first pregnancy or subsequent pregnancies? Can the disease be prevented? What if the man is also Rh-negative?

5. If the allele frequency for Rh-negative is 0.26 in a population, what fraction of first pregnancies would sensitize the mother (assume Hardy-Weinberg equilibrium)? If no prophylaxis were given, what fraction of second pregnancies would be at risk for hemolytic disease of the newborn due to Rh incompatibility?

6. In a population at equilibrium, three genotypes are present in the following proportions: *A/A*, 0.81; *A/a*, 0.18; *a/a*, 0.01.
   a. What are the frequencies of *A* and *a*?
   b. What will their frequencies be in the next generation?
   c. What proportion of all matings in this population are *A/a* × *A/a*?

7. In a screening program to detect carriers of β-thalassemia in an Italian population, the carrier frequency was found to be about 4%. Calculate:
   a. the frequency of the β-thalassemia allele (assuming that there is only one common β-thalassemia mutation in this population);
   b. the proportion of matings in this population that could produce an affected child;
   c. the incidence of affected fetuses or newborns in this population;

   d. the incidence of β-thalassemia among the offspring of couples both found to be heterozygous.

8. Which of the following populations is in Hardy-Weinberg equilibrium?
   a. *A/A*, 0.70; *A/a*, 0.21; *a/a*, 0.09.
   b. MN blood groups: (i) *M*, 0.33; *MN*, 0.34; *N*, 0.33. (ii) 100% *MN*.
   c. *A/A*, 0.32; *A/a*, 0.64; *a/a*, 0.04.
   d. *A/A*, 0.64; *A/a*, 0.32; *a/a*, 0.04.

   What explanations could you offer to explain the frequencies in those populations that are not in equilibrium?

9. You are consulted by a couple, Abby and Andrew, who tell you that Abby's sister Anna has Hurler syndrome (a mucopolysaccharidosis) and that they are concerned that they themselves might have a child with the same disorder. Hurler syndrome is an autosomal recessive condition with a population incidence of about 1 in 90,000 in your community.
   a. If Abby and Andrew are not consanguineous, what is the risk that Abby and Andrew's first child will have Hurler syndrome?
   b. If they are first cousins, what is the risk?
   c. How would your answers to these questions differ if the disease in question were cystic fibrosis instead of Hurler syndrome?

10. In a certain population, each of three serious neuromuscular disorders—autosomal dominant facioscapulohumeral muscular dystrophy, autosomal recessive Friedreich ataxia, and X-linked Duchenne muscular dystrophy—has a population frequency of approximately 1/25,000.
    a. What are the gene frequency and the heterozygote frequency for each of these?
    b. Suppose that each one could be treated, so that selection against it is substantially reduced and affected individuals can have children. What would be the effect on the gene frequencies in each case? Why?

11. As discussed in this chapter, the autosomal recessive condition tyrosinemia type I has an observed incidence of 1/685 individuals in one population in the province of Quebec but an incidence of about 1/100,000 elsewhere. What is the frequency of the mutant tyrosinemia allele in these two groups? Suggest two possible explanations for the difference in allele frequencies between the population in Quebec and populations elsewhere.

Chapter 10

Human Gene Mapping and Disease Gene Identification

This chapter provides an overview of how geneticists use the familial nature of disease to identify the responsible genes and gene variants. Whether a disease is inherited in a recognizable mendelian pattern or just occurs at a higher frequency in relatives of affected individuals, the genetic contribution to disease must result from genotypic differences among family members that either cause disease outright or increase or decrease disease susceptibility. The field of genomics, resting on the foundation of the completed sequence of human DNA provided by the Human Genome Project, has provided geneticists with a complete list of all human genes, knowledge of their location and structure, and a catalogue of some of the millions of variants in DNA sequence found among individuals in different populations. As we saw in Chapter 9, some of these variants are common, others are rare, and still others differ in frequency among different ethnic groups. Whereas some variants clearly have functional consequences, others are certainly neutral. For most, their significance for human health and disease is unknown.

In Chapter 9, we dealt with the effect of mutation, which alters one or more genes or loci to generate variant alleles and polymorphisms. We also outlined the role of selection and drift that affect the frequency of variant alleles in the population. In this chapter, we discuss how the process of meiosis, acting over both time and space, determines the relationships between genes and polymorphic loci with their neighbors.

We first present what the study of the inheritance of genetic variants has taught us about the genetic landscape of the human genome. We then describe two fundamental approaches to disease gene identification. The first approach, **linkage analysis,** is *family-based.* Linkage analysis takes explicit advantage of family pedigrees to follow the inheritance of a disease over a few generations by looking for consistent, repeated inheritance of a *particular region* of the genome whenever the disease is passed on in a family. The second approach, **association analysis,** is *population-based.* Association analysis does not depend explicitly on pedigrees but instead looks for increased or decreased frequency of a *particular allele* or *set of alleles* in a sample of affected individuals taken from the population, compared with a control set of unaffected people. Association analysis takes advantage of the entire history of a population to look for alleles that are found more or less frequently in patients with a disease compared with a control unaffected population.

Use of linkage and association studies to map and identify disease genes has had an enormous impact on our understanding of the pathogenesis and pathophysiology of many diseases. This knowledge will also suggest new methods of prevention, management, and treatment (see Box on next page).

THE GENETIC LANDSCAPE OF THE HUMAN GENOME

A fundamental fact of human biology is that each generation reproduces by combining haploid gametes that are formed through independent assortment of one member of each of the 23 chromosome pairs and recombination of homologous chromosomes during meiosis (see Chapter 2). To understand fully the concepts underlying genetic linkage analysis and tests for association, it is necessary to review briefly the behavior of chromosomes and genes during meiosis. Some of this infor-

▪▪▪ How Does Gene Mapping Contribute to Medical Genetics?

- Disease gene mapping has immediate clinical application by providing information about a gene's location that can be used to develop indirect **linkage** methods for use in **prenatal diagnosis, presymptomatic diagnosis,** and **carrier testing.**
- Disease gene mapping is a critical first step in identifying a disease gene. Mapping the gene focuses attention on a limited region of the genome in which to carry out a systematic analysis of all the genes so we can find the mutations or variants that contribute to the disease (known as **positional cloning**).
- Positional cloning of a disease gene provides an opportunity to characterize the disorder as to the extent of **locus heterogeneity,** the spectrum of **allelic heterogeneity,** the frequency of various disease-causing or predisposing variants in various populations, the **penetrance** and **positive predictive value of mutations,** the fraction of the total genetic contribution to a disease attributable to the variant at any one locus, and the natural history of the disease in asymptomatic at-risk individuals.
- Characterization of a gene and the mutations in it furthers our understanding of **disease pathogenesis** and has applications for the development of specific and sensitive diagnosis by direct detection of mutations, population-based carrier screening to identify individuals at risk for disease in themselves or their offspring, cell and animal models, drug therapy to prevent or ameliorate disease or to slow its progression, and treatment by gene replacement.

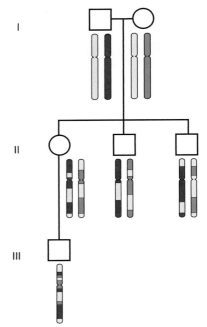

Figure 10-1 ▪ The effect of recombination on the origin of various portions of a chromosome. Because of crossing over in meiosis, the copy of the chromosome the boy (generation III) inherited from his mother is a mosaic of segments of all four of his grandparents' copies of that chromosome.

mation repeats the classic material on gametogenesis presented in Chapter 2, but much new information has become available as a result of the Human Genome Project and its application to the study of human variation.

Independent Assortment and Homologous Recombination in Meiosis

During meiosis I, homologous chromosomes pair and the pairs line up along the meiotic spindle. The paternal and maternal homologues exchange homologous segments by crossing over and creating new chromosomes that are a "patchwork" consisting of alternating portions of the grandmother's chromosomes and the grandfather's chromosomes. Examples of recombined chromosomes are shown in the offspring (generation II) of the couple in generation I in Figure 10-1. Also shown is that the individual in generation III inherits a maternal chromosome that contains segments derived from all four of his maternal grandparents. The creation of such patchwork chromosomes emphasizes the notion of

human genetic individuality: each chromosome inherited by a child from a parent is never exactly the same as either of the two copies of that chromosome in the parent. Rather, each chromosome contains some segments derived from that parent's father and other segments from that parent's mother (the child's grandfather and grandmother).

Since homologous chromosomes generally look identical under the microscope, we must have a way of differentiating them; only then can we trace the grandparental origin of each segment of a chromosome inherited by a particular child to determine if and where recombination events have occurred along the homologous chromosomes. For this purpose, we use **genetic markers,** which are defined as any characteristic located at the same position on a pair of homologous chromosomes that allows us to distinguish one homologous chromosome from the other. In the era of the Human Genome Project, millions of genetic markers are now available that can be readily genotyped by polymerase chain reaction analysis (see Chapter 9).

Alleles at Loci on Different Chromosomes Assort Independently

Assume there are two polymorphic loci, 1 and 2, on different chromosomes, with alleles D and d at locus 1 and alleles M and m at locus 2 (Fig. 10-2). Suppose an individual's genotype at these loci is Dd and Mm, that is, he is heterozygous at both loci, with alleles D and

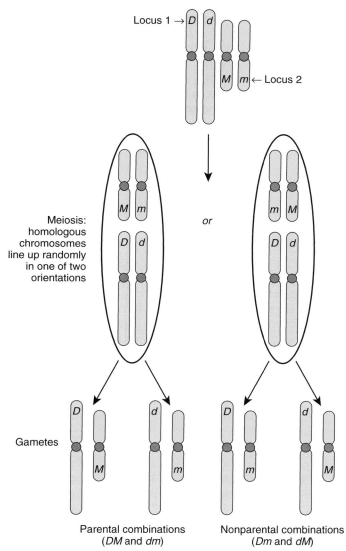

Locus 1 → D d

M m ← Locus 2

Meiosis:
homologous
chromosomes
line up randomly
in one of two
orientations

or

M m   m M

D d   D d

Gametes

D   d   D   d

M   m   m   M

Parental combinations   Nonparental combinations
(*DM* and *dm*)   (*Dm* and *dM*)

Figure 10-2 ■ Independent assortment of alleles at two loci, 1 and 2, when they are located on different chromosomes. Assume that alleles *D* and *M* were inherited from one parent, *d* and *m* from the other.

M inherited from his father and alleles *d* and *m* inherited from his mother. The two different chromosomes will line up on the metaphase plate at meiosis I in one of two orientations with equal likelihood. After meiosis is complete, there will be four possible combinations of alleles, *DM*, *dm*, *Dm*, and *dM*, in a gamete; each combination is as likely to occur as any other, a phenomenon known as **independent assortment**. Since *DM* gametes contain only his paternally derived alleles, and *dm* gametes only his maternally derived alleles, these gametes are designated *parental*. In contrast, *Dm* or *dM* gametes, each containing one paternally derived allele and one maternally derived allele, are *nonparental* gametes. Half (50%) of gametes will be parental (*DM* or *dm*) and 50% nonparental (*Dm* or *dM*).

Alleles at Loci on the Same Chromosome Assort Independently if at Least One Crossover Occurs Between Them in Every Meiosis

Suppose that an individual is heterozygous at two loci 1 and 2, with alleles *D* and *M* paternally derived and *d* and *m* maternally derived, but the loci are on the *same* chromosome (Fig. 10-3). Genes that reside on the same chromosome are said to be **syntenic** (literally, "on the same thread"), regardless of how close together or how far apart they lie on that chromosome. How will these alleles behave during meiosis? We know that between one and four crossovers occur somewhere along every chromosome per meiosis at the four-strand stage, when there are four chromatids per chromosome pair. If *no* crossing over occurs within the segment of the chromatids between the loci (and ignoring whatever happens in segments outside the interval between loci), the chromosomes we see in the gametes will be *DM* and *dm*, which are the same as the original parental chromosomes; a parental chromosome is therefore a **nonrecombinant** chromosome. If crossing over occurs at least once in the segment between the loci, the resulting chromatids may be either nonrecombinant or *Dm* and *dM*, which are *not* the same as the parental chromosomes; such a nonparental chromosome is therefore a **recombinant** chromosome (shown in Fig. 10-3). One, two, or more recombinations occurring between two loci at the four-chromatid stage result in gametes that are 50% nonrecombinant (parental) and 50% recombinant (nonparental), which is precisely the same proportions one sees if the loci were on different chromosomes. Thus, if two syntenic loci are sufficiently far apart on the same chromosome, there is going to be *at least one* crossover between them in every meiosis. As a result, the ratio of recombinant to nonrecombinant genotypes will be, on average, 1 : 1, just as if the loci were on separate chromosomes and assorting independently.

Recombination Frequency and Map Distance

Frequency of Recombination as a Measure of How Far Apart Two Loci Are

Suppose now that two loci are on the same chromosome but are far apart, very close together, or somewhere in between (Fig. 10-4A). When the loci are far apart, at least one crossover occurs in the segment of the chromosome between loci 1 and 2, and both the nonrecombinant genotypes *DM* and *dm* and recombinant genotypes *Dm* and *dM* will be seen, on average, in equal proportions in the offspring. In this case, the loci will appear to be assorting independently. On the other hand, if two loci are so close together on the same chromosome that crossovers never occur between them,

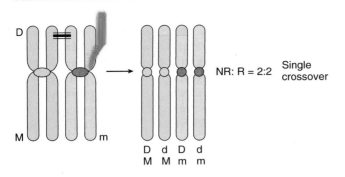

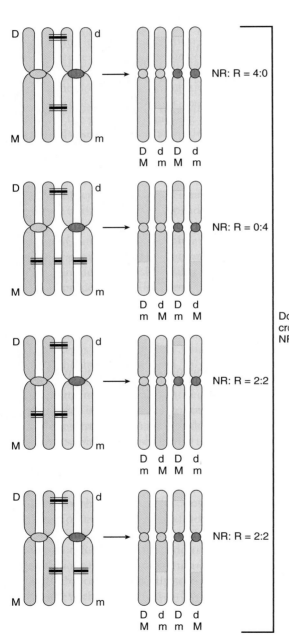

Figure 10-3 ■ Crossing over between homologous chromosomes (*black horizontal lines*) in meiosis is shown in the quadrivalents on the left. Crossovers result in new combinations of maternally and paternally derived alleles on the recombinant chromosomes present in gametes, shown on the right. If no crossing over occurs in the interval between loci 1 and 2, only parental (nonrecombinant) allele combinations, *DM* and *dm*, occur in the offspring. If one or two crossovers occur in the interval between the loci, half the gametes will contain a nonrecombinant combination of alleles and half the recombinant combination. The same is true if more than two crossovers occur between the loci (not illustrated here). NR, nonrecombinant; R, recombinant.

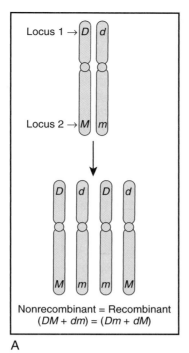
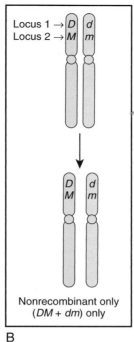
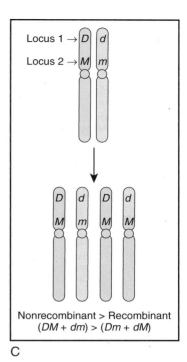

Figure 10-4 ■ Assortment of alleles at two loci, 1 and 2, when they are located on the same chromosome. **A,** The loci are far apart and at least one crossover between them is likely to occur in every meiosis. **B,** The loci are so close together that crossing over between them is very unlikely. **C,** The loci are close together on the same chromosome but far enough apart that crossing over occurs in the interval between the two loci only in some meioses and not in others.

there will be no recombination; the nonrecombinant genotypes (parental chromosomes *DM* and *dm* in Fig. 10-4B) are transmitted together all of the time, and the frequency of the recombinant genotypes *Dm* and *dM* will be 0. In between these two extremes is the situation in which two loci are far enough apart that at least one recombination between them occurs in some meioses but not in others (Fig. 10-4C). In this situation, we will observe nonrecombinant and recombinant combinations of alleles in the offspring, but the frequency of recombinant chromosomes at the two loci will fall between 0% and 50%: *the smaller the recombination frequency, the closer together two loci are.* A common notation for recombination frequency (as a proportion, not a percentage) is the Greek letter theta, θ, where θ varies from 0 (no recombination at all) to 0.5 (independent assortment).

Effect of Heterozygosity and Phase on Detecting Recombination Events

Detecting the recombination events between loci requires that (1) a parent be heterozygous (**informative**) at both loci and (2) we know which allele at locus 1 is on the same chromosome as which allele at locus 2. In an individual who is heterozygous at two syntenic loci, one with alleles *D* and *d,* the other *M* and *m,* which allele at the first locus is on the same chromosome with which allele at the second locus defines what is referred to as the **phase** (Fig. 10-5). Alleles on the same homologue are in **coupling** (or *cis*), whereas alleles on the different homologues are in **repulsion** (or *trans*). Figure 10-6 shows a pedigree of a family with multiple indi-

viduals affected by **retinitis pigmentosa (RP),** a degenerative disease of the retina that causes progressive blindness in association with abnormal retinal pigmentation. As shown, I-1 is heterozygous at both marker locus 1 (with alleles *A* and *a*) and marker locus 2 (with alleles *B* and *b*) as well as being a heterozygote for this autosomal dominant disorder (*D* is the disease allele, *d* is the normal allele). We can trace the inheritance of her disease allele or her normal allele and the alleles at both marker loci easily in her six children. However, if, for example, the mother (I-1) had been homozygous at locus 2, with alleles *bb,* all children would inherit a maternal *b* allele regardless of whether they received a mutant *D* or normal *d* allele at the RP locus. It would then be impossible to determine whether recombination had occurred. Similarly, if the information provided for the family in Figure 10-6 was simply that individual I-1

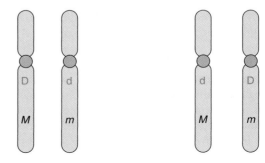

In coupling: *D* and *M* *d* and *m*   In coupling: *d* and *M* *D* and *m*
In repulsion: *d* and *M* *D* and *m*   In repulsion: *D* and *M* *d* and *m*

Figure 10-5 ■ Possible phases of alleles *M* and *m* at a marker locus with alleles *D* and *d* at a disease locus.

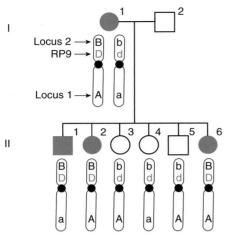

Figure 10-6 ■ Co-inheritance of the gene for an autosomal dominant form of retinitis pigmentosa, RP9, with marker locus 2 and not with marker locus 1. Only the mother's contribution to the children's genotypes is shown. The mother (I-1) is affected with this dominant disease and is heterozygous at the RP9 locus *(Dd)* as well as at loci 1 and 2. She carries the *A* and *B* alleles on the same chromosome as the mutant RP9 allele *(D)*. The unaffected father is homozygous normal *(dd)* at the RP9 locus as well as at the two marker loci *(AA* and *BB)*; his contributions to his offspring are not considered further. All three affected offspring have inherited the *B* allele at locus 2 from their mother, whereas the three unaffected offspring have inherited the *b* allele. Thus, all six offspring are nonrecombinant for RP9 and marker locus 2. However, individuals II-1, II-3, and II-5 are recombinant for RP9 and marker locus 1, indicating that meiotic crossover has occurred between these two loci.

was heterozygous, *Bb*, at locus 2 and heterozygous for an autosomal dominant form of RP, one could not determine which of her children were nonrecombinant between the RP locus and locus 2 and which of her children were recombinant. This is because determination of who is or is not a recombinant requires that we know whether the *B* allele at locus 2 was on the same chromosome as the mutant *D* allele for RP in individual I-1 and whether the *b* allele at locus 2 was on the same chromosome as the normal *d* allele (see Fig. 10-6). The set of alleles whose phase is in coupling at neighboring loci is what we have referred to in Chapters 7 and 9 as the **haplotype.**

Linkage and Recombination Frequency

Linkage is the term used to describe a departure from the independent assortment of two loci, or, in other words, the tendency for alleles at loci that are close together on the same chromosome to be transmitted together, as an intact unit, through meiosis. Analysis of linkage depends on determining the frequency of recombination as a measure of how close different loci are to each other on a chromosome. If two loci are so close together that $\theta = 0$ between them, they are said to be **tightly linked;** if they are so far apart that $\theta = 0.5$, they are assorting independently and are **unlinked.** In

between these two extremes are various degrees of linkage. Suppose that among the offspring of informative meioses (i.e., those in which a parent is heterozygous at both loci), 80% of the offspring are nonrecombinant and 20% are recombinant. At first glance, the recombination frequency is therefore 20% ($\theta = 0.2$). However, the accuracy of this measure of θ depends on the size of the family used to make the measurement. If 20% of the offspring show a recombination and 80% do not, the estimate of $\theta = 0.2$ is accurate only if the number of offspring has been sufficient to be confident that the observed 80 : 20 ratio of nonrecombinants to recombinants is really different from the 50 : 50 ratio expected for unlinked loci. For example, if you are counting only five children and four of the five children were nonrecombinant and one was recombinant, this ratio would not be significantly different from the result expected for two randomly assorting loci. (Would you consider it significant if you flipped a coin five times and it came up heads four of five times? No, because four or more heads out of five coin tosses would be expected to occur at least some of the time by chance alone.) However, if one observes the same 80 : 20 ratio after genotyping 50 children from several families, it would certainly be considered different from 50 : 50, just as you would find it very unusual to flip a coin 50 times and have it come up heads 40 times of 50 (40 or more flips coming up heads out of 50 would happen only about one time in a thousand by chance alone, a very unlikely occurrence!). Measurement of θ therefore requires statistical methods to know how accurate and reliable the measurement is. The statistical method for measuring θ from family data, the **LOD score** method, is the mainstay of linkage analysis. LOD scores are presented in detail later in this chapter.

One additional effect of sample size on measurement of θ needs to be considered. Clearly, when two loci are very close together, such as when θ is 0.01 or less, a very large sample size is required to have any chance of actually seeing the expected single rare recombination event out of 100 or more offspring. Otherwise, θ is simply recorded as 0. In practical terms, θ values below 0.01 are difficult to measure accurately and require vast amounts of data generally available only in a few, very large human genetics studies.

Genetic Maps and Physical Maps

The **map distance** between two loci is a *theoretical* concept that is based on *real* data, the extent of observed recombination, θ, between the loci. Map distance is measured in units called **centimorgans** (cM), defined as the genetic length over which, on average, one crossover occurs in 1% of meioses. (The centimorgan is 1/100 of a morgan, named after Thomas Hunt Morgan, who first observed genetic crossing over in the fruit fly *Drosophila*.) Therefore, a recombination fraction of 1% (θ

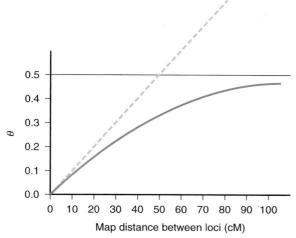

Figure 10-7 ■ The relationship between map distance in centimorgans and recombination fraction, θ. Recombination fraction *(solid line)* and map distance *(dotted line)* are nearly equal, with 1 cM = 0.01 recombination, for values of genetic distance below 10 cM, but they begin to diverge because of double crossovers as the distance between the markers increases. The recombination fraction approaches a maximum of 0.5 no matter how far apart loci are; the genetic distance increases proportionally to the distance between loci.

= 0.01) translates approximately into a map distance of 1 cM (why this value of map distance is only approximate is explained next).

As the map distance between two loci increases, however, the frequency of recombination we observe between them does not increase proportionately (Fig. 10-7). This is because as the distance between two loci increases, the chance that the chromosome carrying these two markers could undergo more than one crossing over event between these loci also increases. As we saw in Figure 10-3, when two loci are far enough apart on a chromosome that at least one crossover occurs with every meiosis, they will assort independently (θ = 0.5) no matter how far apart they are physically. As a rule of thumb, recombination frequency begins to underestimate true genetic distance significantly once θ rises above 0.1.

To measure true genetic map distance between two widely spaced loci accurately, therefore, one has to use markers spaced at short genetic distances in the interval between these two loci and add up the values of θ between the intervening markers, since the values of θ between pairs of closely neighboring markers will be good approximations of the genetic distances between them (Fig. 10-8). As an extreme example, two markers at opposite ends of a chromosome will behave as though they are unlinked, with θ = 0.5. Yet, adding together all the small recombination frequencies between closely spaced markers allows an accurate measurement of the genetic length of individual human chromosomes. Thus, for example, human chromosome 1 is the largest human chromosome in physical length (283 Mb) and also has the greatest genetic length, 270 cM (0.95 cM/

Mb); the q arm of the smallest chromosome, number 21, is 30 Mb in physical length and 62 cM in genetic length (~2.1 cM/Mb). The measurement of map lengths of chromosomes, combined with the complete DNA sequence available from the Human Genome Project, allows a direct comparison of genetic to physical length at the rather coarse scale of entire chromosomes. Overall, the human genome, which is estimated to contain about 3200 Mb, has a genetic length of 3615 cM, for an average of 1.13 cM/Mb. Furthermore, as we will discuss later, the ratio of genetic distance to physical length is not uniform along a chromosome as one looks with finer and finer resolution at recombination versus physical length.

Sex Differences in Map Distances   In the previous discussion, we described measurement of meiotic recombination without reference to whether it is occurring in male or female gametogenesis. Just as male and female gametogenesis shows sex differences in the types of mutations and their frequencies, there are also significant differences in recombination between males and females. Across all chromosomes, the genetic length in females, 4460 cM, is 72% greater than the genetic distance of 2590 cM in males, and it is consistently about 70% greater in females on each of the different autosomes. The reason for increased recombination in females compared with males is unknown, although one might speculate that it has to do with the many years that female gamete precursors remain in meiosis I before ovulation.

Linkage Equilibrium and Disequilibrium

Genetic maps are generally constructed by counting directly how many recombination events occurred between loci in the offspring of parents informative for alleles at these loci. Such measurements are based on a small number of recombinations in a few hundred to a few thousand meioses and therefore provide a level of resolution of approximately 0.5 to 1 cM. To measure smaller genetic distances would require observing even rarer recombination events among many thousands to tens of thousands of meioses, a formidable and imprac-

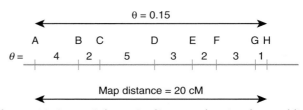

Figure 10-8 ■ Schematic diagram showing how adding together short genetic distances, measured as recombination fraction, θ, between neighboring loci A, B, C, and so on allows accurate determination of genetic distance between the two loci A and H located far apart. The value of θ between A and H is not an accurate measure of genetic distance.

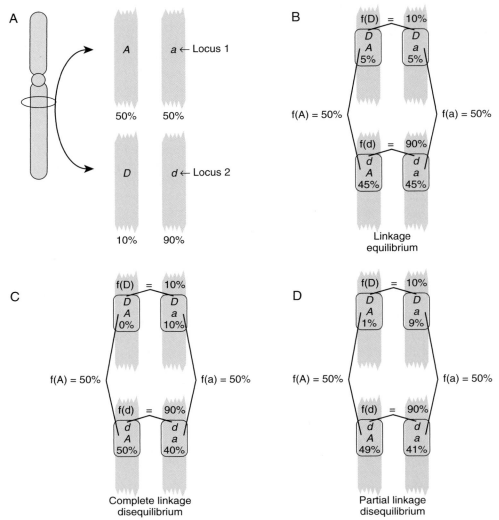

Figure 10-9 ■ Diagram of linkage equilibrium and disequilibrium between alleles at locus 1 and alleles at locus 2. **A,** Loci 1 and 2 are located very close to one another. Allele frequencies of *A* and *a* at locus 1 are both 50%. Allele frequencies of *D* and *d* at locus 2 are 10% and 90%. **B,** Haplotype frequencies under **linkage equilibrium.** Haplotypes containing the *D* allele, *D-A* and *D-a,* each have a frequency of 5% and together constitute 10%, equal to the allele frequency f(D) of the *D* allele. Similarly, haplotypes containing the *A* allele, *D-A* and *d-A,* have frequencies of 5% and 45%, respectively, and together constitute 50%, equal to frequency f(A) of the *A* allele. Similarly, the frequency f(a) of the *a* allele is 5% + 45% = 50%, and f(d) of the *d* allele = 90%. **C,** Haplotype frequencies under **linkage disequilibrium.** The haplotype containing the disease allele *D* is enriched for allele *a* at locus 1; haplotype *D-A* is not present in the population. The frequencies of the remaining haplotypes are such that there is no change in the allele frequencies f(A), f(a), f(D), and f(d), only in the frequencies of the various haplotypes. **D, Partial linkage disequilibrium,** with the haplotype *D-A* rare but not absent from the population.

tical task. There is, however, another characteristic of the genetic landscape, a phenomenon known as **linkage disequilibrium,** that permits a higher resolution map based on inferring recombinations that occurred during millions of meioses over thousands of generations, back to the origins of modern humans.

To understand linkage disequilibrium, we need first to explain its opposite: **linkage equilibrium.** Consider two loci: a polymorphic marker locus 1 with two alleles, *A* and *a,* and a nearby disease locus 2, with disease allele *D* and normal allele *d.* Suppose allele *A* is present on 50% of the chromosomes in a population and allele

a on the other 50% of chromosomes. At locus 2, disease allele *D* is present in 10% of chromosomes and *d* in 90% (Fig. 10-9A). Knowing the allele frequencies for these two loci does not mean that we know how these alleles are distributed into the four possible haplotypes, *A-D, A-d, a-D,* and *a-d.* Shown in Figure 10-9B is the situation in which the population frequency of both haplotypes containing the *A* allele (*A-D* plus *A-d*) is 50%, the same as the allele frequency for *A* in the population. Similarly, the frequency of the two haplotypes containing the *D* allele (*A-D* plus *a-D*) is 10%, the same as the frequency of the *D* allele in the popula-

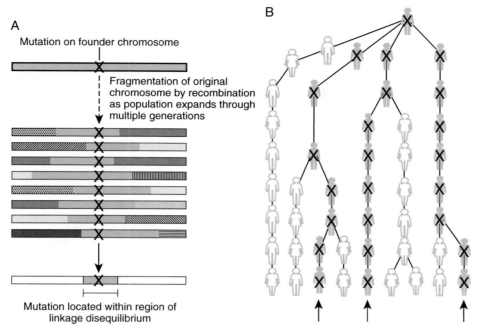

Figure 10-10 ■ **A,** With each generation, meiotic recombination exchanges the alleles that were initially present at polymorphic loci on a chromosome on which a disease-associated mutation arose (▬▬) for other alleles present on the homologous chromosome. Over many generations, the only alleles that remain in coupling phase with the mutation are those at loci so close to the mutant locus that recombination between the loci is very rare. These alleles are in linkage disequilibrium with the mutation and constitute a disease-associated haplotype. **B,** Affected individuals in the current generation (*arrows*) carry the mutation (**X**) in linkage disequilibrium with the disease-associated haplotype (filled-in solid blue symbols). Depending on the age of the mutation and other population genetic factors, a disease-associated haplotype ordinarily spans a region of DNA of a few kb to a few hundred kb. (Modified from original figures of Thomas Hudson, McGill University, Canada.)

tion. When the frequency of each allele within the haplotypes is the same as the frequency of that allele in the population as a whole, the alleles are said to be in **linkage equilibrium.** Indeed, at a low level of resolution of a few centimorgans, it is generally the case that the alleles at two loci of 1 cM or more apart will not show any preferred phase in the population. Each haplotype is as frequent in the population as one would expect simply on the basis of the frequency of the alleles at the loci making up the haplotype.

As we examine haplotypes involving loci that are very close together, however, each haplotype is not always as frequent as one would expect simply on the basis of the frequency of the alleles at the loci making up the haplotype. Why is this the case? When a disease allele first enters the population (by mutation or by immigration of a founder who carries the disease allele), the particular set of alleles at markers linked to the disease locus constitutes a **disease-containing haplotype** in which the disease allele is located (Fig. 10-10). The degree to which this original disease-containing haplotype will persist over time depends on the probability that recombination can move the disease allele *off* of the original haplotype and *onto* chromosomes with different sets of alleles at these linked marker loci. The speed with which recombination will move the disease allele onto a new haplotype is the product of two

factors: (1) the number of generations, and therefore the number of opportunities for recombination, since the mutation first appeared; and (2) the frequency of recombination between the loci. (A third factor, selection for or against particular alleles in a haplotype, could theoretically also play a role, but its effect has been difficult to prove in humans.) Figure 10-11 shows a graph of the theoretical rate at which linkage equilibrium arises as a function of the number of generations and the recombination frequency, θ. The shorter the time since the disease allele appeared and the smaller the value of θ, the greater is the chance that the disease-containing haplotype will persist intact. However, with longer time periods and greater values of θ, shuffling by recombination will go further to completion and the allele frequencies for marker alleles in the haplotype that includes the disease allele *D* will come to equal the frequencies of these marker alleles in all chromosomes in the population. At this point, all the alleles in the haplotype will have reached linkage equilibrium.

Haplotypes that are not in linkage equilibrium are said to be in **linkage disequilibrium (LD).** For example, suppose one discovers that *all* chromosomes carrying allele *D* also have allele *a*, whereas none has allele *A* (see Fig. 10-9C). Then allele *D* and allele *a* are in strong LD. As a final example, suppose the *A-D* haplotype is present on only 1% of chromosomes in the population

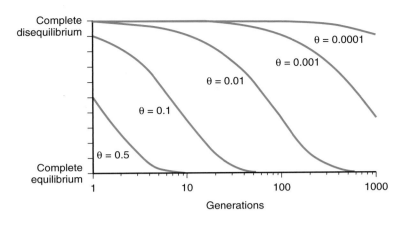

Figure 10-11 ■ Theoretical rate at which initial linkage disequilibrium between alleles at two loci decays and the alleles approach linkage equilibrium as a function of time and various values of recombination frequency, θ, between the markers. (Adapted from original figure by G. Abecasis, University of Michigan. *http://www.sph.umich.edu/csg/abecasis/class/666.03.pdf.*)

(see Fig. 10-9D). The *A-D* haplotype has a frequency much below what one would expect on the basis of the 50% frequency of allele *A* in the population as a whole; the haplotype *a-D* has frequency much greater than expected. In other words, chromosomes carrying the disease allele *D* are enriched for allele *a* at the expense of allele *A*, compared with chromosomes that do not carry the disease allele.

Measure of Linkage Disequilibrium To quantify varying degrees of LD, geneticists often use a measure referred to as D′ (see later). D′ is designed to vary from 0, indicating linkage equilibrium, up to a maximum of 1, indicating very strong LD. Since LD is a result not only of genetic distance but also of the amount of time during which recombination had a chance to occur, different populations with different histories may show different values of D′ between the same two markers in the genome.

The Haplotype Map (HapMap)

One of the biggest human genomics efforts to follow completion of the sequencing is a project designed to create a haplotype map (**HapMap**) of the genome. The goal of the HapMap project is to make LD measurements between a dense collection of millions of single nucleotide polymorphisms (SNPs) throughout the genome to delineate the genetic landscape of the genome on a fine scale. To accomplish this goal, geneticists collected and characterized millions of SNP loci, developed methods to genotype them rapidly and inexpensively, and used them, one pair at a time, to measure LD between neighboring markers throughout the genome. The measurements were made in samples that included both unrelated population samples and samples containing one child and both parents, obtained from four geographically distinct groups: a primarily European population, a West African population, a Han Chinese population, and a population from Japan.

What have we learned from the HapMap? First, the study showed that more than 90% of all SNPs are shared among such geographically disparate populations as West Africans, Europeans, and East Asians, with allele frequencies that are quite similar in the different populations (Fig. 10-12A). This finding indicates that most SNPs are quite old and predate the waves of emigration out of East Africa that populated the rest of the world (Fig. 10-12B). A certain fraction of SNPs, however, may have alleles that are present in some populations and not in others or may show striking differences in frequency between populations originating in different parts of the world. These differences in allele frequencies between populations seen in a small fraction of SNPs may be the result of either genetic drift/founder effect or selection in localized geographical regions after the migrations out of Africa. Such SNPs, termed **ancestry informative markers**, are being applied to studies of human origins, migration, and gene flow. In some cases, they have been used in forensic investigations in which one seeks to determine the likely ethnic background of a perpetrator of a crime for whom the only evidence is DNA left at the crime scene.

Second, when pairwise measurements of linkage disequilibrium were made for neighboring SNPs across the genome, contiguous SNPs could be grouped into clusters of varying size in which the SNPs in any one cluster showed high levels of LD with each other but not with SNPs outside that cluster (Fig. 10-13A). For example, the nine SNPs in cluster 1, shown in Figure 10-13A, has the potential for generating $2^9 = 512$ different haplotypes; yet, only five haplotypes constitute 98% of all haplotypes seen. The values of D′ between SNPs within the cluster are well above 0.8. These clusters of SNPs in high LD, located across segments of a few kilobase pairs to a few dozen kilobase pairs along a chromosome, are termed **LD blocks.** The sizes of individual LD blocks are not identical in all populations. African populations have smaller blocks, averaging 7.3 kb per block, compared with 16.3 kb in Europeans; the Chinese and Japanese block sizes are comparable to each other and are intermediate, averaging 13.2 kb. This difference in block size is almost cer-

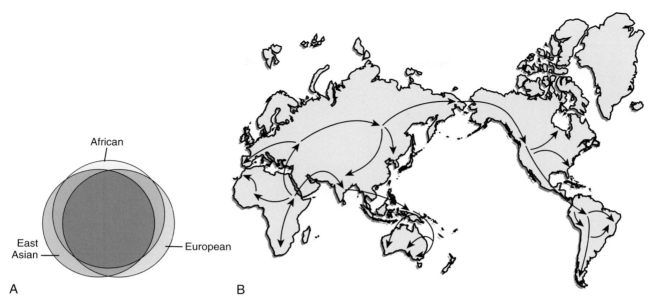

Figure 10-12 ■ **A,** Diagram of polymorphisms found in people living in three broadly defined regions of the globe. The vast majority of all polymorphic alleles are found in all three populations at similar frequencies, but a subset in each population either has not been detected or differs substantially in frequency in one or both of the other populations. **B,** Gene flow of polymorphisms as modern humans migrated from their sites of origin in East Africa. (Modified from diagrams provided by Thomas Hudson, McGill University, Canada.)

tainly the result of the smaller number of generations since the founding of the non-African populations compared with populations in Africa, thereby limiting the time in which there has been opportunity for recombination to break up regions of LD.

Third, when pairwise measurements of recombination were made between closely neighboring SNPs, the ratio of map distance to base pairs, which, as we discussed previously, is a fairly constant ~1 cM/Mb on the scale of entire chromosomes, ranged from far below 0.01 cM/Mb to more than 60 cM/Mb when measured on a very fine scale of a few kilobase pairs (Fig. 10-13B). Such high-resolution measurements of recombination require that many tens of thousands of meioses be examined for recombination. Pedigrees are impractical as a source of such large numbers of meioses. Thus, one must rely on direct measurement of male recombination by genotyping very large numbers of individual sperm (which is labor-intensive and technically demanding and therefore ill-suited for measurements on a genome-wide scale) or by using population genetics methods to estimate how much recombination has occurred over large numbers of meioses across thousands of generations. Thus, what was previously thought to be a fairly uniform rate of recombination between polymorphic markers millions of base pairs of DNA apart is, in fact, the result of an averaging of "hotspots" of recombination interspersed among regions of little or no recombination when viewed on the scale of a few tens of kilobase pairs of DNA. The biological basis for these recombination hotspots is unknown.

Finally, when the HapMap of LD blocks is compared in a few areas of the genome for which genetic maps of extremely high resolution are also available, the boundaries between neighboring LD blocks and regions of markedly increased recombination are often found to coincide (see Fig. 10-13B). The correlation is by no means exact, and many apparent boundaries between LD blocks are not located over apparent recombination hotspots. This lack of perfect correlation is not surprising given what we have already surmised about LD: it is affected not only by how likely a recombination event is (i.e., where the hotspots are) but also by the age of the population and the frequency of the haplotypes present in the founding members of that population.

The purpose of the HapMap was not just to gather basic information about the genetic architecture and history of the human genome. Its primary purpose was to provide a powerful new tool for finding the genetic variants that contribute to human disease. How the HapMap can be applied for this purpose is described later in this chapter.

● MAPPING HUMAN GENES BY LINKAGE ANALYSIS

Determining Whether Two Loci Are Linked

Linkage analysis is a method of mapping genes that uses family studies to determine whether two genes show linkage (are **linked**) when passed on from one generation to the next. To decide whether two loci are

A

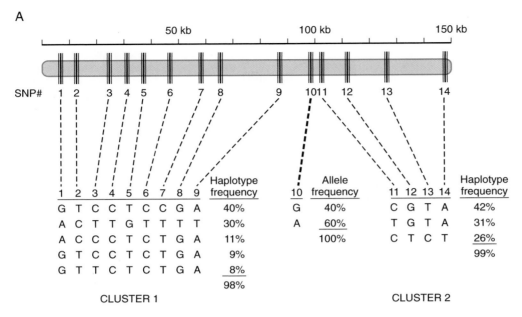

B

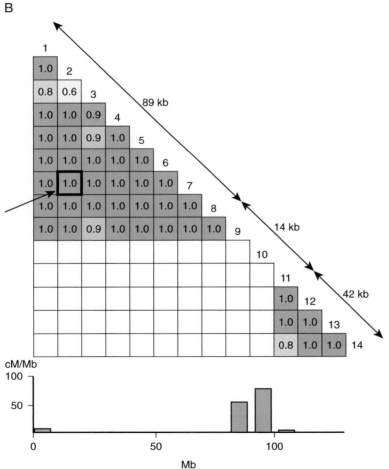

cM/Mb

Figure 10-13 ■ **A,** A 145-kb region of chromosome 4 containing 14 SNPs. In cluster 1, containing SNPs 1 through 9, five of the $2^9 = 512$ theoretically possible haplotypes are responsible for 98% of all the haplotypes in the population, reflecting substantial linkage *disequilibrium* among these SNP loci. Similarly, in cluster 2, only three of the $2^4 = 16$ theoretically possible haplotypes involving SNPs 11 to 14 represent 99% of all the haplotypes found. In contrast, alleles at SNP 10 are found in linkage *equilibrium* with the SNPs in cluster 1 and cluster 2. **B,** A schematic diagram in which each box contains the pairwise measurement of the degree of linkage disequilibrium between two SNPs (e.g., the arrow points to the box, outlined in black, containing the value of D′ for SNPs 2 and 7). The higher the degree of LD, the darker the color in the box, with maximum D′ values of 1.0 occurring when there is complete LD. Two LD blocks are detectable, the first containing SNPs 1 through 9, and the second SNPs 11 through 14. In the first block, pairwise measurements of D′ reveal LD. A similar level of LD is found in block 2. Between blocks, the 14-kb region containing SNP 10 shows no LD with neighboring SNPs 9 or 11 or with any of the other SNP loci. Below is a graph of the ratio of map distance to physical distance (cM/Mb) showing that a recombination hotspot is present in the region around SNP 10 between the two blocks, with values of recombination that are 50- to 60-fold above the average of approximately 1.13 cM/Mb for the genome. (Based on data and diagrams provided by Thomas Hudson, Quebec Genome Center, Montreal, Canada.)

linked, and if so, how close or far apart they are, we rely on two pieces of information. First, we ascertain whether the recombination fraction θ between two loci deviates significantly from 0.5; determining whether two loci are linked is equivalent to asking whether the recombination fraction between them differs significantly from the 0.5 fraction expected for unlinked loci. Second, if θ is less than 0.5, we need to make the best estimate we can of θ since that will tell us how close or far apart the linked loci are. For both of these determinations, we use a statistical tool called the likelihood ratio. Likelihoods are probability values; odds are ratios of likelihoods. One proceeds as follows: examine a set of actual family data, count the number of children who show or do not show recombination between the loci, and finally calculate the likelihood of observing the data at various possible values of θ between 0 and 0.5. Calculate a second likelihood based on the null hypothesis that the two loci are unlinked, that is, $\theta = 0.50$. We take the ratio of the likelihood of observing the family data for various values of θ to the likelihood the loci are unlinked to create an odds ratio. The odds in favor at a given value of θ are therefore:

$$\frac{\text{Likelihood of the data if loci are linked at a particular } \theta}{\text{Likelihood of the data if loci are unlinked } (\theta = 0.50)}$$

The computed odds ratios for different values of θ are usually expressed as the $\log_{10}$ of this ratio and are called a **LOD score** *(Z)* for "*l*ogarithm of the *od*ds." (The use of logarithms allows data collected from different families to be combined by simple addition.)

The odds ratio is important in two ways (see Box). First, it provides a statistically valid method for using the family data to estimate the recombination frequency between the loci. This is because statistical theory tells us that the value of θ that gives the greatest value for Z is, in fact, the best estimate of the recombination fraction you can make given the data. This value of θ is called θ_{max}. If θ_{max} differs from 0.50, you have evidence of linkage. However, even if θ_{max} is the best estimate of θ you can make, how good an estimate is it? The odds ratio also provides you with an answer to this question because *the higher the value of Z, the better an estimate*

θ_{max} *is*. Positive values of Z (odds >1) at a given θ suggest that the two loci are linked, whereas negative values (odds <1) suggest that linkage is less likely than the possibility that the two loci are unlinked. *By convention, a combined LOD score of +3 or greater (equivalent to greater than 1000:1 odds in favor of linkage) is considered definitive evidence that two loci are linked.*

Mapping genes by linkage analysis provides an opportunity to localize medically relevant genes by following inheritance of the condition and the inheritance of alleles at polymorphic markers to see if the disease locus and the polymorphic marker locus are linked. Let us return to the family shown in Figure 10-6. The mother has an autosomal dominant form of retinitis pigmentosa. There are dozens of different forms of this disease, many of which have been mapped to specific sites within the genome and the genes for which have been identified. We do not know which of the forms of RP the mother has. She is also heterozygous for two loci on chromosome 7, one at 7p14 and one at the distal end of the long arm. One can see that transmission of the RP mutant allele *(D)* invariably "follows" that of allele *B* at marker locus 2 from the first generation to the second generation in this family. All three offspring with the disease (who therefore must have inherited their mother's mutant allele *D* at the RP locus) also inherited the *B* allele at marker locus 2. All the offspring who inherited their mother's normal allele, *d*, inherited the *b* allele and will not develop RP. The gene encoding RP, however, shows no tendency to follow the allele at marker locus 1.

Suppose we let θ be the "true" recombination fraction between RP and locus 2, the fraction we would see if we had unlimited numbers of offspring to test. Viewed in this way, θ can be considered to be the probability, in each meiosis, that a recombination will occur between the two loci. Because either a recombination occurs or it does not, the probability of a recombination, θ, and the probability of no recombination must add up to 1. Therefore, the probability that no recombination will occur is $1 - \theta$. In fact, there are only six offspring, all of whom show no recombination. Because each meiosis is an independent event, one multiplies the probability of a recombination, θ, or of no recombination, $(1 - \theta)$, for each child. The likelihood of seeing zero offspring with a recombination and six offspring with no recombination between RP and marker locus 2 is therefore $(\theta)^0(1 - \theta)^6$. The LOD score between RP and marker 2, then, is:

$$Z = \log_{10} \frac{\theta^0 (1 - \theta)^6}{(1/2)^0 (1/2)^6}$$

The maximum value of Z is 1.81, which occurs when $\theta = 0$, and is suggestive of but not definite evidence for linkage because Z is positive but less than 3.

●●● Model-Based Linkage Analysis of Mendelian Diseases

Linkage analysis is called **model-based** (or **parametric**) when it assumes that there is a particular mode of inheritance (autosomal dominant, autosomal recessive, or X-linked) that explains the inheritance pattern.

LOD score analysis allows mapping of genes in which mutations cause diseases that follow mendelian inheritance.

The LOD score gives both:
• a best estimate of the recombination frequency, θ_{max}, between a marker locus and the disease locus; and
• an assessment of how strong the evidence is for linkage at that value of θ_{max}. Values of the LOD score above 3 are considered strong evidence.

Linkage at a particular θ_{max} of a disease gene locus to a marker with known physical location implies that the disease gene locus must be near the marker.

Combining LOD Score Information Across Families

In the same way that each meiosis in a family that produces a nonrecombinant or recombinant offspring is an independent event, so too are the meioses that occur in other families. We can therefore multiply the likelihoods in the numerators and denominators of each family's likelihood odds ratio together. An equivalent but more convenient calculation is to add the $\log_{10}$ of each likelihood ratio, calculated at the various values of θ, to form an overall Z score for all families combined. In the case of RP in Figure 10-6, suppose two other families were studied and one showed no recombination between locus 2 and RP in four children and the third showed no recombination in five children. The individual LOD scores can be generated for each family and added together (Table 10-1). In this case, one could say that the RP gene in this group of families is linked to locus 2. Because the chromosomal location of polymorphic locus 2 was known to be at 7p14, the RP in this family can be mapped to the region around 7p14, which is near *RP9*, an already identified locus for one form of autosomal dominant RP.

If, however, some of the families being used for the study have RP due to mutations at another locus, the LOD scores between families will diverge, with some showing a trend to being positive at small values of θ and others showing strongly negative LOD scores at these values. One can still add the Z scores together, but the result will show a sharp decline in the overall LOD score. Thus, in linkage analysis involving more than one family, unsuspected locus heterogeneity can obscure what may be real evidence for linkage in a subset of families.

Phase in Linkage Analysis

Phase-Known and Phase-Unknown Pedigrees Phase information is important in linkage analysis. Figure 10-14 shows two pedigrees of autosomal dominant neurofibromatosis, type 1 (NF1) (Case 29). In the three-generation family on the left (see Fig. 10-14A), the

Table 10-1

LOD Score Table for Three Families with Retinitis Pigmentosa							
$\theta =$	0.00	0.01	0.05	0.10	0.20	0.30	0.40
Family 1	1.8	1.78	1.67	1.53	1.22	0.88	0.48
Family 2	1.2	1.19	1.11	1.02	0.82	0.58	0.32
Family 3	1.5	1.48	1.39	1.28	1.02	0.73	0.39
Total	4.5	4.45	4.17	3.83	3.06	2.19	1.19

$Z_{max} = 4.5$ at $\theta_{max} = 0$

affected mother, II-2, is heterozygous at both the NF1 locus *(D/d)* and a marker locus *(M/m)*, but we have no genotype information on her parents. Her unaffected husband, II-1, is homozygous both for the normal allele *d* at the NF1 locus and happens to be homozygous for allele *M* at the marker locus. He can only transmit to his offspring a chromosome that has the normal allele *(d)* and the *M* allele. By inspection, then, we can infer which alleles in each child have come from the mother. The two affected children received the *M* alleles along with the *D* disease allele, and the one unaffected has received the *m* allele along with the normal *d* allele. Without knowing the phase of these alleles in the mother, either all three offspring are recombinants or all three are nonrecombinants.

Which of these two possibilities is correct? There is no way to know for certain, and thus we must compare the likelihoods of the two possible results. Given that II-2 is an *M/m* heterozygote, we assume the correct phase on her two chromosomes is *D-m* and *d-M* half of the time and *D-M* and *d-m* the other half (we will discuss why this is a safe assumption later). If the phase of the disease allele is *D-m*, all three children have inherited a chromosome in which *no recombination* occurred between NF1 and the marker locus. If the probability of recombination between NF1 and the marker is θ, the probability of no recombination is $(1 - \theta)$, and the likelihood of having zero recombinant and three nonrecombinant chromosomes is $\theta^0 (1 - \theta)^3$. The contribution to the total likelihood, assuming this

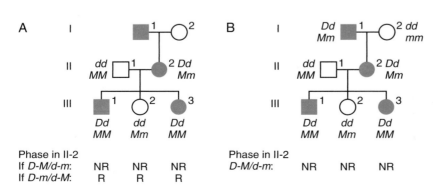

Figure 10-14 ■ Two pedigrees of autosomal dominant neurofibromatosis, type 1 (NF1). **A,** Phase of the disease allele *D* and marker alleles *M* and *m* in individual II-2 is unknown. **B,** Availability of genotype information for generation I allows a determination that the disease allele *D* and marker allele *M* are in coupling in individual II-2. NR, nonrecombinant; R, recombinant.

Table 10-2

Maximum Likelihood Analysis for Linkage Between NF1 and Marker Locus in Pedigrees in Figure 10-14

Type of Pedigree	LOD SCORES (Z) AT VARIOUS VALUES OF θ						
	0.00	0.01	0.05	0.10	0.20	0.30	0.40
Phase unknown $Z_{max} = 0.602$ at $\theta_{max} = 0$	.602	.589	.533	.465	.318	.170	.049
Phase known $Z_{max} = 0.903$ at $\theta_{max} = 0$	.903	.890	.837	.765	.612	.438	.237

phase is correct half the time, is $1/2\ \theta^0(1 - \theta)^3$. The other half of the time, however, the correct phase is *D-M* and *d-m*, which makes each of these three children *recombinants;* the likelihood, assuming this phase is correct half the time, is $1/2\ \theta^3(1 - \theta)^0$. To calculate the overall likelihood of this pedigree, we add the likelihood calculated assuming one phase in the mother is correct to the likelihood calculated assuming the other phase is correct. Therefore, the overall likelihood = $1/2(1 - \theta)^3 + 1/2(\theta^3)$.

On the other hand, if there is no linkage between these loci, one expects independent assortment of the two loci, and the probabilities of a recombinant and a nonrecombinant genotype in the offspring are both equal to 1/2. The probability of having three children with these genotypes, under the assumption of no linkage, is $(1/2)^3$, or 1/8. The relative odds for this pedigree, then, are:

$$\frac{1/2(1 - \theta)^3 + 1/2(\theta^3)}{1/8}$$

By evaluating the relative odds for values of θ from 0 to 0.5, the maximum value of the LOD score, Z_{max}, is found to be $\log_{10}(4) = 0.602$ when θ = 0.0 (Table 10-2). Because this is far short of a LOD score greater than 3, we would need at least five equivalent families to establish linkage (at θ = 0.0) between this marker locus and NF1. With slightly more complex calculations (made much easier by computer programs written to facilitate linkage analysis), one can calculate the LOD scores for other values of θ (see Table 10-2).

Why are the two phases in individual II-2 in the pedigree shown in Figure 10-14A equally likely? First, unless the marker locus and NF1 are so close together as to produce linkage disequilibrium between alleles at these loci, we would expect them to be in linkage equilibrium. Second, as discussed in Chapter 9, new mutations represent a substantial fraction of all the alleles in an autosomal dominant disease with reduced fitness, such as NF1. If new mutations are occurring independently and repeatedly, the alleles that happened to be present at the neighboring linked loci when each muta-

tion occurred in the *NF1* gene will then be the alleles in coupling with the new disease mutation. A group of unrelated families are likely to have many different mutant alleles, each of which is as likely to be in coupling with one polymorphic marker allele at a linked locus as with any other. Thus, it was a safe assumption that in the phase-unknown pedigree in Figure 10-14A, the phase of the alleles in individual II-2 is just as likely to be *D-M* and *d-m* as it is to be *D-m* and *d-M*.

Suppose now that additional genotype information, shown in Figure 10-14B, becomes available in the family in Figure 10-14A. By inspection, it is now clear that the maternal grandfather, I-1, must have transmitted both the NF1 allele *(D)* and the *M* allele to his daughter. This finding does not require any assumption about whether a crossover occurred in the grandfather's germline; all that matters is that we can be sure the paternally derived chromosome in individual II-2 must have been *D-M* and the maternally derived chromosome was *d-m*. The availability of genotypes in the first generation makes this a **phase-known pedigree.** The three children can now be scored definitively as nonrecombinant and we do not have to consider the opposite phase. The probability of having three children with the observed genotypes is now $(1 - \theta)^3$. As in the previous phase-unknown pedigree, the probability of the observed data if there is no linkage between the loci is $(1/2)^3 = 1/8$. Overall, the relative odds for this pedigree are $(1 - \theta)^3 \div 1/8$ in favor of linkage, and the maximum LOD score Z at θ = 0.0 is 0.903 or 8 to 1 (see Table 10-2). Thus, the strength of the evidence supporting linkage (8 to 1) is twice as great in the phase-known situation as in the phase-unknown situation (4 to 1).

Determining Phase from Pedigrees As shown in the pedigree in Figure 10-14B, having grandparental genotypes may be helpful in establishing phase in the next generation. However, depending on what the genotypes are, phase may not always be definitively determined. For example, if the grandmother, I-2, had been an *M/m* heterozygote, it would not be possible to determine the phase in the affected parent, individual II-2. For linkage analysis in X-linked pedigrees, the mother's father's

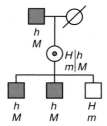

Figure 10-15 ■ Pedigree of X-linked hemophilia. The affected grandfather in the first generation has the disease (mutant allele *h*) and is hemizygous for allele *M* at an X-linked locus. No matter how far apart the marker locus and the factor VIII gene are on the X, there is no recombination involving the X-linked portion of the X chromosome in a male, and he will pass the hemophilia mutation *h* and allele *M* together. The phase in his daughter must be that *h* and *M* are in coupling.

genotype is particularly important because, as illustrated in Figure 10-15, it provides direct information on linkage phase in the mother. Because there can be no recombination between X-linked genes in a male and because the mother always receives her father's only X, any X-linked marker present in her genotype, but not in her father's, must have been inherited from her mother. Knowledge of phase, so important for genetic counseling, can thus be readily ascertained from the appropriate male members of an X-linked pedigree, if they are available for study.

⬤ MAPPING OF COMPLEX TRAITS

Knowing that a disease inherited as a complex trait has a significant hereditary component does not mean that the genes and molecular variants involved are known. Two major approaches have been used to locate and identify genes that predispose to complex diseases or contribute to the genetic variance of quantitative traits. The first is a type of linkage analysis that relies on pairs of family members, such as siblings, who are concordant for the phenotype; this is known as the **affected pedigree member method**. As shown previously in Chapter 8 (see Fig. 8-1), siblings have, on average, one allele of two in common (i.e., the same allele was inherited by both children from their parents) at any one locus. If a region of the genome is shared more frequently than expected by relatives concordant for a particular phenotype, the inference is that alleles predispose to that phenotype at one or more loci in that region. The second approach is known as **association**, which looks for increased frequency of particular alleles in affected compared with unaffected individuals in the population. Both approaches have advantages and disadvantages in particular situations, as described in this section.

Model-Free Linkage Analysis of Complex Disease Traits

Model-based linkage analysis, as described earlier in this chapter, is a powerful method for mapping single-gene disorders, but it is rarely applicable to complex traits. By their very nature, diseases inherited as complex traits are not usually amenable to an analysis that depends on knowing that a mutation in a single gene, inherited in a specific mendelian inheritance pattern, causes the disease. Instead, **model-free** (or **nonparametric**) **methods** have been developed that make no assumption concerning the number of loci at which alleles contribute to the trait (see Box). Such model-free methods depend solely on the assumption that affected relatives will be more likely to have disease-predisposing alleles in common than is expected by chance alone.

Model-Free Linkage Analysis of Qualitative (Disease) Traits

One type of model-free analysis is the **affected sibpair method**. Only siblings concordant for a disease are used, thereby eliminating the problem of determining whether an unaffected individual is a nonpenetrant carrier of the alleles that predispose to disease or simply did not inherit them. No assumptions need be made about the number of loci involved or the inheritance pattern. Instead, sibs are analyzed to determine whether there are loci at which affected sibpairs share alleles more frequently than the 50% expected by chance alone (see Fig. 8-1). In the affected sibpair method,

DNA of affected sibs is systematically analyzed by use of hundreds of polymorphic markers throughout the entire genome (a so-called **genome scan**) in a search for regions that are shared by the two sibs significantly more frequently than is expected on a purely random basis. When elevated degrees of allele-sharing are found at a polymorphic marker, it suggests that a locus involved in the disease is located close to the marker. Whether the degree of allele-sharing diverges significantly from the 50% expected by chance alone can be assessed by use of a maximum likelihood odds ratio to generate a **nonparametric LOD score** for excessive allele sharing, just as model-based linkage analysis uses a LOD score to assess the significance of a recombination frequency between two loci that appears to be less than 50%.

False-Positive Errors The more polymorphic loci across the genome that are analyzed for excessive allele-sharing, the more likely it is that some locus somewhere will show what looks like significantly elevated allele-sharing by chance alone. To understand why, consider the example of coin tossing. Although it is unlikely that a single experiment of tossing a coin five times will give five heads, it is very likely that if the experiment is repeated hundreds of times, at least one of those hundreds of experiments will yield five heads. In a typical genome scan using approximately 400 markers, nonparametric LOD score thresholds for determining significance of increased allele-sharing have been proposed to reduce the risk of inappropriately assigning significance to what is only random fluctuation from expected levels of allele-sharing. In this setting, a LOD score greater than approximately 3.6 for allele-sharing at a locus would occur with a probability of less than 1 in 20 by chance alone; a LOD score greater than 5.4 would occur by chance only once in 1000 studies.

Although the affected sibpair method does not require that one make possibly incorrect assumptions about how many loci are involved and how alleles at these various loci interact to cause disease, it does so at the cost of being insensitive and imprecise. Its insensitivity is reflected in the fact that large numbers of sibpairs are required to detect a significant deviation from the expected 50% allele-sharing. Suppose, for example, an allele at a disease locus has a frequency of 10% in the population and increases disease risk 4-fold in heterozygotes and 16-fold in homozygotes. In this situation, under the best of circumstances, it would take 185 sibpairs to detect an elevation of allele-sharing to nearly 60%. If the locus is a relatively infrequent contributor to the disease or causes much less of an increase in disease risk than 4-fold in heterozygotes, elevation of allele-sharing greater than 50% would be proportionately less. In this case, many, many more sibpairs, numbering in the thousands or tens of thou-

sands, would be needed to detect the locus. Thus, practically speaking, affected sibpair methods are unlikely to identify loci in which there are only a few rare alleles or the alleles make only minor contributions to a disease.

Model-free methods are also imprecise. Because one is not assuming that a single gene or a particular inheritance pattern is involved, one cannot determine definitively whether a recombination has occurred between a possible disease-predisposing locus and the disease phenotype. In model-based linkage strategy for fine mapping of a single-gene disease, the closest markers on either side of the disease gene that *do* recombine at least once with the disease gene define the boundaries of a narrow **critical interval** in which the disease gene must reside. In contrast, model-free methods can identify only broad regions of increased allele-sharing and not a narrow, critical region delimiting the location of a gene contributing to a complex trait. However, when the model-free linkage method has been used to highlight regions of interest, the search for variants in these regions that are in linkage disequilibrium with the disease gene can be used effectively to narrow the region of interest. This combined approach has had some success in finding disease alleles that contribute to such complex diseases as inflammatory bowel disease and age-related macular degeneration (see examples at the end of this chapter).

Model-Free Linkage Analysis of Quantitative Traits

Model-free linkage methods based on allele-sharing can also be used to map loci involved in quantitative complex traits. Although a number of approaches are available, one interesting example is the **highly discordant sibpair method.** Once again, no assumptions need be made about the number of loci involved or the inheritance pattern. Sibpairs with values of a physiological measurement that are at opposite ends of the bell-shaped curve are considered discordant for that quantitative trait and can be assumed to be less likely to share alleles at loci that contribute to the trait. The DNA of highly discordant sibs is then systematically analyzed by use of polymorphic markers throughout the entire genome in a search for regions that are shared by the two sibs significantly *less* frequently than is expected on a purely random basis. When reduced levels of allele-sharing are found at a polymorphic marker, it suggests that the marker is linked to a locus whose alleles contribute to whatever physiological measurement is under study.

Disease Association

An entirely different approach to identification of the genetic contribution to complex disease relies on finding *particular alleles* that are associated with the disease. The presence of a particular allele at a locus at increased or decreased frequency in affected individuals compared with controls is known as a **disease association.** In an association study, the frequency of a *particular allele* (such as for an HLA haplotype or a particular SNP or SNP haplotype) is compared among affected and unaffected individuals in the population (see Chapter 9).

	Patients	Controls	Totals
With allele	a	b	a + b
Without allele	c	d	c + d
Totals	a + c	b + d	

a = number of patients with the allele; b = number of controls with the allele; c = number of patients without the allele; d = number of controls without the allele.

If the study design is a case-control study (see Chapter 17) in which individuals with the disease are selected in the population, a matching group of controls without disease are then chosen, and the genotypes of individuals in the two groups are determined; an association between disease and genotype is then calculated by an **odds ratio.** Odds are ratios. With use of the above table, the odds of an allele carrier's developing the disease is the number of allele carriers that develop the disease (a) divided by the number of allele carriers who do not develop the disease (b). Similarly, the odds of a noncarrier's developing the disease is the number of noncarriers who develop the disease (c) divided by the number of noncarriers who do not develop the disease (d). The disease odds ratio is then the ratio of these odds, that is, a ratio of ratios.

$$\text{Disease Odds Ratio} = \frac{\dfrac{a}{b}}{\dfrac{c}{d}} = \frac{ad}{bc}$$

If the study was designed as a cross-sectional or cohort study (see Chapter 17), in which a random sample of the entire population is chosen and then analyzed both for disease and for the presence of the susceptibility genotype, the strength of an association can be measured by the **relative risk ratio (RRR).** The RRR compares the frequency of disease in all those who carry a susceptibility allele ([a/(a + b)] with the frequency of disease in all those who do not carry a susceptibility allele ([c/(c + d)].

$$\text{RRR} = \frac{\dfrac{a}{a+b}}{\dfrac{c}{c+d}}$$

The RRR is approximately equal to the odds ratio when the disease is rare (i.e., a < b and c < d). (Do not confuse relative risk ratio with λ_r, the **risk ratio in relatives,** which was discussed in Chapter 8. λ_r is the prevalence of a particular disease phenotype in an affected individual's relatives versus that in the general population.)

The **significance** of any association can be assessed in one of two ways. One is simply to ask if the values of a, b, c, and d differ from what would be expected if there were no association by a χ^2 test. The other is determined by a 95% **confidence interval** for the relative risk ratio. This interval is the range in which one would expect the RRR to fall 95% of the time that you genotype a similar group of cases and controls by chance alone. If the frequency of the allele in question were the same in patients and controls, the RRR would be 1. Therefore, when the 95% confidence interval excludes the value of 1, then the RRR deviates from what would be expected for no association with *P* value <0.05.

For example, suppose there were a case-control study in which a group of 120 patients with **cerebral vein thrombosis** (CVT) (discussed in Chapter 8) and 120 matched controls were genotyped for the 20210G > A allele in the prothrombin gene (see Chapter 8).

	Patients with CVT	Controls without CVT	Totals
20210G > A allele present	23	4	27
20210G > A allele absent	97	116	213
Total	120	120	240

There is clearly a significant increase in the number of patients carrying the 20210G > A allele versus controls ($\chi^2 = 15$ with 1 *df*; $P < 10^{-10}$). Since this is a case-control study, we use an odds ratio (OR) to assess the strength of the association.

$$\text{OR} = (23/4)/(97/116) = \sim 6.9$$

Strengths and Weaknesses of Association Studies

Association methods are powerful tools for pinpointing precisely the genes that contribute to genetic disease by demonstrating not only the genes but also the particular alleles responsible. They are also relatively easy to perform because one needs samples only from a set of affected individuals and controls and does not have to carry out laborious family studies and collection of samples from many members of a pedigree.

Association studies must be interpreted with caution, however, because an increased relative risk seen with an allele at a particular locus does not prove that the allele or even the locus at which the allele resides is involved in disease pathogenesis. There are two ways a particular allele may be associated with a disease, without that allele's being actually involved in causing the disease. First, and most serious, is the problem of totally artifactual association caused by **population stratification** (see Chapter 9). If a population is stratified into separate subpopulations (such as by ethnicity or religion) and members of one subpopulation rarely mate with members of other subpopulations, then a disease that happens to be more common in one subpopulation for whatever reason can appear (incorrectly) to be associated with any alleles that also happen to be more common in that subpopulation than in the population as a whole. Factitious association due to population stratification can be minimized, however, by careful selection of controls. Methods have also been developed that do not use a case-control design but that test for association between a disease and particular alleles within families. These methods require not only association but also that the associated allele be at a locus that is linked to the disease locus. Such family-based association methods are not subject to the artifacts caused by stratification.

A second limitation to inferring functional significance when an allele is found to be associated with a disease is that many loci can be in LD. Suppose two closely linked loci have two alleles that are in LD with each other. This means that when one of the alleles is present in a haplotype, the other one also has an increased chance of being present within this haplotype. In fact, *all* alleles in LD with an allele at a locus involved in the disease will show an apparently positive association, whether they have any functional relevance in disease predisposition or not. An association based on LD is still quite useful, however, since the associated alleles must at least be in loci that are close enough to the disease locus to appear associated.

Genome-Wide Association and the Haplotype Map

Up until now, association studies for human disease genes have been limited to particular sets of variants in restricted sets of genes. For example, geneticists might look for association with variants in genes encoding proteins thought to be involved in a pathophysiological pathway in a disease. Many such association studies were undertaken before the Human Genome Project era, with use of the HLA loci (see Chapter 9), because these loci are highly polymorphic and easily genotyped in case-control studies. A more powerful approach, however, would be to test systematically for association genome-wide between the more than 10 million variants in the genome and a disease phenotype, without any preconception of what genes and genetic variants might be contributing to the disease. Although such a massive undertaking is not currently feasible, recent advances in genomics, building on the HapMap (discussed earlier), make possible an approximation to a full-scale genome-wide association that still retains sufficient power to detect significant associations across the entire genome.

How does the HapMap facilitate genome-wide association studies? In discussing the limitations of association studies earlier, we pointed out that LD can lead to an apparent association in a case-control study between an allele and a disease, even when the allele is functionally *not* involved in disease pathogenesis, because the associated allele is in LD with another allele at a nearby locus that *is* functionally involved. Indeed, if the object of the association study is to immediately find *the* specific variant that contributes to the disease, then LD can confound the outcome. However, suppose one has less ambitious goals. A positive association between a disease and even one allele anywhere within an LD block immediately pinpoints the region of the genome located within the LD block as the region containing the disease-associated allele. Consequently, this region will be the place to search for the allelic variant that *is* functionally involved in the disease process itself. This strategy, of relying on LD to reduce the number of polymorphic alleles that need to be used in an association study, was a primary motivation for creation of the HapMap.

Tag SNPs   Once an allele within an LD block is found to be associated with a disease, are some alleles in that LD block better than others to serve as the representative for all the alleles with which it is in LD? By examining all the haplotypes within an LD block and measuring the degree of LD between alleles making up the haplotypes, it is possible to identify the most useful, minimum set of SNP alleles (so-called **tag SNPs**) that are capable of defining most of the haplotypes contained in each LD block with minimum redundancy. In theory, a set of well-chosen tag SNPs constitutes the minimal number of SNPs that need to be genotyped to provide nearly complete information on which haplotypes are present on any chromosome. A careful analysis of the patterns of LD blocks indicates that, in practice, genotyping a few hundred thousand tag SNPs is only a bit less useful for an association study than is genotyping more than 10 million SNP genotypes at every known variant in the genome. Any proposed set of tag SNPs will, however, need to be examined and refined before we know if the results based on the four populations studied in the HapMap project are applicable worldwide.

Limitations of Genome-Wide Association with the HapMap

Success in relying on LD between variants in disease genes and tag SNPs to find disease genes in populations worldwide depends on some fundamental assumptions: the allelic variant that contributes to a disease must (1) be common and (2) not be the result of recurrent independent mutational events. The frequency of the disease gene affects a genome-wide association study that relies on LD with tag SNPs because the haplotypes defined by tag SNPs in the HapMap are only the most common haplotypes in the various populations studied. If only a very small fraction of chromosomes with a particular haplotype contains the disease gene and most do not, individuals without the disease gene but with the haplotype will obscure any association that there might be between the haplotype and the disease. Recurrent mutation will also make it difficult to find an association with use of tag SNPs because if the same variant has occurred as a result of mutation multiple times on different haplotype backgrounds, no single haplotype will be in LD with the disease-associated allele.

The characteristics, strengths, and weaknesses of linkage and association methods for disease gene mapping are summarized in the Box.

● FROM GENE MAPPING TO GENE IDENTIFICATION

The application of gene mapping to medical genetics has met with many spectacular successes. The overall strategy—mapping the location of a disease gene by linkage analysis or other means, followed by attempts to identify the gene on the basis of its map position—is called **positional cloning**. This strategy has led to the identification of the genes associated with hundreds of mendelian disorders and to a small but increasing number of genes associated with genetically complex disorders. In this section, we present the cloning of the gene for cystic fibrosis (CF) and of genes associated with Crohn disease and age-related macular degeneration.

Positional Cloning of an Autosomal Recessive Disorder by Model-Based Linkage Mapping: Cystic Fibrosis

Because of its relatively high frequency, particularly in white populations, and the nearly total lack of understanding of its underlying physiological pathogenesis, CF (Case 10) (see Chapter 12) represented a prime target for positional cloning. DNA samples from nearly 50 CF

●■■ Comparison of Linkage and Association Methods

Linkage	Association
• Follows inheritance of a disease trait and regions of the genome from individual to individual in family pedigrees	• Tests for altered frequency of particular alleles or haplotypes in affected individuals compared with controls in a population
• Looks for regions of the genome harboring disease alleles; uses polymorphic variants only as a way of marking which region an individual has inherited from which parent	• Examines particular alleles or haplotypes for their contribution to the disease
• Uses hundreds to thousands of polymorphic markers across the genome	• Uses anywhere from a few markers in targeted genes to hundreds of thousands of markers for genome-wide analyses
• Not designed to find the specific variant responsible for or predisposing to the disease; can only demarcate where the variant can be found within (usually) one or a few megabases	• Can occasionally pinpoint the variant that is actually functionally responsible for the disease; more frequently, defines a disease-containing haplotype over a 1- to 10-kb interval (usually)
• Relies on recombination events occurring in families during only a few generations to allow measurement of the genetic distance between a disease gene and polymorphic markers on chromosomes	• Relies on finding a set of alleles, including the disease gene, that remained together for many generations because of a *lack* of recombination events among the markers
• Requires sampling of families, not just people affected by the disease	• Can be carried out on case-control or cohort samples from populations
• Loses power when disease has complex inheritance with substantial lack of penetrance	• Is sensitive to population stratification artifact, although this can be controlled by proper case-control designs or the use of family-based approaches
• Most often used to map disease-causing mutations with strong enough effects to cause a mendelian inheritance pattern	• Is the best approach for finding variants with small effect that contribute to complex traits

families were analyzed for linkage between CF and hundreds of DNA markers throughout the genome until linkage of CF to markers on the long arm of chromosome 7 was finally identified. Linkage to additional DNA markers in 7q31 to q32 narrowed the localization of the CF gene to an approximately 500-kb region of chromosome 7.

Linkage Disequilibrium in CF   At this point, however, an important feature of CF genetics emerged: even though the closest linked markers were still some distance from the CF gene, it became clear that there was significant LD between mutant alleles at the CF locus and a particular haplotype at loci tightly linked to the CF locus. Regions with the greatest degree of LD were analyzed for gene sequences, leading to the isolation of the CF gene in 1989. The gene responsible, which was named the cystic fibrosis transmembrane conductance regulator *(CFTR),* showed an interesting spectrum of mutations. A 3-bp deletion (ΔF508) that removed a phenylalanine at position 508 in the protein was found in approximately 70% of all mutant CF genes in northern European populations but never in normal alleles at this locus. Although subsequent studies have demonstrated many hundreds of mutant *CFTR* alleles worldwide, it was the high frequency of the ΔF508 mutation in the families used to map the CF gene and the LD between it and alleles at other polymorphic loci nearby that proved so helpful in the ultimate identification of the *CFTR* gene.

Mapping of the CF locus and cloning of the *CFTR* gene made possible a wide range of research advances and clinical applications, from basic pathophysiology to molecular diagnosis for genetic counseling, prenatal diagnosis, animal models, and finally current ongoing attempts to treat the disorder (see Box).

Positional Cloning of a Complex Disease Gene by Model-Free Linkage Mapping: Inflammatory Bowel Disease (Crohn Disease)

Inflammatory bowel disease (IBD) is a chronic inflammatory disease of the gastrointestinal tract that primarily affects adolescents and young adults. The disease is divided into two major categories: **Crohn disease** (Case 9) and **ulcerative colitis.** Family and twin studies indicate that Crohn disease is a complex genetic disease without a discernible mendelian inheritance pattern (see Chapter 8).

Many genome scans using affected sibpair and other model-free linkage analyses were carried out in families with two or more affected individuals. Among 11 regions of the genome with positive NPL scores, the one with the highest score (>5) showed linkage to Crohn disease only and not to ulcerative colitis; most of the others showed linkage to both forms of IBD. A locus, termed IBD1, was proposed to reside in this region of

---

▪▪▪ The Impact of Gene Mapping: The Example of Cystic Fibrosis

- 1985 — Gene for cystic fibrosis mapped to chromosome 7q31.2 by linkage in families. Linked markers were immediately applied to prenatal diagnosis and carrier testing in families.

- 1989 — Identification of *CFTR* as the one and only gene in which mutations cause cystic fibrosis. Mutational analysis was immediately applied to the diagnosis of affected individuals, prenatal diagnosis, and carrier testing in families.

- 1989 — *CFTR* mutation database established. It grows during the next 18 years to include more than 1400 different variant alleles with information on their frequency among different ethnic groups. Genetic factors in clinical heterogeneity (pancreatic function, congenital absence of vas deferens) are discovered.

- 1992 — Successful preimplantation diagnosis of cystic fibrosis.

- 1992 — First of many mouse models developed with a mutation in the *Cftr* gene.

- 1994 — First of many (and still ongoing) attempts to correct cystic fibrosis in patients by transfer of the normal *CFTR* gene into lung epithelial cells.

- 1997 — National Institutes of Health Consensus Conference recommends introduction of cystic fibrosis carrier screening. Widespread screening for carriers of dozens of mutations soon follows.

- 2003 — Preliminary progress reported on finding drugs with potential utility in cystic fibrosis based on knowledge of the spectrum of *CFTR* mutations, their effect on the expression and function of the CFTR proteins they encode, and the abnormalities in ion and H_2O transport caused by the loss of normal function of *CFTR*.

- 2005 — Modifier genes identified that can affect clinical severity of lung disease in cystic fibrosis, thereby suggesting alternative pathogenic pathways and novel treatments.

---

the highest LOD score, and researchers set about trying to find the gene involved.

The IBD1 Locus Is the *NOD2* Gene   Moving from model-free linkage analysis in IBD1 to use of LD for mapping, one of the markers in the original genome scan was found to be in LD with Crohn disease. Association studies using SNPs in the region of 160 kb around this marker revealed three SNPs with strong evidence for LD with the disease; all three were found to be located in the coding exons of the gene *NOD2* (also known as *CARD15*) and to cause either amino acid substitutions or premature termination of the protein. The NOD2 protein binds to gram-negative bacterial cell walls and participates in the inflammatory response to bacteria by activating the NF-κB transcription factor in mononuclear leukocytes. The three variants all reduce the ability of the NOD2 protein to activate NF-κB, suggesting that the variants in this gene alter the ability of monocytes in intestinal wall to respond to resident bacteria, thereby predisposing to an abnormal, inflammatory response. Thus, NOD2 variants are likely to be the alleles actually responsible for increased susceptibility to Crohn disease at the IBD1 locus. Additional studies in several independent cohorts of patients with Crohn disease have confirmed that these variants are strongly associated with Crohn disease. The genetic contribution of NOD2 variants to Crohn disease is also supported by showing a dosage effect; heterozygotes for the NOD2 variants have a 1.5- to 4-fold increased risk of the disease, whereas homozygotes or compound heterozygotes have a 15- to 40-fold increased risk.

The discovery of NOD2 variants helps explain the complex inheritance pattern in Crohn disease, since the variants are clearly neither necessary nor sufficient to cause Crohn disease. They are not necessary because although half of all white patients with Crohn disease have one or two copies of a NOD2 variant, half do not. NOD2 variants represent, at most, 20% of the genetic contribution to IBD in white patients. Furthermore, the particular variants associated with the disease risk in Europe are not found in Asian or African populations, and Crohn disease in these populations shows no association with NOD2. The variants are also not sufficient to cause the disease. The NOD2 variants are common in Europe; 20% of the population are heterozygous for these alleles and yet show no signs of IBD. Even in the highest risk genotype, those who are homozygotes or compound heterozygotes for the NOD2 variants, penetrance is less than 10%. The low penetrance points strongly to other genetic or environmental factors that act on genotypic susceptibility at the NOD2 locus. The obvious connection between Crohn disease, an inflammatory bowel disease, and structural variants in the NOD2 protein, a modulator of the innate antibacterial inflammatory response, is a strong clue as to what some of these environmental factors might be. The genetic analysis of Crohn disease exemplifies how we now think about the genetic contribution to complex traits and how we might identify these contributions and use them to further our understanding of all the factors, both genetic and environmental, that come together to cause a genetically complex disease.

Positional Cloning of a Complex Disease by Genome-Wide Association: Age-Related Macular Degeneration

Age-related macular degeneration (AMD) is a progressive degenerative disease of the portion of the retina responsible for central vision (Case 2). It causes blindness in 1.75 million Americans older than 50 years. The disease is characterized by the accumulation of extracellular protein deposits, referred to as drusen, behind the retina in the region of the macula. Although there is ample evidence for a genetic contribution to the disease, most individuals with AMD are not in families in which there is a clear mendelian pattern of inheritance. Environmental contributions are also important, as shown by the increased risk of AMD in cigarette smokers compared with nonsmokers.

A case-control genome-wide association study using only 100,000 SNPs revealed association of alleles at two common SNPs with AMD. Both alleles showed a 4-fold increase in the odds ratio for disease in affected individuals who were heterozygous for either of these SNP alleles and an approximately 6-fold to 7-fold increase in the odds ratio for disease in individuals homozygous for either of the risk alleles. Examination of HapMap data revealed that these two SNPs were in linkage disequilibrium with SNPs across an approximately 41-kb LD block on chromosome 1. Both SNPs were located within an intron of the gene encoding complement factor H (CFH), a regulator of the alternative complement pathway involved in inflammation. A search through the SNPs in LD with the two SNPs that showed a positive association revealed a nonsynonymous SNP that substituted a histidine for tyrosine at position 402 of the CFH protein (Tyr402His). The Tyr402His alteration, which has an allele frequency of 26% to 29% in white and African populations, showed an even stronger association with AMD than did the two SNPs that showed an association in the original collection of SNPs used for the genome-wide association study. The association of Tyr402His in the gene encoding CFH has been replicated in other case-control samples with AMD and is estimated to be responsible for 43% of all the genetic contribution to the disease.

Given that drusen contain complement factors and that CFH is found in retinal tissues around drusen, it is believed that the Tyr402His variant is less protective against the inappropriate inflammation that is thought to be responsible for drusen formation and retinal damage. Thus, Tyr402His is likely to be the variant at the CFH locus responsible for increasing the risk for AMD.

With the functional clue provided by the CFH association, variants in other components of the complement system have been investigated as candidate loci for AMD. SNPs in two more complement system genes, factor B and complement factor 2, were found to be strongly protective against AMD; in both cases, some of these SNPs altered amino acid residues and affected the function of the proteins encoded by these genes. Variants at all three of these loci are estimated to account for most of the genetic contribution to this disease.

In the example of AMD, a complex disease, a genome-wide association study led to the identification of strongly associated, common SNPs that in turn were in LD with a common coding SNP in the complement factor H gene that appears to be the functional variant involved in the disease. This discovery, in turn, led to the identification of other SNPs in the complement cascade that can also predispose to or protect against the disease. Taken together, these results give important clues to the pathogenesis of AMD and suggest that the complement pathway might be a fruitful target for novel therapies. We expect that many more genetic variants responsible for complex diseases will be successfully identified by genome-wide association with HapMap markers, thereby providing us with powerful insights and potential therapeutic targets for many of the common diseases that cause so much morbidity and mortality in the population.

● GENERAL REFERENCES

Gibson G, Muse SV: A Primer of Genome Science, 2nd ed. Sunderland, Mass, Sinauer Associates, 2004.

Terwilliger JD, Ott J: Handbook of Human Genetic Linkage. Baltimore, Md, Johns Hopkins University Press, 1994.

The International HapMap Consortium: A haplotype map of the human genome. Nature 437:1299-1320, 2005.

● REFERENCES FOR SPECIFIC TOPICS

Cho JH: Significant role of genetics in IBD: the *NOD2* gene. Rev Gastroenterol Disord 3:S18-S22, 2003.

de Bakker PI, Yelensky R, Pe'er I, et al: Efficiency and power in genetic association studies. Nat Genet 37:1217-1223, 2005.

Gold B, Merriam JE, Zernant J, et al: Variation in factor B *(BF)* and complement component 2 *(C2)* genes is associated with age-related macular degeneration. Nat Genet 38:458-462, 2006. Epub March 5, 2006.

Hugot JP: Inflammatory bowel disease: a complex group of genetic disorders. Best Pract Res Clin Gastroenterol 18:451-462, 2004.

Kerem E: Pharmacological induction of CFTR function in patients with cystic fibrosis: mutation-specific therapy. Pediatr Pulmonol 40:183-196, 2005.

Klein RJ, Zeiss C, Chew EY, et al: Complement factor H polymorphism in age-related macular degeneration. Science 308:385-389, 2005.

Kong A, Gudbjartsson DF, Sainz J, et al: A high-resolution recombination map of the human genome. Nat Genet 31:241-247, 2002.

Kruglyak L: Power tools for human genetics. Nat Genet 37:1299-1300, 2005.

Lander E, Kruglyak L: Genetic dissection of complex traits: guidelines for interpreting and reporting linkage results. Nat Genet 11:241-247, 1995.

Lander ES, Schork NJ: Genetic dissection of complex traits. Science 265:2037-2048, 1994.

Risch N, Merikangas K: The future of genetic studies of complex human diseases. Science 273:1516-1517, 1996.

● USEFUL WEBSITES

GDB Human Genome Database. *http://www.gdb.org/hugo/*
International HapMap Project. *http://www.hapmap.org/*

PROBLEMS

1. The Huntington disease (HD) locus was found to be tightly linked to a DNA polymorphism on chromosome 4. In the same study, however, linkage was ruled out between HD and the locus for the MNSs blood group polymorphism, which also maps to chromosome 4. What is the explanation?

2. Linkage between a polymorphism in the α-globin locus on the short arm of chromosome 16 and an autosomal dominant disease was analyzed in a series of British and Dutch families, with the following data:

θ	0.00	0.01	0.10	0.20	0.30	0.40
LOD scores *(Z)*	−∞	23.4	24.6	19.5	12.85	5.5

$Z_{max} = 25.85$ at $\theta_{max} = 0.05$

How would you interpret these data? What does the value of $Z = -\infty$ at $\theta = 0$ mean?

In a subsequent study, a large family from Sicily with what looks like the same disease was also investigated for linkage to α-globin, with the following results:

θ	0.00	0.10	0.20	0.30	0.40
LOD scores *(Z)*	−∞	−8.34	−3.34	−1.05	−0.02

How would you interpret the data in this second study? What implications do these data have for use of linkage information in presymptomatic diagnosis and genetic counseling?

3. This pedigree was obtained in a study designed to determine whether a mutation in a gene for γ-crystallin, one of the major proteins of the eye lens, may be responsible for an autosomal dominant form of cataract. The filled-in symbols in the pedigree indicate family members with cataracts. The letters indicate three alleles at the polymorphic γ-crystallin locus on chromosome 2. If you examine each affected person who has passed on the cataract to his or her children, how many of these represent a meiosis that is informative for linkage between the cataract and γ-crystallin? In which individuals is the phase known between the cataract mutation and the γ-crystallin alleles? Are there any meioses in which a crossover must have occurred to explain the data? What would you conclude about linkage between the cataract and γ-crystallin from this study? What additional studies might be performed to confirm or reject the hypothesis?

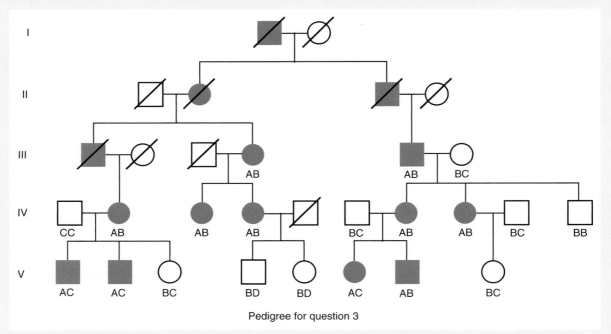

Pedigree for question 3

4. The following pedigree shows an example of molecular diagnosis in Wiskott-Aldrich syndrome, an X-linked immunodeficiency, by use of a linked DNA polymorphism with a map distance of approximately 5 cM between the polymorphic locus and the Wiskott-Aldrich syndrome gene.
    a. What is the likely phase in the carrier mother? How did you determine this? What diagnosis would you make regarding the current prenatal diagnosis if it were a male fetus?
    b. The maternal grandfather now becomes available for DNA testing and shows allele B at the linked locus. How does this finding affect your determination of phase in the mother? What diagnosis would you make now in regard to the current prenatal diagnosis?

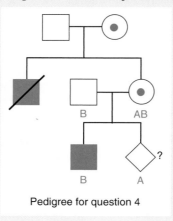

Pedigree for question 4

5. The Duchenne muscular dystrophy gene encoding the protein dystrophin was isolated by positional cloning in the 1980s. What impact has the identification of this gene had on diagnosis, management, treatment, and prevention of this severe childhood muscular dystrophy? Do you think that the impact of the recent finding of the NOD2 gene variants in Crohn disease will have a similar impact on that disease in the next 20 years? How are these two situations similar and different?

6. Estimates are that variants in the complement factor H, complement factor B, and complement component 2 genes can each account for 50%, 35%, and 40%, respectively, of the genetic risk for age-related macular degeneration (AMD). How could the fraction of genetic risk contributed by all three loci add up to more than 100%? Given that the sum of the risk conferred by variants at each of these three genes is so great, do these variants account for all the genetic risk for AMD worldwide?

Clinical Case Studies Illustrating Genetic Principles

These 43 clinical vignettes illustrate genetic principles in the practice of medicine. Each vignette is followed by a brief explanation or description of the disease and its etiology, pathophysiology, phenotype, management, and inheritance risk. These explanations and descriptions are based on current knowledge and understanding; therefore, like most things in medicine and science, they are subject to refinement and change as our knowledge and understanding evolve. The description of each case uses standard medical terminology; student readers, therefore, may need to consult a standard medical dictionary for explanations. Each vignette is also followed by a few questions that are intended to initiate discussion of some basic genetic or clinical principles illustrated by the case. Neither the vignettes nor the ensuing explanations or descriptions are intended to be definitive or comprehensive treatments of a topic.

The cases are not intended to direct medical care or to set a standard of care; they are simply illustrations of the application of genetic principles to the practice of medicine. Although the cases are loosely based on clinical experience, all individuals and medical details presented are fictitious.

Ada Hamosh, MD, MPH
Roderick R. McInnes, MD, PhD
Robert L. Nussbaum, MD
Huntington F. Willard, PhD

CASE PRESENTATIONS

1. Achondroplasia
2. Age-Related Macular Degeneration
3. Alzheimer Disease
4. Beckwith-Wiedemann Syndrome
5. Hereditary Breast and Ovarian Cancer
6. Charcot-Marie-Tooth Disease Type 1A
7. CHARGE Syndrome
8. Chronic Myelogenous Leukemia
9. Crohn Disease
10. Cystic Fibrosis
11. Deafness, Nonsyndromic
12. Duchenne Muscular Dystrophy
13. Familial Adenomatous Polyposis
14. Familial Hypercholesterolemia
15. Fragile X Syndrome
16. Glucose-6-Phosphate Dehydrogenase Deficiency
17. Hereditary Hemochromatosis
18. Hemophilia
19. Hereditary Nonpolyposis Colon Cancer
20. Hirschsprung Disease
21. Holoprosencephaly (Nonsyndromic Form)
22. Huntington Disease
23. Insulin-Dependent Diabetes Mellitus
24. Intrauterine Growth Restriction
25. Long QT Syndrome
26. Marfan Syndrome
27. Miller-Dieker Syndrome
28. Myoclonic Epilepsy with Ragged-Red Fibers
29. Neurofibromatosis 1
30. Non–Insulin-Dependent Diabetes Mellitus
31. Ornithine Transcarbamylase Deficiency
32. Polycystic Kidney Disease
33. Prader-Willi Syndrome
34. Retinoblastoma
35. Rett Syndrome
36. Sex Reversal
37. Sickle Cell Disease
38. Tay-Sachs Disease
39. Thalassemia
40. Thiopurine S-Methyltransferase Deficiency
41. Thrombophilia
42. Turner Syndrome
43. Xeroderma Pigmentosum

1. Achondroplasia

(*FGFR3* Mutation)
Autosomal Dominant

PRINCIPLES

- Gain-of-function mutations
- Advanced paternal age
- De novo mutation

MAJOR PHENOTYPIC FEATURES

- Age at onset: prenatal
- Rhizomelic short stature
- Megalencephaly
- Spinal cord compression

HISTORY AND PHYSICAL FINDINGS

P.S., a 30-year-old healthy woman, was 27 weeks pregnant with her first child. A fetal ultrasound examination at 26 weeks' gestation identified a female fetus with macrocephaly and rhizomelia (shortening of proximal segments of extremities). P.S.'s spouse was 45 years of age and healthy; he had three healthy children from a previous relationship. Neither parent has a family history of skeletal dysplasia, birth defects, or genetic disorders. The obstetrician explained to the parents that their fetus had the features of achondroplasia. The infant girl was delivered at 38 weeks' gestation by cesarean section. She had the physical and radiographic features of achondroplasia including frontal bossing, megalencephaly, midface hypoplasia, lumbar kyphosis, limited elbow extension, rhizomelia, trident hands, brachydactyly, and hypotonia. Consistent with her physical features, DNA testing identified a 1138G>A mutation leading to a glycine to arginine substitution at codon 380 (Gly380Arg) in the fibroblast growth factor receptor 3 gene (*FGFR3*).

BACKGROUND

Disease Etiology and Incidence

Achondroplasia (MIM# 100800), the most common cause of human dwarfism, is an autosomal dominant disorder caused by specific mutations in *FGFR3*; two mutations, 1138G>A (~98%) and 1138G>C (1% to 2%), account for more than 99% of cases of achondroplasia, and both result in the Gly380Arg substitution. Achondroplasia has an incidence of 1 in 15,000 to 1 in 40,000 live births and affects all ethnic groups.

Pathogenesis

FGFR3 is a transmembrane tyrosine kinase receptor that binds fibroblast growth factors. Binding of fibroblast growth factors to the extracellular domain of FGFR3 activates the intracellular tyrosine kinase domain of the receptor and initiates a signaling cascade. In endochondral bone, FGFR3 activation inhibits proliferation of chondrocytes within the growth plate and thus helps coordinate the growth and differentiation of chondrocytes with the growth and differentiation of bone progenitor cells.

The *FGFR3* mutations associated with achondroplasia are gain-of-function mutations that cause ligand-independent activation of FGFR3. Such constitutive activation of FGFR3 inappropriately inhibits chondrocyte proliferation within the growth plate and consequently leads to shortening of the long bones as well as to abnormal differentiation of other bones.

Guanine at position 1138 in the *FGFR3* gene is one of the most mutable nucleotides identified in *any* human gene. Mutation of this nucleotide accounts for nearly 100% of achondroplasia; more than 80% of patients have a de novo mutation. De novo mutations of *FGFR3* guanine 1138 occur exclusively in the father's germline and increase in frequency with advanced paternal age (>35 years) (see Chapter 7).

Phenotype and Natural History

Patients with achondroplasia present at birth with rhizomelic shortening of the arms and legs, relatively long and narrow trunk, trident configuration of the hands, and macrocephaly with midface hypoplasia and prominent forehead. They have a birth length that is usually slightly less than normal although occasionally within the low-normal range; their length or height falls progressively farther from the normal range as they grow.

In general, patients have normal intelligence, although most have delayed motor development. Their delayed motor development arises from a combination of hypotonia, hyperextensible joints (although the elbows have limited extension and rotation), mechanical difficulty balancing their large heads, and, less commonly, foramen magnum stenosis with brainstem compression.

Abnormal growth of the skull and facial bones results in midface hypoplasia, a small cranial base, and small cranial foramina. The midface hypoplasia causes dental crowding, obstructive apnea, and otitis media. Narrowing of the jugular foramina is believed to increase intracranial venous pressure and thereby to cause hydrocephalus. Narrowing of the foramen magnum often causes compression of the brainstem at the craniocervical junction in approximately 10% of patients and results in an increased frequency of hypotonia, quadriparesis, failure to thrive, central apnea, and sudden death. Between 3% and 7% of patients die unexpectedly during their first year of life because of brainstem compression (central apnea) or obstructive apnea. Other medical complications include obesity, lumbar spinal stenosis that worsens with age, and genu varum.

Management

Suspected on the basis of clinical features, the diagnosis of achondroplasia is usually confirmed by radiographic findings. DNA testing for *FGFR3* mutations can be helpful in ambiguous cases but is usually not necessary for the diagnosis to be made.

Throughout life, management should focus on the anticipation and treatment of the complications of achondroplasia. During infancy and early childhood, patients must be monitored for chronic otitis media, hydrocephalus, brainstem compression, and obstructive apnea and treated as necessary. Treatment of patients with brainstem compression by decompression of their craniocervical junction usually results in marked improvement of neurological function. During later childhood and through early adulthood, patients must be monitored for symptomatic spinal stenosis, symptomatic

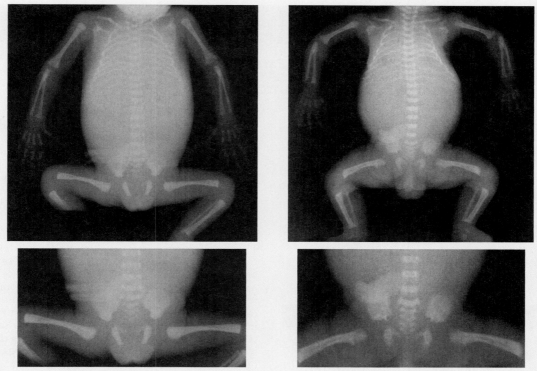

Figure C-1 ■ Radiographs of a normal 34-week fetus *(left)* and a 34-week fetus with achondroplasia *(right)*. Comparison of the upper frames shows rhizomelia and trident positioning of the fingers in the fetus with achondroplasia. Comparison of the lower frames illustrates the caudal narrowing of the interpedicular distance in the fetus with achondroplasia versus the interpedicular widening in the normal fetus. Also, the fetus with achondroplasia has small iliac wings shaped like an elephant's ear and narrowing of the sacrosciatic notch. (Courtesy of S. Unger, R. S. Lachman, and D. L. Rimoin, Cedars-Sinai Medical Center, Los Angeles.)

genu varum, obesity, dental complications, and chronic otitis media and treated as necessary. Treatment of the spinal stenosis usually requires surgical decompression and stabilization of the spine. Obesity is difficult to prevent and control and often complicates the management of obstructive apnea and joint and spine problems.

Both growth hormone therapy and surgical lengthening of the lower legs have been promoted for treatment of the short stature. Both therapies remain controversial.

In addition to management of their medical problems, patients often need help with social adjustment both because of the psychological impact of their appearance and short stature and because of their physical handicaps. Support groups often assist by providing interaction with similarly affected peers and social awareness programs.

INHERITANCE RISK

For normal parents with a child affected with achondroplasia, the risk of recurrence in their future children is low but probably higher than for the general population because mosaicism involving the germline, although extremely rare in achondroplasia, has been documented. For relationships in which one partner is affected with achondroplasia, the risk of recurrence in each child is 50% because achondroplasia is an autosomal dominant disorder with full penetrance. For relationships in which both partners are affected, each child has a 50% risk of having achondroplasia, a 25% risk of having lethal homozygous achondroplasia, and a 25% chance of being of normal stature. Cesarean section is required for a pregnancy in which a baby of normal stature is carried by a mother with achondroplasia.

Prenatal diagnosis before 20 weeks of gestation is available only by molecular testing of fetal DNA, although the diagnosis can be made late in pregnancy by analysis of a fetal skeletal radiograph (Fig. C-1). The features of achondroplasia cannot be detected by prenatal ultrasonography before 24 weeks' gestation, whereas the more severe thanatophoric dysplasia can be detected earlier.

Questions for Small Group Discussion

1. Name other disorders that increase in frequency with increasing paternal age. What types of mutations are associated with these disorders?
2. Discuss possible reasons that the *FGFR3* mutations 1138g>a and 1138g>c arise exclusively during spermatogenesis.
3. Marfan syndrome, Huntington disease, and achondroplasia arise as a result of dominant gain-of-function mutations. Compare and contrast the pathological mechanisms of these gain-of-function mutations.
4. In addition to achondroplasia, *FGFR3* gain-of-function mutations are associated with hypochondroplasia and thanatophoric dysplasia. Explain how phenotypic severity of these three disorders correlates with the level of constitutive FGFR3 tyrosine kinase activity.

REFERENCES

GeneTests. Medical genetics information resource [database online]. University of Washington, Seattle, 1993-2006. Updated weekly. *http://www.genetests.org*

OMIM: Online Mendelian Inheritance in Man. McKusick-Nathans Institute for Genetic Medicine, Johns Hopkins University, and National Center for Biotechnology Information, National Library of Medicine. *http://www.ncbi.nlm.nih.gov/entrez/query.fcgi?db=OMIM*

2. Age-Related Macular Degeneration

(Complement Factor H Variants)

Multifactorial

PRINCIPLES

- Complex inheritance
- Predisposing and resistance alleles, at several loci
- Gene-environment (smoking) interaction

MAJOR PHENOTYPIC FEATURES

- Age at onset: >50 years
- Gradual loss of central vision
- Drusen in the macula
- Changes in the retinal pigment epithelium
- Neovascularization (in "wet" form)

HISTORY AND PHYSICAL EXAMINATION

C.D., a 57-year-old woman, presents to her ophthalmologist for routine eye examination. She has not been evaluated in 5 years. She reports no change in visual acuity but has noticed that it takes her longer to adapt to changes in light level. Her mother was blind from age-related macular degeneration by her 70s. C.D. smokes a pack of cigarettes per day. On retinal examination, she has many drusen, yellow deposits found beneath the retinal pigment epithelium. A few are large and soft. She is told that she has early features of age-related macular degeneration, causing a loss of central vision that may progress to complete blindness over time. Although there is no specific treatment for this disorder, smoking cessation and oral administration of antioxidants (vitamins C and E and beta-carotene) and zinc are recommended as steps she can take to slow the progression of disease.

BACKGROUND

Disease Etiology and Incidence

Age-related macular degeneration (AMD, MIM# 603075) is a progressive degenerative disease of the macula, the region of the retina responsible for central vision, which is critical for fine vision (e.g., reading). It is one of the most common forms of blindness in the elderly. Early signs occur in 30% of all individuals older than 75 years; about one quarter of these individuals have severe disease with significant visual loss. AMD is rarely found in individuals younger than 55 years. Approximately 50% of the population-attributable genetic risk is due to a polymorphic variant, Tyr402His, in the complement factor H (*CFH*) gene. In contrast, polymorphic variants in two other genes in the alternative complement pathway, factor B (*CFB*) and complement component 2 (*C2*), confer a significantly *reduced* risk of AMD (see Chapter 10).

In addition to the polymorphisms in the three complement factor genes, mutations at other loci have been implicated in a small percentage of patients with AMD. In 7 of 402 patients with AMD, different heterozygous missense mutations were identified in the *FBLN5* gene encoding fibulin 5, a component of the extracellular matrix involved in the assembly of elastin fibers. All patients had small circular drusen and

retinal detachments. AMD was also seen among relatives of patients with Stargardt disease, an early-onset recessive form of macular degeneration seen in individuals homozygous for mutations in the *ABCA4* gene. The affected relatives were heterozygous for *ABCA4* mutations. Mutations at each of these loci account for only a small proportion of the large number of individuals with AMD.

Pathogenesis

The pathobiology of AMD is characterized by inflammation. The current view is that inflammatory insults characteristic of aging have a greater impact in the retina of individuals predisposed to AMD because of reduced activity of the alternative complement pathway in limiting the inflammatory response. The inflammation damages the photoreceptors of the macula, causing retinal atrophy. AMD is further divided into "dry" (atrophic) and "wet" (neovascular or exudative) types. Early AMD is usually dry. Dry AMD is characterized by large soft drusen, the clinical and pathological hallmark of AMD. Drusen are localized deposits of extracellular material behind the retina in the region of the macula. Although small "hard" drusen, which are small granular deposits commonly found in normal retinas, are not associated with macular degeneration, large soft drusen are strongly linked with AMD and are harbingers of retinal damage. As AMD progresses, there is thinning and loss of retinal tissue in focal or patchy areas. In about 10% of patients, retinal pigment epithelium remodeling occurs at the site of large, soft drusen. There is invasion of the subretinal space by new blood vessels (neovascularization) that grow in from the choroid. These vessels are fragile, break, and bleed in the retina, resulting in wet AMD.

Drusen contain complement factors, including CFH. Given that CFH is a negative regulator of the alternative complement cascade and the Tyr402His variant is less capable of inhibiting complement activation, Tyr402His is likely to be a functional variant that predisposes to AMD. Importantly, the CFH variants confer increased risk for both the wet and dry forms, suggesting that these two manifestations of the disease have a common basis.

The Leu9His and Arg32Gln variants in factor B and the Glu318Asp and intron 10 variants of component 2 reduce the risk for AMD substantially (odds ratios of 0.45 and 0.36, respectively). The mechanism by which the variants in the factor B and complement component 2 genes decrease the risk for AMD is not yet known but is also likely to occur through their effect on complement activation.

Although it is clear that environmental factors contribute to AMD, the only nongenetic risk factor identified to date is smoking. Interestingly, smoking significantly decreases serum levels of CFH. The reason for the epidemic of AMD in developed countries is unknown.

Phenotype and Natural History

AMD leads to changes in the central retina that are readily apparent by ophthalmoscopy (Fig. C-2). Patients complain of loss of central vision, making reading and driving difficult or impossible. Visual loss is generally slowly progressive in dry AMD. In contrast, the bleeding from neovascularization

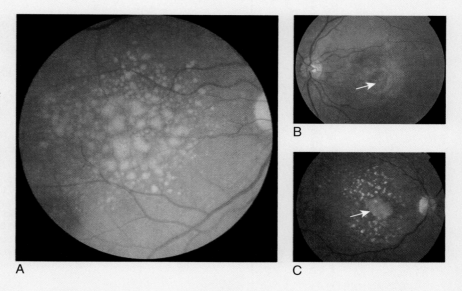

Figure C-2 ■ A, Funduscopic image of numerous large, soft drusen in and around the region of the fovea (dry AMD). B, Neovascularization and scarring in the region of the fovea (*arrow*). C, Area of thinning and loss of retinal tissue at the fovea ("geographic atrophy"; *arrow*), which tends to protect against neovascularization. (Courtesy of Alan Bird, Moorfields Eye Hospital, London.)

can lead to retinal detachment or bleeding under the retina and cause rapid vision loss. Peripheral vision is usually preserved.

Management

There is no specific treatment of the dry type of AMD. Smoking cessation is strongly indicated. Large clinical trials have suggested that for individuals with extensive intermediate-sized drusen or one large drusen, the use of antioxidants (vitamins A and E, beta-carotene) and zinc may slow progression of disease. Beta-carotene should probably not be used by smokers because some studies suggest it increases the risk of lung cancer and coronary heart disease.

For wet-type AMD, thermal laser photocoagulation, photodynamic therapy, and intravitreous injection of a vascular endothelial growth factor inhibitor (pegaptanib) may slow the rate of visual loss.

INHERITANCE RISK

The role of both genetic and environmental influences is demonstrated by twin studies showing concordance in monozygotic twins of 37%, far below the 100% expected for a purely genetic trait but still significantly greater than the 19% concordance in dizygotic twins, indicating there is a prominent genetic contribution to the disorder. First-degree relatives of patients are at a 4.2-fold greater risk for disease compared with the general population. Thus, AMD falls into

the category of a genetically complex disease trait. Despite ample evidence for familial aggregation in AMD, most affected individuals are not in families in which there is a clear mendelian pattern of inheritance.

Questions for Small Group Discussion

1. How could mutations in a complement factor account for a disease limited to the eye?
2. Suggest other types of proteins that could be implicated in AMD.
3. Discuss possible reasons that *ABCR* mutations account for such a small proportion of AMD if they are the main cause of Stargardt disease.
4. How would antibodies against vascular endothelial growth factor help in wet-type AMD? Suggest other diseases for which this treatment might be effective alone or in conjunction with other therapies.

REFERENCES

Arroyo JG: Age-related macular degeneration. UpToDate version 13.3, 2006. *http://uptodate.com*

Kourlas H, Schiller DS: Pegaptanib sodium for the treatment of neovascular age-related macular degeneration: a review. Clin Ther 28:36-44, 2006.

OMIM: Online Mendelian Inheritance in Man. McKusick-Nathans Institute for Genetic Medicine, Johns Hopkins University, and National Center for Biotechnology Information, National Library of Medicine. *http://www.ncbi.nlm.nih.gov/entrez/query.fcgi?db=OMIM*

Pauleikhoff D: Neovascular age-related macular degeneration: natural history and treatment outcomes. Retina 25:1065-1084, 2005.

3. Alzheimer Disease

(Cerebral Neuronal Dysfunction and Death)
Multifactorial or Autosomal Dominant

PRINCIPLES

- Variable expressivity
- Genetic heterogeneity
- Gene dosage
- Toxic gain of function
- Risk modifier

MAJOR PHENOTYPIC FEATURES

- Age at onset: middle to late adulthood
- Dementia
- β-Amyloid plaques
- Neurofibrillary tangles
- Amyloid angiopathy

HISTORY AND PHYSICAL FINDINGS

L.W. was an elderly woman with dementia. Eight years before her death, she and her family noticed a deficit in her short-term memory. Initially, they ascribed this to the forgetfulness of "old age"; her cognitive decline continued, however, and progressively interfered with her ability to drive, shop, and look after herself. L.W. did not have findings suggestive of thyroid disease, vitamin deficiency, brain tumor, drug intoxication, chronic infection, depression, or strokes; magnetic resonance imaging of her brain showed diffuse cortical atrophy. L.W.'s brother, father, and two other paternal relatives had died of dementia in their 70s. A neurologist explained to L.W. and her family that normal aging is not associated with dramatic declines in memory or judgment and that declining cognition with behavioral disturbance and impaired daily functioning suggested a clinical diagnosis of familial dementia, possibly Alzheimer disease. The suspicion of Alzheimer disease was supported by her apolipoprotein E genotype: ε4/ε4. L.W.'s condition deteriorated rapidly during the next year, and she died of malnutrition at 82 years of age. Her autopsy confirmed the diagnosis of Alzheimer disease.

BACKGROUND

Disease Etiology and Incidence

Approximately 10% of persons older than 70 years have dementia, and about half of them have Alzheimer disease (AD, MIM# 104300). AD is a panethnic, genetically heterogeneous disease; less than 5% of patients have early-onset familial disease, 15% to 25% have late-onset familial disease, and 75% have sporadic disease. Approximately 10% of familial AD exhibits autosomal dominant inheritance; the remainder exhibits multifactorial inheritance.

Current evidence suggests that defects of β-amyloid precursor protein metabolism cause the neuronal dysfunction and death observed with AD. Consistent with this hypothesis, mutations associated with early-onset autosomal dominant AD have been identified in the β-amyloid precursor protein gene (APP), the presenilin 1 gene (PSEN1), and the presenilin 2 gene (PSEN2) (see Chapter 12). The prevalence of mutations in these genes varies widely, depending on the inclusion criteria of the study; 20% to 70% of patients with early-onset autosomal dominant AD have mutations in PSEN1, 1% to 2% have mutations in APP, and less than 5% have mutations in PSEN2.

No mendelian causes of late-onset AD have been identified; however, both familial AD and sporadic late-onset AD are strongly associated with allele ε4 at the apolipoprotein E gene (APOE; see Chapter 8). The frequency of ε4 is 12% to 15% in normal controls compared with 35% in all patients with AD and 45% in patients with a family history of dementia.

Pathogenesis

A β-amyloid precursor protein (APP) undergoes endoproteolytic cleavage to produce peptides with neurotrophic and neuroprotective activities. Cleavage of APP within the endosomal-lysosomal compartment produces a carboxyl-terminal peptide of 40 amino acids ($A\beta_{40}$); the function of $A\beta_{40}$ is unknown. In contrast, cleavage of APP within the endoplasmic reticulum or cis-Golgi produces a carboxyl-terminal peptide of 42 or 43 amino acids ($A\beta_{42/43}$). $A\beta_{42/43}$ readily aggregates and is neurotoxic in vitro and possibly in vivo. Patients with AD have a significant increase in $A\beta_{42/43}$ aggregates within their brains. Mutations in APP, PSEN1, and PSEN2 increase the relative or absolute production of $A\beta_{42/43}$. About 1% of all cases of AD occur in patients with Down syndrome, who overexpress APP (the gene for APP is on chromosome 21) and thus $A\beta_{42/43}$. The role of APOE ε4 is clear but the mechanism is uncertain.

AD is a central neurodegenerative disorder, especially of cholinergic neurons of the hippocampus, neocortical association area, and other limbic structures. Neuropathological changes include cortical atrophy, extracellular neuritic plaques, intraneuronal neurofibrillary tangles (Fig. C-3), and amyloid deposits in the walls of cerebral arteries. The neuritic plaques (Fig. C-3) contain many different proteins including $A\beta_{42/43}$ and apolipoprotein E. The neurofibrillary tangles are composed predominantly of hyperphosphorylated tau protein; tau helps maintain neuronal integrity, axonal transport, and axonal polarity by promoting the assembly and stability of microtubules.

Phenotype and Natural History

AD is characterized by a progressive loss of cognitive function including recent memory, abstract reasoning, concentration, language, visual perception, and visual-spatial function. Beginning with a subtle failure of memory, AD is often attributed initially to benign "forgetfulness." Some patients perceive their cognitive decline and become frustrated and anxious, whereas others are unaware. Eventually, patients are unable to work, and they require supervision. Social etiquette and superficial conversation are often retained surprisingly well. Ultimately, most patients develop rigidity, mutism, and incontinence and are bedridden. Other symptoms associated with AD include agitation, social withdrawal, hallucinations, seizures, myoclonus, and parkinsonian features. Death usually results from malnutrition, infection, or heart disease.

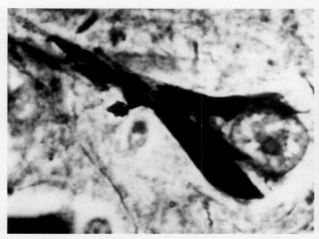 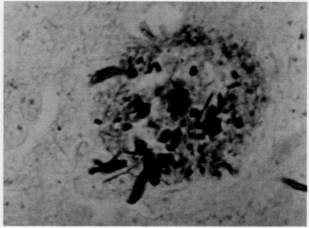

Figure C-3 ■ A neurofibrillary tangle *(left)* and a neuritic plaque *(right)* observed on histopathological examination of the brain of an individual with Alzheimer disease. (Courtesy of D. Armstrong, Baylor College of Medicine and Texas Children's Hospital, Houston.)

Aside from the age at onset, early-onset AD and late-onset AD are clinically indistinguishable. Mutations in *PSEN1* are fully penetrant and usually cause rapidly progressive disease with a mean onset at 45 years. Mutations in *APP* are fully penetrant and cause a rate of AD progression similar to that of late-onset AD; the age at onset ranges from 40s to early 60s. Mutations in *PSEN2* may not be fully penetrant and usually cause slowly progressive disease with onset ranging from 40 to 75 years. In contrast to early-onset AD, late-onset AD develops after 60 to 65 years of age; the duration of disease is usually 8 to 10 years, although the range is 2 to 25 years. For both late-onset AD and AD secondary to *APP* mutations, the *APOE* allele ε4 is a dose-dependent modifier of onset; that is, the age at onset varies inversely with the number of copies of the ε4 allele.

Management

Except for patients in families segregating an AD-associated mutation, patients with dementia can be definitively diagnosed with AD only by autopsy; however, with rigorous adherence to diagnostic criteria, a clinical suspicion of AD is confirmed by neuropathological examination 80% to 90% of the time. The accuracy of the clinical suspicion increases to 97% if the patient is homozygous for allele ε4 of *APOE*.

Because no curative therapies are available for AD, treatment is focused on the amelioration of associated behavioral and neurological problems. Approximately 10% to 20% of patients have a modest decrease in the rate of cognitive decline if they are treated early in the disease course with agents that increase cholinergic activity.

INHERITANCE RISK

Old age, family history, female gender, and Down syndrome are the most important risk factors for AD. In Western populations, the empirical lifetime risk for AD is 5%. If patients have a first-degree relative in whom AD developed after 65 years, they have a 3-fold to 6-fold increase in their risk of AD. If patients have a sibling in whom AD developed before 70 years and an affected parent, their risk is increased 7-fold to 9-fold. *APOE* testing may be used as an adjunct diagnostic test in individuals seeking evaluation for signs and symptoms suggestive of dementia but should not be used for predictive testing for AD in asymptomatic patients.

Patients with Down syndrome have an increased risk for AD. After the age of 40 years, nearly all patients with Down syndrome have neuropathological findings of AD, and approximately 50% experience cognitive decline.

For families segregating autosomal dominant AD, each person has a 50% risk of inheriting an AD-causing mutation. With the exception of some *PSEN2* mutations, full penetrance and relatively consistent age at onset within a family facilitate genetic counseling. Currently, clinical DNA testing is available for *APP, PSEN1,* and *PSEN2;* DNA testing should be offered only in the context of genetic counseling.

Questions for Small Group Discussion

1. Why is the *APOE* genotype not useful for predicting AD in asymptomatic individuals?
2. Why is AD usually a neuropathological diagnosis? What is the differential diagnosis for AD?
3. Mutation of *MAPT,* the gene encoding tau protein, causes frontotemporal dementia; however, *MAPT* mutations have not been detected in AD. Compare and contrast the proposed mechanisms by which abnormalities of tau cause dementia in AD and frontotemporal dementia.
4. Approximately 30% to 50% of the population risk for AD is attributed to genetic factors. What environmental factors are proposed for the remaining risk? What are the difficulties with conclusively identifying environmental factors as risks?

REFERENCES

GeneTests. Medical genetics information resource [database online]. University of Washington, Seattle, 1993-2006. Updated weekly. *http://www.genetests.org*

OMIM: Online Mendelian Inheritance in Man. McKusick-Nathans Institute for Genetic Medicine, Johns Hopkins University, and National Center for Biotechnology Information, National Library of Medicine. *http://www.ncbi.nlm.nih.gov/entrez/query.fcgi?db=OMIM*

4. Beckwith-Wiedemann Syndrome

(Uniparental Disomy and Imprinting Defect)

Chromosomal with Imprinting Defect

PRINCIPLES

- Multiple pathogenic mechanisms
- Imprinting
- Uniparental disomy
- Assisted reproductive technology

MAJOR PHENOTYPIC FEATURES

- Age at onset: prenatal
- Prenatal and postnatal overgrowth
- Macroglossia
- Omphalocele
- Visceromegaly
- Embryonal tumor in childhood
- Hemihyperplasia
- Renal abnormalities
- Adrenocortical cytomegaly
- Neonatal hypoglycemia

HISTORY AND PHYSICAL FINDINGS

A.B., a 27-year-old G1P0 female, presented to a prenatal diagnostic center for level II ultrasonography and genetic counseling after a routine ultrasound examination revealed a large for gestational age male fetus with possible omphalocele. The pregnancy, the first for each of his parents, was undertaken without assisted reproductive technology. After confirmation by level II ultrasonography, the family was counseled that the fetus had a number of abnormalities most consistent with Beckwith-Wiedemann syndrome, although other birth defects were also possible. The couple decided not to undergo amniocentesis. The baby, B.B., was delivered by cesarean section at 37 weeks with a birth weight of 9 pounds, 2 ounces and a notably large placenta. Omphalocele was noted, as were macroglossia and vertical ear lobe creases.

A genetics consultant made a clinical diagnosis of Beckwith-Wiedemann syndrome. When hypoglycemia developed, B.B. was placed in the newborn intensive care unit and was treated with intravenous administration of glucose for 1 week; the hypoglycemia resolved spontaneously. The findings on cardiac evaluation were normal, and the omphalocele was surgically repaired without difficulty. Methylation studies of the KCNQOT1 gene confirmed an imprinting defect at 11p15 consistent with the diagnosis of Beckwith-Wiedemann syndrome. Abdominal ultrasound examination to screen for Wilms tumor was recommended every 3 months until B.B. was 8 years old, and serum alpha-fetoprotein was recommended every 6 weeks as a screen for hepatoblastoma for the first 3 years of life. At a follow-up visit, the family was counseled that in view of their negative family history and normal parental karyotypes, the imprinting defect was consistent with sporadic Beckwith-Wiedemann syndrome and the recurrence risk was low.

BACKGROUND

Disease Etiology and Incidence

Beckwith-Wiedemann syndrome (BWS) (MIM# 130650) is a panethnic syndrome that is usually sporadic but may rarely be inherited as an autosomal dominant. BWS affects approximately one in 13,700 live births.

BWS results from an imbalance in the expression of imprinted genes in the p15 region of chromosome 11. These genes include KCNQOT1 and H19, which are transcribed but are not translated, and CDKN1C and IGF2, which do encode proteins. Normally, these genes are imprinted and expressed from the paternal allele only (IGF2 and KCNQOT1) or the maternal allele only (H19 and CDKN1C). IGF2 encodes an insulin-like growth factor that *promotes* growth; in contrast, CDKN1C encodes a cell cycle suppressor that *constrains* cell division and growth. Transcription of H19 and KCNQOT1 RNA suppresses expression of the maternal copy of IGF2 and the paternal copy of CDKN1C, respectively.

Unbalanced expression of 11p15 imprinted genes can occur through a number of mechanisms. Mutations in the maternal CDKN1C allele are found in 5% to 10% of sporadic cases and in 40% of families with autosomal dominant BWS. The majority of patients with BWS, however, have loss of expression of the maternal CDKN1C allele due to abnormal imprinting, not mutation. In 10% to 20% of individuals with BWS, loss of maternal CDKN1C expression and increased IGF2 expression are caused by paternal isodisomy of 11p15. Because the somatic recombination leading to segmental uniparental disomy occurs after conception, individuals with segmental uniparental disomy are mosaic and may require testing of tissues other than blood to reveal the isodisomy. Another 1% to 2% of BWS patients have a detectable chromosomal abnormality, such as maternal translocation, inversion of chromosome 11, or duplication of paternal chromosome 11p15. Thus, parental karyotyping to rule out a structural abnormality of 11p15 is necessary to guide genetic counseling. Rare microdeletions in KCNQOT1 or H19 that disrupt imprinting have also been found in BWS. In the remaining patients, the abnormalities in imprinting and gene expression are unexplained.

Pathogenesis

During gamete formation and early embryonic development, a different pattern of DNA methylation is established within the KCNQOT1 and H19 genes between males and females. Abnormal imprinting in BWS is most easily detected by analysis of DNA methylation at specific CpG islands in the KCNQOT1 and H19 genes. In 60% of patients with BWS, there is hypomethylation of the maternal KCNQOT1. In another 2% to 7% of patients, *hypermethylation* of the maternal H19 gene decreases its expression, resulting in excess IGF2 expression. Inappropriate IGF2 expression from both parental alleles may explain some of the overgrowth seen in BWS. Similarly, loss of expression of the maternal copy of CDKN1C removes a constraint on fetal growth.

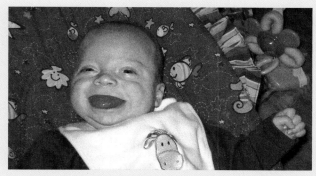

Figure C-4 ■ Characteristic macroglossia in a 4-month-old male infant with Beckwith-Wiedemann syndrome. The diagnosis was made soon after birth on the basis of the clinical findings of macrosomia, macroglossia, omphalocele, a subtle ear crease on the right, and neonatal hypoglycemia. Organomegaly was absent. Karyotype was normal, and molecular studies showed hypomethylation of the *KCNQOT1* gene. (Courtesy of Rosanna Weksberg and Cheryl Shuman, Hospital for Sick Children, Toronto, Canada.)

Phenotype and Natural History

BWS is associated with prenatal and postnatal overgrowth. Up to 50% of affected individuals are premature and large for gestational age at birth. The placentas are particularly large and pregnancies are frequently complicated by polyhydramnios. Additional complications in infants with BWS include omphalocele, macroglossia (Fig. C-4), neonatal hypoglycemia, and cardiomyopathy, all of which contribute to a 20% mortality rate. Neonatal hypoglycemia is typically mild and transient, but some cases of more severe hypoglycemia have been documented. Renal malformations and elevated urinary calcium with nephrocalcinosis and lithiasis are present in almost half of BWS patients. Hyperplasia of various body segments or of selected organs may be present at birth and may become more or less evident over time. Development is typically normal in individuals with BWS unless they have an unbalanced chromosome abnormality.

Children with BWS have an increased risk for development of embryonal tumors, particularly Wilms tumor and hepatoblastoma. The overall risk of neoplasia in children with BWS is approximately 7.5%; the risk is much lower after 8 years of age.

Management

Management of BWS involves treatment of presenting symptoms, such as omphalocele repair and management of hypoglycemia. Special feeding techniques or speech therapy may be required due to the macroglossia. Surgical intervention may be necessary for abdominal wall defects, leg length discrepancies, and renal malformations. If hypercalciuria is present, medical therapy may be instituted to reduce calcium excretion. Periodic screening for embryonal tumors is essential because these are fast-growing and dangerous neoplasias. The current recommendations for monitoring for tumors are an abdominal ultrasound examination every 3 months for the first 8 years of life and measurement of serum alpha-fetoprotein for hepatoblastoma every 6 weeks for the first few years of life.

RECURRENCE RISK

The recurrence risk for siblings and offspring of children with BWS varies greatly with the molecular basis of their condition. See the Table for the recurrence risk for various molecular alterations.

Increased Risk of BWS with Assisted Reproductive Technologies

Assisted reproductive technologies (ART), such as in vitro fertilization (IVF) and intracytoplasmic sperm injection, have become commonplace, accounting now for 1% to 2% of all births in many countries. Retrospective studies demonstrated that ART had been used 10 to 20 times more frequently in the pregnancies that resulted in infants with BWS compared with controls. The risk of BWS after IVF is estimated to be 1 in 4000, which is 9-fold higher than in the general population.

The reason for the increased incidence of imprinting defects with ART is unknown. The incidence of Prader-Willi syndrome (see Case 33), a defect in paternal imprinting, has *not* been shown to be increased with IVF, whereas the frequency of Angelman syndrome, a maternal imprinting defect, *is* increased with IVF, suggesting a specific relationship between ART and maternal imprinting. Since the paternal imprint takes place well before IVF, whereas maternal imprinting takes place much closer to the time of fertilization, a role for IVF itself in predisposing to imprinting defects merits serious study.

DIAGNOSTIC APPROACHES IN BECKWITH-WIEDEMANN SYNDROME

Test Method	Alteration Detected	Detection Rate	Recurrence Risk to Sibs	Recurrence Risk to Offspring
Karyotype, fluorescence in situ hybridization	Cytogenetic duplication (paternal); translocation, inversion (maternal)	1%-2%	Low if sporadic, variable if parental	Variable with abnormality
Methylation studies	*KCNQOT1* (*LIT1*) hypomethylation	50%-60%	Low	Probably low
	H19 hypermethylation	2%-7%		
Microsatellite analysis	11p15 paternal uniparental disomy	10%-20%	Very low	Very low
Sequencing	*CDKN1C* gene mutations	5%-10% sporadic cases	50% if parent has mutation, low if not	50% if patient is female; increased but not defined if male
		40% autosomal dominant families	~50%	50% if patient is female; increased but not defined if male

Questions for Small Group Discussion

1. Discuss possible reasons for embryonal tumors in BWS. Why would these decline in frequency with age?
2. Discuss reasons why imprinted genes frequently affect fetal size. Name another condition associated with uniparental disomy for another chromosome.
3. Besides imprinting defects, discuss other genetic disorders that may cause infertility and yet can be passed on by means of ART.
4. In addition to mutations in the genes implicated in BWS, discuss how a mutation in the imprinting locus control region could cause BWS.

REFERENCES

Allen C, Reardon W: Assisted reproduction technology and defects of genomic imprinting. BJOG 112:1589-1594, 2005.

GeneTests. Medical genetics information resource [database online]. University of Washington, Seattle, 1993-2006. Updated weekly. *http://www.genetests.org*

Maher E: Imprinting and assisted reproductive technology. Hum Mol Genet 14(Spec No 1):R133-R138, 2005.

OMIM: Online Mendelian Inheritance in Man. McKusick-Nathans Institute for Genetic Medicine, Johns Hopkins University, and National Center for Biotechnology Information, National Library of Medicine. *http://www.ncbi.nlm.nih.gov/entrez/query.fcgi?db=OMIM*

5. Hereditary Breast and Ovarian Cancer

(*BRCA1* and *BRCA2* Mutations)

Autosomal Dominant

PRINCIPLES

- Tumor-suppressor gene
- Multistep carcinogenesis
- Somatic mutation
- Incomplete penetrance and variable expressivity
- Founder effect

MAJOR PHENOTYPIC FEATURES

- Age at onset: adulthood
- Breast cancer
- Ovarian cancer
- Prostate cancer
- Multiple primary cancers

HISTORY AND PHYSICAL FINDINGS

S.M., a 27-year-old previously healthy woman, was referred to the cancer genetics clinic by her gynecologist after being diagnosed with breast cancer. She was concerned about her children's risk for development of cancer and about her risk for development of ovarian cancer. Her mother, two maternal aunts, and maternal grandfather had breast cancer; her mother had also had ovarian cancer (Fig. C-5). The genetic counselor explained that the family history of breast cancer was indicative of an inherited predisposition and calculated that the proband's risk for carrying a mutation in the breast cancer susceptibility gene *BRCA1* or *BRCA2* was well above the threshold for considering gene sequencing. On the basis of the ensuing discussion of prognosis and recurrence risks, S.M. chose to pursue DNA sequencing of *BRCA1* and *BRCA2*. This testing showed that she had a premature termination mutation in one *BRCA2* allele that had been previously seen in other patients with early-onset breast cancer. During the discussion of the results, S.M. inquired whether her 6- and 7-year-old girls should be tested. The genetic counselor explained that because the mutations posed little risk in childhood, the decision to have genetic testing was better left until the children were mature enough to decide on the utility of such testing, and S.M. agreed.

Five adult relatives elected to have predictive testing, and four, including one male, were found to be carriers of the mutation; one of these four, a female, pursued prophylactic bilateral mastectomy. The risk for cancers at other sites was also discussed with all mutation carriers.

BACKGROUND

Disease Etiology and Incidence

Mutations of major cancer predisposition genes account for 3% to 10% of cases of breast cancer and have an estimated overall prevalence of 1 in 300 to 1 in 800. Two of these genes are *BRCA1* and *BRCA2*. In the general North American population, the prevalence of *BRCA1* mutations is between 1 in 500 and 1 in 1000; the prevalence of *BRCA2* mutations is approximately twice as high. There are, however, marked differences in ethnic distribution of deleterious mutations among families with two or more cases of breast or ovarian cancer. Mutations of *BRCA1* or *BRCA2* account for approximately 70% to 80% of *familial* breast cancer but only a small fraction of breast cancer overall (see Chapter 16).

Pathogenesis

BRCA1 and *BRCA2* encode ubiquitously expressed nuclear proteins that are believed to maintain genomic integrity by regulating DNA repair, transcriptional transactivation, and the cell cycle.

Despite the ubiquitous expression of *BRCA1* and *BRCA2*, mutation of these genes predisposes predominantly to breast and ovarian neoplasias. Loss of *BRCA1* or *BRCA2* function probably permits the accumulation of other mutations that are directly responsible for neoplasia. Consistent with this hypothesis, breast and ovarian carcinomas from patients with mutations of *BRCA1* or *BRCA2* have chromosomal instability and frequent mutations in other tumor-suppressor genes.

Tumor formation in carriers of *BRCA1* or *BRCA2* germline mutations follows the two-hit hypothesis; that is, both alleles of either *BRCA1* or *BRCA2* lose function in tumor cells (see Chapter 16). Somatic loss of function by the second allele occurs by loss of heterozygosity, intragenic mutation, or promoter hypermethylation. Because of the high frequency with which the second allele of *BRCA1* or *BRCA2* loses function, families segregating a germline *BRCA1* or *BRCA2* mutation exhibit autosomal dominant inheritance of neoplasia.

The population prevalence of *BRCA1* or *BRCA2* germline mutations varies widely and often suggests a founder effect. In Iceland, the *BRCA2* 999del5 mutation occurs on a specific haplotype and has a prevalence of 0.6%. Among Ashkenazi Jews, the *BRCA1* 185delAG and 5382insC mutations and the *BRCA2* 6174delT mutation also occur on specific haplotypes and have prevalences of 1%, 0.4%, and 1.2%, respectively.

Phenotype and Natural History

Patients with *BRCA1* or *BRCA2* germline mutations have an increased risk for several cancers (see Table). In addition to the increased risk of ovarian and female breast cancer, *BRCA1* mutations confer an increased risk for prostate cancer and, possibly, for colon cancer. Similarly, in addition to ovarian and female breast cancer, germline *BRCA2* mutations increase the risk of prostate, pancreatic, bile duct, gallbladder, and male breast cancers.

Among female carriers of a *BRCA1* or *BRCA2* germline mutation, the overall penetrance of breast cancer, ovarian cancer, or both is estimated to be approximately 50% to 80% for *BRCA1* mutations but lower for *BRCA2* mutations (40% for breast cancer and 10% for ovarian cancer). Approximately two thirds of families with a history of breast and ovarian cancer segregate a *BRCA1* mutation, whereas approximately two thirds of families with a history of male *and* female breast cancer segregate a *BRCA2* mutation.

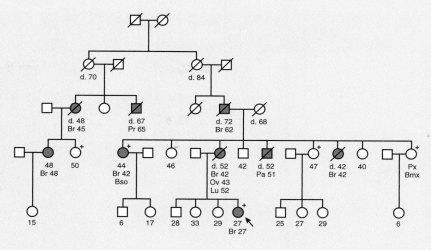

Figure C-5 ■ Family segregating a *BRCA2* C3590G mutation. The proband, S.M., is indicated by an arrow. Blue symbols indicate a diagnosis of cancer. Ages are shown directly below the symbol. A plus sign identifies carriers of the *BRCA2* mutation and a minus sign identifies noncarriers as determined by DNA sequencing. Cancer diagnoses are followed by the age at diagnosis. Cancer abbreviations: Br, breast; Ov, ovarian; Lu, lung; Pa, pancreatic; Pr, prostate. Other abbreviations: Bso, bilateral salpingo-oophorectomy; d., age at death; Px Bmx, prophylactic bilateral mastectomy. (Courtesy of A. Liede and S. Narod, Women's College Hospital and University of Toronto, Canada.)

Management

Current recommendations for women with a germline *BRCA1* or *BRCA2* mutation include frequent breast and ovarian examinations as well as imaging studies. Management of at-risk males includes frequent prostate and breast examinations and laboratory tests for evidence of prostate cancer. In families with known germline mutations, molecular analysis can focus surveillance or prophylaxis on members carrying a mutation. Total bilateral mastectomy may reduce the risk of breast cancer by more than 90%, although the risk is not abolished because some breast tissue often remains. Similarly, bilateral salpingo-oophorectomy may reduce the risk of ovarian cancer by more than 90%.

INHERITANCE RISK

Female gender, age, and family history are the most important risk factors for breast cancer. In Western populations, the cumulative female breast cancer incidence is 1 in 200 at 40 years, 1 in 50 at 50 years, and 1 in 10 by 70 years. If patients have a first-degree relative in whom breast cancer developed after 55 years, they have a 1.6 relative risk for breast cancer, whereas the relative risk increases to 2.3 if the breast cancer developed in the family member before 55 years and to 3.8 if it developed before 45 years. If the first-degree relative had bilateral breast cancer, the relative risk is 6.4.

Children of a patient with a *BRCA1* or *BRCA2* germline mutation have a 50% risk of inheriting that mutation. Because of incomplete penetrance and variable expressivity, the development and onset of cancer cannot be precisely predicted.

CUMULATIVE RISK (%) AT AGE 70 YEARS

	Female		Male	
	Breast Cancer	Ovarian Cancer	Breast Cancer	Prostate Cancer
BRCA1 mutation carriers	40-87	16-63	?	25
BRCA2 mutation carriers	28-84	27	6-14	20
General population	8-10	1.5	<0.1	10

Questions for Small Group Discussion

1. At what age and under what conditions might testing of an at-risk child be appropriate?
2. What is the risk for development of prostate cancer in a son if a parent carries a *BRCA1* germline mutation? a *BRCA2* germline mutation?
3. Currently, sequencing of the coding region of *BRCA1* detects only 60% to 70% of mutations in families with linkage to the gene. What mutations would sequencing miss? How should a report of "no mutation detected by sequencing" be interpreted and counseled? How would testing of an affected family member clarify the testing results?

REFERENCES

GeneTests. Medical genetics information resource [database online]. University of Washington, Seattle, 1993-2006. Updated weekly. *http://www.genetests.org*
Levy-Lahad E, Friedman E: Cancer risks among *BRCA1* and *BRCA2* mutation carriers. Br J Cancer 96(1):11-15, 2007. Review.

6. Charcot-Marie-Tooth Disease Type 1A

(*PMP22* Mutation or Duplication)

Autosomal Dominant

PRINCIPLES

- Genetic heterogeneity
- Gene dosage
- Recombination between repeated DNA sequences

MAJOR PHENOTYPIC FEATURES

- Age at onset: childhood to adulthood
- Progressive distal weakness
- Distal muscle wasting
- Hyporeflexia

HISTORY AND PHYSICAL FINDINGS

During the past few years, J.T., an 18-year-old woman, had noticed a progressive decline in her strength, endurance, and ability to run and walk. She also complained of frequent leg cramps exacerbated by cold and recent difficulty stepping over objects and climbing stairs. She did not recollect a precedent illness or give a history suggestive of an inflammatory process, such as myalgia, fever, or night sweats. No other family members had similar problems or a neuromuscular disorder. On examination, J.T. was thin and had atrophy of her lower legs, mild weakness of ankle extension and flexion, absent ankle reflexes, reduced patellar reflexes, footdrop as she walked, and enlarged peroneal nerves. She had difficulty walking on her toes and could not walk on her heels. The findings from her examination were otherwise normal. As part of her evaluation, the neurologist requested several studies, including nerve conduction velocities (NCVs). J.T.'s NCVs were abnormal; her median NCV was 25 m/sec (normal, >43 m/sec). Results of a subsequent nerve biopsy showed segmental demyelination, myelin sheath hypertrophy (redundant wrappings of Schwann cells around nerve fibers), and no evidence of inflammation. The neurologist explained that these results were strongly suggestive of a demyelinating neuropathy such as type 1 Charcot-Marie-Tooth disease (CMT1), also known as hereditary motor and sensory neuropathy type 1. Explaining that the most common cause of CMT1 is a duplication of the peripheral myelin protein 22 gene (*PMP22*), the neurologist requested testing for this duplication. This test confirmed that J.T. had a duplicated *PMP22* allele and the disease CMT1A.

BACKGROUND

Disease Etiology and Incidence

The CMT disorders are a genetically heterogeneous group of hereditary neuropathies characterized by chronic motor and sensory polyneuropathy. CMT has been subdivided according to patterns of inheritance, neuropathological changes, and clinical features. By definition, CMT1 is an autosomal dominant demyelinating neuropathy; it has a prevalence of approximately 15 in 100,000 and is also genetically heterogeneous. CMT1A, which represents 70% to 80% of CMT1, is caused by increased dosage of PMP22 secondary to dupli-

cation of the *PMP22* gene on chromosome 17. De novo duplications account of 20% to 33% of CMT1A; of these, more than 90% arise during male meiosis.

Pathogenesis

PMP22 is an integral membrane glycoprotein. Within the peripheral nervous system, PMP22 is found in compact but not in noncompact myelin. The function of PMP22 has not been fully elucidated, but evidence suggests that it plays a key role in myelin compaction.

Dominant negative mutations within *PMP22* and increased dosage of PMP22 cause a demyelinating peripheral polyneuropathy. Increased dosage of PMP22 arises by tandem duplication of band p11.2 on chromosome 17. This 1.5-Mb region is flanked by repeated DNA sequences that are approximately 98% identical. Misalignment of these flanking repeat elements during meiosis can lead to unequal crossing over and formation of one chromatid with a duplication of the 1.5-Mb region and another with the reciprocal deletion. (The reciprocal deletion causes the disease hereditary neuropathy with pressure palsies [HNPP]). An individual inheriting a chromatid with the duplication will have three copies of a normal *PMP22* gene and, thus, overexpress PMP22 (see Chapter 6).

Overexpression of PMP22 or expression of dominant negative forms of PMP22 results in an inability to form and to maintain compact myelin. Nerve biopsy specimens from severely affected infants show a diffuse paucity of myelin, and nerve biopsy specimens from more mildly affected patients show segmental demyelination and myelin sheath hypertrophy. The mechanism by which PMP22 overexpression causes this pathological process remains unclear.

The muscle weakness and atrophy observed in CMT1 result from muscle denervation secondary to axonal degeneration. Longitudinal studies of patients have shown an age-dependent reduction in the nerve fiber density that correlates with the development of disease symptoms. In addition, evidence in murine models suggests that myelin is necessary for maintenance of the axonal cytoskeleton. The mechanism by which demyelination alters the axonal cytoskeleton and affects axonal degeneration has not been completely elucidated.

Phenotype and Natural History

CMT1A has nearly full penetrance, although the severity, onset, and progression of CMT1 vary markedly within and among families. Many affected individuals do not seek medical attention, either because their symptoms are not noticeable or because their symptoms are accommodated easily. On the other hand, others have severe disease that is manifested in infancy or in childhood.

Symptoms of CMT1A usually develop in the first two decades of life; onset after 30 years of age is rare. Typically, symptoms begin with an insidious onset of slowly progressive weakness and atrophy of the distal leg muscles and mild sensory impairment (Fig. C-6). The weakness of the feet and legs leads to abnormalities of gait, a dropped foot, and eventually foot deformities (pes cavus and hammer toes) and loss of balance; it rarely causes patients to lose their ability to walk. Weakness of the intrinsic hand muscles usually occurs

Inflammatory peripheral neuropathies are frequently difficult to distinguish from CMT1 and HNPP, and before the advent of molecular testing many patients with inherited neuropathies were treated with immunosuppressants and experienced the associated morbidity without improvement of their neuropathy.

Treatment focuses on symptomatic management because curative therapies are currently unavailable for CMT1. Paralleling disease progression, therapy generally follows three stages: strengthening and stretching exercises to maintain gait and function, use of orthotics and special adaptive splints, and orthopedic surgery. Further deterioration may require use of ambulatory supports such as canes and walkers or, in rare, severely affected patients, a wheelchair. All patients should be counseled to avoid exposure to neurotoxic medications and chemicals.

INHERITANCE RISK

Because the *PMP22* duplication and most *PMP22* point mutations are autosomal dominant and fully penetrant, each child of an affected parent has a 50% chance for development of CMT1A. The variable expressivity of the *PMP22* duplication and *PMP22* mutations, however, makes prediction of disease severity impossible.

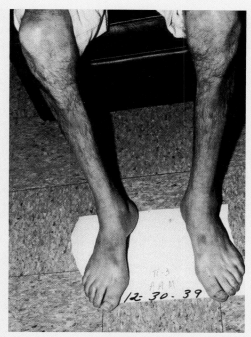

Figure C-6 ■ Distal leg muscle wasting in an elderly man with the *PMP22* duplication. (Courtesy of J. R. Lupski, Department of Molecular and Human Genetics, Baylor College of Medicine, Houston, and C. Garcia, Department of Neurology, Tulane University, New Orleans.)

> **Questions for Small Group Discussion**
> 1. Genomic deletions and duplications frequently arise by recombination between repetitive sequences within the human genome (see Chapter 6). Name three disorders caused by deletion after presumed recombination between repetitive sequences. Which of these deletions are associated with a reciprocal duplication? What does the identification of a reciprocal duplication suggest about the mechanism of recombination? What does the absence of a reciprocal duplication suggest?
> 2. In general, genomic duplications are associated with less severe disease than are genomic deletions. Duplication of a *PMP22* allele, however, usually causes more severe disease than deletion of a *PMP22* allele does. Discuss possible reasons for this.
> 3. Name two other diseases that are caused by a gene dosage effect.

late in the disease course and, in severe cases, causes clawhand deformities due to imbalance between flexor and extensor muscle strength. Other associated findings include decreased or absent reflexes, upper extremity ataxia and tremor, scoliosis, and palpably enlarged superficial nerves. On occasion, the phrenic and autonomic nerves are also involved.

In electrophysiological studies, the hallmark of CMT1A is uniform slowing of NCVs in all nerves and nerve segments as a result of demyelination. The full reduction in NCVs is usually present by 2 to 5 years of age, although clinically apparent symptoms may not be manifested for many years.

Management
Although the diagnosis of CMT1 is suspected because of clinical, electrophysiological, and pathological features, a definitive diagnosis often depends on detection of a mutation.

REFERENCES

GeneTests. Medical genetics information resource [database online]. University of Washington, Seattle, 1993-2006. Updated weekly. *http://www. genetests.org*

OMIM: Online Mendelian Inheritance in Man. McKusick-Nathans Institute for Genetic Medicine, Johns Hopkins University, and National Center for Biotechnology Information, National Library of Medicine. *http://www. ncbi.nlm.nih.gov/entrez/query.fcgi?db=OMIM*

7. CHARGE Syndrome

(*CHD7* Mutation)
Autosomal Dominant

PRINCIPLES

- Pleiotropy
- Haploinsufficiency
- Association versus syndrome

MAJOR PHENOTYPIC FEATURES

- Coloboma of the iris, retina, optic disc, or optic nerve
- *Heart defects*
- *Atresia of the choanae*
- *Retardation of growth and development*
- *Genital abnormalities*
- *Ear anomalies*
- Facial palsy
- Cleft lip
- Tracheoesophageal fistula

HISTORY AND PHYSICAL FINDINGS

Baby girl E.L. was the product of a full-term pregnancy to a 34-year-old gravida 1, para 1 mother after an uncomplicated pregnancy. At birth, it was noted that E.L.'s right ear was cupped and posteriorly rotated. Because of feeding difficulties, she was placed in the neonatal intensive care unit. Placement of a nasogastric tube was attempted but was unsuccessful in the right naris, demonstrating unilateral choanal atresia. A geneticist determined that she may have the CHARGE syndrome. Further evaluation included echocardiography, which revealed a small atrial septal defect, and ophthalmic examination, which revealed a retinal coloboma in the left eye. The atrial septal defect was repaired surgically without complications. She failed the newborn hearing screen and was subsequently diagnosed with mild to moderate sensorineural hearing loss. Testing for mutations in the CHARGE syndrome gene, *CHD7*, demonstrated a 5418C>G heterozygous mutation in exon 26 that results in a premature termination codon (Tyr1806Ter). Mutation analyses in E.L.'s parents were normal, indicating that a de novo mutation had occurred in E.L. Consequently, the family was advised that the recurrence risk in future pregnancies was low. At 1 year of age, E.L. was moderately delayed in gross motor skills and had speech delay. Her height and weight were at the 5th percentile, and head circumference was at the 10th percentile. Yearly follow-up was planned.

BACKGROUND

Disease Etiology and Incidence

CHARGE syndrome (MIM# 214800) is an autosomal dominant condition with multiple congenital malformations caused by mutations in the *CHD7* gene in the majority of individuals tested. Estimated birth prevalence of the condition is 1 in 3,000 to 12,000. However, the advent of genetic testing may reveal *CHD7* mutations in atypical cases, leading to recognition of a higher incidence.

Pathogenesis

The *CHD7* gene, located at 8q12, is a member of the superfamily of chromodomain helicase DNA-binding (CHD) genes. The proteins in this family are predicted to affect chromatin structure and gene expression in early embryonic development. The *CHD7* gene is expressed ubiquitously in many fetal and adult tissues, including the eye, cochlea, brain, central nervous system, stomach, intestine, skeleton, heart, kidney, lung, and liver. Heterozygous nonsense and missense mutations in the *CHD7* gene, as well as deletions in the 8q12 region encompassing *CHD7*, have been demonstrated in patients with CHARGE syndrome, indicating that haploinsufficiency for the gene causes the disease. However, some patients with CHARGE syndrome have no identifiable mutation in *CHD7*, suggesting that mutations in other loci may sometimes underlie the condition.

Phenotype and Natural History

The acronym CHARGE (*c*oloboma, *h*eart defects, *a*tresia of the choanae, *r*etardation of growth and development, *g*enital abnormalities, *e*ar anomalies), encompassing the most common features of the condition, was coined by dysmorphologists as a descriptive name for an association of abnormalities of unknown etiology and pathogenesis seen together more often than would be expected by chance. With the discovery of *CHD7* mutations in CHARGE, the condition is now considered to be a dysmorphic syndrome, a characteristic pattern of causally related anomalies (see Chapter 14). The current major diagnostic criteria are ocular coloboma (affecting the iris, retina, choroid, or disc with or without microphthalmia), choanal atresia (unilateral or bilateral; stenosis or atresia), cranial nerve anomalies (with unilateral or bilateral facial palsy, sensorineural deafness, or swallowing problems), and characteristic ear anomalies (external ear lop or cupshaped ear, middle ear ossicular malformations, mixed deafness, and cochlear defects). A number of other abnormalities are found less often, such as cleft lip or palate, congenital heart defect, growth deficiency, and tracheoesophageal fistula or esophageal atresia. CHARGE syndrome is diagnosable if three or four major criteria or two major and three minor criteria are found (Fig. C-7).

Perinatal or early infant mortality (before 6 months of age) is seen in approximately half of affected patients and appears to be most highly correlated with the most severe congenital anomalies, including bilateral posterior choanal atresia and congenital heart defects. Gastroesophageal reflux is a significant cause of morbidity and mortality. Feeding problems are also common; as many as 50% of adolescent and adult patients require gastrostomy tube placement. Behavioral abnormalities (including hyperactivity, sleep disturbances, and obsessive-compulsive behavior) and delayed puberty are found in the majority of patients with CHARGE syndrome. Developmental delay or mental retardation can range from mild to severe in the majority of individuals, and behavioral abnormalities (including hyperactivity, sleep disturbances, and obsessive-compulsive behavior) are frequent. As *CHD7* mutation testing delineates more individuals with CHARGE, the features of the condition may become more well defined and the phenotypic spectrum widened.

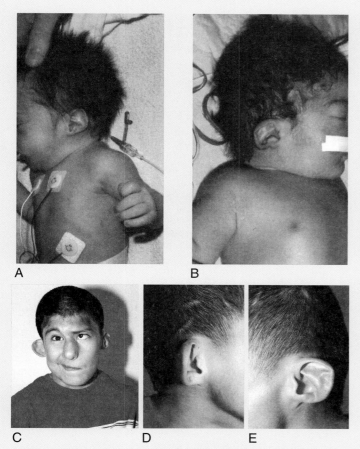

Management consists of surgical correction of malformations and supportive care. Developmental evaluation is an important component of follow-up. With the availability of testing for *CHD7* mutations, a molecular diagnosis can be made in at least 50% of patients.

INHERITANCE RISK

Almost all cases of CHARGE syndrome are due to new dominant mutations, with low recurrence risk in the parents. There has been one known reported instance of monozygotic twins having CHARGE as well as one family with two affected siblings (male and female). The latter situation suggests that germline mosaicism may be present with this condition. If a mutation in *CHD7* is found in an affected individual and both parents test negative for the mutation, the recurrence risk for future offspring would be less than 5%. An affected individual has a 50% recurrence risk to his or her offspring.

Questions for Small Group Discussion
1. Explain the difference between an association and a syndrome. Give an example of a common association.
2. By what mechanism could haploinsufficiency for a chromodomain protein cause the pleiotropic effects of CHARGE syndrome?
3. Why would you counsel the parents of a child with a proven de novo mutation in *CHD7* of a 5% recurrence risk? Would the risk change if their next child were affected?

Figure C-7 ■ Ear and eye anomalies in patients with CHARGE syndrome. (From Jones K: Smith's Recognizable Patterns of Human Malformation, 6th ed. Philadelphia, Elsevier, 2005.)

REFERENCES

Blake KD, Davenport SL, Hall BD, et al: CHARGE association: an update and review for the primary pediatrician. Clin Pediatr (Phila) 37:159-173, 1998.
Lalani SR, Safiullah AM, Fernbach SD, et al: Spectrum of CHD7 mutations in 110 individuals with CHARGE syndrome and genotype-phenotype correlation. Am J Hum Genet 78:303-314, 2006.
OMIM: Online Mendelian Inheritance in Man. McKusick-Nathans Institute for Genetic Medicine, Johns Hopkins University, and National Center for Biotechnology Information, National Library of Medicine. *http://www.ncbi.nlm.nih.gov/entrez/query.fcgi?db=OMIM*

Management

If CHARGE syndrome is suspected, thorough evaluation is warranted for possible choanal atresia or stenosis (unilateral), congenital heart defect, central nervous system abnormalities, renal anomalies, hearing loss, and feeding difficulties.

8. Chronic Myelogenous Leukemia

(*BCR-ABL* Oncogene)
Somatic Mutation

PRINCIPLES

- Chromosomal abnormality
- Oncogene activation
- Fusion protein
- Multi-hit hypothesis
- Therapy targeted to an oncogene

MAJOR PHENOTYPIC FEATURES

- Age at onset: middle to late adulthood
- Leukocytosis
- Splenomegaly
- Fatigue and malaise

HISTORY AND PHYSICAL FINDINGS

E.S., a 45-year-old woman, presented to her family physician for her annual checkup. She had been in good health and had no specific complaints. On examination, she had a palpable spleen tip but no other abnormal findings. Results of her complete blood count unexpectedly showed an elevated white blood cell count of 31×10^9/L and a platelet count of 650×10^9/L. The peripheral smear revealed basophilia and immature granulocytes. Her physician referred her to the oncology department for further evaluation. Her bone marrow was found to be hypercellular with an increased number of myeloid and megakaryocytic cells and an increased ratio of myeloid to erythroid cells. Cytogenetic analysis of her marrow identified several myeloid cells with a Philadelphia chromosome, der(22)t(9;22)(q34;q11.2). Her oncologist explained that she had chronic myelogenous leukemia, which, although indolent now, had a substantial risk of becoming a life-threatening leukemia in the next few years. She was also advised that although the only potentially curative therapy currently available is allogeneic bone marrow transplantation, newly developed drug therapy targeting the function of the oncogene in chronic myelogenous leukemia is able to induce or to maintain long-lasting remissions.

BACKGROUND

Disease Etiology and Incidence
Chronic myelogenous leukemia (CML, MIM# 608232) is a clonal expansion of transformed hematopoietic progenitor cells that increases circulating myeloid cells. Transformation of progenitor cells occurs by expression of the *BCR-ABL* oncogene. CML accounts for 15% of adult leukemia and has an incidence of 1 to 2 per 100,000; the age-adjusted incidence is higher in men than in women (1.3 to 1.7 versus 1.0; see Chapter 16).

Pathogenesis
Approximately 95% of patients with CML have a Philadelphia chromosome; the remainder have complex or variant translocations (see Chapter 16). The Abelson proto-oncogene (*ABL*), which encodes a nonreceptor tyrosine kinase, resides on 9q34, and the breakpoint cluster region gene (*BCR*), which encodes a phosphoprotein, resides on 22q11. During the formation of the Philadelphia chromosome, the *ABL* gene is disrupted in intron 1 and the *BCR* gene in one of three breakpoint cluster regions; the *BCR* and *ABL* gene fragments are joined head to tail on the derivative chromosome 22 (Fig. C-8). The *BCR-ABL* fusion gene on the derivative chromosome 22 generates a fusion protein that varies in size according to the length of the Bcr peptide attached to the amino terminus.

To date, the normal functions of Abl and Bcr have not been clearly defined. Abl has been conserved fairly well throughout metazoan evolution. It is found in both the nucleus and cytoplasm and as a myristolated product associated with the inner cytoplasmic membrane. The relative abundance of Abl in these compartments varies among cell types and in response to stimuli. Abl participates in the cell cycle, stress responses, integrin signaling, and neural development. The functional domains of Bcr include a coiled-coil motif for polymerization with other proteins, a serine-threonine kinase domain, a GDP-GTP exchange domain involved in regulation of Ras family members, and a guanosine triphosphatase–activating domain for regulating Rac and Rho GTPases.

Expression of Abl does not result in cellular transformation, whereas expression of the Bcr-Abl fusion protein does. Transgenic mice expressing Bcr-Abl develop acute leukemia at birth, and infection of normal mice with a retrovirus expressing Bcr-Abl causes a variety of acute and chronic leukemias, depending on the genetic background. In contrast to Abl, Bcr-Abl has constitutive tyrosine kinase activity and is confined to the cytoplasm, where it avidly binds actin microfilaments. Bcr-Abl phosphorylates several cytoplasmic substrates and thereby activates signaling cascades that control growth and differentiation and, possibly, adhesion of hematopoietic cells. Unregulated activation of these signaling pathways results in unregulated proliferation of the hematopoietic stem cell, release of immature cells from the marrow, and ultimately CML.

As CML progresses, it becomes increasingly aggressive. During this evolution, tumor cells of 50% to 80% of patients acquire additional chromosomal changes (trisomy 8, i(17q), or trisomy 19), another Philadelphia chromosome, or both. In addition to the cytogenetic changes, tumor-suppressor genes and proto-oncogenes are also frequently mutated in the progression of CML.

Phenotype and Natural History
CML is a biphasic or triphasic disease. The initial or chronic stage is characterized by an insidious onset with subsequent development of fatigue, malaise, weight loss, and minimal to moderate splenic enlargement. Over time, CML typically evolves to an accelerated phase and then to a blast crisis, although some patients progress directly from the chronic phase to the blast crisis. CML progression includes development of additional chromosomal abnormalities within tumor cells, progressive leukocytosis, anemia, thrombocytosis or thrombocytopenia, increasing splenomegaly, fever, and bone

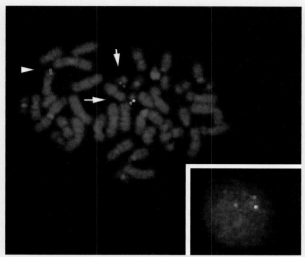

Figure C-8 ■ Fluorescence in situ hybridization of a locus-specific probe to metaphase and interphase *(inset)* cells for the detection of the t(9;22)(q34;q11.2) in CML. The DNA is counterstained with DAPI. The probe is a mixture of DNA probes for the *BCR* gene (red) at 22q11.2 and for the *ABL* gene (green) at 9q34. In normal cells, the green signal is observed on both chromosome 9 homologues, and the red signal is observed on both chromosome 22 homologues. In cells with the t(9;22), a green signal is observed on the normal chromosome 9 *(arrowhead)*, a red signal on the normal chromosome 22 *(short arrow)*, and a yellow fusion signal *(long arrow)* from the presence of both green and red signals together on the Philadelphia chromosome as a result of the translocation of *ABL* to the derivative 22 chromosome. (Courtesy of M. M. LeBeau and H. T. Abelson, University of Chicago.)

lesions. Blast crisis is an acute leukemia in which the blasts can be myeloid, lymphoid, erythroid, or undifferentiated. The accelerated phase is intermediate between the chronic phase and blast crisis.

Approximately 85% of patients are diagnosed in the chronic phase. Depending on the study, the median age at diagnosis ranges from 45 to 65 years, although all ages can be affected. Untreated, the rate of progression from the chronic phase to blast crisis is approximately 5% to 10% during the first 2 years and then 20% per year subsequently. Because blast crisis is rapidly fatal, demise parallels progression to blast crisis.

Management

Recognition of the molecular basis of CML led to the development of a specific Bcr-Abl tyrosine kinase inhibitor, imatinib mesylate (Gleevec). This drug is now the first line of treatment for CML. More than 85% of patients have a clear cytogenetic response after imatinib therapy, with disappearance of the t(9;22) in cells obtained by bone marrow aspirates. Cytogenetic response corresponds to a large reduction in CML disease burden to levels below 10^9 to 10^{10} leukemic cells. Few patients (<5%), however, show no evidence of the *BCR-ABL* fusion gene by polymerase chain reaction analysis, indicating that even in remission, most patients have a residual leukemia burden of at least 10^6 to 10^7 cells. Of patients with complete hematological and cytogenetic remission, more than 95% remained in control for more than 3.5 years. Patients in blast crisis also respond with improved 12-month survival of 32%, but relapses are common. In these patients, imatinib resistance is frequent (60% to 90%), in association with point mutations that render the Abl kinase resistant to the drug or, less commonly, with *BCR-ABL* gene amplification.

Although allogeneic bone marrow transplantation (BMT) is the only known curative therapy, the success of imatinib mesylate has limited the population of patients to whom it is offered to those with the highest success rate (patients younger than 40 years with an HLA-matched sibling donor, in whom BMT success is quoted at 80%) and to those in blast crisis. The success of BMT depends on the stage of CML, the age and health of the patient, the bone marrow donor (related versus unrelated), the preparative regimen, the development of graft-versus-host disease, and the post-transplantation treatment. Much of the long-term success of BMT depends on a graft-versus-leukemia effect, that is, a graft-versus-host response directed against the leukemic cells. After BMT, patients are monitored frequently for relapse by reverse transcriptase polymerase chain reaction to detect *BCR-ABL* transcripts and treated as necessary. If BMT fails, patients often respond to infusion of BMT donor-derived T cells, consistent with a graft-versus-leukemia mechanism of action of BMT for CML.

Patients in blast crisis are usually treated with imatinib mesylate, cytotoxic agents, and, if possible, BMT. Unfortunately, only 30% of patients have a related or unrelated HLA-matched bone marrow donor. The outcome of these therapies for blast crisis remains poor.

INHERITANCE RISK

Because CML arises from a somatic mutation that is not found in the germline, the risk of a patient's passing the disease to his or her children is zero.

Questions for Small Group Discussion
1. What is the multi-hit hypothesis? How does it apply to neoplasia?
2. Discuss two additional mechanisms of proto-oncogene activation in human cancer.
3. Neoplasias graphically illustrate the effects of the accumulation of somatic mutations; however, other less dramatic diseases arise, at least in part, through the accumulation of somatic mutations. Discuss the effect of somatic mutations on aging.
4. Many somatic mutations and cytogenetic rearrangements are never detected because the cells containing them do not have a selective advantage. What advantage does the Philadelphia chromosome confer?
5. Name other cancers caused by fusion genes resulting in oncogene activation. Which others have been successfully targeted?

REFERENCES

Cohen MH, Johnson JR, Pazdur R: U.S. Food and Drug Administration Drug Approval Summary: conversion of imatinib mesylate (STI571; Gleevec) tablets from accelerated approval to full approval. Clin Cancer Res 11:12-19, 2005.

GeneTests. Medical genetics information resource [database online]. University of Washington, Seattle, 1993-2006. Updated weekly. *http://www.genetests.org*

Goldman JM, Melo JV: Chronic myeloid leukemia—advances in biology and new approaches to treatment. N Engl J Med 349:1451-1464, 2003.

Krause DS, Van Etten RA: Tyrosine kinases as targets for cancer therapy. N Engl J Med 353:172-187, 2005.

O'Hare, Cobrin AS, Druker BJ: Targeted CML therapy: controlling drug resistance, seeking cure. Curr Opin Genet Dev 16:92-99, 2006.

OMIM: Online Mendelian Inheritance in Man. McKusick-Nathans Institute for Genetic Medicine, Johns Hopkins University, and National Center for Biotechnology Information, National Library of Medicine. *http://www.ncbi.nlm.nih.gov/entrez/query.fcgi?db=OMIM*

9. Crohn Disease

(Increased Risk from *NOD2* Mutations)
Multifactorial Inheritance

PRINCIPLES

- Multifactorial inheritance
- Autoimmune disease
- Ethnic predilection

MAJOR PHENOTYPIC FEATURES

- Episodic abdominal pain, cramping, and diarrhea
- Occasional hematochezia (blood in the stool)
- May involve any segment of the intestinal tract
- Transmural ulceration and granulomas of the gastrointestinal tract
- Fistulas
- Patchy involvement usually of the terminal ileum and ascending colon
- Extraintestinal manifestations including inflammation of the joints, eyes, and skin

HISTORY AND PHYSICAL FINDINGS

P.L. is a 14-year old white male brought to the emergency department by his mother for severe right lower quadrant pain and nausea without vomiting or fever. His history revealed intermittent non-bloody diarrhea for 1 year, no significant constipation, 1-hour postprandial lower quadrant abdominal pain relieved by defecation, and nocturnal abdominal pain that awakens him from sleep. The patient's developmental history was normal except that his growth was noted to have dropped from the 50th-75th percentile to the 25th percentile during the past 2 years. Family history was significant in that a first cousin on the paternal side also had Crohn disease. Physical examination revealed peritoneal signs, hyperactive bowel sounds, and diffuse lower abdominal pain to palpation without palpable masses or organomegaly. A stool guaiac test was trace positive. Peripheral blood count revealed only a slightly elevated white blood cell count and a slight microcytic hypochromic anemia. Urinalysis and abdominal plain films were unremarkable. A computed tomographic scan showed mucosal inflammation extending from the distal ileum into the ascending colon. Upper endoscopy and colonoscopy with biopsy were performed, revealing transmural ulceration of the distal ileum with moderate to severe ulceration of the ileocecal junction, consistent with Crohn disease.

Subsequent genetic testing identified a Gly908Arg mutation on one allele of the *NOD2* (*CARD15*) gene.

BACKGROUND

Disease Etiology and Incidence

Inflammatory bowel disease (IBD) is a chronic inflammatory disease of the gastrointestinal tract that primarily affects adolescents and young adults. The disease is divided into two major categories, Crohn disease (CD) and ulcerative colitis, each of which occurs with approximately equal frequency in the population. IBD affects 1 in 500 to 1000 individuals, with a 2-fold to 4-fold increased prevalence in individuals of Ashkenazi Jewish backgrounds compared with non–Ashkenazi Jewish whites. Both disorders show substantial familial clustering and increased concordance rates in monozygotic twins, but they do not follow a mendelian inheritance pattern and are therefore classified as multifactorial. Three different common variants in the *NOD2* gene (also known as *CARD15*) have been found to significantly increase the risk for development of CD (but not of ulcerative colitis) with an additive effect; heterozygotes have a 1.5- to 4-fold increased risk, whereas homozygotes or compound heterozygotes have a 15- to 40-fold increased risk. The absolute risk among homozygotes or compound heterozygotes therefore approaches 1% to 2%.

Pathogenesis

Because of inflammation in the intestinal tract, IBD was long thought to be an autoimmune disease. Association studies in whites revealed three single nucleotide polymorphisms with strong evidence for linkage disequilibrium with the disease; all three were found to be in the coding exons of the *NOD2* gene and to cause either amino acid substitutions (Gly908Arg and Arg702Trp) or premature termination of the protein (3020insC). Additional studies in several independent cohorts of CD patients have confirmed that these variants are strongly associated with CD.

The NOD2 protein binds to gram-negative bacterial cell walls and participates in the inflammatory response to bacteria by activating the NF-κB transcription factor in mononuclear leukocytes. The three variants all reduce the ability of the NOD2 protein to activate NF-κB, suggesting that the variants in this gene alter the ability of monocytes in the intestinal wall to respond to resident bacteria, thereby predisposing to an abnormal, inflammatory response. Thus, *NOD2* variants are likely to be the alleles actually responsible for increased susceptibility to CD at the IBD1 locus.

The *NOD2* variants are clearly neither necessary nor sufficient to cause CD. They are not necessary because although half of all white patients with CD have one or two copies of a *NOD2* variant, half do not. Estimates are that the *NOD2* variants account, at most, for 20% of the genetic contribution to IBD in whites. Furthermore, the particular variants associated with disease risk in Europe are not found in Asian or African populations, and CD in these populations shows no association with *NOD2*. The variants are also not sufficient to cause the disease. The *NOD2* variants are common in Europe; 20% of the population are heterozygous for these alleles yet show no signs of IBD. Even in the highest risk genotype, those who are homozygotes or compound heterozygotes for the *NOD2* variants, penetrance is less than 10%. The low penetrance points strongly to other genetic or environmental factors that act on genotypic susceptibility at the *NOD2* locus. The obvious connection between an IBD and structural protein variants in the NOD2 protein, a modulator of the innate antibacterial inflammatory response, is a strong clue that the intestinal microenvironment may be an important environmental factor contributing to pathogenesis.

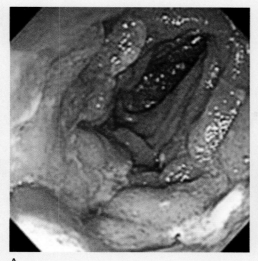
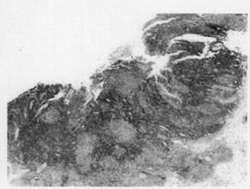

Figure C-9 ■ A, Endoscopic appearance of ileitis in a patient with Crohn disease. B, Multiple granulomas in the wall of the small intestine in a patient with Crohn disease. (Courtesy of Harris Yfantis and Raymond Cross, University of Maryland and Veterans Administration Medical Center, Baltimore.)

A   B

Phenotype and Natural History

Presenting in adolescence or young adulthood, CD most often affects segments of the gastrointestinal tract, such as the terminal small intestine (ileum) and portions of the ascending colon; but it can occur anywhere within the digestive tract, with granulomatous inflammation (Fig. C-9) that penetrates the wall of the intestine and produces narrowing and scarring. Onset is usually insidious with a history of nocturnal abdominal pain, diarrhea, and gradual weight loss.

Fistulous tracks and intra-abdominal abscesses can occur and may be life-threatening. Hospitalization is frequent, and surgery for abscesses may be necessary in CD. Symptoms outside the gastrointestinal tract in CD may include arthritis of the spine and joints, inflammation of the eyes (uveitis), skin involvement (erythema nodosum and pyoderma gangrenosum), primary sclerosing cholangitis, and hypercoagulability. There is also an increased risk of adenocarcinoma of the intestine in long-standing CD, although the risk is not as great as the substantial risk in ulcerative colitis, another type of IBD.

Management

Currently, there is no cure for IBD. The goals of treatment include induction of remission, maintenance of remission, minimization of side effects of treatment, and improvement of the quality of life. Five main categories of drugs are used alone or in combination to treat CD flare-ups: anti-inflammatory medications, corticosteroids, antibiotics, immune modulators, and mixed inflammatory-immune modulators. All of the anti-inflammatory medications are derivatives of mesalamine, and the choice of which anti-inflammatory medication to use is based on side effect profile and location of disease within the intestine. During the acute phase of the disease, corticosteroids are the mainstay of therapy. These medications, combined with dietary modification, are used to decrease the severity of the disease and to prevent flare-ups. Because fiber is poorly digested, its intake should be reduced in patients with CD. As a result of chronic inflammation and scarring, malnutrition is common. Folate, iron, calcium, and vitamin B_{12} commonly need to be supplemented. Surgery to remove diseased bowel, to drain abscesses, and to close fistulous tracks is often necessary.

INHERITANCE RISK

The empirical risk for development of IBD is approximately 1% to 8% in a sibling of an IBD patient and falls to 0.1% to 0.2% in second-degree relatives, findings not compatible with classic autosomal recessive or dominant inheritance. However, this sibling recurrence is still high compared with the risk in the general population (the relative risk ratio, λ_s, for siblings is between 10 and 30) (see Chapter 8). In one large twin registry, monozygotic twins showed a concordance rate for CD of 44%; dizygotic twins were concordant only 4% of the time. Concordance in ulcerative colitis was only 6% in monozygotic twins but still much higher than in dizygotic twins, in whom no concordant twins were observed. Thus, the genetic epidemiological data all strongly support classification of IBD as a disorder with a strong genetic contribution but with complex inheritance.

Questions for Small Group Discussion

1. Discuss possible environmental factors that play a role in CD.
2. How could variation in innate immunity interact with these environmental factors?
3. How should a family member of a patient with CD who is found to have one of the *NOD2* variants be counseled? Should the testing be done? Why or why not?

REFERENCE

Sands BE: Inflammatory bowel disease: past, present, and future. J Gastroenterol 42:16-25, 2007.

10. Cystic Fibrosis

(*CFTR* Mutation)
Autosomal Recessive

PRINCIPLES

- Ethnic variation in mutation frequency
- Variable expressivity
- Tissue-specific expression of mutations
- Genetic modifiers
- Environmental modifiers

MAJOR PHENOTYPIC FEATURES

- Age at onset: neonatal to adulthood
- Progressive pulmonary disease
- Exocrine pancreatic insufficiency
- Obstructive azoospermia
- Elevated sweat chloride concentration
- Growth failure
- Meconium ileus

HISTORY AND PHYSICAL FINDINGS

J.B., a 2-year-old boy, was referred to the pediatric clinic for evaluation of poor growth. During infancy, J.B. had diarrhea and colic that resolved when an elemental formula was substituted for his standard formula. As table foods were added to his diet, he developed malodorous stools containing undigested food particles. During his second year, J.B. grew poorly, developed a chronic cough, and had frequent upper respiratory infections. No one else in the family had poor growth, feeding disorders, or pulmonary illnesses. On physical examination, J.B.'s weight and height plotted less than the 3rd percentile and his head circumference at the 10th percentile. He had a severe diaper rash, diffuse rhonchi, and mild clubbing of his digits. The findings from his examination were otherwise normal. After briefly discussing a few possible causes of J.B.'s illness, the pediatrician requested several tests, including a test for sweat chloride concentration by pilocarpine iontophoresis; the sweat chloride level was 75 mmol/L (normal, <40 mmol/L; indeterminate, 40 to 60 mmol/L), a level consistent with cystic fibrosis. On the basis of this result and the clinical course, the pediatrician diagnosed J.B.'s condition as cystic fibrosis. J.B. and his parents were referred to the cystic fibrosis clinic for further counseling, mutation testing, and treatment.

BACKGROUND

Disease Etiology and Incidence

Cystic fibrosis (CF, MIM# 219700) is an autosomal recessive disorder of epithelial ion transport caused by mutations in the CF transmembrane conductance regulator gene (*CFTR*). Although CF has been observed in all races, it is predominantly a disease of northern Europeans. The live birth incidence of CF ranges from 1 in 313 among the Hutterites of southern Alberta, Canada, to 1 in 90,000 among the Asian population of Hawaii. Among all U.S. whites, the incidence is 1 in 3200.

Pathogenesis

CFTR is a cAMP-regulated chloride channel that regulates other ion channels. CFTR maintains the hydration of secretions within airways and ducts through the transport of chloride and inhibition of sodium uptake (see Chapter 12). Dysfunction of CFTR can affect many different organs, particularly those that secrete mucus, including the upper and lower respiratory tracts, pancreas, biliary system, male genitalia, intestine, and sweat glands.

The dehydrated and viscous secretions in the lungs of patients with CF interfere with mucociliary clearance, inhibit the function of naturally occurring antimicrobial peptides, provide a medium for growth of pathogenic organisms, and obstruct airflow. Within the first months of life, these secretions and the bacteria colonizing them initiate an inflammatory reaction. The release of inflammatory cytokines, host antibacterial enzymes, and bacterial enzymes damages the bronchioles. Recurrent cycles of infection, inflammation, and tissue destruction decrease the amount of functional lung tissue and eventually lead to respiratory failure (Fig. C-10).

Loss of CFTR chloride transport into the pancreatic duct impairs the hydration of secretions and leads to the retention of exocrine enzymes in the pancreas. Damage from these retained enzymes eventually causes fibrosis of the pancreas.

CFTR also regulates the uptake of sodium and chloride from sweat as it moves through the sweat duct. In the absence of functional CFTR, the sweat has an increased sodium chloride content, and this is the basis of the historical "salty baby syndrome" and the diagnostic sweat chloride test.

Phenotype and Natural History

CF classically manifests in early childhood, although approximately 4% of patients are diagnosed in adulthood; 15% to 20% of patients present at birth with meconium ileus, and the remainder present with chronic respiratory complaints (rhinitis, sinusitis, obstructive lung disease) or poor growth, or both, later in life. The poor growth results from a combination of increased calorie expenditure because of chronic lung infections and malnutrition from pancreatic exocrine insufficiency. Five percent to 15% of patients with CF do not develop pancreatic insufficiency. More than 95% of male patients with CF are azoospermic because of congenital bilateral absence of the vas deferens. The progression of lung disease is the chief determinant of morbidity and mortality. Most patients die of respiratory failure and right ventricular failure secondary to the destruction of lung parenchyma and high pulmonary vascular resistance (cor pulmonale); the current median survival is 33 years in North America.

In addition to CF, mutations within *CFTR* have been associated with a spectrum of diseases including obstructive azoospermia, idiopathic pancreatitis, disseminated bronchiectasis, allergic bronchopulmonary aspergillosis, atypical sinopulmonary disease, and asthma. Some of these disorders are associated with mutations within a single *CFTR* allele; others, like CF, are observed only when mutations are present in both *CFTR* alleles. A direct causative role for mutant *CFTR* alleles has been established for some but not all of these disorders.

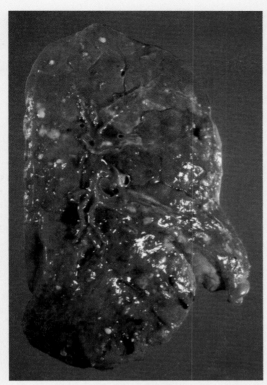

Figure C-10 ■ A median cross section of a lung from a patient with CF. Note the mucous plugs and purulent secretions within the airways. (Courtesy of J. Rutledge, University of Washington and Children's Hospital and Medical Center, Seattle.)

A correlation between particular *CFTR* mutant alleles and disease severity exists only for pancreatic insufficiency. Secondary mutations or polymorphisms within a *CFTR* allele may alter the efficiency of splicing or protein maturation and thereby extend the spectrum of disease associated with some mutations. In addition, some mutations in *CFTR* cause disease manifestations only in certain tissues; for example, some mutations affecting the efficiency of splicing have a greater effect on wolffian duct derivatives than in other tissues because of a tissue-specific need for full-length transcript and protein. Environmental factors, such as exposure to cigarette smoke, markedly worsen the severity of lung disease among patients with CF.

Management

Because more than 1000 different mutations and variants have been described across the *CFTR* gene, the diagnosis of CF in North America is usually based on clinical criteria and sweat chloride concentration. Sweat chloride concentrations are normal in 1% to 2% of patients with CF; in these patients, however, an abnormal nasal transepithelial potential difference measurement is usually diagnostic of CF.

Currently, there are no curative treatments of CF, although improved symptomatic management has increased the average longevity from early childhood to between 30 and 40 years. The objectives of medical therapy for CF are clearance of pulmonary secretions, control of pulmonary infection, pancreatic enzyme replacement, adequate nutrition, and prevention of intestinal obstruction. Although medical therapy slows the progression of pulmonary disease, the only effective treatment of respiratory failure in CF is lung transplantation. Pancreatic enzyme replacement and supplementation of fat-soluble vita-

mins treat the malabsorption effectively; because of increased caloric needs and anorexia, however, many patients also require caloric supplements. Most patients also require extensive counseling to deal with the psychological effects of having a chronic fatal disease.

In 2004, the American College of Medical Genetics, the U.S. Centers for Disease Control and Prevention, and the Cystic Fibrosis Foundation recommended newborn screening for CF because detection in the newborn period prevents the malnutrition seen in clinically undiagnosed pancreatic insufficient patients. Long-term effects on survival and pulmonary disease progression are unclear.

INHERITANCE RISK

A couple's empirical risk for having a child affected with CF varies greatly, depending on the frequency of CF in their ethnic groups. For North Americans who do not have a family history of CF and are of northern European ancestry, the empirical risk for each to be a carrier is approximately 1 in 29, and such a couple's risk of having an affected child is therefore 1 in 3200. For couples who already have a child affected with CF, the risk for future children to have CF is 1 in 4. In 1997, a National Institutes of Health consensus conference recommended offering CF carrier testing to all pregnant women and couples considering a pregnancy in the United States. The American College of Obstetrics and Gynecology adopted those recommendations. As of 2004, up to 25% of pregnant women in the United States underwent CF carrier testing.

Prenatal diagnosis is based on identification of the *CFTR* mutations in DNA from fetal tissue, such as chorionic villi or amniocytes. Effective identification of affected fetuses usually requires that the mutations responsible for CF in a family have already been identified.

Questions for Small Group Discussion

1. Newborn screening for CF can be performed by testing immunoreactive trypsinogen (IRT) alone or by IRT followed by mutation screening. Discuss risks and benefits of adding *CFTR* mutation screening to a newborn screening panel.
2. The most common CF mutation is ΔF508; it accounts for approximately 70% of all mutant *CFTR* alleles worldwide. For a couple of northern European origin, what is their risk of having an affected child if each tests negative for ΔF508? if one tests positive and the other tests negative for ΔF508?
3. What constitutes disease—a mutation in a gene or the phenotype caused by that mutation? Does detection of a mutation in the *CFTR* gene of patients with congenital bilateral absence of the vas deferens mean they have CF?

REFERENCES

Cystic Fibrosis Mutation Database. *http://www.genet.sickkids.on.ca/cftr/*
GeneTests. Medical genetics information resource [database online]. University of Washington, Seattle, 1993-2006. Updated weekly. *http://www.genetests.org*
Grosse SD, Boyle CA, Botkin JR, et al: CDC: Newborn screening for cystic fibrosis: evaluation of benefits and risks and recommendations for state newborn screening programs. MMWR Recomm Rep 53(RR-13):1-36, 2004.
OMIM: Online Mendelian Inheritance in Man. McKusick-Nathans Institute for Genetic Medicine, Johns Hopkins University, and National Center for Biotechnology Information, National Library of Medicine. *http://www.ncbi.nlm.nih.gov/entrez/query.fcgi?db=OMIM*
Watson MS, Cutting GR, Desnick RJ, et al: Cystic fibrosis population carrier screening: 2004 revision of American College of Medical Genetics mutation panel [erratum in Genet Med 6:548, 2004; Genet Med 7:286, 2005]. Genet Med 6:387-391, 2004.
Welsh MJ, Ramsey BW, Accurso F, Cutting GR: Cystic fibrosis. In Scriver CR, Beaudet AL, Sly WS, et al (eds): The Metabolic and Molecular Bases of Inherited Disease, 8th ed. New York, McGraw-Hill, 2001, pp 5121-5188.

11. Deafness (Nonsyndromic)

(*GJB2* Mutation)
Autosomal Dominant and Recessive

PRINCIPLES

- Allelic heterogeneity with both dominant and recessive inheritance patterns
- Newborn screening
- Cultural sensitivity in counseling

MAJOR PHENOTYPIC FEATURES

- Congenital deafness in the recessive form
- Progressive childhood deafness in the dominant form

HISTORY AND PHYSICAL FINDINGS

R.K. and J.K. are a couple referred to the genetics clinic by their ENT specialist because their 6-week-old son, B.K., was diagnosed with congenital hearing loss. The child was initially identified by routine neonatal hearing testing (evoked otoacoustic emissions testing) and then underwent formal auditory brainstem response (ABR) testing, which demonstrated moderate hearing impairment.

B.K. is the child of a healthy couple of European ancestry. Neither parent has a personal or family history of hearing difficulties in childhood, although the father thought that his aunt might have had some hearing difficulties in her old age. B.K. was the product of a full-term, uncomplicated pregnancy.

On examination, B.K. was non-dysmorphic. There was no evidence of craniofacial malformation affecting the pinnae or external auditory canals. Tympanic membranes were visible and normal. Ophthalmoscope examination was limited because of the patient's age, but no abnormalities were seen. There was no goiter. Skin was normal.

Laboratory testing revealed a hearing loss of 60 dB bilaterally in the middle- and high-frequency range (500 to 2000 Hz and >2000 Hz). Electrocardiography was normal. Computed tomography scans of petrous bone and cochlea were normal, without malformation or dilatation of the canals.

DNA from B.K. was examined for mutations in the *GJB2* gene. He was found to be homozygous for the common frameshift mutation 35delG in the *GJB2* gene.

BACKGROUND

Disease Etiology and Incidence

Approximately 1 in 500 to 1000 neonates has clinically significant congenital hearing impairment, which arises either from defects of the conductive apparatus in the middle ear or from neurological defects. It is estimated that approximately a third to a half of congenital deafness has a genetic etiology. Of the hereditary forms, approximately three quarters are nonsyndromic, characterized by deafness alone; one quarter is syndromic, that is, associated with other manifestations.

Among inherited forms of nonsyndromic deafness, mutations of *GJB2* are among the more common causes. They cause DFNB1 (MIM# 220290), which accounts for half of congenital nonsyndromic autosomal recessive deafness, as well as DFNA3 (MIM# 601544), a rare form of childhood-onset progressive autosomal dominant deafness. The mutation 35delG accounts for approximately two thirds of identified autosomal recessive *GJB2* mutations in white populations but not in other ethnic groups. Among the Chinese, for example, 235delC is the predominant mutation in *GJB2* causing DFNB1.

Pathogenesis

The *GJB2* gene encodes connexin26, one of a family of proteins that form gap junctions. Gap junctions create pores between cells, allowing exchange of ions and passage of electrical currents between cells. Connexin26 is highly expressed in the cochlea, the inner ear organ that transduces sound waves to electrical impulses. The failure to form functional gap junctions results in loss of cochlear function but does not affect the vestibular system or auditory nerve.

Phenotype and Natural History

Autosomal recessive deafness due to *GJB2* mutations is congenital and may be mild to profound (Fig. C-11). Cognitive deficits are *not* a component of the disorder if the hearing impairment is detected early and the child is referred for proper management to allow the development of spoken or sign language.

Autosomal dominant deafness due to *GJB2* mutations also occurs. It has an early childhood onset and is associated with progressive, moderate to severe high-frequency sensorineural hearing loss. Like the autosomal recessive disease, it also is not associated with cognitive deficits.

Management

The diagnosis of congenital deafness is usually made through newborn screening. Newborn screening is carried out either by measuring otoacoustic emissions, which are sounds caused by internal vibrations from within a normal cochlea, or by automated ABR, which detects electrical signals in the brain generated in response to sound. With the introduction of universal newborn screening, the average age at diagnosis has fallen to 3 to 6 months, allowing early intervention with hearing aids and other forms of therapy. Infants in whom therapy is initiated before 6 months of age show improvement in language development compared with infants identified at an older age.

As soon as deafness is identified, the child needs to be referred for early intervention, regardless of the etiology of the deafness. By consulting with professionals such as audiologists, cochlear implant teams, otolaryngologists, and speech pathologists about the benefits and the drawbacks of different options, parents can be helped to choose those that seem best for their families. Age-appropriate, intensive language therapy with sign language and spoken language with hearing assistance with hearing aids can be instituted as early as possible. Parents can be offered the option of an early cochlear implant, a device that bypasses the dysfunctioning

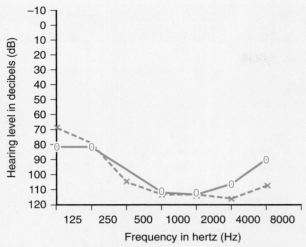

Figure C-11 ■ Profound hearing loss in a child homozygous for mutations in the connexin 26 gene. X and O represent left and right ear, respectively. Normal hearing level is 0 to 20 dB throughout the frequency range. (Audiogram courtesy of Virginia W. Norris, Gallaudet University.)

cochlea. Use of cochlear implants before 3 years of age is associated with better oral speech and language outcomes than in those receiving an implant later in childhood.

During the newborn period, clinically distinguishing between some forms of syndromic deafness and nonsyndromic deafness is difficult because some syndromic features, such as the goiter in Pendred syndrome or the retinitis pigmentosa in the Usher syndromes, may have an onset late in childhood or adolescence. However, a definitive diagnosis is often important for prognosis, management, and counseling; therefore, a careful family history and DNA analysis for mutations in the GJB2 gene and occasionally other genes are key to such a diagnosis. Importantly, distinguishing among nonsyndromic forms of deafness is often critical for selecting proper therapy.

INHERITANCE RISK

The form of severe congenital deafness caused by loss-of-function mutations in GJB2 (DFNB1) is inherited in a typical autosomal recessive manner. Unaffected parents are both carriers of one normal and one altered gene. Two carrier parents have a one chance in four with each pregnancy of having a child with congenital deafness. Prenatal diagnosis by direct detection of the mutation in DNA is available.

Among families segregating nonsyndromic, progressive deafness with childhood onset due to GJB2 mutations (DFNA3), inheritance is autosomal dominant, and the risk for an affected parent to have a deaf child is one in two for each pregnancy.

Questions for Small Group Discussion

1. Why might certain missense mutations in GJB2 cause *dominant*, progressive hearing loss, whereas another mutation (frameshift) results in *recessive*, nonprogressive hearing loss?
2. What special considerations and concerns might arise in providing genetic counseling to a deaf couple about the risk of their having a child with hearing loss? What is meant by the term *Deaf culture*?
3. Mutation testing detects only 95% of the GJB2 mutations among white families known to have autosomal recessive deafness secondary to GJB2 defects. Also, many sequence variations have been detected in the GJB2 gene. If a couple with a congenitally deaf child presented to you and mutation analysis detected a GJB2 sequence variation, not previously associated with disease, in only one parent, how would you counsel them regarding recurrence risk and genetic etiology? Would your counseling be different if the sequence variation had been previously associated with disease, and what would constitute significant association? Would your counseling be different if the child had early childhood onset of progressive deafness?
4. Why might a child with a cochlear implant learn sign language in addition to spoken language?

REFERENCES

GeneTests. Medical genetics information resource [database online]. University of Washington, Seattle, 1993-2006. Updated weekly. *http://www.genetests.org*

Liu Y, Ke X, Qi Y, et al: Connexin26 gene (GJB2): prevalence of mutations in the Chinese population. J Hum Genet 47:688-690, 2002.

Morton CC, Nance WE: Newborn hearing screening: a silent revolution. N Engl J Med 354:2151-2164, 2006.

OMIM: Online Mendelian Inheritance in Man. McKusick-Nathans Institute for Genetic Medicine, Johns Hopkins University, and National Center for Biotechnology Information, National Library of Medicine. *http://www.ncbi.nlm.nih.gov/entrez/query.fcgi?db=OMIM*

12. Duchenne Muscular Dystrophy

(Dystrophin Mutation)

X-Linked

PRINCIPLES

- High frequency of new mutations
- Allelic heterogeneity
- Manifesting carriers
- Phenotypic variability

MAJOR PHENOTYPIC FEATURES

- Age at onset: childhood
- Muscle weakness
- Calf hypertrophy
- Mild intellectual compromise
- Elevated serum creatine kinase level

HISTORY AND PHYSICAL FINDINGS

A.Y., a 6-year-old boy, was referred for mild developmental delay. He had difficulty climbing stairs, running, and participating in vigorous physical activities; he had decreased strength and endurance. His parents, two brothers, and one sister were all healthy; no other family members were similarly affected. On examination, he had difficulty jumping onto the examination table, a Gowers sign (a sequence of maneuvers for rising from the floor; Fig. C-12), proximal weakness, a waddling gait, tight heel cords, and apparently enlarged calf muscles. His serum creatine kinase level was 50-fold higher than normal. Because the history, physical examination findings, and elevated creatine kinase level strongly suggested a myopathy, A.Y. was referred to the neurogenetics clinic for further evaluation. Results of his muscle biopsy showed marked variation of muscle fiber size, fiber necrosis, fat and connective tissue proliferation, and no staining for dystrophin. On the basis of these results, A.Y.'s condition was given a provisional diagnosis of Duchenne muscular dystrophy, and he was tested for deletions of the dystrophin gene; he was found to have a deletion of exons 45 through 48. Subsequent testing showed his mother to be a carrier. The family was counseled, therefore, that the risk for affected sons was 50%, the risk for affected daughters was low but dependent on skewing of X inactivation, and the risk of carrier daughters was 50%. Because her carrier status placed her at a high risk for cardiac complications, the mother was referred for a cardiac evaluation.

BACKGROUND

Disease Etiology and Incidence

Duchenne muscular dystrophy (DMD, MIM# 310200) is a panethnic, X-linked progressive myopathy caused by mutations within the *DMD* gene. It has an incidence of approximately 1 in 3500 male births.

Pathogenesis

DMD encodes dystrophin, an intracellular protein that is expressed predominantly in smooth, skeletal, and cardiac muscle as well as in some brain neurons (see Chapter 12). In skeletal muscle, dystrophin is part of a large complex of sarcolemma-associated proteins that confers stability to the sarcolemma.

DMD mutations that cause DMD include large deletions (60% to 65%), large duplications (5% to 10%), and small deletions, insertions, or nucleotide changes (25% to 30%). Most large deletions occur in one of two hot spots. Nucleotide changes occur throughout the gene, predominantly at CpG dinucleotides. De novo mutations arise with comparable frequency during oogenesis and spermatogenesis; most de novo large deletions arise during oogenesis, whereas most de novo nucleotide changes arise during spermatogenesis.

Mutations causing a dystrophin null phenotype effect more severe muscle disease than do mutant *DMD* alleles expressing partially functional dystrophin. A consistent genotype-phenotype correlation has not been defined for the intellectual impairment.

Phenotype and Natural History

Males

DMD is a progressive myopathy resulting in muscle degeneration and weakness. Beginning with the hip girdle muscles and neck flexors, the muscle weakness progressively involves the shoulder girdle and distal limb and trunk muscles. Although occasionally manifesting in the newborn period with hypotonia or failure to thrive, male patients usually present between the ages of 3 and 5 years with gait abnormalities. By 5 years of age, most patients use a Gowers maneuver and have calf pseudohypertrophy, that is, enlargement of the calf through replacement of muscle by fat and connective tissue. By 12 years of age, most patients are confined to a wheelchair and have or are developing contractures and scoliosis. Most patients die of impaired pulmonary function and pneumonia; the median age at death is 18 years.

Nearly 95% of patients with DMD have some cardiac compromise (dilated cardiomyopathy or electrocardiographic abnormalities, or both), and 84% have demonstrable cardiac involvement at autopsy. Chronic heart failure develops in nearly 50% of patients. Rarely, cardiac failure is the presenting complaint for patients with DMD. Although dystrophin is also present in smooth muscle, smooth muscle complications are rare. These complications include gastric dilatation, ileus, and bladder paralysis.

Patients with DMD have an average IQ approximately 1 standard deviation below the mean, and nearly a third have some degree of mental retardation. The basis of this impairment has not been established.

Females

The age at onset and the severity of DMD in females depend on the degree of skewing of X inactivation (see Chapter 6). If the X chromosome carrying the mutant *DMD* allele is active in most cells, females develop signs of DMD; if the X chromosome carrying the normal *DMD* allele is predomi-

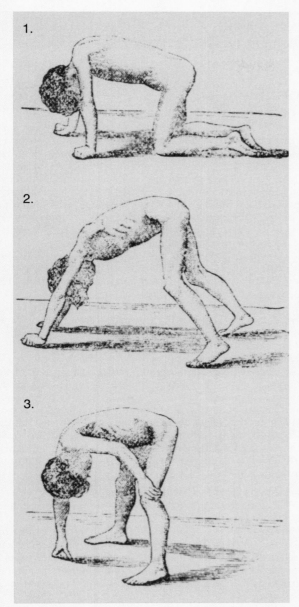

Figure C-12 ■ Drawing of a boy with DMD rising from the ground, that is, the Gowers maneuver. (From Gowers WR: Pseudohypertrophic muscular paralysis. A clinical lecture. London, J. and A. Churchill, 1879.)

nantly active, females have few or no symptoms of DMD. Regardless of whether they have clinical symptoms of skeletal muscle weakness, most carrier females have cardiac abnormalities, such as dilated cardiomyopathy, left ventricle dilatation, and electrocardiographic changes.

Management

The diagnosis of DMD is based on family history and either DNA analysis or muscle biopsy to test for immunoreactivity for dystrophin.

Currently, there are no curative treatments of DMD, although improved symptomatic management has increased the average longevity from late childhood to early adulthood. The objectives of therapy are slowing of disease progression, maintenance of mobility, prevention and correction of contractures and scoliosis, weight control, and optimization of pulmonary and cardiac function. Glucocorticoid therapy can slow the progression of DMD for several years. Several experimental therapies including gene transfer are under investigation. Most patients also require extensive counseling to deal with the psychological effects of having a chronic fatal disease.

INHERITANCE RISK

A third of mothers who have a single affected son will not themselves be carriers of a mutation in the *DMD* gene (see Chapter 19). Determination of carrier status remains difficult, however, because currently available molecular methods do not detect small alterations such as nucleotide changes. Determination of carrier risk in families without identifiable deletions or duplications must rely on linkage analysis, serial serum creatine kinase levels, and mosaic expression of dystrophin in muscle biopsy specimens (due to random X chromosome inactivation). Counseling of recurrence risk must take into account the high rate of germline mosaicism (approximately 14%).

If a mother is a carrier, each son has a 50% risk of DMD and each daughter has a 50% risk of inheriting the *DMD* mutation. Reflecting the random nature of X chromosome inactivation, daughters inheriting the *DMD* mutation have a low risk of DMD; however, for reasons not fully understood, their risk of cardiac abnormalities may be as high as 50% to 60%. If a mother is apparently not a carrier by DNA testing, she still has an approximately 7% risk of having a boy with DMD due to germline mosaicism (see Chapter 7). Counseling and possibly prenatal diagnosis are indicated for these mothers.

Questions for Small Group Discussion
1. Why is DMD considered a genetic lethal condition? What features define a condition as being genetically lethal?
2. Discuss what mechanisms may cause a gender bias in different types of mutation. Name several diseases other than DMD in which this occurs. In particular, discuss the mechanism and high frequency of mutations at CpG dinucleotides during spermatogenesis.
3. How is the rate of germline mosaicism determined for a disease? Name several other diseases with a high rate of germline mosaicism.
4. Contrast the phenotype of Becker muscular dystrophy with DMD. What is the postulated basis for the milder phenotype of Becker muscular dystrophy?

REFERENCES

Davies KE, Nowak KJ: Molecular mechanisms of muscular dystrophies: old and new players. Nat Rev Mol Cell Biol 7:762-773, 2006.
GeneTests. Medical genetics information resource [database online]. University of Washington, Seattle, 1993-2006. Updated weekly. *http://www.genetests.org*
OMIM: Online Mendelian Inheritance in Man. McKusick-Nathans Institute for Genetic Medicine, Johns Hopkins University, and National Center for Biotechnology Information, National Library of Medicine. *http://www.ncbi.nlm.nih.gov/entrez/query.fcgi?db=OMIM*

13. Familial Adenomatous Polyposis

(*APC* Mutation)
Autosomal Dominant

PRINCIPLES

- Tumor-suppressor gene
- Multistep carcinogenesis
- Somatic mutation
- Cytogenetic instability
- Variable expressivity

MAJOR PHENOTYPIC FEATURES

- Age at onset: adolescence through mid-adulthood
- Colorectal adenomatous polyps
- Colorectal cancer
- Multiple primary cancers

HISTORY AND PHYSICAL FINDINGS

R.P., a 35-year-old man, was referred to the cancer genetics clinic by his oncologist. He had just undergone a total colectomy; the colonic mucosa had more than 2000 polyps and pathological changes consistent with adenomatous polyposis coli. In addition to his abdominal scars and colostomy, he had retinal pigment abnormalities consistent with congenital hypertrophy of the retinal pigment epithelium. Several of his relatives had died of cancer. He did not have a medical or family history of other health problems. On the basis of the medical history and suggestive family history, the geneticist counseled R.P. that he most likely had familial adenomatous polyposis. The geneticist explained the surveillance protocol for R.P.'s children and the possibility of using molecular testing to identify those children at risk for familial adenomatous polyposis. Because R.P. did not have contact with his family, linkage analysis was not possible, and R.P. elected to proceed with screening of the adenomatous polyposis coli gene (*APC*); he had a nonsense mutation in exon 15 of one *APC* allele.

BACKGROUND

Disease Etiology and Incidence

At least 50% of individuals in Western populations develop a colorectal tumor, including benign polyps, by the age of 70 years, and approximately 10% of these individuals eventually develop colorectal carcinoma. Approximately 15% of colorectal cancer is familial, including familial adenomatous polyposis (FAP, MIM #175100) and hereditary nonpolyposis colorectal cancer. FAP is an autosomal dominant cancer predisposition syndrome caused by inherited mutations in the *APC* gene. It has a prevalence of 2 to 3 per 100,000 and accounts for less than 1% of colon cancer. Somatic *APC* mutations also occur in more than 80% of sporadic colorectal tumors (see Chapter 16).

Pathogenesis

The APC protein directly or indirectly regulates transcription, cell adhesion, the microtubular cytoskeleton, cell migration, crypt fission, apoptosis, and cell proliferation. It forms complexes with several different proteins including β-catenin.

Both alleles of *APC* must be inactivated for adenoma formation. The high frequency of somatic loss of function in the second *APC* allele defines FAP as an autosomal dominant condition. This somatic loss of function occurs by loss of heterozygosity, intragenic mutation, transcriptional inactivation, and, rarely, dominant negative effects of the inherited mutant allele. More than 95% of intragenic *APC* mutations cause truncation of the APC protein. Loss of functional APC usually results in high levels of free cytosolic β-catenin; free β-catenin migrates to the nucleus, binds to T-cell factor 4, and inappropriately activates gene expression. Consistent with this mechanism, mutations of the β-catenin gene have been identified in some colorectal carcinomas without *APC* mutations.

Although loss of functional APC causes affected cells to form dysplastic foci within intestinal crypts, these cells are not cancerous and must acquire other somatic mutations to progress to cancer (see Chapter 16). This progression is characterized by cytogenetic instability resulting in the loss of large chromosomal segments and, consequently, loss of heterozygosity. Specific genetic alterations implicated in this progression include activation of the Ki-*ras* or N-*ras* oncogenes, inactivation of a tumor-suppressor gene on 18q, inactivation of the *TP53* gene, and alterations in methylation leading to transcriptional silencing of tumor-suppressor genes. As cells accumulate mutations, they become increasingly neoplastic and eventually form invasive and metastatic carcinomas.

Phenotype and Natural History

FAP is characterized by hundreds to thousands of colonic adenomatous polyps (Fig. C-13). It is diagnosed clinically by the presence of either more than 100 colorectal adenomatous polyps or between 10 and 100 polyps in an individual with a relative with FAP. Adenomatous polyps usually appear between 7 and 40 years of age and rapidly increase in number. Untreated, 7% of patients develop colorectal cancer by 21 years of age, 87% by 45 years, and 93% by 50 years.

Although nonpenetrance is very rare, patients with germline mutations of *APC* do not necessarily develop adenomas or colorectal cancer; they are only predisposed. The rate-limiting step in adenoma formation is somatic mutation of the wild-type *APC* allele. Progression of an adenoma to carcinoma requires the accumulation of other genetic alterations. Patients with FAP are at much greater risk than is the general population for development of colorectal carcinoma for two reasons. First, although the average time to progress from adenoma to carcinoma is approximately 23 years, these patients develop adenomas earlier in life and are less likely to die of other causes before the development of carcinoma. Second, although less than 1% of adenomas progress to carcinoma, patients have tens to thousands of adenomas, each with the potential to transform to carcinoma. Thus, the likelihood that at least one adenoma will progress to become an adenocarcinoma is a near certainty.

The penetrance and expressivity of *APC* mutations depend on the particular *APC* mutation, genetic background, and environment. Mutations in different regions of the gene are variously associated with Gardner syndrome (an association of colonic adenomatous polyposis, osteomas, and soft tissue tumors), with congenital hypertrophy of the retinal pigment epithelium, with attenuated adenomatous polyposis coli, or with Turcot syndrome (colon cancer and central nervous system tumors, usually medulloblastoma). Among mice strains with an *APC* mutation, some alleles of phospholipase A_2 modify the number of adenomas; similar modifiers in the human genome may cause patients with identical germline mutations to have dissimilar clinical features. Many studies of sporadic colorectal tumorigenesis identify an enhanced risk for individuals consuming diets high in animal fat; therefore, given the common mechanism of tumorigenesis, diet is likely to play a role in FAP as well.

Management

Early recognition of FAP is necessary for effective intervention, that is, prevention of colorectal cancer. After the development of polyps, definitive treatment is total colectomy with ileoanal pull-through. Recommended surveillance for patients at risk for FAP is colonoscopy every 1 to 2 years beginning at the age of 10 to 12 years. To focus this surveillance, molecular testing is recommended to identify at-risk family members.

INHERITANCE RISK

The empirical lifetime risk for colorectal cancer among Western populations is 5% to 6%. This risk is markedly modified by family history. Patients who have a sibling with adenomatous polyps but no family history of colorectal cancer have a 1.78 relative risk; the relative risk increases to 2.59 if a sibling developed adenomas before the age of 60 years. Patients with a first-degree relative with colorectal cancer have a 1.72 relative risk; this relative risk increases to 2.75 if two or more first-degree relatives had colorectal cancer. If an affected first-degree relative developed colorectal cancer before 44 years of age, the relative risk increases to more than 5.

In contrast to these figures for all colorectal cancer, a patient with FAP or an *APC* germline mutation has a 50% risk of having a child affected with FAP in each pregnancy. The absence of a family history of FAP does not preclude the diagnosis of FAP in a parent because approximately 20% to 30% of patients have a new germline *APC* mutation. Prenatal diagnosis is available by linkage analysis or by testing for the mutation if the mutation in the parent has been defined. Because of intrafamilial variation in expressivity, the severity, time at onset, and associated features cannot be predicted.

Germline *APC* mutations are not detected in between 10% and 30% of individuals with a clinical phenotype of typical FAP and in 90% of individuals with "attenuated" FAP (FAP phenotype except there are fewer than 100 adenomas). Among these patients, 10% are germline homozygotes or compound heterozygotes for a mutation in the DNA repair gene *MYH*; another 10% carry one mutant *MYH* allele in their germline. Heterozygosity for a mutant *MYH* allele increases the risk of colon cancer 3-fold; having both alleles mutant increases risk 50-fold. A patient with FAP and no *APC* mutation should be investigated for *MYH* mutations, particularly if there is a family history suggestive of autosomal recessive inheritance (MIM #608456).

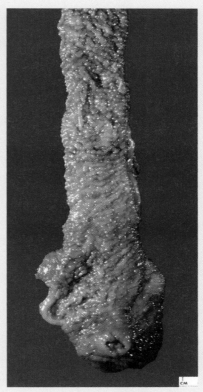

Figure C-13 ■ The mucosa of an ascending colon resected from a patient with FAP. Note the enormous number of polyps. (Courtesy of J. Rutledge, University of Washington and Children's Hospital and Medical Center, Seattle.)

Questions for Small Group Discussion

1. Name additional disorders that demonstrate autosomal dominant inheritance but are recessive at the cellular level. Why do these diseases exhibit autosomal dominant inheritance if two mutations are required for expression of the disease?
2. Discuss some other mendelian disorders that have modeled or provided insights into more common diseases, including at least one for cancer and one for dementia.
3. What does the association of attenuated adenomatous polyposis coli with early truncations of APC suggest about the biochemical basis of attenuated adenomatous polyposis coli compared with classic FAP?

REFERENCES

GeneTests. Medical genetics information resource [database online]. University of Washington, Seattle, 1993-2006. Updated weekly. *http://www.genetests.org*

Jenkins MA, Croitoru ME, Monga N, et al: Risk of colorectal cancer in monoallelic and biallelic carriers of MYH mutations: a population-based case-family study. Cancer Epidemiol Biomarkers Prev 15:312-314, 2006.

OMIM: Online Mendelian Inheritance in Man. McKusick-Nathans Institute for Genetic Medicine, Johns Hopkins University, and National Center for Biotechnology Information, National Library of Medicine. *http://www.ncbi.nlm.nih.gov/entrez/query.fcgi?db=OMIM*

14. Familial Hypercholesterolemia

(Low-density Lipoprotein Receptor Mutation)

Autosomal Dominant

PRINCIPLES

- Environmental modifiers
- Founder effects
- Gene dosage
- Genetic modifiers

MAJOR PHENOTYPIC FEATURES

- Age at onset: heterozygote—early to middle adulthood; homozygote—childhood
- Hypercholesterolemia
- Atherosclerosis
- Xanthomas
- Arcus corneae

HISTORY AND PHYSICAL FINDINGS

L.L., a previously healthy 45-year-old French Canadian poet, was admitted for a myocardial infarction. He had a small xanthoma on his right Achilles tendon. His brother also had coronary artery disease (CAD); his mother, maternal grandmother, and two maternal uncles had died of CAD. In addition to his family history and gender, his risk factors for CAD and atherosclerosis included an elevated level of low-density lipoprotein (LDL) cholesterol, mild obesity, physical inactivity, and cigarette smoking. On the basis of family history, L.L. was believed to have an autosomal dominant form of hypercholesterolemia. Confirming this suspicion, molecular analysis revealed that he was heterozygous for a deletion of the 5′ end of the LDL receptor gene (LDLR), a mutation found in 59% of French Canadians with familial hypercholesterolemia. Screening of his children revealed that two of the three children had elevated LDL cholesterol levels. The cardiologist explained to L.L. that in addition to drug therapy, effective treatment of his CAD required dietary and lifestyle changes, such as a diet low in saturated fat and low in cholesterol, increased physical activity, weight loss, and smoking cessation. L.L. was not compliant with treatment and died a year later of a myocardial infarction.

BACKGROUND

Disease Etiology and Incidence

Familial hypercholesterolemia (FH, MIM# 143890) is an autosomal dominant disorder of cholesterol and lipid metabolism caused by mutations in LDLR (see Chapter 12). FH occurs among all races and has a prevalence of 1 in 500 in most white populations. It accounts for somewhat less than 5% of patients with hypercholesterolemia.

Pathogenesis

The LDL receptor, a transmembrane glycoprotein predominantly expressed in the liver and adrenal cortex, plays a key role in cholesterol homeostasis. It binds apolipoprotein B-100, the sole protein of LDL, and apolipoprotein E, a protein found on very low density lipoproteins, intermediate-density lipoproteins, chylomicron remnants, and some high-density lipoproteins. Hepatic LDL receptors clear approximately 50% of intermediate-density lipoproteins and 66% to 80% of LDL from the circulation by endocytosis; poorly understood LDL receptor–independent pathways clear the remainder of the LDL.

Mutations associated with FH occur throughout LDLR; 2% to 10% are large insertions, deletions, or rearrangements mediated by recombination between Alu repeats within LDLR. Some mutations appear to be dominant negative. Most mutations are private mutations, although some populations—such as Lebanese, French Canadians, South African Indians, South African Ashkenazi Jews, and Afrikaners—have common mutations and a high prevalence of disease because of founder effects.

Homozygous or heterozygous mutations of LDLR decrease the efficiency of intermediate-density lipoprotein and LDL endocytosis and cause accumulation of plasma LDL by increasing production of LDL from intermediate-density lipoproteins and decreasing hepatic clearance of LDL. The elevated plasma LDL levels cause atherosclerosis by increasing the clearance of LDL through LDL receptor–independent pathways, such as endocytosis of oxidized LDL by macrophages and histiocytes. Monocytes, which infiltrate the arterial intima and endocytose oxidized LDL, form foam cells and release cytokines that cause proliferation of smooth muscle cells of the arterial media. Initially, the smooth muscle cells produce sufficient collagen and matrix proteins to form a fibrous cap over the foam cells; because foam cells continue to endocytose oxidized LDL, however, the foam cells eventually rupture through the fibrous cap into the arterial lumen and trigger thrombus formation. Such thrombus formation is a common cause of strokes and myocardial infarction.

Environment, gender, and genetic background modify the effect of LDL receptor mutations on LDL plasma levels and thereby the occurrence of atherosclerosis. Diet is the major environmental modifier of LDL plasma levels; most Tunisian FH heterozygotes have LDL levels in the "normal North American" range and rarely develop cardiovascular disease and xanthomas. Similarly, Chinese FH heterozygotes living in China rarely have xanthomas and cardiovascular disease, whereas Chinese FH heterozygotes living in Western societies have clinical manifestations similar to those of white FH heterozygotes. Dietary cholesterol suppresses the synthesis of LDL receptors and thereby raises plasma LDL levels; this effect of dietary cholesterol is potentiated by saturated fatty acids such as palmitate from dairy products and ameliorated by unsaturated fatty acids such as oleate and linoleate. Because a similar diet does not elevate LDL levels equally among patients, other environmental and genetic factors must also influence LDL metabolism. A few families with FH segregate a different dominant locus that reduces plasma LDL, providing evidence for a genetic modifier.

Phenotype and Natural History

Hypercholesterolemia, the earliest finding in FH, usually manifests at birth and is the only clinical finding through the

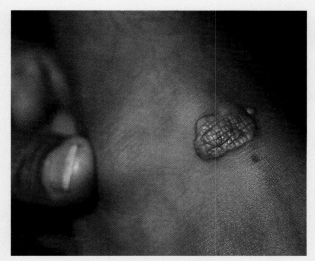

Figure C-14 ■ An Achilles tendon xanthoma from a patient with familial hypercholesterolemia. (Courtesy of M. L. Levy, Department of Dermatology, Baylor College of Medicine, Houston.)

first decade in heterozygous patients; at all ages, the plasma cholesterol concentration is greater than the 95th percentile in more than 95% of patients. Arcus corneae and tendon xanthomas begin to appear by the end of the second decade, and by death, 80% of FH heterozygotes have xanthomas (Fig. C-14). Nearly 40% of adult patients have recurrent nonprogressive polyarthritis and tenosynovitis. As tabulated, the development of CAD among FH heterozygotes depends on age and gender. In general, the untreated cholesterol level is greater than 300 mg/dL.

Homozygous FH presents in the first decade with tendon xanthomas and arcus corneae. Without aggressive treatment, homozygous FH is usually lethal by the age of 30 years. The untreated cholesterol concentration is between 600 and 1000 mg/dL.

Management

Elevated plasma LDL cholesterol and a family history of hypercholesterolemia, xanthomas, or premature CAD strongly suggest a diagnosis of FH. Confirmation of the diagnosis is difficult, however, because it requires quantification of LDL receptor function in the patient's skin fibroblasts or identification of the *LDLR* mutation. In most populations, the plethora of *LDLR* mutations precludes direct DNA analysis unless a particular mutation is strongly suspected. The absence of DNA confirmation does not interfere with management of FH patients, however, because a definitive molecular diagnosis of FH does not provide prognostic or therapeutic information beyond that derived already from the family history and determination of plasma LDL cholesterol.

Regardless of whether they have FH, all patients with elevated LDL cholesterol levels require aggressive normalization of the LDL cholesterol concentration to reduce their risk of CAD; rigorous normalization of the LDL cholesterol concentration can prevent and reverse atherosclerosis. Among FH heterozygotes, rigorous adherence to a low-fat, high-carbohydrate diet usually produces a 10% to 20% reduction in LDL cholesterol. Because this reduction is usually insufficient, patients are often also treated with one or a combination of

AGE- AND SEX-SPECIFIC RATES (%) OF CAD AND DEATH IN FAMILIAL HYPERCHOLESTEROLEMIA HETEROZYGOTES

	Males		Females	
Age	CAD	Death	CAD	Death
30	5	—	0	—
40	20-24	—	0-3	0
50	45-51	25	12-20	2
60	75-85	50	45-57	15
70	100	80	75	30

CAD, coronary artery disease.
From Rader DJ, Hobbs HH: Disorders of lipoprotein metabolism. In Kasper DL, Braunwald E, Fauci AS, et al, eds: Harrison's Principles of Internal Medicine, 16th ed. New York, McGraw-Hill, 2004.

three classes of drugs: bile acid sequestrants, 3-hydroxy-3-methylglutaryl coenzyme A reductase inhibitors, and nicotinic acid (see Chapter 13). Current recommendations are initiation of drug therapy at 10 years of age for patients with an LDL cholesterol level of more than 190 mg/dL and a negative family history for premature CAD and at 10 years of age for patients with an LDL cholesterol level of more than 160 mg/dL and a positive family history for premature CAD. Among FH homozygotes, LDL apheresis can reduce plasma cholesterol levels by as much as 70%. The therapeutic effectiveness of apheresis is increased when it is combined with aggressive statin and nicotinic acid therapy. Liver transplantation has also been used on rare occasions.

INHERITANCE RISK

Because FH is an autosomal dominant disorder, each child of an affected parent has a 50% chance of inheriting the mutant *LDLR* allele. Untreated FH heterozygotes have a 100% risk for development of CAD by the age of 70 years if male and a 75% risk if female. Current medical therapy markedly reduces this risk by normalizing plasma cholesterol concentration.

Questions for Small Group Discussion

1. What insights does FH provide into the more common polygenic causes of atherosclerosis and CAD?
2. Familial defective apolipoprotein B-100 is a genocopy of FH. Why?
3. Vegetable oils are hydrogenated to make some margarines. What effect would eating margarine have on LDL receptor expression compared with vegetable oil consumption?
4. Discuss genetic susceptibility to infection and potential heterozygote advantage in the context of the role of the LDL receptor in hepatitis C infection.

REFERENCES

GeneTests. Medical genetics information resource [database online]. University of Washington, Seattle, 1993-2006. Updated weekly. *http://www.genetests.org*
OMIM: Online Mendelian Inheritance in Man. McKusick-Nathans Institute for Medical Genetics, Johns Hopkins University, and National Center for Biotechnology Information, National Library of Medicine. *http://www.ncbi.nlm.nih.gov/entrez/query.fcgi?db=OMIM*
Rader DJ, Hobbs HH: Disorders of lipoprotein metabolism. In Kasper DL, Braunwald E, Fauci AS, et al, eds: Harrison's Principles of Internal Medicine, 16th ed. New York, McGraw-Hill, 2004.

15. Fragile X Syndrome

(*FMR1* Mutation)
X-Linked

PRINCIPLES

- Triplet repeat expansion
- Somatic mosaicism
- Sex-specific anticipation
- DNA methylation
- Haplotype effect

MAJOR PHENOTYPIC FEATURES

- Age at onset: childhood
- Mental deficiency
- Dysmorphic facies
- Male postpubertal macroorchidism

HISTORY AND PHYSICAL FINDINGS

R.L., a 6-year-old boy, was referred to the developmental pediatrics clinic for evaluation of mental retardation and hyperactivity. He had failed kindergarten because he was disruptive, was unable to attend to tasks, and had poor speech and motor skills. His development was delayed, but he had not lost developmental milestones: he sat by 10 to 11 months, walked by 20 months, and spoke two or three clear words by 24 months. He had otherwise been in good health. His mother and maternal aunt had mild childhood learning disabilities, and a maternal uncle was mentally retarded. The findings from his physical examination were normal except for hyperactivity. The physician recommended several tests, including a karyotype, thyroid function studies, and DNA analysis for fragile X syndrome. The Southern blot analysis of the *FMR1* gene was consistent with fragile X syndrome.

BACKGROUND

Disease Etiology and Incidence

Fragile X syndrome (MIM# 309550) is an X-linked mental retardation disorder that is caused by mutations in the *FMR1* gene on Xq27.3 (see Chapter 12). Fragile X syndrome has an estimated prevalence of 16 to 25 per 100,000 in the general male population and half that in the general female population. Fragile X syndrome accounts for 3% to 6% of mental retardation among boys with a positive family history of mental retardation and no birth defects.

Pathogenesis

The *FMR1* gene product, FMRP, is expressed in many cell types but most abundantly in neurons. FMRP may chaperone a subclass of mRNAs from the nucleus to the translational machinery.

More than 99% of *FMR1* mutations are expansions of a $(CGG)_n$ repeat sequence in the 5' untranslated region of the gene (see Chapter 12). In normal alleles of *FMR1*, the number of CGG repeats ranges from 6 to approximately 50. In disease-causing alleles or full mutations, the number of repeats is more than 200. Alleles with more than 200 CGG repeats usually have hypermethylation of the CGG repeat sequence and the adjacent *FMR1* promoter (Fig. C-15). Hypermethylation inactivates the *FMR1* promoter, causing a loss of FMRP expression.

Full mutations arise from premutation alleles (approximately 59 to 200 CGG repeats) with maternal transmission of a mutant *FMR1* allele but not with paternal transmission; in fact, premutations often shorten with paternal transmission. Full mutations do not arise from normal alleles. Because the length of an unstable CGG repeat increases each generation if it is transmitted by a female, increasing numbers of affected offspring are usually observed in later generations of an affected family; this phenomenon is referred to as genetic anticipation (see Chapter 7).

The risk of premutation expansion to a full mutation increases as the repeat length of the premutation increases (see Fig. 7-31). Not all premutations, however, are equally predisposed to expand. Although premutations are relatively common, progression to a full mutation has been observed only on a limited number of haplotypes; that is, there is a haplotype predisposition to expansion. This haplotype predisposition may relate partly to the presence of a few AGG triplets embedded within the string of CGG repeats; these AGG triplets appear to inhibit expansion of the string of CGG repeats, and their absence in some haplotypes, therefore, may predispose to expansion.

Phenotype and Natural History

Fragile X syndrome causes moderate mental retardation in affected males and mild mental retardation in affected females. Most affected individuals also have behavioral abnormalities, including hyperactivity, hand flapping or biting, temper tantrums, poor eye contact, and autistic features. The physical features of males vary in relation to puberty such that before puberty, they have somewhat large heads but few other distinctive features; after puberty, they frequently have more distinctive features (long face with prominent jaw and forehead, large ears, and macro-orchidism). Because these clinical findings are not unique to fragile X syndrome, the diagnosis depends on molecular detection of mutations. Patients with fragile X syndrome have a normal life span.

Nearly all males and 40% to 50% of females who inherit a full mutation will have fragile X syndrome. The severity of the phenotype depends on repeat length mosaicism and repeat methylation. Because full mutations are mitotically unstable, some patients have a mixture of cells with repeat lengths ranging from premutation to full mutation (repeat length mosaicism). All males with repeat length mosaicism are affected but often have higher mental function than do those with a full mutation in every cell; females with repeat length mosaicism are normal to fully affected. Similarly, some patients have a mixture of cells with and without methylation of the CGG repeat (repeat methylation mosaicism). All males with methylation mosaicism are affected but often have higher mental function than do those with a hypermethylation in every cell; females with methylation mosaicism are normal to fully affected. Very rarely, patients have a full

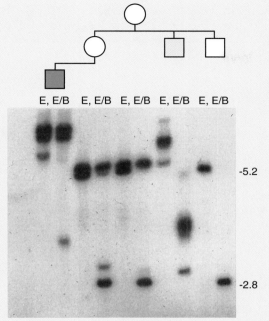

E, E/B E, E/B E, E/B E, E/B E, E/B

-5.2

-2.8

Figure C-15 ■ Southern blot showing a family segregating *FMR1* premutations in the mother and grandmother of the proband and expansion of a premutation into a full mutation in the proband in the third generation.

Using a probe from the 5' end of the *FMR1* gene, a DNA sample digested with the endonuclease *EcoRI* alone (E) normally yields a 5.2 kb band; double digestion with *EcoRI* and *BssH2* (E/B) yields a 2.8 kb band. Because *BssH2* digestion is inhibited by DNA methylation, it does not cut within the methylated CGG repeats of the *FMR1* allele on the inactive X in females or of a methylated *FMR1* full mutation. Thus, the full mutation allele in the affected boy yields larger than normal *EcoRI* fragments (>>5.2 kb) that are mostly resistant to *BssH2*. Note that the unaffected grandmother carries a small amount of premutation, the unaffected mother carries a larger amount of a slightly larger premutation, and the affected boy has a full mutation. The grandmother also has a mildly affected son with a full mutation that is, however, not methylated and an unaffected son with a normal allele. (Courtesy of Peter Ray, The Hospital for Sick Children and University of Toronto, Canada.)

mutation that is unmethylated in all cells; whether male or female, these patients vary from normal to fully affected. In addition, in females, the phenotype is dependent on the degree of skewing of X chromosome inactivation (see Chapter 6).

Female carriers of premutations (but not full mutations) are at a 20% risk of premature ovarian failure. Male premutation carriers are at risk of the fragile X–associated tremor/ataxia syndrome (FXTAS). FXTAS manifests as late-onset, progressive cerebellar ataxia and intention tremor. Affected individuals may also have loss of short-term memory, executive function, and cognition as well as parkinsonism, peripheral neuropathy, proximal lower limb muscle weakness, and autonomic dysfunction. Penetrance of FXTAS is age depen-

dent, manifesting in 17% in the sixth decade, in 38% in the seventh decade, in 47% in the eighth decade, and in three fourths of those older than 80 years. FXTAS may manifest in some female premutation carriers.

Management

No curative treatments are currently available for fragile X syndrome. Therapy focuses on educational intervention and pharmacological management of the behavioral problems.

INHERITANCE RISK

The risk that a woman with a premutation will have an affected child is determined by the size of the premutation, the sex of the fetus, and the family history. Empirically, the risk to a permutation carrier of having an affected child can be as high as 50% for each male child and 25% for each female child but depends on the size of the premutation. On the basis of analysis of a relatively small number of carrier mothers, the recurrence risk appears to decline as the premutation decreases from 100 to 59 repeats. Prenatal testing is available by use of fetal DNA derived from chorionic villi or amniocytes.

Questions for Small Group Discussion

1. Discuss haplotype bias in disease, that is, the effect of haplotype on mutation development (fragile X syndrome), disease severity (sickle cell disease), or predisposition to disease (autoimmune diseases).
2. Fragile X syndrome, myotonic dystrophy, Friedreich ataxia, Huntington disease, and several other disorders are caused by expansion of repeat sequences. Contrast the mechanisms or proposed mechanisms by which expansion of the repeat causes disease for each of these disorders. Why do some of these disorders show anticipation whereas others do not?
3. The sex bias in transmission of *FMR1* mutations is believed to arise because FMRP expression is necessary for production of viable sperm. Compare the sex bias in transmitting fragile X syndrome and Huntington disease. Discuss mechanisms that could explain biases in the transmitting sex for various diseases.
4. What family history and diagnostic information are necessary before prenatal diagnosis is undertaken for fragile X syndrome?
5. How would you counsel a pregnant woman carrying a 46,XY fetus with 60 repeats? a 46,XX fetus with 60 repeats? a 46,XX fetus with more than 300 repeats?

REFERENCES

Garber K, Smith KT, Reines D, Warren ST: Transcription, translation and fragile X syndrome. Curr Opin Genet Dev 16:270-275, 2006.

GeneTests. Medical genetics information resource [database online]. University of Washington, Seattle, 1993-2006. Updated weekly. *http://www.genetests.org*

OMIM: Online Mendelian Inheritance in Man. McKusick-Nathans Institute for Genetic Medicine, Johns Hopkins University, and National Center for Biotechnology Information, National Library of Medicine. *http://www.ncbi.nlm.nih.gov/entrez/query.fcgi?db=OMIM*

Visootsak J, Warren ST, Anido A, Graham JM Jr: Fragile X syndrome: an update and review for the primary pediatrician. Clin Pediatr (Phila) 44:371-381, 2005.

16. Glucose-6-Phosphate Dehydrogenase Deficiency

(*G6PD* Mutation)

X-Linked

PRINCIPLES

- Heterozygote advantage
- Pharmacogenetics

MAJOR PHENOTYPIC FEATURES

- Age at onset: neonatal
- Hemolytic anemia
- Neonatal jaundice

HISTORY AND PHYSICAL FINDINGS

L.M., a previously healthy 5-year-old boy, presented to the emergency department febrile, pale, tachycardic, tachypneic, and minimally responsive; his physical examination was otherwise normal. The morning before presentation, he had been in good health, but during the afternoon, he had abdominal pain, headache, and fever; by late evening, he was tachypneic and incoherent. He had not ingested any medications or known toxins, and results of a urine toxicology screen were negative. Results of other laboratory tests showed massive nonimmune intravascular hemolysis and hemoglobinuria. After resuscitation, L.M. was admitted to the hospital; the hemolysis resolved without further intervention. L.M. was of Greek ethnicity; his parents were unaware of a family history of hemolysis, although his mother had some cousins in Europe with a "blood problem." Further inquiry revealed that the morning before admission, L.M. had been eating fava beans from the garden while his mother was working in the yard. The physician explained to the parents that L.M. probably was deficient for glucose-6-phosphate dehydrogenase (G6PD) and that because of this, he had become ill after eating fava beans. Subsequent measurement of L.M.'s erythrocyte G6PD activity confirmed that he had G6PD deficiency. The parents were counseled concerning L.M.'s risk of acute hemolysis after exposure to certain drugs and toxins and given a list of compounds that L.M. should avoid.

BACKGROUND

Disease Etiology and Incidence

G6PD deficiency (MIM# 305900), a hereditary predisposition to hemolysis, is an X-linked disorder of antioxidant homeostasis that is caused by mutations in the *G6PD* gene. In areas in which malaria is endemic, G6PD deficiency has a prevalence of 5% to 25%; in nonendemic areas, it has a prevalence of less than 0.5% (Fig. C-16). Like sickle cell disease, G6PD deficiency appears to have reached a substantial frequency in some areas because it confers to individuals heterozygous for G6PD deficiency some resistance to malaria and thus a survival advantage (see Chapter 9).

Pathogenesis

G6PD is the first enzyme in the hexose monophosphate shunt, a pathway critical for generating nicotinamide adenine dinucleotide phosphate (NADPH). NADPH is required for the regeneration of reduced glutathione. Within erythrocytes, reduced glutathione is used for the detoxification of oxidants produced by the interaction of hemoglobin and oxygen and by exogenous factors such as drugs, infection, and metabolic acidosis.

Most G6PD deficiency arises because mutations in the X-linked *G6PD* gene decrease the catalytic activity or the stability of G6PD, or both. When G6PD activity is sufficiently depleted or deficient, insufficient NADPH is available to regenerate reduced glutathione during times of oxidative stress. This results in the oxidation and aggregation of intracellular proteins (Heinz bodies) and the formation of rigid erythrocytes that readily hemolyze.

With the more common *G6PD* alleles, which cause the protein to be unstable, deficiency of G6PD within erythrocytes worsens as erythrocytes age. Because erythrocytes do not have nuclei, new G6PD mRNA cannot be synthesized; thus, erythrocytes are unable to replace G6PD as it is degraded. During exposure to an oxidative stress episode, therefore, hemolysis begins with the oldest erythrocytes and progressively involves younger erythrocytes, depending on the severity of the oxidative stress.

Phenotype and Natural History

As an X-linked disorder, G6PD deficiency predominantly and most severely affects males. Rare symptomatic females have a skewing of X chromosome inactivation such that the X chromosome carrying the *G6PD* disease allele is the active X chromosome in erythrocyte precursors (see Chapter 6).

Besides gender, the severity of G6PD deficiency depends on the specific *G6PD* mutation. In general, the mutation common in the Mediterranean basin (i.e., G6PD B⁻ or Mediterranean) tends to be more severe than those mutations common in Africa (i.e., G6PD A⁻ variants) (Fig. C-16). In erythrocytes of patients with the Mediterranean variant, G6PD activity decreases to insufficient levels 5 to 10 days after erythrocytes appear in the circulation, whereas in the erythrocytes of patients with the G6PD A⁻ variants, G6PD activity decreases to insufficient levels 50 to 60 days after erythrocytes appear in the circulation. Therefore, most erythrocytes are susceptible to hemolysis in patients with severe forms of G6PD deficiency, such as G6PD Mediterranean, but only 20% to 30% are susceptible in patients with G6PD A⁻ variants.

G6PD deficiency most commonly manifests as either neonatal jaundice or acute hemolytic anemia. The peak incidence of neonatal jaundice occurs during days 2 and 3 of life. The severity of the jaundice ranges from subclinical to levels compatible with kernicterus; the associated anemia is rarely severe. Episodes of acute hemolytic anemia usually begin within hours of an oxidative stress and end when G6PD-deficient erythrocytes have hemolyzed; therefore, the severity of the anemia associated with these acute hemolytic episodes is proportionate to the deficiency of G6PD and the oxidative stress. Viral and bacterial infections are the most common triggers, but many drugs and toxins can also precipitate hemolysis. The disorder favism results from hemolysis sec-

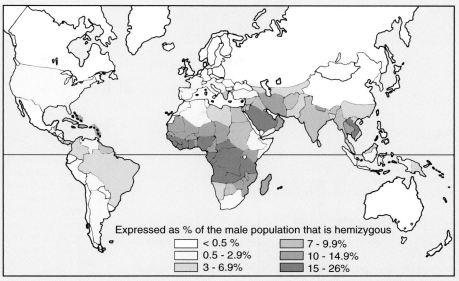

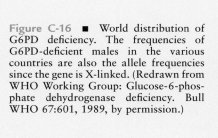

Figure C-16 ■ World distribution of G6PD deficiency. The frequencies of G6PD-deficient males in the various countries are also the allele frequencies since the gene is X-linked. (Redrawn from WHO Working Group: Glucose-6-phosphate dehydrogenase deficiency. Bull WHO 67:601, 1989, by permission.)

Expressed as % of the male population that is hemizygous

□ < 0.5 %	▨ 7 - 9.9%
□ 0.5 - 2.9%	▨ 10 - 14.9%
▨ 3 - 6.9%	▨ 15 - 26%

ondary to the ingestion of fava beans by patients with more severe forms of G6PD deficiency, such as G6PD Mediterranean; fava beans contain β-glycosides, naturally occurring oxidants.

In addition to neonatal jaundice and acute hemolytic anemia, G6PD deficiency rarely causes congenital or chronic nonspherocytic hemolytic anemia. Patients with chronic nonspherocytic hemolytic anemia generally have a profound deficiency of G6PD that causes chronic anemia and an increased susceptibility to infection. The susceptibility to infection arises because the NADPH supply within granulocytes is inadequate to sustain the oxidative burst necessary for killing of phagocytosed bacteria.

Management

G6PD deficiency should be suspected in patients of African, Mediterranean, or Asian ancestry who present with either an acute hemolytic episode or neonatal jaundice. G6PD deficiency is diagnosed by measurement of G6PD activity in erythrocytes; this activity should be measured only when the patient has had neither a recent transfusion nor a recent hemolytic episode. (Because G6PD deficiency occurs primarily in older erythrocytes, measurement of G6PD activity in the predominantly young erythrocytes present during or immediately after a hemolytic episode often gives a false-negative result.)

The key to management of G6PD deficiency is prevention of hemolysis by prompt treatment of infections and avoidance of oxidant drugs (e.g., sulfonamides, sulfones, nitrofurans) and toxins (e.g., naphthalene). Although most patients with a hemolytic episode will not require medical intervention, those with severe anemia and hemolysis may require resuscitation and erythrocyte transfusions. Patients presenting with neonatal jaundice respond well to the same therapies as for other infants with neonatal jaundice (hydration, light therapy, and exchange transfusions).

INHERITANCE RISK

Each son of a mother carrying a *G6PD* mutation has a 50% chance of being affected, and each daughter has a 50% chance of being a carrier. Each daughter of an affected father will be a carrier, but each son will be unaffected because an affected father does not contribute an X chromosome to his sons. The risk that carrier daughters will have clinically significant symptoms is low because sufficient skewing of X chromosome inactivation is relatively uncommon.

Questions for Small Group Discussion

1. The consumption of fava beans and the occurrence of G6PD deficiency are coincident in many areas. What evolutionary advantage might the consumption of fava beans give populations with G6PD deficiency?
2. Several hundred different mutations have been described that cause G6PD deficiency. Presumably, all of these mutations have persisted because of selection. Discuss heterozygote advantage in the context of G6PD deficiency.
3. What is pharmacogenetics? How does G6PD deficiency illustrate the principles of pharmaco-genetics?

REFERENCES

GeneTests. Medical genetics information resource [database online]. University of Washington, Seattle, 1993-2006. Updated weekly. *http://www.genetests.org*

Luzzatto L, Melta A, Vulliamy T: Glucose-6-phosphate dehydrogenase deficiency. In Scriver CR, Beaudet AL, Sly WS, et al (eds): The Metabolic and Molecular Bases of Inherited Disease, 8th ed. New York, McGraw-Hill, 2001, pp 4517-4553.

OMIM: Online Mendelian Inheritance in Man. McKusick-Nathans Institute for Genetic Medicine, Johns Hopkins University, and National Center for Biotechnology Information, National Library of Medicine. *http://www.ncbi.nlm.nih.gov/entrez/query.fcgi?db=OMIM*

17. Hereditary Hemochromatosis

(*HFE* Mutation)
Autosomal Recessive

PRINCIPLES

- Incomplete penetrance and variable expressivity
- Sex differences in penetrance
- Population screening versus at-risk testing
- Molecular versus biochemical testing

MAJOR PHENOTYPIC FEATURES

- Age at onset: 40 to 60 years in males; after menopause in females
- Fatigue, impotence, hyperpigmentation (bronzing), diabetes, cirrhosis, cardiomyopathy
- Elevated serum transferrin iron saturation
- Elevated serum ferritin

HISTORY AND PHYSICAL FINDINGS

S.F. was a 30-year-old healthy white male referred to the genetics clinic for counseling because his 55-year-old father had just been diagnosed with cirrhosis due to hereditary hemochromatosis. History and physical examination findings were normal. His transferrin iron saturation was 48% (normal, 20% to 50%). His serum ferritin level was normal (<300 ng/mL), and liver transaminase activities were normal. Given that S.F. was an obligate carrier for the condition and his mother had an 11% population risk of being a carrier, his prior risk for having inherited two mutant *HFE* alleles was 5.5%. S.F. chose to have his *HFE* gene examined for the two common hemochromatosis variants. Molecular testing revealed that he was homozygous for the Cys282Tyr mutation, putting him at risk for development of hemochromatosis. He was referred to his primary care provider to follow serum ferritin levels every 3 months and to institute therapy as needed.

BACKGROUND

Disease Etiology and Incidence

Hereditary hemochromatosis (MIM# 235200) is a disease of iron overload that occurs in some individuals with homozygous or compound heterozygous mutations in the *HFE* gene. Most patients (90% to 95%) with hereditary hemochromatosis are homozygous for a Cys282Tyr mutation; the remaining 5% to 10% of affected individuals are compound heterozygotes for the Cys282Tyr and another mutation, His63Asp. Homozygosity for His63Asp does not lead to clinical hemochromatosis unless there is an additional cause of iron overload. The carrier rate in the white population of North America is approximately 11% for Cys282Tyr and approximately 27% for His63Asp, which means that about 1 in 330 individuals will be Cys282Tyr homozygotes and an additional 1 in 135 will be compound heterozygotes for *HFE* disease-causing mutations. The frequency of these mutations is far lower in Asians, Africans, and Native Americans.

The penetrance of clinical hereditary hemochromatosis has been difficult to determine; estimates vary from 10% to 70%, depending on whether hereditary hemochromatosis is defined as organ damage due to pathological iron overload or by biochemical evidence of an elevation of ferritin and transferrin saturation. In a family-based study, for example, between 75% and 90% of homozygous relatives of affected individuals were asymptomatic. Population-based studies have provided estimates of penetrance based on biochemical evidence of hereditary hemochromatosis of 25% to 50%, but penetrance may be higher if liver biopsies are performed to find occult cirrhosis. Whatever the penetrance, it is clear that males are affected more frequently than are females and that Cys282Tyr/His63Asp compound heterozygotes are at much lower risk for hereditary hemochromatosis than are Cys282Tyr homozygotes. Although the exact value of the penetrance in Cys282Tyr homozygotes remains to be definitively determined, penetrance is clearly incomplete.

Pathogenesis

Hereditary hemochromatosis is a disorder of iron overload. Body stores of iron are determined largely by dietary iron absorption from enterocytes of the small intestine and release of endogenous iron from macrophages that phagocytose red blood cells. Iron release from enterocytes and macrophages is regulated by a circulating iron response hormone, hepcidin, which is synthesized in the liver and released to block further iron absorption when iron supplies are adequate. Mutant *HFE* interferes with hepcidin signaling, which results in the stimulation of enterocytes and macrophages to release iron. The body therefore continues to absorb and recycle iron, despite an iron-overloaded condition.

Ultimately, a small proportion of individuals with two mutations in the *HFE* gene will develop symptomatic iron overload. Early symptoms include fatigue, arthralgia, decreased libido, and abdominal pain. An additional presentation is the finding of elevated transferrin iron saturation or ferritin on routine screening. Late findings of iron overload include hepatomegaly, cirrhosis (Fig. C-17), hepatocellular carcinoma, diabetes mellitus, cardiomyopathy, hypogonadism, arthritis, and increased skin pigmentation (bronzing). Males develop symptoms between the ages of 40 and 60 years. Women, who are reported to develop symptoms at one-half to one-tenth the rate of men, do not develop symptoms until after menopause. Prognosis is excellent in patients diagnosed and treated before the development of cirrhosis. Patients diagnosed with cirrhosis and treated effectively with phlebotomy still have a 10% to 30% risk of liver cancer years later.

Management

Individuals with an at-risk genotype are monitored with serum ferritin levels annually. If the level is higher than 50 ng/mL, phlebotomy to remove a unit of blood is recommended to maintain normal levels. Phlebotomy is repeated until a normal ferritin concentration is achieved. Failure to achieve a normal ferritin concentration within 3 months of starting phlebotomy is a poor prognostic sign. Once the ferritin concentration is below 50 ng/mL, maintenance phlebotomy is performed every 3 to 4 months for men and every 6 to 12 months for women.

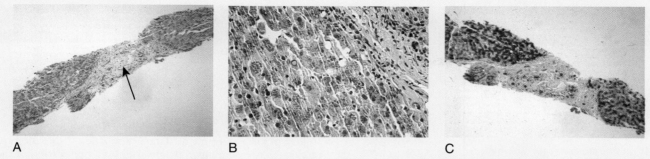

Figure C-17 ■ Liver of patient with hereditary hemochromatosis showing iron deposition and cirrhosis. **A,** Low-power view showing area of fibrosis (*arrow*; hematoxylin and eosin stain). **B,** Higher power view showing iron deposition (brown pigment seen within hepatocytes) next to an area of fibrosis (hematoxylin and eosin stain). **C,** Perl's stain in which iron stains dark blue. Heavy staining in hepatocytes flanks an area of fibrosis with much less iron deposition. (Courtesy of Victor Gordeuk, Howard University, Washington, DC.)

Symptomatic patients with initial ferritin concentrations of more than 1000 ng/mL should undergo liver biopsy to determine if cirrhosis is present. Patients found to have biochemical abnormalities should undergo phlebotomy weekly until the hematocrit is 75% of the baseline and the ferritin concentration is below 50 ng/mL.

INHERITANCE RISK

Hereditary hemochromatosis is an autosomal recessive disorder with reduced penetrance. The sibs of an affected individual have a 25% chance of having two mutations. The child of an affected individual will be a carrier and has a 5% risk of having two mutations if both parents are white. Because of the apparently low penetrance of this disease, universal population screening for *HFE* mutations has not been considered to be indicated. However, because of the prevalence of the disorder, the uncertainty as to the true penetrance, and the availability of easy and effective treatment, one-time screening of serum transferrin iron saturation and ferritin concentrations in adult white, non-Hispanic men of northern European descent may be justified.

Questions for Small Group Discussion
1. Why do women have much lower incidence of hemochromatosis?
2. Besides phlebotomy, what dietary interventions would be indicated to prevent iron overload?
3. Discuss the possible reasons for the high prevalence of the Cys282Tyr mutation among whites.

REFERENCES

Fleming RE, Bacon BR: Orchestration of iron homeostasis. N Engl J Med 352:1741-1744, 2005.

GeneTests. Medical genetics information resource [database online]. University of Washington, Seattle, 1993-2006. Updated weekly. *http://www.genetests.org*

OMIM: Online Mendelian Inheritance in Man. McKusick-Nathans Institute for Genetic Medicine, Johns Hopkins University, and National Center for Biotechnology Information, National Library of Medicine. *http://www.ncbi.nlm.nih.gov/entrez/query.fcgi?db=OMIM*

Yen AW, Fancher TL, Bowlus CL: Revisiting hereditary hemochromatosis: current concepts and progress. Am J Med 119:391-399, 2006.

18. Hemophilia

(*F8* or *F9* Mutation)
X-Linked

PRINCIPLES

- Intrachromosomal recombination
- Transposable element insertion
- Variable expressivity
- Protein replacement therapy

MAJOR PHENOTYPIC FEATURES

- Age at onset: infancy to adulthood
- Bleeding diathesis
- Hemarthroses
- Hematomas

HISTORY AND PHYSICAL FINDINGS

S.T., a healthy 38-year-old woman, scheduled an appointment for counseling regarding her risk of having a child with hemophilia. She had a maternal uncle who had died in childhood from hemophilia and a brother who had had bleeding problems as a child. Her brother's bleeding problems had resolved during adolescence. No other family members had bleeding disorders. The geneticist explained to S.T. that her family history was suggestive of an X-linked abnormality of coagulation such as hemophilia A or B and that her brother's improvement was particularly suggestive of the hemophilia B variant factor IX Leyden. To confirm the diagnosis of hemophilia, the geneticist told S.T. that her brother should be evaluated first because identification of an isolated carrier is difficult. S.T. talked to her brother, and he agreed to an evaluation. Review of his records showed that he indeed had been diagnosed with factor IX deficiency as a child but now had nearly normal plasma levels of factor IX. DNA mutation analysis confirmed that he had a mutation in the *F9* gene promoter, consistent with factor IX Leyden. Subsequent testing of S.T. showed that she did not carry the mutation identified in her brother.

BACKGROUND

Disease Etiology and Incidence

Hemophilia A (MIM# 307600) and hemophilia B (MIM# 306900) are X-linked disorders of coagulation caused by mutations in the *F8* and *F9* genes, respectively. Mutations of *F8* cause deficiency or dysfunction of clotting factor VIII; mutations of *F9* cause deficiency or dysfunction of clotting factor IX.

Hemophilia is a panethnic disorder without racial predilection. Hemophilia A has an incidence of 1 in 5000 to 10,000 newborn males. Hemophilia B is far rarer, with an incidence of 1 in 100,000.

Pathogenesis

The coagulation system maintains the integrity of the vasculature through a delicate balance of clot formation and inhibition. The proteases and protein cofactors composing the clotting cascade are present in the circulation as inactive precursors and must be sequentially activated at the site of injury to form a fibrin clot. Timely and efficient formation of a clot requires exponential activation or amplification of the protease cascade. Clotting factors VIII and IX, which complex together, are key to this amplification; they activate clotting factor X, and active factor X, in turn, activates more factor IX and factor VIII (see Figure 8-5). Factor IX functions as a protease and factor VIII as a cofactor. Deficiency or dysfunction of either factor IX or factor VIII causes hemophilia.

Mutations of *F8* include deletions, insertions, inversions, and point mutations. The most common mutation is an inversion deleting the carboxyl terminus of factor VIII; it accounts for 25% of all hemophilia A and for 40% to 50% of severe hemophilia A. This inversion results from an intrachromosomal recombination between sequences in intron 22 of *F8* and homologous sequences telomeric to *F8*. Another intriguing class of mutation involves retrotransposition of L1 repeats into the gene. For all *F8* mutations, the residual enzymatic activity of the factor VIII–factor IX complex correlates with the severity of clinical disease (see Table).

Many different *F9* mutations have been identified in patients with hemophilia B; but in contrast to the frequent partial inversion of *F8* in hemophilia A, a common *F9* mutation has not been identified for hemophilia B. Factor IX Leyden is an unusual *F9* variant caused by point mutations in the *F9* promoter; it is associated with very low levels of factor IX and severe hemophilia during childhood, but spontaneous resolution of hemophilia occurs at puberty as factor IX levels nearly normalize. For each *F9* mutation, the residual enzymatic activity of the factor VIII–factor IX complex correlates with the severity of clinical disease (see Table).

Phenotype and Natural History

Hemophilia is classically a male disease, although rare females can be affected because of skewed X chromosome inactivation. Clinically, hemophilia A and hemophilia B are indistinguishable. Both are characterized by bleeding into soft tissues, muscles, and weight-bearing joints (Fig. C-18). Bleeding occurs within hours to days after trauma and often continues for days or weeks. Those with severe disease are usually diagnosed as newborns because of excessive cephalohematomas or prolonged bleeding from umbilical or circumcision wounds. Patients with moderate disease often do not develop hematomas or hemarthroses until they begin to crawl or walk and therefore escape diagnosis until that time. Patients with mild disease frequently present in adolescence or adulthood with hemarthroses or prolonged bleeding after surgery or trauma.

CLINICAL CLASSIFICATION AND CLOTTING FACTOR LEVELS	
Classification	% Activity (Factor VIII or IX)
Severe	<1%
Moderate	1%-5%
Mild	5%-25%

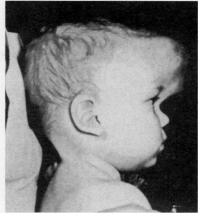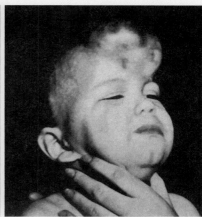

Figure C-18 ■ Subcutaneous hematoma of the forehead in a young boy with hemophilia. The photograph was taken 4 days after a minor contusion. The appearance of the forehead returned to normal in 6 months. (Modified from The Hemorrhagic Disorders: A Clinical and Therapeutic Approach, 1962, Grune & Stratton, p 252, by permission. Photographic restoration courtesy of B. Moseley-Fernandini.)

Hemophilia A and hemophilia B are diagnosed and distinguished by measurement of factor VIII and IX activity levels. For both hemophilia A and hemophilia B, the level of factor VIII or IX activity predicts the clinical severity.

Management

Although current gene therapy trials show promise, no curative treatments are available for hemophilia A and hemophilia B except for liver transplantation (see Chapter 13). Currently, the standard of care is intravenous replacement of the deficient factor. Factor replacement therapy has increased life expectancy from an average of 1.4 years in the early 1900s to approximately 65 years today.

INHERITANCE RISK

If a woman has a family history of hemophilia, her carrier status can be determined by linkage analysis or by identification of the *F8* or *F9* mutation segregating in the family. Routine mutation identification is available only for the common *F8* inversion, however. Carrier detection by enzyme assay is difficult and not widely available.

If a mother is a carrier, each son has a 50% risk of hemophilia, and each daughter has a 50% risk of inheriting the *F8* or *F9* mutation. Reflecting the low frequency of clinically significant skewing of X chromosome inactivation, daughters inheriting an *F8* or *F9* mutation have a low risk of hemophilia.

If a mother has a son with hemophilia but no other affected relatives, her a priori risk of being a carrier depends on the type of mutation. Point mutations and the common *F8* inversions almost always arise in male meiosis; as a result, 98% of mothers of a male with one of these mutations are carriers due to a new mutation in their father (the affected male's maternal grandfather). In contrast, deletion mutations usually arise during female meiosis. If there is no knowledge

of the mutation type, then approximately a third of patients are assumed to have a new mutation in *F8* or *F9*. Through the application of Bayes' theorem, this risk can be modified by considering the number of unaffected sons in the family (see Chapter 19).

Questions for Small Group Discussion

1. What other diseases are caused by recombination between repeated genome sequences? Compare and contrast the recombination mechanism observed with hemophilia A with that observed with Smith-Magenis syndrome and with familial hypercholesterolemia.
2. One of the more unusual mutations in *F8* is insertion of an L1 element into exon 14. What are transposable elements? How do transposable elements move within a genome? Name another disease caused by movement of transposable elements.
3. In patients with hemophilia B due to factor IX Leyden, why does the deficiency of factor IX resolve during puberty?
4. Compare and contrast protein replacement for hemophilia to that for Gaucher disease. Approximately 10% of patients with hemophilia develop a clinically significant antibody titer against factor VIII or IX. Why? Is there a genetic predisposition to development of antibodies against the replacement factors? How could this immune reaction be circumvented? Would gene therapy be helpful for patients with antibodies?
5. Discuss current approaches to gene therapy in hemophilia B.

REFERENCES

GeneTests. Medical genetics information resource [database online]. University of Washington, Seattle, 1993-2006. Updated weekly. *http://www.genetests.org*

OMIM: Online Mendelian Inheritance in Man. McKusick-Nathans Institute for Genetic Medicine, Johns Hopkins University, and National Center for Biotechnology Information, National Library of Medicine. *http://www.ncbi.nlm.nih.gov/entrez/query.fcgi?db=OMIM*

(DNA Mismatch Repair Gene Mutations)
Autosomal Dominant

PRINCIPLES

- Tumor susceptibility genes
- Multistep carcinogenesis
- Somatic mutation
- Microsatellite instability
- Variable expressivity and incomplete penetrance

MAJOR PHENOTYPIC FEATURES

- Age at onset: middle adulthood
- Colorectal cancer
- Multiple primary cancers

HISTORY AND PHYSICAL FINDINGS

P.P., a 38-year-old banker and mother of three children, was referred to the cancer genetics clinic by her physician for counseling regarding her family history of cancer. Her father, brother, nephew, niece, paternal uncle, and paternal grandmother all developed colorectal cancer. P.P. did not have a history of medical or surgical problems. The findings from her physical examination were normal. The geneticist explained to P.P. that her family history was suggestive of hereditary nonpolyposis colon cancer (HNPCC) and that the most efficient and effective way to determine the genetic cause of HNPCC in her family was through molecular testing of a living affected family member. After some discussion with her niece, the only surviving affected family member, P.P. and her niece returned to the clinic for testing. Testing of an archived tumor sample from the niece's resected colon identified microsatellite instability; subsequent sequencing of DNA from a blood sample obtained from the niece revealed a germline mutation in MLH1. P.P. did not carry the mutation; therefore, the geneticist counseled that her risk and her children's risk for development of cancer were similar to that of the general population. Her unaffected brother was found to carry the mutation and continued to have an annual screening colonoscopy.

BACKGROUND

Disease Etiology and Incidence
At least 50% of individuals in Western populations develop a colorectal tumor by the age of 70 years, and approximately 10% of these individuals eventually develop colorectal cancer. HNPCC (MIM# 120435) is a genetically heterogeneous autosomal dominant cancer predisposition syndrome that is often caused by mutations in DNA mismatch repair genes. HNPCC has a prevalence of 2 to 5 per 1000 and accounts for approximately 3% to 8% of colorectal cancer.

Pathogenesis
In most colorectal cancers, including familial adenomatous polyposis, the tumor karyotype becomes progressively more aneuploid (see Chapter 16). Approximately 13% to 15% of colorectal cancers do not have such chromosomal instability but have insertion or deletion mutations in repetitive sequences (microsatellite instability). Microsatellite instability occurs in 85% to 90% of HNPCC tumors. Consistent with this observation, approximately 70% of HNPCC families with carcinomas exhibiting microsatellite instability have germline mutations in one of six DNA mismatch repair genes: MSH2, MSH6, MLH1, MLH3, PMS1, or PMS2.

DNA mismatch repair reduces DNA replication errors by 1000-fold. Errors of DNA synthesis cause mispairing and deform the DNA double helix. A complex of mismatch repair proteins recruits other enzymes to effect repair. By use of the process of long patch excision, this complex excises the errant fragment of the newly synthesized DNA strand and then resynthesizes it.

Both alleles of a DNA mismatch repair gene must lose function to cause microsatellite instability. The high frequency of somatic loss of function in the second allele defines HNPCC as an autosomal dominant disease with approximately 80% penetrance. This somatic loss of function can occur by loss of heterozygosity, intragenic mutation, or hypermethylation.

In HNPCC, an increasing number of microsatellite loci mutate during the progression from adenoma to carcinoma. Inactivation of genes containing microsatellite sequences could play key roles in tumor progression. For example, microsatellite instability induces frameshift mutations in the transforming growth factor receptor II gene (TGFBR2). Mutations within TGFBR2 cause the loss of TGFβRII expression, and because the TGFβ system inhibits the growth of colonic epithelial cells, its loss allows escape from growth control. In support of the role of TGFBR2 in HNPCC, one affected family without mutations in a DNA mismatch repair gene had a germline mutation in TGFBR2. TGFBR2 mutations occur in early HNPCC lesions and may contribute to the growth of adenomas.

Phenotype and Natural History
Although patients with HNPCC develop polyps similar in number to those of the general population, they develop them at younger ages. Their median age at diagnosis with a colorectal adenocarcinoma is younger than 50 years, that is, 10 to 15 years younger than the general population (Fig. C-19). Patients with HNPCC and a defined germline mutation have an 80% lifetime risk for development of colorectal cancer. Sixty percent to 70% of adenomas and carcinomas in HNPCC occur between the splenic flexure and ileocecal junction. By way of contrast, most sporadic colorectal cancers (and cancer in familial adenomatous polyposis) occur in the descending colon and sigmoid. Carcinomas in HNPCC are less likely to have chromosome instability and behave less aggressively than sporadic colon cancer; sporadic cancers and the carcinomas in familial adenomatous polyposis are more likely to be aneuploid and more aggressive. For this reason, patients with HNPCC have a better prognosis when it is adjusted for stage and age than do patients with familial adenomatous polyposis or colorectal tumors with chromosome instability.

In addition to colorectal cancer, HNPCC-associated cancers include cancer of the stomach, small bowel, pancreas, kidney, endometrium, and ovaries; cancers of the lung and breast are not associated with HNPCC (Fig. C-19).

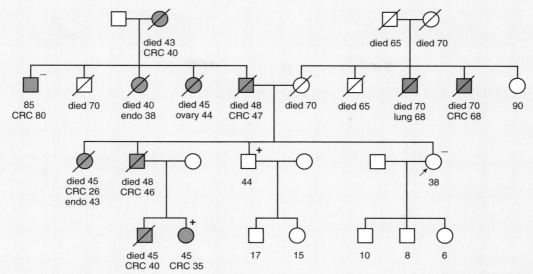

Figure C-19 ■ Family segregating an *MLH1* mutation. Note the frequent occurrence of colon cancer as well as other HNPCC-associated cancers, such as endometrial cancer, pancreatic cancer, and ovarian cancer. Note that one family member had cancers of the colorectum and endometrium and that another had sporadic colon cancer (tested negative for family mutation). The consultand is indicated by an arrow. Shaded symbols indicate a diagnosis of cancer. Ages are shown directly below the symbol. A plus sign identifies carriers of the *MLH1* mutation and a minus sign identifies noncarriers. Cancer diagnoses are followed by the age at diagnosis. Cancer abbreviations: CRC, colorectal cancer; endo, endometrial cancer; ovary, ovarian cancer; lung, lung cancer. (Courtesy of T. Pal and S. Narod, Women's College Hospital and University of Toronto, Canada.)

Patients with HNPCC and a defined germline mutation have a more than 90% lifetime risk for development of colorectal cancer or one of these associated cancers or both.

Management

Family history defines HNPCC; patients do not have distinguishing physical features. The minimal criteria for considering HNPCC are the occurrence of colorectal cancer or another HNPCC-associated tumor in three members of a family, at least two of whom are first-degree relatives, across two or more generations, and the development of colorectal cancer in at least one affected individual before the age of 50 years. In patients without a family history but with early-onset colorectal cancer, DNA analysis of the tumor to detect microsatellite instability and immunohistochemistry for the MLH1 and MSH2 proteins are now used to screen for HNPCC. Early recognition of HNPCC is necessary for effective intervention; surveillance colonoscopy of the proximal colon beginning at the age of 25 years increases life span expectancy by 13.5 years, and prophylactic surgical removal of the colon at the age of 25 years increases life span expectancy by 15.6 years. Surveillance endometrial biopsies and abdominal ultrasound scans for at-risk women have not proved to be effective preventive measures for the uterine cancer seen in this condition. In families with known germline mutations, identification of the DNA mismatch repair gene mutation can focus surveillance on those patients carrying the mutation, but in HNPCC families without an identified germline mutation, the absence of a mutation does not negate the need for frequent surveillance.

INHERITANCE RISK

The empirical Western general population risk for the development of colorectal cancer is 5% to 6%. This risk is markedly modified by family history. Patients with a first-degree relative with colorectal cancer have a 1.7 relative risk; this relative risk increases to 2.75 if two or more first-degree relatives had colorectal cancer. If an affected first-degree relative developed colorectal cancer before 44 years of age, the relative risk increases to more than 5.

In contrast, a patient with a DNA mismatch repair gene germline mutation has a 50% risk of having a child carrying a germline mutation. Each child carrying such a mutation has a lifetime cancer risk of approximately 90%, assuming the 80% penetrance of HNPCC is responsible for a cancer risk over and above the background risk in the general population for colon cancer and the other cancers of the types associated with HNPCC (stomach, small bowel, pancreas, kidney, endometrium, and ovaries). Prenatal diagnosis is highly controversial and not routine but is theoretically possible if the germline mutation has been identified in the parent. Because of incomplete penetrance and variation in expressivity, the severity and onset of HNPCC and the occurrence of associated cancers cannot be predicted.

Questions for Small Group Discussion

1. Compare the mechanisms of tumorigenesis in disorders of nucleotide excision repair, chromosomal instability, and microsatellite instability.
2. How should a patient with a family history of HNPCC be counseled if testing for DNA mismatch repair gene mutations is positive? negative?
3. Discuss the ethics of testing of minors for HNPCC.

REFERENCES

GeneTests. Medical genetics information resource [database online]. University of Washington, Seattle, 1993-2006. Updated weekly. *http://www.genetests.org*

Lynch HT, de la Chapelle A: Hereditary colorectal cancer. N Engl J Med 348:919-932, 2003.

OMIM: Online Mendelian Inheritance in Man. McKusick-Nathans Institute for Genetic Medicine, Johns Hopkins University, and National Center for Biotechnology Information, National Library of Medicine. *http://www.ncbi.nlm.nih.gov/entrez/query.fcgi?db=OMIM*

20. Hirschsprung Disease

(Neurocristopathy)
Autosomal Dominant, Autosomal Recessive, or Multigenic

PRINCIPLES

- Genetic heterogeneity
- Incomplete penetrance and variable expressivity
- Genetic modifiers
- Sex-dependent penetrance

MAJOR PHENOTYPIC FEATURES

- Age at onset: neonatal to adulthood
- Constipation
- Abdominal distention
- Enterocolitis

HISTORY AND PHYSICAL FINDINGS

S.L. and P.L. were referred to the genetics clinic to discuss their risk of having another child with Hirschsprung disease; their daughter had been born with long-segment Hirschsprung disease and was doing well after surgical removal of the aganglionic segment of colon. On examination and by history, the daughter did not have signs or symptoms of other diseases. The mother knew of an uncle and a brother who had died in infancy of bowel obstruction. The genetic counselor explained that in contrast to short-segment Hirschsprung disease, long-segment disease usually segregates as an autosomal dominant trait with incomplete penetrance and is often caused by mutations in the RET (rearranged during transfection) gene, which encodes a cell surface tyrosine kinase receptor. Subsequent testing showed that the affected daughter and the mother were heterozygous for a mutation in RET.

BACKGROUND

Disease Etiology and Incidence

Hirschsprung disease (HSCR, MIM# 142623) is the congenital absence of parasympathetic ganglion cells in the submucosal and myenteric plexuses along a variable length of the intestine (Fig. C-20); aganglionosis extending from the internal anal sphincter to proximal of the splenic flexure is classified as long-segment disease, whereas aganglionosis with a proximal limit distal to the splenic flexure is classified as short-segment disease. About 70% of HSCR occurs as an isolated trait, 12% in conjunction with a recognized chromosomal abnormality, and 18% in conjunction with multiple congenital anomalies.

Isolated or nonsyndromic HSCR is a panethnic, incompletely penetrant, sex-biased disorder with intrafamilial and interfamilial variation in expressivity; it has an incidence from 1.8 per 10,000 live births among Europeans to 2.8 per 10,000 live births among Asians. Long-segment disease, including total colonic aganglionosis, generally segregates as an autosomal dominant low-penetrance disorder; short-segment disease usually exhibits autosomal recessive or multigenic inheritance.

Pathogenesis

The enteric nervous system forms predominantly from vagal neural crest cells that migrate craniocaudally during the fifth to twelfth weeks of gestation. Some enteric neurons also emigrate cranially from the sacral neural crest; however, correct migration and differentiation of these cells depend on the presence of vagal neural crest cells.

HSCR arises from premature arrest of craniocaudal migration of vagal neural crest cells in the hindgut and thus is characterized by absence of parasympathetic ganglion cells in the submucosal and myenteric plexuses of the affected intestine. The genes implicated in HSCR include RET, EDNRB, EDN3, GDNF, and NRTN. How mutations in these genes cause premature arrest of the craniocaudal migration of vagal neural crest cells remains undefined. Regardless of the mechanism, the absence of ganglion cells causes loss of peristalsis and thereby intestinal obstruction.

RET is the major susceptibility gene for isolated HSCR. Nearly all families with more than one affected patient demonstrate linkage to the RET locus. However, mutations in the RET coding sequence can be identified only in approximately 50% of patients with familial HSCR and in 15% to 35% of patients with sporadic HSCR. In addition, within families segregating mutant RET alleles, penetrance is only 65% in males and 45% in females. A common noncoding variant within a conserved enhancer-like sequence in intron 1 of RET has been shown to be associated with HSCR and accounts for incomplete penetrance and sex differences. In addition, the variant is far more frequent in Asians than in whites, explaining the population differences.

Phenotype and Natural History

Patients with HSCR usually present early in life with impaired intestinal motility; however, 10% to 15% of patients are not identified until after a year of life. Approximately 50% to 90% of patients fail to pass meconium within the first 48 hours of life. After the newborn period, patients can present with constipation (68%), abdominal distention (64%), emesis (37%), or occasionally diarrhea; 40% of these patients have a history of delayed passage of meconium.

Untreated, HSCR is generally fatal. Failure to pass stool sequentially causes dilatation of the proximal bowel, increased intraluminal pressure, decreased blood flow, deterioration of the mucosal barrier, bacterial invasion, and enterocolitis. Recognition of HSCR before the onset of enterocolitis is essential to reduce morbidity and mortality.

HSCR frequently occurs as part of a syndrome or complex of malformations. As a neurocristopathy, HSCR is part of a continuum of diseases involving tissues of neural crest origin such as peripheral neurons, Schwann cells, melanocytes, conotruncal cardiac tissue, and endocrine and paraendocrine tissues. An illustration of this continuum is Waardenburg syndrome type IV, which is characterized by HSCR, deafness, and the absence of epidermal melanocytes.

Management

The diagnosis of HSCR requires histopathological demonstration of the absence of enteric ganglion cells in the distal

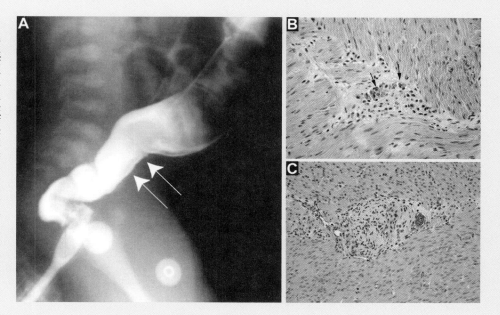

Figure C-20 ■ **A,** Barium enema study of a 3-month-old child with Down syndrome with a history of severe constipation. Note the narrowing of the distal colon, with the transition from dilated to narrowed colon demarcated by arrows; subsequent mucosal biopsy showed an absence of myenteric ganglion cells consistent with Hirschsprung disease. **B,** Normal myenteric ganglion. **C,** Aganglionic distal bowel of Hirschsprung disease. Myenteric ganglion cells (**B,** *arrows*) are located normally in the plexus between the longitudinal and circular layers of the muscularis propria. (**A** courtesy of D. Goodman and S. Sargeant, Department of Radiology, Dartmouth University, Hanover, New Hampshire. **B** and **C** courtesy of Raj Kapur, Department of Pathology, University of Washington, Seattle.)

rectum (Figure C-20C). Biopsy specimens for such testing are usually obtained by suction biopsies of the rectal mucosa and submucosa.

Definitive treatment of HSCR involves removal or bypassing of the aganglionic segment of bowel. The surgical procedure also usually involves the anastomosis of innervated bowel to the anal sphincter rather than a permanent colostomy. The prognosis for surgically treated patients is generally good, and most patients achieve fecal continence; however, a few patients have postoperative problems including enterocolitis, strictures, prolapse, perianal abscesses, and incontinence.

INHERITANCE RISK

Nonsyndromic HSCR has a 4 : 1 predominance in males versus females as well as variable expressivity and incomplete penetrance. The empirical recurrence risk for HSCR in siblings is dependent on the sex of the proband, the length of aganglionosis in the proband, and the sex of the sibling (see Table).

Prenatal counseling is complicated by the incomplete penetrance and variable expressivity. Even if a mutation has been identified in a family, generally neither the prediction of short- or long-segment HSCR nor the prediction of nonsyndromic or syndromic HSCR is possible. Moreover, prenatal diagnosis is currently further complicated by the poor availability of molecular testing.

SEX-DEPENDENT RECURRENCE RISK IN SIBLINGS OF A PROBAND WITH HSCR

Sex of Proband	Sex of Sibling	Proband Phenotype	Recurrence Risk (%)
Male	Male	Long-segment HSCR	17
		Short-segment HSCR	5
	Female	Long-segment HSCR	13
		Short-segment HSCR	1
Female	Male	Long-segment HSCR	33
		Short-segment HSCR	5
	Female	Long-segment HSCR	9
		Short-segment HSCR	3

From Parisi M: Hirschsprung disease overview. In GeneTests. *http://www.genetests.org*

Questions for Small Group Discussion

1. Mutations in the *RET* gene also cause multiple endocrine neoplasia; how do these mutations generally differ from those observed in HSCR disease? On occasion, the same mutation can cause both HSCR and multiple endocrine neoplasia; discuss possible explanations for this.
2. Discuss how stochastic, genetic, and environmental factors can cause incomplete penetrance and give examples of each.
3. Haddad syndrome (congenital central hypoventilation and HSCR) has also been associated with mutations of *RET, GDNF,* and *EDN3.* Describe the developmental relationship and pathology of HSCR and congenital central hypoventilation.
4. Mutations of the transcription factor *SOX10* cause Waardenburg syndrome type IV plus dysmyelination of the central and peripheral nervous system. Mutations of the endothelin pathway cause HSCR and Waardenburg syndrome type IV without dysmyelination. Mutations of *RET* and its ligands cause HSCR but not Waardenburg syndrome type IV or dysmyelination. Discuss what these observations say about the relationship between these three pathways and their regulation of neural crest cells.
5. Compare and contrast the various forms of multigenic inheritance, that is, additive, multiplicative, mixed multiplicative, and epistatic inheritance. (See Nature Genetics 31:11-12, 2002.)

REFERENCES

Emison E, McCallion AS, Cashuk CS, et al: A common sex-dependent mutation in a RET enhancer underlies Hirschsprung disease risk. Nature 434:857-863, 2005.

GeneTests. Medical genetics information resource [database online]. University of Washington, Seattle, 1993-2006. Updated weekly. *http://www.genetests.org*

OMIM: Online Mendelian Inheritance in Man. McKusick-Nathans Institute for Genetic Medicine, Johns Hopkins University, and National Center for Biotechnology Information, National Library of Medicine. *http://www.ncbi.nlm.nih.gov/entrez/query.fcgi?db=OMIM*

21. Holoprosencephaly (Nonsyndromic Form)

(Sonic Hedgehog Mutation)

Autosomal Dominant

PRINCIPLES

- Developmental regulatory gene
- Genetic heterogeneity
- Position-effect mutations
- Incomplete penetrance and variable expressivity

MAJOR PHENOTYPIC FEATURES

- Age at onset: prenatal
- Ventral forebrain maldevelopment
- Facial dysmorphism
- Developmental delay

HISTORY AND PHYSICAL FINDINGS

Dr. D., a 37-year-old physicist, presented to the genetics clinic with his wife because their first child died at birth of holoprosencephaly. The pregnancy had been uncomplicated, and the child had a normal karyotype. Neither he nor his wife reported any major medical problems. Dr. D. had been adopted as a child and did not know the history of his biological family; his wife's family history was not suggestive of any genetic disorders. Careful examination of Dr. D. and his wife showed that he had an absent superior labial frenulum and slight hypotelorism but no other dysmorphic findings. His physician explained to him that the holoprosencephaly in his child and his absent superior labial frenulum and slight hypotelorism were suggestive of autosomal dominant holoprosencephaly. Subsequent molecular testing confirmed that Dr. D. had a mutation in the Sonic hedgehog gene (*SHH*).

BACKGROUND

Disease Etiology and Incidence

Holoprosencephaly (HPE, MIM# 236100), which has a birth incidence of 1 in 10,000 to 1 in 12,000, is the most common human congenital brain defect. It affects twice as many girls as boys.

HPE results from a variety of causes, including chromosomal and single-gene disorders, environmental factors such as maternal diabetes, and possibly maternal exposure to cholesterol-lowering agents (statins). The disorder occurs both in isolation and as a feature of various syndromes, such as Smith-Lemli-Opitz syndrome. Nonsyndromic familial HPE, when inherited, is predominantly autosomal dominant, although both autosomal recessive and X-linked inheritance have been reported. Approximately 25% to 50% of all HPE is associated with a chromosomal abnormality; the nonrandom distribution of chromosomal abnormalities predicts at least 12 different HPE loci including 7q36, 13q32, 2p21, 18p11.3, and 21q22.3.

SHH, the first gene identified with mutations causing HPE, maps to 7q36. *SHH* mutations account for approximately 30% to 40% of familial nonsyndromic autosomal dominant HPE but for less than 5% of nonsyndromic HPE

overall. Other genes implicated in autosomal dominant nonsyndromic HPE are *ZIC2*, accounting for 5%; *SIX3* and *TGIF*, each accounting for 1.3%; and *PTCH*, which has only rarely been found mutated in HPE.

Pathogenesis

SHH is a secreted signaling protein required for developmental patterning in both mammals and insects (see Chapter 14).

Human *SHH* mutations are loss-of-function mutations. Some of the cytogenetic abnormalities affecting *SHH* expression are translocations that occur 15 to 256kb 5' to the coding region of *SHH*. These translocations are referred to as position-effect mutations because they do not mutate the coding sequence but disrupt distant regulatory elements or chromatin structure, or both, and thereby alter *SHH* expression.

Phenotype and Natural History

The prosencephalic malformations of HPE follow a continuum of severity but are usually subdivided into alobar HPE (no evidence of an interhemispheric fissure), semilobar HPE (posterior interhemispheric fissure only), and lobar HPE (ventricular separation and almost complete cortical separation) (Fig. C-21). Among HPE patients with a normal karyotype, 63% have alobar HPE, 28% have semilobar HPE, and 9% have lobar HPE. Other commonly associated central nervous system malformations include undivided thalami, dysgenesis of the corpus callosum, hypoplastic olfactory bulbs, hypoplastic optic bulbs and tracts, and pituitary dysgenesis.

The spectrum of facial dysmorphism in HPE extends from cyclopia to normal and usually reflects the severity of the central nervous system malformations. Dysmorphic features associated with, but not diagnostic of, HPE include microcephaly or macrocephaly, anophthalmia or microphthalmia, hypotelorism or hypertelorism, dysmorphic nose, palatal anomalies, bifid uvula, a single central incisor, and absence of a superior labial frenulum.

Delayed development occurs in nearly all patients with HPE. The severity of delay correlates with the severity of central nervous system malformation; that is, patients with normal brain imaging usually have normal intelligence. In addition to delayed development, patients frequently have seizures, brainstem dysfunction, and sleep dysregulation.

Among HPE patients without chromosomal abnormalities, survival varies inversely with the severity of the facial phenotype. Patients with cyclopia or ethmocephaly usually do not survive a week; approximately 50% of patients with alobar HPE die before 4 to 5 months of age, and 80% before a year. Approximately 50% of patients with isolated semilobar or lobar HPE survive the first year.

Management

Patients with HPE require an expeditious evaluation within the first few days of life. Treatment is symptomatic and supportive. Aside from the medical concerns of the patient, a major part of the management includes counseling and supporting the parents as well as defining the cause of HPE.

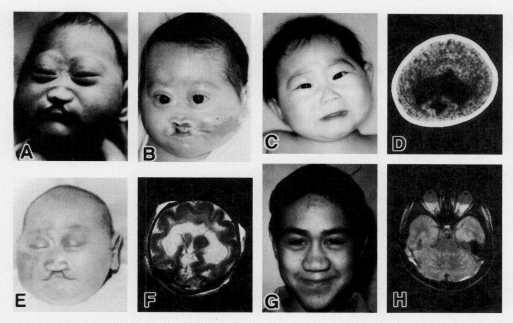

Figure C-21 ■ Holoprosencephaly in patients with *SHH* mutations. **A,** Microcephaly, absence of nasal bones, midline cleft palate, and semilobar HPE. **B,** Semilobar HPE, premaxillary agenesis, and midline cleft lip. **C** and **D,** Mild facial findings with severe semilobar HPE on magnetic resonance imaging. **E** and **F,** Microcephaly, prominent optic globes, premaxillary agenesis, and cleft lip, with semilobar HPE on magnetic resonance imaging. **G** and **H,** Microcephaly, ocular hypotelorism, flat nose without palpable cartilage, midface and philtrum hypoplasia, normal intelligence, and normal brain on magnetic resonance imaging. All patients have *SHH* mutations. Patients **A** and **B** also have mutations of *TGIF*, and patient **C** also has a mutation in *ZIC2*. *TGIF* mutations indirectly decrease SHH expression. (Courtesy of M. Muenke, National Human Genome Research Institute, National Institutes of Health, Bethesda, Maryland. Modified by permission from Nanni L, Ming JE, Bocian M, et al: The mutational spectrum of the sonic hedgehog gene in holoprosencephaly: SHH mutations cause a significant portion of autosomal dominant holoprosencephaly. Hum Mol Genet 8:2479, 1999.)

INHERITANCE RISK

Etiologically, HPE is extremely heterogeneous, and the recurrence risk in a family is dependent on identification of the underlying cause. Diabetic mothers have a 1% risk of having a child with HPE. For parents of a patient with a cytogenetic anomaly, the recurrence risk depends on whether one of them has a cytogenetic abnormality that gave rise to the abnormality in the patient. For parents of patients with syndromic HPE, the recurrence risk depends on the recurrence risk for that syndrome. In the absence of a family history of HPE or a cytogenetic or syndromic cause of HPE, parents and siblings must be examined closely for microforms, subtle features associated with HPE such as an absent frenulum or a single upper incisor. For parents with a negative family history, no identifiable causes of HPE, and no microforms suggestive of autosomal dominant HPE, the empirical recurrence risk is approximately 4% to 5%. In some cases, digenic inheritance may explain the reduced penetrance of some *SHH* mutations.

Although autosomal recessive and X-linked HPE have been reported, most families with an established mode of inheritance exhibit autosomal dominant inheritance. The penetrance of autosomal dominant HPE is approximately 70%. Among obligate carriers of autosomal dominant HPE, the risk of having a child affected with severe HPE is 16% to 21% and with a microform, 13% to 14%. The phenotype of the carrier does not affect the risk of having an affected child, nor does it predict the severity if the child is affected.

Molecular testing for certain of the HPE mutations is currently available as a clinical service. Severe HPE can be detected by prenatal ultrasound examination at 16 to 18 weeks of gestation.

Questions for Small Group Discussion
1. What factors might explain the variable expressivity and penetrance of *SHH* mutations among siblings?
2. Discuss genetic disorders with a sex bias and the mechanisms underlying the sex bias. As examples, consider Rett syndrome to illustrate embryonic sex-biased lethality, pyloric stenosis to illustrate a sex bias in disease frequency, and coronary heart disease in familial hypercholesterolemia to illustrate a sex bias in disease severity.
3. Considering the many loci associated with HPE, discuss why mutations in different genes give rise to identical phenotypes.
4. Considering that *GLI3* is in the signal transduction cascade of SHH, discuss why *GLI3* loss-of-function mutations do not give rise to the same phenotype as *SHH* loss-of-function mutations.
5. Discuss the role of cholesterol in brain morphogenesis.

REFERENCES

GeneTests. Medical genetics information resource [database online]. University of Washington, Seattle, 1993-2006. Updated weekly. *http://www.genetests.org*

Ming JE, Muenke M: Multiple hits during early embryonic development: digenic diseases and holoprosencephaly. Am J Hum Genet 71:1017-1032, 2002.

Muenke M, Beachy PA: Holoprosencephaly. In Scriver CR, Beaudet AL, Sly WS, et al (eds): The Metabolic and Molecular Bases of Inherited Disease, 8th ed. New York, McGraw-Hill, 2001, pp 6203-6230.

OMIM: Online Mendelian Inheritance in Man. McKusick-Nathans Institute for Genetic Medicine, Johns Hopkins University, and National Center for Biotechnology Information, National Library of Medicine. *http://www.ncbi.nlm.nih.gov/entrez/query.fcgi?db=OMIM*

22. Huntington Disease

(*HD* Mutation)
Autosomal Dominant

PRINCIPLES

- Triplet repeat expansion
- Novel property mutation
- Sex-specific anticipation
- Reduced penetrance and variable expressivity
- Presymptomatic counseling

MAJOR PHENOTYPIC FEATURES

- Age at onset: late childhood to late adulthood
- Movement abnormalities
- Cognitive abnormalities
- Psychiatric abnormalities

HISTORY AND PHYSICAL FINDINGS

M.P., a 45-year-old man, presented initially with declining memory and concentration. As his intellectual function deteriorated during the ensuing year, he developed involuntary movements of his fingers and toes as well as facial grimacing and pouting. He was aware of his condition and became depressed. He had been previously healthy and did not have a history of any similarly affected relatives; his parents had died in their 40s in an automobile accident. M.P. had one healthy daughter. After an extensive evaluation, the neurologist diagnosed M.P.'s condition as Huntington disease. The diagnosis of Huntington disease was confirmed by a DNA analysis showing 43 CAG repeats in one of his *HD* alleles (normal, <26). Subsequent presymptomatic testing of M.P.'s daughter showed that she had also inherited the mutant *HD* allele (Fig. C-22). Both received extensive counseling.

BACKGROUND

Disease Etiology and Incidence

Huntington disease (HD, MIM# 143100) is a panethnic, autosomal dominant, progressive neurodegenerative disorder that is caused by mutations in the *HD* gene (see Chapter 12). The prevalence of HD ranges from 3 to 7 per 100,000 among western Europeans to 0.1 to 0.38 per 100,000 among Japanese. This variation in prevalence reflects the variation in distribution of *HD* alleles and haplotypes that predispose to mutation.

Pathogenesis

The *HD* gene product, huntingtin, is ubiquitously expressed. The function of huntingtin remains unknown.

Disease-causing mutations in *HD* usually result from an expansion of a polyglutamine-encoding CAG repeat sequence in exon 1; normal *HD* alleles have 10 to 26 CAG repeats, whereas mutant alleles have more than 36 repeats (see Chapter 12). Approximately 3% of patients develop HD as the result of a new CAG repeat expansion; 97% inherit a mutant *HD* allele from an affected parent. New mutant *HD* genes arise from expansion of a premutation (27 to 35 CAG

repeats) to a full mutation. To date, all patients described have inherited the new full mutation from their father.

Expansion of the huntingtin polyglutamine tract appears to confer a deleterious novel property and appears to be both necessary and sufficient for the induction of an HD-like phenotype. In addition to the diffuse, severe atrophy of the neostriatum that is the hallmark of HD, expression of mutant huntingtin causes neuronal dysfunction, generalized brain atrophy, changes in neurotransmitter levels, and accumulation of neuronal nuclear and cytoplasmic aggregates. Ultimately, expression of mutant huntingtin leads to neuronal death; however, it is likely that clinical symptoms and neuronal dysfunction precede the development of intracellular aggregates and neuronal death. The mechanism by which expression of this expanded polyglutamine tract causes HD remains unclear.

Phenotype and Natural History

The patient's age at disease onset is inversely proportional to the number of *HD* CAG repeats. Patients with adult-onset disease usually have 40 to 55 repeats; those with juvenile-onset disease usually have more than 60 repeats (see Fig. 7-27). Patients with 36 to 41 *HD* CAG repeats exhibit reduced penetrance; that is, they may or may not develop HD in their lifetime. Apart from the relationship to the age at onset, the number of repeats does not correlate with other features of HD.

Instability and expansion of the CAG repeats within mutant *HD* alleles often results in anticipation, that is, progressively earlier ages at onset with succeeding generations. Once the number of CAG repeats is 36 or more, the CAG repeat length generally expands during paternal transmission; expansions during maternal transmission are less frequent and shorter than are expansions during paternal transmission. Because the CAG repeat length is inversely correlated with the age at onset, individuals inheriting a mutation from their father have an increased risk for development of early-onset disease; approximately 80% of juvenile patients inherit the mutant *HD* gene from their father.

Approximately one third of patients present with psychiatric abnormalities; two thirds present with a combination of cognitive and motor disturbances. The mean age of patients at presentation is 35 to 44 years; approximately one quarter of patients develop HD after the age of 50 years, however, and one tenth before the age of 20 years. The median survival after diagnosis is 15 to 18 years, and the mean age at death is 54 to 55 years.

HD is characterized by progressive motor, cognitive, and psychiatric abnormalities. The motor disturbances involve both voluntary and involuntary movement. Initially, these movements interfere little with daily activities but generally become incapacitating as HD progresses. Chorea, which is present in more than 90% of patients, is the most common involuntary movement; it is characterized by nonrepetitive, nonperiodic jerks that cannot be suppressed voluntarily. Cognitive abnormalities begin early in the disease course and affect all aspects of cognition; language is usually affected later than are other cognitive functions. Behavioral distur-

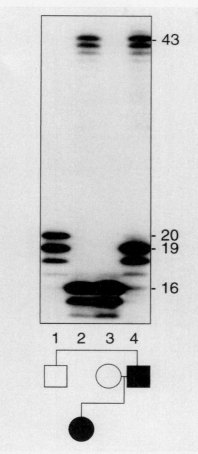

Figure C-22 ■ Segregation of an *HD* gene mutation in a family with Huntington disease—photograph of a Southern blot of polymerase chain reaction products derived from amplification of the CAG repeats in exon 1 of the *HD* gene. Each allele generates a full-length fragment as well as two or more shorter fragments due to difficulties with doing PCR across a triplet repeat. Notice that the affected father and daughter both have an allele with a full mutation (43 CAG repeats) and a normal allele (19 and 16 repeats, respectively). The daughter's unaffected mother and her unaffected paternal uncle have *HD* alleles with a normal number of CAG repeats. (Courtesy of M. R. Hayden, University of British Columbia, Vancouver, Canada.)

bances, which usually develop later in the disease course, include social disinhibition, aggression, outbursts, apathy, sexual deviation, and increased appetite. The psychiatric manifestations, which can develop anytime in the disease course, include personality changes, affective psychosis, and schizophrenia.

In the end stages of HD, patients usually develop such severe motor impairments that they are fully dependent on others. They also experience weight loss, sleep disturbances,

incontinence, and mutism. Their behavioral disturbances decrease as the disease advances.

Management
Currently, no curative treatments are available for HD. Therapy focuses on supportive care as well as pharmacological management of the behavioral and neurological problems.

INHERITANCE RISK

Each child of a parent with HD has a 50% risk of inheriting a mutant *HD* allele. Except for those alleles with incomplete penetrance (36 to 41 CAG repeats), all children inheriting a mutant *HD* allele will develop HD if they have a normal life span.

Children of fathers carrying a premutation have an empirical risk of approximately 3% of inheriting an *HD* allele in which the premutation has expanded to a full mutation. Not all males carrying a premutation, however, are equally likely to transmit a full mutation.

Presymptomatic testing and prenatal testing are available through analysis of the number of CAG repeats within exon 1 of the *HD* gene. Presymptomatic testing and prenatal testing are forms of predictive testing and are best interpreted after confirmation of a CAG expansion in an affected family member.

Questions for Small Group Discussion
1. Patients with heterozygous and homozygous mutations of *HD* have similar clinical expression of HD, whereas individuals with deletion of one *HD* allele on chromosome 4p have a normal phenotype. How can this be explained?
2. Some studies suggest that a father with a premutation and an affected child has a higher risk of transmitting a full mutation than does a father with a premutation and no affected children. Discuss possible mechanisms for this predisposition to transmit *HD* mutations.
3. Expansion of *HD* premutations to full mutations occurs through the male germline, whereas expansion of *FMR1* (fragile X syndrome) premutations to full mutations occurs through the female germline. Discuss possible mechanisms for sex biases in disease transmission.
4. By international consensus, asymptomatic at-risk children are not tested for *HD* mutations because testing removes the child's choice to know or not know, testing results open the child to familial and social stigmatization, and testing results could affect educational and career decisions. When would it be appropriate to test asymptomatic at-risk children? What advances in medicine are necessary to make testing of all asymptomatic at-risk children acceptable? (Consider the reasoning underlying newborn screening.)

REFERENCES
GeneTests. Medical genetics information resource [database online]. University of Washington, Seattle, 1993-2006. Updated weekly. *http://www.genetests.org*

OMIM: Online Mendelian Inheritance in Man. McKusick-Nathans Institute for Genetic Medicine, Johns Hopkins University, and National Center for Biotechnology Information, National Library of Medicine. *http://www.ncbi.nlm.nih.gov/entrez/query.fcgi?db=OMIM*

23. Insulin-Dependent Diabetes Mellitus

(Autoimmune Destruction of Islet β Cells)

Multifactorial

PRINCIPLES

- Polygenic disease
- Environmental trigger
- Susceptibility allele
- Protective allele

MAJOR PHENOTYPIC FEATURES

- Age at onset: childhood through adulthood
- Polyuria, polydipsia, polyphagia
- Hyperglycemia
- Ketosis
- Wasting

HISTORY AND PHYSICAL FINDINGS

F.C., a 45-year-old father with late-onset diabetes mellitus, was referred to the endocrinology clinic for counseling regarding his children's risk for diabetes. F.C. developed glucose intolerance (inability to maintain normal blood glucose levels after ingestion of sugar) at the age of 39 years and fasting hyperglycemia at 45 years. He did not have a history of other medical or surgical problems. The findings from his physical examination were normal except for moderate abdominal obesity; his body mass index [weight in kilograms/(height in meters)^2] was 31.3 with the excess adiposity distributed preferentially around his waist. He had five children by two different partners; a child from each relationship had developed insulin-dependent diabetes mellitus (IDDM) before 10 years of age. His sister developed IDDM as a child and died during adolescence from diabetic ketoacidosis. The geneticist explained that given his family history, F.C. might have a late-onset form of IDDM and that his current non–insulin-dependent diabetes mellitus was probably an antecedent to development of IDDM. After discussing the possible causes of and prognostic factors for the development of IDDM, F.C. elected to enroll himself and his children, who are all minors, in a research protocol studying the prevention of IDDM. As part of that study, he and his children were tested for anti-islet antibodies. Both he and an unaffected daughter had a high titer of anti-islet antibodies; the daughter also had an abnormal glucose tolerance test result but not fasting hyperglycemia. As part of the study protocol, F.C. and his daughter were prescribed low-dose insulin injections.

BACKGROUND

Disease Etiology and Incidence

IDDM (sometimes called type 1 diabetes, MIM# 222100) is usually caused by autoimmune destruction of islet β cells in the pancreas; this autoimmune reaction is triggered by an unknown mechanism. The destruction of islet β cells causes insulin deficiency and thereby dysregulation of anabolism and catabolism, resulting in metabolic changes similar to those observed in starvation (Fig. C-23). Among North American whites, IDDM is the second most common chronic disease of childhood, increasing in prevalence from 1 in 2500 at 5 years of age to 1 in 300 at 18 years of age.

Pathogenesis

IDDM usually results from a genetic susceptibility and subsequent environmental insult (see Chapter 8) and only very rarely from an environmental insult or a genetic mutation alone. Although approximately 90% of IDDM occurs in patients without a family history of diabetes, observations supporting a genetic predisposition include differences in concordance between monozygotic (33% to 50%) and dizygotic twins (1% to 14%), familial clustering, and differences in prevalence among different populations (see Chapter 8). More than 13 different genetic susceptibility loci have been reported in humans, although few have been identified consistently and reproducibly. One of the few confirmed loci is the HLA locus that may account for as much as 30% to 60% of the genetic susceptibility. Approximately 95% of white patients express a DR3 or a DR4 allele, or both, compared with 50% of controls; this association apparently arises not because DR3 and DR4 are susceptibility alleles but because of linkage disequilibrium between DR and DQ. The DQβ1*0201 allele, which segregates with DR3, and DQβ1*0302, which segregates with DR4, appear to be the primary susceptibility alleles. In contrast, DQβ1*602, which segregates with DR2, appears to be a protective allele; that is, it negates the effect of a susceptibility allele when both are present. Both of the DQβ1 susceptibility alleles have a neutral amino acid at position 57, a site within the putative antigen-binding cleft, whereas protective or neutral DQβ1 alleles have an aspartic acid at position 57. This substitution of an uncharged amino acid for aspartic acid is predicted to change the specificity of antigen binding to the DQ molecule.

Evidence supporting an environmental component to the induction of IDDM in genetically susceptible individuals includes a concordance of less than 50% among monozygotic twins, a seasonal variation in incidence, and an increased incidence of diabetes among children with congenital rubella. Proposed environmental triggers include viral infections and early exposure to bovine albumin. Exposure to viruses and bovine albumin could cause autoimmune destruction of β cells by molecular mimicry, that is, sharing of antigenic determinants between β-cell proteins and the virus or bovine albumin. Approximately 80% to 90% of newly diagnosed patients with IDDM have anti–islet cell antibodies. These autoantibodies recognize cytoplasmic and cell surface determinants such as glutamic acid decarboxylase, carboxypeptidase H, ganglioside antigens, islet cell antigen 69 (ICA69), and a protein tyrosine phosphatase. Glutamic acid decarboxylase and ICA69, respectively, share epitopes with coxsackievirus B4 and bovine serum albumin.

In sum, IDDM appears to be an autoimmune disease, although the precise role of islet cell autoantibodies remains uncertain. Additional evidence for an autoimmune mechanism in IDDM includes an increased prevalence of other autoimmune diseases, mononuclear cell infiltrates of islets, and recurrent β-cell destruction after transplantation from a

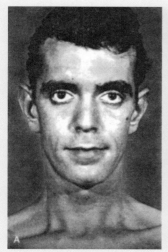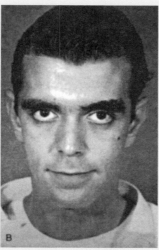

Figure C-23 ■ A 28-year-old man with insulin-dependent diabetes mellitus. **A,** Photograph after 3 weeks of polydipsia and polyuria. **B,** Photograph after 5-kg weight gain with 10 days of insulin replacement. (Modified from Oakley WG, Pyke DA, Taylor KW: Clinical Diabetes and Its Biochemical Basis. Oxford, Blackwell Scientific Publications, 1968, p 258, by permission. Photographic restoration courtesy of B. Moseley-Fernandini.)

monozygotic twin. But two lines of evidence suggest that progression to IDDM involves more than the development of autoantibodies. First, less than 1% of the general population develops diabetes although 10% have islet autoantibodies; and second, first-degree relatives and schoolchildren have remission rates of 10% to 78% for islet cell antibodies.

Phenotype and Natural History

Loss of insulin reserve occurs during a few to many years. The earliest sign of abnormality is the development of islet autoantibodies when blood glucose concentrations, glucose tolerance (ability to maintain normal blood glucose levels after ingestion of sugar), and insulin responses to glucose are normal. This period is followed by a phase of decreased glucose tolerance but normal fasting blood glucose concentration. With continued loss of β cells, fasting hyperglycemia eventually develops but sufficient insulin is still produced to prevent ketosis; during this period, patients have non–insulin-dependent diabetes mellitus. Eventually, insulin production falls below a critical threshold, and patients become dependent on exogenous insulin supplements and have a propensity to ketoacidosis. Younger patients generally progress through these phases more rapidly than do older patients.

Although the acute complications of diabetes can be controlled by administration of exogenous insulin, the loss of endogenous insulin production causes many problems, including atherosclerosis, peripheral neuropathy, renal disease, cataracts, and retinopathy. Approximately 50% of patients eventually die of renal failure. The development and severity of these complications are related to the genetic background and degree of metabolic control. Rigorous control of blood glucose levels reduces the risk of complications by 35% to 75%.

Management

Although pancreatic or islet transplantation can cure IDDM, the paucity of tissue for transplantation and complications of immunosuppression limit this therapy. Management of most patients emphasizes intensive control of blood glucose levels by injection of exogenous insulin.

The development of islet autoantibodies several years before the onset of IDDM has led to the development of studies to predict and prevent IDDM. The administration of insulin or nicotinamide appears to delay the development of IDDM in some patients.

INHERITANCE RISK

The risk of IDDM in the general population is approximately 1 in 300. With one affected sibling, the risk increases to 1 in 14 (1 in 6 if HLA identical, 1 in 20 if HLA haplo-identical). The risk increases to 1 in 6 with a second affected first-degree relative in addition to an affected sibling and to 1 in 3 with an affected monozygotic twin. Children of an affected mother have a 1 in 50 to 1 in 33 risk for development of IDDM, whereas children of an affected father have a 1 in 25 to 1 in 16 risk. This paternity-related increased risk appears to be limited to fathers with an HLA DR4 allele.

Questions for Small Group Discussion

1. Discuss the difficulties of identifying the genetic components of polygenic diseases.
2. How might HLA susceptibility alleles effect susceptibility and protective alleles effect protection?
3. Discuss the underlying mechanisms for prevention of IDDM by exogenous insulin injections.
4. Compare risk counseling for fathers and mothers with IDDM. Discuss the teratogenic risks and mechanisms of maternal diabetes.

REFERENCES

Alemzadeh R, Wyatt DT: Diabetes mellitus. In Behrman RE, Kliegman RM, Jenson HB (eds): Nelson Textbook of Pediatrics, 17th ed. Philadelphia, WB Saunders, 2004, pp 1947-1972.

OMIM: Online Mendelian Inheritance in Man. McKusick-Nathans Institute for Genetic Medicine, Johns Hopkins University, and National Center for Biotechnology Information, National Library of Medicine. *http://www.ncbi.nlm.nih.gov/entrez/query.fcgi?db=OMIM*

24. Intrauterine Growth Restriction

(Abnormal Fetal Karyotype)
Spontaneous Mutation

PRINCIPLES

- Prenatal diagnosis
- Ultrasound screening
- Interstitial deletion
- Cytogenetic analysis
- Genetic counseling
- Pregnancy management options

MAJOR PHENOTYPIC FEATURES

- Age at onset: prenatal
- Intrauterine growth restriction
- Increased nuchal fold
- Dysmorphic facies

HISTORY AND PHYSICAL FINDINGS

A.G. is a 26-year-old gravida 2, para 1 white female referred for ultrasonography for detailed examination of fetal anatomy. A.G. denied any medication, drug, or alcohol exposure in the pregnancy, and both parents were in good health. The biometric parameters from the fetal anatomy study suggested a 17.5-week fetus. On the basis of first-trimester ultrasound dating and the date of the patient's last menstrual period, however, the fetus should have been approximately at 21 weeks of gestation. This discrepancy suggested symmetrical fetal intrauterine growth restriction (IUGR). Further evaluation also revealed increased nuchal fold measurements of 6.1 to 7.3 mm. The couple was counseled regarding the increased risk for fetal aneuploidy, and amniocentesis was performed. The chromosome results revealed an interstitial chromosome 4p deletion, with karyotype 46,XX,del(4)(p15.1p15.32). Parental chromosomes were normal. After extensive genetic counseling, the couple decided to terminate the pregnancy. The autopsy revealed a 19-week fetus by size (22.5 weeks by dates) with bilateral epicanthal folds, low-set and posteriorly rotated ears, prominent nasal bridge, and micrognathia. Redundant posterior nuchal skin was also noted.

BACKGROUND

Disease Etiology and Incidence

IUGR is diagnosed when a fetus or neonate is <10th percentile for weight (<2500 g for a neonate born at term in the United States) (Fig. C-24). An IUGR newborn should be distinguished from a small for gestational age (SGA) newborn, who is also below the 10th percentile in size but is small for physiological reasons, such as the size of the parents. Approximately 7% of pregnancies result in an SGA fetus, of which approximately 1 in 8 is truly IUGR.

IUGR may result from uteroplacental insufficiency, exposure to drugs or alcohol, congenital infections, or intrinsic genetic limitations of growth potential. Fetuses with growth restriction due to nutritional compromise tend to have less retardation of head growth compared to the rest of the body.

Several chromosomal disorders are associated with IUGR, and a finding of early or symmetrical IUGR increases the likelihood that a fetus is affected with a chromosomal abnormality such as trisomy 18, triploidy, or maternal uniparental disomy for chromosome 7 or 14. Nuchal fold measurements of more than 3 mm in the first trimester (11 to 14 weeks) and of 6 mm or more in the second trimester are considered increased, and are associated with a greater risk for Down syndrome (see Fig. 15-4). Approximately 1 in 7 fetuses with a second-trimester nuchal thickening will have Down syndrome. The ultrasound findings in A.G.'s fetus increased the suspicion of aneuploidy and led to the identification of the small interstitial deletion in 4p, which is the likely explanation for the fetal abnormalities.

The etiology and incidence of such a rare deletion are not entirely understood, especially in light of the normal parental chromosomes. Most de novo deletions are considered to originate at meiosis but they may also arise during mitosis, prior to meiosis in gametogenesis, so that a parent is a gonadal mosaic. Gonadal mosaicism cannot be ruled out with any certainty by fibroblast or lymphoblast testing of the parents; consequently, prenatal testing should be offered in future pregnancies.

Pathogenesis

The breakpoints in 46,XX,del(4)(p15.1p15.32) flank a 14.5-Mb deletion of DNA on the short arm of chromosome 4. Analysis of the human genome sequence in this region indicates that 47 known protein-coding genes exist within this deleted region; haploinsufficiency for one or more of these genes is the likely cause of the phenotype of this fetus.

Phenotype and Natural History

All pregnancies regardless of family, medical, or pregnancy history are at an approximate 3% to 5% risk for mental retardation or a birth defect in the infant. Although this couple was not at increased risk, the routine second-trimester ultrasound findings increased the suspicion of fetal aneuploidy. The finding of an interstitial deletion is likely to explain the ultrasound findings. Although this exact deletion has not been reported previously, many deletions of the short arm of chromosome 4 have been associated with birth defects. For example, Wolf-Hirschhorn syndrome is due to a microdeletion of 4p, resulting in both severe mental retardation and physical anomalies. FISH analysis in this fetus revealed that the sequences for the Wolf-Hirschhorn critical region at 4p16.3 were present on both copies of chromosome 4 and that the deletion in this case was more proximal, in band p15. In this case, as with any substantial loss or gain of material on an autosome not previously reported in other patients, the outcome is likely to involve both physical and neurological impairment, the severity of which cannot be predicted.

Management

No curative treatments are available for chromosome abnormalities. The overriding question for many couples regarding the outcome for their unborn child is whether the fetus is at risk for mental retardation or a significant birth defect. In light of the already present ultrasound anomalies and the identified chromosomal abnormality, this fetus will have sequelae, the extent of which is not predictable. In such cases,

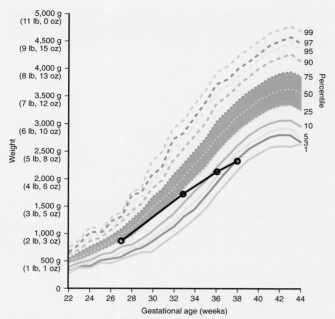

Figure C-24 ■ Intrauterine growth curve for a fetus with trisomy 18, superimposed on a standard intrauterine and postnatal growth chart averaged for both sexes over the U.S. population (shown in blue). The aneuploid fetus' growth curve begins at the 30th percentile at 27 weeks of gestation but then cuts across percentile lines, as shown, culminating in birth at 38 weeks with fetal weight just below the 3rd percentile. Fetal weight during pregnancy is estimated by a formula that combines ultrasound measurements of the distance between the parietal bones of the fetal skull (biparietal diameter), head circumference, abdominal circumference, and femur length. (Reproduced with permission from Peleg D, et al: Am Fam Physician 58:453-460, 466-467, 1998.)

the couple is counseled in detail about the limited information and the inability to conclude with any certainty what the expected outcome of the pregnancy will be. The options include continuation of the pregnancy with expectant management, with or without giving the neonate up for adoption, or termination of pregnancy.

Follow-up ultrasound evaluations can assess fetal growth and development. Long-term progressive IUGR alone suggests a poor prognosis for the fetus. By the late second trimester, the majority of cardiac lesions that would require intervention at birth can usually be identified. Consultation with neonatologists and maternal-fetal medicine specialists can provide information regarding what to expect at delivery and the types of postnatal evaluations that should be considered. There may be advantages to arranging for delivery in a tertiary facility that provides specialized neonatal intensive care and surgery.

Termination of the pregnancy is currently legal in the United States, but not always available. In the second trimester of pregnancy, this procedure can be performed by either dilation and evacuation or induction of labor (prostaglandin induction). The former is usually not performed in pregnancies of more than 24 weeks' gestation. Prostaglandin induction provides the couple with the option of an autopsy, but with a known serious chromosome anomaly, the information from an autopsy provides no additional information that would affect recurrence risk or prenatal testing options in a future pregnancy. The emotional and physical benefits and disadvantages of the two procedures should be outlined in detail before the patient's decision to terminate, should that option be chosen. In the United States, pregnancy terminations are not covered by insurance for federal employees and Medicaid recipients and are only rarely covered by private health insurance, even when the indication is for a severe birth defect diagnosed prenatally. The costs can be in excess of thousands of dollars, and the financial burden of this procedure may affect decision-making in some individuals.

Finally, the parents can be offered the option of giving the neonate up for adoption if they decide that termination is either not an option or unaffordable, or because the anomalies were identified too late in the pregnancy to allow termination.

INHERITANCE RISK

De novo deletions have a low recurrence risk, due to the chance of undetectable gonadal mosaicism in either parent. Prenatal testing, such as chorionic villus sampling or amniocentesis, is available for future pregnancies, although the risk for miscarriage from these procedures may be comparable to the actual empirical risk for a recurrence.

Questions for Small Group Discussion
1. What is the difference between the terms "small for gestational age" (SGA) and "intrauterine growth restriction" (IUGR)?
2. What would be the advantages and disadvantages of performing amniocentesis for karyotype at 24 weeks of gestation in a pregnancy thought to have IUGR even if the societal regulations and family situation preclude a pregnancy termination if the amniocentesis demonstrates a chromosomal abnormality?

REFERENCES

Gardner RJM, Sutherland GR: Chromosome Abnormalities and Genetic Counseling, 3rd ed. New York, Oxford University Press, 2004.
Sanders RC: Structural Fetal Abnormalities: The Total Picture, 2nd ed. St. Louis, Mosby, 2002.
South ST, Corson VL, McMichael JL, et al: Prenatal detection of an interstitial deletion in 4p15 in a fetus with an increased nuchal skin fold measurement. Fetal Diagn Ther 20:58-63, 2005.

25. Long QT Syndrome

(Cardiac Ion Channel Gene Mutations)

Autosomal Dominant or Recessive

PRINCIPLES

- Locus heterogeneity
- Incomplete penetrance
- Genetic susceptibility to medications

MAJOR PHENOTYPIC FINDINGS

- QTc prolongation (>470 msec in males, >480 msec in females)
- Tachyarrhythmias (torsades de pointes)
- Syncopal episodes
- Sudden death

HISTORY AND PHYSICAL FINDINGS

A.B. is a 30-year-old female with long QT (LQT) syndrome who presents to the genetics clinic with her husband because they are contemplating a pregnancy. The couple wants to know the recurrence risks for this condition in their children and the genetic testing and prenatal diagnosis options that might be available to them. She is also concerned about potential risks to her health in carrying a pregnancy. The patient was diagnosed with the LQT syndrome in her early 20s when she was evaluated after the sudden death of her 15-year-old brother. Overall, she is a healthy individual with normal hearing, no dysmorphic features, and an otherwise negative review of systems. She has never had any fainting episodes. Subsequently, electrocardiographic findings confirmed the diagnosis of the syndrome in A.B., her father, and one of her paternal aunts. Molecular testing revealed a missense mutation in *KCNH2*, one that has been previously seen in other families with Romano-Ward syndrome, type LQT2. A.B. was initially prescribed β-blockade medication, which she is continuing, but her cardiologists decided that the less than total efficacy of β blockers in LQT2, and the previous, lethal event in her brother, justified the use of implantable cardioverter-defibrillators in A.B. and her affected relatives. A.B. is the first person in her family to pursue genetic counseling for the LQT syndrome.

BACKGROUND

Disease Etiology and Incidence

The long QT syndromes are a heterogeneous, panethnic group of disorders referred to as channelopathies because they are caused by defects in cardiac ion channels (see Table). The prevalence of LQT disorders is approximately 1 in 5000 to 7000 individuals. Mutations in five known cardiac ion channel genes (*KCNQ1, KCNH2, SCN5A, KCNE1,* and *KCNE2*) are responsible for most cases of LQT.

The genetics underlying LQT syndromes is complex. First, there is locus heterogeneity. The most common of the LQT syndromes, autosomal dominant Romano-Ward syndrome (MIM# 192500), is caused predominantly by mutations in two loci, *KCNQ1* and *KCNH2*, with a third locus,

SCN5A, also contributing. Second, different mutant alleles in the same locus can result in two distinct LQT syndromes, the Romano-Ward syndrome and the autosomal recessive Jervell and Lange-Nielsen syndrome (MIM# 220400).

Pathogenesis

LQT syndrome is caused by repolarization defects in cardiac cells. Repolarization is a controlled process that requires a balance between inward currents of sodium and calcium and outward currents of potassium. Imbalances cause the action potential of cells to increase or to decrease in duration, causing elongation or shortening, respectively, of the QT interval on electrocardiography. Most cases of LQT syndrome are caused by loss-of-function mutations in genes that encode subunits or regulatory proteins for potassium channels (genes whose names begin with *KCN*). These mutations decrease the outward, repolarization current, thereby prolonging the action potential of the cell and lowering the threshold for another depolarization. In other LQT syndrome patients, gain-of-function mutations in a sodium channel gene, *SCN5A,* lead to an increased influx of sodium, resulting in similar shifting of action potential and repolarization effects.

Phenotype and Natural History

The LQT syndromes are characterized by elongated QT interval and T wave abnormalities on electrocardiography (Fig. C-25), including tachyarrhythmia and torsades de pointes, a ventricular tachycardia characterized by a change in amplitude and twisting of the QRS complex. Torsades de pointes is associated with a prolonged QT interval and typically stops spontaneously but may persist and worsen to ventricular fibrillation.

In the most common LQT syndrome, Romano-Ward, syncope due to cardiac arrhythmia is the most frequent symptom; if undiagnosed or left untreated, it recurs and can be fatal in 10% to 15% of cases. However, between 30% and 50% of individuals with the syndrome never show syncopal symptoms. Cardiac episodes are most frequent from the preteen years through the 20s, with the risk decreasing over time. Episodes may occur at any age when triggered by QT-prolonging medications (see list in *http://www.qtdrugs.org*). Nonpharmacological triggers for cardiac events in the Romano-Ward syndrome differ on the basis of the gene responsible. LQT1 triggers are typically adrenergic stimuli including exercise and sudden emotion. Individuals with LTQ2 are at risk with exercise and at rest and with auditory stimuli such as alarm clocks and phones. LQT3 individuals have episodes with slower heart rates during rest periods and sleep. In addition, 40% of LQT1 cases are symptomatic before 10 years of age; in 10% of LTQ2 and rarely in LQT3 do symptoms occur before 10 years of age. LQT5 is rare, and less is known about its natural history and triggers.

The LQT syndrome exhibits reduced penetrance in terms of both electrocardiographic abnormalities and syncopal episodes. As many as 30% of affected individuals can have QT intervals that overlap with the normal range. Variable expression of the disorder can occur within and between families. Due to reduced penetrance, exercise electrocardiography is

THE COMMON LONG QT INTERVAL SYNDROMES

Locus	Gene and Protein	Location	Inheritance	Syndrome (MIM#)	Associated Phenotypes	Induced by
LQT1	KCNQ1 Voltage-gated potassium channel	11p15.5	AD	Romano-Ward* (#192500)	—	Exercise Emotional stress
			AR	Jervell and Lange-Nielsen† (#220400)	Congenital sensorineural deafness Penetrance of arrhythmia only in ~25% of heterozygous carriers	Exercise Emotional stress
LQT2	KCNH2 Voltage-gated potassium channel	7q35-q36	AD	Romano-Ward* (#192500)	—	Rest or sleep Auditory stimuli Emotional stress
LQT3	SCN5A Voltage-gated sodium channel type V	3p21	AD	Romano-Ward (#192500)	—	Rest or sleep
LQT5	KCNE1 Voltage-gated potassium channel (β subunit of KCNQ1)	21q22.1-q22.2	AD	Romano-Ward* (#192500)	—	?
			AR	Jervell and Lange-Nielsen† (#220400)	Congenital sensorineural deafness	?
LQT6	KCNE2 β subunit of KCNH2	21q22.1-q22.2	AD	Romano-Ward (#192500)	—	?

*LQT1 and LQT2 Romano-Ward syndrome is the most common, accounting for more than 80% of all patients. More than 400 mutations are known.
†Jervell and Lange-Nielsen syndrome accounts for 3% to 5% of patients with LQT.
Modified from Modell SM, Lehmann MH: The long QT syndrome family of cardiac ion channelopathies: a HuGE review. Genet Med 8:143-155, 2006.

often necessary for accurate diagnosis of at-risk family members.

LQT syndromes may be accompanied by other findings on physical examination. For example, Jervell and Lange-Nielsen syndrome (MIM# 220400) is characterized by congenital, profound sensorineural hearing loss together with LQT syndrome. It is an autosomal recessive disorder caused by particular mutations within either one of two genes (KCNQ1 and KCNE1) implicated in the autosomal dominant Romano-Ward syndrome. Heterozygous relatives of Jervell and Lange-Nielsen syndrome patients are not deaf but have a 25% risk of LQT syndrome.

Management
Treatment of the LQT syndrome is aimed at prevention of syncopal episodes and cardiac arrest. Optimal treatment is influenced by identification of the gene responsible in a given case. For instance, β-blocker therapy before the onset of symptoms is most effective in LQT1 and, to a somewhat lesser extent, in LQT2, but its efficacy in LQT3 is reduced. β-Blockade therapy must be monitored closely for age-related dose adjustment, and it is imperative that doses are not missed. Pacemakers may be necessary for individuals with bradycardia; access to external defibrillators may be appropriate. Implantable cardioverter-defibrillators may be needed in individuals with LQT3 or in other individuals with the LQT syndrome in whom β-blocker therapy is problematic, such as in patients with asthma, depression, or diabetes and those with a history of cardiac arrest. Medications such as the antidepressant amitriptyline, over-the-counter cold medications such as phenylephrine and diphenhydramine, or anti-

fungal drugs including fluconazole and ketoconazole should be avoided because of their effect on prolonging the QT interval or causing increased sympathetic tone. Activities and sports likely to be associated with intense physical activity, emotion, or stress should also be avoided.

INHERITANCE RISK

Individuals with the Romano-Ward syndrome have a 50% chance of having a child with the inherited gene mutations. Most individuals have an affected (although perhaps asymptomatic) parent, as the rate of de novo mutations is low. A detailed family history and careful cardiac evaluation of family members are extremely important and could be lifesaving. The recurrence risk in siblings of patients with Jervell and Lange-Nielsen syndrome is 25%, as expected with an autosomal recessive condition. The penetrance of LQT alone, without deafness, is 25% in heterozygous carriers in Jervell and Lange-Nielsen syndrome families.

Questions for Small Group Discussion
1. Some genetic syndromes rely on clinical evaluation, even with the availability of molecular testing, for diagnosis. In the case of LQT, how would you proceed with a patient thought to have LQT on family history? Why?
2. Discuss the ethics of testing minors in this condition.
3. You have just diagnosed a child with Jervell and Lange-Nielsen syndrome. What do you counsel the family in regard to recurrence risk and management for other family members?

A

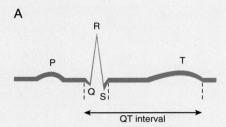

QT interval

Rate-correction formula (Bazett's):

$$QTc\ (msec) = \frac{QT\ (msec)}{\sqrt{RR\ (sec)}}$$

B

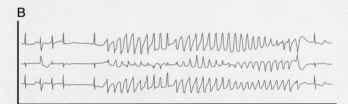

Figure C-25 ■ **A,** Measurement of the QT interval from the electrocardiogram. Diagram depicts the normal electrocardiogram with the P wave representing atrial activation, the QRS complex representing ventricular activation and the start of ventricular contraction, and the T wave representing ventricular repolarization. The QT interval is defined as the distance from the beginning of the Q wave to the end of the T wave. Owing to heart rate sensitivity of the QT interval, this parameter is corrected (normalized) to heart rate (as reflected by the beat-to-beat RR interval), yielding the QTc. QT and QTc can both be expressed in milliseconds or seconds. (Modified with permission from Liu BA, Juurlink DN: Drugs and the QT interval—caveat doctor. N Engl J Med 351:1053-1056, 2004.) **B,** Arrhythmia onset in long QT syndrome. Three simultaneous (and distinct) electrocardiographic channel recordings in a patient with QT prolongation and runs of continuously varying polymorphic ventricular tachycardia (torsades de pointes). Torsades de pointes may resolve spontaneously or progress to ventricular fibrillation and cardiac arrest. (Modified from Chiang C, Roden DM: The long QT syndromes: genetic basis and clinical implications. J Am Coll Cardiol 36:1-12, 2000.)

REFERENCES

GeneTests. Medical genetics information resource [database online]. University of Washington, Seattle, 1993-2006. Updated weekly. *http://www.genetests.org*

Modell SM, Lehmann MH: The long QT syndrome family of cardiac ion channelopathies: a HuGE review. Genet Med 8:143-155, 2006.

Moss AJ, Kass RS: Long QT syndrome: from channels to cardiac arrhythmias. J Clin Invest 115:2018-2024, 2005.

OMIM: Online Mendelian Inheritance in Man. McKusick-Nathans Institute for Genetic Medicine, Johns Hopkins University, and National Center for Biotechnology Information, National Library of Medicine. *http://www.ncbi.nlm.nih.gov/entrez/query.fcgi?db=OMIM*

University of Arizona Center for Education and Research on Therapeutics, Arizona Health Sciences Center—listing of drugs of concern in patients with LQT because these drugs prolong the QT interval or increase the risk of ventricular tachycardia. *http://www.qtdrugs.org*

Wilde AAM, Bezzina CR: Genetics of cardiac arrhythmias. Heart 91:1352-1358, 2005.

26. Marfan Syndrome

(FBN1 Mutation)
Autosomal Dominant

PRINCIPLES

- Dominant negative mutations
- Variable expressivity

MAJOR PHENOTYPIC FEATURES

- Age at onset: early childhood
- Disproportionate tall stature
- Skeletal anomalies
- Ectopia lentis
- Mitral valve prolapse
- Aortic dilatation and rupture
- Spontaneous pneumothorax
- Lumbosacral dural ectasia

HISTORY AND PHYSICAL FINDINGS

J.L., a healthy 16-year-old high school basketball star, was referred to the genetics clinic for evaluation for Marfan syndrome. His physique was similar to that of his father. His father, a tall, thin man, had died during a morning jog; no other family members had a history of skeletal abnormalities, sudden death, vision loss, or congenital anomalies. On physical examination, J.L. had an asthenic habitus with a high arched palate, mild pectus carinatum, arachnodactyly, arm span–height ratio of 1.1, diastolic murmur, and stretch marks on his shoulders and thighs. He was referred for echocardiography; this showed dilatation of the aortic root with aortic regurgitation. An ophthalmological examination showed bilateral iridodonesis and slight superior displacement of the lenses. On the basis of his physical examination and testing results, the geneticist explained to J.L. and his mother that he had Marfan syndrome.

BACKGROUND

Disease Etiology and Incidence

Marfan syndrome (MIM# 154700) is a panethnic, autosomal dominant, connective tissue disorder that results from mutations in the fibrillin 1 gene (FBN1, MIM# 134797). Marfan syndrome has an incidence of about 1 in 10,000. Approximately 25% to 35% of patients have de novo mutations. Mutations leading to Marfan syndrome are scattered across the gene, and each mutation is usually unique to a family.

Pathogenesis

FBN1 encodes fibrillin 1, an extracellular matrix glycoprotein with wide distribution. Fibrillin 1 polymerizes to form microfibrils in both elastic and nonelastic tissues, such as the aortic adventitia, ciliary zonules, and skin.

Mutations affect fibrillin 1 synthesis, processing, secretion, polymerization, or stability. Studies of fibrillin 1 deposition and cell culture expression assays have generally suggested a dominant negative pathogenesis; that is, production of mutant fibrillin 1 inhibits formation of normal microfibrils by normal fibrillin 1 or stimulates inappropriate proteolysis of extracellular microfibrils. More recent evidence in mouse models of Marfan syndrome suggests that half-normal amounts of normal fibrillin 1 are insufficient to initiate effective microfibrillar assembly. Thus, haploinsufficiency may also contribute to disease pathogenesis.

In addition to Marfan syndrome, mutations in FBN1 can cause other syndromes including neonatal Marfan syndrome, isolated skeletal features, autosomal dominant ectopia lentis, and the MASS phenotype (marfanoid signs including mitral valve prolapse or myopia, borderline and nonprogressive aortic enlargement, and nonspecific skeletal and skin findings). In general, the phenotypes are fairly consistent within a family, although the severity of the phenotype may vary considerably. To date, clear genotype-phenotype correlations have not emerged. The intrafamilial and interfamilial variability suggests that environmental and epigenetic factors play a significant role in determining the phenotype.

Recent evidence in mouse models suggests that fibrillin 1 is not simply a structural protein and that Marfan syndrome is not the result of structural weakness of the tissues. Rather, fibrillin 1 microfibrils normally bind and reduce the concentration and activity of growth factors in the TGFβ superfamily. Loss of fibrillin 1 increases signaling by free TGFβ, which contributes significantly to the disorder since TGFβ antagonism is sufficient to rescue the pulmonary and valvular changes seen in fibrillin 1–deficient mice.

Phenotype and Natural History

Marfan syndrome is a multisystem disorder with skeletal, ocular, cardiovascular, pulmonary, skin, and dural abnormalities. The skeletal abnormalities include disproportionate tall stature (arm span–height ratio >1.05; upper to lower segment ratio <0.85 in adults), arachnodactyly, pectus deformities, scoliosis, joint laxity, and narrow palate. The ocular abnormalities include ectopia lentis (Fig. C-26), flat corneas, increased globe length, and hypoplastic irides. The cardiovascular abnormalities include mitral valve prolapse, aortic regurgitation, and dilatation and dissection of the ascending aorta. The pulmonary abnormalities include spontaneous pneumothorax and apical blebs. The skin abnormalities include striae atrophicae and recurrent herniae. The dural abnormalities include lumbosacral dural ectasia.

Many features of Marfan syndrome develop with age. Skeletal anomalies such as anterior chest deformity and scoliosis worsen with bone growth. Subluxation of the lens is often present in early childhood but can progress through adolescence. Retinal detachment, glaucoma, and cataracts show increased frequency in Marfan syndrome. Cardiovascular complications manifest at any age and progress throughout life.

The major causes of premature death in patients with Marfan syndrome are heart failure from valve regurgitation and aortic dissection and rupture. As surgical and medical management of the aortic dilatation have improved, however, so has survival. Between 1972 and 1993, the age at which 50% of patients are predicted to be alive rose from 49 to 74 years for women and from 41 to 70 years for men.

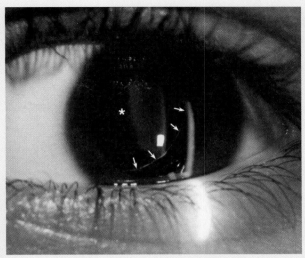

Figure C-26 ■ Ectopia lentis. Slit-lamp view of the left eye of a patient with Marfan syndrome. The asterisk indicates the center of the lens that is displaced superior nasally; normally, the lens is in the center of the pupil. The arrows indicate the edge of the lens that is abnormally visible in the pupil. (Courtesy of A. V. Levin, The Hospital for Sick Children and University of Toronto, Canada.)

Management

Marfan syndrome is a clinical diagnosis defined by the presence of particular features. Confirmation of Marfan syndrome by identification of mutations in *FBN1* is not currently practical because extreme allelic heterogeneity makes identification of the causative mutation in each family prohibitively labor-intensive and because of the lack of reliable genotype-phenotype correlation. Mutational analysis is neither fully sensitive nor specific for Marfan syndrome, limiting clinical utility.

No curative treatments are available for Marfan syndrome; therefore, treatment focuses on prevention and symptomatic management. Ophthalmological management includes frequent examinations, correction of the myopia, and, often, lens replacement. Orthopedic management includes bracing or surgery for scoliosis. Pectus deformity repair is largely cosmetic. Physical therapy or orthotics can compensate for joint instability. Cardiovascular management includes a combination of medical and surgical therapy. Medical therapy attempts to prevent or to slow progression of aortic dilatation by reducing heart rate, blood pressure, and ventricular ejection force with β-adrenergic blockers, and through restriction of participation in contact sports, competitive sports, and isometric exercise. Prophylactic replacement of the aortic root is recommended when aortic dilatation or aortic regurgitation becomes sufficiently severe.

Most patients now receive a valve-sparing aortic root replacement that eliminates the need for chronic anticoagulation.

The hemodynamic changes associated with pregnancy can precipitate progressive aortic enlargement or dissection. The aortic dissections are believed to be secondary to the hormonal, blood volume, and cardiac output changes associated with pregnancy and parturition. Current evidence suggests that there is an intolerable risk of pregnancy if the aortic root measures more than 4 cm. Women can elect to undergo valve-sparing aortic replacement before pregnancy.

INHERITANCE RISK

Patients with Marfan syndrome have a 50% risk of having a child affected with Marfan syndrome. In families segregating Marfan syndrome, at-risk individuals can be identified by detecting the mutation (in those rare circumstances when it happens to be known) or by linkage analysis if markers tightly linked to the *FBN1* locus show obvious linkage with the disease in the proband's family. Prenatal diagnosis is available only for those families in which linkage studies are possible or in which the *FBN1* mutation has been identified.

Questions for Small Group Discussion

1. Homocystinuria has many overlapping features with Marfan syndrome. Why? How can these two disorders be distinguished by medical history? by physical examination? by biochemical testing?
2. Discuss the difference between a prenatal diagnosis made by linkage analysis and one made by identification of a "disease-causing" mutation. What factors influence the accuracy of each diagnosis? How should the results of such testing be presented to prospective parents?
3. What are dominant negative mutations? What are gain-of-function mutations? Contrast the two. Why are dominant negative mutations common in connective tissue disorders?
4. If one wished to design a curative treatment for a disorder caused by dominant negative mutations, what must the therapy accomplish at a molecular level? How is this different from treatment of a disease caused by loss-of-function mutations?

REFERENCES

Dietz HC, Pyeritz RE: Marfan syndrome and related disorders. In Scriver CR, Beaudet AL, Sly WS, et al (eds): The Metabolic and Molecular Bases of Inherited Disease, 8th ed. New York, McGraw-Hill, 2001, pp 5287-5311.

GeneTests. Medical genetics information resource [database online]. University of Washington, Seattle, 1993-2006. Updated weekly. *http://www.genetests.org*

OMIM: Online Mendelian Inheritance in Man. McKusick-Nathans Institute for Genetic Medicine, Johns Hopkins University, and National Center for Biotechnology Information, National Library of Medicine. *http://www.ncbi.nlm.nih.gov/entrez/query.fcgi?db=OMIM*

Robinson PN, Arteaga-Solis E, Baldock C, et al: The molecular genetics of Marfan syndrome and related disorders. J Med Genet 43:769-787, 2006.

27. Miller-Dieker Syndrome

(17p13.3 Hemizygous Deletion)
Chromosomal

PRINCIPLES

- Microdeletion syndrome
- Contiguous gene disorder
- Haploinsufficiency

MAJOR PHENOTYPIC FEATURES

- Age at onset: prenatal
- Lissencephaly type 1 or type 2
- Facial dysmorphism
- Severe global mental deficiency
- Seizures
- Early death

HISTORY AND PHYSICAL FINDINGS

B.B., a 5-day-old boy born at 38 weeks of gestation, was admitted to the neonatal intensive care unit because of marked hypotonia and feeding difficulties. He was the product of an uncomplicated pregnancy; a fetal ultrasound examination at 14 weeks of gestation and a maternal triple screen at 16 weeks of gestation had been normal. B.B. was born by spontaneous vertex vaginal delivery; his Apgar scores were 8 at 1 minute and 9 at 5 minutes. He did not have a family history of genetic, neurological, or congenital disorders. On physical examination, B.B. had hypotonia and mild dysmorphic facial features including bitemporal narrowing, depressed nasal bridge, small nose with anteverted nares, and micrognathia. The findings from the examination were otherwise normal. His evaluation had included normal serum electrolyte values, normal metabolic screen, and normal study results for congenital infections. Brain ultrasound scan showed a hypoplastic corpus callosum, mild ventricular dilatation, and a smooth cortex. In addition to those studies, the genetics consultation team recommended a chromosome analysis, fluorescence in situ hybridization (FISH) for the *LIS1* gene (located in 17p13.3), and magnetic resonance imaging (MRI) of the brain. MRI showed a thickened cerebral cortex, complete cerebral agyria, multiple cerebral heterotopias, hypoplastic corpus callosum, normal cerebellum, and normal brainstem. The G-banded chromosome analysis was normal (46,XY), but FISH showed a deletion of *LIS1* on one chromosome 17. On the basis of these results, the geneticist explained to the parents that B.B. had Miller-Dieker syndrome. The parents declined further measures other than those to keep the baby comfortable, and B.B. died at 2 months of age.

BACKGROUND

Disease Etiology and Incidence

Miller-Dieker syndrome (MDS, MIM# 247200) is a contiguous gene syndrome caused by hemizygous deletion of 17p13.3; the mechanism underlying recurrent deletion of 17p13.3 has not yet been elucidated, but it may (like other microdeletion syndromes; see Chapter 6) involve recombination between low-copy repeated DNA sequences. MDS is a rare disorder of undefined incidence that occurs in all populations.

Pathogenesis

More than 50 genes have been mapped within the MDS deletion region in 17p13.3, but only the *LIS1* gene (MIM# 601545) has been associated with a specific phenotypic feature of MDS; hemizygosity for *LIS1* causes lissencephaly. *LIS1* encodes the brain isoform of the noncatalytic β subunit of platelet-activating factor acetylhydrolase (PAFAH). PAFAH hydrolyzes platelet-activating factor, an inhibitor of neuronal migration. PAFAH also binds to and stabilizes microtubules; preliminary observations suggest that PAFAH may play a role in the microtubule reorganization required for neuronal migration.

Haploinsufficiency of *LIS1* alone, however, does not cause the other dysmorphic features associated with MDS. Mutations within *LIS1* cause isolated lissencephaly sequence (MIM# 607432), that is, lissencephaly without other dysmorphism. Because all patients with MDS have dysmorphic facial features, this dysmorphism must be caused by haploinsufficiency of one or more different genes in the common MDS deletion interval.

Phenotype and Natural History

The features of MDS include brain dysgenesis, hypotonia, failure to thrive, and facial dysmorphism. The brain dysgenesis is characterized by lissencephaly type 1 (complete agyria) or type 2 (widespread agyria with a few sulci at the frontal or occipital poles), a cerebral cortex with four instead of six layers, gray matter heterotopias, and attenuated white matter (see Chapter 14). Some patients also have heart malformations and omphaloceles.

Patients with MDS feed and grow poorly. Smiling, brief visual fixation, and nonspecific motor responses are the only developmental skills most patients acquire. In addition to mental deficiency, patients usually suffer from opisthotonos, spasticity, and seizures. Nearly all patients die by 2 years of age.

Management

A patient's facial features and an MRI finding of lissencephaly often suggest a diagnosis of MDS (Fig. C-27). Confirmation of the diagnosis, however, requires detection of a 17p13.3 deletion by chromosome analysis or by FISH with a *LIS1*-specific probe. Approximately 60% of patients have a visible deletion of the MDS critical region.

MDS is incurable; therefore, treatment focuses on the management of symptoms and palliative care. Nearly all patients require pharmacological management of their seizures. Also, many patients receive nasogastric or gastrostomy tube feedings because of poor feeding and repeated aspiration.

INHERITANCE RISK

Eighty percent of patients have a de novo microdeletion of 17p13.3, and 20% inherit the deletion from a parent who

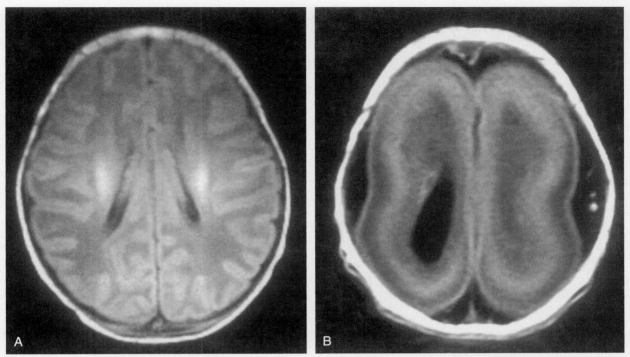

Figure C-27 ■ Brain magnetic resonance images of an infant without lissencephaly (**A**) and an infant with Miller-Dieker syndrome (**B**). Note the smooth cerebral surface, the thickened cerebral cortex, and the classic "figure-8" appearance of the brain of the patient with Miller-Dieker syndrome. (Courtesy of D. Chitayat, The Hospital for Sick Children and University of Toronto, Canada.)

carries a balanced chromosomal rearrangement. Because of the frequency with which the deletion is inherited from a parent with a balanced translocation, karyotype analysis and FISH for *LIS1* should be performed in both parents. A parent with a balanced translocation involving 17p13.3 has approximately one chance in four of having an abnormal liveborn child (MDS or dup17p) and approximately one chance in five of pregnancy loss. In contrast, if a patient has MDS as a result of a de novo deletion, the parents have a low risk for recurrence of MDS in future children.

Although the brain malformations of MDS result from incomplete migration of neurons to the cerebral cortex during the third and fourth months of gestation, lissencephaly is not detected by fetal MRI or ultrasonography until late in gestation. Prenatal diagnosis of MDS requires detection of a 17p13.3 deletion in fetal chorionic villi or amniocytes.

Questions for Small Group Discussion

1. Rubenstein-Taybi syndrome is caused either by deletion of 16p13.3 or by mutation of the *CREBBP* transcription factor. Compare and contrast the relationship of *CREBBP* and Rubenstein-Taybi syndrome with the relationship of *LIS1* and MDS. Why is MDS a contiguous gene deletion syndrome, whereas Rubenstein-Taybi syndrome is not?

2. Mutations of either *LIS1* on chromosome 17 or *DCX* on the X chromosome account for approximately 75% of isolated lissencephaly sequence. What features of the family history and brain MRI can be used to focus testing on *DCX* as opposed to *LIS1*?

3. At 30 weeks of gestation, a woman had a fetal ultrasound examination showing fetal lissencephaly. The pregnancy was otherwise uncomplicated, and fetal ultrasound findings earlier in gestation had been normal. What counseling and evaluation are indicated? Discuss your counseling approach if she and her spouse wish to terminate the pregnancy at 32 weeks of gestation.

REFERENCES

GeneTests. Medical genetics information resource [database online]. University of Washington, Seattle, 1993-2006. Updated weekly. *http://www.genetests.org*

Kato M, Dobyns WB: Lissencephaly and the molecular basis of neuronal migration. Hum Mol Genet 12(Spec No. 1):R89-96, 2003.

28. Myoclonic Epilepsy with Ragged-Red Fibers

(Mitochondrial tRNA^{lys} Mutation)

Matrilineal, Mitochondrial

PRINCIPLES

- Mitochondrial DNA mutations
- Replicative segregation
- Expression threshold
- High mutation rate
- Accumulation of mutations with age
- Heteroplasmy

MAJOR PHENOTYPIC FEATURES

- Age at onset: childhood through adulthood
- Myopathy
- Dementia
- Myoclonic seizures
- Ataxia
- Deafness

HISTORY AND PHYSICAL FINDINGS

R.S., a 15-year-old boy, was referred to the neurogenetics clinic for myoclonic epilepsy; his electroencephalogram was characterized by bursts of slow wave and spike complexes. Before the seizures developed, he had been well and developing normally. His family history was remarkable for a maternal uncle who had died of an undiagnosed myopathic disorder at 53 years; a maternal aunt with progressive dementia who had presented with ataxia at 37 years; and an 80-year-old maternal grandmother with deafness, diabetes, and renal dysfunction. On examination, R.S. had generalized muscle wasting and weakness, myoclonus, and ataxia. Initial evaluation detected sensorineural hearing loss, slowed nerve conduction velocities, and mildly elevated blood and cerebrospinal fluid lactate levels. Results of a subsequent muscle biopsy identified abnormal mitochondria, deficient staining for cytochrome oxidase, and ragged-red fibers—muscle fibers with subsarcolemmal mitochondria that stained red with Gomori trichrome stain. Molecular testing of a skeletal muscle biopsy specimen for mutations within the mitochondrial genome (mtDNA) identified a heteroplasmic mutation (8344G>A, tRNA^{lys} gene), a mutation known to be associated with myoclonic epilepsy with ragged-red fibers (MERRF), in 80% of the mtDNA from muscle. Subsequent testing of blood samples from R.S.'s mother, aunt, and grandmother confirmed that they also were heteroplasmic for this mutation. A review of the autopsy of the deceased uncle identified ragged-red fibers in some muscle groups. The physician counseled the family members (R.S.'s sibs and his mother's sibs) that they were either manifesting or non-manifesting carriers of a deleterious mtDNA mutation compromising oxidative phosphorylation. No other family members chose to be tested for the mutation.

BACKGROUND

Disease Etiology and Incidence

MERRF (MIM# 545000) is a rare panethnic disorder caused by mutations within the mtDNA in the tRNA^{lys} gene. More than 90% of patients have one of three mutations within this gene: 8344G>A accounts for 80% and 8356T>C and 8363G>A together account for an additional 10% (see Fig. 12-28). The disease is inherited maternally because mitochondria are inherited almost exclusively from the mother. MERRF patients are nearly always heteroplasmic for the mutant mitochondria (see Chapters 7 and 12).

Pathogenesis

Mitochondria generate energy for cellular processes by producing adenosine triphosphate through oxidative phosphorylation. Five enzyme complexes, I to V, compose the oxidative phosphorylation pathway. Except for complex II, each complex has some components encoded within the mtDNA and some in the nuclear genome. The mtDNA encodes 13 of the polypeptides in the oxidative phosphorylation complexes as well as 2 rRNAs and 22 tRNAs (see Chapter 12).

In MERRF, the activities of complexes I and IV are usually most severely reduced. The tRNA^{lys} mutations associated with MERRF reduce the amount of charged tRNA^{lys} in the mitochondria by 50% to 60% and thereby decrease the efficiency of translation such that at each lysine codon, there is a 26% chance of termination. Because complexes I and IV have the most components synthesized within the mitochondria, they are most severely affected.

Because each mitochondrion contains multiple mtDNAs and each cell contains multiple mitochondria, a cell can contain normal mtDNAs or abnormal mtDNAs in varying proportions; therefore, expression of the MERRF phenotype in any cell, organ, or individual ultimately depends on the overall reduction in oxidative phosphorylation capacity. The threshold for expression of a deleterious phenotype depends on the balance between oxidative supply and demand. This threshold varies with age and among individuals, organ systems, and tissues.

The threshold for expression of the MERRF phenotype in an individual tissue heteroplasmic for a tRNA^{lys} can be exceeded either by an accumulation of mutations in the normal mtDNA or by increasing the proportion of mutant mtDNAs. Compared to nuclear DNA, mtDNA has a 10-fold higher mutation rate; this may result from exposure to a high concentration of oxygen free radicals from oxidative phosphorylation, a lack of protective histones, and ineffective DNA repair. Because mtDNA has no introns, random mutations usually affect coding sequences. Consistent with this increased mutation rate, mitochondrial efficiency declines gradually throughout adulthood, and as reserve oxidative phosphorylation activity declines, expression of defects in the oxidative phosphorylation pathway becomes increasingly likely.

Increases in the proportion of mutant mtDNA can occur by a combination of inheritance, preferential replication of mutant mtDNA, and selection. First, the children of heteroplasmic mothers have widely varying proportions of mtDNA genotypes because of replicative segregation, that is, random partitioning of mitochondria during expansion of the oogonial population, particularly because of the mitochondrial "genetic bottleneck" that occurs during oogenesis. Second, as heteroplasmic cells within an individual undergo mitosis, the proportion of mtDNA genotypes in daughter cells changes

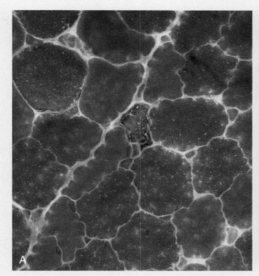
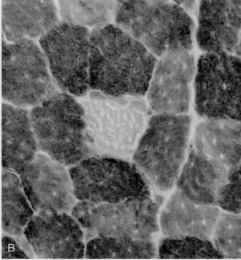

Figure C-28 ■ Quadriceps muscle histology. **A,** Modified Gomori trichrome stain illustrating ragged-red fiber (magnification ×525). **B,** Cytochrome oxidase stain illustrating absence of cytochrome oxidase in an affected muscle fiber, consistent with a mitochondrial DNA defect (magnification ×525). (Courtesy of Annette Feigenbaum, The Hospital for Sick Children, Toronto, Canada.)

from that of the parent cell by replicative segregation. Third, because changes in the proportion of mtDNA genotypes affect the cellular phenotype, the mtDNA is subject to strong selective pressures; the selective pressures vary among tissues and result in different mtDNA populations in different tissues of the same person. Thus, both intercellular and intergenerational mtDNA transmission follow the principles of population genetics.

Phenotype and Natural History

The classic MERRF phenotype includes myoclonic epilepsy and mitochondrial myopathy with ragged-red fibers (Fig. C-28). Other associated findings include abnormal brainstem evoked responses, sensorineural hearing loss, ataxia, renal dysfunction, diabetes, cardiomyopathy, and dementia. Onset of symptoms can be in childhood or adult life, and the course can be slowly progressive or rapidly downhill.

Because mtDNA genetics follows quantitative and stochastic principles, clinical features of affected relatives vary in pattern and severity and do not have an easily defined clinical course. The absence of ragged-red fibers in a muscle biopsy specimen does not exclude MERRF. Within pedigrees, phenotypes generally correlate well with the severity of the oxidative phosphorylation deficit, but correlation with the percentage of mutant mtDNA in skeletal muscle requires adjustment for age. In one pedigree, a young adult with 5% normal mtDNA in skeletal muscle had a severe clinical and biochemical phenotype; other young adults with 15% normal mtDNA had normal phenotypes; and an elderly adult with 16% normal mtDNA had a severe phenotype. This expression pattern demonstrates that symptoms accumulate progressively as oxidative phosphorylation capacity drops below organ expression thresholds and that age-related declines in oxidative phosphorylation play a critical role in the appearance and progression of symptoms.

Management

Treatment is symptomatic and palliative. No specific therapies are currently available. Most patients are given coenzyme Q and L-carnitine supplements to optimize the activity of the oxidative phosphorylation complexes.

INHERITANCE RISK

The risk to children of affected males is zero because, with only one known exception, children do not inherit paternal mtDNA. The risk to children of affected or unaffected females with a MERRF mutation cannot be estimated accurately by prenatal testing because the critical parameters defining disease in the child (replicative segregation, tissue selection, and somatic mtDNA mutations) cannot be predicted in advance.

Similarly, molecular testing of blood samples from at-risk family members is complicated by two general problems. First, because of replicative segregation and tissue selection, the mutation may not be detectable in blood; therefore, a negative result does not exclude a family member as a carrier of the mtDNA mutation. Second, because of replicative segregation, a positive result predicts neither the proportion of mutant mtDNA in other tissues nor the expected severity of disease.

Questions for Small Group Discussion

1. How does a mutant mtDNA molecule, arising de novo in a cell with hundreds of normal molecules, become such a significant fraction of the total that energy-generating capacity is compromised and symptoms develop?
2. How could mitochondrial mutations affecting oxidative phosphorylation accelerate the mutation rate of mtDNA?
3. How would mitochondrial mutations affecting oxidative phosphorylation accelerate aging?
4. In the fetus, oxygen tension is low and most energy is derived from glycolysis. How could this observation affect the prenatal expression of deleterious oxidative phosphorylation mutations?

REFERENCES

GeneTests. Medical genetics information resource [database online]. University of Washington, Seattle, 1993-2006. Updated weekly. *http://www.genetests.org*

OMIM: Online Mendelian Inheritance in Man. McKusick-Nathans Institute for Genetic Medicine, Johns Hopkins University, and National Center for Biotechnology Information, National Library of Medicine. *http://www.ncbi.nlm.nih.gov/entrez/query.fcgi?db=OMIM*

Taylor RW, Turnbull DM: Mitochondrial DNA mutations in human disease. Nat Rev Genet 6:389-402, 2005.

29. Neurofibromatosis 1

(NF1 Mutation)
Autosomal Dominant

PRINCIPLES

- Variable expressivity
- Extreme pleiotropy
- Tumor-suppressor gene
- Loss-of-function mutations
- Allelic heterogeneity
- De novo mutations

MAJOR PHENOTYPIC FEATURES

- Age at onset: prenatal to late childhood
- Café au lait spots
- Axillary and inguinal freckling
- Cutaneous neurofibromas
- Lisch nodules (iris hamartomas)
- Plexiform neurofibromas
- Optic glioma
- Specific osseous lesions

HISTORY AND PHYSICAL FINDINGS

L.M. is a 2-year-old male referred because of five café au lait spots, of which three measured larger than 5 mm in diameter. He had no axillary or inguinal freckling, no osseous malformations, and no neurofibromas. Physical examination of each parent revealed no stigmata of neurofibromatosis. The consulting geneticist informed the parents and referring pediatrician that L.M. did not meet the clinical criteria for neurofibromatosis type 1.

L.M. returned to the genetics clinic at 5 years of age. He now had Lisch nodules in both eyes and 12 café au lait spots, 8 of which measured at least 5 mm in diameter. He also had axillary freckling bilaterally. He was given the diagnosis of neurofibromatosis 1; his parents were told that he had a de novo mutation and the recurrence risk was therefore low, but that gonadal mosaicism could not be excluded.

L.M.'s parents declined both molecular testing in L.M. and prenatal testing during their next pregnancy.

BACKGROUND

Disease Etiology and Incidence

Neurofibromatosis 1 (NF1, MIM# 162200) is a panethnic autosomal dominant condition with symptoms most frequently expressed in the skin, eye, skeleton, and nervous system. NF1 results from mutations in the neurofibromin gene (NF1). The disease has an incidence of 1 in 3500 individuals, making it one of the most common autosomal dominant genetic conditions. Approximately half of patients have de novo mutations; the mutation rate for the NF1 gene is one of the highest known for any human gene, at approximately 1 mutation per 10,000 live births. Approximately 80% of the de novo mutations are paternal in origin, but there is no evidence for a paternal age effect increasing the mutation rate (see Chapter 9).

Pathogenesis

NF1 is a large gene (350 kb and 60 exons) that encodes neurofibromin, a protein widely expressed in almost all tissues but most abundantly in the brain, spinal cord, and peripheral nervous system. Neurofibromin is thought to regulate several intracellular processes, including the activation of Ras GTPase, thereby controlling cellular proliferation and acting as a tumor suppressor.

More than 500 mutations in the NF1 gene have been identified; most are unique to each family. The clinical manifestations result from a loss of function of the gene product; 80% of the mutations cause protein truncation. A disease-causing mutation can be identified for more than 95% of individuals with NF1.

NF1 is characterized by extreme clinical variability, both between and within families. This variability is probably caused by a combination of genetic, nongenetic, and stochastic factors. No clear genotype-phenotype correlations have been recognized, although large deletions are more common in NF1 patients with neurodevelopmental difficulties.

Phenotype and Natural History

NF1 is a multisystem disorder with neurological, musculoskeletal, ophthalmological, and skin abnormalities, and a predisposition to neoplasia (Fig. C-29). A diagnosis of NF1 can be made if an individual meets two or more of the following criteria: six or more café au lait spots measuring at least 5 mm in diameter (if prepubertal) or 15 mm in diameter (if postpubertal); two or more neurofibromas of any type, or one plexiform neurofibroma; axillary or inguinal freckling; optic glioma; two or more Lisch nodules; a distinctive osseous phenotype (sphenoid dysplasia and thinning of the long bone cortex with or without pseudarthrosis); or a first-degree relative with NF1.

Nearly all individuals with NF1 but no family history will meet clinical criteria by the age of 8 years. Children who have inherited NF1 can usually be identified clinically within the first year of life, as they require only one other feature of the disease to be present.

Although penetrance is essentially complete, manifestations are extremely variable. Multiple café au lait spots are present in nearly all individuals, with freckling seen in 90% of cases. Many individuals with NF1 have only cutaneous manifestations of the disease and iris Lisch nodules. Numerous neurofibromas are usually present in adults. Plexiform neurofibromas are less common. Ocular manifestations include optic gliomas (which may lead to blindness) and iris Lisch nodules. The most serious bone complications are scoliosis, vertebral dysplasia, pseudarthrosis, and overgrowth. Stenosis of pulmonic, renal, and cerebral vessels and hypertension are also frequent. The most common neoplasms for children with NF1 (other than neurofibromas) are optic nerve gliomas, brain tumors, and malignant myeloid disorders. About half of all children with NF1 will have a learning disability or attention deficits, which can persist into adulthood.

Individuals with features of NF1 limited to one region of the body, and who have unaffected parents, may be diagnosed with segmental (or regional) NF1. Segmental NF1 may

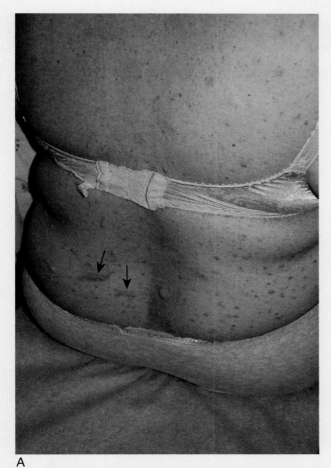

A

B

Figure C-29 ■ **A,** Cutaneous manifestations of NF1 including hundreds of small to medium-sized reddish papular neurofibromas and two large café au lait spots *(arrows).* **B,** Iris showing numerous Lisch nodules (one typical nodule is indicated by the arrow). (Courtesy of K. Yohay, Johns Hopkins School of Medicine, Baltimore, Md.)

represent an unusual distribution of clinical features by chance or somatic mosaicism for an *NF1* gene mutation.

Management

NF1 is a clinical diagnosis. Identification of mutations is not currently done routinely due to the size of the gene and the extreme allelic heterogeneity.

No curative treatments are available, and therefore treatment focuses on symptomatic management. Ongoing surveillance in an individual with NF1 should include an annual physical examination conducted by someone familiar with NF1, annual ophthalmological evaluation in childhood (less frequent as an adult), regular developmental assessments in childhood, and regular blood pressure measurements.

The deformities caused by NF1 are the most distressing disease manifestation. Discrete cutaneous and subcutaneous neurofibromas can be surgically removed if they are disfiguring or inconveniently located. Plexiform neurofibromas causing disfigurement or impingement can also be surgically managed. However, surgical intervention for these neoplasms can be problematic as they are often intimately involved with nerves and have a tendency to grow back at the site of removal.

INHERITANCE RISK

Individuals with NF1 have a 50% risk of having a child affected with NF1, although the features may be different in an affected child. Prenatal diagnosis is available for those families in which a causative *NF1* gene mutation has been identified or in which linkage studies are informative. Although prenatal diagnosis is accurate, it will not provide much prognostic information because of the extreme phenotypic variability of the disease. Parents of an affected child who themselves show no signs of the disease are still at some small elevated recurrence risk in the next pregnancy because of the possibility of germline mosaicism, which has been documented with NF1.

Questions for Small Group Discussion

1. Why is there such clinical variability in NF1? What factors could be influencing this phenotype?
2. Why is a positive family history of NF1 one of the major diagnostic criteria for this condition and not for other autosomal dominant conditions?
3. Review the major points of discussion with a family that desires prenatal testing for NF1 based on a known mutation in one of the parents.
4. How would a treatment of NF1 need to be targeted at the molecular level to specifically address the loss of function seen with this condition? How is that different from a disease caused by a dominant negative mutation?

REFERENCES

Ferner RE: Neurofibromatosis 1. Eur J Hum Genet 15:131-138, 2007.
GeneTests. Medical genetics information resource [database online]. University of Washington, Seattle, 1993-2006. Updated weekly. *http://www.genetests.org*
OMIM: Online Mendelian Inheritance in Man. McKusick-Nathans Institute for Genetic Medicine, Johns Hopkins University, and National Center for Biotechnology Information, National Library of Medicine. *http://www.ncbi.nlm.nih.gov/entrez/query.fcgi?db=OMIM*

30. Non–Insulin-Dependent Diabetes Mellitus

(Insulin Deficiency and Resistance)
Multifactorial

PRINCIPLES

- Polygenic disease
- Environmental modifiers

MAJOR PHENOTYPIC FEATURES

- Age at onset: childhood through adulthood
- Hyperglycemia
- Relative insulin deficiency
- Insulin resistance
- Obesity
- Acanthosis nigricans

HISTORY AND PHYSICAL FINDINGS

M.P. is a 38-year-old healthy male member of the Pima Indian tribe who requested information on his risk for development of non–insulin-dependent diabetes mellitus (NIDDM). Both of his parents had had NIDDM; his father died at 60 years from a myocardial infarction and his mother at 55 years from renal failure. His paternal grandparents and one older sister also had NIDDM, but he and his four younger siblings did not have the disease. The findings from M.P.'s physical examination were normal except for mild obesity; he had a normal fasting blood glucose level but an elevated blood insulin level and abnormally high blood glucose levels after an oral glucose challenge. These results were consistent with early manifestations of a metabolic state likely to lead to NIDDM. His physician advised M.P. to change his lifestyle so that he would lose weight and increase his physical activity. M.P. sharply reduced his dietary fat consumption, began commuting to work by bicycle, and jogged three times per week; his weight decreased 10 kg, and his glucose tolerance and blood insulin level normalized.

BACKGROUND

Disease Etiology and Incidence

Diabetes mellitus (DM) is a heterogeneous disease composed of type 1 (referred to as insulin-dependent DM or IDDM) and type 2 (referred to as non–insulin-dependent or NIDDM) diabetes mellitus (see Table). NIDDM (MIM# 125853) accounts for 80% to 90% of all diabetes mellitus and has a prevalence of 6% to 7% among adults in the United States. For as yet unknown reasons, there is a strikingly increased prevalence of the disease among Native Americans from the Pima tribe in Arizona, in whom the prevalence of NIDDM is nearly 50% by the age of 35 to 40 years. Approximately 5% to 10% of patients with NIDDM have maturity-onset diabetes of the young (MODY, MIM# 606391); 5% to 10% have a rare genetic disorder; and the remaining 70% to 85% have "typical NIDDM," a form of type 2 diabetes mellitus characterized by relative insulin deficiency and resistance. The molecular and genetic bases of typical NIDDM remain poorly defined.

COMPARISON OF TYPE 1 AND TYPE 2 DIABETES MELLITUS

Characteristic	Type 1 (IDDM)	Type 2 (NIDDM)
Sex	Female = male	Female > male
Age at onset	Childhood and adolescence	Adolescence through adulthood
Ethnic predominance	Whites	African Americans, Mexican Americans, Native Americans
Concordance		
Monozygotic twins	33%-50%	69%-90%
Dizygotic twins	1%-14%	24%-40%
Family history	Uncommon	Common
Autoimmunity	Common	Uncommon
Body habitus	Normal to wasted	Obese
Acanthosis nigricans	Uncommon	Common
Plasma insulin	Low to absent	Normal to high
Plasma glucagon	High, suppressible	High, resistant
Acute complication	Ketoacidosis	Hyperosmolar coma
Insulin therapy	Responsive	Resistant or responsive
Oral hypoglycemic therapy	Unresponsive	Responsive

Pathogenesis

NIDDM results from a derangement of insulin secretion and resistance to insulin action. Normally, basal insulin secretion follows a rhythmic pattern interrupted by responses to glucose loads. In patients with NIDDM, the rhythmic basal release of insulin is markedly deranged, responses to glucose loads are inadequate, and basal insulin levels are elevated although low relative to the hyperglycemia of these patients.

Persistent hyperglycemia and hyperinsulinemia develop before NIDDM and initiate a cycle leading to NIDDM. The persistent hyperglycemia desensitizes the islet β cell such that less insulin is released for a given blood glucose level. Similarly, the chronic elevated basal levels of insulin down-regulate insulin receptors and thereby increase insulin resistance. Furthermore, as sensitivity to insulin declines, glucagon is unopposed and its secretion increases; as a consequence of excessive glucagon, glucose release by the liver increases, worsening the hyperglycemia. Ultimately, this cycle leads to NIDDM.

Typical NIDDM, hereafter referred to as NIDDM, results from a combination of genetic susceptibility and environmental factors. Observations supporting a genetic predisposition include differences in concordance between monozygotic and dizygotic twins, familial clustering, and differences in prevalence among populations. Whereas human inheritance patterns suggest complex inheritance, identification of the relevant genes in humans, although made difficult by the effects of age, gender, ethnicity, physical fitness, diet, smoking, obesity, and fat distribution, has met with some success. Genome-wide screens and analyses have shown that an allele of a short tandem repeat polymorphism in the intron for a transcription factor, *TCF7L2*, is significantly associated with NIDDM in the Icelandic population. Heterozygotes (38% of the population) and homozygotes (7% of the population) have an increased relative risk for NIDDM of approximately 1.5- and 2.5-fold, respectively, over noncarriers. The increased risk due to the *TCF7L2* variant has been replicated in both a Danish and a U.S. cohort. The risk for NIDDM attributable to this allele is 21%. *TCF7L2* encodes a transcription factor involved in the expression of the hormone glucagon, which raises the blood glucose concentration and therefore works to oppose the action of insulin in lowering blood glucose. Screens of Finnish and Mexican American groups have identified another predisposition variant, a Pro12Ala mutation in *PPARG*, that is apparently specific to those populations and may account for up to 25% of the population-attributable risk of NIDDM in these populations. The more common proline allele has a frequency of 85% and causes a modest increase in risk (1.25-fold) for diabetes. PPARG is a member of the nuclear hormone receptor family and is important in the regulation of adipocyte function and differentiation.

Evidence for an environmental component includes a concordance of less than 100% in monozygotic twins; differences in prevalence in genetically similar populations; and associations with lifestyle, diet, obesity, pregnancy, and stress. The body of experimental evidence suggests that although genetic susceptibility is a prerequisite for NIDDM, clinical expression of NIDDM is likely to be strongly influenced by environmental factors.

Phenotype and Natural History

NIDDM usually affects obese individuals in middle age or beyond, although an increasing number of children and younger individuals are affected as more become obese and sedentary.

NIDDM has an insidious onset and is diagnosed usually by an elevated glucose level on routine examination. In contrast to patients with IDDM, patients with NIDDM usually do not develop ketoacidosis. In general, the development of NIDDM is divided into three clinical phases. First, the plasma glucose concentration remains normal despite elevated blood levels of insulin, indicating that the target tissues for insulin action appear to be relatively resistant to the effects of the hormone. Second, postprandial hyperglycemia develops despite elevated insulin concentrations. Third, declining insulin secretion causes fasting hyperglycemia and overt diabetes.

In addition to hyperglycemia, the metabolic dysregulation resulting from islet β-cell dysfunction and insulin resistance causes atherosclerosis, peripheral neuropathy, renal disease, cataracts, and retinopathy (Fig. C-30). One in six patients with NIDDM will develop end-stage renal disease or will require a lower extremity amputation for severe vascular disease; one in five will become legally blind from retinopathy. The development of these complications is related to the genetic background and degree of metabolic control. Chronic hyperglycemia can be monitored by means of measurements of the percentage of hemoglobin that has become modified by glycosylation, referred to as HbA_{1c}. Rigorous control of blood glucose levels, as determined by HbA_{1c} levels as close to normal as possible (<7%), reduces the risk of complications by 35% to 75% and can extend the average life expectancy, which now averages 17 years after diagnosis, by a few years.

Management

Weight loss, increased physical activity, and dietary changes help many patients with NIDDM by markedly improving insulin sensitivity and control. Unfortunately, many patients

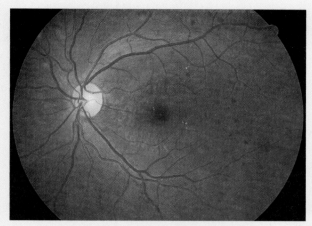

Figure C-30 ■ Nonproliferative diabetic retinopathy in a patient with NIDDM. Note the multiple "dot and blot" hemorrhages, the scattered "bread crumb" patches of intraretinal exudate, and, superonasally, a few cotton-wool patches. (Courtesy of R. A. Lewis, Baylor College of Medicine, Houston.)

are unable or unwilling to change their lifestyle sufficiently to accomplish this control and require treatment with oral hypoglycemic agents, such as sulfonylureas and biguanides. A third class of agent, thiazolidinediones, reduces insulin resistance by binding to PPARG. A fourth category of medication, α-glucosidase inhibitors, which act to slow intestinal absorption of glucose, can also be used. Each of these classes of drugs has been approved as monotherapy for NIDDM. As they fail with progression of disease, an agent from another class can be added. Oral hypoglycemics are not as effective as weight loss, increased physical activity, and dietary changes for achieving glycemic control. To achieve glycemic control and, possibly, reduce the risk of diabetic complications, some patients require treatment with exogenous insulin; however, insulin therapy accentuates insulin resistance by increasing hyperinsulinemia and obesity.

INHERITANCE RISK

The population risk of NIDDM is highly dependent on the population under consideration; in most populations, this risk is 1% to 5%, although it is 6% to 7% in the United States. If a patient has one affected sibling, the risk increases to 10%; an affected sibling and another first-degree relative, the risk is 20%; an affected monozygotic twin, the risk is 50% to 100%. In addition, because some forms of NIDDM are antecedents to IDDM (see Case 23), children of parents with NIDDM have an empirical risk of 1 in 10 for development of IDDM.

Questions for Small Group Discussion

1. How could civil engineering have a major impact on the treatment of patients with NIDDM?
2. What counseling should members, including children, of NIDDM families be given?
3. What factors are contributing to the rising prevalence of NIDDM?

REFERENCES

GeneTests. Medical genetics information resource [database online]. University of Washington, Seattle, 1993-2006. Updated weekly. *http://www.genetests.org*

OMIM: Online Mendelian Inheritance in Man. McKusick-Nathans Institute for Genetic Medicine, Johns Hopkins University, and National Center for Biotechnology Information, National Library of Medicine. *http://www.ncbi.nlm.nih.gov/entrez/query.fcgi?db=OMIM*

Sladek R, Rocheleau G, Rung J, et al: A genome-wide association study identifies novel risk loci for type 2 diabetes. Nature 445:881-885, 2007.

31. Ornithine Transcarbamylase Deficiency

(OTC Mutation)
X-Linked

PRINCIPLES

- Inborn error of metabolism
- X chromosome inactivation
- Manifesting heterozygotes
- Asymptomatic carriers
- Germline mutation rate much greater in spermatogenesis than in oogenesis

MAJOR PHENOTYPIC FEATURES

- Age at onset: hemizygous male with null mutation—neonatal; heterozygous female—with severe intercurrent illness, postpartum, or never
- Hyperammonemia
- Coma

HISTORY AND PHYSICAL FINDINGS

J.S. is a 4-day-old male infant brought to the emergency department because he could not be aroused. The parents reported a history of 24 hours of decreased intake, vomiting, and increasing lethargy. He was the 3-kg full-term product of an uncomplicated gestation born to a healthy 26-year-old primiparous woman. Physical examination showed a comatose, hyperpneic, nondysmorphic male newborn. Initial laboratory evaluation revealed a blood ammonium concentration of 900 micromolar (normal in a newborn is <75) and elevated venous pH of 7.48, with a normal bicarbonate concentration and anion gap. A urea cycle disorder was suspected, so plasma amino acid levels were determined on an emergency basis. Glutamine was elevated at 1700 micromolar (normal, <700), and citrulline was undetectable (normal is 7 to 34) (Fig. C-31). Analysis of urine for organic acids was normal; urinary orotic acid was extremely elevated. Elevated urine orotic acid with low citrulline indicates a diagnosis of ornithine transcarbamylase deficiency pending confirmation by mutation analysis.

Further questioning of J.S.'s mother revealed that she had a lifelong aversion to protein and a brother who died in the first week of life of unknown causes. J.S. was started on intravenous sodium benzoate and sodium phenylacetate (Ammonul) and arginine HCl supplementation. The child was transported by air to a tertiary care center equipped for neonatal hemodialysis. On arrival, his plasma ammonium level had dropped to 700 micromolar. The parents were counseled about the high risk of brain damage from this degree of hyperammonemia. They elected to proceed with hemodialysis, which was well tolerated and resulted in decline of the blood ammonium to less than 200 micromolar after 4 hours. The child was maintained on Ammonul and high calories from intravenous dextrose and intralipids until the ammonium level was normal, at which point he was slowly started on a protein-restricted diet and monitored for hyperammonemia, especially during intercurrent illnesses.

BACKGROUND

Disease Etiology and Incidence

Ornithine transcarbamylase (OTC) deficiency (MIM# 311250) is a panethnic X-linked disorder of urea cycle metabolism caused by a mutation of the gene encoding ornithine transcarbamylase (OTC). It has an incidence of 1 in 30,000 males. The exact incidence of manifesting females is unknown.

Pathogenesis

Ornithine transcarbamylase is an enzyme in the urea cycle (Fig. C-31). The urea cycle is the mechanism by which waste nitrogen is detoxified and excreted. Complete deficiency of any enzyme within the cycle (except arginase) leads to severe hyperammonemia in the neonatal period. For patients with urea cycle defects, arginine becomes an essential amino acid (Fig. C-31). In utero, excess nitrogen is metabolized by the mother. Postnatal accumulation of waste nitrogen in the extremely catabolic period after birth leads to elevation of glutamine and alanine, the body's natural pools for nitrogen, and ultimately to elevated levels of ammonium ion. Plasma ammonium levels above 200 micromolar may cause brain damage; the degree of brain damage is related to how high the concentrations of ammonium and glutamine in the blood rise and how long the elevations persist. Thus, early detection and treatment are critical to outcome.

Males are hemizygous for the OTC gene and are therefore more severely affected by mutations in this gene. Because OTC undergoes random X chromosome inactivation (see Chapter 6), females are mosaic for expression of the mutation and can demonstrate a wide range of enzyme function and clinical severity. Female heterozygotes can be completely asymptomatic and are able to eat as much protein as they wish. Alternatively, if their loss of OTC activity is more significant, they may find themselves avoiding dietary protein and subject to recurrent, symptomatic hyperammonemia.

Phenotype and Natural History

Males with complete OTC deficiency are born normal but begin vomiting, become lethargic, and eventually lapse into coma between 48 and 72 hours of age. Because they have been vomiting, they are usually dehydrated as well. Untreated males with null mutations usually die in the first week of life. Even if the patient with OTC deficiency is promptly and successfully treated in the neonatal period, the risk remains high for recurrent bouts of hyperammonemia, particularly during intercurrent illnesses, because complete control of severe OTC deficiency is difficult even with dietary protein restriction and medications that divert the ammonia to nontoxic pathways (see Chapter 13). With each episode of hyperammonemia, the patient may suffer brain damage or die in a matter of only a few hours after the onset of metabolic decompensation.

Girls (or boys with partial OTC deficiency) are usually asymptomatic in the neonatal period but develop hyperammonemia during intercurrent febrile illnesses, such as influenza, or with excessive dietary protein intake. Other catabolic stresses, such as surgery or long bone fracture, may also

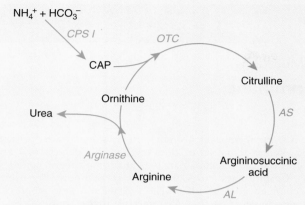

Figure C-31 ■ The urea cycle. CPS I, carbamoyl phosphate synthetase I; CAP, carbamoyl phosphate; OTC, ornithine transcarbamylase; AS, argininosuccinate synthetase; AL, argininosuccinate lyase.

precipitate hyperammonemia. Like affected males, symptomatic females are at risk for brain damage and mental retardation.

OTC deficiency and carbamoyl phosphate synthetase deficiency (Fig. C-31) cannot be detected by newborn screening. Abnormal metabolites that occur in other enzyme deficiencies within the urea cycle, however, can be detected by tandem mass spectrometry of serum amino acids (see Chapter 17).

Management
Plasma ammonium concentration should be measured in any sick neonate. For most urea cycle defects, the pattern of abnormalities on quantitative amino acid determination is diagnostic. To distinguish between OTC deficiency and carbamoyl phosphate synthetase deficiency, both of which are characterized by very low or absent citrulline, it is necessary to measure urine orotic acid, which is elevated in OTC deficiency. Determination of urine organic acids is also important to rule out an organic aciduria, which can also present with hyperammonemia in the newborn period. Molecular testing is available to confirm the diagnosis.

Acutely hyperammonemic patients should be treated with a four-pronged approach: (1) 10% dextrose at twice the maintenance rate, to provide calories in the form of sugar for gluconeogenesis and thereby reduce catabolism of endogenous proteins, and elimination of dietary protein intake; (2) intravenous Ammonul, a solution of sodium benzoate and sodium phenylacetate, both of which provide diversion therapy by driving the excretion of nitrogen independently of the urea cycle (see Chapter 13); (3) intravenous arginine HCl to provide adequate amounts of arginine, an essential amino acid, and to drive any residual enzyme activity by ensuring adequate substrate to the urea cycle; and (4) if a patient does not respond to the initial bolus of these medications, hemodialysis.

Chronic management entails careful control of dietary calories and protein as well as oral phenylbutyrate. Mainte-

nance of a high carbohydrate intake spares endogenous protein from being catabolized for gluconeogenesis; dietary protein restriction reduces the load of ammonia requiring detoxification through the urea cycle. Phenylbutyrate is readily converted to phenylacetate, which promotes non–urea cycle dependent nitrogen excretion. The family must be carefully trained to look for early signs of hyperammonemia, such as irritability, vomiting, and sleepiness, so that the patient can be promptly brought to the hospital for intravenous treatment.

Because of the great difficulty in achieving metabolic control and the substantial risk for brain damage or death within hours of the onset of metabolic decompensation, liver transplantation to provide a functioning urea cycle is recommended as soon as a patient has grown sufficiently (>10 kg) to tolerate the procedure.

INHERITANCE RISK

OTC deficiency is inherited as an X-linked trait. Since OTC deficiency is nearly always a genetic lethal, approximately 67% of the mothers of affected infants would be expected to be carriers, as discussed in Chapter 7. Surprisingly, studies in families with OTC deficiency indicate, in fact, that 90% of the mothers of affected infants are carriers. The reason for this discrepancy between the theoretical and actual carrier rates is that the underlying assumption of equal male and female mutation rates used for the theoretical calculation is incorrect. In fact, mutations in the *OTC* gene are much more frequent (~50-fold) in the male germline than in the female germline. Most of the mothers of an isolated boy with OTC deficiency are carriers as a result of a new mutation inherited on the X chromosome they received from their fathers.

In a woman who is a carrier of a mutant OTC deficiency allele, her sons who receive the mutant allele will be affected and her daughters will be carriers who may or may not be symptomatic, depending on random X inactivation in the liver. Males with partial OTC deficiency who reproduce will have all carrier daughters and no affected sons. When the mutation in the family is known, prenatal testing by examination of the gene is available. Prenatal diagnosis by assay of the OTC enzyme is not practical because the enzyme is not expressed in chorionic villi or amniotic fluid cells.

> **Questions for Small Group Discussion**
> 1. Discuss the Lyon hypothesis and explain the variability of disease manifestations in females.
> 2. Why is arginine an essential amino acid in this disorder? Arginine is ordinarily not an essential amino acid in humans.
> 3. What organic acidurias cause hyperammonemia?

REFERENCES

GeneTests. Medical genetics information resource [database online]. University of Washington, Seattle, 1993-2006. Updated weekly. *http://www. genetests.org*

OMIM: Online Mendelian Inheritance in Man. McKusick-Nathans Institute for Genetic Medicine, Johns Hopkins University, and National Center for Biotechnology Information, National Library of Medicine. *http://www. ncbi.nlm.nih.gov/entrez/query.fcgi?db=OMIM*

32. Polycystic Kidney Disease

(*PKD1* and *PKD2* Mutations)

Autosomal Dominant

PRINCIPLES

- Variable expressivity
- Genetic heterogeneity
- Two-hit hypothesis

MAJOR PHENOTYPIC FEATURES

- Age at onset: childhood through adulthood
- Progressive renal failure
- Renal and hepatic cysts
- Intracranial saccular aneurysms
- Mitral valve prolapse
- Colonic diverticula

HISTORY AND PHYSICAL FINDINGS

Four months ago, P.J., a 35-year-old man with a history of mitral valve prolapse, developed intermittent flank pain. He eventually presented to his local emergency department with severe pain and hematuria. A renal ultrasound scan showed nephrolithiasis and polycystic kidneys consistent with polycystic kidney disease. The findings from his physical examination were normal except for a systolic murmur consistent with mitral valve prolapse, mild hypertension, and a slight elevation of serum creatinine concentration. His father and his sister had died of ruptured intracranial aneurysms, and P.J.'s son had died at 1 year of age from polycystic kidney disease. At the time of his son's death, the physicians had suggested that P.J. and his wife should be evaluated to see whether either of them had polycystic kidney disease; however, the parents elected not to pursue this evaluation because of guilt and grief about their son's death. P.J. was admitted for management of his nephrolithiasis. During this admission, the nephrologists told P.J. that he had autosomal dominant polycystic kidney disease.

BACKGROUND

Disease Etiology and Incidence

Autosomal dominant polycystic kidney disease (ADPKD, MIM# 173900) is genetically heterogeneous. Approximately 85% of patients have ADPKD-1 caused by mutations in the *PKD1* gene; most of the remainder have ADPKD-2 due to mutations of *PKD2*. A few families have not shown linkage to either of these loci, suggesting that there is at least one additional, as yet unidentified locus.

ADPKD is one of the most common genetic disorders and has a prevalence of 1 in 300 to 1 in 1000 in all ethnic groups studied. In the United States, it accounts for 8% to 10% of end-stage renal disease.

Pathogenesis

PKD1 encodes polycystin 1, a transmembrane receptor–like protein of unknown function. *PKD2* encodes polycystin 2, an integral membrane protein with homology to the voltage-activated sodium and calcium α_1 channels. Polycystin 1 and polycystin 2 interact as part of a heteromultimeric complex.

Cyst formation in ADPKD appears to follow a "two-hit" mechanism such as that observed with tumor-suppressor genes and neoplasia (see Chapter 16); that is, both alleles of either *PDK1* or *PDK2* must lose function for cysts to form. The mechanism by which loss of either polycystin 1 or polycystin 2 function causes cyst formation has not been defined but involves mislocalization of cell surface proteins that are normally restricted either to basolateral or epithelial surfaces of developing renal tubular cells (see Chapter 14).

Phenotype and Natural History

ADPKD may manifest at any age but symptoms or signs most frequently appear in the third or fourth decade. Patients present with urinary tract infections, hematuria, urinary tract obstruction (clots or nephrolithiasis), nocturia, hemorrhage into a renal cyst, or complaints of flank pain from the mass effect of the enlarged kidneys (Fig. C-32). Hypertension affects 20% to 30% of children and nearly 75% of adults with ADPKD. The hypertension is a secondary effect of intrarenal ischemia and activation of the renin-angiotensin system. Nearly half of patients have end-stage renal disease by 60 years of age. Hypertension, recurrent urinary tract infections, male sex, and early age of clinical onset are most predictive of early renal failure. Approximately 43% of patients presenting with ADPKD before or shortly after birth die of renal failure within the first year of life; end-stage renal disease, hypertension, or both develop in the survivors by 30 years of age.

ADPKD exhibits both interfamilial and intrafamilial variation in the age at onset and severity. Part of the interfamilial variation is secondary to locus heterogeneity because patients with ADPKD-2 have milder disease than patients with ADPKD-1. Intrafamilial variation appears to result from a combination of environment and genetic background because the variability is more marked between generations than among siblings.

In addition to renal cysts, patients with ADPKD develop hepatic, pancreatic, ovarian, and splenic cysts as well as intracranial aneurysms, mitral valve prolapse, and colonic diverticula. Hepatic cysts are common in both ADPKD-1 and ADPKD-2, whereas pancreatic cysts are generally observed with ADPKD-1. Intracranial saccular aneurysms develop in 5% to 10% of patients with ADPKD; however, not all patients have an equal risk for development of aneurysms because they exhibit familial clustering. Patients with ADPKD have an increased risk of aortic and tricuspid valve insufficiency, and approximately 25% develop mitral valve prolapse. Colonic diverticula are the most common extrarenal abnormality; the diverticula associated with ADPKD are more likely to perforate than are those observed in the general population.

Management

In general, ADPKD is diagnosed by family history and renal ultrasound examination. The detection of renal cysts by ultrasound examination increases with age such that 80% to 90% of patients have detectable cysts by 20 years, and nearly

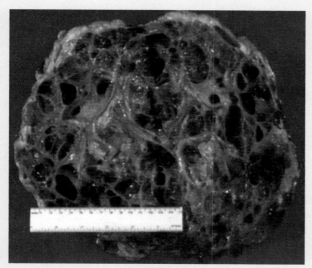

Figure C-32 ■ Cross section of a kidney from a patient with ADPKD showing large cysts and widespread destruction of the normal renal parenchyma. (Courtesy of J. Rutledge, Department of Pathology, University of Washington, Seattle.)

100% have them by 30 years. If necessary for prenatal diagnosis or identification of a related kidney donor, the diagnosis can be confirmed by linkage or mutation detection, or both, in some families.

The management and treatment of patients with ADPKD focus on slowing the progression of renal disease and minimizing its symptoms. Hypertension and urinary tract infections are treated aggressively to preserve renal function. Pain from the mass effect of the enlarged kidneys is managed by drainage and sclerosis of the cysts.

INHERITANCE RISK

Approximately 90% of patients have a family history of ADPKD; only 10% of ADPKD results from de novo mutations of either *PDK1* or *PDK2*. Parents with ADPKD have a 50% risk of having an affected child in each pregnancy. If the parents have had a child with onset of disease in utero, the risk of having another severely affected child is approximately 25%. In general, however, the severity of disease cannot be predicted because of variable expressivity. For families in which the mutation is known or in which linkage analysis is possible, the recurrence risk can be modified by analysis of fetal DNA.

Siblings and parents of patients with ADPKD also have an increased risk of disease. Renal ultrasonography is the recommended method for the screening of family members.

Questions for Small Group Discussion

1. Compare the molecular mechanism of cyst development in ADPKD with the development of neurofibromas in neurofibromatosis type 1.
2. Many mendelian diseases have variable expressivity that might be accounted for by modifier loci. How would one identify such loci?
3. Why is ADPKD frequently associated with tuberous sclerosis? How might this illustrate a contiguous gene deletion syndrome?
4. How can ADPKD be distinguished from autosomal recessive polycystic kidney disease?
5. Linkage analysis of families segregating ADPKD requires the participation of family members in addition to the patient. What should be done if individuals crucial to the study do not want to participate?

REFERENCES

GeneTests. Medical genetics information resource [database online]. University of Washington, Seattle, 1993-2006. Updated weekly. *http://www.genetests.org*

OMIM: Online Mendelian Inheritance in Man. McKusick-Nathans Institute for Genetic Medicine, Johns Hopkins University, and National Center for Biotechnology Information, National Library of Medicine. *http://www.ncbi.nlm.nih.gov/entrez/query.fcgi?db=OMIM*

Wilson PD: Polycystic kidney disease. N Engl J Med 350:151-164, 2004.

33. Prader-Willi Syndrome

(Absence of Paternally Derived 15q11-q13)

Chromosomal, Uniparental Disomy

PRINCIPLES

- Imprinting
- Uniparental disomy
- Microdeletion
- Recombination between repeated DNA sequences

MAJOR PHENOTYPIC FEATURES

- Age at onset: infancy
- Infantile feeding difficulties
- Childhood hyperphagia and obesity
- Hypotonia
- Cognitive impairment
- Sterility
- Dysmorphism

HISTORY AND PHYSICAL FINDINGS

J.T. was born at 38 weeks' gestation after an uncomplicated pregnancy and delivery. He was the second child of nonconsanguineous parents. Shortly after birth, his parents and the nurses noticed that he was hypotonic and feeding poorly. His parents and older sister were in good health; he did not have a family history of neuromuscular, developmental, genetic, or feeding disorders. Review of the medical record did not reveal a history of overt seizures, hypoxic insults, infection, cardiac abnormalities, or blood glucose or electrolyte abnormalities. On examination, J.T. did not have respiratory distress or dysmorphic features except for a hypoplastic scrotum and cryptorchidism; his weight and length were appropriate for gestational age; he was severely hypotonic with lethargy, weak cry, decreased reflexes, and a poor suck. Subsequent evaluation included testing for congenital infections and congenital hypothyroidism, brain magnetic resonance imaging, measurements of blood ammonium, plasma amino acids, and urine organic acids, evaluation for hypothyroidism, and karyotype with fluorescence in situ hybridization (FISH) for deletion of the Prader-Willi syndrome locus (chromosome 15q11-q13; see Chapter 5). The results of the tests were normal except for the FISH assay, which showed a deletion of chromosome 15q11-q13. The geneticist explained to the parents that J.T. had Prader-Willi syndrome. After much discussion and thought, J.T.'s parents decided that they were unable to care for a disabled child and gave him up for adoption.

BACKGROUND

Disease Etiology and Incidence

Prader-Willi syndrome (PWS, MIM# 176270) is a panethnic developmental disorder caused by loss of expression of genes on paternally derived chromosome 15q11-q13. Loss of paternally expressed genes can arise by several mechanisms; approximately 70% of patients have a deletion of 15q11-q13, 25% have maternal uniparental disomy, less than 5% have

mutations within the imprinting control element, and less than 1% have a chromosomal abnormality (see Chapter 5). PWS has an incidence of 1 in 10,000 to 1 in 15,000 live births.

Pathogenesis

Many genes within 15q11-q13 are differentially expressed, depending on whether the region is inherited from the father or the mother. In other words, many genes expressed by paternal 15q11-q13 are not expressed by maternal 15q11-q13, and many genes expressed by maternal 15q11-q13 are not expressed by paternal 15q11-q13. This phenomenon of differential expression of a gene according to whether it is inherited from the father or mother is known as imprinting (see Chapters 5 and 7). Maintenance of correct expression of imprinted genes requires switching of the imprint on passage through the germline; that is, paternal imprints are switched to maternal ones on passage through the maternal germline, and maternal imprints are switched to paternal ones on passage through the paternal germline. Switching of imprinting on passage through the germline is regulated by an imprinting control element and reflected by epigenetic changes in DNA methylation and chromatin that regulate gene expression.

Deletion of 15q11-q13 during male meiosis gives rise to children with PWS because children formed from a sperm carrying the deletion will be missing genes that are active only on the paternally derived 15q11-q13. The mechanism underlying this recurrent deletion is illegitimate recombination between low-copy repeat sequences flanking the deletion interval (see Chapter 6). Less commonly, inheritance of a deletion spanning this region occurs if a patient inherits an unbalanced karyotype from a parent who has a balanced translocation.

Failure to switch the maternal imprints to paternal imprints during male meiosis gives rise to children with PWS because children formed from a sperm with a maternally imprinted 15q11-q13 will not be able to express genes active only on the paternally imprinted 15q11-q13. Imprinting failure arises from mutations within the imprinting control element.

Maternal uniparental disomy also gives rise to PWS because the child has two maternal chromosomes 15 and no paternal chromosome 15. Maternal uniparental disomy is thought to develop secondary to trisomy rescue, that is, loss of the paternal chromosome 15 from a conceptus with chromosome 15 trisomy secondary to maternal nondisjunction.

Despite the observations that loss of a paternally imprinted 15q11-q13 gives rise to PWS and despite the identification of many imprinted genes within this region, the precise cause of PWS is still unknown. PWS has not yet been shown to result from a mutation in any one specific gene.

Phenotype and Natural History

In early infancy, PWS is characterized by severe hypotonia, feeding difficulties, and hypogonadism with cryptorchidism. The hypotonia improves over time, although adults remain mildly hypotonic. The hypogonadism, which is of hypothalamic origin, does not improve with age and usually causes delayed and incomplete pubertal development as well as infertility. The feeding difficulties usually resolve within the first year of life, and between 1 and 6 years, the patients develop extreme hyperphagia and food-seeking behavior (hoarding, foraging, and stealing). This behavior and a low metabolic rate cause marked obesity. The obesity is a major cause of morbidity due largely to cardiopulmonary disease and non–insulin-dependent (type 2) diabetes mellitus. Longevity can be nearly normal if obesity is avoided.

Most children with PWS have delayed motor and language development as well as mild mental retardation (mean IQ, 60 to 80) and severe learning disabilities. They also have behavioral problems including temper tantrums, obsessive-compulsive disorders, and poor adaptation to changes in routine. These behavioral problems continue into adulthood and remain disabling. Approximately 5% to 10% of patients also develop psychoses during early adulthood.

Other anomalies associated with PWS include short stature, scoliosis, osteoporosis, and dysmorphism. Dysmorphic features include a narrow bifrontal diameter, almond-shaped eyes, triangular mouth, and small hands and feet (Fig. C-33). Also, many patients have hypopigmentation of their hair, eyes, and skin.

Management

Although it is often suspected on the basis of history and physical features, a diagnosis of PWS is defined by the absence of a paternally imprinted 15q11-q13. Loss of the paternal imprint is detected by DNA analyses showing that the imprinted genes have only a maternal methylation pattern. If the DNA studies confirm PWS, genetic counseling requires a subsequent karyotype and FISH for 15q11-q13 to determine whether PWS arose from inheritance of a chromosomal translocation.

No medications are currently available to treat the hyperphagia; diet and exercise remain the mainstays for controlling the obesity. Growth hormone replacement can normalize height and improve lean body mass. Sex hormone replacement promotes secondary sexual features but frequently worsens behavioral problems in males and increases the risk of stroke in females. Behavioral management and serotonin reuptake inhibitors are the most effective therapies currently available for the behavioral disorder. Adult patients usually perform best in sheltered living (group homes) and employment environments.

INHERITANCE RISK

The risk for recurrence of PWS in future children of parents is related to the molecular cause. For imprinting defects, the risk can be as high as 50%, whereas for either deletion of 15q11-q13 or maternal uniparental disomy, the recurrence risk is less than 1%. The risk for recurrence if a parent carries a balanced translocation depends on the nature of the translocation but can be as high as 25%; in contrast, all PWS

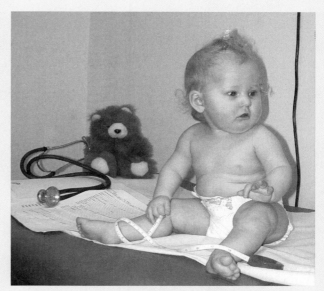

Figure C-33 ■ A 12-month-old girl with Prader-Willi syndrome. Note her fair coloring, narrow bifrontal diameter, almond-shaped eyes, and down-turned mouth. The hyperphagia, with resulting central obesity, generally does not begin until the age of 2 to 6 years. (Courtesy of S. Heeger, University Hospitals of Cleveland.)

patients reported to date with an unbalanced translocation have had a de novo chromosomal rearrangement.

Questions for Small Group Discussion

1. Angelman syndrome also arises from imprinting defects of 15q11-q13. Compare and contrast the phenotypes and causative molecular mechanisms of Prader-Willi syndrome and Angelman syndrome.
2. How might imprinting explain the phenotypes associated with triploidy?
3. Beckwith-Wiedemann syndrome and Russell-Silver syndrome also appear to be caused by abnormal expression of imprinted genes. Explain.
4. J.T.'s parents gave him up for adoption. Should the genetic counseling have been done differently? What is nondirective genetic counseling?

REFERENCES

Eiholzer U, Whitman BY: A comprehensive team approach to the management of patients with Prader-Willi syndrome. J Pediatr Endocrinol Metab 17:1153-1175, 2004.

GeneTests. Medical genetics information resource [database online]. University of Washington, Seattle, 1993-2006. Updated weekly. *http://www.genetests.org*

OMIM: Online Mendelian Inheritance in Man. McKusick-Nathans Institute for Genetic Medicine, Johns Hopkins University, and National Center for Biotechnology Information, National Library of Medicine. *http://www.ncbi.nlm.nih.gov/entrez/query.fcgi?db=OMIM*

34. Retinoblastoma

(RB1 Mutation)
Autosomal Dominant

PRINCIPLES

- Tumor-suppressor gene
- Two-hit hypothesis
- Somatic mutation
- Tumor predisposition
- Cell-cycle regulation
- Variable expressivity

MAJOR PHENOTYPIC FEATURES

- Age at onset: childhood
- Leukocoria
- Strabismus
- Visual deterioration
- Conjunctivitis

HISTORY AND PHYSICAL FINDINGS

J.V., a 2-year-old girl, was referred by her pediatrician for evaluation of right strabismus and leukocoria, a reflection from a white mass within the eye giving the appearance of a white pupil (see Fig. 16-5). Her mother reported that she had developed progressive right esotropia in the month before seeing her pediatrician. She had not complained of pain, swelling, or redness of her right eye. She was otherwise healthy. She had healthy parents and a 4-month-old sister; no other family members had had ocular disease. Except for the leukocoria and strabismus, the findings from her physical examination were normal. Her ophthalmological examination defined a solitary retinal tumor of 8 disc diameters arising near the macula. Magnetic resonance imaging of the head did not show extension of the tumor outside the globe. She received chemotherapy combined with focal irradiation. DNA analysis showed that she had a germline mutation (C to T transition) in one allele of her retinoblastoma (RB1) gene.

BACKGROUND

Disease Etiology and Incidence
Retinoblastoma (MIM# 180200) is a rare embryonic neoplasm of retinal origin (Fig. C-34) that results from germline or somatic mutations, or both, in both alleles of the RB1 gene. It occurs worldwide with an incidence of 1 in 18,000 to 30,000.

Pathogenesis
The retinoblastoma protein (Rb) is a tumor suppressor that plays an important role in regulating the progression of proliferating cells through the cell cycle and the exit of differentiating cells from the cell cycle. Rb effects these two functions by sequestration of other transcription factors and by promoting deacetylation of histones, a chromatin modification associated with gene silencing.

Retinoblastoma-associated RB1 mutations occur throughout the coding region and promoter of the gene. Mutations within the coding region of the gene either desta-

bilize Rb or compromise its association with enzymes necessary for histone deacetylation. Mutations within the promoter reduce expression of normal Rb. Both types of mutations result in a loss of functional Rb.

An RB1 germline mutation is found in 40% of patients with retinoblastoma, but only 10% of all patients have a history of other affected family members. RB1 mutations include cytogenetic abnormalities of chromosome 13q14, single-base substitutions, and small insertions or deletions. Some evidence suggests that the majority of new germline mutations arise on the paternal allele, whereas somatic mutations arise with equal frequency on the maternal and paternal alleles. Nearly half of the mutations occur at CpG dinucleotides. After either the inheritance of a mutated allele or the generation of a somatic mutation on one allele, the other RB1 allele must also lose function (the second "hit" of the two-hit hypothesis; see Chapter 16) for a cell to proliferate unchecked and develop into a retinoblastoma. Loss of a functional second allele occurs by a novel mutation, loss of heterozygosity, or promoter CpG island hypermethylation; deletion or the development of isodisomy occurs most frequently, and promoter hypermethylation occurs least frequently.

Retinoblastoma usually segregates as an autosomal dominant disorder with full penetrance; a few families have been described with reduced penetrance, however. The RB1 mutations identified within these families include missense mutations, in-frame deletions, and promoter mutations. In contrast to the more common null RB1 alleles, these mutations are believed to represent alleles with some residual function.

Phenotype and Natural History
Patients with bilateral retinoblastoma generally present during the first year of life, whereas those with unilateral disease present somewhat later with a peak between 24 and 30 months. Approximately 70% of patients have unilateral retinoblastoma and 30% bilateral retinoblastoma. All patients with bilateral disease have germline RB1 mutations, but not all patients with germline mutations develop bilateral disease. The disease is diagnosed before 5 years of age in 80% to 95% of patients. Retinoblastoma is uniformly fatal if untreated; with appropriate therapy, however, more than 80% to 90% of patients are free of disease 5 years after diagnosis.

As might be expected with mutation of a key cell-cycle regulator, patients with germline RB1 mutations have a markedly increased risk of secondary neoplasms; this risk is increased by environmental factors such as treatment of the initial retinoblastoma with radiotherapy. The most common secondary neoplasms are osteosarcomas, soft tissue sarcomas, and melanomas. There is no increase in second malignant neoplasms in patients with nonhereditary retinoblastoma.

Management
Early detection and treatment are essential for optimal outcome. The goals of therapy are to cure the disease and to preserve as much vision as possible. Treatment is tailored to

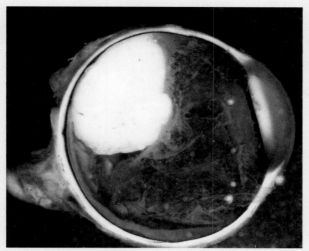

Figure C-34 ■ Midline cross section of an enucleated eye from a patient with retinoblastoma. Notice the large primary tumor in the posterior third of the globe and a few white vitreous seeds. (The brown discoloration of the vitreous is a fixation artifact.) (Courtesy of R. A. Lewis, Baylor College of Medicine, Houston.)

the tumor size and involvement of adjacent tissues. Treatment options for intraocular retinoblastoma include enucleation, various modes of radiotherapy, cryotherapy, light coagulation, and chemotherapy.

If the disease is unilateral at the time of the patient's presentation, the patient needs frequent examinations to detect any new retinoblastomas in the unaffected eye because 30% of apparently sporadic cases are caused by the inheritance of a new germline mutation. Such frequent examinations are usually continued until at least 7 years of age.

To direct follow-up more efficiently, patients should receive molecular testing to identify the mutations in the *RB1* gene. Ideally, a tumor sample is examined first, and then another tissue, such as blood, is analyzed to determine whether one of those mutations is a germline mutation. If neither mutation is a germline mutation, the patient does not require such frequent follow-up.

INHERITANCE RISK

If a parent had bilateral retinoblastoma and thus probably carries a germline mutation, the empirical risk of an affected child is 45%; this reflects the high likelihood of a second, somatic mutation (or "hit") in the second *RB1* allele of the child. On the other hand, if the parent had unilateral disease, the empirical risk of an affected child is 7% to 15%; this reflects the relative proportion of germline mutations versus somatic mutations in patients with unilateral disease. Nearly 90% of children who develop retinoblastoma are the first individuals affected within the family. Interestingly, 1% of unaffected parents of an affected child have evidence of a spontaneously resolved retinoblastoma on retinal examination; for these families, therefore, the risk of an affected child is 45%. Except for the rare situation in which one parent is a nonpenetrant carrier of an *RB1* mutation, families in which neither parent had retinoblastoma have a risk of recurrence equivalent to that of the general population.

Questions for Small Group Discussion

1. What other diseases develop as a result of a high frequency of mutations in CpG dinucleotides? What is the mechanism of mutation at CpG dinucleotides? What could explain the increased frequency of CpG dinucleotide mutations with increasing paternal age?
2. Compare and contrast the type and frequency of tumors observed in Li-Fraumeni syndrome with those observed in retinoblastoma. Both Rb and p53 are tumor suppressors; why are *TP53* mutations associated with a different phenotype than are *RB1* mutations?
3. Discuss four diseases that arise as a result of somatic mutations. Examples should illustrate chromosomal recombination, loss of heterozygosity, gene amplification, and accumulation of point mutations.
4. Both SRY (see Chapter 6) and Rb regulate development by modulating gene expression through the modification of chromatin structure. Compare and contrast the two different mechanisms that each uses to modify chromatin structure.

REFERENCES

Balmer A, Zografos L, Munier F: Diagnosis and current management of retinoblastoma. Oncogene 25:5341-5349, 2006.

GeneTests. Medical genetics information resource [database online]. University of Washington, Seattle, 1993-2006. Updated weekly. *http://www.genetests.org*

OMIM: Online Mendelian Inheritance in Man. McKusick-Nathans Institute for Genetic Medicine, Johns Hopkins University, and National Center for Biotechnology Information, National Library of Medicine. *http://www.ncbi.nlm.nih.gov/entrez/query.fcgi?db=OMIM*

35. Rett Syndrome

(*MEPC2* Mutations)
X-Linked Dominant

PRINCIPLES

- Loss-of-function mutation
- Incomplete penetrance
- Variable expressivity
- Sex-dependent phenotype

MAJOR PHENOTYPIC FEATURES

- Age at onset: neonatal to early childhood
- Neurodevelopmental regression
- Repetitive stereotypic hand movements

HISTORY AND PHYSICAL FINDINGS

P.J. had had normal growth and development until 18 months of age. At 24 months, she was referred for decelerating head growth and progressive loss of language and motor skills. She had lost purposeful hand movements and developed repetitive hand wringing by 30 months. She also had mild microcephaly, truncal ataxia, gait apraxia, and severely impaired expressive and receptive language. No other family members had neurological diseases. On the basis of these findings, the neurologist suggested that P.J. might have Rett syndrome. The physician explained that Rett syndrome is a result of mutations in the methyl-CpG–binding protein 2 gene (*MECP2*) in most patients and that testing for such mutations could help confirm the diagnosis. Subsequent testing of P.J.'s DNA identified a heterozygous *MECP2* mutation; she carried the transition 763C>T, which causes Arg255Ter. Neither parent carried the mutation.

BACKGROUND

Disease Etiology and Incidence

Rett syndrome (MIM# 312750) is a panethnic X-linked dominant disorder with a female prevalence of 1 in 10,000 to 15,000. It is caused by loss of function mutations of the *MECP2* gene. A few males with severe developmental and neurological abnormalities have been described with mutations that cause partial loss of MeCP2 function, but males do not develop typical Rett syndrome unless they have a 47,XXY karyotype or somatic mosaicism. A few patients with atypical Rett syndrome have mutations in one allele of the *CDKL5* gene, which is also X-linked. CDKL5 is a threonine/serine kinase, but little is known of its function.

Pathogenesis

MECP2 encodes a nuclear protein that binds methylated DNA and recruits histone deacetylases to regions of methylated DNA. The precise function of MeCP2 has not been fully defined, but it is hypothesized to mediate transcriptional silencing and epigenetic regulation of genes in these regions of methylated DNA. Accordingly, dysfunction or loss of MeCP2, as observed in Rett syndrome, would be predicted to cause *inappropriate activation* of genes.

The brains of patients with Rett syndrome are small and have cortical and cerebellar atrophy without neuronal loss; Rett syndrome is therefore not a typical neurodegenerative disease. Within much of the cortex and hippocampus, the neurons from Rett patients are smaller and more densely packed than normal and have a simplified dendritic branching pattern. These observations suggest that MeCP2 is important for establishing and maintaining neuronal interactions rather than for neuronal precursor proliferation or neuronal determination.

Phenotype and Natural History

Classic Rett syndrome is a progressive neurodevelopmental disorder occurring almost exclusively in girls (Fig. C-35). After apparently normal development until 6 to 18 months of age, patients enter a short period of developmental slowing and stagnation with decelerating head growth. Subsequently, they rapidly lose speech and acquired motor skills, particularly purposeful hand use. With continued disease progression, they develop stereotypic hand movements, breathing irregularities, ataxia, and seizures. After a brief period of pseudostabilization, usually during the preschool to early school years, the patients deteriorate further to become severely mentally retarded and develop progressive spasticity, rigidity, and scoliosis. Patients usually live into adulthood, but their life span is short due to an increased incidence of unexplained sudden death.

Besides Rett syndrome, *MECP2* mutations cause a broad spectrum of diseases affecting both boys and girls. Among girls, the range extends from severely affected patients who never learn to speak, turn, sit, or walk and develop severe epilepsy, to mildly affected patients who speak and have good gross motor function as well as relatively well-preserved hand function. Among boys, the range encompasses intrauterine death, congenital encephalopathy, mental retardation with various neurological symptoms, and mild mental retardation only; classic Rett syndrome is observed only among boys with somatic mosaicism for a *MECP2* mutation or with an extra X chromosome.

Management

Suspected on the basis of clinical features, the diagnosis of Rett syndrome is usually confirmed by DNA testing; however, current testing detects *MECP2* mutations in only 80% to 90% of patients with typical Rett syndrome. The clinical diagnosis criteria for typical Rett syndrome include normal prenatal and perinatal periods, normal head circumference at birth, relatively normal development through 6 months of age, deceleration of head growth between 6 and 48 months of age, loss of acquired hand skills and purposeful hand movements by 5 to 30 months of age and subsequent development of stereotyped hand movements, impaired expressive and receptive language, severe psychomotor retardation, and development of gait apraxia and truncal ataxia between 12 and 48 months of age.

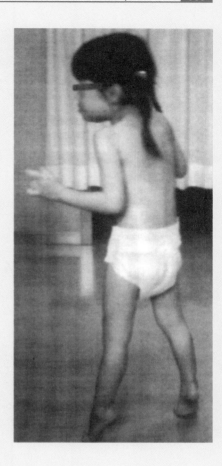

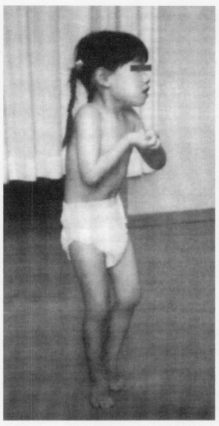

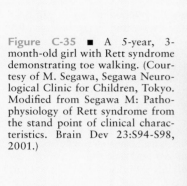

Figure C-35 ■ A 5-year, 3-month-old girl with Rett syndrome demonstrating toe walking. (Courtesy of M. Segawa, Segawa Neurological Clinic for Children, Tokyo. Modified from Segawa M: Pathophysiology of Rett syndrome from the stand point of clinical characteristics. Brain Dev 23:S94-S98, 2001.)

Currently, there are no curative treatments of Rett syndrome, and the management focuses on supportive and symptomatic therapy. Current medical therapy includes anticonvulsants for seizures, serotonin uptake inhibitors for agitation, carbidopa or levodopa for rigidity, and melatonin to ameliorate sleep disturbances. Families often have problems with social adjustment and coping and should therefore be provided with the opportunity to interact with similarly affected families through support groups and referred for professional counseling as needed.

INHERITANCE RISK

Approximately 99% of Rett syndrome is sporadic; most *MECP2* mutations are de novo, although in rare cases they can be inherited from an unaffected or mildly affected mother with skewed X chromosome inactivation. At least 70% of de novo mutations arise in the paternal germline.

If a couple has an affected child but a *MECP2* mutation is not identified in either parent, the risk to future siblings is low, although it is higher than among the general population because of the possibility of undetected germline mosaicism. In contrast, if the mother carries a disease-causing *MECP2* mutation, each daughter and son has a 50% risk of inheriting the mutation. However, the poor genotype-phenotype correlation among patients with *MECP2* mutations generally prohibits prediction of whether a female fetus with a *MECP2* mutation will develop classic Rett syndrome or another *MECP2*-associated disease. Similarly, identification of a *MECP2* mutation in a male fetus does not predict intrauterine demise, the development of congenital encephalopathy, or another *MECP2*-associated disease.

Questions for Small Group Discussion

1. *MECP2* is on the X chromosome. Discuss how this could affect the phenotypic variability observed among females with *MECP2* mutations. Discuss how this might account for the fewer numbers of males with *MECP2* mutations and the differences in disease severity observed generally between males and females.

2. Given that MeCP2 is an epigenetic mediator of gene expression, discuss possible molecular mechanisms by which genetic background, environment, and stochastic factors could cause the phenotypic variability observed among males with *MECP2* mutations.

3. Rett syndrome is a neurodevelopmental disorder without neurodegeneration. Why could the absence of neurodegeneration make this disease more amenable to treatment than Alzheimer disease or Parkinson disease? why less amenable? In this context, also discuss possible molecular mechanisms for the neurodevelopmental regression observed with Rett syndrome.

4. What defines a disease, the molecular mutation or the clinical phenotype?

REFERENCES

GeneTests. Medical genetics information resource [database online]. University of Washington, Seattle, 1993-2006. Updated weekly. *http://www.genetests.org*

Moretti P, Zoghbi HY: *MeCP2 dysfunction in Rett syndrome and related disorders. Curr Opin Genet Dev 16:276-281, 2006.*

OMIM: Online Mendelian Inheritance in Man. McKusick-Nathans Institute for Genetic Medicine, Johns Hopkins University, and National Center for Biotechnology Information, National Library of Medicine. *http://www.ncbi.nlm.nih.gov/entrez/query.fcgi?db=OMIM*

36. Sex Reversal

(SRY Mutation or Translocation)
Y-Linked or Chromosomal

PRINCIPLES

- Sex reversal
- Developmental regulatory gene
- Pseudoautosomal regions of the X and Y chromosomes
- Illegitimate recombination
- Incomplete penetrance
- Fertility loci

MAJOR PHENOTYPIC FEATURES

- Age at onset: prenatal
- Sterility
- Reduced secondary sexual features
- Unambiguous genitalia

HISTORY AND PHYSICAL FINDINGS

Ms. R., a 37-year-old executive, was pregnant with her first child. Because of her age-related risk of having a child with a chromosomal abnormality, she elected to have an amniocentesis to assess the fetal karyotype; the karyotype result was normal 46,XX. At 18 weeks' gestation, however, a fetal ultrasound scan revealed a normal male fetus; a subsequent detailed ultrasound scan confirmed a male fetus. Ms. R. had been in good health before and during the pregnancy with no infections or exposures to drugs during the pregnancy. Neither she nor her partner had a family history of ambiguous genitalia, sterility, or congenital anomalies. Re-evaluation of the chromosome analysis confirmed a normal 46,XX karyotype, but fluorescence in situ hybridization identified a sex-determining region Y gene (SRY) signal on one X chromosome (Fig. C-36). At 38 weeks of gestation, Ms. R. had an uncomplicated spontaneous vaginal delivery of a phenotypically normal male child.

BACKGROUND

Disease Etiology and Incidence

Sex reversal is panethnic and genetically heterogeneous. In patients with complete gonadal dysgenesis, point mutations, deletions, or translocations of SRY are the most common causes of sex reversal (see Chapter 6). Approximately 80% of 46,XX males with complete gonadal dysgenesis have a translocation of SRY onto an X chromosome, and 20% to 30% of 46,XY females with complete gonadal dysgenesis have a mutation or deletion of the SRY gene. The incidence of 46,XX males and 46,XY females is about 1 in 20,000.

Pathogenesis

SRY is a DNA-binding protein that alters chromatin structure by bending DNA. These DNA-binding and DNA-bending properties suggest that SRY regulates gene expression.

During normal human development, SRY is necessary for the formation of male genitalia, and its absence is permissive for the formation of female genitalia. The precise mechanism through which SRY effects development of male genitalia is undefined, although some observations suggest that SRY represses a negative regulator of testicular development.

SRY mutations identified in XY females cause a loss of SRY function. Ten percent to 15% of XY females have a deletion of SRY (SRY⁻ XY females), and 10% to 15% have point mutations within SRY. The point mutations within SRY impair either DNA binding or DNA bending.

The SRY alteration observed in XX males is a translocation of SRY from Yp to Xp (SRY⁺ XX males; Fig. C-36). During male meiosis, an obligatory crossing over occurs between the pseudoautosomal regions of Xp and Yp; this crossing over ensures proper segregation of the chromosomes and maintains sequence identity between the X and Y pseudoautosomal regions. On occasion, however, recombination occurs centromeric to the pseudoautosomal region and results in the transfer of Yp-specific sequences, including SRY to Xp (see Chapter 6).

In addition to SRY, the Y chromosome contains at least three loci (azoospermic factor loci AZFa, AZFb, and AZFc) required for normal sperm development. The absence of these loci at least partially explains the infertility of SRY⁺ XX males.

The X chromosome also contains several loci necessary for ovarian maintenance and female fertility. Oocyte development requires a single X chromosome, but maintenance of those oocytes requires two X chromosomes. Consistent with these observations, XY female fetuses develop oocytes, but their ovarian follicles degenerate by birth or shortly thereafter. The absence of a second X chromosome therefore explains the infertility of XY females (see Chapter 6).

Phenotype and Natural History

SRY⁺ XX males have many features of Klinefelter syndrome (47,XXY), including hypogonadism, azoospermia, hyalinization of seminiferous tubules, and gynecomastia. Despite decreased testosterone production, most patients enter puberty spontaneously, although they may require testosterone supplementation to attain full virilization. In contrast to patients with Klinefelter syndrome, most 46,XX male patients have normal to short stature, normal skeletal proportions, normal intelligence, and fewer psychosocial problems. Patients with an extensive portion of Yp on an X chromosome more closely resemble patients with Klinefelter syndrome.

SRY⁻ XY females have complete gonadal dysgenesis and are usually taller than average for normal women. These patients have physical features of Turner syndrome only when the deletion of SRY is associated with an extensive deletion of Yp. Because these patients have only streak gonads, they do not enter puberty spontaneously.

In contrast to the complete penetrance and relatively uniform expressivity observed with translocation or deletion of SRY, point mutations of SRY exhibit both incomplete penetrance and variable expressivity. Patients with SRY point mutations usually have complete gonadal dysgenesis, are taller than average for normal women, and do not spontaneously develop secondary sexual characteristics. A few SRY

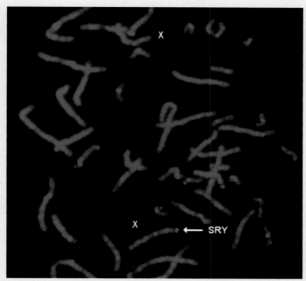

Figure C-36 ■ Fluorescence in situ hybridization of a locus-specific probe to metaphase chromosomes for the detection of the t(X;Y)(p22.3;p11.2) translocation in an *SRY*⁺ XX male. The chromosomes are counterstained with DAPI. The probe for *SRY* is a mixture of locus-specific sequences (red). The centromere of chromosome X is probed with sequences that map to the α-satellite DNA (green). In normal cells, the red signal is observed only on the Y chromosome. In cells with the t(X;Y)(p22.3;p11.2) translocation, a red signal is observed on the abnormal chromosome X and a green signal on both X chromosomes. (Courtesy of B. Bejjani and L. Shaffer, Baylor College of Medicine, Houston.)

point mutations, however, have been associated with both an infertile (complete gonadal dysgenesis) female phenotype and a fertile male phenotype within the same family.

Management

In patients with complete gonadal dysgenesis, the diagnosis of sex reversal usually arises either because of discordance between the fetal ultrasound scan and fetal karyotype or because of absent or incomplete secondary sexual development and infertility. Confirmation that the sex reversal is secondary to an abnormality of *SRY* expression requires demonstration of the appropriate *SRY* alteration.

For *SRY*⁺ XX males, androgen supplementation is usually effective for virilization, but treatment of the azoospermia is not currently possible. Administration of supplemental androgens does not prevent gynecomastia. Patients need surgical treatment if the gynecomastia becomes sufficiently disconcerting or severe.

For *SRY*⁻ XY females and XY females with point mutations of *SRY*, estrogen therapy is usually initiated at about 14 to 15 years of age to promote development of secondary sexual characteristics. Progesterone therapy is added to the regimen to induce menses either at the time of the first vaginal breakthrough bleeding or in the second year of estrogen

therapy. In addition, because of the risk for development of gonadoblastoma, it is recommended that dysgenic gonads be removed once skeletal growth is complete.

As with all disorders of genital ambiguity or of discordance between genetic and phenotypic sex, the psychosocial management and counseling of the family and patient are extremely important. Many families and patients have difficulty understanding the medical data and making appropriate psychosocial adjustments.

INHERITANCE RISK

De novo illegitimate recombination is the most common cause of *SRY*⁺ XX males and *SRY*⁻ XY females; therefore, most couples with an affected child have a low risk of recurrence in future children. Rarely, however, *SRY*⁺ XX males and *SRY*⁻ XY females arise as a result of inheriting an *SRY* deletion or translocation from a father with a balanced translocation between Xp and Yp. If the father is a translocation carrier, all children will be either an *SRY*⁺ XX boy or an *SRY*⁻ XY girl. Because *SRY*⁺ XX males and *SRY*⁻ XY females are invariably sterile, they are at no risk of passing on the disorder.

Most XY females with point mutations in *SRY* have de novo mutations. Parents of an affected child, therefore, usually have a low risk of recurrence in future children; however, because some *SRY* mutations have incomplete penetrance, normal fertile fathers can carry *SRY* mutations that may or may not cause sex reversal among their XY children.

Questions for Small Group Discussion

1. Mutations of other genes, such as *WT1*, *SOX9*, *SF1*, and *DAX1*, can also result in sex reversal. Compare and contrast the phenotypes observed with mutations in the genes with those observed with *SRY* mutations.
2. The association of *SRY* point mutations with an infertile female phenotype and a fertile male phenotype within the same family suggests either stochastic variation dependent on the reduced SRY activity or segregation of another locus that interacts with *SRY*. Why? How could this be resolved?
3. Mutations affecting steroid synthesis or steroid responsiveness are usually associated with ambiguous genitalia, whereas *SRY* mutations are generally associated with reversed but unam-biguous genitalia. Discuss the reasons for this generalization.
4. Discuss genetic, gonadal, phenotypic, and psychological gender and the importance of each to genetic counseling.

REFERENCES

GeneTests. Medical genetics information resource [database online]. University of Washington, Seattle, 1993-2006. Updated weekly. *http://www.genetests.org*

Nikolova G, Vilain E: Mechanisms of disease: transcription factors in sex determination—relevance to human disorders of sex development. Nat Clin Pract Endocrinol Metab 2:231-238, 2006.

OMIM: Online Mendelian Inheritance in Man. McKusick-Nathans Institute for Genetic Medicine, Johns Hopkins University, and National Center for Biotechnology Information, National Library of Medicine. *http://www.ncbi.nlm.nih.gov/entrez/query.fcgi?db=OMIM*

37. Sickle Cell Disease

(β-Globin Glu6Val Mutation)
Autosomal Recessive

PRINCIPLES

- Heterozygote advantage
- Novel property mutation
- Genetic compound
- Ethnic variation in allele frequencies

MAJOR PHENOTYPIC FEATURES

- Age at onset: childhood
- Anemia
- Infarction
- Asplenia

HISTORY AND PHYSICAL FINDINGS

For the second time in 6 months, a Caribbean couple brought their 24-month-old daughter, C.W., to the emergency department because she refused to bear weight on her feet. There was no history of fever, infection, or trauma, and her medical history was otherwise unremarkable; findings from the previous visit were normal except for a low hemoglobin level and a mildly enlarged spleen. Findings from the physical examination were normal except for a palpable spleen tip and swollen feet. Her feet were tender to palpation, and she would not stand up. Both parents had siblings who died in childhood of infection and others who may have had sickle cell disease. In view of this history and the recurrent painful swelling of her feet, her physician tested C.W. for sickle cell disease by hemoglobin electrophoresis. This test result documented sickle cell hemoglobin, Hb S, in C.W.

BACKGROUND

Disease Etiology and Incidence

Sickle cell disease (MIM# 603903) is an autosomal recessive disorder of hemoglobin in which the β subunit genes have a missense mutation that substitutes valine for glutamic acid at amino acid 6. The disease is most commonly due to homozygosity for the sickle cell mutation, although compound heterozygosity for the sickle allele and a hemoglobin C or a β-thalassemia allele can also cause sickle cell disease (see Chapter 11). The prevalence of sickle cell disease varies widely among populations in proportion to past and present exposure to malaria (see Table). The sickle cell mutation appears to confer some resistance to malaria and thus a survival advantage to individuals heterozygous for the mutation.

Pathogenesis

Hemoglobin is composed of four subunits, two α subunits encoded by *HBA* on chromosome 16 and two β subunits encoded by the *HBB* gene on chromosome 11 (see Chapter 11). The Glu6Val mutation in β-globin decreases the solubility of deoxygenated hemoglobin and causes it to form a gelatinous network of stiff fibrous polymers that distort the red blood cell, giving it a sickle shape (see Fig. 11-5). These sickled erythrocytes occlude capillaries and cause infarctions. Initially, oxygenation causes the hemoglobin polymer to dissolve and the erythrocyte to regain its normal shape;

FREQUENCIES OF THE SICKLE CELL MUTATION AMONG CALIFORNIA NEWBORNS		
Ethnicity	Hb SS	Hb AS
African American	1/700	1/14
Asian Indian	0/1600	1/700
Hispanic	1/46,000	1/180
Middle Eastern	0/22,000	1/360
Native American	1/17,000	1/180
White	1/160,000	1/600
Asian	0/200,000	1/1300

repeated sickling and unsickling, however, produce irreversibly sickled cells that are removed from the circulation by the spleen. The rate of removal of erythrocytes from the circulation exceeds the production capacity of the marrow and causes a hemolytic anemia.

As discussed in Chapter 11, allelic heterogeneity is common in most mendelian disorders, particularly when the mutant alleles cause loss of function. Sickle cell disease is an important exception to the rule because one specific mutation is responsible for the unique novel properties of HbS. HbC is also less soluble than HbA, and also tends to crystallize in red cells, decreasing their deformability in capillaries and causing mild hemolysis, but HbC does not form the rod-shaped polymers of HbS. Not surprisingly, other novel property mutations, such as the mutations in *FGFR3* that cause achondroplasia, frequently show a similar lack of allelic heterogeneity when the phenotype depends on there being a specific, unique alteration in protein function.

Phenotype and Natural History

Patients with sickle cell disease generally present in the first two years of life with anemia, failure to thrive, splenomegaly, repeated infections, and dactylitis (the painful swelling of the hands or feet from the occlusion of the capillaries in small bones seen in patient C.W.; see Fig. C-37). Vasoocclusive infarctions occur in many tissues, causing strokes, acute chest syndrome, renal papillary necrosis, autosplenectomy, leg ulcers, priapism, bone aseptic necrosis, and visual loss. Bone vasoocclusion causes painful "crises," and if untreated, these painful episodes can persist for days or weeks. The functional asplenia, from infarction and other poorly understood factors, increases susceptibility to bacterial infections such as pneumococcal sepsis and *Salmonella* osteomyelitis. Infection is a major cause of death at all ages, although progressive renal failure and pulmonary failure are also common causes of death in the fourth and fifth decades. Patients also have a high risk for development of life-threatening aplastic anemia after parvovirus infection because parvovirus infection causes a temporary cessation of erythrocyte production.

Heterozygotes for the mutation (who are said to have sickle cell trait) do not have anemia and are usually clinically normal. Under conditions of severe hypoxia, however, such as ascent to high altitudes, erythrocytes of patients with sickle cell trait may sickle and cause symptoms similar to those observed with sickle cell disease.

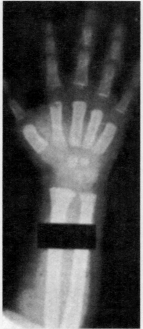
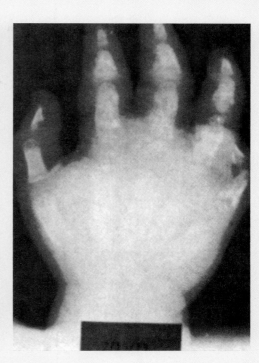

Figure C-37 ■ Acute dactylitis in a child with sickle cell disease. Radiographs of a child's hand during (*left*) and 2 weeks following (*right*) an attack of dactylitis. Note the development of destructive bony lesions. (From Nathan DG, Oski FA: Hematology of Infancy and Childhood. Philadelphia, WB Saunders Company, 1981.)

Management

In a given patient with sickle cell disease, there are no accurate predictors for the severity of the disease course. Although the molecular basis of the disease has been known longer than that of any other single-gene defect, current treatment is only supportive. No specific therapy that prevents or reverses the sickling process in vivo has been identified. Persistence of fetal hemoglobin greatly ameliorates disease severity. Several pharmacological interventions aimed at increasing fetal hemoglobin concentrations are under investigation (see Chapter 13), and hydroxyurea has been approved for this indication. Although gene therapy has the potential to ameliorate and cure this disease (see Chapter 13), effective β globin gene transfer has not been achieved. Allogeneic bone marrow transplantation is the only treatment currently available that can cure sickle cell disease.

Because of the 11% mortality from sepsis in the first 6 months of life, most states in the United States offer newborn screening for sickle cell disease to initiate antibiotic prophylaxis that is maintained through 5 years of age (see Chapter 17).

INHERITANCE RISK

Because sickle cell disease is an autosomal recessive disorder, future siblings of an affected child have a 25% risk of sickle cell disease and a 50% risk of sickle cell trait. With use of fetal DNA derived from chorionic villi or amniocytes, prenatal diagnosis is available by molecular analysis for the sickle cell mutation.

Questions for Small Group Discussion

1. What are the difficulties with gene therapy for this disorder?
2. Name two other diseases that may have become prevalent because of a heterozygote survival advantage. What is the rationale for hypothesizing a heterozygote advantage for those diseases?
3. Although it is always a severe disease, the severity of sickle cell disease is determined partially by the haplotype on which the mutation occurs. How could the haplotype affect disease severity?
4. Using the incidence figures in the Table, what is the risk that an unrelated African American woman and man will have a child affected with sickle cell disease? with sickle cell trait?

REFERENCES

Buchanan GR, DeBaun MR, Quinn CT, Steinberg MH: Hematology, the American Society of Hematology Education Program Book. Washington, DC, American Society of Hematology, 2004, pp 35-47.

GeneTests. Medical genetics information resource [database online]. University of Washington, Seattle, 1993-2006. Updated weekly. *http://www.genetests.org*

Morris CR, Singer ST, Walters MC: Clinical hemoglobinopathies: iron, lungs and new blood. Curr Opin Hematol 13:407-418, 2006.

OMIM: Online Mendelian Inheritance in Man. McKusick-Nathans Institute for Genetic Medicine, Johns Hopkins University, and National Center for Biotechnology Information, National Library of Medicine. *http://www.ncbi.nlm.nih.gov/entrez/query.fcgi?db=OMIM*

38. Tay-Sachs Disease

(*HEXA* Mutation)
Autosomal Recessive

PRINCIPLES

- Lysosomal storage disease
- Ethnic variation in allele frequencies
- Genetic drift
- Pseudodeficiency
- Population screening

MAJOR PHENOTYPIC FEATURES

- Age at onset: infancy through adulthood
- Neurodegeneration
- Retinal cherry-red spot
- Psychosis

HISTORY AND PHYSICAL FINDINGS

R.T. and S.T., an Ashkenazi Jewish couple, were referred to the genetics clinic for evaluation of their risk of having a child with Tay-Sachs disease. S.T. had a sister who died of Tay-Sachs disease as a child. R.T. had a paternal uncle living in a psychiatric home, but he did not know what disease his uncle had. Both R.T. and S.T. had declined screening for Tay-Sachs carrier status as teenagers. Enzymatic carrier testing showed that both R.T. and S.T. had extremely reduced hexosaminidase A activity. Subsequent molecular analysis for *HEXA* mutations predominant in Ashkenazi Jews confirmed that S.T. carried a disease-causing mutation, whereas R.T. had only a pseudodeficiency allele but no disease-causing mutation.

BACKGROUND

Disease Etiology and Incidence

Tay-Sachs disease (MIM# 272800), infantile GM_2 gangliosidosis, is a panethnic autosomal recessive disorder of ganglioside catabolism that is caused by a deficiency of hexosaminidase A (see Chapter 12). In addition to severe infantile-onset disease, hexosaminidase A deficiency causes milder disease with juvenile or adult onset.

The incidence of hexosaminidase A deficiency varies widely among different populations; the incidence of Tay-Sachs disease ranges from 1 in 3600 Ashkenazi Jewish births to 1 in 360,000 non–Ashkenazi Jewish North American births. French Canadians, Louisiana Cajuns, and Pennsylvania Amish have an incidence of Tay-Sachs comparable to that of Ashkenazi Jews. The increased carrier frequency in these four populations appears to be due to genetic drift, although heterozygote advantage cannot be excluded (see Chapter 9).

Pathogenesis

Gangliosides are ceramide oligosaccharides present in all cell surface membranes but most abundant in the brain. Gangliosides are concentrated in neuronal surface membranes, particularly in dendrites and axon termini. They function as receptors for various glycoprotein hormones and bacterial toxins and are involved in cell differentiation and cell-cell interaction.

Hexosaminidase A is a lysosomal enzyme composed of two subunits. The α subunit is encoded by the *HEXA* gene on chromosome 15, and the β subunit is encoded by the *HEXB* gene on chromosome 5. In the presence of activator protein, hexosaminidase A removes the terminal *N*-acetylgalactosamine from the ganglioside GM_2. Mutations of the α subunit or the activator protein cause the accumulation of GM_2 in the lysosome and thereby Tay-Sachs disease of the infantile, juvenile, or adult type. (Mutation of the β subunit causes Sandhoff disease [MIM# 268800].) The mechanism by which the accumulation of GM_2 ganglioside causes neuronal death has not been fully defined, although by analogy with Gaucher disease (see Chapter 13), toxic byproducts of GM_2 ganglioside may cause the neuropathology.

The level of residual hexosaminidase A activity correlates inversely with the severity of the disease. Patients with infantile-onset GM_2 gangliosidosis have two null alleles, that is, no hexosaminidase A enzymatic activity. Patients with juvenile- or adult-onset forms of GM_2 gangliosidosis are usually compound heterozygotes for a null *HEXA* allele and an allele with low residual hexosaminidase A activity.

Phenotype and Natural History

Infantile-onset GM_2 gangliosidosis is characterized by neurological deterioration beginning between the ages of 3 and 6 months and progressing to death by 2 to 4 years. Motor development usually plateaus or begins to regress by 8 to 10 months and progresses to loss of voluntary movement within the second year of life. Visual loss begins within the first year and progresses rapidly; it is almost uniformly associated with a "cherry-red spot" on funduscopic examination (Fig. C-38). Seizures usually begin near the end of the first year and progressively worsen. Further deterioration in the second year of life results in decerebrate posturing, swallowing difficulties, worse seizures, and finally an unresponsive, vegetative state.

Juvenile-onset GM_2 gangliosidosis manifests between 2 and 4 years and is characterized by neurological deterioration beginning with ataxia and incoordination. By the end of the first decade, most patients experience spasticity and seizures; by 10 to 15 years, most develop decerebrate rigidity and enter a vegetative state with death generally in the second decade. Loss of vision occurs, but there may not be a cherry-red spot; optic atrophy and retinitis pigmentosa often occur late in the disease course.

Adult-onset GM_2 gangliosidosis exhibits marked clinical variability (progressive dystonia, spinocerebellar degeneration, motor neuron disease, or psychiatric abnormalities). As many as 40% of patients have progressive psychiatric manifestations without dementia. Vision is rarely affected, and the ophthalmologic examination is generally normal.

Management

The diagnosis of a GM_2 gangliosidosis relies on the demonstration of both absent to nearly absent hexosaminidase A

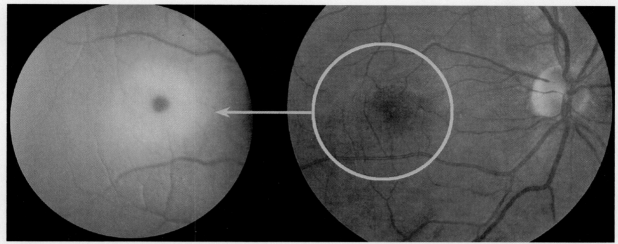

Figure C-38 ■ Cherry-red spot in Tay-Sachs disease. The right frame shows normal retina. The circle surrounds the macula, lateral to the optic nerve. The left frame shows the macula of a child with Tay-Sachs disease. The cherry-red center is the normal retina of the fovea at the center of the macula that is surrounded by macular retina made white by abnormal storage of GM_2 in retinal neurons. (Courtesy of A. V. Levin, The Hospital for Sick Children and University of Toronto, Canada.)

activity in the serum or white blood cells and normal to elevated activity of hexosaminidase B. Mutation analysis of the *HEXA* gene can also be used for diagnosis but is more typically only used to clarify carrier status and for prenatal testing.

Tay-Sachs disease is currently an incurable disorder; therefore, treatment focuses on the management of symptoms and palliative care. Nearly all patients require pharmacological management of their seizures. The psychiatric manifestations of patients with adult-onset GM_2 gangliosidosis are not usually responsive to conventional antipsychotic or antidepressant medications; lithium and electroconvulsive therapy are most effective.

INHERITANCE RISK

For potential parents without a family history of GM_2 gangliosidosis, the empirical risk for having a child affected with GM_2 gangliosidosis depends on the frequency of GM_2 gangliosidosis in their ethnic groups. For most North Americans, the empirical risk of being a carrier is approximately 1 in 250 to 1 in 300, whereas for Ashkenazi Jewish individuals, the empirical risk of being a carrier is approximately 1 in 30. For couples who are each carriers, the risk of having a child with GM_2 gangliosidosis is 1 in 4.

Prenatal diagnosis relies on identification of the *HEXA* mutations or hexosaminidase A deficiency in fetal tissue such as chorionic villi or amniocytes. Effective identification of affected fetuses by *HEXA* mutation analysis usually requires that the mutations responsible for GM_2 gangliosidosis in a family have already been identified.

Screening of high-risk populations for carriers and subsequent prevention has reduced the incidence of Tay-Sachs disease among Ashkenazi Jews by nearly 90% (see Chapters 12 and 17). Traditionally, such screening is performed by determining the serum activity of hexosaminidase A with an artificial substrate. This sensitive assay, however, cannot distinguish between pathological mutations and pseudodefi-

ciency (reduced catabolism of the artificial substrate but normal catabolism of the natural substrate); therefore, carrier status is usually confirmed by molecular analysis of *HEXA*. Two pseudodeficiency alleles and more than 70 pathological mutations have been identified in the *HEXA* gene. Among Ashkenazi Jews who are positive by enzymatic carrier screening, 2% are heterozygous for a pseudodeficiency allele and 95% to 98% are heterozygous for one of three pathological mutations, two causing infantile-onset and one causing adult-onset GM_2 gangliosidosis (see Chapter 12). In contrast, among non-Jewish North Americans who are positive by enzymatic carrier screening, 35% are heterozygous for a pseudodeficiency allele.

Questions for Small Group Discussion

1. Screening for what other diseases is complicated by "pseudodeficiency"?
2. Name two other diseases that exhibit genetic drift. What is genetic drift? What are causes of genetic drift?
3. Should population screening be instituted to identify carriers of other diseases?
4. What diseases are genocopies of adult-onset hexosaminidase A deficiency? Consider psychiatric disorders and adult-onset neuronal ceroid lipofuscinosis. What diseases are genocopies of infantile-onset hexosaminidase A deficiency? Consider GM_2 activator mutations. How would you distinguish between a genocopy and hexosaminidase A deficiency?

REFERENCES

GeneTests. Medical genetics information resource [database online]. University of Washington, Seattle, 1993-2006. Updated weekly. *http://www.genetests.org*

OMIM: Online Mendelian Inheritance in Man. McKusick-Nathans Institute for Genetic Medicine, Johns Hopkins University, and National Center for Biotechnology Information, National Library of Medicine. *http://www.ncbi.nlm.nih.gov/entrez/query.fcgi?db=OMIM*

Ross LF: Heterozygote carrier testing in high schools abroad: what are the lessons for the U.S.? J Law Med Ethics 34:753-764, 2006.

39. Thalassemia

(α- or β-Globin Deficiency)
Autosomal Recessive

PRINCIPLES

- Heterozygote advantage
- Ethnic variation in allele frequencies
- Gene dosage

MAJOR PHENOTYPIC FEATURES

- Age at onset: childhood
- Hypochromic microcytic anemia
- Hepatosplenomegaly
- Extramedullary hematopoiesis

HISTORY AND PHYSICAL FINDINGS

J.Z., a 25-year-old healthy Canadian woman, presented to her obstetrician for routine prenatal care. Results of her complete blood count showed a mild microcytic anemia (hemoglobin, 98 g/L; mean corpuscular volume, 75 μm³). She was of Vietnamese origin, and her spouse, T.Z., was of Greek origin. J.Z. was unaware of any blood disorders in her or T.Z.'s family. Nonetheless, hemoglobin (Hb) electrophoresis showed a mildly elevated Hb A_2 ($\alpha_2\delta_2$) and Hb F ($\alpha_2\gamma_2$), which suggested that J.Z. had β-thalassemia trait; molecular testing detected a nonsense mutation in one β-globin allele and no α-globin deletions. The results of T.Z.'s testing showed that he also had a nonsense mutation of one β-globin allele and no α-globin deletions. After referral to the genetics clinic, the geneticist explained to J.Z. and T.Z. that their risk for a child with β-thalassemia major was 25%. After discussing prenatal diagnosis, J.Z. and T.Z. chose to carry the pregnancy to term without further investigation.

BACKGROUND

Disease Etiology and Incidence

Thalassemias are autosomal recessive anemias caused by deficient synthesis of either α-globin or β-globin. A relative deficiency of α-globin causes α-thalassemia, and a relative deficiency of β-globin causes β-thalassemia (see Chapter 11).

Thalassemia is most common among persons of Mediterranean, African, Middle Eastern, Indian, Chinese, and Southeast Asian descent. Thalassemias appear to have evolved because they confer heterozygote advantage in providing some resistance to malaria (see Chapter 9); the prevalence of thalassemia in an ethnic group therefore reflects past and present exposure of a population to malaria. The prevalence of α-thalassemia trait ranges from less than 0.01% in natives from nonmalarial areas such as the United Kingdom, Iceland, and Japan to approximately 49% among natives of some Southwest Pacific islands; Hb H disease and hydrops fetalis (see Table) are restricted to the Mediterranean and Southeast Asia. The incidence of β-thalassemia trait ranges from approximately 1% to 2% among Africans and African Americans to 30% in some villages of Sardinia.

Pathogenesis

Thalassemia arises from inadequate hemoglobin production and unbalanced accumulation of globin subunits. Inadequate hemoglobin production causes hypochromia and microcytosis. Unbalanced accumulation of globin causes ineffective erythropoiesis and hemolytic anemia. The severity of thalassemia is proportionate to the severity of the imbalance between α-globin and β-globin production.

More than 200 different mutations have been associated with thalassemia, although only a few mutations account for most thalassemia cases. Deletion of α-globin genes accounts for 80% to 85% of α-thalassemia, and approximately 15 mutations account for more than 90% of β-thalassemia. Molecular studies of both α-globin and β-globin mutations strongly suggest that the various mutations have arisen independently in different populations and then achieved their high frequency by selection.

Phenotype and Natural History

The α-globin mutations are separated into four clinical groups that reflect the impairment of α-globin production (see Table).

The phenotypes observed in a population reflect the nature of the α-globin mutations in that population. Chromosomes with deletion of both α-globin genes are observed in

GENOTYPE-PHENOTYPE CORRELATION IN α-THALASSEMIA

Phenotype	No. of Functional Globin Genes	α-Globin/ β-Globin Ratio	α-Globin Genotypes	Hb H Inclusions	Complications
Normal	4	1	αα/αα	None	None
Silent carrier	3	0.8	–α/αα or – –/ααα	Rare	None
α-Thalassemia trait	2	0.6	–α/–α or – –/αα	Many	Mild anemia
Hb H disease	1	0.3	– –/–α	Many	Moderate anemia, jaundice, hepatosplenomegaly, gallstones, increased susceptibility to infection, folic acid deficiency
Hydrops fetalis	0	0.0	– –/– –	Present	Severe anemia, congestive heart failure, fatal in utero or shortly after birth

Southeast Asia and the Mediterranean basin; therefore, Hb H disease and hydrops fetalis usually occur in these populations and not in Africans, who usually have chromosomes with deletion of only one α-globin gene on a chromosome.

The β-globin mutations are also divided into clinical groups reflecting the impairment of β-globin production. β-Thalassemia trait is associated with a mutation in one β-globin allele and β-thalassemia major with mutations in both β-globin alleles. In general, patients with β-thalassemia trait have a mild hypochromic microcytic anemia, mild bone marrow erythroid hyperplasia, and occasionally hepatosplenomegaly; they are usually asymptomatic. Patients with β-thalassemia major present with severe hemolytic anemia when the postnatal production of Hb F decreases. The anemia and ineffective erythropoiesis cause growth retardation, jaundice, hepatosplenomegaly (extramedullary hematopoiesis), and bone marrow expansion (Fig. C-39). Approximately 80% of untreated patients die by 5 years. Patients receiving transfusion therapy alone die before 30 years of infection or hemochromatosis, while patients receiving both transfusion therapy and iron chelation therapy usually survive beyond the third decade. Iron overload from repeated transfusions and increased intestinal absorption causes cardiac, hepatic, and endocrine complications.

Management

Initial screening for α- or β-thalassemia trait is usually done by determination of erythrocyte indices. For patients without iron deficiency anemia, the diagnosis of β-thalassemia trait is usually confirmed by finding increased levels of Hb A_2 ($\alpha_2\delta_2$) and Hb F ($\alpha_2\gamma_2$) (which contain other β-like globin chains from the β-globin cluster), or DNA mutation analysis, or both. In contrast, α-thalassemia trait is not associated with Hb A_2 or Hb F and is confirmed by DNA mutation analysis or demonstration of a high β-globin/α-globin ratio.

Treatment of Hb H disease is primarily supportive. Therapy includes folate supplementation, avoidance of oxidant drugs and iron, prompt treatment of infection, and judicious transfusion. Splenectomy is rarely required.

Treatment of β-thalassemia includes blood transfusions, iron chelation, prompt treatment of infection, and, frequently, splenectomy. Bone marrow transplantation is the only currently available cure. Clinical trials are currently under way for drugs that will increase the expression of fetal hemoglobin, which would ameliorate β-thalassemia (but not α-thalassemia) (see Chapter 13).

INHERITANCE RISK

If each parent has β-thalassemia trait, the couple has a 25% risk of having a child with β-thalassemia major and a 50% risk of having a child with β-thalassemia trait. If one parent has β-thalassemia trait and the other parent a triplication of the α-globin gene, this couple could also have a 25% risk of having a child with β-thalassemia major.

For parents with α-thalassemia trait, their risk for a child with Hb H disease or hydrops fetalis depends on the nature of their α-globin mutations. Parents with α-thalassemia trait can have either the −α/−α or −−/αα genotype; therefore, depending on their genotypes, all their children will have α-thalassemia trait (−α/−α), or they may have a 25% risk of having a child with Hb H disease (−α/−−) or hydrops fetalis (−−/−−).

For both α- and β-thalassemia, prenatal diagnosis is possible by molecular analysis of fetal DNA from either chorionic villi or amniocytes. Molecular prenatal diagnosis of thalassemia is most efficient if the mutations have already been identified in the carrier parents.

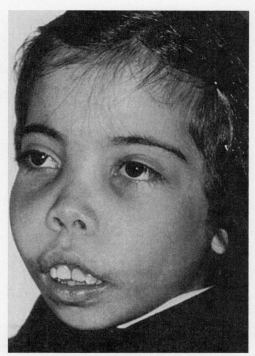

Figure C-39 ■ The typical facial appearance of a child with untreated β-thalassemia. Note the prominent cheekbones and the protrusion of the upper jaw that results from the expansion of the marrow cavity in the bones of the skull and face. (Courtesy of N. Olivieri, The Hospital for Sick Children and University of Toronto, Canada.)

Questions for Small Group Discussion

1. A father has the genotype ααα/α−, β/β and a mother αα/αα, β/−. If their child has the genotype α−/αα, β/−, what is the most likely phenotype? Why? If the child's genotype is ααα/αα, β/−, what is the most likely phenotype? Why?
2. What are the molecular mechanisms of α-globin gene deletion? of α-globin gene triplication?
3. How does expression of γ-globin protect against β-thalassemia?
4. Describe carrier screening for thalassemia. To what ethnic groups should carrier screening be applied? Should individuals from classically low-risk ethnic groups be screened if their partner has α- or β-thalassemia trait? Consider population admixture.
5. α-Thalassemia is the most common single-gene disorder in the world. Three mechanisms can increase the frequency of a mutation in a population: selection, genetic drift, and founder effects. Describe each mechanism and the reason that selection is likely to account for the high frequency of α-thalassemia.

REFERENCES

GeneTests. Medical genetics information resource [database online]. University of Washington, Seattle, 1993-2006. Updated weekly. http://www.genetests.org

OMIM: Online Mendelian Inheritance in Man. McKusick-Nathans Institute for Genetic Medicine, Johns Hopkins University, and National Center for Biotechnology Information, National Library of Medicine. http://www.ncbi.nlm.nih.gov/entrez/query.fcgi?db=OMIM

Orkin S, Nathan D: The thalassemias. In Nathan DG, Orkin SH, Ginsburg D, Look AT (eds): Nathan and Oski's Hematology of Infancy and Childhood, 6th ed. Philadelphia, WB Saunders, 2003.

Quek L, Thein SL: Molecular therapies in beta-thalassaemia. Br J Haematol 136:353-365, 2007.

40. Thiopurine S-Methyltransferase Deficiency

(*TPMT* Polymorphisms)
Autosomal Semidominant

PRINCIPLES

- Pharmacogenetics
- Personalized medicine
- Cancer and immunosuppression chemotherapy
- Ethnic variation

MAJOR PHENOTYPIC FEATURES

- Age at onset: deficiency is present at birth, manifestation requires drug exposure
- Myelosuppression
- Increased risk of brain tumor in TPMT-deficient patients with acute lymphoblastic leukemia receiving brain irradiation

HISTORY AND PHYSICAL FINDINGS

J.B. is a 19-year-old male with ulcerative colitis of long standing. Because he has been refractory to steroid treatment, his physician prescribed azathioprine at a standard dose of 2.5 mg/kg/day. After a few weeks, J.B. developed severe leukopenia. The physician measured TPMT activity in the red cells and found it to be normal. The physician remembered that J.B. had received a red blood cell transfusion 3 weeks previously and decided to determine his *TPMT* genotype. J.B. was found to be a compound heterozygote for the *TPMT*2 and -*3A* alleles. Consequently, he should have been started and maintained on 6%–10% of the standard dose of azathioprine.

BACKGROUND

Disease Etiology and Incidence

Thiopurine methyltransferase (TPMT) is the enzyme responsible for phase II metabolism of 6-mercaptopurine (6-MP) and 6-thioguanine by catalyzing S-methylation and thus inactivating these compounds (see Chapter 18). Azathioprine, a commonly used immunosuppressant, is activated by conversion to 6-mercaptopurine, and so its metabolism is also affected by TPMT activity. These agents are used as immunosuppressants for various systemic inflammatory diseases, such as inflammatory bowel disease and lupus, and to prevent the rejection of solid tumor transplants. 6-MP is a component in standard treatment of acute lymphoblastic leukemia. About 10% of whites carry at least one slow-metabolizer variant that causes accumulation of high levels of toxic metabolites, which can cause fatal hematopoietic toxicity (Fig. C-40). One in 300 whites is homozygous for an allele that causes complete deficiency of TPMT activity. Deficiency is much less common in other ethnic groups.

Phenotype and Natural History

Toxicity from thiopurines was first recognized in patients receiving 6-MP for acute lymphoblastic leukemia. Although patients with 6-MP toxicity had a risk of life-threatening leukopenia, those who survived were noted to have longer periods of leukemia-free survival. Among TPMT-deficient patients with acute lymphoblastic leukemia, there was an increased risk of radiation-induced brain tumors and of chemotherapy-induced acute myelogenous leukemia. Fifteen different mutations in the *TPMT* gene have been associated with decreased activity in red cell assay. The wild-type allele is *TPMT*1. *TPMT*2 is a missense mutation that results in an alanine to proline substitution at codon 80 (Ala80Pro). This rare allele is seen only in whites. The *TPMT*3C allele is a tyrosine to cysteine substitution at codon 240. It is seen in 14.8% of Ghanaians, 2% of Chinese, Koreans, and Japanese. It is rarely present in whites, whose predominant deficiency allele is the *TPMT*3A allele, representing 75% of their deficiency alleles. The *TPMT*3A allele has two mutations in cis, the Tyr240Cys mutation and an alanine to threonine substitution at codon 154 (Ala154Thr). The Ala154Thr mutation has not been seen in isolation and presumably occurred on a chromosome that already carried the Tyr240Cys allele after the European migration.

Testing for the *TPMT* mutations by polymerase chain reaction is inexpensive and accurate and can prevent toxicity by allowing dose adjustment before starting therapy. TPMT testing is the standard of care for acute lymphoblastic leukemia and has a favorable cost-benefit analysis for inflammatory bowel disease. Because TPMT activity is measured in red cells, false negatives are common in patients receiving transfusions as long as 3 months earlier. Direct genotyping of a DNA sample avoids this problem.

Management

Patients with complete TPMT deficiency should receive 6% to 10% of the standard dose of thiopurine medications. Heterozygous patients may start at the full dose but should have a dose reduction to half within 6 months or as soon as any myelosuppression is observed. The example of *TPMT* polymorphism is an instructive example of the clinical importance of pharmacogenetics in personalized medicine (see Chapters 17 and 18).

INHERITANCE RISK

The prior risk of a white individual carrying a *TPMT* deficiency allele is about 10%. In other ethnic groups, it is 2% to 5%. Because this is a simple semidominant trait, siblings of heterozygous individuals have a 50% chance of being heterozygous. Siblings of a deficient individual have a 25% chance of being deficient and a 50% chance of being heterozygous.

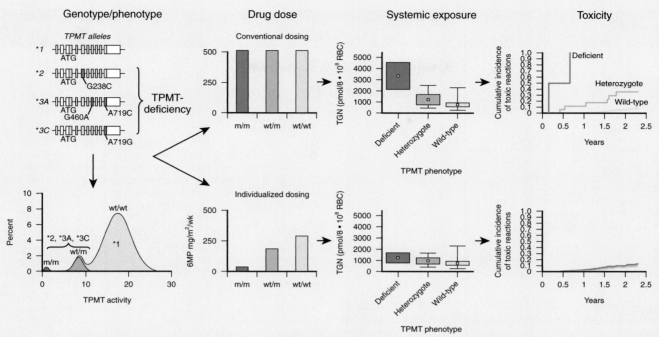

Figure C-40 ■ Genetic polymorphism of thiopurine S-methyltransferase (TPMT) and its role in determining response to thiopurine medications (azathioprine, mercaptopurine, and thioguanine). The left panels depict the predominant *TPMT* mutant alleles causing autosomal semidominant inheritance of TPMT activity in humans. As depicted in the adjacent top three panels, when uniform (conventional) dosages of thiopurine medications are given to all patients, TPMT homozygous mutant patients accumulate 10-fold higher cellular concentrations of the active thioguanine nucleotides (TGN); heterozygous patients accumulate about 2-fold higher TGN concentrations. These differences translate into a significantly higher frequency of toxicity (far right panels). As depicted in the bottom three panels, when genotype-specific dosing is used, similar cellular TGN concentrations are achieved, and all three TPMT phenotypes can be treated without acute toxicity. (Colored bars depict mercaptopurine [6MP] doses that were tolerated in patients who presented with hematopoietic toxicity.) (From Eichelbaum M, et al: Annu Rev Med 57:119-137, 2006.)

Questions for Small Group Discussion

1. *VKORC1* polymorphisms account for significant variation in warfarin metabolism. Name several conditions in which warfarin therapy is commonly used.
2. The P450 enzymes encoded by the *CYP* genes are important to drug metabolism. Which *CYP* genes metabolize selective serotonin reuptake inhibitors? Does this result in toxicity or decreased effect?
3. Why do humans have genes for drug metabolism?
4. Suggest reasons for ethnic variation in these genes.

REFERENCES

OMIM: Online Mendelian Inheritance in Man. McKusick-Nathans Institute for Genetic Medicine, Johns Hopkins University, and National Center for Biotechnology Information, National Library of Medicine. *http://www. ncbi.nlm.nih.gov/entrez/query.fcgi?db=OMIM*

Eichelbaum M, Ingelman-Sundberg M, Evans WE: Pharmacogenomics and individualized drug therapy. Annu Rev Med 57:119-137, 2006.

Pui C-H, Relling MV, Downing JR: Acute lymphoblastic leukemia. N Engl J Med 350:1535-1548, 2004.

41. Thrombophilia

(FV and PROC Mutations)
Autosomal Dominant

PRINCIPLES

- Gain-of-function mutation (Factor V Leiden)
- Loss-of-function mutation (Protein C mutations)
- Incomplete penetrance
- Genetic modifiers
- Environmental modifiers
- Heterozygote advantage
- Founder effect

MAJOR PHENOTYPIC FEATURES

- Age at onset: adulthood
- Deep venous thrombosis

HISTORY AND PHYSICAL FINDINGS

J.J., a 45-year-old businessman of French and Swedish descent, suddenly developed shortness of breath on the day after a trans–Pacific Ocean flight. His right leg was swollen and warm. Subsequent studies identified a thrombus in the popliteal and iliac veins and a pulmonary embolus. Both of his parents had had leg venous thromboses, and his sister had died of a pulmonary embolus during pregnancy. Based on his age and family history, J.J. was believed to have inherited a predisposition to thrombophilia. Screening for inherited causes of thrombophilia identified that J.J. was a carrier of factor V Leiden. Subsequent studies of other family members identified the same heterozygous mutation in J.J.'s father, deceased sister, and unaffected older brother. J.J. and his mother, deceased sister, and unaffected older sister were all found to be heterozygous for a frameshift mutation (3363insC) in PROC, the gene encoding protein C. Thus, J.J. is a double heterozygote for two variants, in two unlinked genes, that predispose to thrombosis.

BACKGROUND

Disease Etiology and Incidence

Venous thrombosis (MIM# 188050) is a panethnic multifactorial disorder (see Chapter 8); its incidence increases with age and varies among races. The incidence is low among Asians and Africans and higher among whites. Major predisposing influences are stasis, endothelial damage, and hypercoagulability. Identifiable genetic factors, present in 25% of unselected patients, include defects in coagulation factor inhibition and impaired clot lysis. Factor V Leiden occurs in 12% to 14%, prothrombin mutations in 6% to 18%, and deficiency of antithrombin III or protein C or S in 5% to 15% of patients with venous thromboses.

Factor V Leiden, an Arg506Gln mutation in the FV gene, has a prevalence of 2% to 15% among healthy European populations; it is highest in Swedes and Greeks and rare in Asians and Africans. Factor V Leiden apparently arose from a mutation in a white founder after the divergence from Africans and Asians.

Protein C deficiency is a panethnic disorder with a prevalence of 0.2% to 0.4%. Mutations of PROC are usually associated with activity levels of less than 55% of normal.

Pathogenesis

The coagulation system maintains a delicate balance of clot formation and inhibition; however, venous thrombi arise if coagulation overwhelms the anticoagulant and fibrinolytic systems. The proteases and protein cofactors of the clotting cascade must be activated at the site of injury to form a fibrin clot and then be inactivated to prevent disseminated coagulation (see Fig. 8-5). Activated factor V, a cofactor of activated factor X, accelerates the conversion of prothrombin to thrombin. Factor V is inactivated by activated protein C, which cleaves activated factor V at three sites (Arg306, Arg506, and Arg679). Cleavage at Arg506 occurs first and accelerates cleavage at the other two sites; cleavage at Arg506 reduces activated factor V function, whereas cleavage at Arg306 abolishes its function. Protein S, a cofactor for protein C, both accelerates the inactivation of activated factor V by protein C and enhances cleavage at Arg306.

The factor V Leiden mutation removes the preferred site for protein C proteolysis of activated factor V, thereby slowing inactivation of activated factor V and predisposing patients to thrombophilia. The risk of thrombophilia is higher for patients homozygous for factor V Leiden; the lifetime risks of venous thrombosis for factor V Leiden heterozygosity and homozygosity are approximately 10% and 80%, respectively.

Inherited deficiency of protein C arises from mutations in the PROC coding and regulatory sequences. Many mutations are sporadic, although some, such as the French-Canadian mutation 3363insC, entered populations through a founder. Unlike the gain-of-function factor V Leiden mutation, PROC mutations impair protein C function, thereby slowing inactivation of activated clotting factors V and VIII and predisposing to thrombus formation. Inheritance of two mutant PROC alleles usually results in purpura fulminans, a form of disseminated intravascular coagulation that is often fatal if it is not treated promptly. Heterozygous protein C mutations predispose to thrombophilia and carry a 20% to 75% lifetime risk of venous thrombosis.

In general, for patients heterozygous for the factor V Leiden polymorphism or a PROC mutation, progression from a hypercoagulable state to venous thrombi requires coexisting genetic or environmental factors. Associated nongenetic factors include pregnancy, oral contraceptive use, surgery, advanced age, neoplasia, immobility, and cardiac disease. Associated genetic abnormalities include other disorders of coagulation factor inhibition and impaired clot lysis.

Phenotype and Natural History

Although thrombi can develop in any vein, most arise at sites of injury or in the large venous sinuses or valve cusp pockets of the legs. Leg thrombi are usually confined to the veins of the calf, but approximately 20% extend into more proximal vessels. Obstruction of the deep leg veins can cause swelling, warmth, erythema, tenderness, distention of superficial veins, and prominent venous collaterals, although many patients are asymptomatic (Fig. C-41).

Once formed, a venous thrombus can propagate along the vein and eventually obstruct other veins, give rise to an embolus, be removed by fibrinolysis, or be organized and possibly recanalized. Embolism is serious and can be acutely fatal if it obstructs the pulmonary arterial system; pulmonary embolism occurs in 5% to 20% of patients presenting initially with deep calf vein thrombosis. In contrast, organization of proximal vein thrombi chronically impedes venous return and causes post-thrombotic syndrome, characterized by leg pain, edema, and frequent skin ulceration.

With the possible exception of an increased risk of recurrence, the symptoms, course, and outcomes of patients with *PROC* mutations and factor V Leiden are similar to those of other thrombophilia patients. In general, untreated patients with proximal vein thrombosis have a 40% risk of recurrent venous thrombosis.

Management

The diagnosis of deep venous thrombosis of the calf is difficult because patients are often asymptomatic and most tests are relatively insensitive until the thrombus extends proximal to the deep calf veins. Duplex venous ultrasonography is used most often to diagnose deep venous thrombosis; the thrombus is detected either by direct visualization or by inference when the vein does not collapse on compressive maneuvers. Doppler ultrasound detects flow abnormalities in the veins.

Factor V Leiden can be diagnosed directly by DNA analysis or can be suspected on the basis of activated protein C resistance. Protein C deficiency is diagnosed by measuring protein C activity; *PROC* mutations are identified by analysis of the *PROC* gene.

Acute treatment focuses on minimizing thrombus propagation and associated complications, especially pulmonary embolism; it usually involves anticoagulation and elevation of the affected extremity. Subsequent therapy focuses on prevention of recurrent venous thrombosis through identification and amelioration of predispositions, and anticoagulant prophylaxis. Treatment recommendations for patients with protein C deficiency and factor V Leiden are still evolving. All patients should receive standard initial therapy followed by at least 3 months of anticoagulant therapy. It is unclear which patients with a single mutant allele should receive prolonged, perhaps lifelong anticoagulation, but long-term anticoagulation is generally reserved for patients with a second episode of deep venous thrombosis. In contrast, homozygous factor V Leiden patients as well as those who are homozygous for other mutations or are combined carriers (like J.J.) are placed on long-term anticoagulation after their initial episode.

INHERITANCE RISK

Each child of a couple in which one parent is heterozygous for factor V Leiden has a 50% risk of inheriting a mutant allele. Assuming 10% penetrance, each child has a 5% lifetime risk for development of a venous thrombosis.

Each child of a couple in which one parent is heterozygous for a *PROC* mutation also has a 50% risk of inheriting a mutant allele. Estimates for penetrance of protein C deficiency range from 20% to 75%; therefore, each child has a 10% to 38% lifetime risk for development of a venous thrombosis.

Because of the incomplete penetrance and availability of effective therapy for factor V Leiden and heterozygous *PROC* mutations, prenatal diagnostic testing is not routinely used except for detection of homozygous or compound heterozygous *PROC* mutations. Prenatal detection of homozygous or compound heterozygous *PROC* mutations is helpful because of the severity of the disease and the need for prompt neonatal treatment.

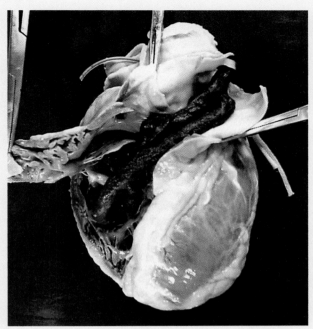

Figure C-41 ■ Autopsy picture of the cardiac right ventricle from a 58-year-old man who had had a cervical laminectomy and decompression. He complained of right calf pain 33 days after surgery, and Homans sign was present. Venous ultrasonography detected a thrombus extending from the post-tibial and popliteal veins into the femoral vein. Despite anticoagulation with heparin, the patient was found 2 days later unresponsive and with a low oxygen saturation; he did not respond to cardiopulmonary resuscitation and died. Autopsy showed a thromboembolus in the right ventricle occluding the pulmonary artery. (Courtesy of H. Meyerson and Robert Hoffman, Department of Pathology, Case Western Reserve University, Cleveland.)

Questions for Small Group Discussion

1. Some studies of oral contraceptives suggest that such drugs decrease the blood levels of protein S. How would this predispose to thrombosis? At a molecular level, why would this be expected to enhance the development of venous thromboses in women with the factor V Leiden mutation? Should such women avoid the use of oral contraceptives? Should women be tested for factor V Leiden before using oral contraceptives?
2. Testing of asymptomatic relatives for the factor V Leiden mutation is controversial. For it to be of clear utility, what should presymptomatic testing allow?
3. Synergism is the multiplication of risk with the co-occurrence of risk factors. Illustrate this with factor V Leiden and protein C deficiency (the family of J.J. is an example), factor V Leiden and oral contraceptive use, and factor V Leiden and hyperhomocystinemia.
4. Factor V Leiden is thought to reduce intrapartum bleeding. How would this lead to a heterozygote advantage and maintenance of a high allele frequency in the population?

REFERENCES

GeneTests. Medical genetics information resource [database online]. University of Washington, Seattle, 1993-2006. Updated weekly. *http://www.genetests.org*

Kyrle PA, Eichinger S: Deep vein thrombosis. Lancet 365:1163-1174, 2005.

OMIM: Online Mendelian Inheritance in Man. McKusick-Nathans Institute for Genetic Medicine, Johns Hopkins University, and National Center for Biotechnology Information, National Library of Medicine. *http://www.ncbi.nlm.nih.gov/entrez/query.fcgi?db=OMIM*

42. Turner Syndrome

(Female Monosomy X)
Chromosomal

PRINCIPLES

- Nondisjunction
- Prenatal selection
- Haploinsufficiency

MAJOR PHENOTYPIC FEATURES

- Age at onset: prenatal
- Short stature
- Ovarian dysgenesis
- Sexual immaturity

HISTORY AND PHYSICAL FINDINGS

L.W., a 14-year-old girl, was referred to the endocrinology clinic for evaluation of absent secondary sexual characteristics (menses and breast development). Although born small for gestational age, she had been in good health and had normal intellect. No other family members had similar problems. Her examination was normal except for short stature, Tanner stage I sexual development, and broad chest with widely spaced nipples. After briefly discussing causes of short stature and delayed or absent sexual development, her physician requested follicle-stimulating hormone (FSH) level, growth hormone (GH) level, bone age study, and chromosome analysis. These tests showed a normal GH level, an elevated FSH level, and an abnormal karyotype (45,X). The physician explained that L.W. had Turner syndrome. L.W. was treated with growth hormone supplements to maximize her linear growth; a year later, she started estrogen and progesterone therapy to induce the development of secondary sexual characteristics.

BACKGROUND

Disease Etiology and Incidence

Turner syndrome (TS) is a panethnic disorder caused by complete or partial absence of a second X chromosome in females. It has an incidence of between 1 in 2000 and 1 in 5000 liveborn girls. About 50% of TS cases are associated with a 45,X karyotype, 25% with a structural abnormality of the second X chromosome, and 25% with 45,X mosaicism (see Chapter 6).

Monosomy for the X chromosome can arise either by the failure to transmit a sex chromosome to one of the gametes or by loss of a sex chromosome from the zygote or early embryo. Failure to transmit a paternal sex chromosome to a gamete is the most common cause of a 45,X karyotype; 70% to 80% of patients with a 45,X karyotype are conceived from a sperm lacking a sex chromosome. Loss of a sex chromosome from a cell in the early embryo is the likely cause of 45,X mosaicism.

Pathogenesis

The mechanism by which X chromosome monosomy causes TS in girls is poorly understood. The X chromosome contains many loci that do not undergo X chromosome inactivation (see Chapter 6), several of which appear to be necessary for ovarian maintenance and female fertility. Although oocyte development requires only a single X chromosome, oocyte maintenance requires two X chromosomes. In the absence of a second X chromosome, therefore, oocytes in fetuses and neonates with TS degenerate, and their ovaries atrophy into streaks of fibrous tissue. The genetic bases for the other features of TS, such as the cystic hygroma, lymphedema, broad chest, cardiac anomalies, renal anomalies, and sensorineural hearing deficit, have not been defined but presumably reflect haploinsufficiency for one or more X-linked genes that do not normally undergo inactivation in the female.

Phenotype and Natural History

Although 45,X conceptuses account for between 1% and 2% of all pregnancies, less than 1% of 45,X conceptions result in a liveborn infant. In view of the mild phenotype observed in patients with TS, this high rate of miscarriage is remarkable and suggests that a second sex chromosome is generally required for intrauterine survival.

All patients with TS have short stature, and more than 90% have ovarian dysgenesis. The ovarian dysgenesis is sufficiently severe that only 10% to 20% of patients have spontaneous pubertal development (breast budding and pubic hair growth) and only 2% to 5% have spontaneous menses. Many individuals also have physical anomalies, such as webbed neck, low nuchal hairline, broad chest, cardiac anomalies, renal anomalies, sensorineural hearing deficit, edema of the hands and feet, and dysplastic nails. Nearly 50% of patients have a bicuspid aortic valve and therefore an increased risk of aortic root dilatation and dissection; nearly 60% have renal anomalies and an increased risk of renal dysfunction.

Most patients have normal intellectual development. Those with intellectual impairment usually have an X chromosome structural abnormality. Socially, individuals with TS tend to be shy and withdrawn (see Chapter 6).

In addition to the complications resulting from their congenital anomalies, women with TS have an increased incidence of osteoporotic fractures, thyroiditis, diabetes mellitus type 1 and type 2, inflammatory bowel disease, and cardiovascular disease. The causes of the diabetes mellitus, thyroid disorders, and inflammatory bowel disease are unclear. Estrogen deficiency is probably largely responsible for the osteoporosis and the increased incidence of atherosclerosis, ischemic heart disease, and stroke, although diabetes mellitus probably accentuates the cardiovascular effects of estrogen deficiency.

Management

When a TS patient's stature falls below the fifth percentile, she is usually treated with GH supplements until her bone age reaches 15 years (Fig. C-42). On average, this treatment results in a gain of 10 cm in predicted height; the improvement in final height is less, however, the later GH therapy is started. Concurrent estrogen therapy decreases the effectiveness of GH.

Estrogen therapy is usually initiated at about 14 to 15 years of age to promote development of secondary sexual characteristics and reduce the risk of osteoporosis. Progesterone therapy is added to the regimen to induce menses either at the time of the first vaginal breakthrough bleeding or in the second year of estrogen therapy.

In addition, medical management usually includes echocardiography to evaluate aortic root dilatation and valvular heart disease, renal ultrasonography to find congenital renal anomalies, and a glucose tolerance test to detect diabetes.

Patients who have complete ovarian dysgenesis do not ovulate spontaneously or conceive children. If they have adequate cardiovascular and renal function, however, women with TS can have children by in vitro fertilization and ovum donation.

INHERITANCE RISK

TS is not associated with advanced maternal or paternal age. Although there have been a few familial recurrences, TS is usually sporadic, and the empirical recurrence risk for future pregnancies is not increased above that of the general population. If TS is suspected on the basis of fetal ultrasound findings, such as a cystic hygroma, the diagnosis should be confirmed by karyotyping of chorionic villi or amniocytes.

Only a few pregnancies have been reported among spontaneously menstruating patients with TS. Among the resulting offspring, one in three has had congenital anomalies, such as congenital heart disease, Down syndrome, and spina bifida. The apparently increased risk of congenital anomalies may be due to ascertainment bias in reporting, since pregnancy is unusual in TS. If the increased risk is a real finding, the cause is unknown.

Questions for Small Group Discussion

1. Some observations have suggested that patients with Turner syndrome who inherit a paternal X chromosome are more outgoing and have better social adaptation than those who inherit a maternal X chromosome. What molecular mechanisms could explain this?
2. X-chromosome monosomy is the only viable human monosomy. Discuss possible reasons.
3. Discuss possible reasons for the high rate of birth defects among the children of women with Turner syndrome.
4. Maternal meiotic nondisjunction gives rise more frequently to Down syndrome and paternal meiotic nondisjunction to Turner syndrome. Discuss possible reasons.
5. Discuss the psychosocial support and counseling that are appropriate and necessary for patients with Turner syndrome.

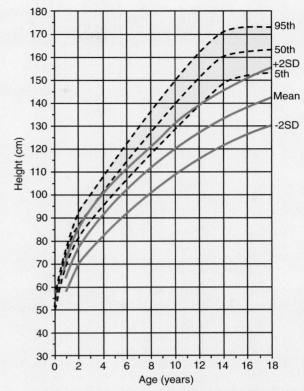

Figure C-42 ■ Growth curves for normal *(shaded dotted lines)* and approximately 350 Turner syndrome girls *(solid lines)*. None of the subjects received hormone treatment. (Modified from Lyon AJ, Preece MA, Grant DB: Growth curve for girls with Turner syndrome. Arch Dis Child 60:932, 1985, by permission.)

REFERENCES

Sybert VP, McCauley E: Turner's syndrome. N Engl J Med 351:1227-1238, 2004.

Saenger P: Turner's syndrome. N Engl J Med 335:1749-1754, 1996.

Zinn AR, Ross JL: Turner syndrome and haploinsufficiency. Curr Opin Genet Dev 8:322-327, 1998.

43. Xeroderma Pigmentosum

(Defect of Nucleotide Excision Repair)
Autosomal Recessive

PRINCIPLES

- Variable expressivity
- Genetic heterogeneity
- Genetic complementation
- Caretaker tumor-suppressor genes

MAJOR PHENOTYPIC FEATURES

- Age at onset: childhood
- Ultraviolet light sensitivity
- Skin cancer
- Neurological dysfunction

HISTORY AND PHYSICAL FINDINGS

W.S., a 3-year-old boy, was referred to the dermatology clinic for evaluation of severe sun sensitivity and freckling. On physical examination, he was photophobic and had conjunctivitis and prominent freckled hyperpigmentation in sun-exposed areas; his development and physical examination were otherwise normal. W.S. was the child of nonconsanguineous Japanese parents; no one else in the family was similarly affected. The dermatologist explained that W.S. had classic features of xeroderma pigmentosum, that is, "parchment-like pigmented skin". To confirm the diagnosis, W.S. had a skin biopsy to evaluate DNA repair and ultraviolet (UV) radiation sensitivity in his skin fibroblasts. The results of this testing confirmed the diagnosis of xeroderma pigmentosum. Despite appropriate preventive measures, W.S. developed metastatic melanoma at 15 years of age and died 2 years later. His parents had two other children; neither was affected with xeroderma pigmentosum.

BACKGROUND

Disease Etiology and Incidence
Xeroderma pigmentosum (XP) is a genetically heterogeneous, panethnic, autosomal recessive disorder of DNA repair that causes marked sensitivity to UV irradiation (see Table). In the United States and Europe, the prevalence is approximately 1 in 1 million, but in Japan, the prevalence is 1 in 100,000.

Pathogenesis
Repair of DNA damaged by UV irradiation occurs by three mechanisms: excision repair, postreplication repair, and photoreactivation. Excision repair mends DNA damage by nucleotide excision repair or base excision repair. Postreplication repair is a damage tolerance mechanism that allows replication of DNA across a damaged template. Photoreactivation reverts damaged DNA to the normal chemical state without removing or exchanging any genetic material.

Nucleotide excision repair is a complex but versatile process involving at least 30 proteins. The basic principle is the removal of a small single-stranded DNA segment containing a lesion by incision to either side of the damaged segment and subsequent gap-filling repair synthesis with use of the intact complementary strand as a template. Within transcribed genes, DNA damage blocks RNA polymerase II

progression. The stalled RNA polymerase II initiates nucleotide excision repair (transcription-coupled repair). In the rest of the genome and on nontranscribed strands of genes, a nucleotide excision repair complex identifies DNA damage by detection of helical distortions within the DNA (global genome repair).

On occasion, nucleotide excision repair will not have repaired a lesion before DNA replication. Because such lesions inhibit the progression of DNA replication, postreplication repair bypasses the lesion, allowing DNA synthesis to continue. DNA polymerase η mediates translesional DNA synthesis; it efficiently and accurately catalyzes synthesis past dithymidine lesions.

XP is caused by mutations affecting the global genome repair subpathway of nucleotide excision repair or by mutations affecting postreplication repair. In contrast, Cockayne syndrome, a related disorder, is caused by mutations affecting the transcription-coupled repair subpathway of nucleotide excision repair. XP and Cockayne syndrome have been separated into 10 biochemical complementation groups; each group reflects a mutation of a different component of nucleotide excision repair or postreplication repair (see Table).

The reduced or absent capacity for global genome repair or postreplication repair represents a loss of caretaker functions required for maintenance of genome integrity and results in the accumulation of oncogenic mutations (see Chapter 16). Cutaneous neoplasms from patients with XP have a higher level of oncogene and tumor-suppressor gene mutations than have tumors from the normal population, and those mutations appear to be highly UV specific.

Phenotype and Natural History
Patients with XP develop symptoms at a median age of 1 to 2 years, although onset after 14 years is seen in approximately 5% of patients. Initial symptoms commonly include easy sunburning, acute photosensitivity, freckling, and photophobia. Continued cutaneous damage causes premature skin aging (thinning, wrinkling, solar lentigines, telangiectasias), premalignant actinic keratoses, and benign and malignant neoplasms (Fig. C-43). Nearly 45% of patients develop basal cell or squamous cell carcinomas, or both, and approximately 5% develop melanomas. Approximately 90% of the carcinomas occur at the sites of greatest UV exposure—the face, neck, head, and tip of the tongue. Before the introduction of preventive measures, the median age for development of cutaneous neoplasms was 8 years, 50 years younger than in the general population, and the frequency of such neoplasms was more than 1000-fold greater than that of the general population.

In addition to cutaneous signs, 60% to 90% of patients experience ocular abnormalities including photophobia, conjunctivitis, blepharitis, ectropion, and neoplasia. Again, the distribution of ocular damage and neoplasms corresponds to the sites of greatest UV exposure.

Approximately 18% of patients experience progressive neuronal degeneration. Features include sensorineural deafness, mental retardation, spasticity, hyperreflexia or areflexia, segmental demyelination, ataxia, choreoathetosis, and supranuclear ophthalmoplegia. The severity of neurological

COMPLEMENTATION GROUPS IN XP AND RELATED DISORDERS

Complementation Group	MIM#	Gene	Process Affected	Phenotype
XPA	278700	XPA	DNA damage recognition	XP
XPB	133510	ERCC3	DNA unwinding	XP-CS, TTD
XPC	2788720	XPC	DNA damage recognition	XP
XPD	278730	ERCC2	DNA unwinding	XP, TTD, XP-CS
XPE	278740	DDB2	DNA damage recognition	XP
XPF	278760	ERCC4	Endonuclease	XP
XPG	278780	ERCC5	Endonuclease	XP, XP-CS
XPV	278750	POLH	Translesional DNA synthesis	XP
CSA	216400	ERCC8	Transcription-coupled repair	CS
CSB	133540	ERCC6	Transcription-coupled repair	CS

CS, Cockayne syndrome; TTD, trichothiodystrophy; XP-CS, combined XP and Cockayne syndrome phenotype.

symptoms is usually proportionate to the severity of the nucleotide excision repair deficit. The neurodegeneration may result from an inability to repair DNA damaged by endogenously generated oxygen free radicals.

Nucleotide excision repair also corrects DNA damage from many chemical carcinogens, such as cigarette smoke, charred food, and cisplatin. Consequently, patients have a 10- to 20-fold increase in the incidence of internal neoplasms, such as brain tumors, leukemia, lung tumors, and gastric carcinomas.

Patients with XP have a shortened life span; without preventive protection, their life span is about 30 years shorter than that of individuals without XP. Metastatic melanoma and squamous cell skin carcinoma are the most common causes of death.

Two related disorders, Cockayne syndrome and trichothiodystrophy, are also caused by defects in other components of the cellular mechanism for repair of UV-induced DNA damage. Both are characterized by poor postnatal growth, diminished subcutaneous tissue, joint contractures, thin papery skin with photosensitivity, mental retardation, and neurological deterioration. Children with Cockayne syndrome also have retinal degeneration and deafness; children with trichothiodystrophy have ichthyosis and brittle hair and nails. In both syndromes, affected patients rarely live past the second decade. Interestingly, neither syndrome shows an increase in the frequency of skin cancers. However, defects in some repair genes (ERCC2, ERCC3, and ERCC5) produce phenotypes that combine characteristics of XP and either Cockayne syndrome or both Cockayne syndrome and trichothiodystrophy (see Table).

Management

Confirmation of the diagnosis of XP relies on functional tests of DNA repair and UV sensitivity; such tests are usually performed on cultured skin fibroblasts. Diagnostic confirmation by identification of mutations in an XP-associated gene is not currently clinically available.

The management of patients with XP includes avoidance of exposure to sunlight, protective clothing, physical and chemical sunscreens, and careful surveillance for and excision of cutaneous malignant neoplasms. No curative treatments are currently available.

INHERITANCE RISK

Because XP is an autosomal recessive disease, many patients do not have a family history of the disease. For parents who already have a child affected with XP, the risk for future children to have XP is 1 in 4. Prenatal diagnosis is possible by functional testing of DNA repair and UV sensitivity in cultured amniocytes or chorionic villi.

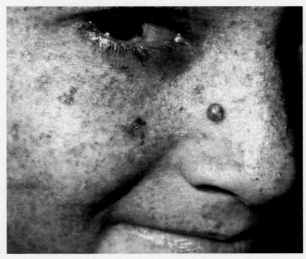

Figure C-43 ■ Cutaneous and ocular findings of xeroderma pigmentosum. Note the freckled hyperpigmentation, the papillomatous and verrucous lesions on the skin, and the conjunctivitis. (Courtesy of M. L. Levy, Baylor College of Medicine and Texas Children's Hospital, Houston.)

Questions for Small Group Discussion

1. Define complementation groups and explain their use for defining the biochemical basis of disease.
2. Compare and contrast XP and Cockayne syndrome. Why is Cockayne syndrome not associated with an increased risk of neoplasia?
3. Patients with XP have a defect of cutaneous cellular immunity. How could the sensitivity of patients with XP to UV irradiation explain this immunodeficiency? How could this immunodeficiency contribute to cancer susceptibility?
4. Werner syndrome, Bloom syndrome, XP, ataxia-telangiectasia, and Fanconi anemia are inherited diseases of genomic instability. What are the molecular mechanisms underlying each of these disorders? What types of genomic instability are associated with each disorder?

REFERENCES

de Boer J, Hoeijmakers JHJ: Nucleotide excision repair and human syndromes. Carcinogenesis 21:453-460, 2000.

GeneTests. Medical genetics information resource [database online]. University of Washington, Seattle, 1993-2006. Updated weekly. http://www.genetests.org

OMIM: Online Mendelian Inheritance in Man. McKusick-Nathans Institute for Genetic Medicine, Johns Hopkins University, and National Center for Biotechnology Information, National Library of Medicine. http://www.ncbi.nlm.nih.gov/entrez/query.fcgi?db=OMIM

Chapter 11

Principles of Molecular Disease: Lessons from the Hemoglobinopathies

A molecular disease is one in which the primary disease-causing event is a mutation, either inherited or acquired. This chapter outlines the basic genetic and biochemical mechanisms underlying genetic disease, using disorders of hemoglobin—the hemoglobinopathies—as examples. This overview of mechanisms is expanded in Chapter 12 to include other genetic diseases that are important because they illustrate additional principles of genetics in medicine.

Knowledge of molecular pathology is the foundation of rational therapy and management for genetic diseases. Moreover, such knowledge is also often instructive about normal function. The study of phenotype at the level of proteins, biochemistry, and metabolism constitutes the discipline of **biochemical genetics.** A genetic disease occurs when an alteration in the DNA of an essential gene changes the amount or function, or both, of the gene products—messenger RNA (mRNA) and protein. Single-gene disorders almost always result from mutations that alter the function of a protein. The few known exceptions to this generalization are mutations found in genes for RNAs that do not encode proteins, including mitochondrial genes that encode transfer RNAs (tRNAs); these mitochondrial tRNA mutations can lead to serious neurological conditions affecting muscle or brain (see Chapter 12).

Understanding the pathogenesis of a genetic disease is not possible without knowledge of the primary biochemical abnormalities that result from the alteration in gene function. By 2007, the online version of *Mendelian Inheritance in Man* (OMIM) listed just over 3900 diseases (both autosomal and X-linked) with mendelian patterns of inheritance. Of these, 3310 or about 85% are known to be caused by mutations in over 1990 genes, and new disease gene identifications

are being made weekly. Although it is impressive that the basic molecular defect has been found in so many disorders, it is sobering to realize that the pathophysiological process is not entirely understood for *any* genetic disease. **Sickle cell disease** (Case 37), discussed later in this chapter, is among the best characterized of inherited disorders, but even here, knowledge is incomplete—despite its being the first molecular disease to be recognized more than 50 years ago. Nevertheless, the study of genetic disease at its various phenotypic levels (gene, protein, cell, tissue, whole body) has not only greatly informed medicine but also, as described in Chapter 13, led to increasingly promising treatment, including protein and gene therapy, of inherited disorders.

● THE EFFECT OF MUTATION ON PROTEIN FUNCTION

Mutations have been found to cause disease through one of four different effects on protein function (Fig. 11-1). The most common effect by far is a **loss of function** of the protein. Many important conditions arise, however, from one of three other mechanisms: a **gain of function**; the acquisition of a **novel property** by the mutant protein; or the expression of a gene at the wrong time (**heterochronic expression**) or in the wrong place (**ectopic expression**), or both.

Loss-of-Function Mutations

The loss of function of a gene may result from alteration of its coding, regulatory, or other critical sequences due to the introduction of nucleotide substitutions,

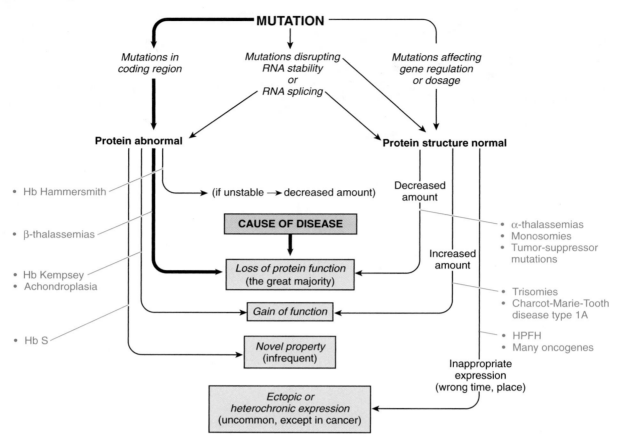

Figure 11-1 ■ A general outline of the mechanisms by which disease-causing mutations produce disease. Mutations in the coding region result in structurally abnormal proteins that have a loss or gain of function or a novel property that causes disease. Mutations in noncoding sequences are of two general types: those that alter the stability or splicing of the mRNA, and those that disrupt regulatory elements or change gene dosage. Mutations in regulatory elements alter the abundance of the mRNA or the time or cell type in which the gene is expressed. Mutations in either the coding region or regulatory domains can decrease the amount of the protein produced. HPFH, hereditary persistence of fetal hemoglobin.

deletions, insertions, or rearrangements. A loss of function due to deletion, leading to a reduction in gene dosage, is exemplified by the α-thalassemias (Case 39), which are most commonly due to deletion of α-globin genes (see later discussion); by chromosome-loss diseases (Case 24), such as monosomies like Turner syndrome (see Chapters 5 and 6 and Case 42); and by acquired somatic mutations—often deletions—that occur in tumor-suppressor genes in many cancers (such as retinoblastoma (Case 34); see Chapter 16). Many other types of mutations can also lead to a complete loss of function. These include the introduction of a premature stop codon or of a missense or other mutation in the coding sequence that abolishes or impairs protein function, or that renders the protein unstable, thereby reducing its abundance. All of these classes of mutation, and others, are illustrated by the β-thalassemias (Case 39) (see later discussion), a group of hemoglobinopathies that result from a reduction in the abundance of β-globin, one of the major adult hemoglobin proteins in red blood cells. As might be expected,

the severity of a disease that results from loss-of-function mutations can generally be correlated to the amount of function lost. In many instances, the retention of a small degree of residual function by the mutant protein greatly reduces the severity of the disease, a situation illustrated by the enzyme defects associated with hyperphenylalaninemia, the most severe form of which is phenylketonuria (see Chapter 12).

Gain-of-Function Mutations

Mutations may also alter the biochemical phenotype by enhancing one or more of the normal functions of a protein. In a biological system, more is not necessarily better, however, and disease may result. A gain in protein function may be due to either an increase in the abundance of the protein, usually from an increase in its expression or that of its cognate gene, or an increase in the ability of each protein molecule to perform one or more normal functions. It is critical to recognize when a disease is due to a gain-of-function mutation because treatment of the resulting disease must necessarily differ from disorders that arise from other mechanisms, such as loss-of-function mutations. Moreover, gain-of-function mutations often provide insight into the regulation of the expression of the affected gene or protein and the molecular mechanism of the protein's function.

Mutations That Enhance One Normal Function of a Protein   Rarely, a mutation in the coding region may increase the ability of each protein molecule to perform a normal function even though it is detrimental to the overall physiological activity of the protein. Once again, mutations in globin genes are among the best understood of mutations of this type and include missense mutations such as **hemoglobin Kempsey,** which locks hemoglobin in its high oxygen affinity state, thereby reducing oxygen delivery to tissues. Another example of this phenomenon occurs in the form of short stature called **achondroplasia** (Case 1) . Mutations of this type, which lead to the increase of a *normal* function, should be distinguished from novel property mutations (see later), which result in the acquisition of a completely *new* function by the mutant protein.

Mutations That Increase Production of a Normal Protein   Some mutations cause disease by increasing the synthesis of a normal protein in cells in which the protein is *normally present* (in contrast to *ectopic expression*). The most common mutations of this type are due to increased gene dosage, as with the presence of three or more copies of an autosomal gene, which is generally the result of the duplication of part or all of a chromosome, as in **trisomy 21** (**Down syndrome;** see Chapter 6). Other important diseases that arise from the increased dosage of single genes include one form of familial Alzheimer disease, which is due to a duplication of the amyloid precursor protein (βAPP) gene (see Chapter 12), and the peripheral nerve degeneration **Charcot-Marie-Tooth disease type 1A** (Case 6) , which generally results from duplication of only one gene, the gene for peripheral myelin protein 22 *(PMP22).* Increases in gene dosage are also prevalent as somatic mutations in cancer cells, where they result from increased copies of part or all of a chromosome; mutations of this type more often contribute to tumor progression than to initiation (discussed in Chapter 16).

Novel Property Mutations

In a few diseases, a change in the amino acid sequence causes disease by conferring a novel property on the protein, without necessarily altering its normal functions. The classic example is **sickle cell disease** (Case 37) (see later discussion), which is due to an amino acid substitution that has *no* effect on the ability of sickle hemoglobin to transport oxygen. Rather, unlike normal hemoglobin, sickle hemoglobin chains aggregate when they are deoxygenated to form polymeric fibers that deform red blood cells. This behavior has not been observed with any other hemoglobin mutant. That novel property mutations are infrequent is not surprising because most amino acid substitutions are either neutral or detrimental to the function or stability of a protein that has been finely tuned by evolution. Only rarely does a mutation introduce a new property of pathological significance.

The difficulty in placing every type of mutation into one or another of the classes discussed in this section is demonstrated by a recently discovered group of mutations, those that lead to **gains of glycosylation.** In disorders of this type, a mutation in the coding sequence creates a novel N-glycosylation site in the mutant protein, conferring on it a *novel property,* the ability to be N-glycosylated. However, the increased glycosylation leads to a *loss of function* of the mutant protein, as has been documented in some individuals with mutations in the R2 subunit of the interferon-γ receptor, leading to a **mendelian susceptibility to mycobacterial infection** (see Chapter 12).

Mutations Associated with Heterochronic or Ectopic Gene Expression

An interesting and important class of mutations includes those that alter the regulatory regions of a gene to cause its inappropriate expression, at an abnormal time or place. One of the most common genetic diseases, cancer, is frequently due to the abnormal expression of a gene that normally promotes cell proliferation—an **oncogene**—in cells in which the gene is not normally expressed, resulting in malignant neoplasia (see Chapter 16). Comparably, some mutations in hemoglobin regulatory elements lead to the continued expression in the adult of the γ-globin gene, which is normally expressed at high levels only in fetal life. Such γ-globin gene mutations lead to a phenotype called the **hereditary persistence of fetal hemoglobin** (see later discussion).

⊙ HOW MUTATIONS DISRUPT THE FORMATION OF BIOLOGICALLY NORMAL PROTEINS

For development of a biologically active protein, information must be transcribed from the nucleotide sequence of the gene to the mRNA and then translated into the polypeptide, which then undergoes progressive stages of maturation (see Chapter 3). Mutations can disrupt any of these steps (Table 11-1). Abnormalities in five of these stages are illustrated by various hemoglobinopathies; the others are exemplified by diseases presented in Chapter 12.

Table 11-1

The Eight Steps at Which Mutations Can Disrupt the Production of a Normal Protein

Step	Disease Example
Transcription	**Thalassemias** due to reduced or absent production of a globin mRNA because of deletions or mutations in regulatory or splice sites of a globin gene
	Hereditary persistence of fetal hemoglobin, which results from increased postnatal transcription of one or more γ-globin genes
Translation	**Thalassemias** due to nonfunctional or rapidly degraded mRNAs with nonsense or frameshift mutations
Polypeptide folding	More than 70 **hemoglobinopathies** are due to abnormal hemoglobins with amino acid substitutions or deletions that lead to unstable globins that are prematurely degraded, e.g., Hb Hammersmith
Post-translational modification	**I-cell disease,** a lysosomal storage disease that is due to a failure to add a phosphate group to mannose residues of lysosomal enzymes. The mannose 6-phosphate residues are required to target the enzymes to lysosomes.
Assembly of monomers into a holomeric protein	Types of **osteogenesis imperfecta** in which an amino acid substitution in a procollagen chain impairs the assembly of a normal collagen triple helix
Subcellular localization of the polypeptide or the holomer	**Familial hypercholesterolemia mutations** (class 4), in the carboxyl terminus of the LDL receptor, that impair the localization of the receptor to clathrin-coated pits, preventing the internalization of the receptor and its subsequent recycling to the cell surface
Cofactor or prosthetic group binding to the polypeptide	Types of **homocystinuria** due to poor or absent binding of the cofactor (pyridoxal phosphate) to the cystathionine synthase apoenzyme
Function of a correctly folded, assembled, and localized protein produced in normal amounts	Diseases in which the mutant protein is normal in nearly every way, except that one of its critical biological activities is altered by an amino acid substitution; e.g., in **Hb Kempsey,** impaired subunit interaction locks hemoglobin into its high oxygen affinity state

● THE HEMOGLOBINS

Disorders of human hemoglobins, referred to as hemoglobinopathies, occupy a unique position in medical genetics. They are the most common single-gene diseases in humans, and they cause substantial morbidity. The World Health Organization has estimated that more than 5% of the world's population are carriers of genes for clinically important disorders of hemoglobin. Moreover, because hemoglobin was one of the first protein structures to be deduced and because the human globin genes were the first disease-related genes to be cloned, their molecular and biochemical pathology is better understood than perhaps that of any other group of genetic diseases. The globins also cast light on the process of evolution at both the molecular and the population levels and provide a model of gene action during development. Before the hemoglobinopathies are discussed in depth, it is important to briefly introduce the normal aspects of the globin genes and hemoglobin biology.

Structure and Function of Hemoglobin

Hemoglobin is the oxygen carrier in vertebrate red blood cells. The molecule contains four subunits: two α chains and two β chains. Each subunit is composed of a polypeptide chain, globin, and a prosthetic group, heme, which is an iron-containing pigment that combines with oxygen to give the molecule its oxygen-transporting ability (Fig. 11-2).

The hemoglobin molecule consists of two each of two different types of polypeptide chains. In normal

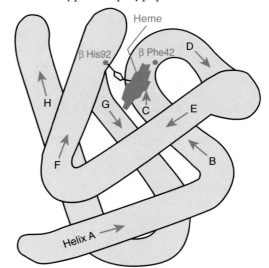

Figure 11-2 ■ The structure of a hemoglobin subunit. Each subunit has eight helical regions, designated A to H. The two most conserved amino acids are shown: at His92, the histidine to which the iron of heme is covalently linked, and at Phe42, the phenylalanine that wedges the porphyrin ring of heme into the heme "pocket" of the folded protein. See discussion of Hb Hammersmith and Hb Hyde Park, which have substitutions for Phe42 and His92, respectively, in the β-globin molecule.

adult hemoglobin, hemoglobin A (Hb A), these globin chains are designated α and β (the structure of the β-globin gene is described in Chapter 3). The four chains are folded and fitted together to form a globular tetramer with a molecular weight of approximately 64,500, a structure that, for Hb A, is abbreviated $\alpha_2\beta_2$. The two types of chains are almost equal in length; the α chain has 141 amino acids, and the β chain has 146. The chains resemble one another markedly both in amino acid sequence (primary structure) and in three-dimensional configuration (tertiary structure; see Fig. 11-2).

The major features of globin structure have been highly conserved during evolution and are central to an understanding of the hemoglobinopathies. Above all, the *tertiary structure* of the globin polypeptide has been remarkably preserved: virtually all globins examined have seven or eight helical regions (depending on the chain). In contrast, only two amino acid residues have been conserved in all globins throughout nature, and not surprisingly, mutations in either of these residues are associated with disease (see Fig. 11-2).

The study of the structure of hemoglobin allows one to predict which types of mutations are likely to be pathogenic. Thus, a mutation that alters globin conformation, substitutes a highly conserved amino acid, or replaces one of the nonpolar residues forming the hydrophobic shell that excludes water from the interior of the molecule, is likely to cause a hemoglobinopathy. Like all proteins, globin has "sensitive areas," in which mutations cannot occur without affecting function, and "insensitive areas," in which variation is more freely tolerated.

The Human Hemoglobin Genes In addition to Hb A, there are five other normal human hemoglobins, each of which has a tetrameric structure comparable to that of Hb A in consisting of two α or α-like chains and two non-α chains (Fig. 11-3A). The genes for the α and α-like chains are clustered in a tandem arrangement on chromosome 16, and those for the β and β-like chains are on chromosome 11. There are two identical α-globin genes, designated $\alpha 1$ and $\alpha 2$, on each copy of chromosome 16. Within the β-globin gene complex, a close homology exists between the different genes. For example, the β- and δ-globins differ in only 10 of their 146 amino acids. All of the globin genes undoubtedly arose from a common ancestral gene.

Developmental Expression of Globin Genes and Globin Switching

The change in the expression during development of the various globin genes, sometimes referred to as **globin switching** (Fig. 11-3B), is a classic example of the ordered regulation of developmental gene expression (see Chapter 14). Note that the genes in the α and β clusters are arranged in the same transcriptional orientation and, remarkably, that the genes in each cluster are situated in the same order in which they are expressed during development. There is equimolar production of the α-like and β-like globin chains.

Interestingly, the temporal switches of globin synthesis are accompanied by changes in the major site of erythropoiesis (Fig. 11-3B). Embryonic globin synthesis occurs in the yolk sac from the third to eighth weeks of gestation, but at about the fifth week of gestation, the major site of hematopoiesis begins to move from the yolk sac to the fetal liver. Hb F ($\alpha_2\gamma_2$) is the predominant hemoglobin throughout fetal life and constitutes approximately 70% of total hemoglobin at birth, but in adult life, Hb F represents less than 1% of the total hemoglobin.

Although β chains can be detected in early gestation, their synthesis becomes significant only near the time of birth; by 3 months of age, almost all the hemoglobin present is of the adult type, Hb A. Synthesis of the δ chain also continues after birth, but Hb A_2 ($\alpha_2\delta_2$) never accounts for more than about 2% of adult hemoglobin. Unfortunately, the small amounts of δ-globin (and therefore Hb A_2) and γ-globin (and therefore Hb F) that are found normally in adult blood are insufficient to compensate for the reduced amounts of β-globin (and therefore Hb A) that are found in diseases such as β–thalassemia (discussed later). Consequently, knowledge of the mechanisms that regulate globin-chain production is of potential therapeutic importance (see Chapter 13). Many of the transcription factors that control the expression of the globin genes have been identified, and treatments that aim to increase the synthesis of the δ- and γ-globins are promising (see Chapter 13).

The Developmental Regulation of β-Globin Gene Expression: The Locus Control Region

As with many other areas of medical genetics, an understanding of the mechanisms that control the expression of the globin genes has provided insight into both normal and pathological biological processes. The expression of the β-globin gene has been found to be only partly controlled by the promoter and two enhancers in the immediate flanking DNA (see Chapter 3). A critical requirement for additional regulatory elements was first suggested by the identification of a unique group of patients who had no gene expression from *any* of the genes in the β-globin cluster, even though the genes themselves (including their individual regulatory elements) were intact. These informative patients were found to have large deletions upstream of the β-globin complex, deletions that removed an approximately 20-kb domain called the **locus control region (LCR)**, which begins approximately 6 kb upstream of the ϵ-globin gene

A

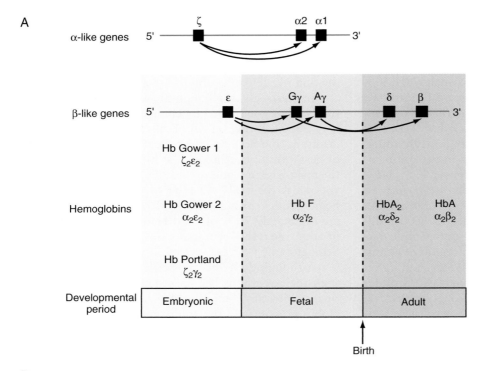

B

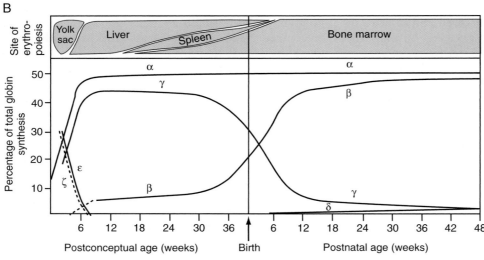

Figure 11-3 ■ **A,** Organization of the human globin genes and hemoglobins produced in each stage of human development. The curved arrows refer to the switches in gene expression during development. **B,** Development of erythropoiesis in the human fetus and infant. Types of cells responsible for hemoglobin synthesis, organs involved, and types of globin chain synthesized at successive stages are shown. (**A** redrawn from Stamatoyannopoulos G, Nienhuis AW: Hemoglobin switching. In Stamatoyannopoulos G, Nienhuis AW, Leder P, Majerus PW [eds]: The Molecular Basis of Blood Diseases. Philadelphia, WB Saunders, 1987. **B** redrawn from Wood WG: Haemoglobin synthesis during fetal development. Br Med Bull 32:282-287, 1976.)

(Fig. 11-4). The resulting disease, εγδβ-thalassemia, is described later. These patients demonstrate that the LCR is required for the expression of all the genes in the β-globin cluster on chromosome 11 (see Fig. 11-3A).

The LCR is defined by five DNase 1 hypersensitive sites (see Fig. 11-4) required for the maintenance of an open chromatin configuration of the locus, a configuration that gives transcription factors access to the regulatory elements that mediate the expression of each gene in the β-globin complex (see Chapter 3). The LCR, along with associated DNA-binding proteins, interacts with the genes of the locus to form a nuclear compartment called the **active chromatin hub,** the

compartment where β-globin gene expression takes place. The sequential switching of gene expression that occurs among the five members of the β-globin gene complex during development results from the sequential association of the active chromatin hub with the different genes in the cluster as the hub moves from the most 5′ gene in the complex (the embryonically expressed ε-globin gene) to the δ- and β-globin genes in adults.

The clinical significance of the LCR is 3-fold. First, as mentioned, patients with deletions of the LCR fail to express the genes of the β-globin cluster. Second, components of the LCR are likely to be essential in gene

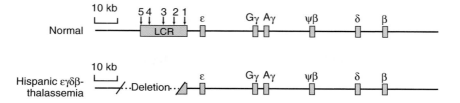

Figure 11-4 ■ The β-globin locus control region (LCR). Each of the five regions of open chromatin *(arrows)* contains several consensus binding sites for both erythroid-specific and ubiquitous transcription factors. The precise mechanism by which the LCR regulates gene expression is unclear. Also shown is a deletion of the LCR that has led to εγδβ-thalassemia, which is discussed in the text. (Redrawn from Kazazian HH Jr, Antonarakis S: Molecular genetics of the globin genes. In Singer M, Berg P [eds]: Exploring Genetic Mechanisms. Sausalito, California, University Science Books, 1997.)

therapy (see Chapter 13) for disorders of the β-globin cluster. Third, knowledge of the molecular mechanisms that underlie globin switching may make it feasible, for example, to up-regulate the expression of the γ-globin gene in patients with β-thalassemia (who have mutations in the β-globin gene), since Hb F ($\alpha_2\gamma_2$) is an effective oxygen carrier in adults who lack Hb A ($\alpha_2\beta_2$) (see Chapter 13).

Gene Dosage, Ontogeny, and Clinical Disease

The differences in gene dosage (four α-globin and two β-globin genes per diploid genome) and ontogeny of the α- and β-globins are important to an understanding of the pathogenesis of many hemoglobinopathies. Mutations in the β-globin gene are more likely to cause disease than are α-chain mutations because a single β-globin gene mutation affects 50% of the β chains, whereas a single α-chain mutation affects only 25% of the α chains. On the other hand, β-globin mutations have no prenatal consequences because γ-globin is the major β-like globin before birth, and Hb F constitutes three quarters of the total hemoglobin at term. Because α chains are the only α-like components of all hemoglobins 6 weeks after conception (see Fig. 11-3B), α-globin mutations cause severe disease in both fetal and postnatal life.

● THE HEMOGLOBINOPATHIES

The hereditary disorders of hemoglobin can be divided into three broad groups, depending on whether the mutation alters the globin protein, its synthesis, or globin developmental switching:

1. **structural variants,** which alter the globin polypeptide without affecting its rate of synthesis;
2. **thalassemias,** in which there is decreased synthesis (or, rarely, extreme instability) of one or more of the globin chains, resulting in an imbalance in the relative amounts of the α and β chains; and

3. **hereditary persistence of fetal hemoglobin,** a group of clinically benign conditions that are of interest because they impair the perinatal switch from γ-globin to β-globin synthesis.

Hemoglobin Structural Variants

Most variant hemoglobins result from point mutations in one of the globin structural genes, but a few are formed by other, more complex molecular mechanisms. More than 400 abnormal hemoglobins have been described, and approximately half of these are clinically significant. The hemoglobin structural variants can be separated into three classes, depending on the clinical phenotype (Table 11-2):

1. Variants that cause **hemolytic anemia.** The great majority of mutant hemoglobins that cause hemolytic anemia make the hemoglobin tetramer unstable. However, two of the best-known variants associated with hemolysis, sickle cell globin and Hb C, are not unstable but cause the mutant globin proteins to assume unusual rigid structures.
2. Mutants with **altered oxygen transport,** due to increased or decreased oxygen affinity or to the formation of methemoglobin, a form of globin incapable of reversible oxygenation.
3. Variants due to mutations in the coding region that cause **thalassemia** because they reduce the abundance of the globin polypeptide. Most of these mutations impair the rate of synthesis of the mRNA or the protein. Some rare variants cause gross instability of the hemoglobin monomer, greater instability than that associated with the variants leading to hemolytic anemia.

The structural mutants described in this chapter are presented either because they are common and representative of one of these three groups or because they illustrate the dramatic and variable biochemical and clinical consequences of mutations.

Table 11-2

The Major Classes of Hemoglobin Structural Variants

Variant Class*	Molecular Basis of Mutation	Change in Polypeptide	Pathophysiological Effect of Mutation	Inheritance
Variants Causing Hemolytic Anemia				
HEMOGLOBINS WITH NOVEL PHYSICAL PROPERTIES				
Hb S	Single nucleotide substitution	β chain: Glu6Val	Deoxygenated Hb S polymerizes → sickle cells → vascular occlusion and hemolysis	AR
Hb C	Single nucleotide substitution	β chain: Glu6Lys	Oxygenated Hb C tends to crystallize → less deformable cells → mild hemolysis. The disease in Hb S/Hb C compounds is like mild sickle cell disease.	AR
UNSTABLE HEMOGLOBINS				
Hb Hammersmith	Single nucleotide substitution	β chain: Phe42Ser	An unstable Hb → Hb precipitation → hemolysis; also low oxygen affinity	AD
Hemoglobins with Altered Oxygen Transport				
Hb Hyde Park (a Hb M)	Single nucleotide substitution	β chain: His92Tyr	The substitution makes oxidized heme iron resistant to methemoglobin reductase → Hb M, which cannot carry oxygen → cyanosis (asymptomatic)	AD
Hb Kempsey	Single nucleotide substitution	β chain: Asp99Asn	The substitution keeps the Hb in its high oxygen affinity structure → less oxygen to tissues → polycythemia	AD
Variants with Thalassemia Phenotypes†				
Hb E	Single nucleotide substitution	β chain: Glu26Lys	The mutation → an abnormal Hb *and* decreased synthesis (abnormal RNA splicing) → mild thalassemia (see Fig. 11-12)	AR

*Hemoglobin variants are often named after the hometown of the first patient described.
†Additional β-chain structural variants that cause β-thalassemia are depicted in Table 11-4.
AD, autosomal dominant; AR, autosomal recessive.
Hb M, methemoglobin; see text.

Hemolytic Anemias

Hemoglobins with Novel Physical Properties: Sickle Cell Disease Sickle cell hemoglobin (Hb S) was the first abnormal hemoglobin to be detected and is of great clinical importance. It is due to a single nucleotide substitution that changes the codon of the sixth amino acid of β-globin from glutamic acid to valine (GAG → GTG: Glu6Val; see Table 11-2). Homozygosity for this mutation is the cause of **sickle cell disease** (Case 37), a serious disorder that is common in some parts of the world. The disease has a characteristic geographical distribution, occurring most frequently in equatorial Africa and less commonly in the Mediterranean area and India and in countries to which people from these regions have migrated. About 1 in 600 African

Americans is born with this disease, which may be fatal in early childhood, although longer survival is becoming more common.

Clinical Features Sickle cell disease is a severe autosomal recessive hemolytic condition characterized by a tendency of the red blood cells to become grossly abnormal in shape (i.e., to sickle) under conditions of low oxygen tension (Fig. 11-5). Heterozygotes, who are said to have **sickle cell trait,** are generally clinically normal, but their red cells sickle when they are subjected to very low oxygen pressure in vitro. Occasions when this might occur in vivo are uncommon, although heterozygotes appear to be at risk for splenic infarction, especially when flying at high altitudes in airplanes with reduced cabin pressure. The heterozygous state is present in approximately 8% of African Americans, but

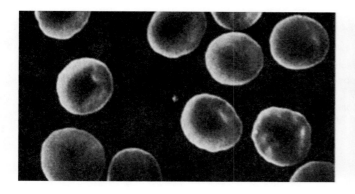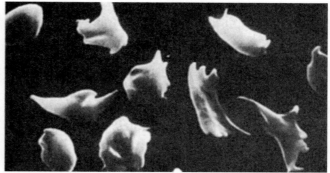

Figure 11-5 ■ Scanning electron micrographs of red cells from a patient with sickle cell disease. Oxygenated cells are round and full *(left)*. The classic sickle cell shape is produced only when the cells are in the deoxygenated state *(right)*. (From Kaul DK, Fabry ME, Windisch P, et al: Erythrocytes in sickle cell anemia are heterogeneous in their rheological and hemodynamic characteristics. J Clin Invest 72:22, 1983.)

in areas where the gene frequency is high (e.g., West Central Africa), up to 25% of the newborn population are heterozygotes.

The Molecular Pathology of Hb S Some 50 years ago, Ingram discovered that the abnormality in sickle cell hemoglobin was a replacement of one of the 146 amino acids in the β chain of the hemoglobin molecule. All the clinical manifestations of sickle cell hemoglobin are consequences of this single change in the β-globin gene. This was the first demonstration *in any organism* that a mutation in a structural gene could cause an amino acid substitution in the corresponding protein. Because the abnormality of Hb S is localized in the β chain, the formula for sickle cell hemoglobin may be written as $\alpha_2\beta_2^S$ or, more precisely, $\alpha_2^A\beta_2^S$. A heterozygote has a mixture of the two types of hemoglobin, A and S, summarized as $\alpha_2^A\beta_2^A$, $\alpha_2^A\beta_2^S$, as well as a hybrid hemoglobin tetramer, written as $\alpha_2^A\beta^A\beta^S$.

Sickling and Its Consequences The molecular and cellular pathology of sickle cell disease is summarized in Figure 11-6. Hemoglobin molecules containing the

mutant β-globin subunits are normal in their ability to perform their principal function of binding oxygen (provided they have not polymerized, as described next), but in deoxygenated blood, they are only one fifth as soluble as normal hemoglobin. The relative insolubility of deoxyhemoglobin S is the physical basis of the sickling phenomenon. Under conditions of low oxygen tension, the sickle hemoglobin molecules aggregate in the form of rod-shaped polymers or fibers, which distort the erythrocyte to a sickle shape. These misshapen erythrocytes are less deformable than normal and, unlike normal red blood cells, cannot squeeze in single file through capillaries, thereby blocking blood flow and causing local ischemia.

Multiple Origins of the Hb S Mutation The normal β-globin gene is contained within a 7.6-kb restriction fragment of DNA in most individuals of African origin (Fig. 11-7). In contrast, the sickle globin allele is frequently found in a fragment of 13 kb in certain parts of Africa, such as Ghana (see Fig. 11-7), and in nearly 70% of African Americans. The frequent association

Figure 11-6 ■ The pathogenesis of sickle cell disease. (Redrawn from Ingram V: Sickle cell disease: molecular and cellular pathogenesis. In Bunn HF, Forget BG [eds]: Hemoglobin: Molecular, Genetic, and Clinical Aspects. Philadelphia, WB Saunders, 1986.)

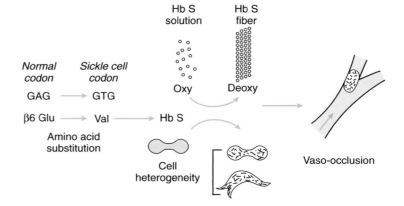

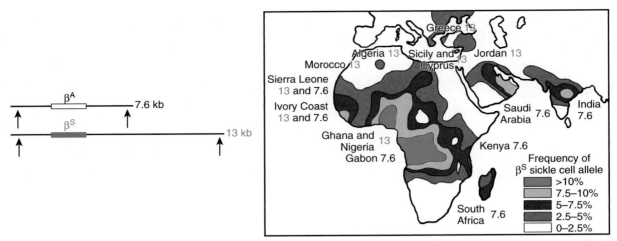

Figure 11-7 ■ The *Hpa*I restriction fragment length polymorphism adjacent to the β^S gene and the geographical distribution of the sickle cell gene in relation to *Hpa*I fragments 7.6 kb and 13 kb in length. The mutation associated with the 13-kb fragment originated in West Africa and spread from there. The mutation associated with the 7.6-kb fragment arose separately and probably had multiple origins. (From Kan YW: Hemoglobin abnormalities: molecular and evolutionary studies. Harvey Lect 76:75-93, 1980-1981.)

of sickle globin with the 13-kb fragment is a striking example of linkage disequilibrium, discussed in Chapter 10. In other parts of Africa (e.g., Kenya), the sickle cell mutation is typically associated with the 7.6-kb fragment (see Fig. 11-7). These findings imply that the sickle mutation arose in West Africa on a chromosome that contained the β-globin gene on the 13-kb fragment and that it occurred independently elsewhere, at least once. The protection that the sickle cell gene confers against malaria in heterozygotes accounts for the high frequency that the gene has reached in malarial areas of the world (see Chapter 9).

Hemoglobins with Novel Physical Properties: Hb C
Hb C was the second hemoglobin variant to be identified, and coincidentally, like Hb S, it is also due to a substitution at the sixth position of the β chain, the glutamic acid being replaced by lysine (Glu6Lys; see Table 11-2). Hb C is less soluble than Hb A and thus tends to crystallize in red blood cells, reducing their deformability in capillaries and causing a mild hemolytic disorder.

The β^C allele is frequent in West Africa and in descendants of people of this region (about 1% of African Americans are carriers). Thus, it is not uncommon to find individuals with Hb C who have a β^S allele or a thalassemia allele at the other β-globin locus. Persons who are **compound heterozygotes** for the β^C and β^S mutations (Hb SC disease) have a hemolytic disorder that is milder than sickle cell anemia and may have no clinical problems until, unexpectedly, a serious complication develops as a result of vascular occlusion, particularly in the retina.

Unstable Hemoglobins   The unstable hemoglobins are generally due to point mutations that cause denatur-

ation of the hemoglobin *tetramer* in mature red blood cells. The denatured globin tetramers are insoluble and precipitate to form inclusions (Heinz bodies) that contribute to damage of the red cell membrane and cause the hemolysis of mature red blood cells in the vascular tree. The instability of hemoglobin *tetramers*, which are prone to denature and to form damaging Heinz body inclusions, is much less pronounced than that of the rare variants which destabilize the globin *monomer* so severely that tetramers fail to form within red cell precursors in the bone marrow, causing chain imbalance and thalassemia (see following text).

The amino acid substitution in the unstable hemoglobin **Hb Hammersmith** (β-chain Phe42Ser; see Table 11-2) is particularly noteworthy because the substituted phenylalanine residue (see Fig. 11-2) is one of the two amino acids that are conserved in all globins. It is therefore not surprising that substitutions at this position produce serious disease. The role of the bulky phenylalanine is to wedge the heme into its pocket in β-globin. Its replacement with serine, a smaller residue that leaves a gap, allows the heme to drop out of its pocket. In addition to its instability, Hb Hammersmith has a low oxygen affinity, which causes cyanosis.

Variants with Altered Oxygen Transport

Mutations that alter the ability of hemoglobin to transport oxygen, although rare, are of general interest because they illustrate how a mutation can impair one set of functions of a protein (in this case, oxygen binding and release) that is the responsibility of one domain of the protein, and yet leave the other properties of the molecule relatively intact; for example, the mutations that affect oxygen transport generally have little or no effect on hemoglobin stability.

Methemoglobins Oxyhemoglobin is the form of hemoglobin that is capable of reversible oxygenation; its heme iron is in the reduced (or ferrous) state. The heme iron tends to oxidize spontaneously to the ferric form, and the resulting molecule, referred to as methemoglobin, is incapable of reversible oxygenation. If significant amounts of methemoglobin accumulate in the blood, cyanosis results. Maintenance of the heme iron in the reduced state is the role of the enzyme methemoglobin reductase. In several mutant globins (either α or β), substitutions in the region of the heme pocket affect the heme-globin bond in a way that makes the iron resistant to the reductase. Although heterozygotes for these mutant hemoglobins are cyanotic, they are asymptomatic. The homozygous state is presumably lethal. One example of a β-chain methemoglobin is **Hb Hyde Park** (see Table 11-2), in which the conserved histidine (His92 in Fig. 11-2) to which heme is covalently bound has been replaced by tyrosine (His92Tyr).

Hemoglobins with Altered Oxygen Affinity Mutations that alter oxygen affinity are of significance because they demonstrate the importance of subunit interaction for the normal function of a multimeric protein such as hemoglobin. In the Hb A tetramer, the α : β interface has been highly conserved throughout evolution because it is subject to significant movement between the chains when the hemoglobin shifts from the oxygenated (relaxed) to the deoxygenated (tense) form of the molecule. Predictably, substitutions in residues at this interface, exemplified by the β-globin mutant **Hb Kempsey** (see Table 11-2), have serious pathological effects because they prevent the oxygen-related movement between the chains. In Hb Kempsey (β-chain Asp99Asn), the mutation "locks" the hemoglobin into the relaxed structure, which has high oxygen affinity, causing polycythemia.

Thalassemia: An Imbalance of Globin-Chain Synthesis

The thalassemias, collectively the most common human single-gene disorders, are a heterogeneous group of diseases of hemoglobin synthesis in which mutations reduce the synthesis or stability of either the α-globin or β-globin chain to cause α-**thalassemia** or β-**thalassemia,** respectively. The resulting imbalance in the ratio of the α : β chains underlies the pathophysiological process. The chain that is produced at the normal rate is in relative excess; in the absence of a complementary chain with which to form a tetramer, the excess normal chains eventually precipitate in the cell, damaging the membrane and leading to premature red blood cell

destruction. The defect in hemoglobin synthesis also results in a hypochromic, microcytic anemia.

The name "thalassemia" is derived from the Greek word for sea, *thalassa,* and signifies that the disease was first discovered in persons of Mediterranean origin. Both α-thalassemia and β-thalassemia, however, have a high frequency in many populations, although α-thalassemia is more prevalent and widely distributed. The frequency of thalassemia is due to the protective advantage against malaria that it confers on carriers, analogous to the heterozygote advantage (see Chapter 9) of sickle hemoglobin carriers. There is a characteristic distribution of the thalassemias in a band around the Old World: in the Mediterranean, the Middle East, and parts of Africa, India, and Asia. In most countries, thalassemia carriers are sufficiently numerous to pose the important problem of differential diagnosis from iron deficiency anemia, and to be a relatively common source of referral for homozygote detection in prenatal diagnosis.

An important clinical consideration is that it is not unusual for alleles for both types of thalassemia, as well as for structural hemoglobin abnormalities, to coexist in an individual. As a result, clinically important interactions may occur among different alleles of the same gene or among mutant alleles of different globin genes.

The α-Thalassemias

Genetic disorders of α-globin production affect the formation of *both* fetal and adult hemoglobins (see Fig. 11-3) and therefore cause intrauterine as well as postnatal disease. In the absence of α-globin chains with which to associate, the chains from the β-globin cluster are free to form a homotetrameric hemoglobin. Hemoglobin with a γ_4 composition is known as Hb Bart's, and the β_4 tetramer is called Hb H. Because neither of these hemoglobins is capable of releasing oxygen to tissues in normal conditions, they are completely ineffective oxygen carriers. Consequently, infants with severe α-thalassemia and high levels of Hb Bart's suffer severe intrauterine hypoxia and are born with massive generalized fluid accumulation, a condition called **hydrops fetalis.** In milder α-thalassemias, an anemia develops because of the gradual precipitation of the Hb H in the erythrocyte. This leads to the formation of inclusions in the mature red blood cell, and the removal of these inclusions by the spleen damages the cells, leading to their premature destruction.

Deletions of the α-Globin Genes The most common forms of α-thalassemia are the result of deletions. The reason for the frequency of this type of abnormality in mutants of the α chain and not the β chain is revealed by comparison of these genes and their local chromo-

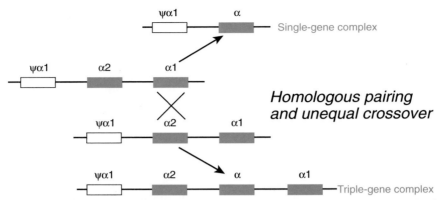

Figure 11-8 ■ The probable mechanism underlying the most common form of α-thalassemia, which is due to deletions of one of the two α-globin genes on a chromosome. Misalignment, homologous pairing, and recombination between the α1 gene on one chromosome and the α2 gene on the homologous chromosome result in the deletion of one α gene. (Redrawn from Orkin SH: Disorders of hemoglobin synthesis: the thalassemias. In Stamatoyannopoulos G, Nienhuis AW, Leder P, Majerus PW [eds]: The Molecular Basis of Blood Diseases. Philadelphia, WB Saunders, 1987, pp 106-126.)

somal contexts (see Fig. 11-3). Not only are there two identical α genes on each chromosome 16, but the intron sequences around the two α genes are also similar.

The arrangement of tandem regions of homology in and around the α genes facilitates misalignment due to homologous pairing and subsequent recombination between the α1 gene domain on one chromosome and the corresponding α2 gene region on the other (Fig. 11-8). Evidence that this explanation for the deletions is correct is provided by reports of rare normal individuals with a triplicated α gene complex. Deletions or other alterations of one, two, three, or all four of these genes cause a correspondingly severe hematological abnormality (Table 11-3).

Although the α-thalassemias are distributed throughout the world, the homozygous deletion type of α-thalassemia leading to hydrops fetalis is largely restricted to Southeast Asia. The high gene frequency in this population (up to 15% in some regions) can be explained by the nature of the deletion. The loss of two α genes, called α-thalassemia trait (two normal and two mutant α genes), can result from either of two genotypes (−α/−α or −−/αα). The latter is relatively common among Southeast Asians, and offspring may consequently receive two −−/−− chromosomes. In other groups, however, α-thalassemia trait is usually the result of the −α/−α genotype, from which there is virtually no possibility of transmitting the hydrops fetalis phenotype.

In addition to α-thalassemia mutations that result in deletion of the α genes, mutations that delete only the LCR of the α-globin complex (see Fig. 11-3A) have also been found to cause α-thalassemia. In fact, such deletions first indicated the existence of this regulatory element.

Other Forms of α-Thalassemia Other forms of α-thalassemia occur much less commonly than the deletion genotypes just described and are therefore of less overall significance. Two other forms of α-thalassemia, however, illustrate important disease mechanisms. In one instance, the α-thalassemia is due to a mutation, the ZF deletion, which leads to the transcription of an antisense RNA that silences the α2-globin gene. In the second instance, the **ATR-X syndrome,** both α-thalassemia and syndromic mental retardation result from mutations in the X-linked *ATRX* gene, which encodes a chromatin remodeling protein required for the normal expression of the α-globin complex.

In two affected individuals from a family segregating α-thalassemia trait, a unique deletion (termed the α-ZF deletion after the family member in whom it was first identified) removed the α1-globin gene and approximately 18 kb of sequence downstream of it (Fig. 11-9). Importantly, the deleted sequences also included the normal transcription termination site of the *LUC7L* gene, which lies immediately 3′ of the α-globin gene complex but is transcribed from the opposite strand to the α-globin genes. (The LUC7L protein is a widely expressed component of the U1–small nuclear ribonuclear protein complex but plays no role in the α-thalassemia in this family).

In individuals carrying the α-ZF deletion, expression of the α2-globin gene was silenced, despite the fact that the gene and all of its local and remote *cis*-regulatory elements remained intact. Silencing of the α2-globin gene is due to the generation of antisense RNAs from the truncated *LUC7L* gene, RNAs that fail to terminate normally and instead extend across the α-ZF breakpoint into the α2-globin CpG island. In carriers of the α-ZF deletion, the LUC7L–α2-globin fusion anti-sense RNA led to the loss of expression of the α2-globin

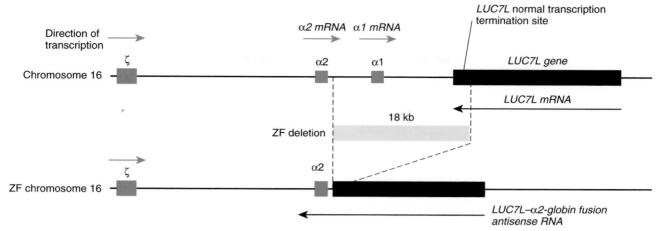

Figure 11-9 ■ The ZF deletion that leads to α-thalassemia. The ZF deletion removes the 3' end of the *LUC7L* gene, including its transcription termination site, leading to the formation of a mutant hybrid RNA composed of the LUC7L mRNA and an antisense α2-globin RNA. The antisense RNA contains sequences corresponding to the α2-globin CpG island. The antisense transcription is consistently associated with methylation of the α2-globin CpG island and silencing of α2-globin gene expression. (Based a figure provided by D. R. Higgs, University of Oxford, Cambridge, England.)

gene on the deleted chromosome in association with complete methylation of the α2-globin CpG island.

The pathological activity of the α-ZF deletion antisense RNA is comparable to the important gene-silencing activity of wild-type antisense transcripts that participate in normal development. For example, antisense transcripts to CpG islands have been shown to mediate the methylation and silencing of a number of maternally imprinted genes (see Chapters 6 and 7), and antisense transcripts from *XIST,* the X chromosome inactivation locus, participate in inactivation of the X chromosome (see Chapter 6). Other examples of pathogenic antisense RNAs that result from mutation will undoubtedly be identified as the molecular basis of disease continues to be explored.

Mutations in the ATRX Chromatin Remodeling Protein In all the classes of α-thalassemia described before, mutations in the α-globin genes or in their *cis*-acting sequences account for the reduction of α-globin synthesis. In contrast, one type of α-thalassemia, the ATR-X syndrome, results from mutations in the *ATRX* gene, leading to reduced activity or expression of a

chromatin remodeling protein, ATRX, that functions in *trans* to activate the expression of the α-globin genes.

The ATR-X syndrome was first thought to be a unique disorder because of the occurrence of Hb H (a β_4 tetramer) disease in three northern European families, α-thalassemia being uncommon in individuals of European origin. In addition, all affected individuals were males who also had severe X-linked mental retardation together with a wide range of other defects including characteristic facial features, skeletal abnormalities, and urogenital malformations. This diversity of phenotypes suggests that ATRX regulates the expression of numerous other genes besides the α-globins, but these other targets are presently unknown.

Although its precise mechanism of action is uncertain, ATRX belongs to a family of chromatin remodeling proteins that typically function within large multiprotein complexes to mediate changes in DNA topology. These topological changes drive the formation of remodeled nucleosomal states. Abnormalities in the DNA methylation patterns of patients with ATR-X

Table 11-3

Clinical States Associated with α-Thalassemia Genotypes

Clinical Condition	Number of Functional α Genes	α-Globin Gene Genotype	α-Chain Production
Normal	4	αα/αα	100%
Silent carrier	3	αα/α–	75%
α-Thalassemia trait (mild anemia, microcytosis)	2	α–/α– or αα/– –	50%
Hb H (β_4) disease (moderately severe hemolytic anemia)	1	α–/– –	25%
Hydrops fetalis or homozygous α-thalassemia (Hb Bart's: γ_4)	0	– –/– –	0%

syndrome indicate that ATRX appears to be required to establish or to maintain the pattern of methylation in certain domains of the genome, perhaps by modulating the access of the methylase to its binding sites. This finding is noteworthy because mutations in the gene encoding another chromatin remodeling protein cause **Rett syndrome** (Case 35) by disrupting the epigenetic regulation of genes in regions of methylated DNA, leading to neurodevelopmental regression.

All the mutations identified to date in the *ATRX* gene are partial loss-of-function mutations. That ATRX is absolutely required for α-globin expression in vivo is not apparent from the study of patients with ATR-X syndrome, who have modest reductions in α-globin synthesis and mild hematological defects compared with those found in the classic forms of α-thalassemia. However, a key role for ATRX in α-globin expression has been revealed by the discovery that patients with an acquired disorder, **myelodysplasia associated with α-thalassemia,** have *somatic* mutations in the *ATRX* gene. In the most severe cases of α-thalassemia myelodysplasia syndrome, these mutations abolish α-chain synthesis almost completely, a consequence that would be developmentally lethal—causing Hb Bart's and hydrops fetalis (see earlier)—if it resulted from an inherited mutation.

The β-Thalassemias

The β-thalassemias share many features with α-thalassemia. Decreased β-globin production causes a hypochromic, microcytic anemia, and the imbalance in globin synthesis leads to precipitation of the excess α chains, which in turn leads to damage of the red cell membrane. In contrast to α-globin, however, the β chain is important only in the postnatal period (see Fig. 11-3). Consequently, the onset of β-thalassemia is not apparent until a few months after birth, when β-globin normally replaces γ-globin as the major non-α chain, and only the synthesis of the major adult hemoglobin, Hb A, is reduced. The excess α chains are insoluble, so that they precipitate in red cells and their precursors (Fig. 11-10), leading to destruction of the red cells and ineffective erythropoiesis. Because the δ gene is intact, Hb A$_2$ production continues, and in fact, elevation of the Hb A$_2$ level is unique to β-thalassemia heterozygotes. The level of Hb F is also increased, not because of a reactivation of the γ-globin gene expression that was switched off at birth, but because of selective survival and perhaps also increased production of the minor population of adult red blood cells that contain Hb F.

In contrast to α-thalassemia, the β-thalassemias are usually due to single–base pair substitutions rather than to deletions (Table 11-4). In many regions of the world where β-thalassemia is common, there are so

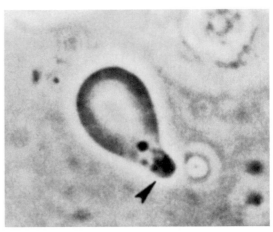

Figure 11-10 ■ Visualization of one pathological effect of the deficiency of β chains in β-thalassemia: the precipitation of the excess normal α chains to form a Heinz body in the red blood cell. Phase microscopy of a wet preparation of scrapings from the spleen of a patient with homozygous β-thalassemia shows an α chain inclusion body *(arrow)* within a teardrop-shaped red blood cell. Such inclusions are removed from the erythrocyte by reticuloendothelial cells, damaging the cell membrane and causing premature destruction of the cell. (From Nathan DG: Thalassemia. N Engl J Med 286:586-594, 1972.)

many different β-thalassemia mutations that persons carrying two β-thalassemia alleles are more likely to be **genetic compounds** than to be true homozygotes for one allele. Most individuals with two β-thalassemia alleles have **thalassemia major,** a condition characterized by severe anemia and the need for lifelong medical management. When the β-thalassemia alleles allow so little production of β-globin that no Hb A is present, the condition is designated β^0 thalassemia. If some Hb A is detectable, the patient is said to have β$^+$ thalassemia. Although the severity of the clinical disease depends on the combined effect of the two alleles present, survival into adult life was, until recently, unusual.

Infants with homozygous β-thalassemia present with anemia once the postnatal production of Hb F decreases, generally before 2 years of age. The red cells in peripheral blood are all markedly hypochromic and variable in size and shape. At present, treatment of the thalassemias is based on correction of the anemia and the increased marrow expansion by blood transfusion, and on control of the consequent iron accumulation by the administration of chelating agents. Bone marrow transplantation is effective, but this is an option only if an HLA-matched family member can be found.

Carriers of one β-thalassemia allele are clinically well and are said to have **thalassemia minor.** Such individuals have hypochromic, microcytic red blood cells and may have a slight anemia that can be misdiagnosed initially as iron deficiency. The diagnosis of thalassemia minor can be supported by hemoglobin electrophoresis, which generally reveals an increase in the level of Hb A$_2$ ($\alpha_2\delta_2$).

β-Thalassemia, Complex Thalassemias, and Hereditary Persistence of Fetal Hemoglobin   Almost every type of mutation known to reduce the synthesis of an mRNA or protein has been identified as a cause of β-thalassemia. The following overview of these genetic defects is therefore instructive about mutational mechanisms in general, describing in particular the molecular basis of one of the most common and severe genetic diseases in the world. Mutations of the β-globin complex are separated into two broad groups with different clinical phenotypes. One group of defects, which accounts for the great majority of patients, impairs the production of β-globin alone and causes **simple β-thalassemia.** The second group of mutations is one in which large deletions cause the **complex thalassemias,** in which the β-globin gene as well as one or more of the other genes—or the LCR—in the β-globin cluster is removed. Some deletions within the β-globin cluster do not cause thalassemia but rather a fascinating phenotype termed the **hereditary persistence of fetal hemo-globin** (i.e., the persistence of γ-globin gene expression throughout adult life).

The Molecular Basis of Simple β-Thalassemia   Simple β-thalassemia results from many different types of molecular abnormalities, predominantly point mutations, in the β-globin gene (Table 11-4 and Fig. 11-11). The only common β-globin deletion in any racial group is a 619-bp partial deletion of the 3' end of the gene in patients of Asian Indian origin. Most mutations causing simple β-thalassemia lead to a decrease in the abundance of the β-globin mRNA and include promoter mutants, RNA splicing mutants (the most common), mRNA capping or tailing mutants, and frameshift or nonsense mutations that introduce premature termination codons within the coding region of the gene. A few hemoglobin structural variants also impair processing of the β-globin mRNA, as exemplified by Hb E, described later.

RNA Splicing Mutations   The majority of β-thalassemia patients with a decreased abundance of β-globin mRNA have abnormalities in RNA splicing. More than two dozen defects of this type have been described, and their combined clinical burden is substantial. These

Table 11-4

The Molecular Basis of Simple β-Thalassemia

Type	Example	Phenotype	Affected Population
DELETIONS*			
β-globin gene deletions	619-bp deletion	β^0	Indian
DEFECTIVE mRNA SYNTHESIS			
RNA splicing defects (see Fig. 11-12)	Abnormal acceptor site of intron 1: **AG → GG**	β^0	Black
Promoter mutants	Mutation in the ATA box −31 −30 −29 −28 −31 −30 −29 −28 **A T A A → G T A A**	β$^+$	Japanese
Abnormal RNA cap site	A → C transversion at the mRNA cap site	β$^+$	Asian
Polyadenylation signal defects	AATAAA → AAC**A**AA	β$^+$	Black
NONFUNCTIONAL mRNAS			
Nonsense mutations	codon 39 gln → stop CAG → **U**AG	β^0	Mediterranean (especially Sardinia)
Frameshift mutations	codon 16 (1-bp deletion) *normal* trp gly lys val asn 15 16 17 18 19 UGG GGC AAG GUG AAC UGG GCA AGG UGA *mutant* trp ala arg stop	β^0	Indian
CODING REGION MUTATIONS THAT ALSO ALTER SPLICING*			
Synonymous mutations	codon 24 gly → gly GG**U** → GG**A**	β$^+$	Black

*One other hemoglobin structural variant that causes β-thalassemia is shown in Table 11-2.

Derived in part from Weatherall DJ, Clegg JB, Higgs DR, Wood WG: The hemoglobinopathies. In Scriver CR, Beaudet AL, Sly WS, Valle D (eds): The Metabolic and Molecular Bases of Inherited Disease, 7th ed. New York, McGraw-Hill, 1995, pp 3417-3484; and Orkin SH: Disorders of hemoglobin synthesis: the thalassemias. In Stamatoyannopoulos G, Nienhuis AW, Leder P, Majerus PW (eds): The Molecular Basis of Blood Diseases. Philadelphia, WB Saunders, 1987, pp 106-126.

mutations have also acquired high visibility because their effects on splicing are often unexpectedly complex, and analysis of the mutant mRNAs has contributed extensively to knowledge of the sequences critical to normal RNA processing (introduced in Chapter 3). The splice defects are separated into three groups (Fig. 11-12), depending on the region of the unprocessed RNA in which the mutation is located.

Group 1, splice junction mutations, includes mutations at the 5′ donor or 3′ acceptor splice junctions of the introns or in the consensus sequences surrounding the junctions. The critical nature of the conserved GT dinucleotide at the 5′ intron donor site and of the AG at the 3′ intron acceptor site (see Chapter 3) is apparent from the complete loss of normal splicing that results from mutations in these dinucleotides (Fig. 11-12B). The inactivation of the normal acceptor site elicits the use of other acceptor-like sequences elsewhere in the RNA precursor. These alternative sites are termed **cryptic splice sites** because they are normally not used by the splicing apparatus when the correct site is available. Cryptic donor or acceptor splice sites can be found in either exons or introns and may be used alone or in competition with other cryptic sites or the normal splice site.

The importance of the consensus sequences adjacent to the donor or acceptor dinucleotides is also illustrated by the effect of mutations. Thus, substitution of the fifth or sixth nucleotide of the donor sequence of intron 1 reduces the effectiveness of the normal splice event, but because some normal splicing still occurs, phenotypes are those of β⁺-thalassemia.

Group 2, intron mutations, result from mutations within an intron cryptic splice site that enhance the use of that site by making it more similar or identical to the normal splice site. An activated cryptic site then competes with the normal site, with variable effectiveness, thereby reducing the abundance of the normal mRNA by decreasing splicing from the correct site, which remains perfectly intact (Fig. 11-12C). Cryptic splice site mutations are often "leaky," which means that some use of the normal site occurs, producing a β⁺ thalassemia phenotype.

Group 3, coding sequence changes that also affect splicing, result from mutations in the open reading frame that may or may not alter the amino acid sequence but that activate a cryptic splice site in an exon. For example, a mild form of β⁺ thalassemia results from a mutation in codon 24 (see Table 11-4) that activates a cryptic splice site but does not change the encoded amino acid (both GGT and GGA code for glycine [see Table 3-1]); this is an example of a **synonymous mutation** that is not neutral in its effect. The structural variant Hb E (see later) demonstrates how both a splicing defect and a change in the coding sequence may result from a single mutation (Fig. 11-12D).

Nonfunctional mRNAs   Some mRNAs are nonfunctional and cannot direct the synthesis of a complete polypeptide because the mutation generates a premature stop codon, which prematurely terminates translation. Two β-thalassemia mutations near the amino terminus exemplify this effect (see Table 11-4). In one (Gln39Stop), the failure in translation is due to a single nucleotide substitution that creates a **nonsense muta-**

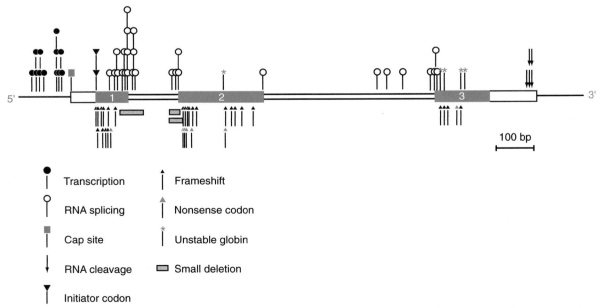

Figure 11-11 ■ Representative point mutations that cause β-thalassemia. Note the distribution of mutations throughout the gene and that the mutations affect virtually every process required for the production of normal β-globin. More than 100 different β-globin point mutations are associated with simple β-thalassemia. (Redrawn from Kazazian HH: The thalassemia syndromes: molecular basis and prenatal diagnosis in 1990. Semin Hematol 27:209-228, 1990.)

A **Normal splicing pattern**

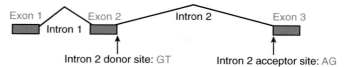

Figure 11-12 ■ Examples of mutations that disrupt normal splicing of the β-globin gene to cause β-thalassemia. **A,** Normal splicing pattern. **B,** An intron 2 mutation (IVS2-2A>G) in the normal splice acceptor site aborts normal splicing. This mutation results in the use of a cryptic acceptor site in intron 2. The cryptic site conforms perfectly to the consensus acceptor splice sequence (where Y is either pyrimidine, T or C). Because exon 3 has been enlarged at its 5′ end by inclusion of intron 2 sequences, the abnormal alternatively spliced mRNA made from this mutant gene has lost the correct open reading frame and cannot encode β-globin. **C,** An intron 1 mutation (G > A in base pair 110 of intron 1) activates a cryptic acceptor site by creating an AG dinucleotide and increasing the resemblance of the site to the consensus acceptor sequence. The globin mRNA thus formed is elongated (19 extra nucleotides) at the 5′ side of exon 2; a premature stop codon is introduced into the transcript. A β⁺ thalassemia phenotype results because the correct acceptor site is still used, although at only 10% of the wild-type level. **D,** In the Hb E defect, the missense mutation (Glu26Lys) in codon 26 in exon 1 activates a cryptic donor splice site in codon 25 that competes effectively with the normal donor site. Moderate use is made of this alternative splicing pathway, but the majority of RNA is still processed from the correct site, and mild β⁺ thalassemia results.

B **Mutation destroying a normal splice acceptor site and activating a cryptic site**

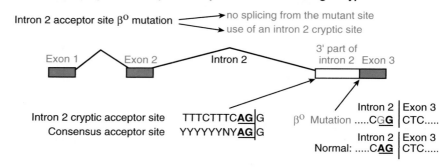

C **Mutation creating a new splice acceptor site in an intron**

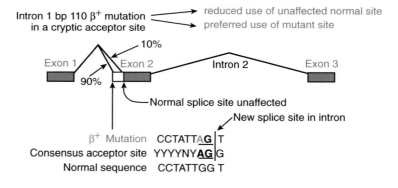

D **Mutation enhancing a cryptic splice donor site in an exon**

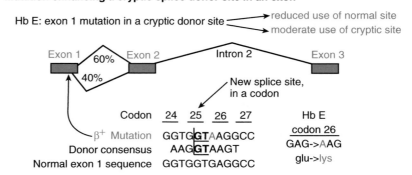

tion. In the other, a **frameshift mutation** results from a single–base pair deletion early in the open reading frame that removes the first nucleotide from codon 16, which normally encodes glycine; in the mutant reading frame that results, a premature stop codon is quickly encountered downstream, well before the normal termination signal. Because no β-globin is made, both of these types of nonfunctional mRNA mutations cause β⁰ thalassemia. In contrast, frameshifts near the carboxyl terminus of the protein allow most of the mRNA to be translated normally or to produce elongated globin chains, resulting in a variant hemoglobin rather than β⁰-thalassemia.

In addition to ablating the production of the β-globin polypeptide, nonsense codons, including the two described above, often lead to a reduction in the abundance of the mutant mRNA; indeed, the mRNA may be undetectable. The mechanisms underlying this phenomenon, called **nonsense-mediated mRNA decay,** are incompletely understood, but the effect appears to be restricted to nonsense codons located more than 50 base pairs 5′ to the final exon-exon junction.

Defects in Capping and Tailing of β-Globin mRNA   Two β⁺-thalassemia mutations highlight the critical nature of the post-transcriptional modifications of all mRNAs, the capping of the RNA at its extreme 5′ end (at the cap site) and the polyadenylation of the 3′ end of the mRNA (see Table 11-4). One patient was discovered to have an A to C transversion in the first nucleotide of the mRNA (the cap site is a purine in 90% of eukaryotic mRNAs). This mutation may impair the addition of the cap, thus exposing the RNA to degradation. The polyadenylation of mRNA occurs after its enzymatic cleavage, and the signal for the cleavage site, AAUAAA, is found near the 3′ end of most eukaryotic mRNAs. A patient with a substitution that changed the signal sequence to AACAAA produced only a minor fraction of β-globin mRNA that was polyadenylated at the normal position.

Variant Hemoglobins with Thalassemia Phenotypes

Hemoglobin E   Hb E is a β-globin structural variant (Glu26Lys) that causes thalassemia because the mutant β chain is synthesized at a reduced rate. It is probably the most common structurally abnormal hemoglobin in the world, occurring at high frequency in Southeast Asia, where there are at least 1 million homozygotes and 30 million heterozygotes. This allele is noteworthy for several reasons: its frequency, its allelic interaction with other β-globin mutants, and its effect on RNA splicing (see Table 11-2). Although Hb E homozygotes are asymptomatic and only mildly anemic, individuals who are genetic compounds with an Hb E mutation and various β-thalassemia alleles have abnormal pheno-

types that are largely determined by the severity of the other allele. Hb E is another example of a coding sequence mutation that also affects splicing through the activation of a cryptic splice site (Fig. 11-12D).

Complex Thalassemias and the Hereditary Persistence of Fetal Hemoglobin

The large deletions that cause the **complex thalassemias** remove the β-globin gene plus one or more other genes—or the LCR—from the β-globin cluster. Thus, affected individuals have reduced expression of β-globin and one or more of the other β-like chains. These disorders are named according to the genes deleted, that is, δβ⁰-thalassemia or $^A\gamma\delta\beta^0$-thalassemia, and so on. Deletions that remove the β-globin LCR start approximately 50 to 100 kb upstream of the β-globin gene cluster and extend 3′ to varying degrees (Fig. 11-13). Although some of these deletions (such as the Hispanic deletion) leave all or some of the genes at the β-globin locus completely intact, they ablate expression from the entire cluster to cause εγδβ-thalassemia. Such mutations demonstrate the total dependence on the LCR of gene expression from the β-globin gene cluster (see Fig. 11-4).

A second group of large β-globin gene cluster deletions of medical significance are those that leave at least one of the γ genes intact (such as the English deletion in Fig. 11-13). Patients carrying such mutations have one of two clinical manifestations, depending on the deletion: δβ⁰-thalassemia; or hereditary persistence of fetal hemoglobin (HPFH), a benign condition due to disruption of the perinatal switch from γ-globin to β-globin synthesis. Homozygotes with either of these conditions are viable because the remaining γ gene or genes are still active after birth, instead of switching off as would normally occur. As a result, Hb F ($\alpha_2\gamma_2$) synthesis continues postnatally at a high level, compensating for the absence of Hb A.

The clinically innocuous nature of HPFH is due to a substantial production of γ chains, producing a higher level of Hb F in heterozygotes (17% to 35% Hb F) than is generally seen in heterozygotes for δβ⁰-thalassemia (5% to 18% Hb F). The deletions that cause δβ⁰-thalassemia overlap with those that cause HPFH (see Fig. 11-13), and it is not clear why patients with HPFH have higher levels of γ gene expression. One possibility is that some HPFH deletions bring enhancers closer to the γ-globin genes (see Fig. 11-13). Insight into the mechanism leading to the high postnatal γ gene expression in patients with HPFH may make it possible to express Hb F at high levels in patients with β-thalassemia, a switch that would treat the disorder (see Chapter 13).

A few patients with HPFH have single–base pair substitutions in the upstream regulatory region of either the $^A\gamma$ or $^G\gamma$ genes. In Greek $^A\gamma$ HPFH, for example, there

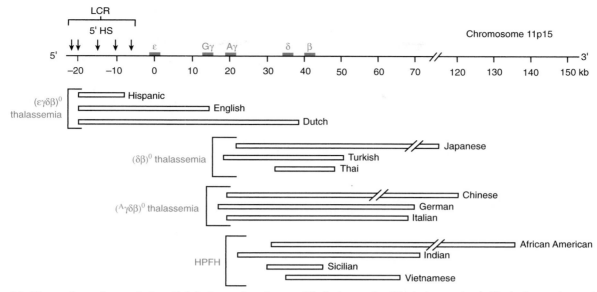

Figure 11-13 ■ Location and size of deletions of various εγδβ-thalassemia, δβ-thalassemia, ^Aγδβ-thalassemia, and HPFH mutants. Note that deletions of the locus control region (LCR) abrogate the expression of all genes in the β-globin cluster. The deletions responsible for δβ-thalassemia, ^Aγδβ-thalassemia, and HPFH overlap (see text). HPFH, hereditary persistence of fetal hemoglobin; HS, hypersensitive sites. (Redrawn from Stamatoyannopoulos G, Grosveld F: Hemoglobin switching. In Stamatoyannopoulos G, Majerus PW, Perlmutter RM, Varmus H [eds]: The Molecular Basis of Blood Diseases. Philadelphia, WB Saunders, 2001.)

is a G > A change a few bases 5′ to a CCAAT box (a promoter element; see Chapter 3) of the ^Aγ gene. These mutations are presumed to alter the affinity of regulatory (DNA-binding) proteins required for the postnatal repression of γ gene expression. Individuals with nondeletion HPFH are clinically normal; their genetic condition is recognized incidentally during hematological studies undertaken for other reasons.

Public Health Approaches to Preventing Thalassemia

Large-Scale Population Screening The clinical severity of many forms of thalassemia, combined with their high frequency, imposes a tremendous health burden on many societies. In Thailand alone, for example, the World Health Organization has determined that there are between half and three quarters of a million children with severe forms of thalassemia. To reduce the high incidence of the disease in some parts of the world, thalassemia control programs have been introduced, with considerable success. For example, in many parts of the Mediterranean, the birth rate of affected newborns has been reduced by as much as 90% through programs of education directed both to the general population and to health care givers. In Sardinia, a program of voluntary screening, followed by testing of the extended family once a carrier is identified, was initiated in 1975. In extended families at risk, the use

of carrier detection and prenatal diagnosis (see Chapter 15) reduced the birth of β-thalassemic newborns after 1999 from more than 100 per year (1 in 250 births) to fewer than 5 per year. Remarkably, these results were achieved by screening only about 11% of the population of the island (about 100,000 individuals), testifying to the efficacy of the screening strategy.

Screening Restricted to Extended Families In developing countries, the initiation of screening programs for thalassemia is a major economic and logistical challenge. Recent work in Pakistan, however, has demonstrated the effectiveness of a screening strategy that may be broadly applicable in countries where consanguineous marriages are common. In the Rawalpindi region of Pakistan, β-thalassemia was found to be largely restricted to a specific group of families with an affected proband. In 10 extended families with an index case, testing of almost 600 persons established that about 8% of the married couples examined consisted of two carriers, whereas no couple at risk was identified among 350 randomly selected pregnant women and their partners outside these 10 families. All carriers reported that the information provided was used to avoid further pregnancy if they already had two or more healthy children or, in the case of couples with only one or no healthy children, for prenatal diagnosis. Although the long-term impact of this program must be established, extended family screening of this type may contribute importantly to the control of recessive diseases in parts of the world where a cultural preference for consanguineous marriage is present. In other words, because of consanguinity, disease gene variants are "trapped" within extended families, so that an affected child is a marker of a group at high risk for the disease.

The initiation of carrier testing and prenatal diagnosis programs for thalassemia requires not only the education of the public and of physicians but also the establishment of skilled central laboratories and the consensus of the population to be screened. Whereas population-wide programs to control thalassemia are inarguably less expensive than the cost of caring for a large population of affected individuals over their lifetime, the temptation for governments or physicians to pressure any population into accepting such programs must be avoided, and the cultural and religious views of each community must be respected.

● GENERAL REFERENCES

Bunn FH: Human hemoglobins: sickle hemoglobin and other mutants. In Stamatoyannopoulos G, Majerus PW, Perlmutter RM, Varmus H (eds): The Molecular Basis of Blood Diseases, 3rd ed. Philadelphia, WB Saunders, 2001, pp 227-273.

Rachmilewitz E, Rund D: Beta-thalassemia. N Engl J Med 353:1135-1146, 2005.

Stamatoyannopoulos G, Grosveld F: Hemoglobin switching. In Stamatoyannopoulos G, Majerus PW, Perlmutter RM, Varmus H (eds): The Molecular Basis of Blood Diseases, 3rd ed. Philadelphia, WB Saunders, 2001, pp 135-182.

Weatherall DJ, Clegg JB, Higgs DR, Wood WG: The hemoglobinopathies. In Scriver CR, Beaudet AL, Sly WS, Valle D (eds): The Metabolic and Molecular Bases of Inherited Disease, 7th ed. New York, McGraw-Hill, 2001, pp 4571-4636.

● REFERENCES FOR SPECIFIC TOPICS

Ahmed S, Saleem M, Modell B, Petrou M: Screening extended families for genetic hemoglobin disorders in Pakistan. N Engl J Med 347:1162-1168, 2002.

Gibbons RJ, Higgs DR: Molecular-clinical spectrum of the ATR-X syndrome. Am J Med Genet 97:204-212, 2000.

Gibbons RJ, Pellagatti A, Garrick D, et al: Identification of acquired somatic mutations in the gene encoding chromatin-remodeling factor ATRX in the α-thalassemia myelodysplasia syndrome (ATMDS). Nat Genet 34:446-449, 2003.

Ingram VM: Specific chemical difference between the globins of normal human and sickle-cell anemia hemoglobin. Nature 178:792-794, 1956.

Patrinos GP, de Krom M, de Boer E, et al: Multiple interactions between regulatory regions are required to stabilize an active chromatin hub. Genes Dev 18:1495-1509, 2004.

Pauling L, Itano HA, Singer SJ, Wells IG: Sickle cell anemia, a molecular disease. Science 110:543-548, 1949.

Tufarelli C, Sloane Stanley JA, Garrick D, et al: Transcription of antisense RNA leading to gene silencing and methylation as a novel cause of human genetic disease. Nat Genet 34:157-165, 2003.

Vogt G, Chapgier A, Yang K, et al: Gains of glycosylation comprise an unexpectedly large group of pathogenic mutations. Nat Genet 37:692-700, 2005.

Weatherall DJ: The thalassemias: the role of molecular genetics in an evolving global health problem. Am J Hum Genet 74:385-392, 2004.

● USEFUL WEBSITES

OMIM: Online Mendelian Inheritance in Man. *http://www.ncbi.nim.nih.gov/entrez/query.fcgi?db=OMIM*

The Globin Gene Server (including a Hemoglobin Mutation database). *http://globin.cse.psu.edu*

PROBLEMS

1. A child dies of hydrops fetalis. Draw a pedigree with genotypes that illustrates to the carrier parents the genetic basis of the infant's thalassemia. Explain why a Melanesian couple whom they met in the hematology clinic, who both also have the α-thalassemia trait, are unlikely to have a similarly affected infant.

2. Why are most β-thalassemia patients likely to be genetic compounds? In what situations might you anticipate that a patient with β-thalassemia would be likely to have two identical β-globin alleles?

3. Tony, a young Italian boy, is found to have moderate β-thalassemia, with a hemoglobin concentration of 7 g/dL (normal amounts are 10 to 13 g/dL). When you perform a Northern blot of his reticulocyte RNA, you unexpectedly find three β-globin mRNA bands, one of normal size, one larger than normal, and one smaller than normal.

   What mutational mechanisms could account for the presence of three bands like this in a patient with β-thalassemia? In *this* patient, the fact that the anemia is mild suggests that a significant fraction of normal β-globin mRNA is being made. What types of mutation would allow this to occur?

4. A man is heterozygous for Hb M Saskatoon, a hemo-globinopathy in which the normal amino acid His is replaced by Tyr at position 63 of the β chain. His mate is heterozygous for Hb M Boston, in which His is replaced by Tyr at position 58 of the α chain. Hetero-zygosity for either of these mutant alleles produces met-hemoglobinemia. Outline the possible genotypes and phenotypes of their offspring.

5. A child has a paternal uncle and a maternal aunt with sickle cell disease; both of her parents do not. What is the probability that the child has sickle cell disease?

6. A woman has sickle cell trait and her mate is heterozy-gous for Hb C. What is the probability that their child has no abnormal hemoglobin?

7. Match the following:

   _____ complex β-thalassemia
   _____ β⁺-thalassemia
   _____ number of α-globin genes missing in Hb H disease
   _____ two different mutant alleles at a locus
   _____ ATR-X syndrome
   _____ insoluble β chains
   _____ number of α-globin genes missing in hydrops fetalis with Hb Bart's
   _____ locus control region
   _____ α–/α– genotype
   _____ increased Hb A₂

   1. detectable Hb A
   2. three
   3. β-thalassemia
   4. α-thalassemia
   5. high-level β-chain expression
   6. α-thalassemia trait
   7. compound heterozygote
   8. δβ genes deleted
   9. four
   10. mental retardation

8. Mutations in noncoding sequences change the number of protein molecules produced, but each protein mole-cule made will generally have a normal amino acid sequence. Give examples of some exceptions to this rule and describe how the alterations in the amino acid sequence are generated.

9. What are some possible explanations for the fact that thalassemia control programs, such as the successful one in Sardinia, have not reduced the birth rate of newborns with severe thalassemia to zero? For example, in Sardinia from 1999 to 2002, approximately two to five such infants were born each year.

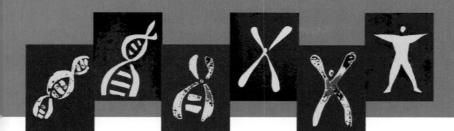

Chapter 12

The Molecular, Biochemical, and Cellular Basis of Genetic Disease

In this chapter, we extend the examination of the molecular and biochemical basis of genetic disease beyond the hemoglobinopathies to include other proteins and their corresponding diseases. In Chapter 11, we presented an outline of the general mechanisms by which mutations cause disease (see Fig. 11-1) and reviewed the steps at which mutations can disrupt the synthesis or function of a protein (see Table 11-1). Those outlines provide a framework for understanding the pathogenesis of all genetic disease. Although the hemoglobinopathies have taught us much about genetic disease, mutations in other classes of proteins often disrupt cell and organ function by processes that differ from those illustrated by the hemoglobinopathies.

To illustrate these other types of disease mechanisms, we generally use well-known disorders such as **phenylketonuria, cystic fibrosis, familial hypercholesterolemia, Duchenne muscular dystrophy,** and **Alzheimer disease.** In some instances, less common disorders are included because they best demonstrate a specific principle. The importance of selecting representative disorders becomes apparent when one considers that the genes associated with more than 1900 single-gene disorders have now been identified. It would be impossible to remember the molecular pathology and pathophysiology of each condition or even of every biochemical category of disease. Moreover, there are more than 2800 other suspected or known single-gene diseases in which the affected gene defect remains to be identified, and many more of the approximately 25,000 genes in the human genome will undoubtedly be shown, in the coming decades, to be associated with both monogenic and genetically complex diseases.

● DISEASES DUE TO MUTATIONS IN DIFFERENT CLASSES OF PROTEINS

Proteins carry out an astounding number of different functions, some of which are presented in Figure 12-1. Mutations in virtually every functional class of protein can lead to genetic disorders. The recognition that a disease results from abnormality in a protein of a particular class is often useful in understanding its pathogenesis and inheritance and in devising therapy. In this chapter, we describe important genetic diseases that affect representative proteins selected from the groups shown in Figure 12-1; many other of the proteins listed in Figure 12-1, and the diseases associated with them, are described in the Case Studies section.

Housekeeping Proteins, Specialty Proteins, and Genetic Disease

Proteins can be separated into two general classes on the basis of their pattern of expression: *housekeeping proteins,* which are present in virtually every cell and have fundamental roles in the maintenance of cell structure and function; and tissue-specific *specialty proteins,* which are produced in only one or a limited number of cell types and have unique functions that contribute to the individuality of the cells in which they are expressed. Most cell types of higher eukaryotes, such as humans, express 10,000 to 15,000 genes. In general, as many as 90% of the messenger RNA (mRNA) species found in a tissue are also present in many other tissues and encode shared housekeeping proteins. The remaining 10% or so encode the specialty

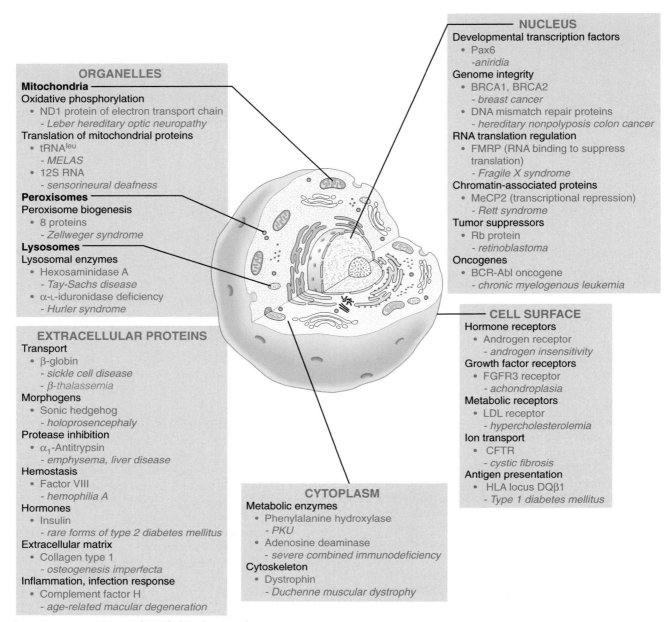

Figure 12-1 ■ Examples of the classes of proteins associated with diseases with a strong genetic component (most are monogenic), and the part of the cell in which those proteins normally function.

proteins of the tissue. Knowledge of the tissues in which a protein is expressed, and of the tissues in which it is expressed at high levels, is often useful in understanding the pathogenesis of a disease.

Two broad generalizations can be made about the relationship between the site of a protein's expression and the site of disease. First, mutation in a tissue-specific protein most often produces a disease restricted to that tissue, although there may be secondary effects on other tissues. However, the relationship between the site at which a protein is expressed and the site of pathological change in a genetic disease may, in some cases, be unpredictable. For example, mutation in a

tissue-specific protein may lead primarily to abnormalities in cells and organs that do not normally express the protein at all; ironically, the tissue expressing the mutant protein may be left entirely unaffected by the pathological process. This situation is exemplified by **phenylketonuria,** discussed later. Phenylketonuria is due to the absence of phenylalanine hydroxylase activity in the liver, but the brain (which does not express this enzyme), not the liver, is damaged by the high blood levels of phenylalanine due to the lack of hepatic phenylalanine hydroxylase. Consequently, one cannot necessarily infer that disease in an organ results from a mutation in a gene expressed

Table 12-1

The Various Types of Heterogeneity Associated with Genetic Disease

Type of Heterogeneity	Definition	Examples
Genetic heterogeneity Allelic heterogeneity	The occurrence of more than one allele at a locus	β-Thalassemia mutations in β-globin Phenylalanine hydroxylase mutations in PKU Perinatal lethal osteogenesis imperfecta (type II), from mutations in the α1 collagen gene
Locus heterogeneity	The association of more than one locus with a specific clinical phenotype	Biopterin metabolism defects causing hyperphenylalaninemia
Clinical or phenotypic heterogeneity	The association of more than one phenotype with mutations at a single locus	Phenylalanine hydroxylase mutations causing PKU, variant PKU, or non-PKU hyperphenylalaninemia α-L-Iduronidase mutations causing Hurler syndrome or Scheie syndrome

principally or only in that organ, or in that organ at all.

Second, although housekeeping proteins are by definition expressed in most or all tissues, genetic diseases that affect these proteins rarely cause pathological changes in every tissue. (Mutations in genes that are essential to every tissue, such as actin or DNA polymerase, are, in most instances, not likely to be compatible with live birth.) Rather, the clinical effects of mutations in housekeeping proteins are frequently limited to one or a few tissues. In principle, there are at least two reasons for the restricted impact on some tissues. In some instances, there may be **genetic redundancy,** a situation in which other genes with overlapping biological activities are expressed in a tissue and lessen the impact of the loss of function of the mutant gene to a subclinical level. Alternatively, a specific tissue may be affected because the protein in question is expressed abundantly there and serves a specialty function in that tissue. As we will see later, this situation is illustrated by **Tay-Sachs disease;** the mutant enzyme in this disorder is hexosaminidase A, an enzyme expressed in virtually all cells, but whose absence leads to a fatal neurodegeneration, leaving non-neuronal cell types unscathed.

The Relationship Between Genotype and Phenotype in Genetic Disease

Variation in the clinical phenotype observed in an inherited disease may be due to one of three types of genetic variation: allelic heterogeneity, locus heterogeneity, or the effect of modifier genes.

Allelic Heterogeneity As discussed in Chapter 7, genetic heterogeneity is most commonly due to the presence of multiple alleles at a locus, a situation referred to as allelic heterogeneity (Table 12-1). In many instances, there is a clear **genotype-phenotype** correlation between a specific allele and a specific phenotype. The most common explanation for the effect of allelic

heterogeneity on the clinical phenotype is that alleles that confer more **residual function** are often associated with a milder form of the principal phenotype associated with the disease. In other instances, however, alleles that confer some residual protein function are associated with only one or a subset of the complete set of phenotypes seen with a null allele. This situation prevails with certain variants of the major cystic fibrosis gene (the *CFTR* gene); these variants lead to **congenital absence of the vas deferens** but not the other manifestations of cystic fibrosis (see later).

A second explanation for allele-based variation in phenotype is that the variation may reflect the specific subfunction of the protein most perturbed by the mutation. In this case, some alleles may be associated with remarkably distinct clinical phenotypes. This situation is well illustrated by **Hb Kempsey,** a β-globin allele that maintains the hemoglobin in a high oxygen affinity structure (see Table 11-2), causing polycythemia because the reduced peripheral delivery of oxygen is misinterpreted by the hematopoietic system as being due to an inadequate production of red blood cells. Specific phenotypes, such as the polycythemia seen with Hb Kempsey, are often so different from the phenotypes associated with severe loss-of-function alleles (e.g., the thalassemias associated with a greatly reduced production of globin chains) that it is not at all obvious, from a clinical perspective, that these diseases result from mutations in the same protein.

Finally, the biochemical and clinical consequences of a specific mutation in a protein are often unpredictable. Thus, no one would have foreseen that the allele most commonly associated with α_1-**antitrypsin deficiency** (the Z allele) would lead to liver disease because the mutation causes the protein to form intracellular aggregates in hepatocytes (see later). Moreover, although rarely, a disease may be uniquely associated with only one or a few alleles, sickle cell disease being the classic example; this disorder has been observed only when the Glu6Val mutation is found on at least one β-globin

Table 12-2

The Locus Heterogeneity of the Hyperphenylalaninemias

Biochemical Defect	Incidence/ 10⁶ Births	Enzyme Affected	Gene Location	Inheritance	Treatment
Mutations in the Gene Encoding Phenylalanine Hydroxylase					
Classic PKU	5-350	PAH	12q24.1	AR	Low-phenylalanine diet*
Variant PKU	Less than classic PKU	PAH	12q24.1	AR	Low-phenylalanine diet (less restrictive than that required to treat PKU*)
Non-PKU hyperphenylalaninemia	15-75	PAH	12q24.1	AR	None, or less restrictive low-phenylalanine diet*
Mutations in Genes Encoding Enzymes of Tetrahydrobiopterin Metabolism					
Impaired BH₄ recycling	1-2	PCD	10q22	AR	Low-phenylalanine diet + L-dopa, 5-HT, carbidopa
		DHPR	4p15.31	AR	Low-phenylalanine diet + L-dopa, 5-HT, carbidopa + folinic acid
Impaired BH₄ synthesis	Rare	GTP-CH	14q22	AR	Low-phenylalanine diet + L-dopa, 5-HT, carbidopa + folinic acid, and pharmacologic doses of BH4
		6-PTS	11q22.3-23.3	AR	As with GTP-CH deficiency

*BH₄ supplementation may increase the PAH activity of some patients in each of these three groups.

AR, autosomal recessive; BH₄, tetrahydrobiopterin; DHPR, dihydropteridine reductase; GTP-CH, guanosine triphosphate cyclohydrolase; 5-HT, 5-hydroxytryptophan; PAH, phenylalanine hydroxylase; PCD, pterin 4α-carbinolamine dehydratase; PKU, phenylketonuria; 6-PTS, 6-pyruvoyltetrahydropterin synthase.

allele. Other alleles may lead to other clinical conditions, as we saw in Chapter 11, but not to sickle cell disease.

Locus Heterogeneity Genetic heterogeneity also arises from the association of more than one locus with a specific clinical condition, a situation termed locus heterogeneity (see Table 12-1 and Chapter 7). This phenomenon is illustrated by the discovery that mutations in any one of five genes can lead to hyperphenylalaninemia (Table 12-2). Once locus heterogeneity has been documented, careful comparison of the phenotype associated with each gene commonly reveals that the phenotype is not as homogeneous as initially believed.

Modifier Genes Sometimes even the most robust genotype-phenotype relationships are found not to hold for a specific patient. Such phenotypic variation can, in principle, be ascribed to environmental factors or to the action of other genes, termed modifier genes (see Chapter 8). To date, few modifier genes for human monogenic disorders have been identified. One example of a well-characterized modifier gene is the amelioration of disease in β-thalassemia homozygotes who also inherit an α-thalassemia allele, which in this case acts as a modifier gene. These β-thalassemia homozygotes sometimes have less severe β-thalassemia; the imbalance of globin chain synthesis that occurs in β-thalassemia, due to the relative excess of α chains, is ameliorated by the decrease in α-chain production that results from the α-thalassemia mutation. In another

example, patients with **cystic fibrosis** who are homozygous for the most common mutation have highly variable lung disease, and this variation has also been shown to be at least partly due to at least one modifier gene.

DISEASES INVOLVING ENZYMES

Enzymes are the biological catalysts that mediate, with great efficiency, the conversion of a substrate to a product. The diversity of substrates on which enzymes act is huge and is reflected in the fact that the human genome contains more than 5000 genes that encode enzymes. Not surprisingly, therefore, there are hundreds of human enzyme defects, or enzymopathies. We first discuss one of the best-known groups of inborn errors of metabolism, the hyperphenylalaninemias, which arise from deficient activity of phenylalanine hydroxylase. Several other enzyme defects of significance are then briefly examined. In a summary section, general features of the pathophysiology of enzymopathies are presented.

Aminoacidopathies

The Hyperphenylalaninemias

The abnormalities that lead to an increase in the blood level of phenylalanine, most notably phenylalanine hydroxylase deficiency or phenylketonuria, illustrate

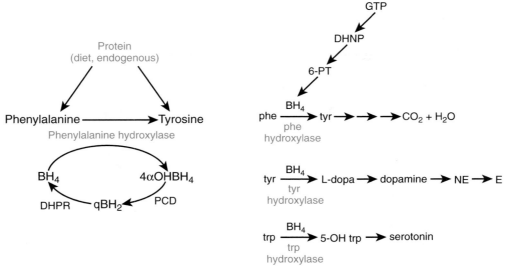

Figure 12-2 ■ The biochemical pathways affected in the hyperphenylalaninemias. BH$_4$, tetrahydrobiopterin; 4αOHBH$_4$, 4α hydroxytetrahydrobiopterin; qBH$_2$, quininoid dihydrobiopterin, the oxidized product of the hydroxylation reactions, which is reduced to BH$_4$ by dihydropteridine reductase (DHPR); PCD, pterin 4α-carbinolamine dehydratase; phe, phenylalanine; tyr, tyrosine; trp, tryptophan; GTP, guanosine triphosphate; DHNP, dihydroneopterin triphosphate; 6-PT, 6-pyruvoyltetra-hydropterin; L-dopa, L-dihydroxyphenylalanine; NE, norepinephrine; E, epinephrine; 5-OH trp, 5-hydroxytryptophan.

almost every principle of biochemical genetics of relevance to enzyme defects. The biochemical causes of hyperphenylalaninemia are illustrated in Figure 12-2, and the principal features of the disease associated with mutations at the five hyperphenylalaninemia loci are presented in Table 12-2. All of the genetic abnormalities of phenylalanine metabolism are due to loss-of-function mutations in the gene encoding phenylalanine hydroxylase (PAH) or in genes required for the synthesis or reutilization of its cofactor, tetrahydrobiopterin (BH$_4$).

Phenylketonuria   Classic phenylketonuria (PKU) has been justifiably termed the epitome of inborn errors of metabolism. It is an autosomal recessive disorder of phenylalanine catabolism, resulting from mutations in the gene encoding PAH, the enzyme that converts phenylalanine to tyrosine (see Fig. 12-2 and Table 12-2). The discovery of PKU by Følling in 1934 marked the first demonstration of a genetic defect as a cause of mental retardation. Because of their inability to degrade phenylalanine, patients with PKU accumulate this amino acid in body fluids. The hyperphenylalaninemia damages the developing central nervous system in early childhood and interferes with the function of the mature brain. A small fraction of total phenylalanine is metabolized by alternative pathways, producing increased amounts of phenylpyruvic acid (a keto acid and the compound responsible for the name of the disease) and other minor metabolites, which are excreted in the urine. Ironically, although the enzymatic defect has been known for decades, the exact neuropathological

mechanism by which the increase in phenylalanine damages the brain is still unknown. Importantly, the neurological damage due to the metabolic block in classic PKU may be largely avoided by dietary modifications that prevent phenylalanine accumulation. The management of PKU is a paradigm of the treatment of many metabolic diseases whose outcome can be improved by preventing accumulation of an enzyme substrate and its derivatives; this concept is described further in Chapter 13.

Newborn Screening   Population screening of newborns for PKU is done widely. PKU is the prototype of genetic diseases for which mass newborn screening is justified (see Chapter 17); the disorder is relatively common in some populations (up to about 1/2900 live births). Treatment, if it is begun early in life, is effective; without treatment, severe retardation is inevitable. The screening test is performed a few days after birth. A droplet of blood is obtained from a heel prick, dried on filter paper, and sent to a central laboratory for assay of blood phenylalanine levels and of the phenylalanine-to-tyrosine ratio. In the past, samples were collected before an infant left the hospital. The trend toward short post-delivery hospitalizations for mothers and newborns has modified that practice, however. The test is preferably not done before 24 hours of age because the phenylalanine level in PKU increases after birth. Positive test results must be confirmed quickly because delays beyond 4 weeks postnatally in the initiation of treatment have profound effects on the intellectual outcome of patients with PKU.

Variant Phenylketonuria and Non-Phenylketonuria Hyperphenylalaninemia Whereas PKU results from a virtual absence of PAH activity (less than 1% of that in controls), less severe phenotypes, designated non-PKU hyperphenylalaninemia and variant PKU (see Table 12-2), result when the mutant PAH enzyme has some residual activity.

Non-PKU hyperphenylalaninemia is defined by plasma phenylalanine concentrations below 1 mM when the patient is receiving a normal diet. This degree of hyperphenylalaninemia is only about 10-fold above normal, lower than the concentrations found in classic PKU (>1 mM). The moderate increase in phenylalanine in non-PKU hyperphenylalaninemia is less damaging to the brain or may even be benign if the increase is small (<0.4 mM), and affected individuals come to clinical attention only because they are identified by newborn screening. Their normal phenotype has been the best indication of the "safe" level of plasma phenylalanine that must not be exceeded in the treatment of patients with classic PKU. **Variant PKU** is a category that includes patients with phenylalanine tolerance intermediate between that of classic PKU and non-PKU hyperphenylalaninemia; such patients require some phenylalanine restriction in their diet but less than that required by patients with classic PKU. The association of these three clinical phenotypes with mutations in the *PAH* gene is a clear example of clinical heterogeneity (see Table 12-1).

The Hyperphenylalaninemias: Allelic and Locus Heterogeneity

The Molecular Defects in the Phenylalanine Hydroxylase Gene A striking degree of allelic heterogeneity at the *PAH* locus—more than 400 different mutations worldwide—has been identified in patients with hyperphenylalaninemia associated with classic PKU, variant PKU, and non-PKU hyperphenylalaninemia (see Table 12-2). The great majority of *PAH* alleles are individually rare mutations that impair PAH enzymatic activity and lead to hyperphenylalaninemia, although benign polymorphisms or less common benign variants have also been identified. Six different mutations account for about two thirds of known mutant chromosomes in populations of European descent (Fig. 12-3). Notably, six other mutations are responsible for slightly more than 80% of *PAH* mutations in Asian populations (see Fig. 12-3). The remaining disease-causing mutations are individually rare. To record and make this information publicly available, a *PAH* database has been developed by an international consortium.

In all populations, there is substantial genetic heterogeneity in the *PAH* mutant population. Owing to the high degree of allelic heterogeneity at the locus, most PKU patients in most populations are **compound**

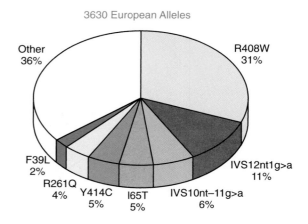

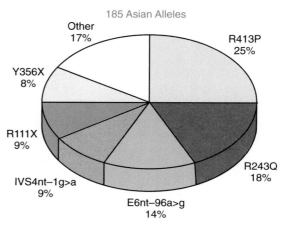

Figure 12-3 ■ The nature and identity of *PAH* mutations in populations of European and Asian descent (the latter from China, Korea, and Japan). The one-letter amino acid code is used (see Table 3-1), and mutation nomenclature is as described in Chapter 9. (Derived from Nowacki PM, Byck S, Prevost L, Scriver CR: PAH mutation analysis consortium database: 1997. Prototype for relational locus-specific mutation databases. Nucl Acids Res 26:220-225, 1998, by permission of Oxford University Press.)

heterozygotes (i.e., they have two different disease-causing alleles), a finding entirely in agreement with the enzymatic and phenotypic heterogeneity observed (see Table 12-1) in PAH defects. Although it first seemed that knowledge of the *PAH* genotype would reliably predict details of the phenotype, this expectation has not fully been borne out, although broad correlations between *PAH* genotype and biochemical phenotype have been identified. In general, mutations that eliminate or dramatically reduce the activity of the PAH enzyme cause classic PKU, whereas mutations that allow greater residual enzyme activity are associated with milder phenotypes. However, certain *PAH* mutations in homozygous patients have been associated with phenotypes ranging all the way from classic PKU to non-PKU hyperphenylalaninemia. Thus, it is now clear that other unidentified biological variables—undoubtedly including modifier genes—generate variation in the phenotype seen with a specific genotype. This observation, which has now been recognized to be a common feature of many single-gene diseases, highlights the fact that even monogenic traits like PKU are not genetically simple disorders.

Defects in Tetrahydrobiopterin Metabolism It was initially believed that all children with hereditary hyperphenylalaninemia had a primary deficiency of PAH. It is now clear, however, that in about 1% to 3% of these patients, the *PAH* gene is normal, and their hyperphenylalaninemia is the result of a genetic defect in any one of several different genes involved in the formation or recycling of the cofactor of PAH, BH_4 (see Fig. 12-2 and Table 12-2). The association of a single phenotype, such as hyperphenylalaninemia, with mutations in different genes is an example of locus heterogeneity (see Table 12-1). As illustrated by mutations in the genes encoding the PAH protein and the biopterin cofactor pathways (see Fig. 12-2), the proteins encoded by genes that manifest locus heterogeneity generally act at different steps in a single biochemical pathway. BH_4-deficient patients were first recognized because, despite the successful administration of a low-phenylalanine diet, they developed profound neurological problems in early life. This poor outcome is due in part to the requirement for the BH_4 cofactor of two other enzymes, tyrosine hydroxylase and tryptophan hydroxylase. Both of these hydroxylases are critical for the synthesis of monoamine neurotransmitters such as dopa, norepinephrine, epinephrine, and serotonin (see Fig. 12-2). BH_4-deficient patients have defects either in one of the steps in the biosynthesis of BH_4 from guanosine triphosphate or in the regeneration of BH_4 (see Fig. 12-2). Like classic PKU, these disorders are inherited as autosomal recessive traits.

It is critical to distinguish patients with a defect in BH_4 metabolism from subjects with mutations in *PAH* because their treatment differs markedly. First, since the PAH enzyme of individuals with BH_4 defects is normal, its activity can be restored if these patients are given large doses of oral BH_4, leading to a reduction in their plasma phenylalanine levels. Consequently, the severity of the phenylalanine restriction in the diet of patients with defects in BH_4 metabolism can be significantly reduced, and some of these patients can actually tolerate a normal (i.e., phenylalanine-unrestricted) diet. Second, one must also try to normalize the neurotransmitters in the brains of these patients by administering the products of tyrosine hydroxylase and tryptophan hydroxylase, L-dopa and 5-hydroxytryptophan, respectively (see Fig. 12-2 and Table 12-2). For these reasons, all hyperphenylalaninemic infants must be screened to determine whether their hyperphenylalaninemia is the result of an abnormality in BH_4 metabolism.

Tetrahydrobiopterin Responsiveness in *PAH* Mutations Many hyperphenylalaninemia patients with mutations in the *PAH* gene itself, rather than in BH_4 metabolism, will also respond with a substantial decrease in plasma phenylalanine levels when they are given large oral doses of the BH_4 cofactor of PAH. The patients most likely to respond are those with significant residual PAH activity (i.e., patients with variant PKU and non-PKU hyperphenylalaninemia), but even a minority of patients with classic PKU are also responsive. The presence of some residual PAH activity does not, however, necessarily guarantee an effect of BH_4 administration on plasma phenylalanine levels. Rather, the degree of BH_4 responsiveness will depend on the specific properties of each mutant PAH protein, reflecting the allelic heterogeneity underlying *PAH* mutations. BH_4 supplementation has been shown to exert its beneficial effect through one or more mechanisms, all of which result from the increased amount of the cofactor that is brought into contact with the mutant PAH apoenzyme. These mechanisms include stabilization of the mutant enzyme, protection of the enzyme from degradation by the cell, increase in the cofactor supply for an enzyme that has a low affinity for BH_4, and other beneficial effects on the kinetic and catalytic properties of the enzyme. The provision of increased amounts of a cofactor is a general strategy that has been employed in the treatment of many inborn errors of enzyme metabolism, as discussed further in Chapter 13.

Maternal Phenylketonuria The generally successful treatment of PKU allows affected homozygotes to lead an independent life and have nearly normal prospects for parenthood. In the past, the low-phenylalanine diet was discontinued for most patients with PKU in mid-childhood on the assumption (now shown to be incorrect) that function of the mature nervous system would not be impaired by the return of hyperphenylalaninemia. Subsequently, it was discovered that almost all the offspring of women with PKU not receiving treatment are abnormal; most of these children are mentally retarded, and many have microcephaly, growth impairment, and malformations, particularly of the heart. As predicted by principles of mendelian inheritance, all of these children are heterozygotes. Thus, their retardation is not due to their own genetic constitution but to the highly teratogenic effect of elevated levels of phenylalanine in the maternal circulation. Accordingly, it is imperative that women with PKU who are planning pregnancies commence a low-phenylalanine diet before conceiving.

Lysosomal Storage Diseases

Lysosomes are membrane-bound organelles containing an array of hydrolytic enzymes involved in the degradation of a variety of biological macromolecules. Genetic defects of these hydrolases lead to the accumulation of

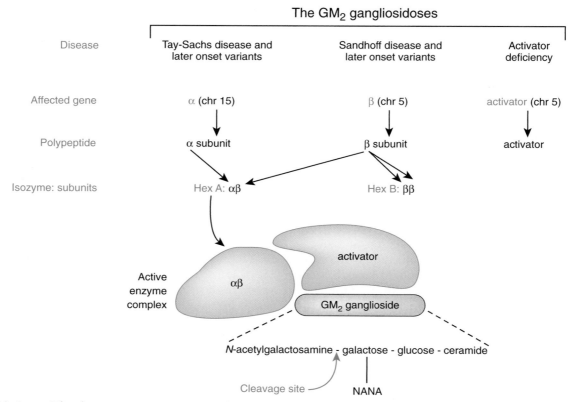

Figure 12-4 ■ The three-gene system required for hexosaminidase A activity and the diseases that result from defects in each of the genes. The function of the activator protein is to bind the ganglioside substrate and present it to the enzyme. NANA, *N*-acetyl neuraminic acid. (Modified from Sandhoff K, Conzelmann E, Neufeld EF, et al: The GM₂ gangliosidoses. In Scriver CR, Beaudet AL, Sly WS, Valle D [eds]: The Metabolic Bases of Inherited Disease, 6th ed. New York, McGraw-Hill, 1989, pp 1807-1839.)

their substrates inside the lysosome, resulting in cellular dysfunction and, eventually, cell death. The gradual accumulation of the substrate is responsible for the one uniform clinical feature of these diseases—their unrelenting progression. In most of these conditions, substrate storage is manifested clinically as an increase in the mass of the affected tissues and organs. When the brain is affected, however, as is often the case, the picture is one of neurodegeneration. The clinical phenotypes often make the diagnosis of a storage disease straightforward and usually suggest the class of storage disease, if not the specific disorder. More than 50 lysosomal hydrolase or lysosomal membrane transport deficiencies, almost all of which are autosomal recessive, have been described. Until recently, these diseases have generally not been amenable to treatment. However, the emergence of **enzyme replacement therapy** as a treatment (see Chapter 13) has dramatically improved the long-term prognosis of patients with some of these conditions.

Tay-Sachs Disease

Tay-Sachs disease (Case 38) is one of a group of heterogeneous lysosomal storage diseases, the GM₂ ganglio-sidoses, that result from the inability to degrade a sphingolipid, GM₂ ganglioside (Fig. 12-4). The biochemical lesion is a marked deficiency of hexosaminidase A (hex A). Although the enzyme is ubiquitous, the disease has its clinical impact almost solely on the brain, the predominant site of GM₂ ganglioside synthesis. Catalytically active hex A is the product of a three-gene system (see Fig. 12-4). These genes encode the α and β subunits of the enzyme (the *HEXA* and *HEXB* genes, respectively) and an activator protein that must associate with the substrate and the enzyme before the enzyme can cleave the terminal N-acetyl-β-galactos-amine residue from the ganglioside.

The clinical manifestations of defects in the three genes are indistinguishable, but they can be differentiated by enzymatic analysis. Mutations in the *HEXA* gene affect the α subunit and disrupt hex A activity to cause Tay-Sachs disease (or less severe variants of hex A deficiency). Tay-Sachs disease alleles lead to a profound deficiency of the α subunit mRNA and of hex A activity (Table 12-3). Defects in the *HEXB* gene or in the gene encoding the activator protein impair the activity of both hex A and hex B (see Fig. 12-4) to produce Sandhoff disease and activator protein deficiency (which is very rare), respectively.

```
                          ... − Arg − Ile − Ser − Try − Gly − Pro − Asp − ...
      Normal HEXA allele
                          ... CGT  ATA  TCC  TAT  GCC  CCT  GAC ...


                          ... CGT  ATA  TCT  ATC  CTA  TGC  CCC  TGA  C ...
      Tay-Sachs allele
                          ... − Arg − Ile − Ser − Ile − Leu − Cys − Pro − Stop

                                              Altered reading
                                                  frame
```

Figure 12-5 ■ Four-base insertion (TATC) in the hexosaminidase A gene in Tay-Sachs disease, leading to a frameshift mutation. This mutation is the major cause of Tay-Sachs disease in Ashkenazi Jews (see Table 12-3). No detectable hex A protein is made, accounting for the complete enzyme deficiency observed in these infantile-onset patients.

The clinical course of Tay-Sachs disease is particularly tragic. Affected infants appear normal until about 3 to 6 months of age but then gradually undergo progressive neurological deterioration until death at 2 to 4 years. The effects of neuronal cell death can be seen directly in the form of the so-called cherry-red spot in the retina, which is the prominent red fovea centralis surrounded by a pale macula. In contrast, *HEXA* alleles associated with some residual activity lead to later onset forms of neurological disease or, in the case of the pseudodeficiency alleles (discussed later), do not cause disease at all. In the later onset variants, the manifestations commonly include lower motor neuron dysfunction and ataxia due to spinocerebellar degeneration, but in contrast to the infantile disease, vision and intelligence usually remain normal, although psychosis develops in one third of these patients.

Population Genetics In many single-gene diseases, some alleles are found at higher frequency in some populations than in others (see Chapter 9). This situation is illustrated by Tay-Sachs disease, in which three alleles account for 99% of the Ashkenazi Jewish alleles, whereas two other alleles, neither of which is common in the Ashkenazi population, account for about 50% of the alleles in other populations (see Table 12-3). Approximately 1 in 27 Ashkenazi Jews is a carrier of a Tay-Sachs allele, and the incidence of affected infants is 100 times higher than in other populations. Either a founder effect

or heterozygote advantage is considered to be the most likely explanation for this high frequency. Because most carriers will have one of the three common alleles, a practical benefit of the molecular characterization of the disease in this population is the degree to which carrier screening has been facilitated.

Hex A Pseudodeficiency Alleles and Their Clinical Significance An unexpected consequence of screening for Tay-Sachs carriers in the Ashkenazi Jewish population was the discovery of a unique class of hex A alleles, the pseudodeficiency alleles. As their name implies, the two pseudodeficiency alleles are clinically benign. Individuals identified as pseudodeficient in screening tests are genetic compounds with pseudodeficiency alleles on one chromosome and a common Tay-Sachs mutation on the other chromosome. These individuals have a low level of hex A activity (in leukocytes, about 20% that of controls) that is still adequate to prevent the accumulation of the GM_2 ganglioside substrate in the brain. The importance of hex A pseudodeficiency alleles is 2-fold. First, they complicate prenatal diagnosis because a pseudodeficient fetus may be incorrectly diagnosed as affected. More generally, the recognition of the hex A pseudodeficiency alleles indicates that screening programs for other genetic diseases must recognize that comparable alleles may exist at other loci and may confound the correct characterization of individuals in screening or diagnostic tests.

Table 12-3

Nature and Frequency of Some Hexosaminidase A Alleles in Ashkenazi Jewish and Other Populations

Mutation	Effect on Gene Product	Estimated Frequency in Ashkenazi Jews	Frequency in Non-Ashkenazi	Homozygous Phenotype
4-bp insertion (exon 11); see Fig. 12-5	Premature stop codon	80%	16%-20%	Tay-Sachs disease
Exon 12 splice junction: G > C	Defective mRNA splicing	10%-15%	<1%	Tay-Sachs disease
Gly269Ser plus abnormal splicing	<3% residual activity	2%-3%	<1%	Adult-onset GM_2 gangliosidosis
Pseudodeficiency alleles	~20% residual activity	<1%	43%	Normal

Derived largely from Triggs-Raine BL, Feigenbaum ASJ, Natowicz M, et al: Screening for carriers of Tay-Sachs disease among Ashkenazi Jews. N Engl J Med 323:6-12, 1990; and Gravel RA, Clarke JTR, Kaback MM, et al: The GM_2 gangliosidoses. In Scriver CR, Beaudet AL, Sly WS, Valle D (eds): The Molecular and Metabolic Bases of Inherited Disease, 7th ed. New York, McGraw-Hill, 1995, pp 2839-2879.

Table 12-4

Examples of Mucopolysaccharidoses

Syndrome	Clinical Features	Enzyme Defect	Genetics	Comment
Hurler	Diagnosed early (<18 months), corneal clouding, skeletal changes, hepatosplenomegaly, coarse facies, death before the age of 10 years	α-L-Iduronidase	AR	Due to alleles that greatly impair enzyme activity
Scheie	Onset after the age of 5 years, normal intelligence and life span, corneal clouding, valvular heart disease	α-L-Iduronidase	AR	Apparently due to alleles that confer some residual enzyme activity
Hunter	Similar to Hurler syndrome, but with slower progression	Iduronate sulfatase	XR	A milder phenotype with variable central nervous system disease

AR, autosomal recessive; XR, X-linked recessive.
Modified from Neufeld EF, Muenzer J: The mucopolysaccharidoses. In Scriver CR, Beaudet AL, Sly WS, Valle D (eds): The Molecular and Metabolic Bases of Inherited Disease, 7th ed. New York, McGraw-Hill, 1995, pp 2465-2494.

The Mucopolysaccharidoses

Mucopolysaccharides, or glycosaminoglycans, are polysaccharide chains synthesized by connective tissue cells as normal constituents of many tissues. They are made up of long disaccharide repeating units; the nature of the two sugar molecules is the distinguishing feature of a specific glycosaminoglycan. The degradation of these macromolecules occurs in the lysosome and requires the stepwise removal of the monosaccharide unit at the end of the chain by an enzyme specific to the monosaccharide and the bond involved. A series of enzymes is thus required for the degradation of any one glycosaminoglycan, and a single enzyme often participates in the catabolism of more than one glycosaminoglycan.

The mucopolysaccharidoses are a heterogeneous group of more than a dozen storage diseases in which mucopolysaccharides accumulate in lysosomes as a result of a deficiency of one of the enzymes required for their degradation. In a specific mucopolysaccharidosis, one or more glycosaminoglycans may accumulate if the defective enzyme is required for their catabolism. The undegraded glycosaminoglycans appear in the urine, in which they can be detected by screening tests.

The first two mucopolysaccharidoses to be recognized were X-linked recessive **Hunter syndrome** and the more severe autosomal recessive **Hurler syndrome** (Table 12-4). Each of these conditions was originally called gargoylism because of the coarseness of the facial features of affected individuals (Fig. 12-6). Affected children are mentally retarded, have skeletal abnormalities and short stature, and manifest other abnormalities listed in Table 12-4.

Hurler syndrome is due to a severe deficiency of α-L-iduronidase. A clinically distinct disorder, **Scheie syndrome**, was originally thought to involve a different locus, principally because of its much milder phenotype. However, the Scheie and Hurler syndromes were found to be allelic, and the α-L-iduronidase mutations

that cause Scheie syndrome appear to be associated with higher residual activity.

The different patterns of inheritance of the autosomal Hurler and X-linked Hunter syndromes indicated that they were due to mutations in different genes. This difference has also been demonstrated in cell culture. Although fibroblasts from patients of either disease

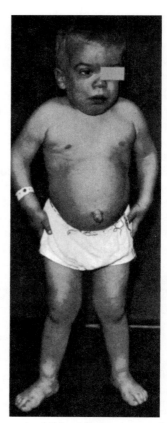

Figure 12-6 ■ A child with Hurler syndrome, showing the typical coarse facial features. At 5 years of age, he is only as tall as a typical 3-year-old. (From Smith DW: Recognizable Patterns of Human Malformation, 3rd ed. Philadelphia, WB Saunders, 1982.)

accumulate mucopolysaccharides in the culture medium, the accumulation is corrected by co-cultivation of both cell types in the same culture dish. The correction is due to the uptake by the α-L-iduronidase–deficient Hurler syndrome fibroblasts of normal α-L-iduronidase released by the Hunter syndrome fibroblasts; the converse phenomenon occurred in the cultured Hunter syndrome cells. This simple experiment was a powerful illustration of the fact that the two diseases affected different proteins. The demonstration that a product from the genome of one mutant is able to correct the biochemical defect in another mutant is termed **genetic complementation,** and studies used to determine whether genetic complementation can occur are termed **complementation analysis.**

The ability of a cell to take up the lysosomal enzyme that it lacks, from the extracellular fluid, is one mechanism by which the transplantation of normal cells (that would secrete the enzyme) into patients with storage diseases may correct, or complement, the biochemical defect in the rest of the body. Dramatic therapeutic benefits have been obtained by treatment of some patients with mucopolysaccharidoses, including Hurler syndrome, with bone marrow transplantation (see Chapter 13). The ability of cells to take up lysosomal enzymes from the extracellular fluid also provided the rationale for enzyme replacement therapy for many of these diseases, a strategy that has proved to be remarkably effective in many instances (see Chapter 13).

Altered Protein Function due to Abnormal Post-Translational Modification

A Loss of Glycosylation: I-Cell Disease

How do proteins get to their correct locations inside the cell? Many proteins have information contained in their primary amino acid sequence that directs them to their subcellular residence. Other proteins, however, are localized on the basis of post-translational modifications. This is true of the acid hydrolases found in lysosomes, but this form of cellular trafficking was unrecognized until **I-cell disease,** a severe autosomal recessive lysosomal storage disease, was investigated in the early 1970s. The disorder has a range of phenotypic effects involving facial features, skeletal changes, severe growth retardation, and mental retardation. Affected children typically survive for only 5 to 7 years. Cultured skin fibroblasts of patients with I-cell disease contain numerous abnormal lysosomes, or inclusions, throughout the cytoplasm (hence, inclusion cells or I cells).

In I-cell disease, many of the acid hydrolases normally present in lysosomes are found in excess in body fluids; their cellular levels are severely diminished. This unusual situation arises because the lysosomal hydro-

lases in these patients are abnormal secondary to a failure to be post-translationally modified. A typical hydrolase is a glycoprotein, the sugar moiety including mannose residues, some of which are phosphorylated. The mannose 6-phosphate residues are essential for recognition of the hydrolases by receptors on the cell and lysosomal membrane surface. In I-cell disease, there is a defect in the enzyme that transfers a phosphate group to the mannose residues. The fact that many enzymes are affected is consistent with the diversity of clinical abnormalities seen in these patients.

Gains of Glycosylation: Mutations That Create New (Abnormal) Glycosylation Sites

In contrast to the failure of protein glycosylation exemplified by I-cell disease, it has been shown that an unexpectedly high proportion (approximately 1.5%) of the missense mutations that cause human disease may be associated with abnormal gains of N-glycosylation due to mutations creating new consensus N-glycosylation sites in the mutant proteins. That such novel sites can actually lead to inappropriate glycosylation of the mutant protein, with pathogenic consequences, was revealed by the investigation of some individuals with a rare autosomal recessive disorder, **mendelian susceptibility to mycobacterial disease (MSMD).** Patients with MSMD may have defects in any one of a number of genes, including interferon receptors, that regulate the defense against infection. The consequence is that they are susceptible to disseminated infections on exposure to moderately virulent mycobacterial species, such as the bacillus Calmette-Guérin (BCG) used throughout the world as a vaccine against tuberculosis, or to nontuberculous environmental bacteria that do not normally cause illness. In a small subset of MSMD patients, the disease results from missense mutations in the gene for interferon-γ receptor 2 (IFNGR2) that generate novel N-glycosylation sites in the mutant IFNGR2 protein. These novel sites lead to the synthesis of an abnormally large, overly glycosylated receptor. The mutant receptors reach the cell surface but fail to respond to interferon-γ. Because removal of the new carbohydrate chains restores responsiveness, the loss of function of the receptor can be attributed to the increased glycosylation rather than to any other effect of the missense mutations that caused the disease. Mutations leading to gains of glycosylation have also been found to lead to a loss of protein function in the several other monogenic disorders.

An analysis of the Human Gene Mutation Database (see the URL among the references at the end of this chapter) reveals that missense mutations predicted to lead to gains of N-glycosylation are overrepresented among all missense mutations, suggesting that many

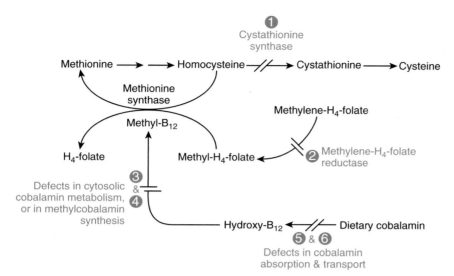

Figure 12-7 ■ The six types of genetic defects that can cause homocystinuria. (1) Classic homocystinuria is due to defective cystathionine synthase. (2) In methylene-H_4-folate reductase defects, the decrease in methyl-H_4-folate impairs the function of methionine synthase. (3) Several different defects in the intracellular metabolism of cobalamins lead to a secondary decrease in the synthesis of methylcobalamin (methyl-B_{12}) and thus in the function of methionine synthase. (4) Some disorders directly affect methylcobalamin formation. (5) Cobalamin intestinal absorption is abnormal in some patients. (6) Other patients have abnormalities in the major extracellular transport protein, transcobalamin II. Hydroxy-B_{12}, hydroxycobalamin.

inherited diseases may result from such mutations. It seems likely that mutations that increase O-glycosylation are also pathogenic. In contrast, mutations predicted to lead to a loss of N-glycosylation are underrepresented in the Human Gene Mutation Database, suggesting that, unlike the situation in I-cell disease, not all glycosylation events are critical for protein function. Finally, the discovery that removal of the abnormal polysaccharides restored function to the mutant IFNGR2 proteins associated with MSMD offers hope that disorders of this type may be amenable to chemical therapies that reduce the excessive glycosylation.

Loss of Protein Function due to Impaired Binding or Metabolism of Cofactors

Some proteins acquire biological activity only after they associate with cofactors, such as tetrahydrobiopterin in the case of phenylalanine hydroxylase, discussed earlier. Mutations that interfere with cofactor binding, synthesis, transport, or removal from a protein (when ligand binding is covalent) are also known. For many of these mutant proteins, an increase in the intracellular concentration of the cofactor is frequently capable of restoring some residual activity to the mutant enzyme, for example, by increasing the stability of the mutant protein. Consequently, enzyme defects of this type are among the most responsive of genetic disorders to specific biochemical therapy because the cofactor or its precursor is often a water-soluble vitamin that can be administered safely in large amounts.

Homocystinuria due to Cystathionine Synthase Deficiency: Impaired Cofactor Binding

Homocystinuria due to cystathionine synthase deficiency (Fig. 12-7) was one of the first aminoacidopa-

thies to be recognized. The clinical phenotype of this autosomal recessive condition is often dramatic. The most common features include dislocation of the lens, mental retardation, osteoporosis, long bones, and thromboembolism of both veins and arteries, a phenotype that can be confused with **Marfan syndrome,** a disorder of connective tissue (Case 26). The accumulation of homocysteine is believed to be central to much if not all of the pathological process.

Homocystinuria was one of the first genetic diseases shown to be vitamin-responsive; pyridoxal phosphate is the cofactor of the enzyme, and the administration of large amounts of pyridoxine, the vitamin precursor of the cofactor, often ameliorates the biochemical abnormality and the clinical disease (see Chapter 13). In many patients, the affinity of the mutant enzyme for pyridoxal phosphate is reduced, indicating that altered conformation of the protein impairs cofactor binding.

Disorders due to Abnormalities in the Metabolism of Cofactors

The loss of a protein's function is sometimes secondary to the decreased availability of an essential associated molecule, such as the cofactor for an enzyme. Dietary vitamin deficiencies—such as that of vitamin B_{12} (cobalamin), causing anemia and neurological disease, and vitamin D–deficiency rickets—exemplify acquired disorders of this type, but inherited disorders affecting the metabolism of the vitamin also cause disease. Not surprisingly, the phenotypes of the acquired and genetic diseases of vitamin cofactors frequently overlap. In other words, the acquired vitamin deficiency may be a partial or complete **phenocopy** of the genetic disorder. Thus, vegans are prone to acquired vitamin B_{12} deficiency, and if they become vitamin B_{12} deficient, they may have biochemical abnormalities similar to those associated with homocystinuria resulting from mutations, in a variety of genes that impair the provision of the vitamin B_{12} cofactor, methylcobalamin, to the enzyme methionine synthase (see Fig. 12-7).

Methionine synthase remethylates homocysteine to form methionine (see Fig. 12-7), and a loss of methionine synthase activity leads to homocystinuria. Numerous inherited disorders of vitamin B_{12} (cobalamin) transport or metabolism reduce the availability of methylcobalamin and therefore impair, secondarily, the

activity of methionine synthase. Several inherited defects of vitamin B_{12} metabolism reduce the intestinal absorption of cobalamin or its transport to other cells; others disrupt specific steps in cobalamin metabolism (see Fig. 12-7). The clinical manifestation of these disorders is variable but includes megaloblastic anemia, developmental delay, and failure to thrive. These conditions, all of which are autosomal recessive, are often partially or completely treatable with high doses of vitamin B_{12}.

●●● Enzyme Deficiencies and Disease: General Concepts

The following concepts are fundamental to the understanding and treatment of enzymopathies.

● **Enzymopathies are almost always recessive** (see Chapter 7).

Most enzymes are produced in quantities significantly in excess of minimal biochemical requirements, so that heterozygotes with about 50% of residual activity are clinically normal. In fact, many enzymes may maintain normal substrate and product levels with activities of less than 10% (e.g., hexosaminidase A). The enzymes of porphyrin synthesis are exceptions (see discussion of acute intermittent porphyria in main text, later).

● **Substrate accumulation or product deficiency**

Because the function of an enzyme is to convert a substrate to a product, all of the pathophysiological consequences of enzymopathies can be attributed to the accumulation of the substrate, to the deficiency of the product, or to some combination of the two (Fig. 12-8).

● **Diffusible versus macromolecular substrates**

An important distinction can be made between enzyme defects in which the substrate is a "small" molecule, such as phenylalanine, which can be readily distributed throughout body fluids by diffusion or transport, and defects in which the substrate is a macromolecule, such as a mucopolysaccharide, that remains trapped within its organelle or cell. The pathological change of the macromolecular diseases is confined to the tissues in which the substrate accumulates, whereas the site of the disease in the small molecule disorders is often unpredictable because the unmetabolized substrate, or its derivatives, can move freely throughout the body, damaging cells that may normally have no relationship to the affected enzyme.

● **Loss of multiple enzyme activities**

A patient with a single-gene defect may have a loss of function in more than one enzyme. There are several possible mechanisms: the enzymes may use the same cofactor (e.g., BH_4 deficiency); the enzymes may share a common subunit or an activating, processing, or stabilizing protein (e.g., the GM_2 gangliosidoses); the enzymes may be pro-

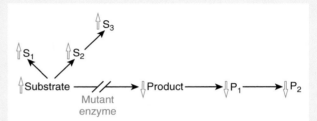

Figure 12-8 ■ A model metabolic pathway showing that the potential effects of an enzyme deficiency include accumulation of the substrate (S) or derivatives of it (S_1, S_2, S_3) and deficiency of the product (P) or compounds made from it (P_1, P_2). In some cases, the substrate derivatives are normally only minor metabolites that are formed at increased rates when the substrate accumulates (e.g., phenylpyruvate in phenylketonuria).

cessed by a common modifying enzyme, and in its absence, they may be inactive, or their uptake into an organelle may be impaired (e.g., I-cell disease, in which failure to add mannose 6-phosphate to many lysosomal enzymes abrogates the ability of cells to recognize and import the enzymes); and a group of enzymes may be absent or ineffective if the organelle in which they are normally found is not formed or is abnormal (e.g., the disorders of peroxisome biogenesis).

● **Phenotypic homology**

The pathological and clinical features resulting from an enzyme defect are often shared by diseases due to deficiencies of other enzymes that function in the same area of metabolism (e.g., the mucopolysaccharidoses) and by the different phenotypes that can result from partial versus complete defects of one enzyme. Partial defects often present with clinical abnormalities that are a subset of those found with the complete deficiency, although the etiological relationship between the two diseases may not be immediately obvious. For example, partial deficiency of the purine enzyme hypoxanthine guanine phosphoribosyltransferase causes only hyperuricemia, whereas a complete deficiency causes hyperuricemia as well as a profound neurological disease, Lesch-Nyhan syndrome, that resembles cerebral palsy.

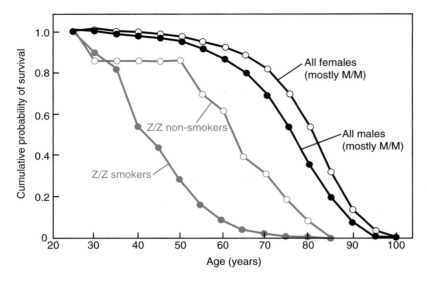

Figure 12-9 ■ The effect of smoking on the survival of patients with α₁-antitrypsin deficiency. The curves show the cumulative probability of survival to specified ages of smokers, with or without α₁-antitrypsin deficiency. (Redrawn from Larson C: Natural history and life expectancy in severe α₁-antitrypsin deficiency, PiZ. Acta Med Scand 204:345-351, 1978.)

α₁-Antitrypsin Deficiency: Mutations of an Enzyme Inhibitor

α₁-Antitrypsin (α1AT) deficiency is an important autosomal recessive condition associated with a substantial risk of chronic obstructive lung disease (emphysema) (Fig. 12-9) and cirrhosis of the liver. The α1AT protein belongs to a major family of protease inhibitors, the *seri*ne *p*rotease *in*hibitors or serpins. Although α1AT inhibits a wide spectrum of proteases, and despite its name, its principal role is to bind and inhibit elastase, particularly elastase released from neutrophils in the lower respiratory tract.

In white populations, α1AT deficiency affects about 1 in 5000 persons, and 2% are carriers. A dozen or so α1AT alleles are associated with an increased risk of lung or liver disease, but only the Z allele (Glu342Lys) is relatively common. The reason for the relatively high frequency of the Z allele in white populations is unknown, but analysis of DNA haplotypes suggests a single origin with subsequent spread in northern Europe. Given the increased risk of emphysema, α1AT deficiency is an important public health problem, affecting an estimated 60,000 persons in the United States alone.

The *α1AT* gene is expressed principally in the liver, which normally secretes α1AT into plasma. About 17% of Z/Z homozygotes present with neonatal jaundice, and approximately 20% of this group subsequently develop cirrhosis. The liver disease associated with the Z allele is thought to result from a novel property of the mutant protein—its tendency to aggregate, trapping it within the rough endoplasmic reticulum of hepatocytes. The molecular basis of the Z protein aggregation is a consequence of structural changes in the Z protein that predispose to the formation of long bead-like necklaces of mutant α1AT polymers. Thus, like the sickle cell disease mutation in β-globin (see Chapter 11), the

Z allele of α1AT is a clear example of a mutation that confers a novel property (in both of these examples, a tendency to aggregate) on the protein (see Fig. 11-1).

Both sickle cell disease and α1AT deficiency associated with homozygosity for the Z allele are examples of inherited **conformational diseases.** Inherited conformational diseases occur when a mutation causes the shape or size of a protein to change in a way that predisposes it to self-association and tissue deposition. In these disorders, some fraction of the mutant protein is invariably correctly folded, and this is indeed the case with α1AT deficiency. Note that not all conformational diseases are single-gene disorders, as illustrated, for example, by nonfamilial Alzheimer disease (discussed later) and prion diseases.

The lung disease associated with the Z allele of α1AT deficiency is due to the alteration of the normal balance between elastase and α1AT, which allows progressive degradation of the elastin of alveolar walls (Fig. 12-10). Two mechanisms contribute to the elastase:α1AT imbalance. First, the block in the hepatic secretion of the Z-mutated protein, although not complete, is severe, and Z/Z patients have only about 15% of the normal plasma concentration of α1AT. Second, α1AT with the Z mutation has only about 20% of the ability of the normal α1AT protein to inhibit neutrophil elastase. The infusion of normal α1AT is used in some patients to augment the level of α1AT in the plasma, to rectify the elastase:α1AT imbalance. This protein replacement strategy has been shown to be clinically beneficial in selected patients with this genetic disease, as discussed in Chapter 13.

α₁-Antitrypsin Deficiency as an Ecogenetic Disease

The development of lung or liver disease in subjects with α1AT deficiency is highly variable, and although

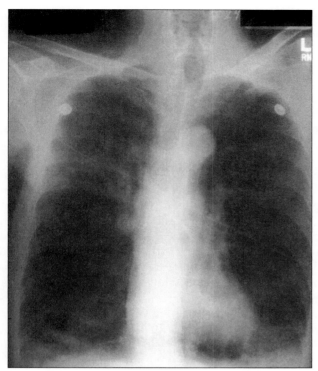

Figure 12-10 ■ A posteroanterior chest radiograph of an individual carrying two *Z* alleles of the *α1AT* gene, showing the hyperinflation and basal hyperlucency characteristic of emphysema. (From Stoller JK, Aboussouan LS: α₁-Antitrypsin deficiency. Lancet 365:2225-2236, 2005.)

the phenotype of a genetic disease. Thus, for persons with the *Z/Z* genotype, survival after 60 years of age is approximately 60% in nonsmokers but only about 10% in smokers (see Fig. 12-9). One molecular explanation for the effect of smoking is that the active site of α1AT, at methionine 358, is oxidized by both cigarette smoke and inflammatory cells, thus reducing its affinity for elastase by 2000-fold.

The field of **ecogenetics**, illustrated by α1AT deficiency, is concerned with the interaction between environmental factors and different human genotypes. This area of medical genetics is likely to be one of increasing importance as genotypes are identified that entail an increased risk of disease on exposure to certain environmental agents (e.g., drugs, foods, industrial chemicals, and viruses). In addition, genetic variation that may not by itself produce disease will be subject to increasing scrutiny in the search for the genetic contribution to nonmendelian disorders, such as diabetes mellitus (see Chapter 8). At present, the most highly developed area of ecogenetics is that of pharmacogenetics, which is discussed in Chapter 18.

Acute Intermittent Porphyria: A Defect in the Regulation of Gene Expression

Acute intermittent porphyria is an autosomal dominant disease associated with intermittent neurological dysfunction. The primary defect in acute intermittent porphyria is a deficiency of porphobilinogen deaminase, an enzyme in the biosynthetic pathway of heme (Fig. 12-11), and as we will describe, altered regulation of the genes that control the synthesis of heme is responsible for the pathophysiological features. All patients with acute intermittent porphyria, whether their disease is clinically latent, as in 90% of patients throughout

no modifier genes have yet been identified, a major environmental variable, cigarette smoke, has been found to dramatically influence the likelihood of development of emphysema. The impact of smoking on the progression of the emphysema is a powerful example of the effect that environmental factors may have on

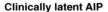

Clinically latent AIP

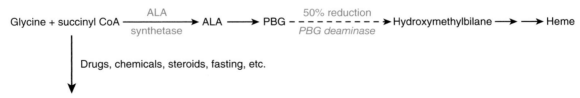

Clinically expressed AIP: post-pubertal neurologic symptoms

Figure 12-11 ■ The pathogenesis of acute intermittent porphyria (AIP). Patients with AIP who are either clinically latent or clinically affected have about half the control levels of porphobilinogen (PBG) deaminase. When the activity of hepatic δ-aminolevulinic acid (ALA) synthase is increased in carriers by exposure to inducing agents (e.g., drugs, chemicals), the synthesis of ALA and PBG is increased. The residual PBG deaminase activity (approximately 50% of controls) is overloaded, and the accumulation of ALA and PBG causes clinical disease. (Redrawn from Kappas A, Sassa S, Galbraith RA, Nordmann Y: The porphyrias. In Scriver CR, Beaudet AL, Sly WS, Valle D [eds]: The Metabolic Bases of Inherited Disease, 6th ed. New York, McGraw-Hill, 1989, pp 1305-1365.)

their lifetime, or clinically expressed, as in about 10%, have an approximately 50% reduction in the enzymatic activity of porphobilinogen deaminase. This reduction is consistent with the autosomal dominant inheritance (see Chapter 7).

Clinical expression of the disease occurs in response to events that decrease the concentration of heme in the liver cell. These precipitating factors include drugs (most prominently the barbiturates, and to this extent, acute intermittent porphyria is a pharmacogenetic disease; see Chapter 18), some steroid hormones (clinical disease is rare before puberty or after menopause), and catabolic states including reducing diets, intercurrent illnesses, and surgery. Exposure to the precipitating factors increases the synthesis of hepatic cytochromes P450, a class of heme-containing proteins discussed in Chapter 18. As a result, the cellular level of heme falls, reducing the feedback inhibition of heme on δ-aminolevulinic acid synthase, the rate-limiting step in the heme synthesis pathway (see Fig. 12-11). The increased expression of the synthase is achieved by both transcriptional and translational mechanisms. Thus, the relative heme deficiency caused by the reduction in porphobilinogen deaminase and the consequent decrease in heme pools is responsible for a *secondary* increase in the synthase to levels greater than the normal range. The fact that half of the normal activity of porphobilinogen deaminase is inadequate to cope with the metabolic load in some situations accounts for both the dominant expression of the condition and the episodic nature of the clinical illness. The pathogenesis of the nervous system disease is uncertain, but it may be mediated by the increased levels of the porphyrin precursors δ-aminolevulinic acid and porphobilinogen (see Fig. 12-11). The peripheral, autonomic, and central nervous systems are all affected, and the clinical manifestations are diverse. Indeed, this disorder is one of the great mimics in clinical medicine, with manifestations ranging from acute abdominal pain to psychosis.

● DEFECTS IN RECEPTOR PROTEINS

The recognition of a class of diseases due to defects in receptor molecules began with the identification, by Goldstein and Brown in 1974, of the low-density lipoprotein (LDL) receptor as the polypeptide affected in the most common form of familial hypercholesterolemia. This disorder, which leads to a greatly increased risk of myocardial infarction, is characterized by elevation of plasma cholesterol carried by LDL, the principal cholesterol transport protein in plasma. Goldstein and Brown's discovery has cast much light on normal cholesterol metabolism and on the biology of cell surface receptors in general. LDL receptor deficiency is repre-

sentative of a number of disorders now recognized to result from receptor defects.

Familial Hypercholesterolemia: A Genetic Hyperlipidemia

Familial hypercholesterolemia belongs to a group of metabolic disorders called the hyperlipoproteinemias, which are characterized by elevated levels of plasma lipids (cholesterol, triglycerides, or both) and specific plasma lipoproteins. Other monogenic hyperlipoproteinemias, each with distinct biochemical and clinical phenotypes, have also been recognized.

In addition to mutations in the LDL receptor, abnormalities in three other genes have also been found to lead to familial hypercholesterolemia (Fig. 12-12 and Table 12-5). Remarkably, all four of the genes associated with familial hypercholesterolemia disrupt either the function or abundance of the LDL receptor at its correct cell surface location, or apoprotein B-100, the protein component of the LDL ligand of the receptor. Accordingly, it is not surprising that the clinical phenotypes of individuals carrying mutations in these four genes are difficult to distinguish. Because of its particular importance, we will review here familial hypercholesterolemia due to mutations in the LDL receptor. We also discuss mutations in the *PCSK9* protease gene; although some mutations in this gene cause hypercholesterolemia, the greater importance of *PCSK9* lies in the fact that several of its common sequence variants *lower* the plasma LDL cholesterol level in the general population, conferring substantial *protection* from coronary heart disease.

Familial Hypercholesterolemia due to Mutations in the LDL Receptor

Mutations in the gene encoding the LDL receptor are the most common cause of familial hypercholesterolemia (see Table 12-5) (Case 14). The receptor is a cell surface protein responsible for binding LDL and delivering it to the cell interior. Both heterozygotes and homozygotes develop premature heart disease as a result of atheromas (deposits of LDL-derived cholesterol in the coronary arteries), xanthomas (cholesterol deposits in skin and tendons; see Fig. 7-13), and arcus corneae (deposits of cholesterol around the periphery of the cornea). Few diseases have been as thoroughly characterized; the sequence of pathological events from the affected locus to its effect on individuals and populations has been meticulously documented.

Genetics   Familial hypercholesterolemia due to mutations in the LDL receptor is inherited as an autosomal semi-dominant trait. Both homozygous and heterozygous phenotypes are known, and a clear gene dosage effect is evident; the disease manifests earlier and much

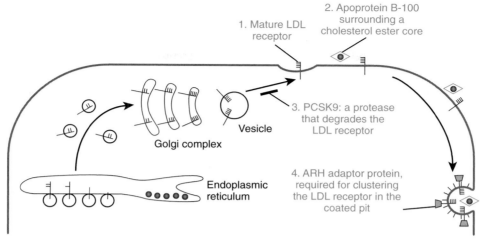

Figure 12-12 ■ The four proteins associated with familial hypercholesterolemia. The LDL receptor binds apoprotein B-100. Mutations in the LDL receptor binding domain of apoprotein B-100 impair LDL binding to its receptor, reducing the removal of LDL cholesterol from the circulation. Clustering of the LDL receptor–apoprotein B-100 complex in clathrin-coated pits requires the ARH adaptor protein, which links the receptor to the endocytic machinery of the coated pit. Homozygous mutations in the ARH protein impair the internalization of the LDL:LDL receptor complex, thereby impairing LDL clearance. PCSK9 protease activity leads to degradation of the LDL receptor (see text).

more severely in homozygotes than in heterozygotes (see Fig. 7-13), reflecting the greater reduction in the number of LDL receptors and the greater elevation in plasma LDL cholesterol (Fig. 12-13). Homozygotes may have clinically significant coronary heart disease in childhood, and few live beyond the third decade. The heterozygous form of the disease, with a population frequency of about 1 in 500, is one of the most common human single-gene disorders. Heterozygotes have levels of plasma cholesterol that are about twice those of controls (see Fig. 12-13). Because of the inherited nature of familial hypercholesterolemia, it is important to make the diagnosis in the approximately 5% of survivors of myocardial infarction that are heterozygotes for an LDL receptor defect. However, only about 1 in 20 individuals in the general population with increased plasma cholesterol and a hyperlipoproteinemia pattern

like that seen with heterozygous deficiency of the LDL receptor has familial hypercholesterolemia; most such individuals have an uncharacterized hypercholesterolemia of multifactorial origin (see Chapter 8).

Cholesterol Uptake by the LDL Receptor Normal cells obtain cholesterol from either de novo synthesis or the uptake from plasma of exogenous cholesterol bound to LDL. The uptake is mediated by the LDL receptor, which recognizes apoprotein B-100, the protein moiety of LDL. LDL receptors on the cell surface are localized to invaginations (coated pits) lined by the protein clathrin (Fig. 12-12). Receptor-bound LDL is brought into the cell by endocytosis of the coated pits, which ultimately evolve into lysosomes in which LDL is hydrolyzed to release free cholesterol. The increase in free intracellular cholesterol reduces endogenous cholesterol

Table 12-5

The Four Genes Associated with Familial Hypercholesterolemia

Mutant Gene Product	Pattern of Inheritance	Prevalence	Effect of Disease-Causing Mutations	Typical LDL Cholesterol Level (Normal Adults: ~120 mg/dL)
LDL receptor	Autosomal dominant	Heterozygotes: 1/500 Homozygotes: 1/million	Loss of function	Heterozygotes: 350 mg/dL Homozygotes: 700 mg/dL
Apoprotein B-100	Autosomal dominant	Heterozygotes: 1/1000* Homozygotes: 1/million*	Loss of function	Heterozygotes: 270 mg/dL Homozygotes: 320 mg/dL
ARH adaptor protein	Autosomal recessive	Very rare†	Loss of function	Homozygotes: 470 mg/dL
PCSK9 protease	Autosomal dominant	Very rare	Gain of function	Heterozygotes: 225 mg/dL

*Principally in individuals of European descent.
†Principally in individuals of Italian and Middle Eastern descent.
Partly modified from Goldstein JL, Brown MS: The cholesterol quartet. Science 292:1310-1312, 2001.

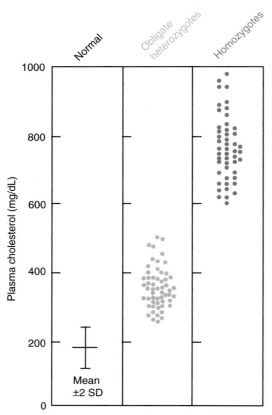

Figure 12-13 ■ Gene dosage in LDL deficiency: the distribution of total plasma cholesterol levels in 49 patients homozygous for deficiency of the LDL receptor, in their parents (obligate heterozygotes), and in normal controls. (Redrawn from Goldstein JL, Brown MS: Familial hypercholesterolemia. In Scriver CR, Beaudet AL, Sly WS, Valle D [eds]: The Metabolic Bases of Inherited Disease, 6th ed. New York, McGraw-Hill, 1989, pp 1215-1250.)

formation by suppressing the rate-limiting enzyme of the synthetic pathway (3-hydroxy-3-methylglutaryl coenzyme A reductase). Cholesterol not required for cellular metabolism or membrane synthesis may be re-esterified for storage as cholesteryl esters, a process stimulated by the activation of acyl coenzyme A:cholesterol acyltransferase. The increase in intracellular cholesterol also reduces synthesis of the receptor (see Fig. 12-14).

Classes of Mutations in the LDL Receptor   More than 700 different mutations have been identified in the LDL receptor gene, and these are distributed throughout the sequence. (It is often unclear whether all of these variant sequences are actually pathogenic or whether some are normal variants with no phenotypic effect.) The great majority of alleles are single nucleotide substitutions, small insertions, or deletions; structural rearrangements account for only 2% to 10% of the LDL receptor alleles in most populations. The mature LDL receptor has five distinct structural domains that for the most part have distinguishable functions (Fig. 12-15). Analysis of the effect on the receptor of mutations in each domain has played an important role in defining the function of each domain. These studies exemplify the important contribution that genetic analysis can make in determining the structure-function relationships of a protein.

Fibroblasts cultured from affected patients have been used to characterize the mutant receptors and the resulting disturbances in cellular cholesterol metabolism. Mutations in the LDL receptor gene can be grouped into six classes, depending on which step of the normal cellular itinerary of the receptor is disrupted by the mutation (see Fig. 12-14). Class 1 mutations are null alleles that prevent the synthesis of any detectable receptor; they are the most common type of disease-causing mutations at this locus. In the remaining five classes, the receptor is synthesized normally, but its function is impaired.

Mutations in classes 2, 4, and 6 (see Fig. 12-14) define features of the polypeptide critical to its subcellular localization. The relatively common class 2 mutations are designated *transport-deficient* because the LDL receptors accumulate at the site of their synthesis, the endoplasmic reticulum, instead of being transported to the Golgi complex. These alleles are predicted to prevent proper folding of the protein, an apparent requisite for exit from the endoplasmic reticulum. Class 3 mutant receptors reach the cell surface but are incapable of binding LDL (see Fig. 12-14). Consequently, these alleles have enabled researchers to identify the LDL-binding domain (see Fig. 12-15). Class 4 mutations impair localization of the receptor to the coated pit, and consequently the bound LDL is not internalized (see Fig. 12-14). These mutations alter or remove the cytoplasmic domain at the carboxyl terminus of the receptor, demonstrating that this region normally targets the receptor to the coated pit. Class 5 mutations are recycling-defective alleles (see Fig. 12-14). Receptor recycling requires the dissociation of the receptor and the bound LDL in the endosome. Mutations in the epidermal growth factor precursor homology domain (see Fig. 12-15) prevent the release of the LDL ligand. This failure leads to degradation of the receptor, presumably because an occupied receptor cannot return to the cell surface.

The PCSK9 Protease and Its Relationship to LDL Cholesterol

Gain-of-function missense mutations in the gene encoding the PCSK9 protease have been found to be a rare cause of autosomal dominant familial hypercholesterolemia. Experimental work indicates that increased PCSK9 protease activity leads to degradation of the LDL receptor (although whether the receptor is the

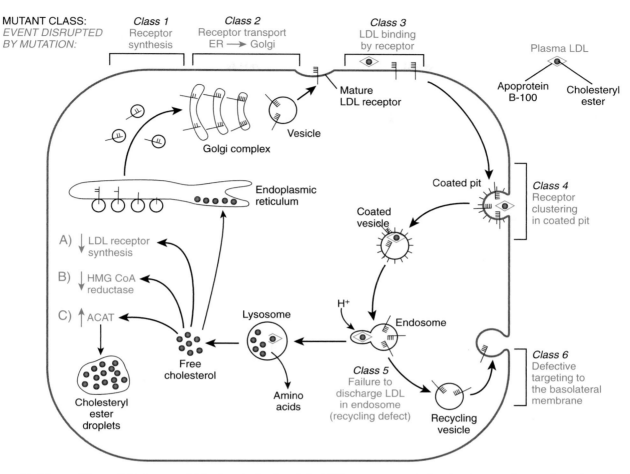

Figure 12-14 ■ The cell biology and biochemical role of the LDL receptor and the six classes of mutations that alter its function. After synthesis in the endoplasmic reticulum (ER), the receptor is transported to the Golgi apparatus and subsequently to the cell surface. Normal receptors are localized to clathrin-coated pits, which invaginate, creating coated vesicles and then endosomes, the precursors of lysosomes. Normally, intracellular accumulation of free cholesterol is prevented because the increase in free cholesterol (A) decreases the formation of LDL receptors, (B) reduces de novo cholesterol synthesis, and (C) increases the storage of cholesteryl esters. The biochemical phenotype of each class of mutant is discussed in the text. ACAT, acyl coenzyme A:cholesterol acyltransferase; HMG CoA reductase, 3-hydroxy-3-methylglutaryl coenzyme A reductase. (Modified from Brown MS, Goldstein JL: The LDL receptor and HMG-CoA reductase—two membrane molecules that regulate cholesterol homeostasis. Curr Top Cell Regul 26:3-15, 1985.)

direct target is unclear), thereby regulating the level of the receptor in hepatocytes (see Fig. 12-12). Consequently, the protease acts as a counterregulatory mechanism to lower receptor levels and prevent the excessive uptake of cholesterol as would be required, for example, in subjects on a low-cholesterol diet. The missense mutations in the PCSK9 protease that are associated with familial hypercholesterolemia appear to cause the disease by increasing protease activity, thereby reducing the levels of the LDL receptor to abnormally low levels. The gain-of-function mutations in the *PCSK9* gene that cause familial hypercholesterolemia indicated that the PCSK9 protease is a major regulator of LDL cholesterol metabolism.

Some *PCSK9* Sequence Variants Protect Against Coronary Heart Disease   The link between familial hyper-

cholesterolemia and the *PCSK9* gene suggested that common sequence variants in *PCSK9* might be linked to very high or very low LDL cholesterol levels in the general population (despite the fact that, disappointingly, common variants in other genes—including the three others associated with familial hypercholesterolemia—have *not* been shown convincingly to be associated with variations in plasma cholesterol levels in the general population). Importantly, several *PCSK9* sequence variants have now been found to be strongly linked to low levels of plasma LDL cholesterol (Table 12-6). For example, in the African American population with very low levels of LDL cholesterol, one of two *PCSK9* nonsense variants is found in 2.6% of all subjects; the presence of either variant is associated with a mean reduction in LDL cholesterol of 40%. This reduction in LDL cholesterol has a powerful protective effect

**Domain of the
LDL receptor protein**

**Effect of mutations
in each domain**

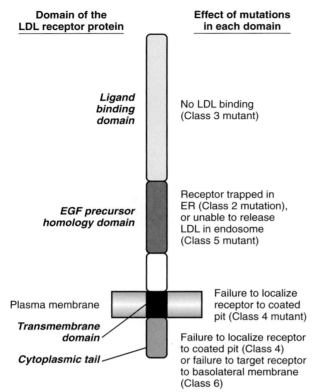

**Ligand
binding
domain**

No LDL binding
(Class 3 mutant)

**EGF precursor
homology domain**

Receptor trapped in
ER (Class 2 mutation),
or unable to release
LDL in endosome
(Class 5 mutant)

Plasma membrane

Failure to localize
receptor to coated
pit (Class 4 mutant)

**Transmembrane
domain**

Cytoplasmic tail

Failure to localize receptor
to coated pit (Class 4)
or failure to target receptor
to basolateral membrane
(Class 6)

Figure 12-15 ■ The structure of the LDL receptor gene showing its five domains and the effect on the receptor of mutations in these domains that lead to familial hypercholesterolemia. EGF, epidermal growth factor. (Based on a figure from Hobbs HH, Russell DW, Brown MS, Goldstein JL: The LDL receptor locus and familial hypercholesterolemia: mutational analysis of a membrane protein. Annu Rev Genet 24:133-170, 1990.)

against coronary artery disease, reducing the risk by about 90%; only about 1% of black subjects carrying one of the nonsense variants developed coronary artery disease in a 15-year study period, compared with almost 10% of individuals without either of these two mutations. Another allele (Arg46Leu) was more common (3.2% of subjects) in white people but conferred a 15% reduction in LDL cholesterol levels and, surprisingly, a 50% reduction in coronary heart disease. These findings have major public health implications because they suggest that modest but lifelong reductions in plasma

LDL cholesterol of 20 to 40 mg/dL would significantly decrease the incidence of coronary heart disease in the population. Finally, these discoveries illustrate how the investigation of rare genetic disorders can lead to important new knowledge about the genetic contribution to common genetically complex diseases.

Pathogenesis of Atherosclerotic Plaques in Familial Hypercholesterolemia Despite more than 30 years of research contributing to the impressive knowledge of the biology of the LDL receptor and the family of molecular defects that lead to familial hypercholesterolemia, the mechanisms by which the elevation in LDL leads to formation of atherosclerotic plaques in arteries are still not clear. In homozygotes, the increased LDL is cleared from the extracellular fluid by alternative "scavenger-type" receptors, on cells such as macrophages. Studies of macrophages in vitro show that excess cholesterol is stored as cholesteryl ester droplets, producing the foam cell appearance typically seen in xanthomas and atherosclerotic plaques, but the in vivo relevance of this work is uncertain at present.

Finally, the elucidation of the biochemical basis of familial hypercholesterolemia has had a profound impact on the treatment of the vastly more common forms of sporadic hypercholesterolemia by leading to the development of the statin class of drugs that inhibit de novo cholesterol biosynthesis (see Chapter 13).

● TRANSPORT DEFECTS

Cystic Fibrosis

Since the 1960s, cystic fibrosis (CF) has been one of the most publicly visible of all human monogenic diseases (see Case 10). It is the most common fatal autosomal recessive genetic disorder of children in white populations, with an incidence of approximately 1 in 2500 white births and a carrier frequency of about 1 in 25. The positional cloning (see Chapter 10) of the CF gene (called *CFTR*, for *CF transmembrane regulator*) in 1989 and the isolation of the Duchenne muscular dystrophy gene 3 years previously were the first illustrations of the power of molecular genetic approaches to identify disease genes. Shortly after the CF gene was cloned, physiological analyses demonstrated that the

Table 12-6

Common *PCSK9* Variants Associated with Low LDL Cholesterol Levels

Sequence Variant	Population Frequency of Heterozygotes	Mean Reduction in LDL Cholesterol	Impact on Incidence of Coronary Heart Disease
Tyr142Stop or Cys679Stop	African Americans: 2.6%	28% (38 mg/dL)	90% reduction
Arg46Leu	Whites: 3.2%	15% (20 mg/dL)	50% reduction

Derived from Cohen JC, Boerwinkle E, Mosley TH, Hobbs H: Sequence variants in *PCSK9*, low LDL, and protection against coronary heart disease. N Engl J Med 354:1264-1272, 2006.

protein encoded by the *CFTR* gene is a regulated chloride channel located in the apical membrane of the epithelial cells affected by the disease.

The Phenotypes of Cystic Fibrosis The lungs and exocrine pancreas are the major organs affected by the disease, but a major diagnostic feature is increased sweat sodium and chloride concentrations (often first noted when parents kiss their infants). In most patients with CF, the diagnosis can be based on the pulmonary or pancreatic findings and on an elevated level of sweat chloride. Less than 2% of patients have normal sweat chloride concentration despite an otherwise typical clinical picture; in these cases, molecular analysis can be used to ascertain whether they have mutations in the *CFTR* gene.

The pulmonary disease of CF develops as a result of thick secretions and recurrent infection; it is initially characterized by chronic obstructive lung disease and later by bronchiectasis. Although intense management of the lung disease prolongs life, death ultimately results from pulmonary failure and infection. At present, about half of patients survive to 33 years of age, but the clinical course is variable. The pancreatic defect in CF is a maldigestion syndrome due to the deficient secretion of pancreatic enzymes (lipase, trypsin, chymotrypsin). Normal digestion and nutrition can be largely restored by pancreatic enzyme supplements. About 5% to 10% of patients with CF have enough residual pancreatic exocrine function for normal digestion and are designated *pancreatic sufficient*. Moreover, patients with CF who are pancreatic sufficient have better growth and overall prognosis than do the majority, who are *pancreatic insufficient*. The clinical heterogeneity of the pancreatic disease is at least partly due to allelic heterogeneity, as discussed later.

Many other phenotypes are observed in patients with CF. For example, postnatal lower intestinal tract obstruction (**meconium ileus**) occurs in 10% to 20% of newborns with CF; its presence requires that the diagnosis of CF be excluded. The genital tract is also affected. Although females with CF have some reduction in fertility, more than 95% of males with CF are infertile because they lack a vas deferens, a phenotype known as **congenital bilateral absence of the vas deferens** (CBAVD). In a striking example of allelic heterogeneity giving rise to a partial phenotype, it has been found that some infertile males who are otherwise well (i.e., have no pulmonary or pancreatic disease) have CBAVD associated with specific mutant alleles in the CF gene. Similarly, some individuals with **idiopathic chronic pancreatitis** carry mutations in the *CFTR* gene yet lack other clinical signs of CF.

The *CFTR* Gene and Protein *CFTR*, the gene in chromosome 7q31 associated with CF, spans about 190 kb of DNA; the coding region, with 27 exons, is predicted to encode a large integral membrane protein of about 170 kD (Fig. 12-16). On the basis of its predicted function, the protein encoded by *CFTR* was named the CF transmembrane conductance regulator (CFTR). Its hypothesized structure indicates that it belongs to the so-called ABC (ATP [adenosine triphosphate]–binding cassette) family of transport proteins. At least 18 ABC transporters have been implicated in mendelian disorders and complex trait phenotypes.

The CFTR chloride channel has five domains, shown in Figure 12-16: two membrane-spanning domains, each with six transmembrane sequences; two nucleotide (ATP)–binding domains; and a regulatory domain with multiple phosphorylation sites. The importance of each domain is demonstrated by the identification of CF-causing missense mutations in each of them (see Fig. 12-16). The pore of the chloride channel is formed by the 12 transmembrane segments. ATP is bound and hydrolyzed by the nucleotide-binding domains, and the energy released is used to open and close the channel. Regulation of the channel is mediated, at least in part, by phosphorylation of the regulatory domain.

The Pathophysiology of Cystic Fibrosis CF is due to abnormal fluid and electrolyte transport across epithelial apical membranes. This abnormality leads to disease in the lung, pancreas, intestine, hepatobiliary tree, and male genital tract. The physiological abnormalities have been most clearly elucidated for the sweat gland. The loss of CFTR function means that chloride in the duct of the sweat gland cannot be reabsorbed, leading to a reduction in the electrochemical gradient that normally drives sodium entry across the apical membrane. This defect leads, in turn, to the increased chloride and sodium concentrations in sweat. The effects on electrolyte transport due to the abnormalities in the CFTR protein have also been carefully studied in airway and pancreatic epithelia. In the lung, the hyperabsorption of sodium and reduced chloride secretion lead to a depletion of airway surface liquid. Consequently, the mucus layer of the lung may become adherent to cell surfaces, disrupting the cough and cilia-dependent clearance of mucus and providing a niche favorable to *Pseudomonas aeruginosa*, the major cause of chronic pulmonary infection in CF.

The Genetics of Cystic Fibrosis

Mutations in the CFTR Polypeptide The first CF mutation identified, a deletion of a phenylalanine residue at position 508 (ΔF508) in the first ATP-binding fold (NBD1; see Fig. 12-16), is the most common defect, accounting for about 70% of all CF alleles in white populations. In these populations, only seven other mutations are more frequent than 0.5%, and the remainder are therefore rare. Mutations of all types

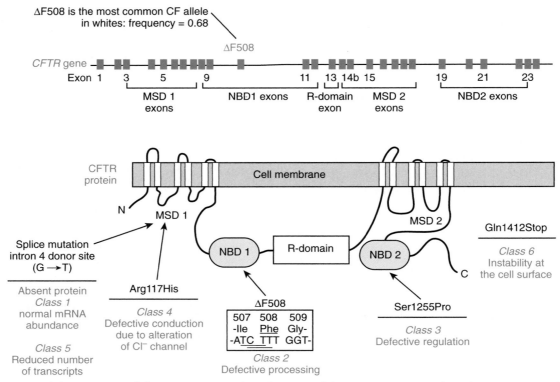

Figure 12-16 ■ The structure of the *CFTR* gene and a schematic of the CFTR protein. Selected mutations are shown. The exons, introns, and domains of the protein are not drawn to scale. MSD, membrane-spanning domain; NBD, nucleotide-binding domain; R-domain, regulatory domain. ΔF508 results from the deletion of TCT or CTT, replacing the Ile codon with ATT, and deleting the Phe codon. (Based on Zielinski J: Genotype and phenotype in cystic fibrosis. Respiration 67:117-133, 2000.)

have been identified, but the largest single group (nearly half) are missense substitutions. The remainder are point mutations of other types, and less than 1% are genomic rearrangements. Although more than 1200 CF gene sequence variants have been associated with disease, the actual number of missense mutations that are disease-causing is somewhat uncertain because few have been subjected to functional analysis.

Although the biochemical abnormalities associated with most CF mutations are not known, four general mechanisms of protein dysfunction have been described. Alleles representative of each of these six classes of dysfunction are shown in Figure 12-16. Class 1 mutations are those that have a defect in protein production, such as those associated with premature stop codons or mutations that generate unstable RNAs. Because CFTR is a glycosylated membrane-spanning protein, it must be processed in the endoplasmic reticulum and Golgi to be glycosylated and secreted; class 2 mutations are a result of defective protein processing due to misfolding of the protein. The ΔF508 mutant typifies this class; this mutant protein does not fold normally enough to allow exit from the endoplasmic reticulum. However, the ΔF508 mutant protein phenotype is complex, since the protein also exhibits defects in stability and activation in addition to impaired folding.

The essential functions of the nucleotide-binding domains and the regulatory domain (see Fig. 12-16) are illustrated by the occurrence of CF-causing mutations that disrupt regulation of the protein (class 3 mutations). Class 4 mutations are located in the membrane-spanning domains and, consistent with this localization, have defective chloride conduction. Class 5 mutations reduce the number of *CFTR* transcripts. Class 6 mutant proteins are synthesized normally but are unstable at the cell surface.

A CF Genocopy: Mutations in the Epithelial Sodium Channel Gene *SCNN1* Although *CFTR* is the only gene that has been linked to classic CF, several families with nonclassic presentations (including CF-like pulmonary infections, less severe intestinal disease, elevated sweat chloride levels) have been found to carry mutations in the epithelial sodium channel gene *SCNN1*. This finding is consistent with the functional interaction between the CFTR protein and the epithelial sodium channel. Its main clinical significance, at present, is the demonstration that patients with nonclassic CF display locus heterogeneity and that if *CFTR* mutations are not present, abnormalities in *SCNNI* must be considered.

Genotype-Phenotype Correlations in Cystic Fibrosis Because all patients with the classic form of CF appear to have mutations in the CF gene, clinical heterogeneity in CF must arise from allelic heterogeneity, the effects of other modifying loci, or nongenetic factors. Two generalizations have emerged from the genetic and clinical analysis of patients with CF. First, the *CFTR* genotype is a good predictor of exocrine pancreatic function. For example, patients homozygous for the common ΔF508 mutation or for predicted null alleles (such as premature stop codons) generally have pancreatic insufficiency. On the other hand, alleles that allow the synthesis of a partially functional CFTR protein, such as Arg117His (see Fig. 12-16), tend to be associated with pancreatic sufficiency. Second, the *CFTR* genotype is a poor predictor of the severity of pulmonary disease. For example, among patients homozygous for the ΔF508 mutation, the severity of lung disease is variable. The reasons for this poor pulmonary genotype-phenotype correlation are not clear. A modifier gene for CF lung disease, the gene encoding transforming growth factor β1 (TGFβ1), has recently been reported. Two variants of TGFβ1 were found to be associated with more severe CF lung disease. If this finding proves to be robust, it may provide insight into the pathological mechanisms underlying the lung disease and suggest therapeutic opportunities.

The Cystic Fibrosis Gene in Populations At present, it is not possible to account for the high *CFTR* mutant allele frequency of 1 in 50 that is observed in white populations (see Chapter 9). The disease is much less frequent in non-whites, although it has been reported in Native Americans, African Americans, and Asians (e.g., approximately 1 in 90,000 Hawaiians of Asian descent). The ΔF508 allele is the only one found to date that is common in virtually all white populations. Haplotype analysis of white populations indicates that the ΔF508 allele probably has a single origin. The frequency of this allele, among all mutant alleles, varies significantly in different European populations, from 88% in Denmark to 45% in southern Italy.

In populations in which the ΔF508 allele frequency is approximately 70% of all mutant alleles, about 50% of patients are homozygous for the ΔF508 allele; an additional 40% have genetic compound genotypes for ΔF508 and another mutant allele. In addition, approximately 70% of CF carriers have the ΔF508 mutation. Except for ΔF508, the CF mutations at the *CFTR* locus are rare, although in specific populations, other alleles may be common.

Population Screening The complex issues that are raised by considering population screening for diseases such as CF are discussed in Chapter 17. At present, CF meets most of the criteria for a newborn screening program, except it is not yet clear that early identification of affected infants significantly improves long-term prognosis. Nevertheless, the advantages of early diagnosis (such as improved nutrition from the provision of pancreatic enzymes) have led some jurisdictions to implement newborn screening programs. Although it is generally agreed that universal screening for carriers should not be considered until at least 90% of the mutations can be detected (the current figure is about 85%), population screening for couples has been under way in the United States, at the level of private medical practices, for several years.

Genetic Analysis of Families of Patients and Prenatal Diagnosis The high frequency of the ΔF508 allele is useful when CF patients without a family history present for DNA diagnosis. The identification of the ΔF508 allele, in combination with a panel of 22 less common but not rare mutations suggested by the American College of Medical Genetics, can be used to predict the status of family members for confirmation of disease (e.g., in a newborn or a sibling with an ambiguous presentation), carrier detection, and prenatal diagnosis. Given the vast knowledge of CF mutations in many populations, direct mutation detection is the method of choice for genetic analysis. If linkage is used in the absence of knowing the specific mutation, accurate diagnosis is possible in virtually all families.

For fetuses with a 1-in-4 risk, prenatal diagnosis by DNA analysis at 10 to 12 weeks, with tissue obtained by chorionic villus biopsy, is the method of choice (see Chapter 15). Biochemical methods of prenatal diagnosis based on the measurement of intestinal enzymes (e.g., intestinal alkaline phosphatase) in amniotic fluid have a high false-positive rate and are no longer used.

Molecular Genetics and the Treatment of Cystic Fibrosis At present, the treatment of CF is directed toward controlling pulmonary infection and improving nutrition. Increasing knowledge of the molecular pathogenesis may make it possible to design pharmacological interventions that would directly correct the abnormal biochemical phenotype. Alternatively, gene transfer therapy may be possible in CF, but there are many difficulties. Potential treatments of CF are discussed in Chapter 13.

● DISORDERS OF STRUCTURAL PROTEINS

Duchenne and Becker Muscular Dystrophies: Defects in Dystrophin

Like cystic fibrosis, **Duchenne muscular dystrophy** (DMD) has long received attention from the general and medical communities because it is a severe, currently untreatable, relatively common disorder associated with relentless clinical deterioration (Case 12). The isolation of the gene affected in this X-linked disorder

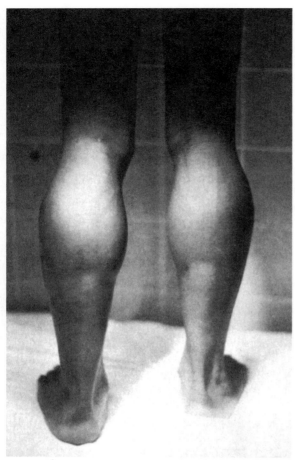

Figure 12-17 ■ Pseudohypertrophy of the calves due to the replacement of normal muscle tissue with connective tissue and fat in an 8-year-old boy with Duchenne muscular dystrophy. (Courtesy of R. H. A. Haslam, The Hospital for Sick Children, Toronto.)

and the characterization of its protein (named dystrophin because of its association with DMD) have given insight into every aspect of the disease, greatly improved the genetic counseling of affected families, and suggested strategies for treatment.

The Clinical Phenotype of Duchenne Muscular Dystrophy Affected boys are normal for the first year or two of life but develop muscle weakness at the age of 3 to 5 years (Fig. 12-17), when they begin to have difficulty climbing stairs and rising from a sitting position. The child is confined to a wheelchair by the age of 12 years and is unlikely to survive beyond the age of 20 years. Patients die of respiratory failure or, because the myocardial muscle is also affected, of cardiac failure. In the preclinical and early stages of the disease, the serum level of creatine kinase is grossly elevated (50 to 100 times the upper limit of normal) because of its release from diseased muscle. The brain is also affected; on average, there is a modest decrease in IQ of about 20 points.

Becker Muscular Dystrophy Becker muscular dystrophy (BMD) is also due to mutations in the dystrophin gene, but the Becker alleles produce a phenotype that is much milder. Patients are said to have BMD if they are still walking at the age of 16 years. There is significant variability in the progression of the disease, and some patients remain ambulatory for many years. In general, patients with BMD carry mutated alleles that maintain the reading frame of the protein and thus express some dystrophin, albeit often an altered product at reduced levels. The presence of dystrophin in the muscle of patients with BMD is generally demonstrable both on Western blots (see Fig. 4-13) and by immunofluorescence (Fig. 12-18; see also Fig. 7-16). In contrast, patients with DMD have little or no detectable dystrophin by either technique.

The Genetics of Duchenne Muscular Dystrophy and Becker Muscular Dystrophy

Inheritance DMD has an incidence of about 1 in 3300 live male births, with a calculated mutation rate of 10^{-4}, an order of magnitude higher than the rate observed in genes involved in most other genetic diseases. In fact, given a production of about 8×10^7 sperm per day, a normal male produces a sperm with a new mutation in the *DMD* gene every 10 to 11 seconds! In Chapter 7, DMD was presented as a typical X-linked recessive disorder that is lethal in males, so that one third of cases are predicted to be new mutants and two thirds of patients have carrier mothers (see also Chapter 19). The great majority of carrier females have no clinical manifestations, although about 70% have slightly elevated levels of serum creatine kinase. In accordance with random inactivation of the X chromosome (see Chapter 7), however, the normal X chromosome appears to be inactivated in a critical proportion of cells in some female heterozygotes; about 19% of adult female carriers have some muscle weakness and, in 8%, life-threatening cardiomyopathy and serious proximal muscle disability. In rare instances, females have been described with DMD (Table 12-7); some have X;autosome translocations (see Chapter 6), others have only one X chromosome (Turner syndrome) with a *DMD* mutation on that chromosome, and a rare group consists of heterozygous monozygotic twins.

BMD accounts for about 15% of the mutations at the locus. An important genetic distinction between these allelic phenotypes is that whereas DMD is a genetic lethal, the reproductive fitness of males with BMD is high (up to about 70% of normal), so that they can transmit the gene to their daughters. Consequently, a high proportion of BMD cases are inherited, and few (only about 10%) represent new mutations.

The *DMD* Gene and Its Product The most remarkable feature of the *DMD* gene is its size, estimated to

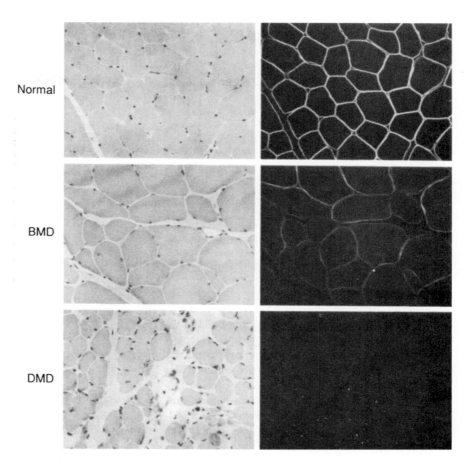

Figure 12-18 ■ Microscopic visualization of the effect of mutations in the dystrophin gene in a patient with Becker muscular dystrophy (BMD) and a patient with Duchenne muscular dystrophy (DMD). Left column, hematoxylin and eosin staining of muscle. Right column, immunofluorescence microscopy staining with an antibody specific to dystrophin. Note the localization of dystrophin to the myocyte membrane in normal muscle, the reduced quantity of dystrophin in BMD muscle, and the complete absence of dystrophin from the myocytes of the DMD muscle. The amount of connective tissue between the myocytes in the DMD muscle is increased. (Courtesy of K. Arahata, National Institute of Neuroscience, Tokyo.)

Table 12-7

Mechanisms of Mutation in Duchenne or Becker Muscular Dystrophy

Molecular or Genetic Defect	Frequency	Phenotype
IN AFFECTED MALES		
Gene deletion (1 exon to whole gene)	~60%	DMD or BMD
Point mutations	~34%	DMD or BMD
Partial duplication of the gene	~6%	DMD or BMD
Contiguous gene deletion	Rare	DMD plus other phenotypes, depending on other genes deleted
IN AFFECTED FEMALES		
Nonrandom X inactivation	Rare	DMD
Turner syndrome (45,X)	Rare	DMD
X;autosome translocation	Rare	DMD

BMD, Becker muscular dystrophy; DMD, Duchenne muscular dystrophy.

be 2300 kb, or 1.5% of the X chromosome. This huge gene, like the gene for neurofibromatosis, type 1 *(NF1)* and a few others, is among the largest known in any species, by an order of magnitude. The high mutation rate can therefore be at least partly explained by the fact that the locus is a large target for mutation. The *DMD* gene is structurally complex, with 79 exons, 7 tissue-specific promoters, and differential splicing giving rise to tissue-specific, developmentally regulated isoforms. In muscle, the primary site of disease, the large (14-kb) dystrophin transcript encodes a huge 427-kD protein (Fig. 12-19). In accordance with the clinical phenotype of the disease, this protein is most abundant in skeletal and cardiac muscle and the brain, although most tissues express at least one dystrophin isoform.

Dystrophin is a structural protein that anchors a large protein complex at the cell membrane. The dystrophin protein complex is a veritable constellation of polypeptides associated with genetically distinct muscular dystrophies (Fig. 12-20). The composition of this complex can vary significantly depending on the protein isoforms, both of dystrophin itself and of other components, particularly the sarcoglycans, that are present. The dystrophin complex serves several major functions. First, it is thought to be essential for the maintenance

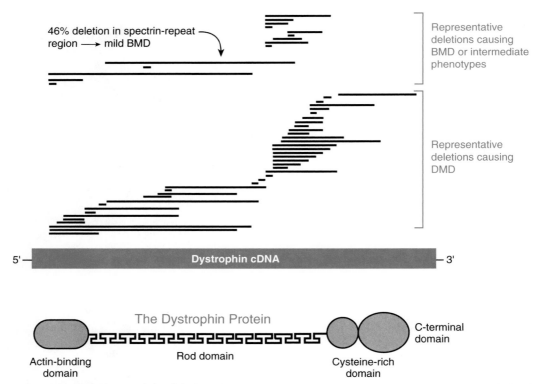

Figure 12-19 ■ A representation of the full-length dystrophin protein, the corresponding cDNA, and the distribution of representative deletions in patients with Becker muscular dystrophy (BMD) and Duchenne muscular dystrophy (DMD). The actin-binding domain links the protein to the filamentous actin cytoskeleton. The rod domain presumably acts as a spacer between the N-terminal and C-terminal domains. The cysteine-rich domain mediates protein-protein interactions. The C-terminal domain, which associates with a large transmembrane glycoprotein complex (see Fig. 12-20), is also found in three dystrophin-related proteins (DRPs): utrophin (DRP-1), DRP-2, and dystrobrevin. The protein domains are not drawn to scale.

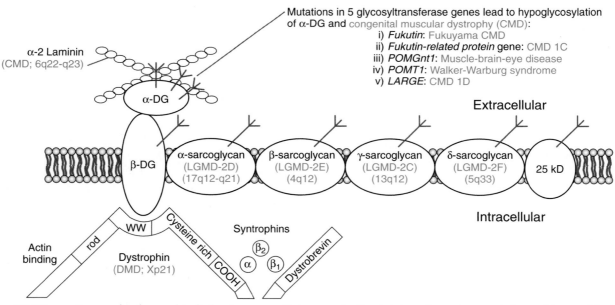

Figure 12-20 ■ In muscle, dystrophin links the extracellular matrix (laminin) to the actin cytoskeleton. Dystrophin interacts with a multimeric complex composed of the dystroglycans (DG), the sarcoglycans, the syntrophins, and dystrobrevin. The α,β-dystroglycan complex is a receptor for laminin and agrin in the extracellular matrix. The function of the sarcoglycan complex is uncertain, but it is integral to muscle function; mutations in the sarcoglycans have been identified in limb girdle muscular dystrophies (LGMD) type 2C, 2D, 2E, and 2F. Mutations in laminin type 2 (merosin) cause a congenital muscular dystrophy (CMD). The branched structures represent glycans. The WW domain of dystrophin is a tryptophan-rich protein binding motif.

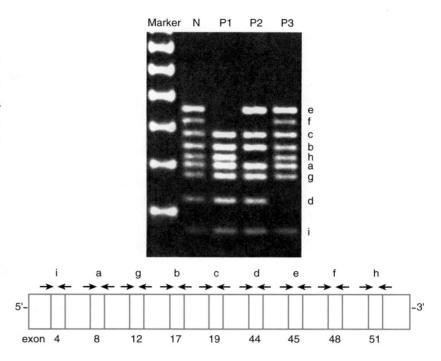

Figure 12-21 ■ Diagnosis of Duchenne muscular dystrophy involves screening for deletions and duplications by a procedure called multiplex polymerase chain reaction (PCR). With use of primer sets *(pairs of arrows)* that amplify various regions of the gene (a to i) in a single reaction, patient DNA is analyzed for aberrant or missing bands by gel electrophoresis. Lane 2 shows the nine PCR products from a normal individual (N), indicating the presence of the corresponding exons. Patient 1 (lane P1) is missing bands e and f, which identifies a deletion encompassing exons 45 to 48. Patient 2 (lane P2) is missing bands f and h, which indicates a deletion involving exons 48 to 51. Patient 3 (lane P3) is missing band d and therefore has a deletion involving exon 44. (Courtesy of P. N. Ray, The Hospital for Sick Children, Toronto.)

of muscle membrane integrity, by linking the actin cytoskeleton to the extracellular matrix. Second, it is required to position the proteins in the complex so that they function correctly. For example, the dystrophin complex is required at the neuromuscular junction for proper acetylcholine clustering during development. The complex may also contain ion channels and signaling molecules, suggesting that it may participate in cell-cell or cell-substratum recognition. Although the function of many of the proteins in the complex is unknown, their association with diseases of muscle indicates that they are essential components of the complex. Thus, as indicated in Figure 12-20, mutations in several of the proteins in the dystrophin glycoprotein complex are responsible for autosomal recessive forms of Duchenne-like muscular dystrophy, limb girdle muscular dystrophies, and other muscular dystrophies.

Post-translational Modification of the Dystrophin Complex   Of special interest are the five diseases that result from mutations in glycosyltransferases, whose loss of function results in hypoglycosylation of α-dystroglycan (see Fig. 12-20). The fact that five proteins are required for the post-translational modification of one other polypeptide testifies to the importance of post-translational modifications to the normal function of most proteins and to the critical nature of glycosylation to the function of α-dystroglycan in particular.

Molecular Analysis of Duchenne Muscular Dystrophy and Becker Muscular Dystrophy   The most common molecular defects in patients with DMD are deletions (60% of alleles) (Fig. 12-21; see also Fig. 12-19 and Table 12-7). The distribution of the deletions in the

gene is not random; they are clustered in one of two regions within the gene, in the 5′ half or in a central region that appears to encompass a deletion hotspot (see Fig. 12-19). The mechanism of deletion in this central region is unknown, but it appears to involve the tertiary structure of the DNA and in some cases recombination between *Alu* repeat sequences (see Chapter 2) in large central introns. Point mutations account for approximately one third of the alleles and are randomly distributed throughout the gene.

The Clinical Application of Molecular Genetics to Muscular Dystrophy

Prenatal Diagnosis and Carrier Detection   With modern molecular techniques, accurate carrier detection and prenatal diagnosis are available for most families with a history of DMD. In the 60% to 70% of families in whom the mutation results from a deletion or duplication, the presence or absence of the defect can be assessed on examination of fetal DNA by simple or quantitative multiplexed polymerase chain reaction analysis (see Fig. 12-21). In other families, point mutations can be identified by sequencing of the coding region and intron-exon boundaries. Because of the large size of the *DMD* gene, sequencing is expensive and time-consuming, but with automated sequencing, it is an economically feasible medical test. In those families in whom direct analysis does not identify a mutation, linked markers allow prenatal diagnosis (see Chapter 19) with an accuracy of 95%. The major obstacle in carrier detection and prenatal diagnosis is that current methods are restricted to families with a history of DMD. Because the disease has a high frequency of new mutations and is manifest in only a minority of carrier females, approximately 80% of Duchenne boys are born into families with no previous history of the disease (see Chapter 7). Thus, the incidence of DMD will not decrease substantially until universal prenatal screening for the disease is possible.

Maternal Mosaicism   If a boy with DMD is the first affected member of his family, and if his mother is not found to carry the mutation in her lymphocytes, the usual explanation is that he has a new mutation at the *DMD* locus. However, about 5% to 15% of such cases appear to be due to maternal germline mosaicism, in which case the recurrence risk is significant (see Chapter 7).

Therapy   At present, only symptomatic treatment is available for DMD. The possibilities for rational therapy for DMD have greatly increased with the isolation of the dystrophin gene and the understanding of its normal role in the myocyte. Some of the therapeutic considerations are discussed in Chapter 13.

Osteogenesis Imperfecta: Mutations in Collagen Structural Genes

Osteogenesis imperfecta (OI) is a group of inherited disorders that predispose to easy fracturing of bones, even with little trauma, and to skeletal deformity (Fig. 12-22). A remarkable range of clinical variation has been recognized, from a lethal perinatal form to only a mild increase in fracture frequency. The four major phenotypes are outlined in Table 12-8. About 90% of affected individuals have mutations in the two genes, *COL1A1* and *COL1A2*, that encode the chains of type I collagen, the major protein in bone. The clinical heterogeneity can be at least partly explained by locus and allelic heterogeneity; the phenotypes vary according to which chain of type I procollagen is affected and according to the type and location of the mutation in the locus. In addition, other genetic loci harbor the primary mutations in some forms. The combined incidence of all forms of the disease is about 1 in 15,000.

Normal Collagen Structure in Relation to Osteogenesis Imperfecta   It is important to appreciate the major features of normal type I collagen to understand the pathogenesis of OI. Type I collagen is the major structural protein of bone and other fibrous tissues. The type I procollagen molecule is formed from two proα1(I) chains (encoded on chromosome 17 by *COL1A1*) and one similar but distinct proα2(I) chain (encoded on chromosome 7 by *COL1A2*) (Fig. 12-23).

   Proteins composed of subunits, like collagen, are often subject to mutations that prevent subunit association by altering the subunit interfaces. The triple helical

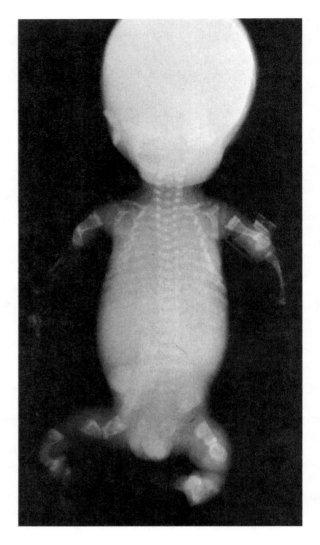

Figure 12-22 ■ Radiograph of a premature (26 weeks' gestation) infant with the perinatal lethal form (type II) of osteogenesis imperfecta. The skull is relatively large and unmineralized and was soft to palpation. The thoracic cavity is small, the long bones of the arms and legs are short and deformed, and the vertebral bodies are flattened. All the bones are undermineralized. (Courtesy of T. Costa, The Hospital for Sick Children, Toronto.)

(collagen) section is composed of 338 tandemly arranged Gly-X-Y repeats; proline is often in the X position, and hydroxyproline or hydroxylysine is often in the Y position. Glycine, the smallest amino acid, is the only residue compact enough to occupy the axial position of the helix, and consequently, mutations that substitute other residues for those glycines are highly disruptive to the helical structure.

   Several features of procollagen maturation are of special significance to the pathophysiology of OI. First, the assembly of the individual proα chains into the trimer begins at the carboxyl terminus, and triple helix formation progresses toward the amino terminus. Con-

Table 12-8

A Summary of the Genetic, Biochemical, and Molecular Features of the Types of Osteogenesis Imperfecta

Type	Phenotype	Inheritance	Biochemical Defect	Gene Defect
Defective Production of Type I Collagen*				
I	**Mild:** blue sclerae, brittle bones but no bone deformity	Autosomal dominant	*Common:* All the collagen made is normal (from the normal allele), but the quantity is *reduced* by half	*Common:* Null alleles that impair the production of proα1(I) chains, such as defects that interfere with mRNA synthesis
Structural Defects in Type I Collagen				
II	**Perinatal lethal:** severe skeletal abnormalities (fractures, deformities), dark sclerae, death within 1 month (see Fig. 12-22)	Autosomal dominant (new mutation)	*Common:* Production of *abnormal* collagen molecules due to substitution of the glycine in Gly-X-Y of the triple helical domain, with some bias toward the C-terminal half of the protein (see Fig. 12-25)	*Common:* Missense skeletal mutations in the glycine codons of the genes for the α1 and α2 chains
III	**Progressive deforming:** fractures, often at birth; progressive bone deformity, limited growth, blue sclerae	Autosomal dominant[†]	Abnormal collagen molecules: glycine substitutions of many types in the triple helix; located throughout the protein (see Fig. 12-25)	Missense mutations in the glycine codons of the genes for the α1 or α2 chains
IV	**Normal sclerae, deforming:** mild to moderate bone deformity, short stature, fractures	Autosomal dominant	Abnormal collagen molecules: glycine substitutions of many types in the triple helix; located throughout the protein	Missense mutations in the glycine codons of the genes for the α1 or α2 chains

*A few patients with type I disease have substitutions of glycine in one of the type I collagen chains (see Fig. 12-25).
[†]Rare cases are autosomal recessive.
Modified from Byers PH: Disorders of collagen biosynthesis and structure. In Scriver CR, Beaudet AL, Sly WS, Valle D (eds): The Metabolic Basis of Inherited Disease, 6th ed. New York, McGraw-Hill, 1989, pp 2805-2842; and Byers PH: Brittle bones–fragile molecules: disorders of collagen structure and expression. Trends Genet 6:293-300, 1990.

sequently, mutations that alter residues in the carboxyl-terminal part of the triple helical domain are more disruptive because they interfere earlier with the propagation of the triple helix (Fig. 12-24). Second, the post-translational modification (e.g., proline or lysine hydroxylation; glycosylation) of procollagen continues on any part of a chain not assembled into the triple helix. Thus, when triple helix assembly is slowed by a mutation, the unassembled sections of the chains amino-terminal to the defect are modified excessively,

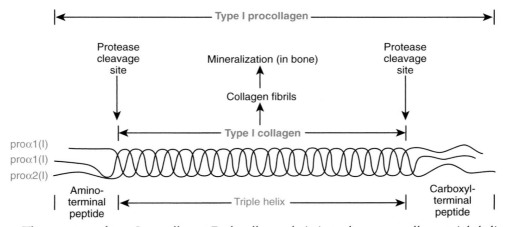

Figure 12-23 ■ The structure of type I procollagen. Each collagen chain is made as a procollagen triple helix that is secreted into the extracellular space. The amino- and carboxyl-terminal domains are cleaved extracellularly to form collagen; mature collagen fibrils are then assembled and, in bone, mineralized. Note that type I procollagen is composed of two proα1(I) chains and one proα2(I) chain. (Redrawn from Byers PH: Disorders of collagen biosynthesis and structure. In Scriver CR, Beaudet AL, Sly WS, Valle D [eds]: The Metabolic Bases of Inherited Disease, 6th ed. New York, McGraw-Hill, pp. 2805-2842, 1989.)

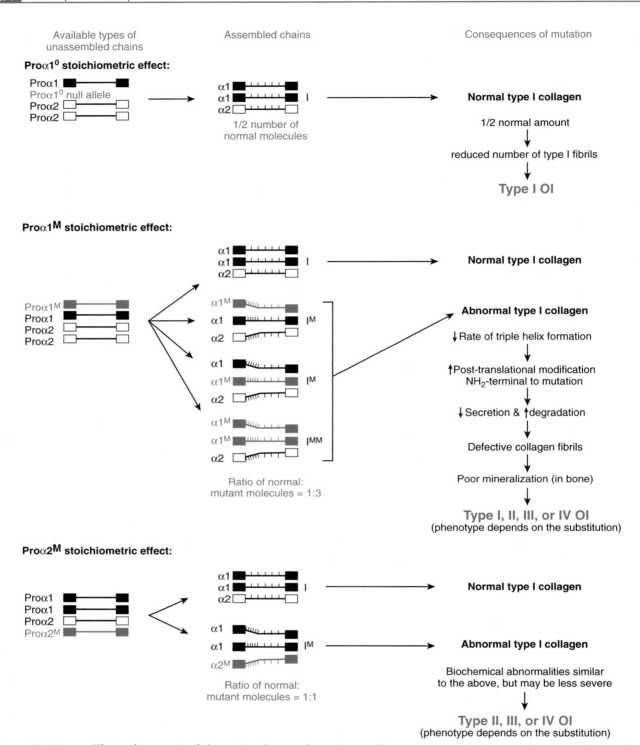

Figure 12-24 ■ The pathogenesis of the major classes of type I procollagen mutants. Column 1: the types of procollagen chains available for assembly into a triple helix. Although there are two α1 and two α2 collagen genes/genome, as implied in the left column, twice as many α1 collagen molecules are produced, compared to α2 collagen molecules, as shown in the central column. Column 2: the effect of type I procollagen stoichiometry on the ratio of normal to defective collagen molecules formed in mutants with proα1 chain versus proα2 chain mutations. The small vertical bars on each procollagen chain indicate post-translational modifications *(see text)*. Column 3: the effect of mutations on the biochemical processing of collagen. Proα1^M, a proα1 chain with a missense mutation; Proα2^M, a proα2 chain with a missense mutation; Proα1^0, a proα1 chain null allele.

which slows their secretion into the extracellular space. Overmodification may also interfere with the formation of collagen fibrils. As a result of all of these abnormalities, the number of secreted collagen molecules is reduced, and many of them are abnormal. In bone, the abnormal chains and their reduced number lead to defective mineralization of collagen fibrils (see Fig. 12-22).

Molecular Abnormalities of Collagen in Osteogenesis Imperfecta

More than 800 different mutations affecting the synthesis or structure of type I collagen have been found in individuals with OI. The clinical heterogeneity of this disease reflects even greater heterogeneity at the molecular level (see Table 12-8). The mutations fall into two general classes, those that reduce the amount of type I procollagen made and those that alter the structure of the molecules assembled. To some extent, it is now possible to predict the phenotype that will result from a specific type of molecular defect (Fig. 12-25).

Type I: Diminished Type I Collagen Production Most individuals with OI type I have mutations that result in production by cells of about half the normal amount of type I procollagen. Most of these mutations result in premature termination codons in one *COL1A1* allele that render the mRNA from that allele highly unstable. Because type I procollagen molecules must have two proα1(I) chains to form, loss of half the mRNA leads to production of half the normal quantity of type I procollagen molecules, although these molecules are normal (see Fig. 12-23). Missense mutations give rise to this milder form of OI when the amino acid change is located in the amino terminus because substitutions at this location tend to be less disruptive of collagen chain assembly (see Fig. 12-25).

Types II, III, and IV: Structurally Defective Collagens The type II, III, and IV phenotypes of OI result from mutations that produce structurally abnormal proα1 chains (see Figs. 12-24 and 12-25); substitutions in the proα2 chain have a comparable effect. Most of these patients have substitutions in the triple helix that replace a glycine with a more bulky residue. The specific collagen affected, the location of the substitution, and the nature of the substituting residue are all important phenotypic determinants, but some generalizations about the phenotype likely to result from a specific substitution are nevertheless possible. Thus, substitutions in the proα1(I) chain are more prevalent in patients with OI types III and IV and are more often lethal. In either chain, replacement of glycine (a neutral residue) with aspartate (an acidic residue) is usually very disruptive and more often associated with a severe (type II) phenotype (see Fig. 12-25). Sometimes, a specific sub-stitution is associated with more than one phenotype, an outcome that is likely to reflect the influence of powerful modifier genes of this monogenic disorder.

Novel Forms of Osteogenesis Imperfecta That Do Not Result from Collagen Mutations

In the last few years, three additional forms of OI have been recognized (types V, VI, and VII) that do not result from mutations in type I collagen genes. The causative genes have not been identified, although a locus for OI type VII has been mapped to the short arm of chromosome 3 and is inherited as a recessive trait. The other forms are dominantly inherited and have distinctive clinical features or bone disease but overall are similar to OI type IV.

The Genetics of Osteogenesis Imperfecta

Most of the mutations in type I collagen genes that cause OI are dominantly acting, but a few are recessive. At least some of the mechanisms by which different patterns of inheritance arise from different mutations in a single molecule have been revealed by characterization of the biochemical defects. More generally, this disease illustrates the genetic complexities that result when mutations alter structural proteins, particularly those composed of multiple different subunits.

The relatively mild phenotype and dominant inheritance of OI type I are consistent with the fact that although only half the normal number of molecules is made, they are of normal quality (see Fig. 12-24). The more severe consequences of producing structurally defective proα1(I) chains (compared with producing no chains) partly reflect the stoichiometry of type I collagen, which contains two proα1 chains to one proα2 chain (see Fig. 12-24). Accordingly, if half the proα1(I) chains are abnormal, three of four type I molecules have at least one abnormal chain; in contrast, if half the proα2(I) chains are defective, only one in two molecules is affected. Mutations such as the proα1(I) missense allele (proα1^M) shown in Figure 12-24 are thus **dominant negative alleles** because they impair the contribution of both the normal proα1 chains and the normal proα2 chains. In other words, the effect of the mutant allele is amplified because of the polymeric nature of the collagen molecule. Consequently, in dominantly inherited diseases such as OI, it is actually better to have a mutation that generates *no* gene product than one that produces an *abnormal* gene product.

Although mutations that produce structurally abnormal proα2 chains reduce the number of normal type I collagen molecules by half (versus three quarters in structurally abnormal proα1 chains; see Fig. 12-24), this reduction is nevertheless sufficient, in the case of

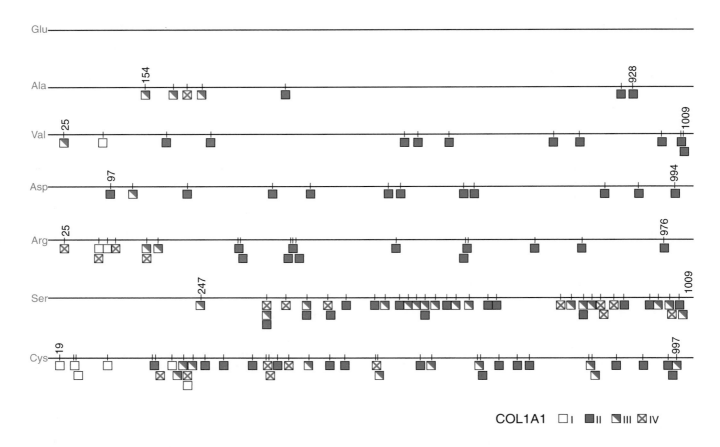

Figure 12-25 ■ The phenotypic effect of substitutions in the proα1 chain of type I collagen. I, II, III, and IV are types I to IV osteogenesis imperfecta. The numbers above the linear representation of the collagen molecules are the glycine residues that have been substituted by the amino acid noted to the left of each line. Note that in general, the phenotypic effect of substitutions near the carboxyl terminus (*on the right*) is more severe but that the effect also depends on the nature of the residue that replaces glycine. (Redrawn from Byers PH: Brittle bones–fragile molecules: disorders of collagen structure and expression. Trends Genet 6:293-300, 1990.)

some mutations, to cause the severe perinatal lethal phenotype (see Table 12-8). Most infants with OI type II, the perinatal lethal form, have a *new* dominant mutation, and consequently, the likelihood of recurrence in the family is very low. In occasional families, however, more than one sibling is affected with OI type II. Such recurrences are usually due to parental germline mosaicism (see pedigree in Fig. 7-24). Strong documentation of autosomal recessive forms of OI type II has not been presented, but a few examples of recessive OI type III have been recognized.

Clinical Management and Prenatal Diagnosis If a patient's molecular defect can be determined, increasing knowledge of the correlation between OI genotypes and phenotypes has made it possible often to predict, at least to some extent, the natural history of the disease. In addition, the demonstration that a defect is inherited from an affected parent (autosomal domi-

nant), from an unaffected parent (with germline mosaicism), from two unaffected but heterozygous parents (autosomal recessive), or as a new mutation will allow accurate recurrence risks to be calculated. Prenatal diagnosis in OI type II, the perinatal lethal form, may be performed by examination of skull and limb length by ultrasonography in the second trimester. For at-risk pregnancies, prenatal diagnosis requires the analysis of collagen synthesized by cells cultured from chorionic villus biopsy specimens or direct analysis of a mutation previously identified in the family.

Although the treatment of OI had been restricted to general medical and surgical measures, this situation is changing because of the discovery that bisphosphonates, a class of drugs that act by decreasing bone resorption, may increase bone density in some affected individuals. The more critical issue, whether bisphosphonates reduce the frequency and severity of fractures in OI, is under study but looks promising.

• NEURODEGENERATIVE DISORDERS

Alzheimer Disease

Until recently, the biochemical mechanisms underlying almost all adult-onset neurodegenerative diseases were completely obscure. One of the most common of these conditions is **Alzheimer disease** (AD) (Case 3). AD generally manifests in the sixth to ninth decades, but there are monogenic forms that often present earlier, sometimes as soon as the third decade. The clinical picture of AD is characterized by a progressive deterioration of memory and of higher cognitive functions, such as reasoning, in addition to behavioral changes. These abnormalities reflect degeneration of neurons in specific regions of the cerebral cortex and hippocampus. AD affects about 1.4% of persons in developed countries and is responsible for 100,000 deaths per year in the United States alone.

The Genetics of Alzheimer Disease   First-degree relatives of patients with AD have a 38% final risk of acquiring the disease by 85 years of age. Consequently, it appears that most cases with familial aggregation have a complex genetic contribution (see Chapter 8). This contribution may come from one or more incompletely penetrant genes that act independently, from multiple interacting genes, or from some combination of genetic and environmental factors. About 7% to 10% of patients have a monogenic highly penetrant form of AD that is inherited in an autosomal dominant manner. In the 1990s, four genes associated with AD were identified (Table 12-9). Mutations in three of these genes, encoding the β-amyloid precursor protein (βAPP), presenilin 1, and presenilin 2, lead to autosomal dominant AD. The fourth gene, *APOE*, encodes apolipoprotein E, the protein component of several plasma lipoproteins. Mutations in *APOE* are not associated with monogenic AD. Rather, the ε4 allele of *APOE* modestly increases susceptibility to nonfamilial AD and influences the age at onset of at least some of the monogenic forms (see later).

The identification of the four genes associated with AD has provided great insight not only into the pathogenesis of monogenic AD but also, as is commonly the case in medical genetics, into the mechanisms that underlie the more common form, nonfamilial or "sporadic" AD. Indeed, the overproduction of one proteolytic product of βAPP, called the Aβ peptide, appears to be at the center of AD pathogenesis, and the currently available experimental evidence suggests that the βAPP, presenilin 1, and presenilin 2 proteins all play a direct role in the pathogenesis of AD.

The Pathogenesis of Alzheimer Disease: β-Amyloid Peptide and Tau Protein Deposits   The most impor-

tant pathological abnormalities of AD are the deposition in the brain of two fibrillary proteins, β-amyloid peptide (Aβ) and tau protein. The Aβ peptide is generated from the larger βAPP protein (see Table 12-9), as discussed later, and is found in extracellular amyloid or senile plaques in the extracellular space of AD brains. Amyloid plaques contain other proteins besides the Aβ peptide, notably apolipoprotein E (see Table 12-9). Tau is a microtubule-associated protein expressed abundantly in neurons of the brain. Hyperphosphorylated forms of tau compose the neurofibrillary tangles that, in contrast to the extracellular amyloid plaques, are found *within* AD neurons. The tau protein normally promotes the assembly and stability of microtubules, functions that are diminished by phosphorylation. Although the formation of tau neurofibrillary tangles appears to be one of the causes of the neuronal degeneration in AD, mutations in the tau gene are associated not with AD but with another autosomal dominant dementia, frontotemporal dementia.

The Amyloid Precursor Protein Gives Rise to the β-Amyloid Peptide   The major features of the βAPP and its corresponding gene are summarized in Table 12-9. βAPP is a single-pass transmembrane protein that is subject to three distinct proteolytic fates, depending on the relative activity of three different proteases: α-secretase and β-secretase, which are cell surface proteases; and γ-secretase, which is an atypical protease that cleaves membrane proteins within their transmembrane domains (Fig. 12-26). The predominant fate of approximately 90% of βAPP is cleavage by the α-secretase (Fig. 12-27), an event that precludes the formation of the Aβ peptide, since α-secretase cleaves within the Aβ peptide domain (see Fig. 12-26). The other approximately 10% of βAPP is cleaved by the β- and γ-secretases to form either the nontoxic $A\beta_{40}$ peptide or the $A\beta_{42}$ peptide, which is recognized to be neurotoxic. The $A\beta_{42}$ peptide is thought to be neurotoxic because it is more fibrillogenic than its $A\beta_{40}$ counterpart, a feature that makes AD a conformational disease like α1AT deficiency (see previous discussion). Normally, little $A\beta_{42}$ peptide is produced, and the factors that determine whether γ-secretase cleavage will produce the $A\beta_{40}$ or $A\beta_{42}$ peptide are not well defined. In monogenic AD due to missense substitutions in the gene encoding βAPP, however, several mutations in the βAPP gene selectively increase the production of the $A\beta_{42}$ peptide. This increase leads to accumulation of the neurotoxic $A\beta_{42}$, an event that appears to be the central pathogenic event of all forms of AD, monogenic or sporadic. Consistent with this model is the fact that patients with Down syndrome, who possess three copies of the βAPP gene (which is on chromosome 21), typically develop the neuropathological changes of AD by 40 years of age. Moreover, muta-

Table 12-9

The Genes and Proteins Associated with Inherited Susceptibility to Alzheimer Disease

Gene	Protein	Normal Function	Role in FAD	Gene Location	Percentage of FAD	Pattern of Inheritance
APP	Amyloid precursor protein (βAPP): a transmembrane protein found in endosomes, lysosomes, ER, and Golgi. Normally, βAPP is cleaved endoproteolytically within the transmembrane domain, so that little of the β-amyloid peptide (Aβ) is formed.	Unknown	β-Amyloid peptide (Aβ) is the principal component of senile plaques. Increased Aβ production, especially of the Aβ_{42} form, is a key pathogenic event. About 10 mutations have been identified in FAD.	21q21.3	1–2%	AD
PSEN1	Presenilin 1 (PS1): a 5 to 10 membrane-spanning domain protein found in cell types both inside and outside the brain	Unknown, but required for γ-secretase cleavage of βAPP	May participate in the abnormal cleavage at position 42 of βAPP and its derivative proteins. More than 100 mutations identified in Alzheimer disease.	14q24.3	50%	AD
PSEN2	Presenilin 2 (PS2): structure similar to PS1, maximal expression outside brain	Unknown, likely to be similar to PS1	At least 5 missense mutations identified.	1q42.1	1–2%	AD
APOE	Apolipoprotein E (ApoE): a protein component of several plasma lipoproteins (e.g. VLDL). The ApoE mRNA is not transcribed in neurons; the protein is imported into the cytoplasm from the extracellular space.	Normal function in neurons is unknown. Outside the brain, ApoE participates in lipid transport between tissues and cells. Loss of function causes one form (type III) of hyperlipoproteinemia.	An Alzheimer disease susceptibility gene (see Table 12-10). ApoE is a component of senile plaques.	19q13	Not applicable	See Table 12-10

AD, autosomal dominant; ER, endoplasmic reticulum; FAD, familial Alzheimer disease; VLDL, very low density lipoprotein.

Data derived from St. George Hyslop PH, et al: Alzheimer's disease and the fronto-temporal dementias: diseases with cerebral deposition of fibrillar proteins. In Scriver CR, Beaudet AL, Sly WS, Valle D (eds): The Molecular and Metabolic Bases of Inherited Disease, 8th ed. New York, McGraw-Hill, 2000; and Martin JB: Molecular basis of the neurodegenerative disorders. N Engl J Med 340:1970-1980, 1999.

tions in the AD genes presenilin 1 and presenilin 2 (see Table 12-9 and Fig. 12-27) also lead to increased production of Aβ_{42}. Notably, the amount of the neurotoxic Aβ_{42} peptide is increased in the serum of individuals with mutations in the βAPP, presenilin 1, and presenilin 2 genes, and in cultured cell systems, the expression of mutant βAPP, presenilin 1, and presenilin 2 genes increases the relative production of Aβ_{42} peptide by 2-fold to 10-fold.

The Presenilin 1 and 2 Genes   The genes encoding presenilin 1 and presenilin 2 (see Table 12-9) were identified by positional cloning strategies in families with autosomal dominant AD. Presenilin 1 is required for γ-secretase cleavage of βAPP derivatives. Indeed, some evidence suggests that presenilin 1 is a critical cofactor protein of γ-secretase. The mutations in presenilin 1 associated with AD, through a mechanism that is presently unclear, increase production of the Aβ_{42} peptide. The presenilin 2 protein is 60% identical in sequence to presenilin 1, suggesting that the two polypeptides have related functions. A major difference between presenilin 1 and presenilin 2 mutations is that the age at onset with the latter is much more variable

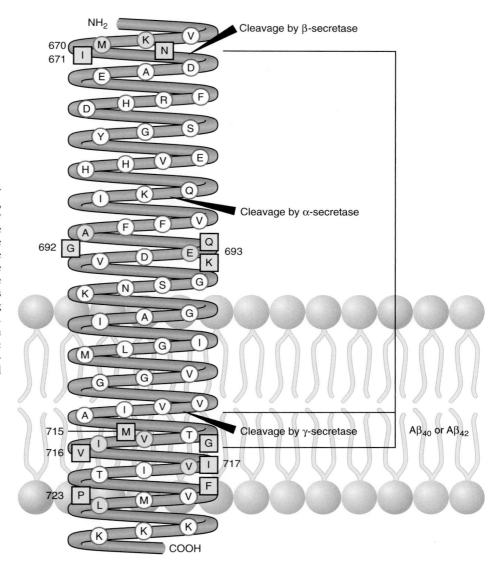

Figure 12-26 ■ The topology of the amyloid precursor protein, its nonamyloidogenic cleavage by α-secretase, and its alternative cleavage by putative β-secretase and γ-secretase to generate the amyloidogenic β-amyloid peptide (Aβ). The amino acids inside squares represent substitutions that interfere with the processing of the β-amyloid precursor protein. (Reproduced with permission from Nussbaum RL, Ellis CE: Alzheimer's disease and Parkinson's disease. N Engl J Med 348:1356-1364, 2003.)

(presenilin 1, 35 to 60 years; presenilin 2, 40 to 85 years), and in one family, an asymptomatic octogenarian carrying a presenilin 2 mutation transmitted the disease to his offspring. The basis of this variation is partly dependent on the number of *APOE* ε4 alleles (see Table 12-9 and later discussion) carried by individuals with a presenilin 2 mutation; two ε4 alleles are associated with an earlier age at onset than one allele, and one confers an earlier onset than other *APOE* alleles.

The *APOE* Gene Is an Alzheimer Disease Susceptibility Locus One allele of the *APOE* gene, the ε4 allele, is a major risk factor for the development of AD. The role for *APOE* as a major susceptibility locus in AD was suggested by four independent lines of evidence: linkage analyses in late-onset families with an aggregation of

AD, increased association of the ε4 allele with AD patients compared with controls, the discovery that the *APOE* protein is a component of the AD amyloid plaques, and the finding that apolipoprotein E binds to the Aβ peptide. The *APOE* protein has three common forms encoded by corresponding *APOE* alleles (Table 12-10). The ε4 allele is significantly overrepresented in patients with AD (~40% vs. ~15% in the general population) and is associated with an early onset of AD (for ε4 allele homozygotes, the age at onset of AD is about 10 to 15 years earlier than in the general population). Moreover, the relationship between the ε4 allele and the disease is dose dependent; two copies of ε4 are associated with an earlier age at onset (mean onset before 70 years) than with one copy (mean onset after 70 years) (see Fig. 8-7 and Table 8-7). In contrast, the ε2 allele has a protective effect and correspondingly is

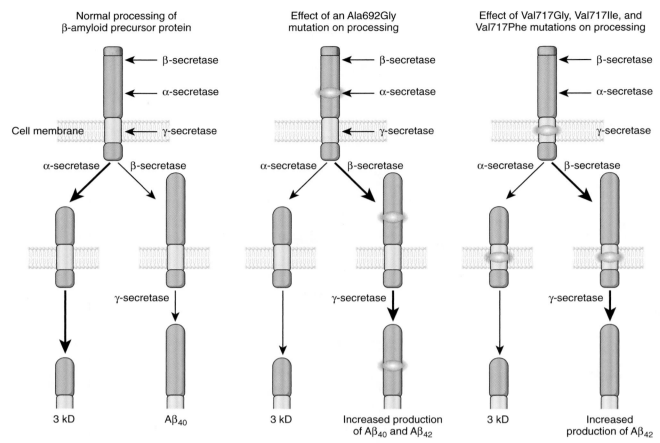

Normal processing of
β-amyloid precursor protein

Effect of an Ala692Gly
mutation on processing

Effect of Val717Gly, Val717Ile, and
Val717Phe mutations on processing

Figure 12-27 ■ The normal processing of β-amyloid precursor protein and the effect on processing of missense mutations in the *βAPP* gene associated with familial Alzheimer disease. The gray ovals show the locations of the missense mutations. (Reproduced, with permission from Nussbaum RL, Ellis CE: Alzheimer's disease and Parkinson's disease. N Engl J Med 348:1356-1364, 2003.)

more common in elderly subjects who are unaffected by AD (see Table 12-10). The mechanisms underlying these effects are not known, but apolipoprotein E polymorphisms may influence the processing of βAPP and the density of amyloid plaques in AD brains. For example, mice without apolipoprotein E have a dramatic reduction in the deposition of Aβ peptide generated from a βAPP mutant allele associated with familial AD. Other mechanisms have been proposed, such as altered response to injury, since the *APOE* gene is upregulated in the brain by injury and repair. It is also important to note that the *APOE* ε4 allele is not

Table 12-10

The Amino Acid Substitutions Underlying the Three Common Apolipoprotein E Polymorphisms

Allele	ε2	ε3	ε4
Residue 112	Cys	Cys	Arg
Residue 158	Cys	Arg	Arg
Frequency in white populations	10%	65%	25%
Frequency in patients with Alzheimer disease	2%	58%	40%
Effect on Alzheimer disease	Protective	None known	30%-50% of the genetic risk of Alzheimer disease

These figures are estimates, with differences in allele frequencies that vary with ethnicity in control populations, and with age, gender, and ethnicity in AD subjects.

Data derived from St. George Hyslop PH, et al: Alzheimer's disease and the fronto-temporal dementias: diseases with cerebral deposition of fibrillar proteins. In Scriver CR, Beaudet AL, Sly WS, Valle D (eds): The Molecular and Metabolic Bases of Inherited Disease, 8th ed. New York, McGraw-Hill, 2000, and P.H. St. George Hyslop, personal communication.

uniquely associated with an increased risk of AD. Thus, carriers of ε4 alleles have poorer neurological outcomes after head injury, stroke, and other neuronal insults. Although carriers of the ε4 allele of *APOE* have a clearly increased risk for development of AD, there is currently no role for screening for the presence of this allele in healthy individuals; such testing has poor positive and negative predictive values and would therefore generate highly uncertain estimates of future risk of AD (see Chapter 17).

Other AD Genes   Statistical analyses suggest that an additional four to eight genes may significantly modify the risk of AD. The identity of these genes remains obscure. In addition, case-control association studies (Chapter 10) have implicated a long list of candidate genes (>100) in AD, but few if any of these assignments have been replicated, and their role in the genetic specification of risk for AD is unclear.

Diseases of Mitochondrial DNA (mtDNA)

The mtDNA Genome and the Genetics of mtDNA Diseases

The characteristics of the mtDNA genome, and the features of the inheritance of disorders caused by mutations in this genome, are described in Chapters 2 and 7 but reviewed briefly here. The circular mtDNA chromosome of 16.5 kb is located inside mitochondria and contains 37 genes (Fig. 12-28). Most cells have at least 1000 mtDNA molecules, distributed among hundreds of individual mitochondria, with multiple copies of mtDNA per mitochondrion. In addition to encoding two types of rRNA and 22 transfer RNAs, mtDNA encodes 13 proteins that are subunits of oxidative phosphorylation. Mutations in mtDNA can be inherited (maternally; see Chapter 7) or acquired as somatic mutations. However, the other 74 polypeptides of the oxidative phosphorylation complex are encoded by the nuclear genome, which encodes most of the estimated 1500 mitochondrial proteins. Thus, diseases of oxidative phosphorylation arise not only from mutations in the mitochondrial genome but also from mutations in nuclear genes that encode oxidative phosphorylation components. Furthermore, the nuclear genome encodes up to 200 factors required for the maintenance and expression of mtDNA or for the assembly of oxidative phosphorylation protein complexes. Mutations in many of these nuclear genes can also lead to disorders with the phenotypic characteristics of mtDNA diseases, but of course the patterns of inheritance are those typically seen with nuclear genome mutations.

The diseases that result from mutations in mtDNA show distinctive patterns of inheritance due to three features of mitochondrial chromosomes: replicative segregation, homoplasmy and heteroplasmy, and maternal inheritance (discussed in greater detail in Chapter 7). **Replicative segregation** refers to the fact that the multiple copies of mtDNA in each mitochondrion in a cell replicate and sort randomly among newly synthesized mitochondria, which are distributed randomly between the daughter cells. **Homoplasmy** is the situation in which a cell contains a pure population of normal mtDNA or of mutant mtDNA, whereas **heteroplasmy** describes the presence of a mixture of mutant and normal mtDNA molecules within a cell. Thus, the phenotype associated with a mtDNA mutation will depend on the relative proportion of normal and mutant mtDNA in the cells of a particular tissue (see Fig. 7-34). As a result, mitochondrial disorders are generally characterized by reduced penetrance, variable expression, and pleiotropy. The **maternal inheritance** of mtDNA reflects the fact that sperm mitochondria are generally eliminated from the embryo, so that mtDNA is almost always inherited entirely from the mother; paternal inheritance of mtDNA disease has been documented in only one instance.

Mutations in mtDNA and Disease

The first pathogenic mutations in mtDNA were identified in the early 1990s. Unexpected and still unexplained is the fact that the mtDNA genome mutates at a rate about 10-fold greater than does nuclear DNA. The range of clinical disease resulting from mtDNA mutations is diverse (Fig. 12-29), although neuromuscular disease predominates. More than 100 different rearrangements and about 100 different point mutations that are disease-related have been identified in mtDNA. The prevalence of mtDNA mutations has been shown, in at least one white population, to be approximately 1 in 8000. Representative mutations and the diseases associated with them are presented in Figure 12-28 and Table 12-11. Three types of mutations have been identified in mtDNA: (1) missense mutations in the coding regions of genes that alter the activity of an oxidative phosphorylation protein; (2) point mutations in tRNA or rRNA genes that impair mitochondrial protein synthesis; and (3) rearrangements that generate deletions or duplications of the mtDNA molecule. The deletions in mtDNA that are associated with disease are generally somatic in origin, although a small proportion is inherited, in some diseases.

Heteroplasmy confers three other characteristics on genetic disorders of mtDNA that are of importance to their pathogenesis. First, the risk of transmission to offspring of deleted mtDNA molecules, a common class of mtDNA mutation, is low; the mechanism underlying this low risk is discussed later. In contrast, female car-

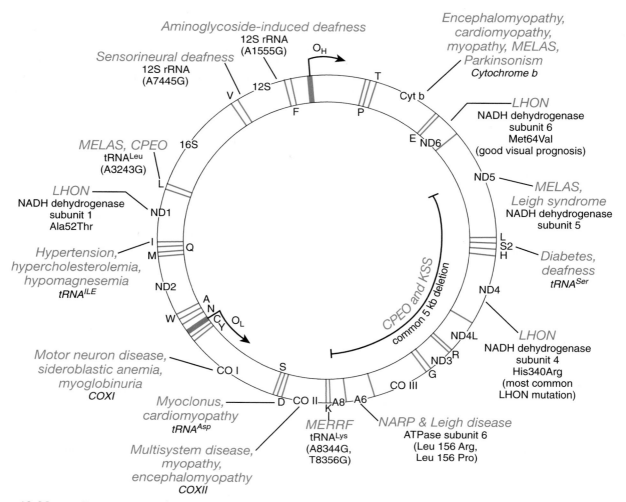

Figure 12-28 ■ Representative disease-causing mutations and deletions in the human mtDNA genome, shown in relation to the location of the genes encoding the 22 tRNAs, 2 rRNAs, and 13 proteins of the oxidative phosphorylation complex. Specific alleles are indicated when they are the predominant or only alleles associated with the phenotype or particular features of it. O_H and O_L are the origins of replication of the two DNA strands, respectively; 12S, 12S ribosomal RNA; 16S, 16S ribosomal RNA. The locations of each of the tRNAs are indicated by the single letter code for their corresponding amino acids. The 13 oxidative phosphorylation polypeptides encoded by mtDNA include components of complex I: NADH dehydrogenase (ND1, ND2, ND3, ND4, ND4L, ND5, and ND6); complex III: cytochrome *b* (cyt *b*); complex IV: cytochrome *c* oxidase I or cytochrome *c* (COI, COII, COIII); and complex V: ATPase 6 and 8 (A6, A8). The disease abbreviations used in this figure (e.g., MELAS, MERRF, LHON) are explained in Table 12-11. (Modified in part from Shoffner JM, Wallace DC: Oxidative phosphorylation disease. In Scriver CR, Beaudet AL, Sly WS, Valle D [eds]: The Metabolic and Molecular Bases of Inherited Disease, 7th ed. New York, McGraw-Hill, 1995. The location of some of the disorders is taken from DiMauro S, Schon EA: Mitochondrial respiratory-chain diseases. N Engl J Med 348:2656-2568, 2003.)

riers of heteroplasmic mtDNA point mutations, or of mtDNA duplications, usually transmit some mutant mtDNAs to their offspring. Second, the number of mtDNA molecules within each oocyte is reduced before being subsequently amplified to the huge total seen in mature oocytes. This restriction and subsequent amplification of mtDNA during oogenesis is termed the **mitochondrial genetic bottleneck.** Consequently, the variability in the percentage of mutant mtDNA molecules seen in the offspring of a mother carrying a mtDNA mutation arises, at least in part, from the sam-

pling of only a subset of the mtDNAs during oogenesis. Third, despite the variability in the degree of heteroplasmy arising from the bottleneck, mothers with a high proportion of mutant mtDNA molecules are more likely to have clinically affected offspring than are mothers with a lower proportion, as one would predict from the random sampling of mtDNA molecules through the bottleneck. Nevertheless, even women carrying low proportions of pathogenic mtDNA molecules have some risk of having an affected child because the bottleneck can lead to the sampling and subsequent

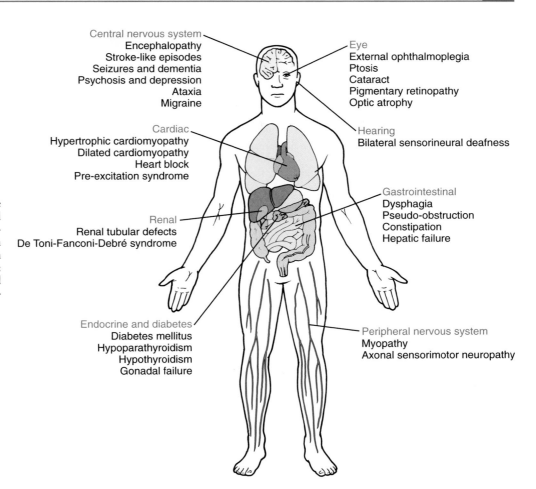

Central nervous system
Encephalopathy
Stroke-like episodes
Seizures and dementia
Psychosis and depression
Ataxia
Migraine

Eye
External ophthalmoplegia
Ptosis
Cataract
Pigmentary retinopathy
Optic atrophy

Cardiac
Hypertrophic cardiomyopathy
Dilated cardiomyopathy
Heart block
Pre-excitation syndrome

Hearing
Bilateral sensorineural deafness

Renal
Renal tubular defects
De Toni-Fanconi-Debré syndrome

Gastrointestinal
Dysphagia
Pseudo-obstruction
Constipation
Hepatic failure

Endocrine and diabetes
Diabetes mellitus
Hypoparathyroidism
Hypothyroidism
Gonadal failure

Peripheral nervous system
Myopathy
Axonal sensorimotor neuropathy

Figure 12-29 ■ The range of affected tissues and clinical phenotypes associated with mutations in mtDNA. (Modified from Chinnery PF, Turnbull DM: Mitochondrial DNA and disease. Lancet 354:SI17-SI21, 1999.)

expansion, by chance, of even a rare mutant mtDNA species.

Deletions of mtDNA and Disease In contrast to the maternal inheritance of most mtDNA diseases, most cases of the **Kearns-Sayre syndrome** and **Pearson syndrome** (see Table 12-11) are due to sporadic somatic mutations; only about 5% of cases result from maternal transmission of the deletions. The reason for the low frequency of transmission is uncertain, but it may simply reflect the fact that women with a high proportion of the deleted mtDNAs in their germ cells have a severe phenotype (**Kearns-Sayre syndrome**) and rarely reproduce.

The importance of deletions in mtDNA as a cause of disease has recently been highlighted by the discovery that *somatic* mtDNA deletions are common in dopaminergic neurons of the substantia nigra, both in normal aging individuals and perhaps to a greater extent in individuals with **Parkinson disease.** The deletions that have occurred in individual neurons from individual aging healthy persons and from Parkinson disease patients have been shown to be unique, indicating that clonal expansion of the different mtDNA deletions occurred in each cell. These findings indicate that

somatic deletions of the mtDNA are an important cause of the loss of dopaminergic neurons in the aging substantia nigra, and raise the possibility that the common sporadic form of Parkinson disease may result from a greater than normal accumulation of deleted mtDNA molecules in the substantia nigra, with a consequently more severe impairment of oxidative phosphorylation. At present, the mechanisms leading to the deletions and the clonal expansions are entirely unclear.

The Phenotypes of Mitochondrial Disorders

Oxidative Phosphorylation and mtDNA Diseases Mitochondrial mutations generally affect those tissues that depend on intact oxidative phosphorylation to satisfy high demands for metabolic energy. This phenotypic focus reflects the central role of the oxidative phosphorylation complex in the production of cellular energy. Consequently, decreased production of ATP characterizes many diseases of mtDNA and is likely to underlie the cell dysfunction and cell death that occur in mtDNA diseases. The evidence that mechanisms other than decreased energy production contribute to the pathogenesis of mtDNA diseases is either indirect or weak, but the

Table 12-11

Representative Examples of Disorders due to Mutations in Mitochondrial DNA and Their Inheritance

Disease	Phenotypes—Largely Neurological	Most Frequent Mutation in mtDNA Molecule	Homoplasmy vs. Heteroplasmy	Inheritance
Leber hereditary optic neuropathy (LHON)	Rapid onset of blindness in young adult life due to optic nerve atrophy; some recovery of vision, depending on the mutation. Strong sex bias: ~50% of male carriers have visual loss vs. ~10% of females	Substitution 1178A>G in the ND4 subunit of complex I of the electron transport chain; this mutation, with two others, accounts for more than 90% of cases; 14459T>A, in the ND1 subunit, is the most severe mutation, with less sex bias	Largely homoplasmic	Maternal
NARP	Neuropathy, ataxia, retinitis pigmentosa; developmental delay, mental retardation, lactic acidemia	Point mutations in the ATPase subunit 6 gene	Heteroplasmic	Maternal
Leigh syndrome	Early-onset progressive neurodegeneration with hypotonia, developmental delay, optic atrophy, and respiratory abnormalities	Point mutations in the ATPase subunit 6 gene	Heteroplasmic	Maternal
MELAS	Myopathy, mitochondrial encephalomyopathy, lactic acidosis, and stroke-like episodes; may present only as diabetes mellitus and deafness	Point mutations in tRNA$^{leu(UUR)}$, a mutation hotspot, most commonly 3243A>G	Heteroplasmic	Maternal
MERRF (Case 28)	Myoclonic epilepsy with ragged-red muscle fibers, myopathy, ataxia, sensorineural deafness, dementia	Point mutations in tRNA^{lys}, most commonly 8344A>G	Heteroplasmic	Maternal
Deafness	Progressive sensorineural deafness, often induced by aminoglycoside antibiotics; nonsyndromic sensorineural deafness	1555A>G mutation in the 12S rRNA gene 7445A>G mutation in the 12S rRNA gene	Homoplasmic Homoplasmic	Maternal Maternal
Chronic progressive external ophthalmoplegia (CPEO)	Progressive atrophy of extraocular muscles, ptosis	The common MELAS point mutation in tRNA$^{leu(UUR)}$; large deletions similar to KSS	Heteroplasmic	Maternal with point mutations, sporadic with deletions
Pearson syndrome	Pancreatic insufficiency, pancytopenia, lactic acidosis, KSS in second decade	Large deletions	Heteroplasmic	Generally sporadic, due to somatic mutations
Kearns-Sayre syndrome (KSS)	Progressive myopathy, progressive external ophthalmoplegia of early onset, cardiomyopathy, heart block, ptosis, retinal pigmentation, ataxia, diabetes	The ~5 kb large deletion (see Fig. 12-28)	Heteroplasmic	Generally sporadic, due to somatic mutations

generation of reactive oxygen species as a byproduct of oxidative phosphorylation may also contribute to the pathology of mtDNA disorders. A substantial body of evidence indicates that there is a **phenotypic threshold effect** associated with mtDNA heteroplasmy; a critical threshold in the proportion of mtDNA molecules carrying the detrimental mutation must be exceeded in cells from the affected tissue before clinical disease becomes apparent. The threshold appears to be about 60% for disorders due to deletions in the mtDNA and about 90% for diseases due to other types of mutations.

The neuromuscular system is most commonly affected by mutations in mtDNA; the consequences include encephalopathy, myopathy, ataxia, retinal degeneration, and loss of function of the external ocular muscles. Mitochondrial myopathy is characterized by so-called ragged-red (muscle) fibers, a histological phenotype due to the proliferation of structurally and biochemically abnormal mitochondria in muscle fibers. The spectrum of mitochondrial disease is broad and, as illustrated in Figure 12-29, may include liver dysfunction, bone marrow failure, pancreatic islet cell deficiency and diabetes, deafness, and other disorders.

Unexplained and Unexpected Phenotypic Variation in mtDNA Diseases Heteroplasmy is the rule for almost all mtDNA diseases, with the exception of Leber hereditary optic neuropathy (LHON; see Table 12-11), which is generally homoplasmic. Heteroplasmy, which leads to an unpredictable and variable fraction of mutant mtDNA being present in any particular tissue, undoubtedly accounts for much of the pleiotropy and variable expressivity of mtDNA mutations (see Table 12-11). Thus, in a single kindred, a specific mutant mtDNA can be associated with diabetes and deafness in one individual and severe encephalopathy with seizures in another. Another example is provided by what appears to be the most common mtDNA mutation, the 3243A>G substitution in the tRNA$^{leu(UUR)}$ gene (the nomenclature refers to the normal nucleotide at position 3243 in the mtDNA molecule, followed by the substituted nucleotide). The 3243A>G substitution is most commonly associated with the phenotype referred to as **MELAS,** an acronym for *m*itochondrial *e*ncephalomyopathy with *l*actic *a*cidosis and *s*troke-like episodes (see Fig. 12-28 and Table 12-11). In some families, however, this mutation leads predominantly to diabetes and deafness, whereas in others it is associated with **chronic progressive external ophthalmoplegia** (see Table 12-11); in yet others, affected individuals present with cardiomyopathy or myopathy. In addition, a very small fraction (<1%) of diabetes mellitus in the general population, particularly in Japanese, has been attributed to the 3243A>G substitution.

Mutations in tRNA and rRNA Genes of the Mitochondrial Genome Mutations in the nonprotein-coding tRNA and rRNA genes of mtDNA are of general significance because they illustrate that not all disease-causing mutations in humans occur in genes that encode proteins. More than 90 pathogenic mutations have been identified in 20 of the 22 tRNA genes of the mtDNA, and they are the most common cause of oxidative phosphorylation abnormalities in humans (see Fig. 12-28 and Table 12-11). The resulting phenotypes are generally those associated with mtDNA defects. Included in the diverse set of tRNA mutations are 18 substitutions in the tRNA$^{leu(UUR)}$ gene, some of which cause MELAS, like the 3243A>G mutation, and others that do not, being associated predominantly with myopathy. Similarly, some substitutions in the 12S rRNA gene, when homoplasmic, cause sensorineural prelingual deafness after exposure to aminoglycoside antibiotics (see Fig. 12-28).

Elucidation of the different effects of the mutations in the tRNA$^{leu(UUR)}$ gene associated with MELAS compared with those causing only myopathy has provided one of the first explanations for the relationship between a genotype and a phenotype in diseases of mtDNA. Many of the tRNA$^{leu(UUR)}$ gene mutations that cause MELAS have been found to prevent, by mechanisms unknown, a key biochemical modification of a wobble base U in the tRNA, whereas those substitutions that lead only to myopathy do not impair the modification of the wobble base (Fig. 12-30). A wobble base is present in the third position of many codons and is so named because it tolerates a mismatch. The wobble base is important in codon recognition and codon-anticodon binding; in the absence of the biochemical modifications, the ability of the anticodon containing the unmodified wobble base to decode some codons is disrupted (see Fig. 12-30).

Parenthetically, only one example of mutation in an RNA gene in the nuclear genome has been recognized to date. Allelic mutations in the *RMRP* gene, which encodes the untranslated RNA subunit of the ribonucleoprotein endoribonuclease RNase MRP, cause three different short stature syndromes, including the autosomal recessive disorder **cartilage hair hypoplasia.**

Interactions Between the Mitochondrial and Nuclear Genomes Because both the nuclear and mitochondrial genomes contribute polypeptides to oxidative phosphorylation, it is not surprising that the phenotypes associated with mutations in the nuclear genes are often indistinguishable from those due to mtDNA mutations. Moreover, mtDNA has been referred to as "the slave of nuclear DNA" because mtDNA depends on many nuclear genome–encoded proteins for its replication and the maintenance of its integrity. Genetic evidence has highlighted the direct nature of the relationship between the nuclear and mtDNA genomes. The first indication of this interaction was provided by

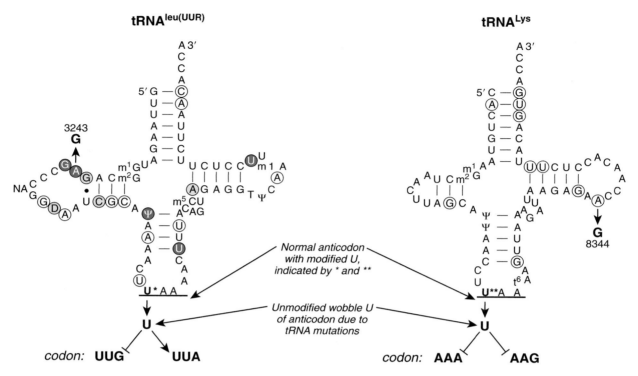

Figure 12-30 ■ The secondary structures of two tRNAs commonly affected by mutations in the mtDNA genome, tRNA^leu(UUR) and tRNA^lys. The wobble base of the tRNA^leu(UUR) is subject to one modification, indicated by an asterisk, whereas that of tRNA^lys is modified twice, as indicated by two asterisks. The most prevalent mutations, at position 3243 in tRNA^leu(UUR) and position 8344 in tRNA^lys, are shown. Circled bases are those subject to pathogenic mutations. Some mutations (dark blue) in the tRNA^leu(UUR) prevent the modification of the wobble base and cause the MELAS phenotype. Other mutations (light blue) that do not disrupt the wobble base modification cause only myopathy. The effect of mutations in the other bases subject to mutation (unshaded circles) has not been examined. Unmodified wobble bases in the anticodon of tRNA^leu(UUR) prevent decoding of the UUG codon for leucine and decrease the efficiency of decoding of the UUA codon, whereas loss of wobble modifications in tRNA^lys impairs the decoding of both of the two lysine codons, AAA and AAG. (Modified from Shoubridge EA, Sasarman F: Mitochondrial translation and human disease. In Mathews MB, Sonenberg N, Hershey JWB [eds]: Translational Control in Biology and Medicine. Cold Spring Harbor, NY, Cold Spring Harbor Laboratory Press, 2007.)

the identification of the syndrome of **autosomally transmitted deletions in mtDNA,** whose phenotype resembles chronic progressive external ophthalmoplegia (see Table 12-11). Mutations in at least two genes have been associated with this phenotype. The protein encoded by one of these genes, amusingly called Twinkle, appears to be a DNA primase or helicase. The product of the second gene is a mitochondrial-specific DNA polymerase γ whose loss of function is associated with both dominant and recessive multiple deletion syndromes.

A second autosomal disorder, the **mtDNA depletion syndrome,** is the result of mutations in any of six nuclear genes (which appear to account for only a minority of affected individuals) that lead to a reduction in the number of copies of mtDNA (both per mitochondrion and per cell) in various tissues. Several of the affected genes encode proteins required to maintain nucleotide pools, or to metabolize nucleotides appropriately, in the mitochondrion. For example, both myopathic and hepatocerebral phenotypes result from mutations in the genes for mitochondrial thymidine kinase and deoxyguanosine kinase. Another disorder, **mitochondrial gastrointestinal encephalomyopathy,** is the result of mutations in thymidine phosphorylase, which, although not a mitochondrial protein, appears to be particularly important for the maintenance of mitochondrial nucleotide pools. Apart from the insights that these rare disorders provide into the biology of the mitochondrion, the identification of the affected genes facilitates genetic counseling and prenatal diagnosis in some families and suggests, in some instances, potential treatments. For example, the blood thymidine level is markedly increased in thymidine phosphorylase deficiency, suggesting that lowering thymidine levels might have therapeutic benefits.

Nuclear Genes Can Modify the Phenotype of mtDNA Diseases Although heteroplasmy is a major source of phenotypic variability in mtDNA diseases, additional factors, including genes at nuclear loci, must also play a role. Strong evidence for the existence of such factors is provided by families carrying mutations associated

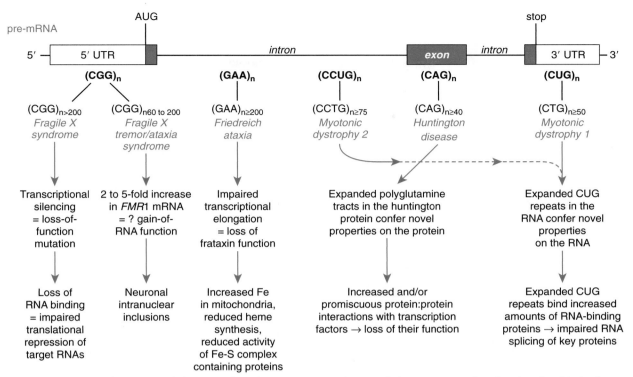

Figure 12-31 ■ The locations of the trinucleotide repeat expansions and the sequence of each trinucleotide in five representative trinucleotide repeat diseases, shown on a schematic of a generic pre-mRNA. The minimal number of repeats in the DNA sequence of the affected gene associated with the disease is also indicated. The effect of the expansion on the mutant RNA or protein is also indicated. (Based partly on an unpublished figure of John A. Phillips III, Vanderbilt University.)

with LHON; in this condition, the mutations are generally homoplasmic (and therefore the phenotypic variation cannot be explained by heteroplasmy). LHON is expressed phenotypically as rapid, painless bilateral loss of central vision due to optic nerve atrophy in young adults (see Table 12-11 and Fig. 12-28). Depending on the mutation, there is often some recovery of vision, but the pathogenic mechanisms of the optic nerve damage are unclear. Affected individuals may be male or female, but there is a striking and unexplained increase in the penetrance of the disease in males; about 50% of male carriers but only about 10% of female carriers of a LHON mutation develop symptoms. The variation in penetrance and the male bias of the phenotype have been shown to be determined by a haplotype on the short arm of the X chromosome. The gene at this nuclear-encoded modifier locus has not yet been identified, but it is contained within an X chromosomal haplotype that is common—and likely ancient—in the general population. When this variant is transmitted to individuals who have inherited the LHON mtDNA mutation from their generally unaffected mother, the phenotype is substantially modified. For example, males carrying alleles other than that associated with the most severe LHON phenotype (see Table 12-11) are 35-fold more likely to develop visual failure if they carry the high-risk X-linked haplotype. These observations are of general significance because they demonstrate that it is indeed possible to identify modifier loci of monogenic diseases, this X-linked locus being one of the few such modifiers documented to date in the human genome.

Diseases due to the Expansion of Unstable Repeat Sequences: Biochemical and Cellular Mechanisms

The inheritance pattern of diseases due to unstable repeat expansions is presented in Chapter 7, with emphasis on the unusual genetics of this unique group of almost 20 disorders. These features include the unstable **dynamic** nature of the mutations, which are due to the expansion, within the *transcribed* region of the affected gene, of repeated sequences such as the codon for glutamine (CAG) in **Huntington disease** and most of a group of neurodegenerative disorders called the **spinocerebellar ataxias** (for which there are at least nine loci), or of trinucleotides in noncoding regions of RNAs, including CGG in **fragile X syndrome**, GAA in **Friedreich ataxia**, and CTG in **myotonic dystrophy 1** (Fig. 12-31; see Table 7-3).

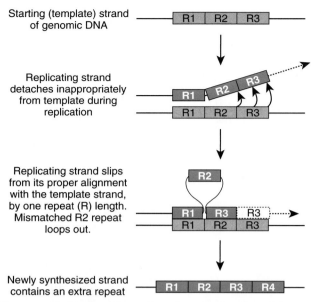

Starting (template) strand
of genomic DNA

Replicating strand
detaches inappropriately
from template during
replication

Replicating strand slips
from its proper alignment
with the template strand,
by one repeat (R) length.
Mismatched R2 repeat
loops out.

Newly synthesized strand
contains an extra repeat

Figure 12-32 ■ The slipped mispairing mechanism thought to underlie the expansion of unstable repeats, such as the (CAG)$_n$ repeat found in Huntington disease and the spinocerebellar ataxias. An insertion occurs when the newly synthesized strand aberrantly dissociates from the template strand during replication synthesis. When the new strand reassociates with the template strand, the new strand may slip back to align out of register with an incorrect repeat copy. Once DNA synthesis is resumed, the misaligned molecule will contain one or more extra copies of the repeat (depending on the number of repeat copies that slipped out in the misalignment event).

Although the initial nucleotide repeat diseases to be described are all due to the expansion of three nucleotide repeats, others disorders have now been found to result from the expansion of longer repeats; these include a tetranucleotide (CCTG) in **myotonic dystrophy 2** (a close genocopy of myotonic dystrophy 1) and a pentanucleotide (ATTCT) in spinocerebellar atrophy 10. As the affected gene is passed from generation to generation, the number of repeats may expand to a degree that is pathogenic, ultimately interfering with normal gene expression and function. The intergenerational expansion of the repeats accounts for the phenomenon of **anticipation,** the appearance of the disease at an earlier age as it is transmitted through a family. The biochemical mechanism most commonly proposed to underlie the expansion of unstable repeat sequences is slipped mispairing (Fig. 12-32). Remarkably, the repeat expansions appear to occur both in proliferating cells such as spermatogonia (during meiosis) and in nonproliferating somatic cells such as neurons. Consequently, expansion can occur, depending on the disease, during both DNA replication (as shown in Fig. 12-32) and genome maintenance (i.e., DNA repair).

The clinical phenotypes of Huntington disease, fragile X syndrome, myotonic dystrophy, and Fried-

reich ataxia are presented in Chapter 7. For reasons that are not at all apparent, diseases due to the expansion of unstable repeats are primarily neurological; the clinical presentations include ataxia, cognitive defects, dementia, nystagmus, parkinsonism, and spasticity. Nevertheless, other systems are sometimes involved, as illustrated by some of the diseases discussed here.

The Pathogenesis of Diseases due to Unstable Repeat Expansions

Diseases of unstable repeat expansion are diverse in their pathogenic mechanisms and can be divided into three classes.

- **Class 1: diseases due to the expansion of noncoding repeats that cause a loss of protein function** by impairing transcription of the preRNA from the affected gene. Examples: fragile X syndrome and Friedreich ataxia.
- **Class 2: disorders resulting from expansions of noncoding repeats that confer novel properties** on the RNA. Examples: myotonic dystrophy 1 and 2, fragile X–associated tremor/ataxia syndrome.
- **Class 3: diseases due to repeat expansion of a codon** (such as CAG for glutamine) that confers novel properties on the affected protein. Examples: Huntington disease, the spinocerebellar ataxias.

Class 1: Diseases due to the Expansion of Noncoding Repeats That Cause a Loss of Protein Function

Fragile X Syndrome In the X-linked fragile X syndrome (Case 15), the expansion of the CGG repeat in the 5′ UTR of the *FMR1* gene, to more than 200 copies, leads to excessive methylation of cytosines in the promoter, an epigenetic modification of the DNA that silences transcription from the gene (see Fig. 12-31). Consequently, loss of the normal function of the FMRP protein is the cause of the mental retardation and learning deficits and the non-neurological features of the clinical phenotype, including macroorchidism and connective tissue dysplasia. FMRP is an RNA-binding protein that associates with polyribosomes to suppress the translation of proteins from its RNA targets. These targets appear to be involved in cytoskeletal structure, synaptic transmission, and neuronal maturation, and the disruption of these processes is likely to underlie the mental retardation and learning abnormalities seen in fragile X patients. For example, FMRP appears to regulate the translation of proteins required for the formation of synapses, since the brains of individuals with the fragile X syndrome have increased density of abnormally long immature dendritic spines. Moreover, FMRP localizes to dendritic spines, where at least one of its roles is to regulate synaptic plasticity, the capacity to alter the strength of a synaptic connection, a process critical to learning and memory.

Friedreich Ataxia Friedreich ataxia, the most common inherited spinocerebellar ataxia, with a prevalence of 2 to 4/100,000 among Europeans and individuals from the Middle East and India, is an autosomal recessive disease that is also characterized by cardiomyopathy and type 2 diabetes. It results from the expansion, to more than 200 and up to 1700 copies, of a GAA repeat in the first intron of the *FRDA* gene (see Fig. 12-31). The greater the number of repeats, the more severe is the disease. As with fragile X syndrome, the expansion impairs gene function, in this case by inhibiting transcriptional elongation. The molecular pathogenesis of Friedreich ataxia reflects the loss of the normal functions of the affected protein, frataxin. Although these functions are not precisely known, its proposed roles include acting as an iron-binding protein, an essential factor in the formation of heme and in the synthesis and integrity of Fe-S clusters (a combination of iron and sulfur found in some proteins, particularly oxidoreductases such as complexes I to IV of the electron transport chain that are associated with diseases of the mitochondrial genome, discussed earlier). Accordingly, the loss of frataxin activity is associated with increased levels of mitochondrial iron, impaired heme synthesis (although interestingly, not in red blood cells), and reduced activity of Fe-S–containing proteins such as complexes I to III of the mitochondrial respiratory transport chain.

Class 2: Disorders Resulting from Expansions of Noncoding Repeats That Confer Novel Properties on the RNA

Myotonic Dystrophy Myotonic dystrophy 1 (DM1) is an autosomal dominant condition with the most pleiotropic phenotype of all the unstable repeat expansion disorders. In addition to myotonia, it is characterized by muscle weakness and wasting, cardiac conduction defects, testicular atrophy, insulin resistance, and cataracts; there is also a congenital form with mental retardation. The disease results from a CTG expansion in the 3′ UTR of the *DMPK* gene, which encodes a protein kinase (see Fig. 12-31). Myotonic dystrophy 2 (DM2) is also an autosomal dominant trait and shares most of the clinical features of DM1, except that there is no associated congenital presentation. DM2 is due to the expansion of a CCTG tetranucleotide in the first intron of the gene encoding zinc finger protein 9 (see Fig. 12-31). The strikingly similar phenotypes of DM1 and DM2 suggest that they have a common pathogenesis. Since the unstable expansions occur within the noncoding regions of two different genes that encode unrelated proteins, the CUG trinucleotide expansion itself is thought to underlie an RNA-mediated pathogenesis.

What is the mechanism by which large tracts of the CUG trinucleotide, in the noncoding region of genes, lead to the DM1 and DM2 phenotypes? The pathogenesis appears to result from the binding of the CUG repeats to RNA-binding proteins. Consequently, the pleiotropy that typifies the disease may reflect the broad array of RNA-binding proteins to which the CUG repeats bind. Many of the RNA-binding proteins "quenched" by the excessive number of CUG repeats are regulators of splicing, and indeed more than a dozen distinct pre-mRNAs have been shown to have splicing alterations in DM1, including cardiac troponin T (which might account for the cardiac abnormalities) and the insulin receptor (which may explain the insulin resistance). Even though our knowledge of the abnormal processes underlying DM1 and DM2 is still incomplete, these molecular insights offer the hope that a rational small molecule therapy might be developed.

Fragile X–Associated Tremor/Ataxia Syndrome Remarkably, the pathogenesis of disease in individuals with 60 to 200 CGG repeats in the *FMR1* gene, causing the clinically distinct **fragile X tremor/ataxia syndrome (FXTAS)**, is entirely different from that of the fragile X syndrome itself. Although decreased translational efficiency impairs the expression of the FMRP protein in FXTAS, this reduction cannot be responsible for the disease, since males with full mutations and virtually complete loss of function of the *FMR1* gene never develop FXTAS. Rather, the evidence suggests that FXTAS results from the twofold to fivefold increased levels of the *FMR1* mRNA present in these patients, representing a gain-of-function mutation. This pathogenic RNA leads to the formation of intranuclear neuronal inclusions, the cellular signature of the disease.

Class 3: Diseases due to Repeat Expansion of a Codon

Huntington Disease Huntington disease is an autosomal dominant neurodegenerative disorder associated with chorea, athetosis, loss of cognition, and psychiatric abnormalities (Case 22). The pathological process is caused by the expansion—to more than 40 repeats—of the codon CAG in the *HD* gene, resulting in long polyglutamine tracts in the mutant protein, huntingtin. It appears that the mutant proteins with expanded polyglutamine sequences are novel property mutants (see Chapter 11), the expanded tract conferring novel features on the protein that damage specific populations of neurons and produce neurodegeneration by a unique toxic mechanism. The most striking cellular hallmark of the disease is the presence of insoluble aggregates of the mutant protein, and other polypeptides, clustered in nuclear inclusions. The aggregates are thought to result from normal cellular responses to the misfolding of huntingtin that results from the polyglutamine expansion. Dramatic as these inclusions are, however, it appears that their formation is actually protective rather than pathogenic.

Although a unifying model of the neuronal death mediated by polyglutamine expansion in huntingtin is not at hand, the soluble nonaggregated form of mutant huntingtin has recently emerged as the focal point of the pathogenesis. The toxic effects of the polyglutamine tract occur only when the tract is situated within its natural "host" protein (in this case huntingtin). For example, neurodegeneration is not induced by a fragment of huntingtin composed only of the polyglutamine tract and adjacent sequences. Several lines of evidence indicate that the mutant polyglutamine tract fosters interactions with a number of transcriptional regulators including, for example, the TATA box (see Chapter 3) binding protein. The consequent alterations in the transcription of many proteins may be central to the pathological process. It seems likely that similar processes underlie the pathogenesis of the spinocerebellar ataxias, each of which is also due to a CAG expansion.

Despite the remarkable progress in our understanding of the molecular events that underlie the pathology of the unstable repeat expansion diseases, we are only beginning to dissect the pathogenic complexity of these important conditions. It is clear that the study of animal models of these disorders is providing critical insights into these disorders, insights that will undoubtedly lead to therapies to prevent or to reverse the pathogenesis of these slowly evolving disorders in the near future.

● GENERAL REFERENCES

Cooper DN, Krawczak M: Human Gene Mutation. Oxford, England, Bios Scientific Publishers, 1993.

Lupski JR, Stankiewicz P (eds): Genomic Disorders: The Genomic Basis of Disease. Totowa, NJ, Humana Press, 2006.

McKusick VA: Online Mendelian Inheritance in Man: Catalogs of Autosomal Dominant, Autosomal Recessive, and X-linked Phenotypes. Available at <http://www3.ncbi.nlm.nih.gov>.

Rimoin DL, Connor JM, Pyeritz RE: Emery and Rimoin's Principles and Practice of Medical Genetics, 4th ed. Philadelphia, WB Saunders, 2001.

Scriver CR, Beaudet AL, Sly WS, Valle D (eds): The Metabolic and Molecular Bases of Inherited Disease, 8th ed. New York, McGraw-Hill, 2001.

Strachan T, Read AP: Human Molecular Genetics, 3rd ed. New York, Garland Science, 2004.

● REFERENCES FOR SPECIFIC TOPICS

Blau N, Erlandsen H: The metabolic and molecular bases of tetrahydrobiopterin-responsive phenylalanine hydroxylase deficiency. Mol Genet Metab 82:101-111, 2004.

Byers PH: Disorders of collagen biosynthesis and structure. In Scriver CR, Beaudet AL, Sly WS, Valle D (eds): The Metabolic and Molecular Bases of Inherited Disease, 8th ed. New York, McGraw-Hill, 2001, pp 5241-5286.

Carrell RW, Lomas DA: Conformational disease. Lancet 350:134-138, 1997.

Chan DC: Mitochondria: dynamic organelles in disease, aging, and development. Cell 125:1241-1252, 2006.

Chillon M, Casals T, Mercier B, et al: Mutations in the cystic fibrosis gene in patients with congenital absence of the vas deferens. N Engl J Med 332:1475-1480, 1995.

Cohen JC, Boerwinkle E, Mosley TH, Hobbs H: Sequence variants in PCSK9, low LDL, and protection against coronary heart disease. N Engl J Med 354:1264-1272, 2006.

Crowther DC, Belorgey D, Miranda E, et al: Practical genetics: α_1-antitrypsin deficiency and the serinopathies. Eur J Hum Genet 12:167-172, 2004.

Cox DW: α_1-Antitrypsin deficiency. In Scriver CR, Beaudet AL, Sly WS, Valle D (eds) The Metabolic and Molecular Bases of Inherited Disease, 8th ed. McGraw-Hill, New York, 2001, pp 5559-5586.

DiMauro S, Schon EA: Mitochondrial respiratory-chain diseases. N Engl J Med 349:1293-1294, 2003.

Drumm ML, Konstat MW, Schluchter MD, et al: Genetic modifiers of lung disease in cystic fibrosis. N Engl J Med 353:1443-1453, 2005.

Gatchel JR, Zoghbi HY: Diseases of unstable repeat expansion: mechanisms and common principles. Nat Rev Gen 6:743-755, 2005.

Goldstein JL, Brown MS: Molecular medicine: the cholesterol quartet. Science 292:1310-1312, 2001.

Goldstein JL, Hobbs HH, Brown MS: Familial hypercholesterolemia. In Scriver CR, Beaudet AL, Sly WS, Valle D (eds): The Metabolic and Molecular Bases of Inherited Disease, 8th ed. New York, McGraw-Hill, 2001, pp 2863-2914.

Lapidos KA, Kakkar R, McNally EM: The dystrophin glycoprotein complex. Circulation 94:1023-1031, 2004.

Lautenschlager NT, Cupples LA, Rao VS, et al: Risk of dementia among relatives of Alzheimer disease patients in the MIRAGE study: what is in store for the oldest old? Neurology 46:641, 1996.

Manfredi G: mtDNA clock runs out for dopaminergic neurons. Nat Genet 38:507-508, 2006.

Montau AC, Roschinger W, Habich M, et al: Tetrahydrobiopterin as an alternative treatment for mild phenylketonuria. N Engl J Med 347:2122-2132, 2002.

Nussbaum RL, Ellis CE: Alzheimer's disease and Parkinson's disease. N Engl J Med 348:1356-1364, 2003.

Pearson CE, Edamura KN, Cleary JD: Repeat instability: mechanisms of dynamic mutations. Nat Rev Genet 6:729-755, 2005.

Rogaeva E, Kawarai T, St. George-Hyslop P: Genetic complexity of Alzheimer's disease: successes and challenges. J Alzheimers Dis 9(Suppl):381-387, 2006

Rowe SM, Miller S, Sorscher EJ: Cystic fibrosis. N Engl J Med 352:1992-2001, 2005.

Schwartz M, Vissing J: Paternal inheritance of mitochondrial DNA. N Engl J Med 347:576-580, 2002.

Scriver CR, Kaufman S: The hyperphenylalaninemias: phenylalanine hydroxylase deficiency. In Scriver CR, Beaudet AL, Sly WS, Valle D (eds): The Metabolic and Molecular Bases of Inherited Disease, 8th ed. New York, McGraw-Hill, 2001, pp 1667-1724.

Scriver CR, Waters PJ: Monogenic traits are not simple: lessons from phenylketonuria. Trends Genet 15:267-272, 1999.

Sheridan MB, Fong P, Groman JD, et al: Mutations in the beta-subunit of the epithelial Na^+ channel in patients with a cystic fibrosis–like syndrome. Hum Mol Genet 14:3493-3498, 2005.

St. George-Hyslop PH, Farrer LA, Goedert M: Alzheimer's disease and the fronto-temporal dementias: diseases with cerebral deposition of fibrillar proteins. In Scriver CR, Beaudet AL, Sly WS, Valle D (eds): The Metabolic and Molecular Bases of Inherited Disease, 8th ed. New York, McGraw-Hill, 2001, pp 5875-5902.

Stoller JK, Aboussouan LS: α_1-Antitrypsin deficiency. Lancet 365:2225-2236, 2005.

Tall AR: Protease variant, LDL, and coronary heart disease. N Engl J Med 354:1310-1312, 2006.

Taylor RW, Turnbull DM: Mitochondrial DNA mutations in human disease. Nat Rev Genet 6:389-402, 2005.

Wallace DC, Lott MT, Brown MD, Kerstann K: Mitochondria and neuro-ophthalmologic diseases. In Scriver CR, Beaudet AL, Sly WS, Valle D (eds): The Metabolic and Molecular Bases of Inherited Disease, 8th ed. New York, McGraw-Hill, 2001, pp 2425-2512.

Welsh MJ, Ramsey BW, Accurso F, Cutting GR: Cystic fibrosis. In Scriver CR, Beaudet AL, Sly WS, Valle D (eds): The Metabolic and Molecular Bases of Inherited Disease, 8th ed. New York, McGraw-Hill, 2001, pp 5121-5188.

Worton R: Muscular dystrophies: diseases of the dystrophin-glyco-protein complex. Science 270:755-756, 2000.

Worton RG, Molnan MJ, Brais B, Karpati G: The muscular dystrophies. In Scriver CR, Beaudet AL, Sly WS, Valle D (eds): The Metabolic and Molecular Bases of Inherited Disease, 8th ed. New York, McGraw-Hill, 2001, pp 5493-5524.

Zielinski J: Genotype and phenotype in cystic fibrosis. Respiration 67:117-133, 2000.

Zielinski J, Corey M, Rozmahel R, et al: Detection of a cystic fibrosis modifier locus for meconium ileus on human chromosome 19q13. Nat Genet 22:128-129, 1999.

● USEFUL WEBSITES

Mutation Databases

The Human Gene Mutation Database.
  http://www.hgmd.cf.ac.uk/ac/index.php
Collagen mutation database.
  http://www.le.ac.uk/genetics/collagen/
Cystic fibrosis and CFTR gene mutation database.
  http://www.genet.sickkids.on.ca/cftr/
Human mitochondrial genome database.
  http://www.gen.emory.edu/mitomap.html
OMIM: Online Mendelian Inheritance in Man.
  http://www.ncbi.nim.nih.gov/entrez/query.fcgi?db=OMIM
Phenylalanine hydroxylase mutation database.
  http://www.pahdb.mcgill.ca

PROBLEMS

1. One mutant allele at the LDL receptor locus (leading to familial hypercholesterolemia) encodes an elongated protein that is about 50,000 daltons larger than the normal 120,000-dalton receptor. Indicate at least three mechanisms that could account for this abnormality. Approximately how many extra nucleotides would need to be translated to add 50,000 daltons to the protein?

2. In discussing the nucleotide changes found to date in the coding region of the CF gene, we stated that some of the changes (the missense changes) found so far are only "putative" disease-causing mutations. What criteria would one need to fulfill before knowing that a nucleotide change is pathogenic and not a benign polymorphism?

3. Johnny, 2 years of age, is failing to thrive. Investigations show that although he has clinical findings of CF, his sweat chloride concentration is normal. The sweat chloride concentration is normal in less than 2% of patients with CF. His pediatrician and parents want to know if DNA analysis can determine whether he indeed has CF.
   a. Would DNA analysis be useful in this case? Briefly outline the steps involved in obtaining a DNA diagnosis for CF.
   b. If he has CF, what is the probability that he is homozygous for the ΔF508 mutation? (Assume that 85% of CF mutations could be detected at the time you are consulted and that his parents are from northern Europe, where the ΔF508 allele has a frequency of 0.70.)
   c. If he does not have the ΔF508 mutation, does this disprove the diagnosis? Explain.

4. James is the only person in his kindred affected by DMD. He has one unaffected brother, Joe. DNA analysis shows that James has a deletion in the *DMD* gene and that Joe has received the same maternal X chromosome but without a deletion. What genetic counseling would you give the parents regarding the recurrence risk of DMD in a future pregnancy?

5. *DMD* has a high mutation rate but shows no ethnic variation in frequency. Use your knowledge of the gene and the genetics of DMD to suggest why this disorder is equally common in all populations.

6. In patients with osteogenesis imperfecta, explain why the missense mutations at glycine positions in the triple helix of type I collagen are confined to a limited number of other amino acid residues (Ala, Ser, Cys, Arg, Val, Asp).

7. Glucose-6-phosphate dehydrogenase (G6PD) is encoded by an X-linked gene. G6PD loss-of-function mutations can lead to hemolysis on exposure to some drugs, fava beans, and other compounds (see Chap. 18). Electrophoresis of red blood cell hemolysates shows that some females have two G6PD bands, but males have a single band. Explain this observation and the possible pathological and genetic significance of the finding of two bands in an African American female.

8. A 2-year-old infant, the child of first-cousin parents, has unexplained developmental delay. A survey of various biochemical parameters indicates that he has a deficiency of four lysosomal enzymes. Explain how a single autosomal recessive mutation might cause the loss of function of four enzyme activities. Why is it most likely that the child has an autosomal recessive condition, if he has a genetic condition at all?

9. The effect of a dominant negative allele illustrates one general mechanism by which mutations in a protein cause dominantly inherited disease. What other mechanism is commonly associated with dominance in genes encoding the subunits of multimeric proteins?

10. The clinical effects of mutations in a housekeeping protein are frequently limited to one or a few tissues, often tissues in which the protein is abundant and serves a specialty function. Identify and discuss examples that illustrate this generalization, and explain why they fit it.

11. The relationship between the site at which a protein is expressed and the site of pathological change in a genetic disease may be unpredictable. In addition, the tissue that lacks the mutant protein may even be left unaffected by disease. Give examples of this latter phenomenon and discuss them.

12. The two pseudodeficiency alleles of hex A are Arg-247Trp and Arg249Trp. What is the probable reason that the missense substitutions of these alleles are so close together in the protein?

13. Why are gain-of-function mutations in proteins, as seen with the autosomal dominant *PCSK9* mutations that cause hypercholesterolemia, almost always missense mutations?

14. What are the possible explanations for the presence of three predominant alleles for Tay-Sachs disease in Ashkenazi Jews? Does the presence of three alleles, and the relatively high frequency of Tay-Sachs disease in this population, necessarily accord with a heterozygote advantage hypothesis or a founder effect hypothesis?

15. Propose a molecular therapy that might counteract the effect of the CUG expansions in the RNAs of myotonic dystrophy 1 and 2 and that would reduce the binding of RNA-binding proteins to the CUG repeats. Anticipate some possible undesirable effects of your proposed therapy.

Chapter 13

The Treatment of Genetic Disease

The understanding of genetic disease at a molecular level, as reviewed in Chapters 11 and 12, is the foundation of rational therapy. In the coming decades, knowledge of the human genome sequence and the catalogue of human genes, together with advances in molecular biology, protein engineering, and bioengineering, will have an enormous impact on the treatment of genetic and other disorders. In this chapter, we review established therapies for genetic disease and also outline new strategies still under investigation that seem likely to be employed in the future. In particular, we emphasize therapies that reflect the genetic approach to medicine.

The objective in treating genetic disease is to eliminate or ameliorate the effects of the disorder, not only on the patient but also on his or her family. In addition, the family must be informed about the risk that the disease may occur in other members. This responsibility, genetic counseling, is a major component of the management of hereditary disorders and is dealt with separately, in Chapter 19.

For single-gene disorders due to loss-of-function mutations, treatment is directed to replacing the defective protein, improving its function, or minimizing the consequences of its deficiency. Replacement of the defective protein may be achieved by direct administration, cell or organ transplantation, or gene therapy. In principle, gene therapy will be the preferred mode of treatment of some and perhaps many single-gene diseases, once it becomes routinely safe and effective. However, even when copies of a normal gene can be transferred into the patient to effect permanent cure, the family will need ongoing genetic counseling, carrier testing, and prenatal diagnosis, in many cases for several generations.

The era of **molecular medicine** promises exciting and dramatic therapies for genetic disease, as demonstrated by the remarkable advances of the last 5 years described in this chapter. These achievements include the first cures of an inherited disorder (severe combined immunodeficiency) by gene therapy; the ability to manipulate gene expression with apparently safe nucleotide analogues (a finding of great significance for the treatment of many hemoglobinopathies, the most common single-gene diseases in the world); and the ability to prevent the clinical manifestations of previously lethal disorders, including lysosomal storage diseases, by enzyme replacement therapy.

● THE CURRENT STATE OF TREATMENT OF GENETIC DISEASE

Genetically Complex Diseases

For most multifactorial diseases (see Chapter 8), which typically manifest in adolescence or adult life, both the environmental and genetic components of the etiology are poorly understood. When an environmental contribution is recognized, an opportunity for effective intervention is available because exposure to the environmental factor can often be modified. Indeed, environmental interventions, such as medications and lifestyle or diet changes, may have a greater impact on the management of genetically complex diseases than such interventions can have for single-gene diseases. For example, cigarette smoking is an environmental factor that all patients with age-related macular degeneration or emphysema should strictly avoid. Cigarette

Table 13-1

The Effect of Intensive Insulin Replacement Therapy on the Rates of Three Common Complications of Type 1 Diabetes Mellitus

	RATE/100 PATIENT-YEARS		
	Conventional Treatment	Intensive Treatment	Risk Reduction
Retinopathy	4.7	1.2	76%
Albuminuria	3.4	2.2	34%
Neuropathy	9.8	3.1	69%

From the Diabetes Control and Complications Trial Research Group: The effect of intensive treatment of diabetes on the development and progression of long-term complications in insulin-dependent diabetes mellitus. N Engl J Med 329:977-986, 1993. Modified from Scriver CR, Treacy EP: Is there treatment for "genetic" disease? Mol Genet Metab 68:93-102, 1999.

smoke oxidizes the critical methionine residue at the active site of α_1-antitrypsin (α1AT), reducing its ability to inhibit elastase by 2000-fold, thereby literally creating a phenocopy of inherited α1AT deficiency (see Chapter 12).

Although most genetically complex diseases are amenable to some form of medical or surgical treatment, such treatment may not be particularly "genetic" in its approach. A striking example of a complex disorder for which standard medical therapy is increasingly successful is type 1 diabetes mellitus, in which intensive insulin replacement therapy greatly improves the outcome (Table 13-1). Surgical treatment of multifactorial disorders can also be highly successful. For example, three structural abnormalities (congenital heart defects, cleft lip and palate, and pyloric stenosis)

affect nearly 1.5% of all liveborn infants and make up approximately 30% of all newborns with genetic disease. In about half of these patients, the diseases are curable by a single operation, a form of phenotypic modification; a cure is therefore possible in at least 10% to 15% of infants with a genetically determined disorder. Admittedly, the treatment of inherited disease is often not so beneficial, although it frequently improves the quality of life.

Single-Gene Diseases

Although powerful advances are being made, the overall treatment of single-gene diseases is presently deficient. A survey of 372 mendelian disorders showed that current therapy is completely effective in 12%, partially effective in 54%, and of no benefit in 34% (Fig. 13-1). An encouraging trend is that treatment is more likely to be successful if the basic biochemical defect is known. In one study, for example, treatment increased life span in only 15% of single-gene diseases studied, but in a subset of 65 inborn errors in which the cause was known, life span was greatly improved in 32%; similar increases were observed for other phenotypes, including growth, intelligence, and social adaptation. Thus, research to elucidate the genetic and biochemical basis of hereditary disease has a dramatic impact on the clinical outcome.

The current unsatisfactory state of treatment of genetic disease is due to numerous factors, including the following:

1. **Gene not identified or pathogenesis not understood.** The mutant locus is unknown in more than 50% of

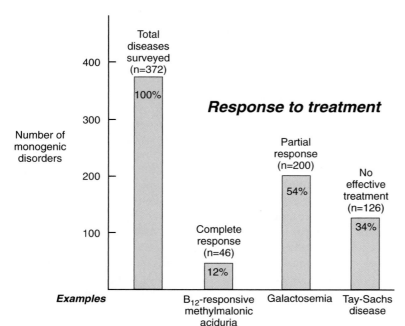

Figure 13-1 ■ The effect of treatment on 372 genetic diseases in which the affected gene or biochemical function is known and for which sufficient information was available for analysis in 1999. The fraction of treatable diseases will have increased to a small extent since this 1999 survey because of the success of enzyme replacement and a few other therapies. B_{12}-responsive methylmalonic aciduria and Tay-Sachs disease are discussed in Chapter 12, and galactosemia is described in this chapter. (Modified from Scriver CR, Treacy EP: Is there treatment for "genetic" disease? Mol Genet Metab 68:93-102, 1999.)

Table 13-2

Examples of Prenatal Treatment of Inherited and Congenital Disorders

PRENATAL MEDICAL TREATMENT		PRENATAL SURGICAL TREATMENT	
Disease	Treatment	Disease	Treatment
Biotinidase deficiency	Maternal biotin administration	Urinary obstruction due to urethral valves → hydronephrosis	Percutaneous catheter or vesicostomy
Vitamin B_{12}–responsive methylmalonic aciduria	Maternal vitamin B_{12} administration	Diaphragmatic hernia → lung hypoplasia	Fetal tracheal occlusion by a balloon*
Congenital adrenal hyperplasia	Dexamethasone, a cortisol analogue*	Twin-twin transfusion syndrome → vascular steal → fetal hydrops	Fetoscopic laser ablation of communicating placental vessels

*Experimental therapy, still being evaluated.

genetic diseases. Even when the gene in known, however, knowledge of the pathophysiological mechanism is often inadequate. In phenylketonuria (PKU), for example, despite years of study, the mechanisms by which the elevation in phenylalanine impairs brain development and function are still poorly understood (see Chapter 12).

2. **Prediagnostic fetal damage.** Some mutations act early in development or cause irreversible pathological changes before they are diagnosed. These problems can sometimes be anticipated if there is a family history of a genetic disease or if carrier screening identifies couples at risk. In such cases, prenatal treatment is sometimes possible for both medical and surgical conditions; examples of prenatal treatments are outlined in Table 13-2.

3. **Severe phenotypes are less amenable to intervention.** The initial cases of a disease to be recognized are usually the most severely affected, but they are often less amenable to treatment. One reason is that in severely affected individuals, the mutation frequently leads to the absence of the encoded protein or to a severely compromised mutant protein with no residual activity. When the effect of the mutation is less disruptive, the mutant protein may retain some residual function. In that case, it may be possible to increase the small amount of function sufficiently to have a therapeutic effect, as described later.

● SPECIAL CONSIDERATIONS IN TREATING GENETIC DISEASE

Long-Term Assessment of Treatment Is Critical

In genetic disease, perhaps more than in other areas of medicine, treatment initially judged as successful may eventually be shown to be imperfect. There are at least three facets to this problem. First, treatment may initially appear to be successful, only to be shown by longer observation to have subtle inadequacies. Thus, although well-managed children with PKU have escaped

severe retardation and have normal or nearly normal IQs (see later), they often manifest subtle learning disorders and behavioral disturbances that impair their academic performance in later years.

Second, successful treatment of the pathological changes in one organ may be followed by unexpected problems in tissues not previously observed to be clinically involved because the patients did not survive long enough. The detection of the later manifestations may require many years of observation after the initial therapy. **Galactosemia,** a well-known inborn error of carbohydrate metabolism, illustrates this point. This disorder results from the inability to metabolize galactose, a monosaccharide that is a component of lactose (milk sugar). Individuals with this autosomal recessive disease completely lack the enzyme galactose-1-phosphate uridyltransferase (GALT), which normally catalyzes the conversion of galactose 1-phosphate to uridine diphosphogalactose (UDPG):

$$\text{Galactose-1-phosphate} \xrightarrow{\text{GALT}} \text{UDPG}$$

Infants with galactosemia are usually normal at birth but begin to develop gastrointestinal problems, cirrhosis of the liver, and cataracts in the weeks after they are given milk. If not recognized, galactosemia causes severe mental retardation and is often fatal. Complete removal of milk from the diet, however, can protect against most of the harmful consequences of GALT deficiency, although, as with PKU, learning disabilities are now recognized to be common even in well-treated galactosemia patients. In addition, despite conscientious treatment, most females with galactosemia have ovarian failure that appears to result from continued galactose toxicity.

Another example is provided by hereditary retinoblastoma (Case 34), due to germline mutations in the **retinoblastoma** *(RB1)* gene (see Chapter 16). Patients successfully treated for the eye tumor in the first years of life are at increased risk for development of an independent malignant neoplasm, osteosarcoma, after the first decade. Ironically, therefore, treatment that successfully prolongs life provides a new opportunity for the clinical expression of the basic defect.

And last, therapy that is believed to be free of side effects in the short term may be associated with serious problems in the long term. For example, clotting factor infusion in hemophilia (Case 18) sometimes results in the formation of antibodies to the infused protein, and blood transfusion in thalassemia (Case 39) invariably produces iron overload, which must then be managed by the administration of the iron chelating agents deferiprone and deferoxamine, discussed later.

Genetic Heterogeneity and Treatment

The optimal treatment of single-gene defects requires an unusual degree of diagnostic precision; often one must determine not only the specific locus involved but also the particular class of allele at the locus. Thus, it is not sufficient merely to determine that a patient has clinically significant hyperphenylalaninemia. One must first establish whether the hyperphenylalaninemia is due to mutations in the phenylalanine hydroxylase (PAH) gene itself or in one of the genes that encode the enzymes required for the synthesis of tetrahydrobiopterin (BH_4), the cofactor of PAH, since as discussed in Chapter 12, the treatment is entirely different. If a mutation in the *PAH* gene is the cause, one must then determine whether the particular allele leads to the formation of a mutant enzyme whose activity is increased by the administration of high doses of the BH_4 cofactor (which might then be the only treatment required) or whether BH_4 administration has no effect (in which case a phenylalanine-restricted diet would be mandatory).

Allelic heterogeneity has additional implications for therapy. Some alleles produce a protein that is decreased in abundance but has some residual function. As stated before, strategies designed to increase the expression or stability of the partially functional protein may be effective in correcting the biochemical defect. In contrast, nothing will be gained by increasing the abundance of a mutant protein with no residual function.

● TREATMENT STRATEGIES

Genetic disease can be treated at many levels, at various steps away from the mutant gene (Fig. 13-2). In the remainder of this chapter, we describe the rationale used or proposed for treatment at each of these levels. The current treatments are not necessarily mutually exclusive, although successful gene therapy would render other therapies superfluous. For diseases in which the biochemical or genetic defect is known, the frequency with which the different strategies are currently used is shown in Figure 13-3.

In treating genetic disease, it is important to emphasize the importance of educating the patient—not only to achieve understanding of the disease, its genetic implications, and its treatment but also to ensure compliance with therapy that may be inconvenient and lifelong.

Therapy Directed at the Clinical Phenotype

Treatment at the level of the clinical phenotype (see Fig. 13-2) includes all the medical or surgical interventions that are not unique to the management of genetic disease. Often, this is the only therapy available and, in some cases, may be all that is necessary.

Treatment of Metabolic Abnormalities

The most successful disease-specific approach to the treatment of genetic disease has been at the level of a metabolic abnormality. The principal strategies used to manipulate metabolism in the treatment of inborn errors are listed in Table 13-3. The necessity for patients with pharmacogenetic diseases, such as glucose-6-phosphate dehydrogenase deficiency, to avoid certain drugs and chemicals is described in Chapter 18.

Dietary Restriction

Dietary restriction is one of the oldest and most effective methods of managing genetic disease. Diseases involving more than several dozen loci are currently managed in this way. The advantage of this approach is that it can be highly effective; its drawback is that it usually requires lifelong compliance with a restricted and often artificial diet. The dietary constraint is onerous for the family as well as for the patient, especially in adolescence. Many of the diseases treatable in this manner involve amino acid catabolic pathways, and therefore severe restriction of normal dietary protein is usually necessary. Essential nutrients such as amino acids, however, cannot be withheld entirely; their intake must be sufficient for anabolic needs. For that group of patients who have mild enzymatic defects (i.e., "leaky" mutant alleles), some small amount of the offending compound can often be tolerated; consequently, the diet is less restrictive, and compliance may be better. If the dietary precursor of the offending substrate is not an essential nutrient, it can be eliminated from the diet altogether. An example of such a compound is galactose, which the body can synthesize from glucose in amounts adequate for the small requirements of normal biochemical processes, such as the synthesis of mucopolysaccharides.

A diet restricted in phenylalanine largely circumvents the neurological damage in classic PKU (see Chapter 12). Phenylketonuric children are normal at birth because the maternal enzyme protects them during prenatal life. The results of treatment are best when the diagnosis is made soon after birth and treatment is

Figure 13-2 ■ The various levels of treatment that are relevant to genetic disease, with the corresponding strategies used at each level. For each level, a disease discussed in the text is given as an example. All the therapies listed are used clinically in many centers, unless indicated otherwise. (Modified from Valle D: Genetic disease: an overview of current therapy. Hosp Pract 22:167-182, 1987.)

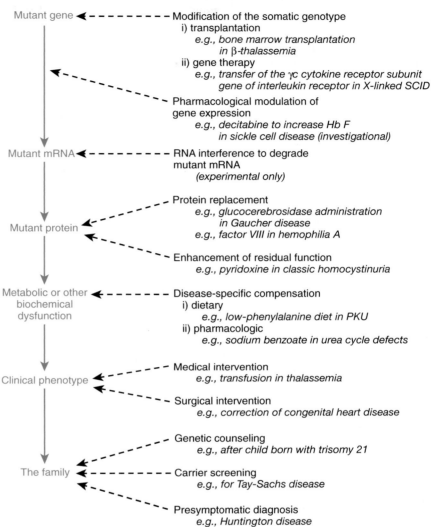

Level of intervention   *Treatment strategy*

Mutant gene ◄ – – – – – – – Modification of the somatic genotype
　　　　　　　　　　　　i) transplantation
　　　　　　　　　　　　　　e.g., bone marrow transplantation
　　　　　　　　　　　　　　　in β-thalassemia
　　　　　　　　　　　　ii) gene therapy
　　　　　　　　　　　　　　e.g., transfer of the γc cytokine receptor subunit
　　　　　　　　　　　　　　　gene of interleukin receptor in X-linked SCID

　　　　　　　　　　　　Pharmacological modulation of
　　　　　　　　　　　　gene expression
　　　　　　　　　　　　　　e.g., decitabine to increase Hb F
　　　　　　　　　　　　　　　in sickle cell disease (investigational)

Mutant mRNA ◄ – – – – – – RNA interference to degrade
　　　　　　　　　　　　mutant mRNA
　　　　　　　　　　　　　　(experimental only)

　　　　　　　　　　　　Protein replacement
　　　　　　　　　　　　　　e.g., glucocerebrosidase administration
　　　　　　　　　　　　　　　in Gaucher disease
Mutant protein ◄　　　　　　*e.g., factor VIII in hemophilia A*

　　　　　　　　　　　　Enhancement of residual function
　　　　　　　　　　　　　　e.g., pyridoxine in classic homocystinuria

Metabolic or other ◄ – – – – – Disease-specific compensation
biochemical　　　　　　　i) dietary
dysfunction　　　　　　　　　*e.g., low-phenylalanine diet in PKU*
　　　　　　　　　　　　ii) pharmacologic
　　　　　　　　　　　　　　e.g., sodium benzoate in urea cycle defects

Clinical phenotype ◄　　　　Medical intervention
　　　　　　　　　　　　　　e.g., transfusion in thalassemia

　　　　　　　　　　　　Surgical intervention
　　　　　　　　　　　　　　e.g., correction of congenital heart disease

　　　　　　　　　　　　Genetic counseling
　　　　　　　　　　　　　　e.g., after child born with trisomy 21

The family ◄ – – – – – – – Carrier screening
　　　　　　　　　　　　　　e.g., for Tay-Sachs disease

　　　　　　　　　　　　Presymptomatic diagnosis
　　　　　　　　　　　　　　e.g., Huntington disease

Figure 13-3 ■ The frequency with which various therapeutic and management strategies are presently used in the treatment of 372 metabolic disorders (the same group of disorders referred to in Fig. 13-1). If a disorder is treated by, for example, two strategies, the impact of each strategy on the total treatment was estimated and allocated between each approach. (From Scriver CR, Treacy EP: Is there treatment for "genetic" disease? Mol Genet Metab 68:93-102, 1999.)

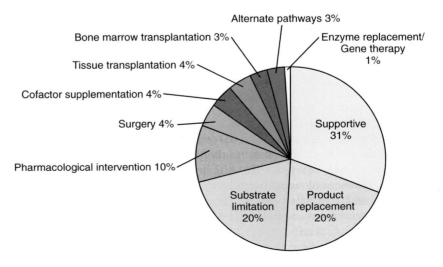

Alternate pathways 3%
Bone marrow transplantation 3%
Enzyme replacement/ Gene therapy 1%
Tissue transplantation 4%
Cofactor supplementation 4%
Surgery 4%
Supportive 31%
Pharmacological intervention 10%
Substrate limitation 20%
Product replacement 20%

Table 13-3

Treatment of Genetic Disease by Metabolic Manipulation

Type of Metabolic Intervention	Substance or Technique	Disease
Avoidance	Antimalarial drugs	Glucose-6-phosphate dehydrogenase deficiency
	Isoniazid	Slow acetylators
Dietary restriction	Phenylalanine	Phenylketonuria
	Galactose	Galactosemia
Replacement	Thyroxine	Congenital hypothyroidism
	Biotin	Biotinidase deficiency
Diversion	Sodium benzoate	Urea cycle disorders
	Oral resins that bind bile acids	Familial hypercholesterolemia heterozygotes
	Drugs that block the intestinal absorption of cholesterol	
Inhibition	Statins	Familial hypercholesterolemia heterozygotes
Depletion	LDL apheresis (direct removal of LDL from plasma)	Familial hypercholesterolemia homozygotes

Modified from Rosenberg LE: Treating genetic diseases: lessons from three children. Pediatr Res 27:S10-S16, 1990.

begun promptly. If the child is fed a normal diet in the first months of life, irreversible mental retardation occurs; the degree of intellectual deficit is directly related to the delay in the institution of the low-phenylalanine diet. It is now recommended that patients with PKU remain on a low-phenylalanine diet for life because neurological and behavioral abnormalities develop in many (although perhaps not all) patients if the diet is stopped. Even in patients who have been treated throughout life and have normal intelligence as measured by IQ tests, however, neuropsychological deficits (e.g., in conceptual, visual-spatial, and language skills) are often present. Nonetheless, treatment produces results vastly superior to the outcome without treatment.

Replacement

The provision of essential metabolites, cofactors, or hormones whose deficiency is due to a genetic disease is simple in concept and often simple in application. Some of the most successfully treated single-gene defects belong to this category. An important example is provided by **congenital hypothyroidism,** 10% to 15% of which is monogenic in origin. This disorder results from a variety of defects in the formation of the thyroid gland or of its major product, thyroxine. Because congenital hypothyroidism is common (about 1/4000 neo-

nates) and treatment can prevent the associated mental retardation, neonatal screening is conducted in many countries so that thyroxine administration may be initiated as soon as possible after birth to prevent the severe intellectual defects that are otherwise inevitable (see Chapter 17).

Diversion

Diversion therapy is the enhanced use of alternative metabolic pathways to reduce the concentration of a harmful metabolite. A successful application of diversion therapy is in the treatment of the **urea cycle disorders** (Fig. 13-4). The function of the urea cycle is to convert ammonia, which is neurotoxic, to urea, which is a benign end product that is excreted. If the cycle is disrupted by an enzyme defect such as **ornithine transcarbamylase deficiency (Case 31)**, the consequent hyperammonemia can be only partially controlled by dietary protein restriction. The ammonia can be reduced to normal levels by diversion to metabolic pathways that are normally of minor significance, leading to synthesis of harmless compounds. Thus, the administration of large quantities of sodium benzoate forces its ligation with glycine to form hippurate, which is excreted in the urine (see Fig. 13-4). Glycine synthesis is thereby increased, and for each mole of glycine formed, one mole of ammonia is consumed.

A similar approach has been successful in helping to reduce the cholesterol level in heterozygotes for **familial hypercholesterolemia (Case 14)** (see Chapter 12). By the diversion of an increased fraction of cholesterol to bile acid synthesis, the single normal low-density lipoprotein (LDL) receptor gene of these patients can be stimulated to produce more hepatic receptors for LDL-bound cholesterol (Fig. 13-5). This treatment achieves significant reductions in plasma cholesterol because 70% of all LDL receptor–mediated uptake of cholesterol is by the liver. The increase in bile acid synthesis is achieved by the oral administration of nonabsorbable resins such as cholestyramine, which

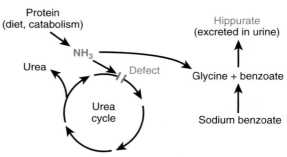

Figure 13-4 ■ The strategy of metabolite diversion. In this example, ammonia cannot be removed by the urea cycle because of a genetic defect of a urea cycle enzyme. The administration of sodium benzoate diverts ammonia to glycine synthesis, and the nitrogen moiety is subsequently excreted as hippurate.

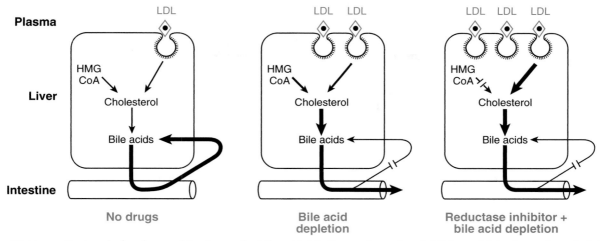

Figure 13-5 ■ Rationale for the combined use of a bile acid–binding resin and an inhibitor of 3-hydroxy-3-methylglutaryl coenzyme A reductase (HMG CoA reductase) in the treatment of familial hypercholesterolemia heterozygotes. (From Brown MS, Goldstein JL: A receptor-mediated pathway for cholesterol homeostasis. Science 232:4, 1986. Copyright by the Nobel Foundation.)

bind bile acids in the intestine and increase their fecal excretion. This example illustrates clearly an important principle: autosomal dominant diseases may sometimes be treated by increasing the expression of the normal allele.

Inhibition

The pharmacological inhibition of enzymes is sometimes used to modify the metabolic abnormalities of inborn errors. Familial hypercholesterolemia also illustrates this principle. When the cholesterol load is decreased by diverting it to other compounds or by removing it with physical methods, the liver tries to compensate for the decreased cholesterol intake by up-regulating cholesterol synthesis. Consequently, the treatment of familial hypercholesterolemia heterozygotes is more effective if hepatic cholesterol synthesis is simultaneously inhibited by a statin, a class of drugs that are powerful inhibitors of 3-hydroxy-3-methylglutaryl coenzyme A reductase, the rate-limiting enzyme of cholesterol synthesis. High doses of a statin typically effect a 40% to 60% decrease in plasma LDL cholesterol levels in familial hypercholesterolemia heterozygotes; when a statin is used together with cholestyramine (see Fig. 13-5), the effect is synergistic, and even greater decreases can be achieved.

Depletion

Genetic diseases characterized by the accumulation of a harmful compound are sometimes treated by direct removal of the compound from the body. This principle is exemplified by the use of phlebotomy to alleviate the iron accumulation that occurs in **hemochromatosis** (Case 17).

THE MOLECULAR TREATMENT OF DISEASE

During the past decade, the growth in knowledge of the molecular pathophysiology of monogenic disease has been accompanied by an encouraging increase in molecular therapies that have had a profound impact on patients with many of these disorders. An overview of the molecular treatment of single-gene diseases is presented in Figure 13-6. Each of these treatments, many of them unimaginable a decade ago, is discussed here. These molecular therapies represent one facet of the important paradigm embraced by the concept of **molecular medicine**. Molecular medicine is a general term used to describe the diagnosis, prevention, and treatment of a disease based on an understanding of the molecular mechanisms that underlie its etiology and pathogenesis.

Treatment at the Level of the Protein

In many instances, if a mutant protein product is made, it may be possible to increase its function. For example, the activity of some mutant polypeptides can be enhanced by improving their ability to "fold"—to adopt their normal secondary and tertiary structure. In other cases, the stability of a mutant protein with some residual function may be increased. Alternatively, it may be possible to augment the residual working capacity of each abnormal protein molecule. With **enzymopathies**, the improvement in function obtained by this approach is usually very small, on the order of a few percent, but this increment is often all that is required to restore biochemical homeostasis. Of course, mutations that

THE MOLECULAR TREATMENT OF GENETIC DISEASE

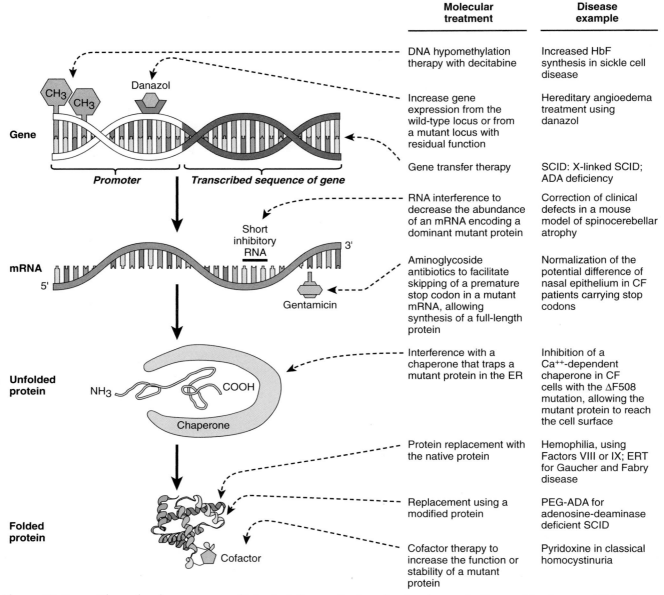

	Molecular treatment	Disease example
	DNA hypomethylation therapy with decitabine	Increased HbF synthesis in sickle cell disease
	Increase gene expression from the wild-type locus or from a mutant locus with residual function	Hereditary angioedema treatment using danazol
	Gene transfer therapy	SCID: X-linked SCID; ADA deficiency
	RNA interference to decrease the abundance of an mRNA encoding a dominant mutant protein	Correction of clinical defects in a mouse model of spinocerebellar atrophy
	Aminoglycoside antibiotics to facilitate skipping of a premature stop codon in a mutant mRNA, allowing synthesis of a full-length protein	Normalization of the potential difference of nasal epithelium in CF patients carrying stop codons
	Interference with a chaperone that traps a mutant protein in the ER	Inhibition of a Ca^{++}-dependent chaperone in CF cells with the $\Delta F508$ mutation, allowing the mutant protein to reach the cell surface
	Protein replacement with the native protein	Hemophilia, using Factors VIII or IX; ERT for Gaucher and Fabry disease
	Replacement using a modified protein	PEG-ADA for adenosine-deaminase deficient SCID
	Cofactor therapy to increase the function or stability of a mutant protein	Pyridoxine in classical homocystinuria

Figure 13-6 ■ The molecular treatment of inherited disease. Each molecular therapy is discussed in the text. ADA, adenosine deaminase; CF, cystic fibrosis; ER, endoplasmic reticulum; ERT, enzyme replacement therapy; PEG, polyethylene glycol; SCID, severe combined immunodeficiency.

prevent the synthesis of any functional protein are not amenable to this approach.

Enhancement of Mutant Protein Function with Small Molecule Therapy

Small molecules are that class of compounds with molecular weights in the few hundreds to thousands. They are usually synthesized by organic chemists or isolated from nature. Vitamins, nonpeptide hormones, and indeed most drugs are classified as small molecules. The vast amount of pharmacological information

compiled during the past century concerning the absorption, metabolism, excretion, and physiological effects of drugs consists primarily of studies of the behavior and biological activity of small molecules.

Vitamin-Responsive Inborn Errors of Metabolism The biochemical abnormalities of a number of metabolic diseases may respond, sometimes dramatically, to the administration of large amounts of the vitamin cofactor of the enzyme impaired by the mutation (Table 13-4). In fact, the vitamin-responsive inborn errors are among the most successfully treated of all genetic diseases. The

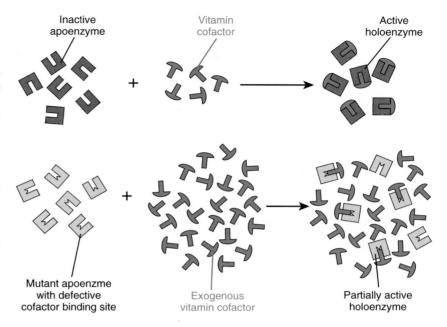

Figure 13-7 ■ The mechanism of the response of a mutant apoenzyme to the administration of its cofactor at high doses. Vitamin-responsive enzyme defects are often due to mutations that reduce the normal affinity (*top*) of the enzyme protein (apoenzyme) for the cofactor needed to activate it. In the presence of the high concentrations of the cofactor that result from the administration of up to 500 times the normal daily requirement, the mutant enzyme acquires a small amount of activity sufficient to restore biochemical normalcy. (Redrawn from Valle D: Genetic disease: an overview of current therapy. Hosp Pract 22:167-182, 1987.)

vitamins used are remarkably nontoxic, generally allowing the safe administration of amounts 100 to 500 times greater than those required for normal nutrition. In **homocystinuria** due to cystathionine synthase deficiency (Fig. 13-7), for example, about 50% of patients respond to the administration of high doses of pyridoxine (vitamin B$_6$, the precursor of pyridoxal phosphate); in most of these patients, homocystine disappears from the plasma. The increase in hepatic enzyme activity is only a few-fold, in one patient, for example, from 1.5% to only 4.5% of control activity. The increased pyridoxal phosphate concentrations may overcome reduced affinity of the mutant enzyme for the cofactor (see Fig. 13-7) or stabilize the mutant enzyme. In any case, pyridoxine treatment substantially improves the clinical course of the disease in responsive patients. Nonresponsive patients generally have no residual cystathionine synthase activity to augment.

Table 13-4

Treatment of Genetic Disease at the Level of the Mutant Protein

Strategy	Example	Status
Enhancement of Mutant Protein Function		
Cofactor administration to increase enzyme activity	Pyridoxine-responsive homocystinuria	Treatment of choice in the 50% of patients who are responsive
Small molecule therapy to allow normal folding of mutant polypeptides	Curcumin for the ΔF508 mutation of cystic fibrosis	Investigational: successful in a mouse model
Aminoglycoside antibiotics to allow translational "skipping" over mutant stop codons	Gentamicin in cystic fibrosis patients with *CFTR* stop codon mutations	Investigational: successful in correcting the nasal epithelial ion transport defect in cystic fibrosis patients carrying stop mutations
Protein Augmentation		
Replacement of an extracellular protein	Factor VIII in hemophilia A α$_1$-antitrypsin in α1AT deficiency	Well-established, effective Established: intravenous infusion to raise serum and lung levels; biochemically and clinically beneficial in many patients; aerosol therapy may supplant intravenous infusion
Extracellular replacement of an intracellular protein	Polyethylene glycol–modified adenosine deaminase (PEG-ADA) in ADA deficiency	Well-established, safe and effective, but costly
Replacement of an intracellular protein: cell targeting	Modified glucocerebrosidase in Gaucher disease	Established; biochemically and clinically effective; expensive

Small Molecules to Increase the Folding of Mutant Polypeptides   Many mutations disrupt the ability of the mutant polypeptide to fold normally. If the folding defect could be overcome, the mutant protein would often be able to resume its normal activity. During the past decade, there has been an increasing awareness that the administration of small molecules may be used to overcome a folding defect. Folding mutants of membrane proteins, for example, fail to pass normally through the endoplasmic reticulum and get "stuck" there, leading to their degradation. Perhaps the best known example of such a mutation is the ΔF508 mutation of the **cystic fibrosis** protein (Case 10) (see Chapter 12). The mutant ΔF508 polypeptide is recognized by a calcium-dependent chaperone protein in the endoplasmic reticulum, retained there, and degraded (see Fig. 13-6). An extraordinary correction of this defect has been obtained in mice carrying the ΔF508 mutation by the administration of curcumin, a nontoxic mixture of compounds derived from turmeric, a spice found in curry. Curcumin inhibits a calcium pump in the endoplasmic reticulum, thereby impairing the binding of the mutant ΔF508 protein by the calcium-dependent chaperone. The treated mice had a normalization of chloride transport in the gut and nasal epithelium and dramatically increased rates of survival. Clinical trials of this seemingly innocuous therapy are planned, but irrespective of their success, this example highlights the potential of small molecule therapy for the treatment of monogenic diseases at the level of the mutant protein.

Small Molecule Therapy to Allow Skipping over Mutant Stop Codons   Nonsense mutations represent a common (about 11%) class of defects in the human genome. For example, approximately 60% of Ashkenazi Jewish patients with cystic fibrosis carry at least one *CFTR* allele with a premature stop codon (e.g., Arg553Stop). Aminoglycoside antibiotics, such as the commonly prescribed gentamicin, encourage the translational apparatus to "skip over" a premature stop codon and instead to misincorporate an amino acid that has a codon comparable to that of the termination codon. In this way, for example, Arg553Stop is converted to 553Tyr, a substitution that generates a CFTR peptide with nearly normal properties. Gentamicin administration is able to normalize the potential difference of the nasal epithelium of cystic fibrosis patients carrying premature stop codons and to increase the amount of the CFTR protein delivered to the surface of nasal epithelial cells. Whether these effects can lead to sustained clinical improvement without substantial toxicity remains to be demonstrated. Nevertheless, because nonsense mutations are so common, patients who carry such alleles may benefit if this principle can be more widely applied. Consequently, large numbers of small molecules are being examined in laboratories and by drug companies around the world to identify novel nontoxic compounds that facilitate the skipping of stop codons.

Protein Augmentation

The principal types of protein augmentation used to date are summarized in Table 13-4. Protein augmentation is part of the routine therapeutic repertoire in only a few diseases, all involving proteins whose principal site of action is in the plasma or extracellular fluid. The prevention or arrest of bleeding episodes in patients with **hemophilia** (Case 18) by the infusion of plasma fractions enriched for factor VIII is the prime example. The years of experience with this disease also illustrate the problems that can be anticipated as new strategies for replacing other, particularly intracellular, polypeptides are attempted. The problems include the difficulty and cost of procuring sufficient amounts of the protein to treat all patients at the optimal frequency, the need to administer the protein at a frequency consistent with its half-life (only 8 to 10 hours for factor VIII), the formation of neutralizing antibodies in some patients (5% of classic hemophiliacs), and the contamination of the protein with foreign agents, particularly viruses (hepatitis, human immunodeficiency virus).

Augmentation of an Extracellular Protein: α₁-Antitrypsin Deficiency   There are approximately 40,000 α1AT-deficient patients in North America alone; thus, α1AT deficiency is a significant cause of premature death in the adult population. In addition to the avoidance of smoking, as discussed earlier, the object of treatment is to redress the imbalance between elastase and α1AT by delivering α1AT to the pulmonary epithelium and alveolar interstitial fluid. Human α1AT can be infused intravenously in doses sufficiently large to maintain the interstitial fluid α1AT concentration at an effective inhibitory level for 1 week or even longer. A clinically significant effect is observed only in patients with moderate impairment of lung function (between 30% and 65% of normal) before treatment; more severely affected patients have no significant slowing of the loss of pulmonary function. An alternative approach still being studied involves the delivery of α1AT directly to the lungs by aerosol inhalation. This route of administration is more attractive, since it requires only 10% of the intravenous dose of α1AT. Despite these promising results, these treatments have yet to be evaluated in placebo-controlled, randomized, blinded, or masked trials designed to document their effectiveness in ameliorating or preventing the lung disease.

Enzyme Replacement Therapy: Extracellular Augmentation of an Intracellular Enzyme

Adenosine Deaminase Deficiency   Adenosine deaminase (ADA) is a critical enzyme of purine metabolism

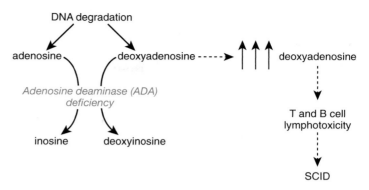

Figure 13-8 ■ Adenosine deaminase (ADA) converts adenosine to inosine and deoxyadenosine to deoxyguanosine. In ADA deficiency, deoxyadenosine accumulation in lymphocytes is lymphotoxic, killing the cells by impairing DNA replication and cell division to cause severe combined immunodeficiency (SCID).

that catalyzes the deamination of adenosine to inosine and of deoxyadenosine to deoxyinosine (Fig. 13-8). The pathology of ADA deficiency, an autosomal recessive disease, results entirely from the accumulation of toxic purines, particularly deoxyadenosine, in lymphocytes. A profound failure of both cell-mediated (T-cell) and humoral (B-cell) immunity results, making ADA deficiency one cause of **severe combined immunodeficiency.** Untreated patients die of infection within the first 2 years of life. As discussed later, successful gene therapy for ADA deficiency has been reported. The current treatment of choice, however, is bone marrow transplantation from a fully HLA-compatible donor. In the absence of an appropriate bone marrow donor, administration of the bovine ADA enzyme has been shown to be effective.

Modified Adenosine Deaminase The infusion of bovine ADA modified by the covalent attachment of an inert polymer, polyethylene glycol (PEG), has been found to be superior to the use of the unmodified ADA enzyme, in several ways. First, PEG-ADA elicits a neutralizing antibody response (that would remove it from plasma) in only a small minority of patients. Second, the modified enzyme remains in the extracellular fluid where it can degrade toxic purines. Third, the plasma half-life of PEG-ADA is 3 to 6 days, much longer than the half-life of unmodified ADA predicted from animal studies. PEG-ADA replacement therapy almost normalizes the metabolic abnormalities in purine metabolism. Although PEG-ADA does not completely correct immune function (most patients remain T lymphopenic), immunoprotection is restored, and dramatic clinical improvement occurs. The efficacy of this treatment, when it is continued for a lifetime, remains to be established, but this approach represents an important therapeutic strategy.

The general principles exemplified by the use of PEG-ADA are that (1) proteins can be chemically modified to improve their effectiveness as pharmacological reagents and (2) an enzyme that is normally located inside the cell can be effective extracellularly if its substrate is in equilibrium with the extracellular fluid and if its product can be taken up by the cells that require

it. As illustrated in the following section, the strategy of modification can be extended to proteins that can function only intracellularly, by targeting the protein to a specific cell type.

Enzyme Replacement Therapy: Targeted Augmentation of an Intracellular Enzyme

Enzyme replacement therapy (ERT) is now established therapy for two lysosomal storage diseases, Gaucher disease and Fabry disease, and it is the subject of clinical trials in six other lysosomal storage diseases. The limitations of ERT are presently twofold. First, on the basis of animal studies, it appears that insufficient amounts of infused enzyme can cross the blood-brain barrier to effectively treat the forms of these diseases that affect the brain, such as the minority of Gaucher patients with neurological degeneration. Second, as with PEG-ADA therapy, ERT is expensive. Here we discuss the success with Gaucher disease, but the effects of ERT in Fabry disease, an X-linked disorder that leads to premature death of affected men by the fourth or fifth decade, if untreated, are equally impressive.

Gaucher Disease The feasibility of directing a polypeptide to a specific cell and a particular intracellular compartment has been demonstrated for Gaucher disease, the most prevalent lysosomal storage disorder, affecting up to 1/450 Ashkenazi Jews and 1/40,000 to 1/100,000 individuals in other populations. This autosomal recessive condition is due to a deficiency of the enzyme glucocerebrosidase. Its substrate, glucocerebroside, is a complex lipid normally degraded in the lysosome. The disease results from glucocerebroside accumulation, particularly in the lysosomes of macrophages in the reticuloendothelial system, leading to gross enlargement of the liver and spleen. In addition, bone marrow is slowly replaced by lipid-laden macrophages ("Gaucher cells") that ultimately compromise the production of erythrocytes and platelets, producing anemia and thrombocytopenia. Bone lesions cause episodic pain, osteonecrosis, and substantial morbidity.

Glucocerebrosidase ERT in Gaucher disease illustrates the challenges in targeting a protein both to a

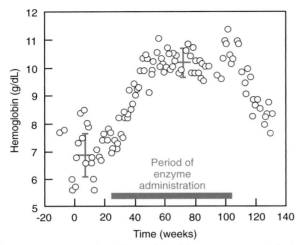

Figure 13-9 ■ The effect of weekly intravenous infusions of modified glucocerebrosidase on the hemoglobin concentration of a child with Gaucher disease without neurological involvement. A review of the response of more than 1000 patients indicates that this response is representative. Treatment was begun at 4 years of age and continued for 18 months. The therapy was accompanied by an increased platelet count and radiological improvement in the bone abnormalities. The hematological parameters returned to pretreatment levels when the infusions were stopped. (Redrawn from Barton NW, Furbish FS, Murray GJ, et al: Therapeutic response to intravenous infusions of glucocerebrosidase in a patient with Gaucher disease. Proc Natl Acad Sci USA 87:1913-1916, 1990.)

particular type of cell and to a specific intracellular address, in this case the macrophage and the lysosome, respectively. Gaucher disease is an excellent model for protein targeting, for several reasons. First, because the central nervous system is not involved in most patients, the enzyme needs to be delivered only to the peripheral reticuloendothelial system. Second, the only alternative therapy at present is bone marrow transplantation, a relatively high risk procedure. Third, the human enzyme is available in abundance, purified either from human placentas or from cultured cells carrying the gene. Finally, the biology of the macrophage is sufficiently well understood to have suggested a strategy for targeting the enzyme to it.

More than 2500 patients with Gaucher disease are now being treated worldwide with glucocerebrosidase ERT, with dramatic clinical benefits. The increase in the hemoglobin level of one patient, a response representative of that seen in more than 1000 affected individuals, is shown in Figure 13-9. Overall, this therapy also reduces the enlargement of liver and spleen, increases the platelet count, accelerates growth, and improves the characteristic skeletal abnormalities. This success depended on a modification of the carbohydrates that normally decorate this glycoprotein: terminal sugars are removed to expose core α-mannosyl residues. The exposed mannose sugars target the

enzyme to the macrophage, through a mannose receptor on the plasma membrane. Once bound, the enzyme is internalized and delivered to the lysosome. This strategy documents the feasibility of directing an intracellular enzyme to its physiologically relevant location to produce clinically significant effects.

Modulation of Gene Expression

A decade ago, the idea that one might treat a genetic disease through the use of drugs that modulate gene expression would have seemed fanciful. Increasing knowledge of the normal and pathological basis of gene expression, however, has made this approach feasible. Indeed, it seems likely that this strategy will become only more widely used as our understanding of gene expression, and how it might be manipulated, increases.

Increasing Gene Expression from the Wild-type or Mutant Locus

Therapeutic effects can be obtained by increasing the amount of messenger RNA transcribed from the wild-type locus associated with a dominant disease or from a mutant locus, if the mutant protein retains some function (Table 13-5). An effective therapy of this type is used to manage a rare but potentially fatal disorder, **hereditary angioedema,** an autosomal dominant condition due to mutations in the gene encoding complement 1 (C1) esterase inhibitor. Affected individuals are subject to unpredictable episodes, of widely varying severity, of submucosal and subcutaneous edema. Attacks that involve the upper respiratory tract can be fatal. Because of the rapid and unpredictable nature of the attacks, long-term prophylaxis with attenuated androgens, particularly danazol, is often employed. Danazol significantly increases the abundance of the C1 inhibitor mRNA, presumably from both the normal and mutant loci. In the great majority of patients, the frequency of serious attacks is dramatically reduced, although long-term androgen administration is not free of side effects.

Increasing Gene Expression from a Locus Not Affected by the Disease

A related therapeutic strategy is to increase the expression of a normal gene that compensates for the effect of mutation at another locus. This approach looks extremely promising in the management of sickle cell disease (Case 37) and β-thalassemia (Case 39), for which drugs that induce **DNA hypomethylation** are being used to increase the abundance of fetal hemoglobin (Hb F), which normally constitutes less than 1% of total hemoglobin in adults. Sickle cell disease causes illness because of both the anemia and the sickling of red

Table 13-5

Treatment by Modification of the Genome or Its Expression

Type of Modification	Example	Status
Pharmacological modulation of gene expression	Decitabine therapy to stimulate γ-globin (and thus Hb F) synthesis in sickle cell disease	Investigational
RNA interference (RNAi) to reduce the abundance of a toxic or dominant negative protein	RNAi gene therapy to suppress polyglutamine-induced neurodegeneration in a mouse model of spinocerebellar ataxia	Experimental
Partial modification of the somatic genotype		
By transplantation	Bone marrow transplantation in β-thalassemia	Curative with HLA-matched donor; good results overall
	Bone marrow transplantation in storage diseases, e.g., Hurler syndrome	Excellent results in some diseases, even if the brain is affected, such as Hurler syndrome
	Cord blood stem cell transplantation for presymptomatic Krabbe disease and Hurler syndrome	Excellent results for these two disorders
	Liver transplantation in α_1-antitrypsin deficiency	Up to 80% survival for 5 years in genetic liver disease
By gene transfer into somatic tissues	X-linked severe combined immunodeficiency	Apparent cure in 9 patients in one trial, but 3 developed a leukemia-like disorder; apparent cure in 4 patients in a second trial, with no evidence of malignant disease
	Severe combined immunodeficiency due to adenosine deaminase deficiency	Apparent cure of 2 patients, with no complications reported

blood cells (see Chapter 11 and Case 37). The increase in the level of Hb F ($\alpha_2\gamma_2$) benefits these patients because Hb F is a perfectly adequate oxygen carrier in postnatal life and because the polymerization of deoxyhemoglobin S is inhibited by Hb F.

The normal postnatal decrease in the expression of the γ-globin gene is at least partly due to methylation of CpG residues (see Chapter 5) in the 5′ promoter region of the gene. Methylation of the promoter can be inhibited if cytidine analogues, such as decitabine (5-aza-2′-deoxycytidine), are incorporated into DNA instead of cytidine. The inhibition of methylation is associated with substantial increases in γ-globin gene expression and, accordingly, in the proportion of Hb F in blood. Sickle cell patients treated with decitabine uniformly display increases in Hb F (Fig. 13-10) to levels that are likely to have a significant impact on morbidity and mortality. Large trials to assess the long-term efficacy and safety of decitabine are under way not only for sickle cell disease, but also for β-thalassemia, since increased Hb F is beneficial for that hemoglobinopathy as well.

Reducing the Expression of a Dominant Mutant Gene Product: RNA Interference

The pathological changes of some dominantly inherited diseases result either from the production of a gene product that is toxic to the cell, as seen with the proteins of the unstable repeat expansion diseases, such as

Huntington disease (Case 22), or from the diminished contribution from the wild-type allele of the normal protein, as with the dominant negative effect of some abnormal collagen chains in some forms of osteogenesis imperfecta (see Chapter 12). In either situation, the goal of therapy is to diminish the amount of the mutant protein made, without disrupting the production of the protein from the normal allele. One example of how this goal might be reached is provided by a technology called **RNA interference (RNAi)**. RNAi can be used to degrade a specific target RNA, such as that encoding the mutant huntingtin protein in Huntington disease. Briefly, short RNAs that correspond to specific sequences of the targeted RNA (see Fig. 13-6) are introduced into cells by, for example, viral gene transfer (discussed later). Strands of the interfering RNA bind to the target RNA and initiate its degradation. Even though the evolution of RNAi therapy is still at a very early stage, impressive results have been obtained in correcting the pathological changes of some single-gene diseases in animal models. These early findings demonstrate clearly the potential of this technology for treating human illness.

Modification of the Somatic Genome by Transplantation

Transplanted cells retain the genotype of the donor, and consequently, transplantation can be regarded as a

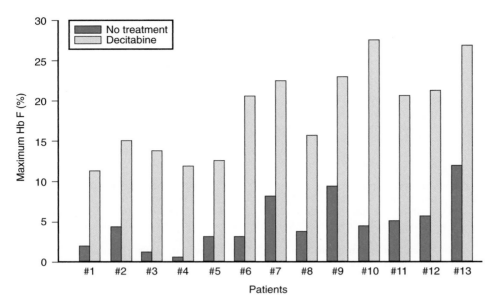

Figure 13-10 ■ The effect of the cytosine analogue decitabine, a DNA hypomethylating agent, on the percentage of hemoglobin F (Hb F) in 13 patients with sickle cell disease, compared with their level of Hb F without any treatment. Note the wide variation between patients in the levels of Hb F without treatment. Every patient shown had a significant increase in Hb F during decitabine therapy. (Modified from Saunthararajah Y, Lavelle D, DeSimone J: DNA hypomethylating reagents and sickle cell disease. Br J Haematol 126:629-636, 2004.)

form of gene transfer therapy because it leads to a modification of the somatic genome. There are two general indications for the use of transplantation in the treatment of genetic disease. First, cells or organs may be transplanted to introduce wild-type copies of a gene into a patient with mutations in that gene. This indication has the ironic consequence that a grossly normal organ is sometimes removed because its biochemical dysfunction is damaging another tissue. This is the case, for example, in homozygous familial hypercholesterolemia, for which liver transplantation is an effective but high-risk procedure. As experience with partial transplantation grows, however, and once gene transfer therapy is successful, whole organ transplants performed for this indication should become less frequent. The second and more common indication is for cell replacement, to compensate for an organ damaged by genetic disease (e.g., a liver that has become cirrhotic in α1AT deficiency). Some examples of the uses of transplantation in genetic disease are provided in Table 13-5.

Stem Cell Transplantation

Stem cells are self-renewing cells defined by two properties: (1) their ability to proliferate to form the differentiated cell types of a tissue in vivo and (2) their ability to self-renew—to form another stem cell. Embryonic stem cells, which can give rise to the whole organism, are discussed in Chapter 14. The use of embryonic stem cells for the treatment of disease is currently a topic of great scientific, ethical, and political controversy. However, if embryonic stem cells can be made to differentiate into cell types that could be used to replace cells missing or damaged by disease, society's view of such treatment might change.

Nuclear Transplantation

Nuclear transplantation (also referred to as nuclear transfer or nuclear cloning) is a new technology that has great potential for regenerative medicine, but also engenders tremendous controversy because of daunting ethical problems associated with its use. Nuclear transplantation refers to the transfer of a diploid nucleus from an adult donor somatic cell, such as a skin fibroblast, into an oocyte cytoplasm (i.e., an oocyte whose own nucleus has been removed) to generate a cloned embryo.

Therapeutic cloning is the use of embryonic stem cells generated by nuclear transplantation to form differentiated cell types of the body in culture. Because the cells derived from this technique are genetically identical to the donor nucleus, they could be used for cell transplantation to the donor without fear of immune rejection, a concept encompassed by the term nuclear transplantation therapy or therapeutic cloning. Cells obtained by therapeutic cloning could, in principle, be used to treat myriad human diseases, both monogenic and genetically complex. Experimental work in animal models has established that this therapy is capable of correcting disease.

At present, however, a large number of difficulties prevent the application of this technology. First, there are serious biological constraints to the application of this technology, including the fact that gene expression in cloned cells is often highly aberrant. Second, the use of human embryos for therapeutic cloning, no matter what the therapeutic benefits might be, is rejected by many on ethical grounds.

Reproductive cloning, in contrast, refers to the process of reimplanting an embryo obtained by nuclear transplantation into the uterus of a surrogate mother, with the purpose of allowing the embryo to develop

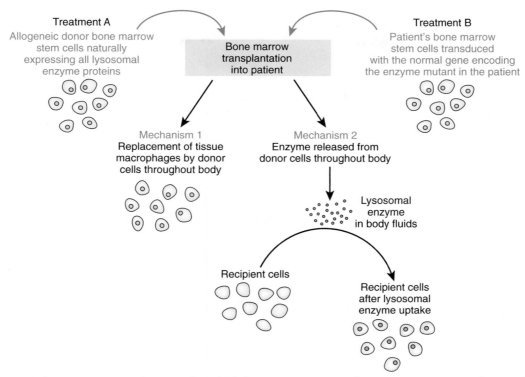

Figure 13-11 ■ The two major mechanisms by which bone marrow transplantation or gene transfer into bone marrow may reduce the substrate accumulation in lysosomal storage diseases. In the case of either treatment, bone marrow transplantation from an allogeneic donor (A) or genetic correction of the patient's own bone marrow stem cells by gene transfer (B), the bone marrow stem cell progeny, now expressing the relevant lysosomal enzyme, expand to repopulate the monocyte-macrophage system of the patient (Mechanism 1). In addition, lysosomal enzymes are released from the bone marrow cells derived from the donor or from the genetically modified marrow cells of the patient and taken up by enzyme-deficient cells from the extracellular fluid (Mechanism 2).

into a human clone of the donor from whom the somatic nucleus was obtained. Reproductive cloning is banned in all countries because of the complex ethical issues related to the creation of human clones.

Stem Cells from Human Donors

Only two types of stem cells are in clinical use at present: **hematopoietic stem cells,** which can reconstitute the blood system after bone marrow transplantation; and **corneal stem cells,** which are used to regenerate the corneal epithelium. The possibility that other types of stem cells will be used clinically in the future is enormous because stem cell research is one of the most active and promising areas of biomedical investigation. Stem cells have been identified in many different adult tissues, including, for example, skin and brain, in both humans and animals, and the hope is that these cells will be capable of regenerating missing or damaged tissue of the cell type from which they are derived. Although it is easy to overstate the potential of such treatment, optimism about the long-term future of stem cell therapy is justified.

Hematopoietic Stem Cell Transplantation in Nonstorage Diseases In addition to its extensive application

in the management of cancer, hematopoietic stem cell transplantation with use of bone marrow stem cells is also the treatment of choice for a selected group of monogenic immune deficiency disorders, including severe combined immunodeficiency of any type. Its role in the management of genetic disease in general, however, is less certain and under careful evaluation. For example, excellent outcomes have been obtained with bone marrow transplantation in the treatment of β-thalassemia patients younger than 16 years. Nevertheless, for each disease that bone marrow transplantation might benefit, its outcomes must be evaluated for many years and weighed against the results obtained with other therapies.

Hematopoietic Stem Cell Transplantation for Lysosomal Storage Diseases

Transplantation of Hematopoietic Stem Cells from Bone Marrow Bone marrow stem cell transplants are effective in correcting lysosomal storage in many tissues including, in some diseases, the brain, through the two mechanisms depicted in Figure 13-11. First, the transplanted cells are a source of lysosomal enzymes that can be transferred to other cells through the extracellular fluid, as initially shown by co-cultiva-

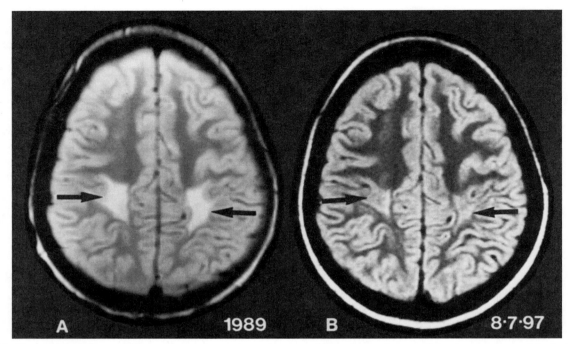

Figure 13-12 ■ The effect of bone marrow transplantation on white matter abnormalities in a patient with the late-onset form of globoid cell leukodystrophy. Eight years after transplantation, the increased white matter signal seen before treatment is greatly reduced. (From Krivit W, Shapiro EG, Peters C, et al: Hematopoietic stem-cell transplantation in globoid-cell leukodystrophy. N Engl J Med 338:1119-1126, 1998.)

tion experiments with Hurler and Hunter syndrome cells (see Chapter 12). Because bone marrow–derived cells constitute about 10% of the total cell mass of the body, the quantitative impact of enzymes transferred from them may be significant. Second, the mononuclear phagocyte system in most if not all tissues is derived from bone marrow stem cells, so that, after bone marrow transplantation, this system is of donor origin throughout the body. Of special note are the brain perivascular microglial cells, whose marrow origin may partially account for the correction of nervous system abnormalities by bone marrow transplantation in some storage disorders, for example, Krabbe disease, discussed later.

Bone marrow transplantation corrects or reduces the visceral abnormalities of many storage diseases including, for example, Gaucher disease. A normalization or reduction in the size of the liver, spleen, and heart is also achieved in Hurler syndrome, and improvements in upper airway obstruction, joint mobility, and corneal clouding are also obtained. Most rewarding, however, has been the impact of transplantation on the neurological component of the disease. Patients who have good developmental indices before transplantation, and who receive transplants before 24 months of age, continue to develop cognitively after transplantation, in contrast to the inexorable loss of intellectual function that otherwise occurs. Interestingly, a gene

dosage effect is manifested in the donor marrow; children who receive cells from homozygous normal donors appear to be more likely to retain fully normal intelligence than the recipients of heterozygous donor cells.

An even more dramatic effect on the neurological pathology of a storage disease has been observed after bone marrow transplantation of patients with the late-onset form of **globoid cell leukodystrophy** (or **Krabbe disease**), a white matter degenerative disorder. Patients with the late-onset form of this disease, which is due to a deficiency of the enzyme galactocerebrosidase, have a clinical onset at 0.5 to 3 years. Untreated, the disorder is characterized by relentless degeneration of central and peripheral myelin, spasticity, dementia, and peripheral neuropathy. Transplant recipients have experienced not only an arrest of the disease process but also actual improvement or normalization of tremors, ataxia, motor incoordination, and other abnormalities. Impressively, the white matter structural defects in the brains of treated patients are often reversible (Fig. 13-12).

Transplantation of Hematopoietic Stem Cells from Placental Cord Blood   The discovery that placental cord blood is a rich source of hematopoietic stem cells is beginning to make a substantial impact on the treatment of genetic disease. The use of placental cord blood has three great advantages over bone marrow as

COGNITIVE DEVELOPMENT

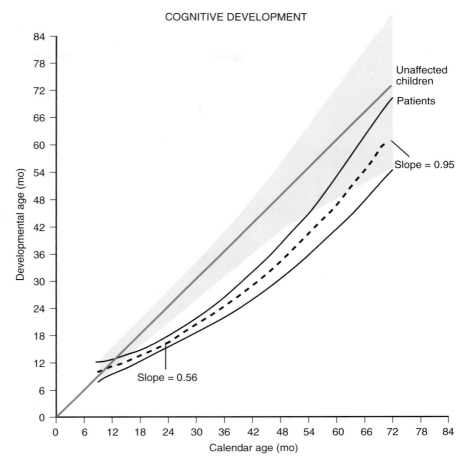

Figure 13-13 ■ Preservation of neurocognitive development in children with Hurler syndrome treated by cord blood transplantation. The figure displays the mean cognitive growth curve for transplanted patients compared with unaffected children. The thin black lines represent the 95% confidence interval for transplanted patients. (From Staba SL, Escolar ML, Poe M, et al: Cord-blood transplantation from unrelated donors in patients with Hurler's syndrome. N Engl J Med 350: 1960-1969, 2004.)

a source of transplantable hematopoietic stem cells. First, recipients are more tolerant of histoincompatible placental blood than of other allogeneic donor cells. Thus, engraftment occurs even if as many as three HLA antigens, cell surface markers encoded by the major histocompatibility complex (see Chapter 9), are mismatched between the donor and the recipient. Second, the wide availability of placental cord blood, together with the increased tolerance of histoincompatible donor cells, greatly expands the number of potential donors for any recipient. This feature is of particular significance to patients from minority ethnic groups, for whom the pool of potential donors is relatively small. Third, the risk of graft-versus-host disease is substantially reduced with use of placental cord blood cells.

Cord blood transplantation from unrelated donors appears to be as effective as bone marrow transplantation from a matched donor for the treatment of Hurler syndrome (Fig. 13-13). In the neonatal form of Krabbe disease, cord blood transplantation has a special role, since cognitive development can be rescued only if patients are transplanted very early in life (perhaps before 45 days of age), while they are still asymptomatic. Because the window of therapeutic opportunity in

neonatal Krabbe disease is so narrow, the ready availability and efficacy of cord blood stem cells—in contrast to the difficult and time-consuming effort to find a well-matched donor for a bone marrow transplant—represent a major therapeutic advance.

Liver Transplantation

For some metabolic liver diseases, liver transplantation is the only treatment of known benefit. For example, the chronic liver disease associated with cystic fibrosis or α1AT deficiency can be treated only by liver transplantation, and together these two disorders account for a large fraction of all the liver transplants performed in the pediatric population. Liver transplantation has now been undertaken for more than two dozen genetic diseases. At present, the 5-year survival rate of all children who receive liver transplants is in the range of 70% to 85%. For almost all of these patients, the quality of life is generally much improved, the specific metabolic abnormality necessitating the transplant is corrected, and in those conditions in which hepatic damage has occurred (such as α1AT deficiency), the provision of healthy hepatic tissue restores growth and normal pubertal development.

The Problems and the Future of Transplantation

Two major problems limit the wider use of transplantation for the treatment of genetic disease. First, the mortality after transplantation is significant, and the morbidity from superimposed infection due to the requirement for immunosuppression and graft-versus-host disease is substantial. The ultimate goal of transplantation research—transplantation without immunosuppression—comes incrementally closer. The increased tolerance of the recipient to cord blood transplants, compared with bone marrow–derived donor cells, exemplifies the advances in this area. The second problem with transplantation is the finite supply of organs, cord blood being a singular exception. For example, for all indications, including genetic disease, between 4000 and 5000 liver transplants may be needed annually in the United States alone. In addition, it remains to be demonstrated that transplanted organs are generally capable of functioning normally for a lifetime.

One solution to these difficulties involves the combination of stem cell and gene therapy. Here, a patient's own stem cells would be cultured in vitro, transfected by gene therapy with the gene of interest, and returned to the patient to repopulate the affected tissue with genetically restored cells. The identification of stem cells in a variety of adult human tissues and recent advances in gene transfer therapy offer great hope for this strategy.

Gene Therapy

Recombinant DNA technology (see Chapter 4) raised the exciting possibility that genetic disease might be treated at its most fundamental level, the gene. In concept, gene therapy is simple: one introduces a gene into a cell to achieve a therapeutic effect. For inherited diseases, the most common application by far will be the introduction of functional copies of the relevant gene into the appropriate target cells of a patient with a loss-of-function mutation (since most genetic diseases result from such mutations). Correction of the *reversible* features of a genetic disease should thereby be possible for many conditions.

In reality, this simple and now decades-old concept has proved to be unexpectedly difficult to apply, but the first successes of gene therapy in humans have been provided by the long-term correction (>5 years) of two forms of **severe combined immunodeficiency** in children (discussed later) and in large animal models of a few other diseases. In this section, we outline the potential, methods, and probable limitations of gene transfer for the treatment of human genetic disease. The minimal requirements that must be met before the use of gene

transfer can be considered for the treatment of a genetic disorder are presented in the Box on the next page.

General Considerations for Gene Therapy

The goal of gene therapy is to improve a patient's health by correction of the mutant phenotype. For this purpose, the delivery of the normal gene to appropriate somatic cells is required. Quite apart from the ethical and technical difficulties involved, it is neither necessary nor desirable to alter the germline of the patient being treated for a genetic disease. One concern is that any effort to integrate a normal copy of a gene into the germline (or into a fertilized egg) would carry a substantial risk of introducing new mutation.

The introduction of a gene into somatic cells may serve one of three purposes (Fig. 13-14). First, gene therapy may be able to correct for a loss-of-function mutation. Here, the introduction of normal functional copies of a gene would suffice to correct a reversible phenotype, such as the increased phenylalanine level in PKU (in this case, the patient's mutant gene or genes are left in place). In these instances, it would generally not be important where in the genome of a cell the transferred gene inserts. In some long-lived types of cells, stable long-term expression may not require integration of the introduced gene into the host genome. For example, if the transferred DNA is stabilized in the form of an **episome** (a stable nuclear but nonchromosomal DNA molecule, such as that formed by an adeno-associated viral vector, discussed later), and if the target cell is long-lived (e.g., neurons, myocytes, hepatocytes), then long-term expression can occur without integration. To function in cells into which it is introduced, the product of the transferred gene must have access to appropriate cofactors or other molecules essential for its function. For example, the cofactor for phenylalanine hydroxylase, BH_4 (see Chapter 12), would have to be given orally if this enzyme were introduced into bone marrow or muscle cells, which do not normally synthesize BH_4.

Second, gene therapy may be undertaken to replace or to inactivate a dominant mutant allele whose abnormal product causes the generally dominant disease. In Huntington disease, for example, one would want to replace the disease gene containing the expanded CAG repeat or at least most of the CAG expansion itself. Alternatively, one could try to degrade the mutant RNA rather than remove the gene that encodes it. For example, selective degradation of a mutant mRNA encoding a dominant negative proα1(I) collagen that causes osteogenesis imperfecta (see Chapter 12) should, in principle, lessen the bone abnormalities of this condition. Therapeutic genes that encode small interfering RNAs, as mentioned earlier, can also be used to degrade

---

◾◾◽ Essential Requirements of Gene Therapy for an Inherited Disorder

- **Identity of the molecular defect**

  The identity of the affected gene, or at least of the biochemical basis of the disorder, must be known.

- **A functional copy of the gene**

  A complementary DNA (cDNA) clone of the gene or the gene itself must be available. If the gene or cDNA is too large for the current generation of vectors, a functional version of the gene from which nonessential components have been removed to reduce its size may suffice.

- **Knowledge of the pathophysiological mechanism**

  Knowledge of the pathophysiological mechanism of the disease must be sufficient to suggest that the gene transfer will ameliorate or correct the pathological process and prevent, slow, or reverse critical phenotypic abnormalities. Loss-of-function mutations require replacement with a functional gene; for diseases due to dominant negative alleles, inactivation of the mutant gene or its products will be necessary.

- **Favorable risk-to-benefit ratio**

  A substantial disease burden and a favorable risk-to-benefit ratio, in comparison with alternative therapy, must be present.

- **Appropriate regulatory components for the transferred gene**

  Tight regulation of the level of gene expression is relatively unimportant in some diseases and critical in others. In thalassemia, for example, overexpression of the transferred gene would cause a new imbalance of globin chains in red blood cells, whereas low levels of expression would be ineffective. In some enzymopathies, a few per cent of normal expression may be therapeutic, and abnormally high levels of expression may have no adverse effect.

- **An appropriate target cell**

  Ideally, the target cell must have a long half-life or good replicative potential in vivo. It must also be accessible for direct introduction of the gene, or alternatively, it must be possible to deliver sufficient copies of the gene to it (e.g., through the blood stream) to attain a therapeutic benefit. The feasibility of gene therapy is often enhanced if the target cell can be cultured in vitro to facilitate gene transfer into it; in this case, it must be possible to introduce a sufficient number of the recipient cells into the patient and have them functionally integrate into the relevant organ.

- **Strong evidence of efficacy and safety**

  Cultured cell and animal studies must indicate that the vector and gene construct are both effective and safe. The ideal precedent is to show that the gene therapy is effective, benign, and enduring in a large animal genetic model of the disease in question. At present, however, large animal models exist for only a few monogenic diseases. Genetically engineered or spontaneous mutant mouse models are much more widely available.

- **Regulatory approval**

  Protocol review and approval by an Institutional Review Board is essential. In most countries, human gene therapy trials are also subject to oversight by a governmental agency.

---

only the mRNA from the mutant allele and have shown promise in laboratory studies.

Third, gene therapy may eventually be most widely used to achieve a pharmacological effect. For example, patients with cancer are likely to benefit from this approach (see Fig. 13-14B to D).

Gene Transfer Strategies

An appropriately engineered gene may be transferred into target cells by one of two general strategies (Fig. 13-15). The first involves ex vivo (i.e., outside the body) introduction of the gene into cells that have been cultured from the patient and then reintroduced after the gene transfer. In the second approach, the gene is injected directly in vivo into the tissue or extracellular fluid of interest (from which it is selectively taken up by the target cells). Targeting of this type is usually achieved

by modifying the coat of a viral vector so that only the designated cells bind the viral particles.

The Target Cell

The ideal target cells are stem cells (which are self-replicating) or progenitor cells with substantial replication potential. Introduction of the gene into stem cells can result in the expression of the transferred gene in a large population of daughter cells. At present, bone marrow is the only tissue for which stem cells or progenitor cells have been used successfully as recipients of transferred genes. Genetically modified bone marrow stem cells have been used to cure two forms of severe combined immunodeficiency, as discussed later, and they could in principle also be used for other diseases affecting blood cells, such as thalassemia and sickle cell disease. In addition, genetically modified bone marrow could also

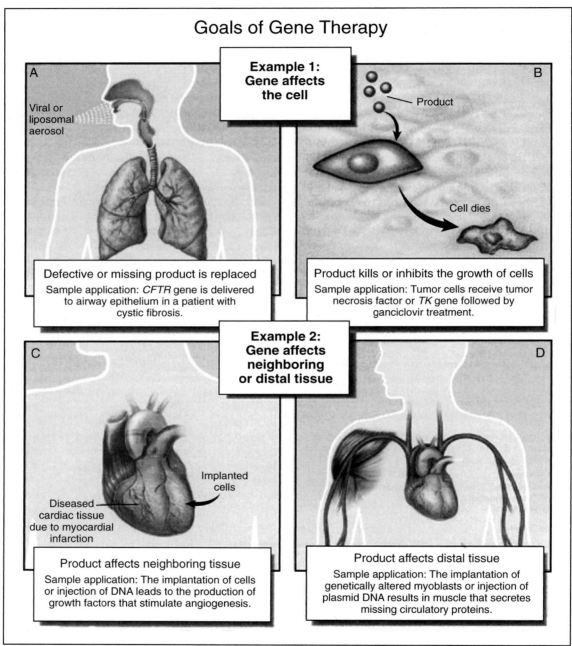

Goals of Gene Therapy

A

Viral or liposomal aerosol

Example 1: Gene affects the cell

B

Product

Cell dies

Defective or missing product is replaced

Sample application: *CFTR* gene is delivered to airway epithelium in a patient with cystic fibrosis.

Product kills or inhibits the growth of cells

Sample application: Tumor cells receive tumor necrosis factor or *TK* gene followed by ganciclovir treatment.

Example 2: Gene affects neighboring or distal tissue

C

Implanted cells

Diseased cardiac tissue due to myocardial infarction

D

Product affects neighboring tissue

Sample application: The implantation of cells or injection of DNA leads to the production of growth factors that stimulate angiogenesis.

Product affects distal tissue

Sample application: The implantation of genetically altered myoblasts or injection of plasmid DNA results in muscle that secretes missing circulatory proteins.

Figure 13-14 ■ Four types of gene therapy. Note that the sample applications presented here are theoretical, and the only human gene therapy corrections of an inherited disease, to date, have been for two forms of severe combined immunodeficiency, X-linked severe combined immunodeficiency and adenosine deaminase deficiency, each of which exemplify (A), the replacement of a defective or missing product (see text). *CFTR* denotes the gene for the cystic fibrosis transmembrane conductance regulator. *TK* denotes herpes simplex thymidine kinase, which confers ganciclovir sensitivity on cells. (From Blau HM, Springer ML: Gene therapy—a novel form of drug delivery. N Engl J Med 333:1204-1207, 1995.)

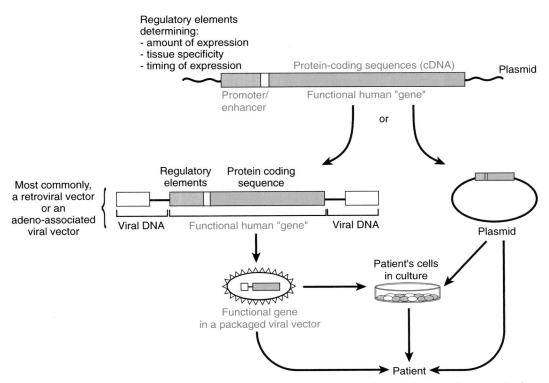

Figure 13-15 ■ The two major strategies used to transfer a gene to a patient. For patients with a genetic disease, the most common approach is to construct a viral vector containing the human cDNA of interest and to introduce it directly into the patient or into cells cultured from the patient that are then returned to the patient. The viral components at the ends of the molecule are required for the integration of the vector into the host genome. In some instances, the gene of interest is placed in a plasmid, which is then used for the gene transfer.

be used for diseases that do not involve the blood system per se, such as PKU. In this case, the circulation would deliver the phenylalanine to the enzyme now expressed in the marrow. Gene transfer therapy into blood stem cells is also likely to be effective for the treatment of storage diseases for which bone marrow transplantation has been effective, as discussed earlier.

If the target cell cannot divide extensively in culture and then be reimplanted in the patient, or if it does not have identifiable stem or progenitor cells in the mature animal, other approaches are needed. For example, hepatocytes can be briefly maintained in primary culture, transfected with a gene, and then returned to the animal. Endothelial cells may prove to be particularly useful targets for gene transfer because they line the walls of blood vessels; the protein product of a gene expressed in endothelial cells can be released into the circulation to achieve a systemic effect. An important logistical consideration arises with all of these approaches: the number of cells into which the gene must be introduced may be very large. Thus, to treat PKU, the approximate number of liver cells into which the phenylalanine hydroxylase gene would have to be transferred is about 5% of the hepatocyte mass, or approximately 10^{10} cells (assuming that the level of

expression of the transferred gene is similar to wild type).

DNA Transfer into Cells: Viral Vectors

The ideal vector for gene therapy would be safe, readily made, and easily introduced into the appropriate target tissue, and it would express the gene of interest for life. At present, no vector—viral or nonviral—has been identified that fulfills all of these criteria. Indeed, no single vector is likely to be satisfactory in all respects for all types of gene therapy (see Fig. 13-14), and a repertoire of vectors will probably be required. Here, we briefly review three of the most widely used classes of viral vectors, those derived from **retroviruses, adenoviruses,** and **adeno-associated viruses.** A major advantage of viral vectors is that they are capable of entering virtually every cell in the target population.

One of the most widely used classes of vectors is derived from retroviruses, simple RNA viruses with only three structural genes that can be removed and replaced with the gene to be transferred (see Fig. 13-15). The current generation of retroviral vectors has been engineered to render them incapable of replication. Their other merits include that they are nontoxic to the cell, that only a low number of copies of the viral DNA (with the transferred gene) integrate into the host genome, that the integrated DNA is stable, and that retroviral vectors can accommodate up to 8 kb of added DNA, commodious enough for many genes that might be transferred. A major limitation of many retroviral vectors is that the target cell must undergo division for integration of the virus into the host DNA, limiting the use of such vectors in nondividing cells such as neurons. **Lentiviruses,** however, the class of retroviruses that includes the human immunodeficiency virus, are capable of DNA integration in many slowly dividing or nondividing cells, including neurons. These vectors may indeed be suitable for the treatment of neurological disorders.

Adeno-associated viruses have the great advantage of having no adverse effects in humans, being widespread in human populations. Moreover, they infect dividing or nondividing cells and can exist either episomally or stably integrated into a host chromosome. A disadvantage is that the current adeno-associated virus vectors can accommodate inserts of up to only 5 kb.

Adenoviral vectors have the advantages that they can be obtained at high titer; that they will infect a wide variety of cell types, dividing or nondividing; and that they can accommodate inserts of 30 to 35 kb. However, in addition to other limitations, they have recently been associated with at least one death in a gene therapy trial through the elicitation of a strong immune response. Consequently, their use in gene therapy is presently being reexamined.

DNA Transfer into Cells: Nonviral Vectors

In principle, nonviral vectors are attractive because they lack the biological risks (e.g., viral contamination) associated with viral vectors and because their preparation, at least theoretically, is more straightforward. Nonviral vectors under development are of four general types:

1. **naked DNA,** for example, a cDNA with regulatory elements in a plasmid; or RNA, such as a small interfering RNA (siRNA);
2. **DNA packaged in liposomes,** a continuous lipid bilayer encasing an aqueous volume;
3. **protein-DNA conjugates,** in which DNA is complexed to a protein—such as a peptide that binds to a cell surface receptor—that facilitates entry of the complex into cells or into a subcellular compartment; and
4. **artificial chromosomes,** in which the minimal functional components of a natural chromosome (see Chapter 3) are combined with a cDNA or gene of interest, with appropriate regulatory elements.

Although the potential of nonviral vectors is substantial, their overall success has been limited. The major difficulties are that DNA introduced by these vectors tends to be taken up by lysosomes and degraded, and DNA that escapes this fate is not taken up efficiently by the nucleus. In addition, each nonviral system has specific problems. For example, the delivery of naked DNA is highly inefficient, although it may be very useful if it can be injected directly into the tissue of interest and when only a transient effect is required, as, for example, in the treatment of malignant disease. Overall, the technology and biology of nonviral vectors are still at too early a stage of development to give a true picture of their potential for the treatment of disease.

Risks of Gene Therapy

Gene therapy for the treatment of human disease has both demonstrated and theoretical risks that are of three general types.

Adverse Response to the Vector or Vector-Disease Combination   Principal among the concerns is that the patient will have an adverse reaction to the vector or the transferred gene. Such problems should be largely anticipated with appropriate animal and preliminary human studies. At least one patient has died, however, apparently from an adverse immune response to the adenoviral vector with which he was injected. An additional consideration in this unfortunate instance is that the immune response appears to have elicited a catabolic response in this subject. Since his genetic disease was a urea cycle defect, his ability to tolerate catabolism was poor. The general lesson from this important example is that the pathophysiological features of the specific disorder must be considered in selecting the appropriate vector; a patient tolerant of catabolism might have survived the immune response to the adenovirus.

Insertional Mutagenesis Causing Malignant Neoplasia   The second concern is insertional mutagenesis, that is, that the transferred gene will integrate into the patient's DNA and activate a proto-oncogene or disrupt a tumor-suppressor gene, leading possibly to malignant neoplasia (see Chapter 16). The illicit expression of an oncogene is less likely to occur with the current generation of viral vectors, which have been altered to minimize the ability of their promoters to activate the expression of adjacent host genes. Insertional inactivation of a tumor-suppressor gene is likely to be infrequent and, as such, is an acceptable risk in diseases for which there is no therapeutic alternative. An unexpected mechanism of oncogenesis in gene therapy was revealed by the occurrence of a lymphoproliferative disorder in some patients receiving gene therapy for X-linked severe combined immunodeficiency, discussed later. In these individuals, it appears that the transgene itself may have contributed to promotion of the malignant disease. Consequently, the biological impact of the transferred gene, when it is expressed from ectopic chromosomal locations and outside its normal biological context, must be anticipated as fully as possible.

Insertional Inactivation of an Essential Gene   A third risk—that insertional inactivation could disrupt a gene essential for viability—will, in general, be without significant effect because such lethal mutations are expected to be rare and will kill only single cells. Although vectors appear to somewhat favor insertion into transcribed genes, and retroviruses are predisposed to insert into the 5′ end of genes, the chance that the same gene will be disrupted in more than a few cells is extremely low; for example, most individual cell types express about 10,000 genes. The one exception to this statement applies to the germline; an insertion into a gene in the germline could create a dominant disease-causing mutation that might manifest in the treated patient's offspring. Such events, however, are likely to be rare and the risk acceptable because it would be difficult to justify withholding, on this basis, carefully planned and reviewed trials of gene therapy from patients who have no other recourse. Moreover, the problem of germline modification by disease treatment is not confined to gene therapy. For example, most chemotherapy used in the treatment of malignant disease is mutagenic, but this risk is accepted because of the therapeutic benefits.

Ethical Considerations

As with any new treatment, proposals for trials of gene transfer into patients must be subjected to rigorous scrutiny by regulatory agencies and hospital ethics committees. However, virtually all governmental and religious agencies that have examined proposals for human gene therapy for the treatment of genetic disease have agreed that this therapeutic opportunity should be pursued. In contrast to the transfer of genes into the germline, somatic gene therapy raises few ethical issues that are not routinely considered when other novel therapy is evaluated (e.g., a new anticancer drug).

Diseases That Have Been or Are Likely to Be Amenable to Gene Therapy

In addition to the two forms of severe combined immunodeficiency (SCID) that have been successfully treated with gene therapy, a large number of other single-gene disorders are potential candidates for correction by this approach. These other diseases include retinal degenerations; hematopoietic conditions, such as hemophilia

and thalassemia; and disorders affecting liver proteins, such as PKU, urea cycle disorders, familial hypercholesterolemia, and α1AT deficiency. Additional considerations relevant to the use of gene therapy for two important disorders are outlined here.

X-linked SCID   The severe combined immunodeficiencies are a group of disorders due to mutations in genes required for lymphocyte maturation. In the absence of treatment, affected individuals fail to thrive and die early in life of infection, since they lack functional B and T lymphocytes. One form of the disease, X-linked SCID, results from mutations in the X-linked gene encoding the γc-cytokine receptor subunit of several interleukin receptors. The receptor deficiency causes an early block in T- and natural killer–lymphocyte growth, survival, and differentiation. This condition was chosen for a gene therapy trial for two principal reasons. First, bone marrow transplantation cures the disease, indicating that the restoration of lymphocyte expression of the γc cytokine receptor can reverse the pathophysiological changes. Second, it was believed that cells carrying the transferred gene would have a selective survival advantage over untransduced cells. (Cells into which a viral vector has been introduced are said to be "transduced.")

The outcome of trials of X-linked SCID has been dramatic and resulted, in 2000, in the first gene therapy cure of a patient with a genetic disease. Subsequent confirmation has been obtained in eight patients in this initial trial. Bone marrow stem cells from the patients were infected in culture (ex vivo) with a retroviral vector that expressed the γc subunit cDNA. A selective advantage was conferred on the transduced cells by the gene transfer. Transduced T cells and natural killer cells populated the blood of treated patients, and the T cells appeared to behave normally. Although the frequency of transduced B cells was low, adequate levels of serum immunoglobulin and antibody levels were obtained. Most significantly, dramatic clinical improvement occurred, with resolution of protracted diarrhea and skin lesions and restoration of normal growth and development.

This remarkable outcome, however, has come at the cost of induction of a leukemia-like disorder in at least three of these patients, who developed an extreme lymphocytosis. In two subjects, the malignant disease is thought to have at least partially resulted from the insertion of the retroviral vector into the *LMO2* locus on chromosome 11. This integration was associated with aberrant expression of the *LMO2* transcript in the monoclonal T-cell population. Notably, the *LMO2* gene has been previously implicated in T-cell leukemia, suggesting that the retroviral insertion caused the lymphoproliferation in these patients. In a second gene therapy trial for X-linked SCID, none of the 10 subjects

Table 13-6

Three Diseases with Special Prospects or Problems for Gene Therapy

Disease	Affected Gene	Specific Considerations
Hemophilia B	Factor IX	An encouraging recent human trial using an adeno-associated virus (AAV) vector delivered to the liver achieved therapeutic levels of factor IX, but a T-cell response to the viral capsid terminated expression after several weeks. Patients with preexisting immunity to AAV may not have this response.
Leber congenital amaurosis (blindness), an early-onset photoreceptor degeneration	Mutations in more than 10 genes cause this phenotype, but RPE65 is the current focus	The RPE65 protein is required for the cycling of retinoids (vitamin A metabolites) to photoreceptors. Adeno-associated virus–mediated gene therapy has restored vision, for at least 6 years, to dogs with RPE65 mutations, after a single dose of the vector into the retina. No side effects were observed. Human clinical trials are under way.
Duchenne muscular dystrophy	Dystrophin	Progress here is hampered by the large size of the cDNA and the logistical barrier posed by trying to place the gene into a therapeutically significant fraction of the huge number of myocytes in the body. A minigene, lacking many of the highly repetitive sequences in the rod domain of dystrophin (see Fig. 12-19), is functional and may surmount the first problem.

treated have manifested leukemic complications. Whether the outcome of this second trial is truly different from the first one or merely reflects the small number of patients treated is presently unclear. It is possible that differences in the protocols in the second study, including vector design and the methods used for transduction of the cells, may account for the absence of lymphoproliferation in the second group of patients.

These initial trials demonstrate the great potential of gene therapy for the correction of inherited disease, even though the current strategies and techniques of gene therapy for X-linked SCID are being reassessed. At this point, bone marrow stem cell transplantation remains the treatment of choice for those children with X-linked SCID fortunate enough to have a donor with an HLA-identical match. For patients without such a match, most authorities would recommend haploidentical bone marrow stem cell transplantation over gene therapy, reserving gene transfer for those who fail haploidentical transplantation.

SCID due to Adenosine Deaminase Deficiency This disorder was selected for a gene therapy trial because of the success of PEG-ADA administration (discussed earlier) in treating it and, as with X-linked SCID, because the transduced cells were likely to have a survival advantage over untransduced cells. In the small but successful trial that has illustrated the powerful impact that gene therapy can have on this condition, bone marrow stem cells were transduced ex vivo with a retroviral vector expressing an ADA cDNA. The transduced cells were transplanted into the patients whose bone marrow had been partially ablated to improve engraftment of the gene-modified marrow. The result, in two children, was excellent sustained engraftment by the ADA-transduced cells, which had a clear survival advantage over the untreated cells. The engrafted hematopoietic stem cells differentiated into multiple lymphocyte lineages, resulting in increased lymphocyte counts, improved immune function, and a reduction of the levels of toxic deoxynucleotides in lymphocytes (see Fig. 13-8). Prolonged follow-up suggests that this treatment is both effective and safe. In particular, there has been no evidence of leukemic transformation of the treated lymphocytes, but additional patients must be treated to demonstrate that this outcome does not simply reflect the small sample size of this first trial.

The Future for Gene Therapy Early clinical trials or animal studies have suggested that two other diseases, hemophilia B due to factor IX deficiency and an early-onset form of photoreceptor degeneration, Leber congenital amaurosis, may be amenable to gene therapy (Table 13-6), and great effort is being invested in many other disorders. One disease that exemplifies some of the problems that must be resolved is Duchenne muscular dystrophy (see Table 13-6).

As of 2007, more than 1200 clinical gene therapy trials were underway worldwide to evaluate both the safety and efficacy of this marvelously promising technology. However, the major conclusions of a 1995 National Institutes of Health panel on the status and promise of gene therapy still hold: progress in this field has been slow, the research emphasis has not always been appropriate, and early claims of efficacy were overstated. Nevertheless, the panel concluded that gene therapy will ultimately be successful in many diseases, despite the numerous difficulties that must be overcome. The exciting results obtained in the last few years with gene therapy for the two forms of human SCID corroborate this optimism, despite the serious concerns about the oncogenic potential of the treatment. It is to be hoped that during the next few decades, gene therapy for both monogenic and genetically complex diseases will transform the management of many disorders, both common and rare.

● GENERAL REFERENCES

Copelan EA: Hematopoietic stem-cell transplantation. N Engl J Med 354:1813-1826, 2006.

Hayes A, Costa T, Scriver CR, Childs B: The effect of mendelian disease on human health. II: Response to treatment. Am J Med Genet 21:243-255, 1985.

Hochelinger K, Jaenisch R: Nuclear transplantation, embryonic stem cells, and the potential for cell therapy. N Engl J Med 349:275-286, 2003.

Körbling M, Estrov Z: Adult stem cells for tissue repair—a new therapeutic concept? N Engl J Med 349:570-582, 2003.

O'Connor TP, Crystal RG: Genetic medicines: treatment strategies for hereditary disorders. Nat Rev Genet 7:261-276, 2006.

Thomas CR, Ehrhardt A, Kay MA: Progress and problems with the use of viral vectors for gene therapy. Nat Rev Genet 4:346-358, 2003.

Treacy EP, Childs B, Scriver CR: Response to treatment in hereditary metabolic disease: 1993 survey and 10-year comparison. Am J Hum Genet 56:359-367, 1995.

Treacy EP, Valle D, Scriver CR: Treatment of genetic disease. In Scriver CR, Beaudet AL, Sly WS, Valle D (eds): The Metabolic and Molecular Bases of Inherited Disease, 8th ed. New York, McGraw-Hill, 2001.

Weissman IL: Translating stem and progenitor cell biology to the clinic: barriers and opportunities. Science 287:1442-1446, 2000.

● REFERENCES FOR SPECIFIC TOPICS

Acland GM, Aguirre GD, Ray J, et al: Gene therapy restores vision in a canine model of childhood blindness. Nat Genet 28:92-95, 2001.

Acland GM, Aguirre GD, Bennett J, et al: Long-term restoration of rod and cone vision by single dose rAAV-mediated gene transfer to the retina in a canine model of childhood blindness. Mol Ther 12:1072-1082, 2005.

Aiuti A, Slavin S, Aker M, et al: Correction of ADA-SCID by stem cell gene therapy combined with nonmyeloablative conditioning. Science 296:2410-2413, 2002.

Cavazzana-Calvo M, Lagresle C, Hacein-Bey-Abina S, Fischer A: Gene therapy for severe combined immunodeficiency. Annu Rev Med 56:585-602, 2005.

Chan B, Wara D, Hershfield MS, et al: Long-term efficacy of enzyme replacement therapy for adenosine deaminase (ADA)–deficient severe combined immunodeficiency (SCID). Clin Immunol 117:133-143, 2005.

Desnick RJ: Enzyme replacement and enhancement therapies for lysosomal diseases. J Inherit Metab Dis 27:385-410, 2004.

Gaspar HB, Parsley KL, Howe S, et al: Gene therapy of X-linked severe combined immunodeficiency by use of a pseudotyped gammaretroviral vector. Lancet 364:2181-2187, 2004.

Goldstein JL, Hobbs HH, Brown MS: Familial hypercholesterolemia. In Scriver CR, Beaudet AL, Sly WS, Valle D (eds): The Metabolic and Molecular Bases of Inherited Disease, 8th ed. New York, McGraw-Hill, 2001.

High K: The risks of germline gene transfer. Hastings Center Rep 33:3, 2003.

Hollon T: Researchers and regulators reflect on first gene therapy death. Nat Med 6:6, 2000.

Kelly DA: Current results of evolving indications for liver transplantation in children. J Pediatr Gastroenterol Nutr 27:214-221, 1998.

Krivit W, Shapiro EG, Peters C, et al: Hematopoietic stem cell transplantation in globoid-cell leukodystrophy. N Engl J Med 338:1119-1126, 1998.

Lukacs GL, Durie PR: Pharmacologic approaches to correcting the basic defect in cystic fibrosis. N Engl J Med 349:1401-1404, 2003.

Manno CS, Arruda VR, Pierce GF, et al: Successful transduction of liver in hemophilia by AAV–factor IX and limitations imposed by the host immune response. Nat Med 12:342-347, 2006.

Muenzer J, Fisher A: Advances in the treatment of mucopolysaccharidosis type 1. N Engl J Med 350:1932-1934, 2004.

Pellegrini G: Changing the cell source in cell therapy. N Engl J Med 351:1170-1172, 2004.

Sandhaus RA: α_1-Antitrypsin deficiency: new and emerging treatments for α_1-antitrypsin deficiency. Thorax 59:904-909, 2004.

Sauntharararajah Y, Lavelle D, DeSimone J: DNA hypomethylating reagents and sickle cell disease. Br J Haematol 126: 629-636, 2004.

Schrier SL, Angelucci E: New strategies in the treatment of the thalassemias. Annu Rev Med 56:157-171, 2005.

Scriver CR, Kaufman S: The hyperphenylalaninemias: phenylalanine hydroxylase deficiency. In Scriver CR, Beaudet AL, Sly WS, Valle D (eds): The Metabolic and Molecular Bases of Inherited Disease, 8th ed. New York, McGraw-Hill, 2001.

Staba SL, Escolar ML, Poe M, et al: Cord-blood transplantation from unrelated donors in patients with Hurler's syndrome. N Engl J Med 350:1960-1969, 2004.

Starzl TE, Demetris AJ: Liver transplantation: a 31-year perspective. Part I. Curr Probl Surg 27:49-116, 1990.

Stevenson M: Therapeutic potential of RNA interference. N Engl J Med 351:1772-1777, 2004.

Stuart MJ, Nagel RL: Sickle cell disease. Lancet 364:1343-1360, 2004.

Weinberg KI: Early use of drastic therapy. N Engl J Med 352:214-2126, 2005.

Weinreb NJ, Charrow J, Andersson HC, et al: Effectiveness of enzyme replacement therapy in 1028 patients with type 1 Gaucher disease after 2 to 5 years of treatment: a report from the Gaucher Registry. Am J Med 113:112-119, 2002.

Wilcox WR, Banikazemi M, Guffon N, et al: Long-term safety and efficacy of enzyme replacement therapy for Fabry disease. Am J Hum Genet 75:65-74, 2004.

Xia H, Mao Q, Eliason SL, et al: RNAi suppresses polyglutamine-induced neurodegeneration in a model of spinocerebellar ataxia. Nat Med 10:816-820, 2004.

Zeitlin P: Can curcumin cure cystic fibrosis? N Engl J Med 351:606-608, 2004.

● USEFUL WEBSITES

Clinical Trials in Human Gene Transfer. *http://www.gemcris.od.nih.gov/Contents/GC_home.asp*

Gene Therapy Clinical Trials Worldwide. *http://www.wiley.co.uk/genetherapy/clinical*

Online Mendelian Inheritance in Man (OMIM). *www.ncbi.nlm.nih.gov/entrez/query.fcgi?db=OMIM*

PROBLEMS

1. X-linked chronic granulomatous disease (CGD) is an uncommon disorder characterized by a defect in host defense that leads to severe, recurrent, and often fatal pyogenic infections beginning in early childhood. The X-linked CGD locus encodes the heavy chain of cytochrome *b*, a component of the oxidase that generates superoxide in phagocytes. Because interferon-γ (IFN-γ) is known to enhance the oxidase activity of normal phagocytes, IFN-γ was administered to boys with X-linked CGD to see whether their oxidase activity increased. Before treatment, the phagocytes of *some* less severely affected patients had small but detectable bursts of oxidase activity (unlike those of severely affected patients), suggesting that increased activity in these less severely affected subjects is the result of greater production of cytochrome *b* from the affected locus. In these less severe cases, IFN-γ increased the cytochrome *b* content, superoxide production, and killing of *Staphylococcus aureus* in the granulocytes. The IFN-γ effect was associated with a definite increase in the abundance of the cytochrome *b* chain. Presumably, the cytochrome *b* polypeptide of these patients is partially functional, and increased expression of the residual function improved the physiological defect. Describe the genetic differences that might account for the fact that the phagocytes of some patients with X-linked CGD respond to IFN-γ in vitro and others do not.

2. Identify some of the restrictions on the types of proteins that can be considered for extracellular replacement therapy, as exemplified by PEG-ADA. What makes this approach inappropriate for phenylalanine hydroxylase deficiency? for Hurler syndrome? for Lesch-Nyhan syndrome? If Tay-Sachs disease caused only liver disease, would this strategy succeed? If not, why?

3. A 3-year-old girl, Rhonda, has familial hypercholesterolemia due to a deletion of the 5′ end of the gene. The mutation removed the promoter and the first two exons of each allele. (Rhonda's parents are second cousins.) You explain to the parents that she will require plasma exchange therapy every 1 to 2 weeks for years. At the clinic, however, they meet another family with a 5-year-old boy with the same disease. The boy has been treated with drugs with some success. Rhonda's parents want to know why she has not been offered similar pharmacological therapy. Explain.

4. What classes of mutations are likely to be found in homocystinuric patients who are not responsive to the administration of large doses (1000 mg/day) of pyridoxine (vitamin B_6)? How might you explain the fact that Tom is completely responsive, whereas his first cousin Allan has only a partial reduction in plasma homocystine when he is given the same amount of vitamin B_6?

5. You have just cloned the gene for phenylalanine hydroxylase and wish ultimately to introduce it into patients with PKU. Your approach will be to culture cells from the patient, introduce a functional version of the gene into the cells, and reintroduce the cells into the patient.
   a. What DNA components do you need to make a functional phenylalanine hydroxylase protein in a gene transfer experiment?
   b. Which tissues would you choose in which to express the enzyme, and why? How does this choice affect your gene construct in (a)?
   c. You introduce your version of the gene into fibroblasts cultured from a skin biopsy specimen from the patient. Northern (RNA) blot analysis shows that the messenger RNA is present in normal amounts and is the correct size. However, no phenylalanine hydroxylase protein can be detected in the cells. What kinds of abnormalities in the transferred gene would explain this finding?
   d. You have corrected all the problems identified in (c). On introducing the new version of the gene into the cultured cells, you now find that the phenylalanine hydroxylase protein is present in great abundance, and when you harvest the cells and assay the enzyme (in the presence of all the required components), normal activity is obtained. However, when you add ^{3}H-labeled phenylalanine to the cells in culture, no ^{3}H-labeled tyrosine is formed (in contrast, some cultured liver cells produce a large quantity of ^{3}H-labeled tyrosine in this situation). What are the most likely explanations for the failure to form ^{3}H-tyrosine? How does this result affect your gene therapy approach to patients?
   e. You have developed a method to introduce your functional version of the gene directly into a large proportion of the hepatocytes of patients with phenylalanine hydroxylase deficiency. Unexpectedly, you find that much lower levels of phenylalanine hydroxylase enzymatic activity are obtained in patients in whom significant amounts of the inactive phenylalanine hydroxylase homodimer were detectable in hepatocytes before treatment than in patients who had no detectable phenylalanine hydroxylase polypeptide before treatment. How can you explain this result? How might you overcome the problem?

6. Both alleles of a gene that is mutant in your patient produce a protein that is decreased in abundance but has residual function. What therapeutic strategies might you consider in such a situation?

7. A patient has a dominant disease due to a mutation that introduces a premature stop codon. Immunoblots of the affected cells confirm that none of the mutant protein is present. The patient is treated with gentamicin to facilitate skipping of the premature stop, allowing a full-length protein to be synthesized, as confirmed by repeated immunoblot analysis after the treatment. However, no protein function can be detected. What is the most likely explanation for this disappointing outcome?

Chapter 14

Developmental Genetics and Birth Defects

A knowledge of developmental genetics, including the mechanisms responsible for normal human development in utero, is essential for the practitioner who seeks to develop a rational approach to the diagnostic evaluation of a patient with a birth defect. With an accurate diagnostic assessment in hand, the practitioner can make predictions about prognosis, recommend management options, and provide an accurate recurrence risk for the parents and other relatives of the affected child. In this chapter, we provide an overview of the branch of medicine concerned with birth defects and review basic mechanisms of embryological development, with examples of some of these mechanisms in detail. Next, we describe examples of birth defects that result from abnormalities in these processes. Finally, we show how an appreciation of developmental biology is essential for understanding prenatal diagnosis (see Chapter 15) and stem cell therapy as applied to regenerative medicine (see Chapter 13).

● DEVELOPMENTAL BIOLOGY IN MEDICINE

The Public Health Impact of Birth Defects

The medical impact of birth defects is considerable. In 2002, the most recent year for which final statistics are available, more than 20% of infant deaths were attributed to birth defects, that is, abnormalities (often referred to as **anomalies**), which are present at birth, in the development of organs or other structures. Another 20% of infant deaths may be attributed to complica-tions of prematurity, which can be considered a failure of maintenance of the maternal-fetal developmental environment. Therefore, nearly half of the deaths of infants are caused by derangements of normal developmental processes. In addition to mortality, congenital anomalies are a major cause of long-term morbidity, mental retardation, and other dysfunctions that limit the productivity of affected individuals.

Developmental anomalies certainly have a major impact on public health. Genetic counseling and prenatal diagnosis, with the option to continue or to terminate a pregnancy, are important for helping individuals faced with a risk of serious birth defects in their offspring improve their chances of having healthy children (see Chapter 15). Physicians and other health care professionals must be careful, however, not to limit the public health goal of reducing disease solely to preventing the birth of children with anomalies through voluntary pregnancy termination. Primary prevention of birth defects can be accomplished. For example, recommendations to supplement prenatal folic acid intake, which markedly reduces the incidence of neural tube defects, and public health campaigns that focus on preventing teratogenic effects of alcohol during pregnancy, are successful public health approaches to prevention of birth defects that do not depend on prenatal diagnosis and elective abortion.

Clinical Dysmorphology

Dysmorphology is the study of congenital birth defects that alter the shape or form of one or more parts of the body of a newborn child. The research goals of the

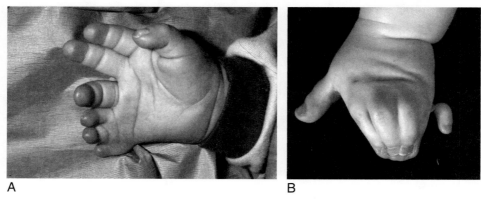

A   B

Figure 14-1 ■ Polydactyly and syndactyly malformations. **A,** Insertional polydactyly. This patient has heptadactyly with insertion of a digit in the central ray of the hand and a supernumerary postaxial digit. This malformation is typically associated with metacarpal fusion of the third and fourth digits. Insertional polydactyly is common in patients with Pallister-Hall syndrome. **B,** Postaxial polydactyly with severe cutaneous syndactyly of digits two through five. This type of malformation is seen in patients with Greig cephalopolysyndactyly syndrome. (Images courtesy of Dr. Leslie Biesecker, Bethesda, Maryland.)

dysmorphologist are to understand the contribution of both abnormal genes and nongenetic, environmental influences to birth defects. The clinical objectives of the dysmorphologist are to diagnose a child with a birth defect, to suggest further diagnostic evaluations, to give prognostic information about the range of outcomes that could be expected, to develop a plan to manage the expected complications, to provide the family with an understanding of the causation of the malformation, and to give recurrence risks to the parents and other relatives. To accomplish these diverse and demanding objectives, the clinician must acquire and organize data from the patient, the family history, and published clinical and basic science literature. Dysmorphologists work closely with specialists in pediatric surgery, neurology, rehabilitation medicine, and the allied health professions to provide ongoing care for children with serious birth defects.

Malformations, Deformations, and Disruptions

Dysmorphologists divide birth defects into three major categories: **malformations, deformations,** and **disruptions.** We will illustrate the difference between these three categories with examples of three distinct birth defects, all involving the limbs.

Malformations result from intrinsic abnormalities in one or more genetic programs operating in development. An example of a malformation is the extra fingers in the disorder known as **Greig cephalopolysyndactyly** (discussed later in the chapter). Greig cephalopolysyndactyly (Fig. 14-1) results from loss-of-function mutations in a gene for a transcription factor, GLI3, which is one component of a complex network of transcription factors and signaling molecules that interact to

cause the distal end of the human upper limb bud to develop into a hand with five digits. Because malformations arise from intrinsic defects in genes that specify a series of developmental steps or programs, and because such programs are often used more than once in different parts of the embryo or fetus at different stages of development, a malformation in one part of the body is often but not always associated with malformations elsewhere as well.

In contrast to malformations, deformations are caused by extrinsic factors impinging physically on the fetus during development. They are especially common during the second trimester of development when the fetus is constrained within the amniotic sac and uterus. For example, contractions of the joints of the extremities, known as **arthrogryposes,** in combination with deformation of the developing skull, occasionally accompany constraint of the fetus due to twin or triplet gestations or prolonged leakage of amniotic fluid (Fig. 14-2). Most deformations apparent at birth either resolve spontaneously or can be treated by external fixation devices to reverse the effects of the instigating cause.

Disruptions, the third category of birth defect, result from destruction of irreplaceable normal fetal tissue. Disruptions are more difficult to treat than deformations because they involve actual loss of normal tissue. Disruptions may be the result of vascular insufficiency, trauma, or teratogens. One example is **amnion disruption,** the partial amputation of a fetal limb associated with strands of amniotic tissue. Amnion disruption is often recognized clinically by the presence of partial and irregular digit amputations in conjunction with constriction rings (Fig. 14-3).

The pathophysiological concepts of malformations, deformations, and disruptions are useful clinical guides to the recognition, diagnosis, and treatment of birth

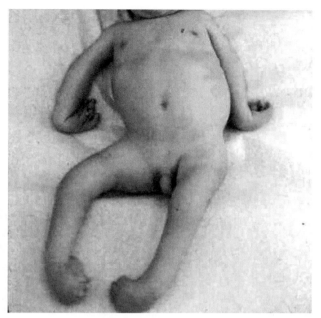

Figure 14-2 ■ Deformation known as congenital arthrogryposis seen with a condition referred to as amyoplasia. There are multiple, symmetrical joint contractures due to abnormal muscle development caused by severe fetal constraint in a pregnancy complicated by oligohydramnios. Intelligence is generally normal, and orthopedic rehabilitation is often successful. (Image courtesy of Judith Hall, University of British Columbia, Vancouver, BC, Canada.)

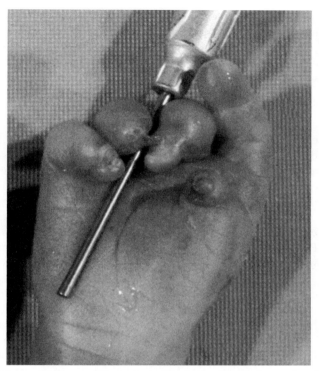

Figure 14-3 ■ Disruption of limb development associated with amniotic bands. This 26-week fetus shows nearly complete disruption of the thumb with only a nubbin remaining. The third and fifth fingers have constriction rings of the middle and distal phalanges, respectively. The fourth digit is amputated distally with a small fragment of amnion attached to the tip. (Image courtesy of Dr. Mason Barr, Jr., University of Michigan, Ann Arbor, Michigan.)

defects, but they sometimes overlap. For example, vascular malformations may lead to disruption of distal structures, and urogenital malformations that cause oligohydramnios can cause fetal deformations. Thus, a given constellation of birth defects in an individual may represent combinations of malformations, deformations, and disruptions.

Genetic and Environmental Causes of Malformations

Malformations have many causes (Fig. 14-4). Chromosome imbalance accounts for about 25%, of which autosomal trisomies for chromosomes 21, 18, and 13 (see Chapter 6) are some of the most common. An additional 20% are caused by mutations in a single gene. Some malformations are inherited as autosomal dominant traits, such as **achondroplasia** or **Waardenburg syndrome**. Many heterozygotes with birth defects, however, represent new mutations that are so severe that they are genetic lethals and are therefore often found to be isolated cases within families (see Chapter 7). Other malformation syndromes are inherited in an autosomal or X-linked recessive pattern, such as the **Smith-Lemli-Opitz syndrome** or the **Lowe syndrome**, respectively. Another approximately 50% of major birth defects have no identifiable cause but recur in families of affected children with a greater frequency

than would be expected on the basis of the population frequency and are considered to be multifactorial diseases (see Chapter 8). This category includes well-recognized birth defects such as cleft lip with or without cleft palate, and congenital heart defects. The remaining 5% of malformations are thought to result from exposure to certain environmental agents—drugs,

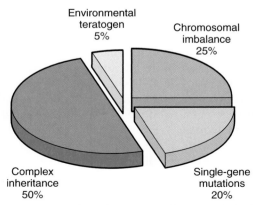

Figure 14-4 ■ The relative contribution of single-gene defects, chromosome abnormalities, and teratogens to birth defects.

infections, chemicals, or radiation—called **teratogens** (derived, inelegantly, from the Greek word for monster plus *-gen,* meaning cause) because of their ability to cause birth defects (discussed later in this chapter).

Pleiotropy: Syndromes and Sequences

In their study of birth defects, clinical dysmorphologists are continually challenged to explain the phenomenon of **pleiotropy** (see Chapter 7). A birth defect demonstrates pleiotropy when a single underlying causative agent results in abnormalities of more than one organ system in different parts of the embryo or in multiple structures that arise at different times during intrauterine life. The agent responsible for the malformation could be either a mutant gene or a teratogen. Pleiotropic birth defects come about in two different ways, depending on the mechanism by which the causative agent produces its effect. When the causative agent causes multiple abnormalities in parallel, the collection of abnormalities is referred to as a **syndrome.** If, however, a mutant gene or teratogen affects only a single organ system at one point in time and it is the perturbation of that organ system that causes the rest of the constellation of pleiotropic defects to occur as secondary effects, the malformation is referred to as a **sequence.**

The autosomal dominant **branchio-oto-renal dysplasia syndrome** exemplifies pleiotropic syndromes. It has long been recognized that patients with branchial arch anomalies affecting development of the ear and neck structures are at high risk for having renal anomalies. The branchio-oto-renal dysplasia syndrome, for example, consists of abnormal cochlear and external ear development, cysts and fistulas in the neck, renal dysplasia, and renal collecting duct malformations. The mechanism of this association is that a conserved set of genes and proteins are used by mammals to form both the ear and the kidney. The syndrome is caused by mutations in one such gene, *EYA1,* which encodes a protein phosphatase that functions in both ear and kidney development. Similarly, the **Rubenstein-Taybi syndrome,** caused by loss of function in a transcriptional coactivator, *CREBBP,* results in abnormalities in transcription of many genes that depend on this coactivator being present in a transcription complex for normal expression (Fig. 14-5).

In contrast, an example of a sequence is the U-shaped cleft palate and small mandible referred to as the **Robin sequence** (Fig. 14-6). This sequence comes about because a restriction of mandibular growth before the ninth week of gestation causes the tongue to lie more posteriorly than is normal, interfering with normal closure of the palatal shelves, thereby causing a cleft palate. The Robin sequence can be an isolated birth defect of unknown cause or can be due to extrinsic impingement on the developing mandible by a twin

in utero. This phenotype can also be one of several features of a condition known as **Stickler syndrome,** in which mutations in the gene encoding a subunit of type II collagen result in an abnormally small mandible as well as other defects in stature, joints, and eyes. The Robin sequence in the Stickler syndrome is a sequence because the mutant collagen gene itself is not responsible for the failure of palatal closure; the cleft palate is secondary to the primary defect in jaw growth. Whatever the cause, a cleft palate due to the Robin sequence must be distinguished from a true primary cleft palate, which has other causes with differing prognoses and implications for the child and family. Knowledge of dysmorphology and developmental genetic principles is necessary to properly diagnose each condition and to recognize that different prognoses are associated with the different primary causes.

These and many other examples serve to illustrate the principle that the clinical practice of dysmorphology rests on a foundation of the basic science of developmental biology. For this reason, it behooves practitioners to have a working knowledge of some of the basic principles of developmental biology and to be familiar with the ways that abnormal function of genes and pathways affect development and, ultimately, their patients.

● INTRODUCTION TO DEVELOPMENTAL BIOLOGY

Developmental biology is concerned with a single, unifying question: How can a single cell transform itself into a mature animal? In humans, this transformation occurs each time a single fertilized egg develops into a human being with more than 10^{13} to 10^{14} cells, several hundred recognizably distinct cell types, and dozens of tissues. This process must occur in a reliable and predictable pattern and time frame.

Developmental biology has its roots in embryology, which was based on observing and surgically manipulating developing organisms. Early embryological studies, carried out in the 19th and early 20th centuries with readily accessible amphibian and avian embryos, determined that embryos developed from single cells and defined many of the fundamental processes of development. Much later, the application of molecular biology and genetics to embryology transformed the field by allowing scientists to study and manipulate development by a broad range of powerful biochemical and molecular techniques.

Development and Evolution

A critically important theme in developmental biology is its relationship to the study of evolution. Early in

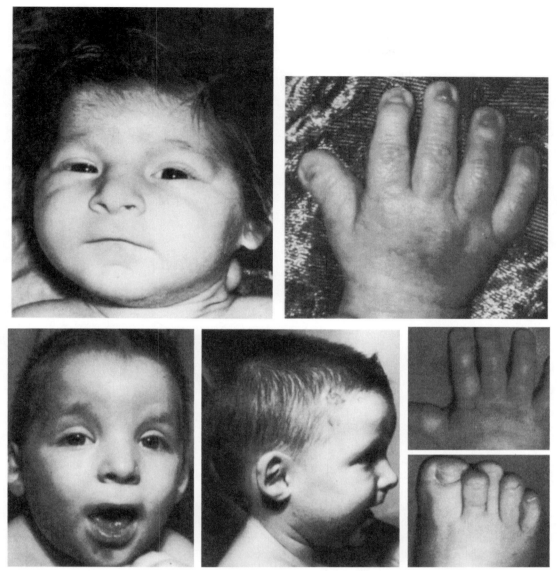

Figure 14-5 ■ Loss-of-function mutations in a transcriptional coactivator cause the Rubinstein-Taybi syndrome. Locus heterogeneity exists in that a mutation in either of two closely related coactivator genes, *CREBBP* or *EP300*, can cause this highly variable and pleiotropic syndrome of mental retardation, broad thumbs and large toes, distinctive facial appearance, and congenital heart defects. (Reprinted with permission from Jones KL: Smith's Recognizable Patterns of Human Malformation. Philadelphia, WB Saunders, 1998.)

development, the embryos of many species look similar. As development progresses, the features shared between species are successively transformed into more specialized features that are, in turn, shared by successively fewer but more closely related species. A comparison of embryological characteristics among and within evolutionarily related organisms shows that developmental attributes (such as fingers) specific to certain groups of animals (for example, primates) are built on a foundation of less specific attributes common to a larger group of animals (for example, mammals), which are in turn related to structures seen in an even larger group of animals (such as the vertebrates). Structures in different

organisms are termed **homologous** if they evolved from a structure present in a common ancestor (Fig. 14-7). In the case of the forelimb, the various ancestral lineages of the four species shown in Figure 14-7, tracing all the way back to their common predecessor, share a common attribute: a functional forelimb. The molecular developmental mechanism that created those limb structures is shared across all four of the contemporary species.

Not all similarity is due to homology, however. Evolutionary studies also recognize the existence of **analogous** structures, those that appear similar but arose independently of one another, through different

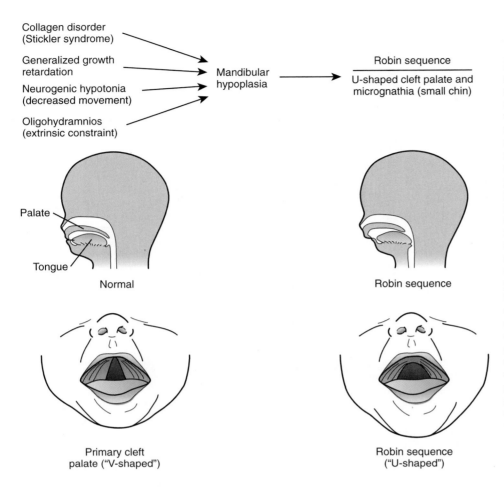

Collagen disorder
(Stickler syndrome)

Generalized growth
retardation

Neurogenic hypotonia
(decreased movement)

Oligohydramnios
(extrinsic constraint)

Mandibular
hypoplasia

Robin sequence

U-shaped cleft palate and
micrognathia (small chin)

Palate

Tongue

Normal

Robin sequence

Primary cleft
palate ("V-shaped")

Robin sequence
("U-shaped")

Figure 14-6 ■ The Robin sequence. Different primary abnormalities can lead to a restriction of mandibular growth in which posterior displacement of the tongue obstructs palatal closure, leading to the constellation of small chin and a U-shaped cleft palate involving the soft palate and extending into the hard palate. In contrast, primary cleft palate resulting from failure of closure of maxillary ridges is a malformation that begins in the anterior region of the maxilla and extends posteriorly to involve first the hard palate and then the soft palate, and it is often V-shaped. If the primary cause of the small chin in children with Robin sequence is external deformation, such as a deficiency of amniotic fluid during pregnancy (oligohydramnios), the mandible often shows postnatal "catch-up" growth. (Adapted in modified form from Wolpert L: Principles of Development. New York, Oxford University Press, 2002.)

lineages that cannot be traced back to a common ancestor with that structure. The molecular pathways that generate analogous structures are unlikely to be evolutionarily conserved. In the example shown in Figure 14-7, the wing structures of the bat and the birds arose independently in evolution to facilitate the task of aerial movement. The evolutionary lineages of these two animals do not share a common ancestor with a primitive wing-like structure from which both bats and birds inherited wings. On the contrary, one can readily see that the birds developed posterior extensions from the limb to form a wing, whereas bats evolved wings through spreading the digits of their forelimbs and connecting them with syndactylous tissue. This situation is termed **convergent evolution.**

The evolutionary conservation of developmental processes is critically important to studies of human development because the vast majority of such research cannot be performed in humans, for obvious ethical reasons (see Chapter 20). Thus, to understand a developmental observation, the scientist uses animal models to investigate normal and abnormal developmental processes. The ability to extend the results to the human is completely dependent on the evolutionary conservation of mechanisms of development and homologous structures.

GENES AND ENVIRONMENT IN DEVELOPMENT

Developmental Genetics

Development results from the action of genes interacting with cellular and environmental cues. The gene products involved include transcriptional regulators, diffusible factors that interact with cells and direct them toward specific developmental pathways, the receptors for such factors, structural proteins, intracellular signaling molecules, and many others. It is therefore not surprising that most of the numerous developmental disorders that occur in humans are caused by genome, chromosome, or gene mutations. However, even though the genome is clearly the primary source of information that controls and specifies human development, the role of genes in development is often described, mistakenly, as a "master blueprint." In fact,

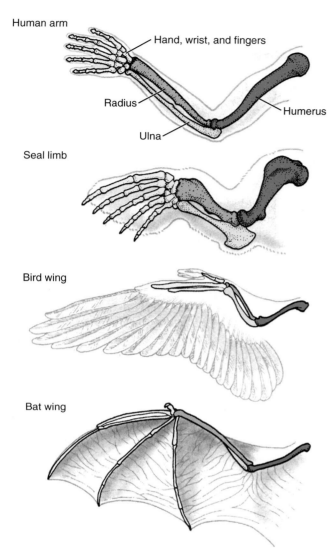

Figure 14-7 ■ Diagram of the upper limb of four species: human, seal, bird, and bat. Despite the superficially dissimilar appearance of the human arm and hand, the seal's flipper, the avian wing, and the bat wing, the similarity in their underlying bone structure and functionality reveals the homology of the forelimbs of all four species. In contrast, the two superficially similar wings in the bird and bat are analogous, not homologous structures. Although both the bird and bat wings are used for flying, they are constructed quite differently and did not evolve from a wing-like structure in a common ancestor. (Reprinted with permission from Gilbert SF: Developmental Biology, 7th ed. Sunderland, Mass, Sinauer Associates, 2003, p 15.)

the genome does not resemble an architect's blueprint that specifies precisely how the materials are to be used, how they are to be assembled, and their final dimensions; it is not a literal description of the final form that all embryological and fetal structures will take. Rather, the genome specifies a set of interacting proteins and noncoding RNAs (see Chapter 3) that set in motion the processes of growth, migration, differentiation, and apoptosis that ultimately result, with a high degree of

probability, in the correct mature structures. Thus, for example, there are no genetic instructions directing that the phalanx of a digit adopt an hourglass shape or that the eye be spherical. These shapes arise as an implicit consequence of developmental processes, thereby generating correctly structured cells, tissues, and organs.

Probability

Although genes are the primary regulators of development, other processes must also play a role. That development is regulated but not determined by the genome is underscored by the important role that probability plays in normal development. For example, in the mouse, a mutation in the formin gene produces **renal aplasia** in only about 20% of the carriers of the mutation, even when the mutation is carried by inbred strains of animals. Given that inbred strains of mice are identical genetically at all the other loci in their genomes, the 20% penetrance of the same formin mutation cannot be explained by different modifying gene variants in the mice affected with renal agenesis versus the mice who are unaffected. Instead, the most likely explanation for this phenomenon is that the formin mutation shifts the balance of some developmental process by increasing the probability that a threshold for causing renal aplasia is exceeded. Thus, carrying a formin mutation will not always lead to renal aplasia but it sometimes will, and neither the rest of the genome nor nongenetic factors are responsible for development of the defect in only a minority of animals. Probabilistic processes provide a rich source of interindividual variation that does not always lead to normal development. Thus, it is not the case in development that "nothing is left to chance."

Environmental Factors

As indicated earlier, the local environment in which a cell or tissue finds itself plays a central role in providing a normal developmental context. It is therefore not unexpected that drugs or other agents introduced from the environment can be teratogens, often because they interfere with intrinsic molecules that mediate the actions of genes. Identification of the mechanism of teratogens has obvious implications not only for clinical medicine and public health but also for basic science; understanding how teratogens cause birth defects can provide insight into the underlying developmental pathways that have been disturbed and result in a defect.

Because the molecular and cellular pathways used during development are often unique and not employed after adulthood, teratogens that cause serious birth defects may have few or no side effects in adult patients because the pathways in question no longer function or have a different purpose in the adult. One important example is **fetal retinoid syndrome** seen in fetuses of pregnant women who took the drug isotretinoin during pregnancy. Isotretinoin is an oral retinoid that is used systemically for the treatment of severe acne. It causes severe birth defects when it is taken by a pregnant woman because it mimics the action of endogenous retinoic acid, a substance that in the developing embryo and fetus diffuses through tissues and interacts with cells, causing them to follow particular developmental pathways.

Different teratogens often cause very specific patterns of birth defects, the risk of which depends critically on the gestational age at the time of exposure, the vulnerability of different tissues to the teratogen, and the level of exposure during pregnancy. One of the best examples is **thalidomide syndrome.** Thalidomide, a sedative widely used in the 1950s, was later found to cause a high incidence of malformed limbs in fetuses exposed between 4 and 8 weeks of gestation because of its effect on the vasculature of the developing limb. Another example is the **fetal alcohol syndrome.** Alcohol causes a particular pattern of birth defects involving primarily the central nervous system because it is relatively more toxic to the developing brain and related craniofacial structures than to other tissues.

Some teratogens, such as x-rays, are also mutagens. A fundamental distinction between teratogens and mutagens is that mutagens cause damage by creating heritable alterations in genetic material, whereas teratogens act directly and transiently on developing embryonic tissue. Thus, fetal exposure to a mutagen can cause an increased risk of birth defects or other diseases (such as cancer) throughout the life of the exposed individual and even in his offspring, whereas exposure to a teratogen increases the risk of birth defects for current but not for subsequent pregnancies.

● BASIC CONCEPTS OF DEVELOPMENTAL BIOLOGY

Overview of Embryological Development

Developmental biology has its own set of core concepts and terminology that may be confusing or foreign to the student of genetics. We therefore provide a brief summary of a number of key concepts and terms used in this chapter (see Box).

●■■ Core Concepts and Terminology in Human Developmental Biology

Blastocyst: the next stage in **embryogenesis** after the **morula,** in which cells on the outer surface of the morula secrete fluid and form a fluid-filled internal cavity within which is a separate group of cells, the **inner cell mass.** The outer cells of the blastocyst will form the **chorion,** part of the placenta and sac in which the **fetus** develops; the **inner cell mass** will become the **fetus** itself (see Fig. 14-10).

Chimera: an embryo made up of two or more cell lines that differ in their genotype. Contrast with **mosaic.**

Chorion: membrane that develops from the outer cells of the **blastocyst** and goes on to form the placenta and the outer layer of the sac in which the **fetus** develops.

Determination: the stage in development in which cells are irreversibly committed to forming a particular tissue.

Dichorionic twins: monozygotic twins arising from splitting of the embryo into two parts, before formation of the blastocyst, so that two independent blastocysts develop.

Differentiation: the acquisition by a cell of novel characteristics specific for a particular cell type or tissue.

Ectoderm: the primary embryonic **germ layer** that gives rise to the nervous system and skin.

Embryo: the stage of a developing human organism between fertilization and 9 weeks of gestation, when separation into placental and embryonic tissues occurs. **Morphogenesis,** to produce the basic structures and body plan, and **organogenesis** are accomplished during this stage.

Embryogenesis: the development of the **embryo.**

Embryonic stem cells: cells derived from the **inner cell mass** that under appropriate conditions can differentiate into all of the cell types and tissues of an **embryo** and form a complete, normal fetus.

Endoderm: the primary embryonic **germ layer** that gives rise to many of the visceral organs and lining of the gut.

Epiblast: the portion of the inner cell mass that gives rise to the embryo proper.

Fate: the ultimate destination for a cell that has traveled down a developmental pathway.

Fetus: the stage of the developing human between 9 weeks of gestation and birth. Further growth and maturation of organs occur.

Gastrulation: the stage of development just after implantation in which the cells of the **inner cell mass** rearrange themselves into the three **germ layers. Regulative development** ceases at gastrulation.

Germ layers: three distinct layers of cells that arise in the inner cell mass, the **ectoderm, mesoderm,** and **endoderm,** which develop into distinctly different tissues in the embryo.

Hypoblast: the portion of the inner cell mass that contributes to fetal membranes (amnion).

Inner cell mass: a group of cells inside the **morula** destined to become the **fetus.**

••• Core Concepts and Terminology in Human Developmental Biology–cont'd

Mesoderm: the primary embryonic **germ layer** that gives rise to connective tissue, muscles, bones, vasculature, and the lymphatic and hematopoietic systems.

Monoamniotic twins: monozygotic twins resulting from cleavage of part of the inner cell cell mass (epiblast) but without cleavage of the part of the inner cell mass that forms the amniotic membrane (hypoblast).

Monochorionic twins: monozygotic twins resulting from cleavage of the inner cell mass without cleavage of the cells on the outside of the **blastocyst**.

Monozygotic twins: twins arising from a single fertilized egg, resulting from cleavage during embryogenesis in the interval between the first cell division of the zygote and gastrulation.

Morphogen: a substance produced by cells in a particular region of an **embryo** that diffuses from its point of origin through the tissues of the embryo to form a concentration gradient. Cells undergo **specification** and then **determination** to different **fates**, depending on the concentration of morphogen they experience.

Morphogenesis: the creation of various structures during **embryogenesis**.

Morula: a compact ball of 16 cells produced after four cell divisions of the **zygote**.

Mosaic: an individual who develops from a single fertilized egg but in whom mutation after conception results in cells with two or more genotypes. Contrast with **chimera**.

Mosaic development: a stage in development in which

cells have already become committed to the point that removal of a portion of an embryo will not allow normal embryonic development.

Multipotent stem cell: a **stem cell** capable of self-renewal as well as of developing into many different types of cells in a tissue, but not an entire organism. Often called adult stem cells or tissue progenitor cells.

Organogenesis: the creation of individual organs during **embryogenesis**.

Progenitor cell: a cell that is traversing a developmental pathway on its way to becoming a fully differentiated cell.

Regulative development: a stage in development in which cells have not yet become determined so that the cells that remain after removal of a portion of an embryo can still form a complete organism.

Specification: a step along the path of differentiation in which cells acquire certain specialized attributes characteristic of a particular tissue but can still be influenced by external cues to develop into a different type of cell or tissue.

Stem cell: a cell that is capable both of generating another stem cell (self-renewal) and of differentiating into specialized cells within a tissue or an entire organism.

Totipotent cell: an early **stem cell** capable of self-renewal as well as of becoming any cell in any tissue. **Embryonic stem cells** are totipotent.

Zygote: the fertilized egg, the first step in embryogenesis.

Cellular Processes During Development

During development, cells divide (**proliferate**), acquire novel functions or structures (**differentiate**), move within the embryo (**migrate**), and undergo programmed cell death (often through **apoptosis**). These four basic cellular processes act in various combinations and in different ways to allow **growth** and **morphogenesis** (literally the "creation of form"), thereby creating an embryo of normal size and shape, containing organs of the appropriate size, shape, and location, and consisting of tissues and cells with the correct architecture, structure, and function.

Although growth may seem too obvious to discuss, growth itself is carefully regulated in mammalian development, and unregulated growth is disastrous. The mere doubling (one extra round of cell division) of cell number (hyperplasia) or the doubling of cell size (hypertrophy) of an organism is likely to be fatal. Dysregulation of growth of segments of the body can cause severe deformity and dysfunction, such as in hemihy-

perplasia and other segmental overgrowth disorders (Fig. 14-8). Furthermore, the exquisite differential regulation of growth can change the shape of a tissue or an organ.

Morphogenesis is accomplished in the developing organism by a number of mechanisms, such as differential growth, differentiation, regulated apoptosis, and cell migration. In some contexts, morphogenesis is used as a general term to describe all of development, but this is formally incorrect as morphogenesis has to be coupled to the process of growth discussed here to generate a normally shaped and functioning tissue or organ.

Human Embryogenesis

This description of human development begins where Chapter 2 ends, with fertilization. After fertilization, the embryo undergoes a series of cell divisions without overall growth, termed cleavage. The single fertilized

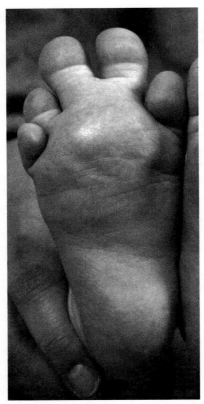

Figure 14-8 ■ The clinical consequences of dysregulated growth. The foot of a patient with **congenital segmental overgrowth** of a small portion of the body, here just several toes. This overgrowth pattern is specifically caused by developmental dysregulation, as the overgrown body parts in this disorder grow proportionately to the rest of the body in the postnatal period. The difference in cell number in these overgrown tissues is likely to be only 2-fold, demonstrating the precision with which growth is controlled in normal development. (Image courtesy of Dr. Leslie Biesecker, Bethesda, Maryland.)

egg undergoes four divisions to yield the 16-cell morula by day 3 (Fig. 14-9). At day 4, the embryo transitions to become a **blastocyst,** in which cells that give rise to the placenta form a wall, inside of which the cells that will make the embryo itself aggregate to one side into what is referred to as the **inner cell mass.** This is the point at which the embryo acquires its first obvious manifestation of polarity, an axis of asymmetry that divides the inner cell mass (most of which goes on to form the mature organism) from the embryonic tissues that will go on to form the chorion, an extraembryonic tissue (placenta, and so on) (Fig. 14-10). The inner cell mass then separates again into the **epiblast,** which will make the embryo proper, and the **hypoblast,** which goes to make the amniotic membrane.

The embryo implants in the endometrial wall of the uterus in the interval between days 7 and 12 after fertilization. After implantation, gastrulation occurs, in which cells rearrange themselves into a structure consisting of three cellular compartments, termed the **germ layers,** comprising ectoderm, mesoderm, and endoderm. The three germ layers give rise to different structures. The endodermal lineage forms the central visceral core of the organism. This includes the cells lining the main gut cavity, the airways of the respiratory system, and other similar structures. The mesodermal lineage gives rise to kidneys, heart, vasculature, and structural or supportive functions in the organism. Bone and muscle are nearly exclusively mesodermal and have the two main functions of structure (physical support) and providing the necessary physical and nutritive support of the hematopoietic system. The ectoderm gives rise to the central and peripheral nervous systems and the skin.

The next major stages of development involve the initiation of the nervous system, establishment of the basic body plan, and then **organogenesis,** which occupies weeks 4 to 8. The position and basic structures of all of the organs are now established, and the cellular components necessary for their full development are now in place.

The **fetal phase** of development is generally considered to include weeks 9 to 40 and is concerned primarily with the maturation and further differentiation of the components of the organs. For some organ systems, development does not cease at birth. For example, the brain undergoes substantial postnatal development, and limbs undergo epiphyseal growth and ultimately closure after puberty.

The Germ Cell: Transmitting Genetic Information

In addition to growth and differentiation of somatic tissues, the organism must also specify which cells will go on to become the gametes of the mature adult. The germ cell compartment serves this purpose. As described in Chapter 2, cells in the germ cell compartment become committed to undergoing gametogenesis and meiosis in order that the species can pass on its genetic complement and facilitate the recombination and random assortment of chromosomes. In addition, the sex-specific epigenetic imprint that certain genes require must be reset within the germ cell compartment (see Chapters 5 and 7).

The Stem Cell: Maintaining Regenerative Capacity in Tissues

In addition to specifying the program of differentiation that is necessary for development, the organism must also set aside tissue-specific **stem cells** that can regenerate differentiated cells during adult life. The best-

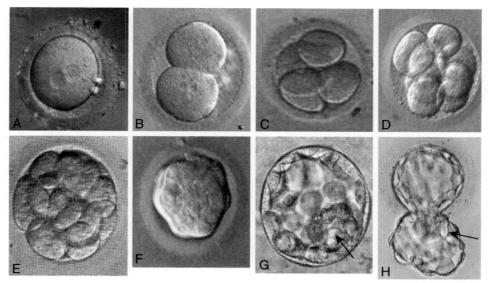

Figure 14-9 ■ Human development begins with cleavage of the fertilized egg. **A,** The fertilized egg at day 0 with two pronuclei and the polar bodies. **B,** A two-cell embryo at day 1 after fertilization. **C,** A four-cell embryo at day 2. **D,** The eight-cell embryo at day 3. **E,** The 16-cell stage later in day 3, followed by the phenomenon of compaction, whereby the embryo is now termed a morula (**F,** day 4). **G** shows the formation of the blastocyst at day 5, with the inner cell mass indicated by the arrow. Finally, the embryo (*arrow*) hatches from the zona pellucida (**H**). (Reproduced, with permission, from Ogilvie CM, Braude PR, Scriven PN: Preimplantation diagnosis—an overview. J Histochem Cytochem 53:255-260, 2005.)

characterized example of these cells is in the hematopoietic system. Among the 10^{11} to 10^{12} nucleated hematopoietic cells in the adult organism are about 10^4 to 10^5 cells that have the potential to generate any of the more specialized blood cells on a continuous basis during a lifetime. Hematopoietic stem cells can be transplanted to other humans and completely reconstitute the hematopoietic system (see Chapter 13). A system of interacting gene products maintains a properly sized pool of hematopoietic stem cells. These regulators permit a balance between the maintenance of stem cells through self-replication and the generation of committed precursor cells that can go on to develop into the various mature cells of the hematopoietic system (Fig. 14-11).

Fate, Specification, and Determination

As an undifferentiated cell undergoes the process of differentiation, it moves through a series of discrete steps in which it manifests various distinct functions or attributes until it reaches its ultimate destination, referred to as its **fate** (e.g., when a precursor cell becomes an erythrocyte, a keratinocyte, or a cardiac myocyte). In the developing organism, these attributes not only vary across the recognizable cell types but also change over time. Early during differentiation, a cell undergoes **specification** when it acquires specific characteristics but can still be influenced by environmental cues (sig-

naling molecules, positional information) to change its ultimate fate. These environmental clues are primarily derived from neighboring cells by direct cell-cell contact or by signals received at the cell surface from soluble substances, including positional information derived from where a cell sits in a gradient of various **morphogens.** Eventually, a cell either irreversibly acquires attributes or has irreversibly been committed to acquire those attributes (referred to as **determination**). With the exception of the germ cell and stem cell compartments, all cells undergo specification and determination to their ultimate developmental fate.

Specification and determination involve the stepwise acquisition of a stable cellular phenotype of gene expression specific to the particular fate of each cell—nerve cells make synaptic proteins but do not make hemoglobin, whereas red blood cells do not make synaptic proteins but must make hemoglobin. With the exception of lymphocyte precursor cells undergoing DNA rearrangements in the T-cell receptor or immunoglobulin genes (see Chapter 3), the particular gene expression profile responsible for the differentiated cellular phenotype does not result from permanent changes in DNA sequence. Instead, the regulation of gene expression depends on **epigenetic** changes, such as stable transcription complexes, modification of histones in chromatin, and methylation of DNA (see Chapter 3). The epigenetic control of gene expression is responsible for the loss of developmental plasticity, as we discuss next.

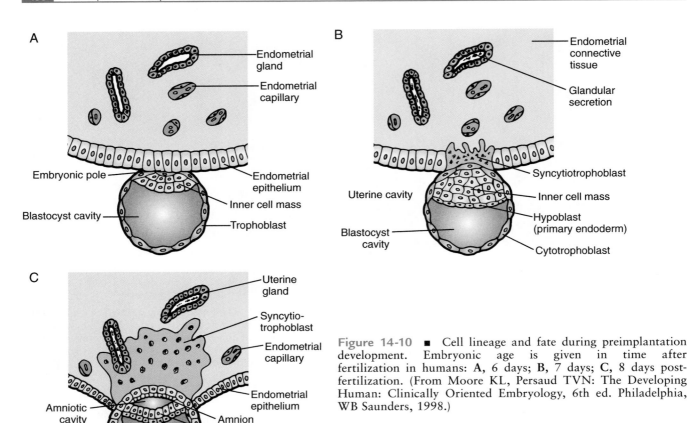

A

Endometrial gland

Endometrial capillary

Embryonic pole

Endometrial epithelium

Inner cell mass

Blastocyst cavity

Trophoblast

B

Endometrial connective tissue

Glandular secretion

Uterine cavity

Syncytiotrophoblast

Inner cell mass

Blastocyst cavity

Hypoblast (primary endoderm)

Cytotrophoblast

C

Uterine gland

Syncytio-trophoblast

Endometrial capillary

Endometrial epithelium

Amniotic cavity

Amnion

Exocoelomic cavity

Epiblast

Hypoblast

Cytotrophoblast

Exocoelomic membrane

Figure 14-10 ■ Cell lineage and fate during preimplantation development. Embryonic age is given in time after fertilization in humans: **A,** 6 days; **B,** 7 days; **C,** 8 days post-fertilization. (From Moore KL, Persaud TVN: The Developing Human: Clinically Oriented Embryology, 6th ed. Philadelphia, WB Saunders, 1998.)

Regulative and Mosaic Development

Early in development, cells are functionally equivalent and subject to dynamic processes of specification, a phenomenon known as **regulative** development. In regulative development, removal or ablation of part of an embryo can be compensated for by the remaining similar cells. In contrast, later in development, each of the cells in some parts of the embryo has a distinct fate, and in each of those parts, the embryo only appears to be homogeneous. In this situation, known as **mosaic** development, loss of a portion of an embryo would lead to the failure of development of the final structures that those cells were fated to become. Thus, the developmental plasticity of the embryo generally declines with time.

Regulative Development and Twinning

That early development is primarily regulative has been demonstrated by basic embryological experiments and confirmed by observations in clinical medicine. Identical (**monozygotic**) twins are the natural experimental evidence that early development is regulative. The most common form of identical twinning occurs in the second half of the first week of development, effectively splitting the inner cell mass in half, each of which develops into a normal fetus (Fig. 14-12). Were the embryo even partly regulated by mosaic development at this stage, the twins would develop only partially and consist of complementary parts. This is clearly not the case, since twins are generally completely normally developed and eventually attain normal size through prenatal and postnatal growth.

The various forms of monozygotic twinning demonstrate regulative development at several different stages. **Dichorionic twins** result from cleavage at the four-cell stage. **Monochorionic twins** result from a cleaved inner cell mass. **Monoamniotic twins** result from an even later cleavage, in this case within the bilayered embryo, which then forms two separate embryos but only one extraembryonic compartment that goes on to make the single amnion. All of these twinning events demonstrate that these cell populations can reprogram their development to form complete embryos from cells that, if cleavage had not occurred, would have contributed to only part of an embryo.

The successful application of the technique of **preimplantation diagnosis** also illustrates that early human development is regulative. In this procedure, male and

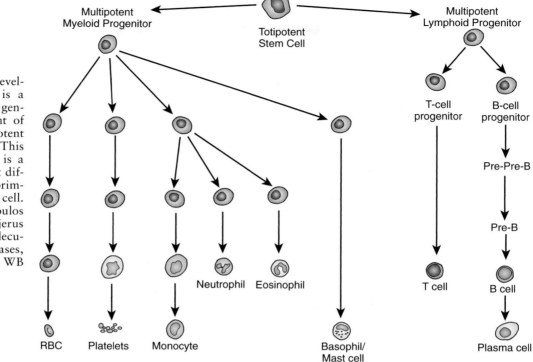

Figure 14-11 ■ The development of blood cells is a continuous process that generates a full complement of cells from a single, totipotent hematopoietic stem cell. This hematopoietic stem cell is a committed stem cell that differentiated from a more primitive mesodermal stem cell. (From Stamatoyannopoulos G, Nienhuis AW, Majerus PW, Varmus H: The Molecular Basis of Blood Diseases, 2nd ed. Philadelphia, WB Saunders, 1987.)

female gametes are harvested from the presumptive parents and fertilized in vitro (Fig. 14-13). When these fertilized embryos have reached the eight-cell stage (at day 3), a biopsy microneedle is used to remove some of the cells of the developing blastocyst. The isolated cell with its clearly visible nucleus is then subjected to FISH analysis for aneuploidy. Alternatively, the genomic DNA can be isolated and used for PCR of specific gene sequences to determine if the embryo has inherited disease-causing alleles from the parents (see Chapter 4).

Embryos comprised of the remaining seven cells that are not affected by the disease can then be selected and implanted in the mother. The capacity of the embryo to recover from the biopsy of one of its eight cells is attributable to regulative development. Were those cells removed by biopsy fated to form a particular part or segment of the body (i.e., governed by mosaic development), one would predict that these parts of the body would be absent or defective in the mature individual. Instead, the embryo has compensatory mechanisms to

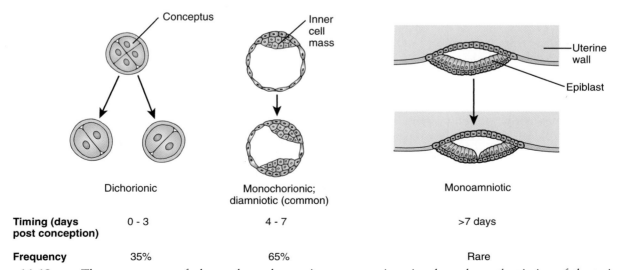

Timing (days post conception)	0 - 3	4 - 7	>7 days
Frequency	35%	65%	Rare

Figure 14-12 ■ The arrangement of placental membranes in monozygotic twins depends on the timing of the twinning event. Dichorionic twins result from a complete splitting of the entire embryo, leading to duplication of all extraembryonic tissues. Monochorionic diamniotic twins are caused by division of the inner cell mass at the blastocyst stage. Monoamniotic twins are caused by division of the epiblast but not the hypoblast.

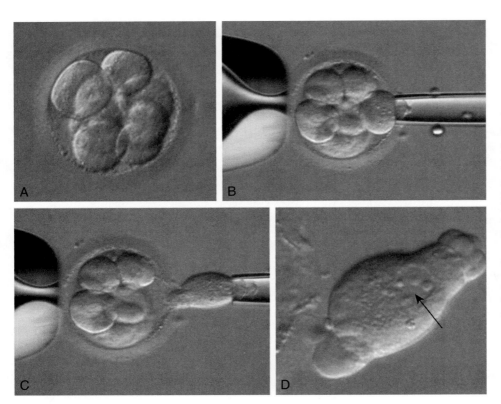

Figure 14-13 ■ Blastomere biopsy of a human cleavage-stage embryo. **A,** Eight-cell embryo, day 3 after fertilization. **B,** Embryo on holding pipette (left) with biopsy pipette (right) breaching the zona pellucida. C, Blastomere removal by suction. **D,** Blastomere removed by biopsy with a clearly visible single nucleus (indicated by arrow). (Reproduced, with permission, from Ogilvie CM, Braude PR, Scriven PN: Preimplantation diagnosis—an overview. J Histochem Cytochem 53:255-260, 2005.)

replace those cells, which then undergo normal development as specified by their neighboring cells.

Mosaic Development

Embryonic development generally proceeds from more regulative to more mosaic development. Normal identical twinning was mentioned earlier as an example of regulative development. However, later embryo cleavage events demonstrate mosaic development because these cleavage events result in the formation of **conjoined twins,** which are two fetuses that share body structures and organs because the cleavage occurred after the transition from regulative to mosaic development, too late to allow complete embryos. Interestingly, in some adult nonhuman species, ablation of a specific tissue may not limit development. For example, the mature salamander can regenerate an entire tail when it is cut off, apparently retaining a population of cells that can re-establish the developmental program for the tail after trauma. One of the goals of developmental biology is to understand this process in other species and potentially harness it in practice for human regenerative medicine.

Axis Specification and Pattern Formation

A critical function of the developing organism is to specify the spatial relationships of structures within the embryo. In early development, the organism must determine the relative orientation of a number of body segments and organs. For example, the head to tail axis, which is termed the **cranial-caudal** or **anterior-posterior** axis, is established very early in embryogenesis (and referred to as the rostral-caudal axis later in development) and is probably determined by the entry position of the sperm that fertilizes the egg. **Dorsal-ventral** axis is the second dimension, and here, too, a series of interacting proteins and signaling pathways are responsible for determining dorsal and ventral structures. The morphogen Sonic hedgehog (discussed later) participates in setting up the axis of dorsal-ventral polarity along the spinal cord. Finally, a **left-right** axis must be established. The left-right axis is essential for proper heart development and positioning of viscera; for example, an abnormality in the X-linked gene *ZIC3*, involved in left-right axis determination, is associated with cardiac anomalies and **situs inversus,** in which some thoracic and abdominal viscera are on the wrong side of the chest and abdomen.

The three axes that must be specified in the whole embryo must also be specified early in the developing limb. Within the limb, the organism must specify the proximal-distal axis (shoulder to fingertip), the anterior-posterior axis (thumb to fifth finger), and the dorsal-ventral axis (dorsum to palm). On a cellular scale, individual cells also develop an axis of polarity, for example, the basal-apical axis of the proximal renal tubular cells or the axons and dendrites of a neuron. Thus, specifying axes in the whole embryo, in limbs, and in cells is a fundamental process in development.

Once an organismal axis is determined, the embryo then overlays a patterning program onto that axis. Conceptually, if axis formation can be considered as

▪▪▪ Embryonic Stem Cell Technology

Inner cell mass cells are believed to be capable of forming any tissue in the body. This is suspected of being true in humans and has been proved to be true in mice. The full developmental potential of inner cell mass cells is the basis of the experimental field of **embryonic stem cell** technology in mice, a technology that is crucial for generating animal models of human genetic disease (Fig. 14-14). In this technique, mouse inner cell mass cells are grown in culture as embryonic stem cells and undergo genetic manipulation to introduce a given mutation into a specific gene. These cells are then injected into the inner cell mass of another early mouse embryo. The mutated cells are incorporated into the inner cell mass of the recipient embryo and contribute to many tissues of that embryo, forming a **chimera** (a single embryo made up of cells from two different sources). If the mutated cells contribute to the germline in a chimeric animal, the offspring of that animal can inherit the engineered mutations. The ability of the recipient embryo to tolerate the incorporation of these totipotent, nonspecified cells, which then undergo specification and can contribute to any tissue in a living mouse, is the converse of regulative development, the ability of an embryo to tolerate removal of some cells.

Human stem cells (HSCs) made from unused fertilized embryos are the subject of intensive research as well as ethical controversy. Although the use of HSCs for cloning an entire human being is considered highly unethical and universally banned, current research is directed toward generating particular cell types from HSCs to repair damaged tissues and organs, a goal of regenerative medicine.

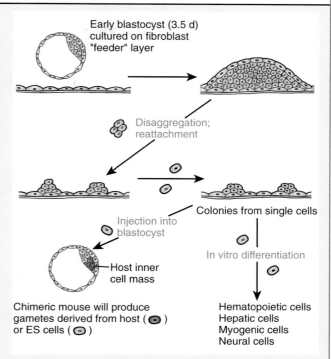

Figure 14-14 ▪ Embryonic stem (ES) cells are derived directly from the inner cell mass or primitive ectoderm, are often euploid, and can contribute to the germline. Cultured embryonic stem cells differentiated in vitro can give rise to a variety of different cell types.

the drawing of a line through an undeveloped mass of cells and specifying which end is to be the head and which end the tail, then patterning is the division of the embryo into segments and the assignment to these segments of an identity, such as head, thorax, abdomen, and so on. The *HOX* genes (see below) have major roles in determining the different structures that develop along the anterior-posterior axis. The end result of these pattern specification programs is that cells or groups of cells are assigned an identity related primarily to their position within the organism. This identity is subsequently used by the cells as an instruction to specify how development should proceed.

Pattern Formation and the HOX Gene System

The **homeobox** *(HOX)* gene system, first described in the fruit fly *Drosophila melanogaster,* constitutes a paradigm in developmental biology. *HOX* genes are so named because the proteins they encode are transcription factors that contain a conserved DNA-binding motif called the homeodomain. (The segment of the gene encoding the homeodomain is called a *homeobox,* thus giving the gene family its name, *HOX.*) Many

species of animals have *HOX* genes, and the homeodomains encoded by these genes are similar; however, different species contain different numbers of *HOX* genes; for example, fruit flies contain 8 and humans nearly 40. The 40 human *HOX* genes are organized into four clusters, A, B, C, and D, on four different chromosomes. The order of the individual genes within the clusters is conserved across species. The human *HOX* gene clusters were generated by a series of gene duplication events (Fig. 14-15). Initially, ancient events duplicated the original ancestral *HOX* gene in tandem along a single chromosome. Subsequent duplications of this single set of *HOX* genes and relocation of the new gene set to other locations in the genome resulted in four unlinked *HOX* gene clusters in humans (and other mammals) named *HOXA, HOXB, HOXC,* and *HOXD.*

Unique combinations of *HOX* gene expression in small groups of cells, located in particular regions of the embryo, help determine the developmental fate of those regions. Just as specific combinations of *HOX* genes from the single *HOX* gene cluster in the fly are expressed along the anterior-posterior axis of the body and regulate different patterns of gene expression and

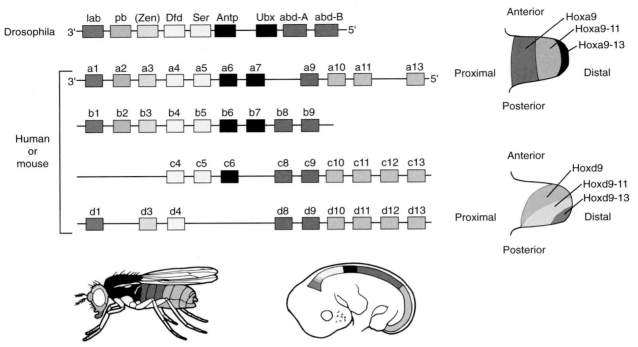

Figure 14-15 ■ Action and arrangement of *HOX* genes. An ancestral *HOX* gene cluster in a common ancestor of vertebrates and invertebrates has been quadruplicated in mammals, and individual members of the ancestral cluster have been lost. The combination of *HOX* genes expressed in adjacent regions along the anteroposterior axis of developing embryos selects a unique developmental fate (as color-coded in the segments of the fly and human embryo shown at bottom). In the developing limbs (*top right*), different combinations of *HOXA* and *HOXD* genes are expressed in adjacent zones that help select developmental fate along the proximal-distal and anterior-posterior axes. (From Wolpert L, Beddington R, Brockes J, et al: Principles of Development. New York, Oxford University Press, 1998. Copyright 1998, Oxford University Press.)

therefore different body structures (see Fig. 14-15), mammals use a number of *HOX* genes from different clusters to accomplish similar tasks. Early, in the whole embryo, HOX transcription factors specify the anterior-posterior axis: the *HOXA* and *HOXB* clusters, for example, act along the rostral-caudal axis to determine the identity of individual vertebrae and somites. Later in development, the *HOXA* and *HOXD* clusters determine regional identity along the axes of the developing limb.

One interesting aspect of *HOX* gene expression is that the order of the genes in a cluster parallels the position in the embryo in which that gene is expressed and the time in development when it is expressed (see Fig. 14-15). In other words, the position of a *HOX* gene in a cluster is co-linear with both the timing of expression and the location of expression along the anterior-posterior axis in the embryo. For example, in the *HOXB* cluster, the genes expressed first and in the anterior portion of the embryo are at one end of the cluster; the order of the rest of the genes in the cluster parallels the order in which they are expressed, both by location along the anterior-posterior axis of the embryo and by timing of expression. Although this gene organization is distinctly unusual and is not a general feature of gene organization in the genome (see Chapter 3), a similar phenomenon is seen within another

developmentally regulated human gene family, the globin gene clusters (see Chapter 11).

The *HOX* gene family illustrates several important principles of developmental biology and evolution. First, a group of genes functions together to accomplish similar general tasks at different times and places in the embryo. Second, homologous structures are generated by sets of homologous transcription factors derived from common evolutionary predecessors. For example, flies and mammals have a similar basic body plan (head anterior to the trunk, with limbs emanating from the trunk, cardiorespiratory organs anterior to digestive), and that body plan is specified by a set of genes that were passed down through common evolutionary predecessors. Third, although it is not usually the case with genes involved in development, the *HOX* genes show a remarkable genomic organization within a cluster that correlates with their function during development.

● CELLULAR AND MOLECULAR MECHANISMS IN DEVELOPMENT

In this section, we review the basic cellular and molecular mechanisms that regulate development (see Box). We illustrate each mechanism with a human birth

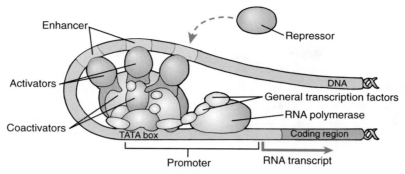

Figure 14-16 ■ General transcription factors, shown in blue, and RNA polymerase bind to *cis*-acting sequences closely adjacent to the mRNA transcriptional start site; these *cis*-acting sequences are collectively referred to as the promoter. More distal enhancer or silencer elements bind specialized and tissue-specific transcription factors. Coactivator proteins facilitate a biochemical interaction between specialized and general transcription factors. (From Tjian R: Molecular machines that control genes. Sci Am 272:54-61, 1995.)

> ●●● **Fundamental Mechanisms Operating in Development**
>
> - Gene regulation by transcription factors
> - Cell-cell signaling by direct contact and by morphogens
> - Induction of cell shape and polarity
> - Cell movement
> - Programmed cell death

defect or disease that results from the failure of each of these normal mechanisms.

Gene Regulation by Transcription Factors

Transcription factors control development by controlling the expression of other genes, some of which are also transcription factors. Groups of transcription factors that function together are referred to as **transcriptional regulatory modules,** and the functional dissection of these modules is an important task of the developmental geneticist. Some transcription factors activate target genes and others repress them. Still other transcription factors have both activator and repressor functions (so-called bifunctional transcription factors). Regulatory modules control development by causing different combinations of transcription factors to be expressed at different places and at different times to direct the spatiotemporal regulation of development. By directing differential gene expression across space and time, various transcriptional regulatory modules are a central element of the development of the embryo.

A transcriptional regulatory complex consists of a large number of general transcription factors joined with the specific transcription factors that are responsible for creating the selectivity of a transcriptional complex (Fig. 14-16). Most general transcription factors are found in thousands of transcriptional complexes throughout the genome, and although each is essential, their roles in development are nonspecific. Specific transcription factors also participate in forming transcription factor complexes, but only in specific cells or at specific times in development, thereby providing the regulation of gene expression that allows developmental processes to be exquisitely controlled.

The importance of transcription factors in normal development is illustrated by an unusual mutation of *HOXD13* that causes **synpolydactyly,** an incompletely dominant condition in which heterozygotes have interphalangeal webbing and extra digits in their hands and feet. Rare homozygotes have similar but more severe abnormalities and also have bone malformations of the hands, wrists, feet, and ankles (Fig. 14-17). The *HOXD13* mutation responsible for synpolydactyly is caused by expansion of a polyalanine tract in the amino-terminal domain of the protein; the normal protein contains 15 alanines, whereas the mutant protein contains 22 to 24 alanines. Heterozygosity for a *HOXD13* loss-of-function mutation has only a mild effect on limb development, characterized by a rudimentary extra digit between the first and second metatarsals and between the fourth and fifth metatarsals of the feet. The polyalanine expansion that causes synpolydactyly is therefore likely to act by a gain-of-function mechanism (see Chapter 11). Regardless of the exact mechanism, this condition demonstrates that a general function for *HOX* genes is to determine regional identity along specific body axes during development.

Morphogens and Cell-to-Cell Signaling

One of the hallmarks of developmental processes is that cells must communicate with each other to develop proper spatial arrangements of tissues and cellular

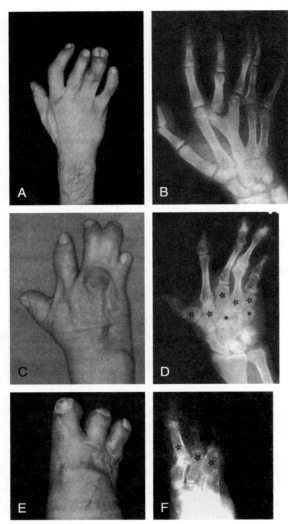

Figure 14-17 ■ An unusual gain-of-function mutation in *HOXD13* creates an abnormal protein with a dominant negative effect. Photographs and radiographs show the syn-polydactyly phenotype. **A** and **B**, Hand and radiograph of an individual heterozygous for a *HOXD13* mutation. Note the branching metacarpal III and the resulting extra digit IIIa. The syndactyly between digits has been partially corrected by surgical separation of III and IIIa-IV. **C** and **D**, Hand and radiograph of an individual homozygous for a *HOXD13* mutation. Note syndactyly of digits III, IV, and V and their single knuckle; the transformation of metacarpals I, II, III, and V to short carpal-like bones *(stars);* two additional carpal bones *(asterisks);* and short second phalanges. The radius, ulna, and proximal carpal bones appear normal. **E** and **F**, Foot and radiograph of the same homozygous individual. Note the relatively normal size of metatarsal I, the small size of metatarsal II, and the replacement of metatarsals III, IV, and V with a single tarsal-like bone *(stars).* (Reprinted with permission from Muragaki Y, Mundlos S, Upton J, Olsen B: Altered growth and branching patterns in synpolydactyly caused by mutations in *HOXD13.* Science 272:548-551, 1996. Copyright 1996, American Association for the Advancement of Science.)

subtypes. This communication occurs through cell signaling mechanisms. These cell-cell communication systems are commonly composed of a cell surface receptor and the molecule, called a **ligand,** that binds to it. On ligand binding, receptors transmit their signals through intracellular signaling pathways. One of the common ligand-receptor pairs are the fibroblast growth factors and their receptors. There are 23 recognized members of the fibroblast growth factor gene family in the human, and many of them are important in development. The fibroblast growth factors serve as ligands for tyrosine kinase receptors. Abnormalities in fibroblast growth factor receptors cause diseases such as **achondroplasia** (Case 1) (see Chapter 7) and certain syndromes that involve abnormalities of craniofacial development, referred to as **craniosynostoses** because they demonstrate premature fusion of cranial sutures in the skull.

One of the best examples of a developmental morphogen is **hedgehog,** originally discovered in *Drosophila* and named for its ability to alter the orientation of epidermal bristles. Diffusion of the hedgehog protein creates a gradient in which different concentrations of the protein cause surrounding cells to assume different fates. In humans, several genes closely related to *Drosophila* hedgehog also encode developmental morphogens; one example is the gene regrettably named Sonic hedgehog *(SHH).* Although the specific programs controlled by hedgehog in *Drosophila* are very different from those controlled by its mammalian counterparts, the underlying themes and molecular mechanisms are similar. For example, secretion of Sonic hedgehog protein (SHH) by the notochord and the floorplate of the developing neural tube generates a gradient that induces and organizes the different types of cells and tissues in the developing brain and spinal cord (Fig. 14-18A). SHH is also produced by a small group of cells in the limb bud to create what is known as the **zone of polarizing activity,** which is responsible for the asymmetrical pattern of digits within individual limbs (Fig. 14-18B).

Mutations that inactivate the *SHH* gene in humans cause birth defects that may be inherited as autosomal dominant traits, which demonstrates that a 50% reduction in gene expression is sufficient to produce an abnormal phenotype, presumably by altering the magnitude of the hedgehog protein gradient. Affected individuals usually exhibit **holoprosencephaly,** or failure of the midface and forebrain to develop, leading to cleft lip and palate, hypotelorism (eyes that are closely spaced together), and absence of forebrain structures. On occasion, however, the clinical findings are mild or subtle, such as, for example, a single central incisor or partial absence of the corpus callosum (Fig. 14-19). Because variable expressivity has been observed in members of the same family, it cannot be due to different mutations

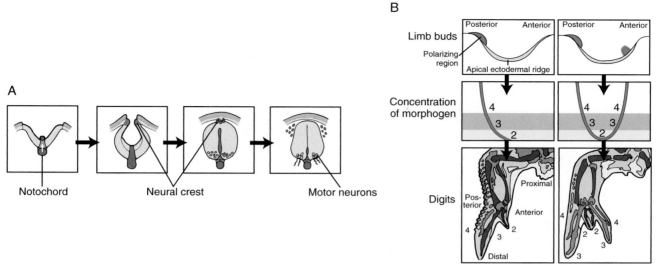

Figure 14-18 ■ **A,** Transverse section of the developing neural tube. Sonic hedgehog protein released from the notochord diffuses upward to the ventral portion of the developing neural tube (dark gray); high concentrations immediately above the notochord induce the floorplate, whereas lower concentrations more laterally induce motor neurons. Ectoderm above (dorsal to) the neural tube releases bone morphogenetic proteins that help induce neural crest development at the dorsal edge of the closing neural tube (dark blue). (From Lumsden A, Graham A: Neural patterning: a forward role for hedgehog. Curr Biol 5:1347-1350, 1995. Copyright 1995, Elsevier Science.) **B,** Morphogenetic action of the Sonic hedgehog protein during limb bud formation. SHH is released from the zone of polarizing activity (labeled polarizing region in **B**) in the posterior limb bud to produce a gradient (shown with its highest levels as 4 declining to 2). Mutations or transplantation experiments that create an ectopic polarizing region in the anterior limb bud cause a duplication of posterior limb elements. (From Wolpert L, Beddington R, Brockes J, et al: Principles of Development. New York, Oxford University Press, 1998. Copyright 1998, Oxford University Press.)

and instead must reflect the action of modifier genes at other loci, or chance, or both.

Cell Shape and Organization

Cells must organize themselves with respect to their position and polarity in their microenvironment. For example, kidney epithelial cells must undergo differential development of the apical and basal aspects of their organelles to effect reabsorption of solutes. The acquisition of polarity by a cell can be viewed as the cellular version of axis determination discussed before with respect to the development of the overall embryo. Under normal circumstances, each renal tubular cell elaborates on its cell surface a filamentous structure, known as a primary cilium. The primary cilium is designed to sense fluid flow in the developing kidney tubule and signal the cell to stop proliferating and to polarize. Adult **polycystic kidney disease** (Case 32) is caused by loss of function of one of two protein components of primary cilia, polycystin 1 or polycystin 2, so that the cells fail to sense fluid flow. As a result, they continue

Figure 14-19 ■ Variable expressivity of an *SHH* mutation. The mother and her daughter carry the same missense mutation in *SHH,* but the daughter is severely affected with microcephaly, abnormal brain development, hypotelorism, and a cleft palate, whereas the only manifestation in the mother is a single central upper incisor. (From Roessler E, Belloni E, Gaudenz K, et al: Mutations in the human Sonic hedgehog gene cause holoprosencephaly. Nat Genet 14:357-360, 1996. Copyright 1996, Macmillan Ltd.)

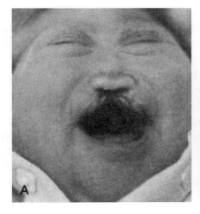
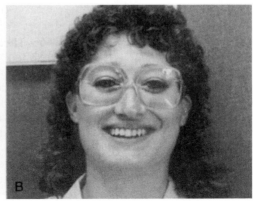

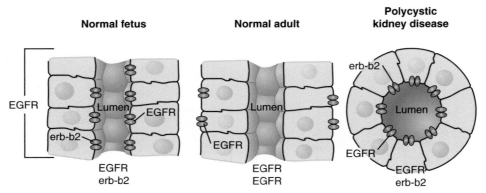

Figure 14-20 ■ Polarization of epidermal growth factor receptor (EGFR) in epithelium from a normal fetus, a normal adult, and a patient with polycystic kidney disease. Fetal cells and epithelial cells from patients with polycystic kidney disease express a heterodimer of EGFR and erb-b2 at apical cell membranes. In normal adults, tubular epithelia express homodimeric complexes of EGFR at the basolateral membrane. (Modified from Wilson PD: Polycystic kidney disease. N Engl J Med 350:151-164, 2004. Copyright 2004, Massachusetts Medical Society.)

to proliferate and do not undergo the appropriate developmental program of polarization in which they stop dividing and display polarized expression of certain proteins, on either the apical or basal aspect of the tubular epithelial cells (Fig. 14-20). The continued cell division leads to the formation of cysts, fluid-filled spaces lined by renal tubular cells. Many of the malformations we have discussed so far result from the failure of progenitor cells to respond appropriately to chemical cues in their environment, such as growth factors or morphogens. Adult polycystic kidney disease is a striking example of a tissue malformation that results from the failure of renal tubular progenitor cells to respond to a physical cue in their environment.

Cell Migration

Programmed cell movement is critical in development, and nowhere is it more important than in the central nervous system. The central nervous system is developed from the neural tube, a cylinder of cells created during weeks 4 to 5 of embryogenesis. Initially, the neural tube is only a few cell layers thick. Neural stem cells, which form the ventricular cell layer situated adjacent to the ventricle, divide to generate new neural stem cells as well as committed neuronal precursors that then migrate outwards toward the pial surface along a radial scaffold of glia. The central nervous system is built by waves of migration of these neuronal precursors. The neurons that populate the inner layers of the cortex migrate earlier in development, and each successive wave of neurons passes through the previously deposited, inner layers to form the next outer layer (Fig. 14-21).

Lissencephaly ("smooth brain") is a severe abnormality of brain development causing profound mental retardation. This developmental defect is one component of the **Miller-Dieker syndrome** (Case 27), which is caused by a 17p contiguous gene deletion syndrome that involves one copy of the *LIS1* gene. When there is loss of *LIS1* function, the progressive waves of migration of cortical neurons do not occur. The result is a thickened, hypercellular cerebral cortex with undefined cellular layers and poorly developed gyri, thereby making the surface of the brain appear smooth.

In addition to the neuronal migrations described, another remarkable example of cell migration involves the neural crest, a population of cells that arises from the dorsolateral aspect of the developing neural tube (see Figure 14-18A). Neural crest cells must migrate from their original location at the dorsal and lateral surface of the neural tube to remarkably distant sites, such as the ventral aspect of the face, the ear, the heart, the gut, and many other tissues, including the skin, where they differentiate into pigmented melanocytes. Population of the gut by neural crest progenitors gives rise to the autonomic innervation of the gut; failure of that migration leads to the aganglionic colon seen in **Hirschsprung disease** (Case 20). The genetics of Hirschsprung disease are complex (see Chapter 8), but a number of key signaling molecules have been implicated. One of the best characterized is the *RET* proto-oncogene. Mutations in *RET* have been identified in about 50% of patients with Hirschsprung disease. Another example of defects in neural crest development is the group of birth defects known as the **Waardenburg syndrome,** which includes defects in skin and hair pigmentation, coloration of the iris, and colon innervation

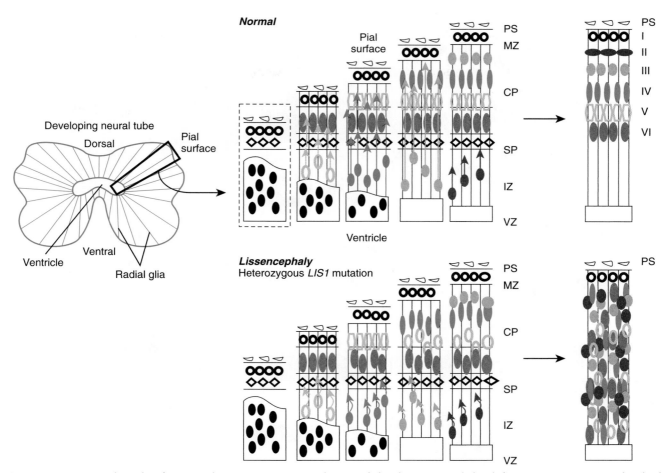

Figure 14-21 ■ The role of neuronal migration in normal cortical development and the defective migration in individuals heterozygous for an *LIS1* mutation causing lissencephaly. *Top:* A radial slice is taken from a normal developing neural tube, showing the progenitor cells at the ventricular zone (VZ). These cells divide, differentiate into postmitotic cells, and migrate radially along a scaffold made up of glia. The different shapes and colors represent the cells that migrate and form the various cortical layers: IZ, intermediate zone; SP, subplate; CP, cortical plate; MZ, marginal zone; PS, pial surface. The six distinguishable layers of the normal cortex (molecular, external granular, external pyramidal, internal granular, internal pyramidal, multiform) that occupy the region of the cortical plate are labeled I through VI. *Bottom:* Aberrant migration and failure of normal cortical development seen in lissencephaly. (Diagram modified from Gupta A, Tsai L-H, Wynshaw-Boris A: Life is a journey: a genetic look at neocortical development. Nat Rev Genet 3:342-355, 2002.)

(Fig. 14-22). This syndrome can be caused by mutations in at least four different transcription factors, all resulting in abnormalities in neural crest development.

Programmed Cell Death

Programmed cell death is a critical function in development and is necessary for the morphological development of many structures. It occurs wherever tissues need to be remodeled during morphogenesis, as during the separation of the individual digits, in perforation of the anal and choanal membranes, or in the establishment of communication between the uterus and vagina. One major form of programmed cell death is **apoptosis.**

Studies of mice with loss-of-function mutations in the *Foxp1* gene indicate that apoptosis is required for the remodeling of the tissues that form portions of the ventricular septum and cardiac outflow tract (**endocardial cushions**), to ensure the normal positioning of the origins of the aortic and pulmonary vessels. By eliminating certain cells, the relative position of the cushions is shifted into their correct location. It is also suspected that defects of apoptosis underlie some other forms of human congenital heart disease (see Chapter 8), such as the conotruncal heart defects of DiGeorge syndrome caused by deletion of the *TBX1* gene located in 22q11. Apoptosis also occurs during development of the immune system to eliminate lymphocyte lineages that react to self, thereby preventing autoimmune disease.

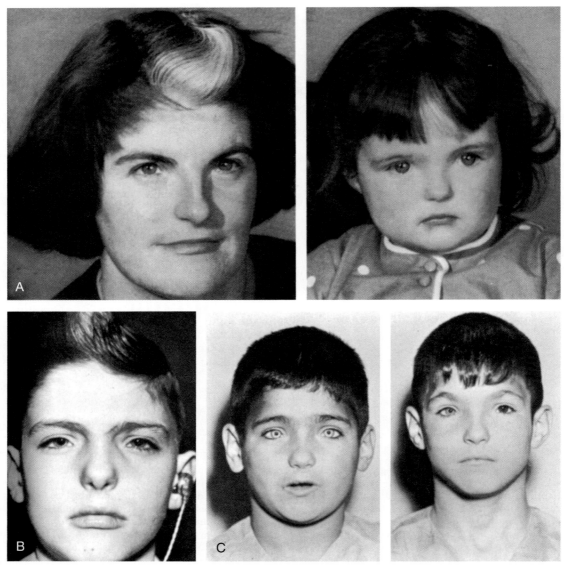

Figure 14-22 ■ Patients with type I Waardenburg syndrome. **A**, Mother and daughter with white forelocks. (From Partington MW: Arch Dis Child 34:1542, 1959.) **B**, A 10-year-old with congenital deafness and white forelock. (From DiGeorge AM, et al: J Pediatr 57:649, 1960.) **C**, Brothers, one of whom is deaf. There is no white forelock, but the boy on the right has heterochromatic irides. Mutations of *PAX3*, which encodes a transcription factor involved in neural crest development, cause type I Waardenburg syndrome. (From Jones KL: Smith's Recognizable Patterns of Human Malformation. Philadelphia, WB Saunders, 1998.)

⬤ INTERACTION OF DEVELOPMENTAL MECHANISMS IN EMBRYOGENESIS

Embryogenesis requires the coordination of multiple developmental processes in which proliferation, differentiation, migration, and apoptosis all play a part. For example, many processes must occur to convert a mass of mesoderm into a heart or a layer of neuroectoderm into a spinal cord. To understand how these processes interact and work together, developmental biologists typically study embryogenesis in a model organism, such as worms, flies, or mice. The general principles elucidated by these simpler, more easily manipulated

systems can then be applied to understanding developmental processes in humans.

The Limb as a Model of Organogenesis

The vertebrate limb is a relatively simple and well-studied product of developmental processes. There is no genomic specification for a human arm to be approximately 1 m long, with one proximal bone, two bones in the forelimb, and 27 bones in the hand. Instead, the limb results from a series of regulated processes that specify development along three axes, the proximal-

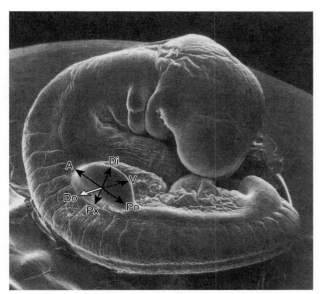

Figure 14-23 ■ This scanning electron micrograph of a 4-week human embryo illustrates the early budding of the forelimb. Overlaid onto the bud are the three axes of limb specification: Do-V, dorsal-ventral (dorsal comes out of the plane of the photo, ventral goes into the plane of the photo); Px-Di, proximal-distal; and A-Po, anterior-posterior. (From Carlson BM: *Human Embryology and Developmental Biology*, 3rd ed. Philadelphia, Mosby, 2004.)

distal axis, the dorsal-ventral axis, and the anterior-posterior axis (Fig. 14-23).

Limbs begin as protrusions of proliferating cells, the **limb buds,** along the lateral edge of the mesoderm of the human embryo in the fourth week of development. The location of each limb bud along the anterior-posterior axis of the embryo (head to tail axis) is associated with the expression of a specific transcription factor at each location, Tbx4 for the hindlimbs and Tbx5 for the forelimbs, whose expression is induced by various combinations of fibroblast growth factor ligands. Thus, the primarily proliferative process of limb bud outgrowth is activated by growth factors and transcription factors.

The limb bud grows primarily in an outward, lateral expansion of the proximal-distal axis of the limb (see Fig. 14-18B). Whereas proximal-distal expansion of the limb is the most obvious process, the two other axes are established soon after the onset of limb bud outgrowth. The anterior-posterior axis is set up soon after limb bud outgrowth, with the thumb considered to be an anterior structure, since it is on the edge of the limb facing the upper body. The fifth finger is a posterior structure because it is on the side of the limb bud oriented toward the lower part of the body. During limb formation, the morphogen Sonic hedgehog (SHH) is expressed in the posterior aspect of the developing limb bud, and its expression level forms a gradient that is primarily responsible for setting up the anterior-posterior axis in the developing limb (see Fig. 14-18B).

Defects in anterior-posterior patterning in the limb cause excessive digit patterning, manifested as polydactyly, or failure of complete separation of developing digits, manifested as syndactyly. The dorsal-ventral axis is also established, resulting in a palm or sole on the ventral side of the hand and foot, respectively.

One can now begin to understand the mechanisms underlying birth defect syndromes by applying knowledge from molecular developmental biology to human disorders. For example, mutations in the *GLI3* transcription factor gene cause two pleiotropic developmental anomaly syndromes, the **Greig cephalopolysyndactyly syndrome** (GCPS) and the **Pallister-Hall syndrome.** These two syndromes comprise distinct combinations of limb, central nervous system, craniofacial, airway, and genitourinary anomalies that are caused by perturbed balance in the production of two variant forms of GLI3, referred to as GLI3 and GLI3R, as shown in Figure 14-24. GLI3 is part of the SHH signaling pathway. SHH signals, in part, through a cell

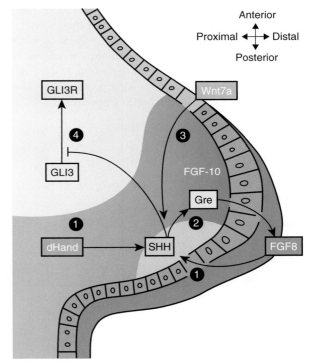

Figure 14-24 ■ Schematic diagram of the anterior-posterior and proximal-distal axes of the limb bud and its molecular components. In this diagram, the anterior aspect is up and the distal aspect is to the right. SHH expression occurs in the zone of polarizing activity of the posterior limb bud, and SHH is activated by the *dHand* gene. SHH inhibits conversion of the GLI3 transcription factor to GLI3R in the posterior regions of the limb bud. However, SHH activity does not extend to anterior regions of the bud. The absence of SHH allows GLI3 to be converted to GLI3R (a transcriptional repressor) in the anterior limb bud. By this mechanism, the anterior-posterior axis of the limb bud is established with a gradient of GLI3 versus GLI3R. (Modified from Gilbert SF: *Developmental Biology*, 7th ed. Sunderland, Mass, Sinauer Associates, 2003, p 538.)

surface receptor encoded by a gene called *PTCH1*. Mutations in *PTCH1* cause the **nevoid basal cell carcinoma syndrome,** or Gorlin syndrome. This syndrome comprises craniofacial anomalies and occasional polydactyly that are similar to those seen in GCPS, but in addition, Gorlin syndrome also manifests dental cysts and susceptibility to basal cell carcinoma. By considering Gorlin syndrome and GCPS, one can appreciate that the two disorders share phenotypic manifestations precisely because the genes that are mutated in the two disorders have overlapping effects in the same developmental genetic pathway. A third protein in the SHH signaling pathway, the CREB binding protein, or CBP, is a transcriptional coactivator of the GLI3 transcription factor. Mutations in *CREBBP* cause the **Rubenstein-Taybi syndrome,** which also shares phenotypic manifestations with GCPS and Gorlin syndrome.

Many other examples of this phenomenon could be cited, but the key points to emphasize are that genes are the primary regulators of developmental processes, their protein products function in developmental genetic pathways, and these pathways are employed in related developmental processes in a number of organ systems. Understanding the molecular basis of gene function, how those functions are organized into modules, and how abnormalities in those modules cause and correlate with malformations and pleiotropic syndromes, forms the basis of the modern clinical approach to human birth defects.

GENERAL REFERENCES

Carlson BM: Human Embryology and Developmental Biology, 3rd ed. Philadelphia, Mosby, 2004.

Dye FJ: Dictionary of Developmental Biology and Embryology. New York, Wiley-Liss, 2002.

Epstein CJ, Erickson RP, Wynshaw-Boris AJ (eds): Inborn Errors of Development: The Molecular Basis of Clinical Disorders of Morphogenesis. New York, Oxford University Press, 2004.

Gilbert SF: Developmental Biology, 7th ed. Sunderland, Mass, Sinauer Associates, 2003.

Wolpert L, Beddington R, Jessell T, et al: Principles of Development, 2nd ed. New York, Oxford University Press, 2002.

REFERENCES FOR SPECIFIC TOPICS

Anderson RN, Smith BL: Deaths: leading causes for 2002. Natl Vital Stat Rep 53:1-89, 2005.

Biesecker LG: What you can learn from one gene: *GLI3*. J Med Genet 43:465-469, 2006.

Davies JA, Fisher CE: Genes and proteins in renal development. Exp Nephrol 10:102-113, 2002.

Gilbert SF, Opitz JM, Raff RA: Resynthesizing evolutionary and developmental biology. Dev Biol 173:357-372, 1996.

Kato M, Dobyns WB: Lissencephaly and the molecular basis of neuronal migration. Hum Mol Genet 12(Spec No 1):R89-R96, 2003.

Mirkes PE: 2001 Warkany Lecture: To die or not to die, the role of apoptosis in normal and abnormal mammalian development. Teratology 65:228-239, 2002.

Mitchell LE, Adzick NS, Melchionne J, et al: Spina bifida. Lancet 364:1885-1895, 2004.

Ogilvie CM, Braude PR, Scriven PN: Preimplantation diagnosis—an overview. J Histochem Cytochem 53:255-260, 2005.

Sells JM, Jaffe KM, Hall JG: Amyoplasia, the most common type of arthrogryposis: the potential for good outcome. Pediatrics 97:225-231, 1996.

USEFUL WEBSITE

GeneReviews. *http://www.geneclinics.org/* Website for reviews of many disorders mentioned in this chapter including: Gorlin syndrome, Greig cephalopolysyndactyly syndrome, Hirschsprung disease, Lowe syndrome, Pallister-Hall syndrome, Rubenstein-Taybi syndrome, Smith-Lemli-Opitz syndrome, Stickler syndrome, velocardiofacial (DiGeorge) syndrome, Waardenberg syndrome.

PROBLEMS

1. What is the difference between regulative and mosaic development? What is the significance of these two stages of development for reproductive genetics and prenatal diagnosis?

2. Match the terms in the left-hand column with the terms that best fit in the right-hand column.

   a. erasure of imprinting during germ cell development
   b. position-dependent development
   c. regulative development
   d. embryonic stem cells

   1. totipotency
   2. morphogen
   3. epigenetic regulation of gene expression
   4. monozygotic twinning

3. Match the terms in the left-hand column with the terms that best fit in the right-hand column.

   a. amniotic band
   b. polydactyly
   c. inadequate amniotic fluid
   d. limb reduction
   e. Robin sequence

   1. U-shaped cleft palate
   2. thalidomide
   3. *GLI3* mutation
   4. disruption
   5. deformation

4. What type of diploid cells would not be appropriate nucleus donors in an animal cloning experiment and why?

5. For discussion: Why do some mutations in transcription factors result in developmental defects even when they are present in the heterozygous state?

Chapter 15

Prenatal Diagnosis

Prenatal diagnosis had its beginning in 1966, when Steele and Breg showed that the chromosome constitution of a fetus could be determined by analysis of cultured cells from the amniotic fluid. Because the association between late maternal age and an increased risk of Down syndrome was already well known, their report led directly to the development of prenatal diagnosis as a medical service. Prenatal diagnosis has already been referred to in the context of many specific genetic disorders, and in this chapter, its scope, methodology, and limitations are considered in further detail.

Some couples may seek prenatal diagnosis because they know from their family history or from carrier testing that they are at substantially elevated risk for having a child with a specific genetic disorder. For others, prenatal diagnosis is performed because of the increased risk conferred simply by advanced maternal age or by a screening test done as part of routine prenatal care, as occurs with autosomal trisomies, such as trisomy 21, or for a neural tube defect. In any case, the ultimate goal of prenatal diagnosis is to inform couples about the risk of a birth defect or genetic disorder in their pregnancy and to provide them with informed choices on how to manage that risk. Some couples known to be at risk of having a child with a specific birth defect, who might otherwise forego having children, use prenatal diagnosis to undertake a pregnancy with the knowledge that the presence or absence of the disorder in the fetus can be confirmed by testing. Many couples at risk of having a child with a severe genetic disorder have been able to have healthy children because of the availability of prenatal diagnosis and the option of terminating the pregnancy if necessary. In some, prenatal testing can reassure and reduce anxiety, especially among high-risk groups. For still other couples,

prenatal diagnosis allows physicians to plan prenatal treatment of a fetus with a genetic disorder or birth defect or, if prenatal treatment is not possible, to arrange for appropriate management for the impending birth of an affected child in terms of psychological preparation of the family, pregnancy and delivery management, and postnatal care.

● INDICATIONS FOR PRENATAL DIAGNOSIS BY INVASIVE TESTING

There are a number of well-accepted indications for prenatal testing by invasive procedures such as **chorionic villus sampling (CVS)** and **amniocentesis** (see Box). By far, the leading indication for prenatal diagnosis is **advanced maternal age.** In North America and western Europe, according to statistical data for maternal age at the time of birth in comparison with the number of prenatal diagnoses, at least half of all pregnant women older than 35 years elect to use CVS or amniocentesis for fetal karyotyping. In the United States, courts have considered a physician to be negligent if he or she fails to offer prenatal diagnosis to women considered to be of advanced maternal age. In addition to maternal age as an indication, there are more than 600 genetic disorders for which prenatal testing by amniocentesis or CVS can be offered to couples known to be at risk. The generally accepted criterion for eligibility for prenatal diagnosis by amniocentesis or CVS is that the risk for fetal abnormality is at least as great as the risk of miscarriage or other complication from the procedure itself.

The chief condition for which pregnant women of advanced age are at risk is **Down syndrome** (see Chapter 6). Despite the widespread availability of prenatal diag-

••• Principal Indications for Prenatal Diagnosis by Invasive Testing

- **Advanced maternal age**

  The definition of advanced maternal age varies somewhat among prenatal genetics centers but is usually at least 35 years at the expected date of confinement. This age had been selected because at 35 years, the risk of a fetus with a chromosome abnormality was thought to be equal to the risk of miscarriage associated with amniocentesis (~1/250) (see Table 15-1).

- **Previous child with de novo chromosomal aneuploidy**

  Although the parents of a child with chromosomal aneuploidy may have normal chromosomes themselves, in some situations there may still be an increased risk of a chromosomal abnormality in a subsequent child. For example, if a woman at 30 years of age has a child with Down syndrome, her recurrence risk for *any* chromosomal abnormality is about 1/100, compared with the age-related population risk of about 1/390. Parental mosaicism is one possible explanation of the increased risk, but in the majority of cases, the mechanism of the increase in risk is unknown.

- **Presence of structural chromosome abnormality in one of the parents**

  Here, the risk of a chromosome abnormality in a child varies according to the type of abnormality and sometimes the parent of origin. The greatest risk, 100% for Down syndrome, occurs only if either parent has a 21q21q Robertsonian translocation or isochromosome (see Chapter 6).

- **Family history of a genetic disorder that may be diagnosed or ruled out by biochemical or DNA analysis**

  Most of the disorders in this group are caused by single-gene defects with 25% or 50% recurrence risks. Cases in which the parents have been diagnosed as carriers after a population screening test, rather than after the birth of an affected child, are also in this category. Even before DNA analysis became available, numerous biochemical disorders could be identified prenatally, and DNA analysis has greatly increased this number. Mitochondrial disorders pose special challenges for prenatal diagnosis.

- **Family history of an X-linked disorder for which there is no specific prenatal diagnostic test**

  When there is no alternative method, the parents of a boy affected with an X-linked disorder may use fetal sex determination to help them decide whether to continue or to terminate a subsequent pregnancy because the recurrence risk may be as high as 25%. For X-linked disorders, such as Duchenne muscular dystrophy and hemophilia A and B, however, for which prenatal diagnosis by DNA analysis is available, the fetal sex is first determined and DNA analysis is then performed if the fetus is male. In either of the situations mentioned, **preimplantation genetic diagnosis** (see text) may be an option for allowing the transfer to the uterus of only those embryos determined to be unaffected for the disorder in question.

- **Risk of a neural tube defect**

  First-degree relatives (and second-degree relatives at some centers) of patients with neural tube defects are eligible for amniocentesis because of an increased risk of having a child with a neural tube defect (see Table 8-9); many open neural tube defects, however, can now be detected by other noninvasive tests, as described in this chapter.

- **Maternal serum screening and ultrasound examination**

  Genetic assessment and further testing are recommended when fetal abnormalities are suspected on the basis of routine screening by maternal serum screening and fetal ultrasound examination.

---

nosis to older women, however, most fetuses with Down syndrome are not identified prenatally. This is because the majority of all pregnancies, including those with a Down syndrome fetus, are in mothers younger than 35 years, who are at a lower risk for Down syndrome in their fetus than are women older than 35 years (Table 15-1) and thus were too young to be offered *invasive* testing such as amniocentesis or CVS on a routine basis. For women younger than 35 years, however, *noninvasive* testing is now recommended for all pregnancies, independent of risk. Such noninvasive testing includes first- and second-trimester **maternal serum screening** together with ultrasonographic examination to screen for fetuses with a variety of birth defects, in particular Down syndrome (and other autosomal trisomies) and neural tube defects (NTDs); these screening tests are described later. However, invasive prenatal diagnosis cannot be used to rule out all possible fetal abnormalities. It is limited to determining whether the fetus has (or probably has) a designated condition for which an increased risk is indicated by late maternal age, family history, a positive screening test result, or other well-defined risk factors.

● METHODS OF PRENATAL DIAGNOSIS

The methods currently used for prenatal diagnosis, both invasive and noninvasive, are shown in Table 15-2. Both amniocentesis and CVS are invasive procedures associ-

Table 15-1

Incidence of Down Syndrome in Liveborns and Fetuses in Relation to Maternal Age*

Maternal Age (Years)	At Birth	At Amniocentesis (16 Weeks)	At Chorionic Villus Sampling (9-11 Weeks)
15-19	1/1250	—	—
20-24	1/1400	—	—
25-29	1/1100	—	—
30	1/900	—	—
31	1/900	—	—
32	1/750	—	—
33	1/625	1/420	1/370
34	1/500	1/333	1/250
35	1/385	1/250	1/250
36	1/300	1/200	1/175
37	1/225	1/150	1/175
38	1/175	1/115	1/115
39	1/140	1/90	1/90
40	1/100	1/70	1/80
41	1/80	1/50	1/50
42	1/65	1/40	1/30
43	1/50	1/30	1/25
44	1/40	1/25	1/25
45 and older	1/25	1/20	1/15

*Figures have been rounded and are approximate.
Data from Benn PA, Hsu LYF: Prenatal diagnosis of chromosome abnormalities through amniocentesis. In Milunsky A: Genetic Disorders and the Fetus: Diagnosis, Prevention, and Treatment, 5th ed. Baltimore, Johns Hopkins University Press, 2004; and Gardner RJM, Sutherland GR: Chromosome Abnormalities and Genetic Counseling, 3rd ed. New York, Oxford University Press, 2003.

ated with a small risk of fetal loss. Thus, the use of amniocentesis or CVS is indicated for only a small percentage of pregnant women, those who meet the criteria for prenatal diagnosis as outlined earlier. In contrast, a combination of maternal serum screening (discussed later) and ultrasonographic scanning can be used for fetal evaluation in low-risk (as well as in some high-risk) pregnancies because both are noninvasive and without risk to the fetus. Maternal serum screening can help identify fetuses at increased risk of open NTDs, some chromosomal abnormalities including Down syndrome, and other disorders, as described later in this chapter. Ultrasonography has many uses in obstetrical genetics, including determining gestational age and fetal growth, screening for specific fetal abnormalities associated with autosomal trisomies, and providing high-resolution images for the diagnosis of a number of morphological abnormalities, many of which are genetic in origin, at early gestational ages (see later).

Invasive Testing

Amniocentesis

Amniocentesis refers to the procedure of inserting a needle into the amniotic sac and removing a sample of amniotic fluid transabdominally by syringe (Fig. 15-1A). The amniotic fluid contains cells of fetal origin that can be cultured for diagnostic tests. Before amniocentesis, ultrasonographic scanning is routinely used to assess fetal viability, gestational age (by measuring the fetal biparietal diameter and femoral length), number of fetuses, volume of amniotic fluid, normality of fetal anatomical structures, and position of the fetus and placenta to allow the optimal position for needle insertion. Amniocentesis is performed on an outpatient basis typically at the 15th to 16th week after the first day of the last menstrual period; however, the procedure has been performed at a much earlier stage in pregnancy, as early as 10 to 14 weeks in some centers, but with some increase in the rate of complications (see later). In addition to fetal chromosome analysis, the concentration of **alpha-fetoprotein (AFP)** can be assayed in amniotic fluid to detect open NTDs. AFP is a fetal glycoprotein produced mainly in the liver, secreted into the fetal circulation, and excreted through the kidneys into the amniotic fluid by fetal urine. AFP enters the maternal blood stream through the placenta, amniotic membranes, and maternal-fetal circulation. It can therefore be assayed either in amniotic fluid (AFAFP) or in maternal serum (MSAFP). Both assays are extremely useful in prenatal diagnosis, chiefly for assessing the risk of an open NTD but also for other reasons (see later discussion).

AFP concentration is measured by immunoassay, a relatively simple and inexpensive method that can be applied to all amniotic fluid samples regardless of the specific indication for the amniocentesis. To interpret an AFAFP, one compares the level to the normal range for each gestational age. If the AFAFP is elevated, one must look for a cause other than an open NTD. Factors potentially leading to abnormally high concentrations of AFP in amniotic fluid are shown in Table 15-3. When the AFAFP assay is used in conjunction with ultrasonographic scanning at 18 to 19 weeks' gestation, about 99% of fetuses with open spina bifida and virtually all fetuses with anencephaly can be identified.

Table 15-2

Methods of Prenatal Diagnosis and Screening

INVASIVE TESTING

    Amniocentesis
    Chorionic villus sampling
    Cordocentesis
    Preimplantation genetic diagnosis

NONINVASIVE TESTING

    Maternal serum alpha-fetoprotein
    First- and second-trimester maternal serum screening
    Ultrasonography
    Isolation of fetal cells from maternal circulation

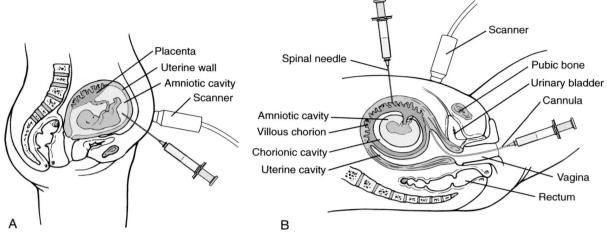

Figure 15-1 ■ **A,** Amniocentesis. A needle is inserted transabdominally into the amniotic cavity, and a sample of amniotic fluid (usually about 20 mL) is withdrawn by syringe for diagnostic studies (e.g., chromosome studies, enzyme measurements, or DNA analysis). Ultrasonography is routinely performed before or during the procedure. **B,** Chorionic villus sampling. Two alternative approaches are drawn: transcervical (by means of a flexible cannula) and transabdominal (with a spinal needle). In both approaches, success and safety depend on use of ultrasound imaging (scanner). (From Moore KL, Persaud TVN: The Developing Human: Clinically Oriented Embryology, 6th ed. Philadelphia, WB Saunders, 1998.)

The major complication associated with midtrimester amniocentesis at 15 to 16 weeks of gestation is a 1 in 1600 risk of inducing miscarriage over the baseline risk of approximately 1% to 2% for any pregnancy at this stage of gestation. Other complications are rare, including leakage of amniotic fluid, infection, and injury to the fetus by needle puncture. As mentioned previously, amniocentesis can be performed as early as 10 to 14 weeks. One randomized study comparing the safety and fetal outcome of early amniocentesis versus midtrimester amniocentesis demonstrated a 3-fold increased risk of spontaneous abortion in the early group versus the midtrimester group. Amniotic fluid leakage was also more common with early amniocentesis. The only congenital anomaly found to be increased

with early amniocentesis is talipes equinovarus (clubfeet), with an incidence of 1.3% versus the general population risk of 0.1% to 0.3% (a risk that is not increased with midtrimester amniocentesis). Most of the increase was in amniocenteses done before 13 weeks of gestation and may be due to the limited amount of amniotic fluid present at this early stage in pregnancy.

If amniocentesis is performed for any reason, both the concentration of AFP in the amniotic fluid and the karyotype of amniotic fluid cells are determined to screen for open NTDs and chromosomal abnormalities, respectively. Other tests are performed only for specific indications.

Chorionic Villus Sampling

CVS involves the biopsy of tissue from the villous area of the chorion transcervically or transabdominally, generally between the 10th and 12th weeks of pregnancy (Fig. 15-1B). A brief review of the early development of the chorionic villi helps to clarify the basis of the CVS technique (Fig. 15-2). The villi are derived from the trophoblast, the extraembryonic part of the blastocyst. During implantation, the trophoblast differentiates into the cytotrophoblast and the syncytiotrophoblast. The syncytiotrophoblast invades the uterine wall and eventually forms lacunae in which maternal blood is pooled. At the end of the second week, the **primary chorionic villi** are formed as proliferations of the cytotrophoblast that protrude into the syncytiotrophoblast. The villi soon begin to branch, and mesenchyme grows into them to form a core; the formation of a core characterizes the **secondary villi.** Networks of capillaries develop in the mesenchymal

---

Table 15-3

Causes of Elevated Amniotic Fluid Alpha-Fetoprotein Other than NTD

Fetal blood contamination

Fetal death

Twin pregnancy

Fetal abnormalities, including omphalocele and at least one form of congenital nephrosis as well as other rare problems

Other unexplained variation in the normal AFP concentration of amniotic fluid

False-positive elevation due to overestimation of gestational age. Since the AFP concentration is normally highest at around the 14th week of pregnancy and falls by 10% to 15% per week after that, a 12- to 14-week gestation that is mistakenly thought to be 16 weeks will appear to have elevated AFP if the normal range for a 16-week gestation is applied.

Note: Some of these causes of an elevated AFAFP level can be confirmed or ruled out by ultrasonographic examination.

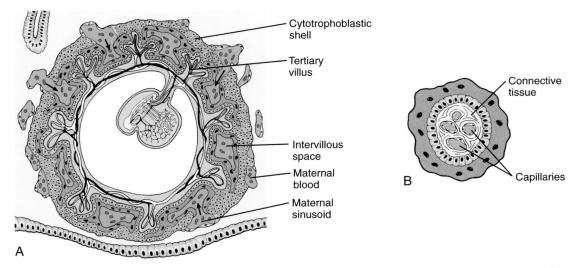

Figure 15-2 ■ Development of the tertiary chorionic villi and placenta. **A,** Cross section of an implanted embryo and placenta at about 21 days. **B,** Cross section of a tertiary villus showing establishment of circulation in mesenchymal core, cytotrophoblast, and syncytiotrophoblast. (From Moore KL: The Developing Human: Clinically Oriented Embryology, 4th ed. Philadelphia, WB Saunders, 1988.)

core, and circulation is established; the villi are then **tertiary villi.** The tertiary villi branch profusely, and by the end of the eighth week, they cover the entire surface of the chorionic sac as the **chorion frondosum.** Part of the chorion subsequently becomes the **smooth chorion (chorion laeve)** as the villi in that area degenerate. The villi that are sampled for prenatal diagnosis are tertiary villi from the chorion frondosum and are composed of mesenchymal core, cytotrophoblast, and an outer layer of syncytiotrophoblast.

The major advantage of CVS compared with midtrimester amniocentesis is that CVS allows the results to be available at an early stage of pregnancy, thus reducing the period of uncertainty and allowing termination, if it is elected, to be performed in the first trimester and on an outpatient basis. However, AFP cannot be assayed at this stage (in contrast, it *can* be done at 15 to 16 weeks when amniocentesis is performed), and screening for open NTDs should be performed by maternal serum screening at approximately 16 weeks of gestation. As with amniocentesis, ultrasonographic scanning is used before CVS to determine the best approach for sampling. The increase in the rate of fetal loss due to CVS is approximately 1% in addition to the baseline risk of 2% to 5% in any pregnancy that is 7 to 12 weeks of gestation. Although there were initial reports of an increase in the frequency of birth defects, particularly limb reduction defects, after CVS, this increase has not been confirmed in large series of CVS procedures performed after 10 weeks of gestation by experienced physicians. The success of chromosome analysis is the same as with amniocentesis (i.e., more than 99%). However, about 2% of CVS samplings yield ambiguous results because of chromosomal mosaicism (including true

mosaicism and pseudomosaicism, see later); in these situations, follow-up with amniocentesis is recommended to establish whether the fetus has a chromosomal abnormality.

To prevent Rh immunization of the mother (see Chapter 9), administration of Rh immune globulin is routine for Rh-negative women after any invasive procedure (including amniocentesis and CVS).

Noninvasive Testing

Screening for Neural Tube Defects

Because an estimated 95% of infants with NTDs are born into families with no known history of this malformation, a relatively simple screening test, such as the noninvasive MSAFP, constitutes an important tool for prenatal diagnosis, prevention, and management. When the fetus has an open NTD, the concentration of AFP is likely to be higher than normal in the maternal serum as well as in the amniotic fluid. This observation is the basis for the use of MSAFP measurement at 16 weeks as a screening test for open NTDs. There is considerable overlap between the normal range of MSAFP and the range of concentrations found when the fetus has an open NTD (Fig. 15-3). An elevated MSAFP is by no means specific to a pregnancy with an open NTD, but many of the other causes that are not NTDs can be distinguished from open NTDs by fetal ultrasonography (Table 15-4). MSAFP is also not perfectly sensitive. If an elevated concentration is defined as two multiples of the median, one can estimate that 20% of fetuses with open NTDs remain undetected. Lowering the cutoff to improve sensitivity would be at the expense of reduced specificity.

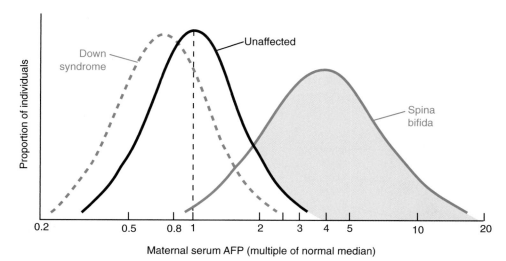

Figure 15-3 ■ Maternal serum alpha-fetoprotein (AFP) concentration, expressed as multiples of the median, in normal fetuses, fetuses with open neural tube defects, and fetuses with Down syndrome. (Redrawn from Wald NJ, Cuckle HS: Recent advances in screening for neural tube defects and Down syndrome. In Rodeck C [ed]: Prenatal Diagnosis. London, Bailliére Tindall, 1987, pp 649-676.)

The combined use of the MSAFP assay with detailed diagnostic ultrasonography (see later discussion) approaches the accuracy of AFAFP and ultrasonography for the detection of open NTDs. Because the assay of MSAFP is not invasive, its measurement, together with ultrasonography, another noninvasive form of testing, is preferred for the diagnosis of open NTDs in many centers. Thus, first-degree, second-degree, or more remote relatives of patients with NTDs may have an MSAFP assay (at 16 weeks) followed by detailed ultrasound examination (at 18 weeks) rather than amniocentesis.

Preventing Neural Tube Defects

Periconceptional supplementation with folic acid (i.e., at least 1 month before conception and continuing through the first trimester of pregnancy) has been shown to decrease the incidence of NTDs by nearly 75% (see Chapter 8). A 40% reduction in the incidence of orofacial clefting has also been demonstrated with periconceptional folic acid supplementation. The recommended dosage of folic acid increases with the estimated risk for NTD (i.e., a higher dose is given to women at increased risk based on a positive family history).

Screening for Down Syndrome and Other Aneuploidies by MSAFP and Ultrasonography

The leading indication for invasive fetal testing by amniocentesis or CVS is the increased risk for chromosomal aneuploidies because of advanced maternal age. Unfortunately, more than 70% of all children with major autosomal trisomies, such as trisomy 21 (Down syndrome), are born to women younger than 35 years, for whom invasive testing is not generally recommended or offered. A solution to this problem was first suggested by the unexpected finding that MSAFP, measured during the second trimester as a screening test for NTD, was depressed in many pregnancies later discovered to have an autosomal trisomy, particularly trisomy 21. MSAFP alone has far too much overlap between unaffected pregnancies and Down syndrome pregnancies to be a useful screening tool on its own (see Fig. 15-3). However, a battery of maternal serum protein markers have now been developed that in combination with specific ultrasound measurements have the necessary sensitivity and specificity to be useful for screening. These batteries of tests are now recommended for noninvasive screening, although not for definitive diagnosis, during the first and second trimesters of all pregnancies regardless of maternal age.

First-trimester screening is ideally performed between 11 and 13 weeks of gestation. It relies on (1) quantifying the levels of certain substances in maternal serum and (2) measuring subcutaneous edema of the

Table 15-4

Causes of Elevated Maternal Serum Alpha-Fetoprotein	
Gestational age older than calculated	Sacrococcygeal teratoma
Spina bifida	Renal anomalies
Anencephaly	Urinary obstruction
Congenital skin defects	Polycystic kidney
Pilonidal cysts	Absent kidney
Abdominal wall defects	Congenital nephrosis
Gastrointestinal defects	Osteogenesis imperfecta
Obstruction	Low birth weight
Liver necrosis	Oligohydramnios
Cloacal exstrophy	Multiple gestation
Cystic hygroma	Decreased maternal weight

Cunningham FG, MacDonald PC, Gant NF, et al: Williams Obstetrics, 20th ed. Stamford, Connecticut, Appleton & Lange, 1997, p 972.

Table 15-5

Elevation and Depression of Parameters Used in First- and Second-Trimester Screening Tests

	FIRST-TRIMESTER SCREEN			SECOND-TRIMESTER SCREEN			
	Nuchal Translucency	PAPP-A	Free β-hCG	uE₃	AFP	Free β-hCG	Inhibin A
Trisomy 21	↑	↓	↑	↓	↓	↑	↑
Trisomy 18	↑	↓	↓	↓	↓	↓	—
Trisomy 13	↑	↓	↓	↓	↓	↓	—
Neural tube defect	—	—	—	—	↑	—	—

AFP, alpha-fetoprotein; β-hCG, human chorionic gonadotropin β subunit; PAPP-A, pregnancy-associated plasma protein A; uE₃, unconjugated estriol.

fetal neck by a highly targeted ultrasonographic examination. The maternal serum substances measured are **pregnancy-associated plasma protein A (PAPP-A)** and the hormone **human chorionic gonadotropin (hCG)**, either as total hCG or as its free β subunit. PAPP-A is depressed below the normal range in all trisomies; hCG (or free β-hCG) is elevated in trisomy 21 but depressed in the other trisomies (Table 15-5).

The primary ultrasonographic examination used in first-trimester screening for trisomies relies on detecting an abnormal excess of fluid in the soft tissue in the neck. The thickness of the echo-free space between the skin and the soft tissue overlying the dorsal aspect of the cervical spine, referred to as **nuchal translucency**, is increased by edema in the first trimester (10 to 14 weeks), a common occurrence in trisomies 21, 13, and 18 and in 45,X fetuses (Fig. 15-4). Nuchal translucency must be determined with reference to gestational age since it varies with age of the fetus. The average nuchal translucency is 0.12 cm at 11 weeks of gestation (95th percentile up to 2 mm) and 0.15 cm at 14 weeks of gestation (95th percentile up to 2.6 mm). Measurement of nuchal translucency requires highly skilled operators with specialized ultrasonography training who participate in ongoing proficiency monitoring. Deviation of these three parameters beyond a cutoff chosen to keep false positives at about 5% makes the sensitivity of first-trimester screening approximately 84% (Table 15-6).

Second-trimester screening is usually accomplished by measuring three substances in the mother's serum: MSAFP, free β-hCG, and **unconjugated estriol**. This battery of tests is referred to as a **triple screen**. Some laboratories offer a **quadruple screen** consisting of the triple screen plus measurement of a fourth substance, **inhibin A.** All of these substances are depressed below the normal range in all trisomies with the exception of free β-hCG, which is elevated in trisomy 21 but depressed in the other trisomies, and inhibin A, which is elevated in trisomy 21 but not significantly affected in the other trisomies (see Table 15-5). Second-trimester triple and quadruple screens provide detection rates for

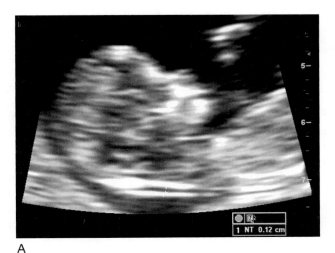

A

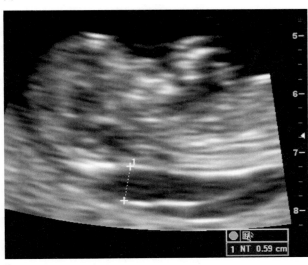

B

Figure 15-4 ■ Nuchal translucency measurements at 11 weeks of gestation. Nuchal translucency is a dark, echo-free zone beneath the skin in an ultrasonographic "sagittal section" through the fetus and is marked by two + signs connected by a dotted line. **A,** Nuchal translucency of 0.12 cm in a normal 11-week fetus, the average for a normal fetus at this gestational age. **B,** Increased nuchal translucency of 0.59 cm, which is nearly 20 standard deviations above the mean, consistent with a diagnosis of Down syndrome. (Courtesy of Evelyn M. Karson, Bethesda, Maryland.)

Table 15-6

Sensitivity and False-Positive Rate of Screening Tests for Autosomal Trisomies

Screening Test	Sensitivity for Trisomy 21	False-Positive Rate
FIRST TRIMESTER		
PAPP-A, hCG, and NT	84%	5%
SECOND TRIMESTER		
Triple screen	72%	5%
Quadruple screen	81%	5%
Stepwise sequential testing	95%	5%

PAPP-A, pregnancy-associated plasma protein A; hCG, human chorionic gonadotropin; NT, nuchal translucency.
Data from Reddy UM, Mennuti MT: Incorporating first-trimester Down syndrome studies into prenatal screening: executive summary of the National Institute of Child Health and Human Development workshop. Obstet Gynecol 107:167-173, 2006.

autosomal trisomies of approximately 72% and 81%, respectively (see Table 15-6). The concentration of unconjugated estriol is also reduced in women who are smokers and, in general, in cases of fetal immaturity; extremely low levels may be indicative of steroid sulfatase deficiency or the Smith-Lemli-Opitz syndrome.

Given the sensitivity and specificity of first- and second-trimester screening by themselves, obstetricians have developed strategies for combining the results of first-trimester and second-trimester testing to increase the ability to detect pregnancies with autosomal trisomies, particularly trisomy 21. These strategies have the advantage of giving couples found to be at significantly increased risk on the basis of first-trimester testing alone the choice of invasive testing early. The most common strategy is to combine the risk as determined from first- and second-trimester screening tests in a sequential manner. In the stepwise sequential strategy, couples are identified as "screen positive" for Down syndrome once an ultrasound examination has confirmed fetal age and the estimated risk is equivalent to or greater than the risk for a 35-year-old woman. At that point, the couple can be offered invasive prenatal testing since their risk for autosomal trisomy has reached the level of a woman with advanced maternal age, for which invasive testing is routinely offered.

The remaining couples with lesser degrees of elevated risk are then offered second-trimester testing, and the combined results from both their first- and second-trimester testing are used to determine whether invasive testing is indicated. This strategy can detect up to 95% of all Down syndrome cases with an approximately 5% false-positive rate. Alternative strategies are being developed to refine the sequential approach to reduce the number and cost of screening tests while maintaining or even improving on the 95% sensitivity and 5% false-positive rate. For example, an additional ultraso-

nographic method is being actively investigated as a screening tool for trisomy 21—absence of the nasal bone. Three quarters of trisomy 21 fetuses have a nasal bone that is undetectable by ultrasonography at the gestational age of 11 to 14 weeks, compared with far less than 1% of normal fetuses. Demonstrating an absence of the nasal bone, together with increased nuchal translucency, may provide a sensitivity and specificity for prenatal Down syndrome screening equivalent to nuchal translucency plus first-trimester biochemical markers.

As with any screening test in medicine, it is critical for couples to be informed that screening for trisomies with maternal serum markers and ultrasound scanning is not a definitive diagnostic tool. Equally important, women whose screening test result is considered to be "negative" must also be counseled that their risk of having a child with Down syndrome or another autosomal trisomy or NTD, although greatly reduced, is not zero.

Prenatal Diagnosis by Ultrasonography

High-resolution, real-time scanning is increasingly important for general assessment of fetal age, multiple pregnancies, and fetal viability as well as for the detection of specific morphological anomalies (Figs. 15-5 and 15-6). It can even be used in midtrimester to identify fetal sex with a high degree of accuracy. Transabdominal ultrasonography, the traditional method, is now supplemented with increasing frequency by transvaginal ultrasonography to evaluate fetal viability and gestational dating and, in the first trimester, to detect several major types of anomalies, such as anencephaly, meningomyelocele (see Fig. 15-5), and cystic hygroma (Table 15-7). Thus, many malformations are now detectable in the first instance by routine ultrasonography, even without a family history to indicate an increased risk. Long-term follow-up assessments have failed to provide any evidence that ultrasonography is harmful to the fetus or the mother.

A number of fetal abnormalities detectable by ultrasound examination are associated with chromosomal aneuploidy. Several common ultrasound abnormalities are typically associated with trisomy 21, trisomy 18, trisomy 13, or 45,X as well as with many other abnormal karyotypes (Table 15-8). These abnormalities may also occur as isolated findings in a chromosomally normal fetus. Table 15-8 compares the prevalence of fetal chromosome defects in fetuses when one of these common ultrasound abnormalities is present as an isolated finding versus when it is one of multiple abnormalities. The likelihood of a chromosomally abnormal fetus increases dramatically when a fetal abnormality detected by ultrasound examination is only one of many abnormalities.

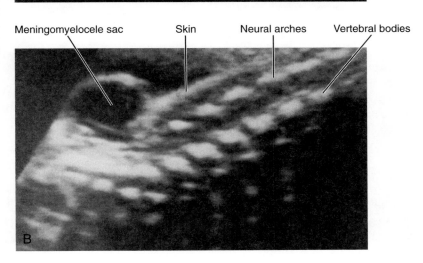

Figure 15-5 ■ Ultrasonograms of spinal canal and neural tube. **A,** Normal fetus at 24 weeks of gestation; longitudinal midline view, with the sacrum to the left, thoracic spine to the right. Note the two parallel rows of white echoes that represent the neural arches. Also shown are echoes of the vertebral bodies and the overlying intact skin. **B,** Fetus with a neural tube defect, clearly showing the meningomyelocele sac protruding through the skin. Compare with Figure 8-8. (Courtesy of A. Toi, Toronto General Hospital, Toronto, Canada.)

Prenatal Ultrasonography for Single-Gene Disorders

In some cases for which DNA testing is possible but a blood or tissue sample is unavailable for DNA or protein studies, diagnostic ultrasonography can be useful for prenatal diagnosis. For example, Figure 15-6B shows an abnormal fetal hand detected by ultrasound examination in a pregnancy at 50% risk for **Holt-Oram syndrome,** an autosomal dominant disorder characterized by congenital heart disease in association with hand anomalies.

Ultrasonography can also be used when the risk for a genetic disorder is uncertain because of insufficient history and laboratory testing to indicate that a fetus is definitively at risk for a particular disorder, but the parents have some valid cause for concern. For example, a woman may present at 16 weeks' gestation stating that her previous pregnancy resulted in a stillbirth with features highly suggestive of the severe bone disorder osteogenesis imperfecta, type II (see Chapter 12); no

tissue samples are available from the stillbirth. Osteogenesis imperfecta, type II, is usually due to a new dominant mutation, with an empirical recurrence risk of 6% due to germline mosaicism. In approximately 5% of families, however, the condition may be inherited in an autosomal recessive manner with 25% recurrence risk. Given that there is an increased recurrence risk of the disorder for this woman's current pregnancy, diagnostic ultrasonography is indicated. The finding of a normal fetus would be reassuring, whereas the identification of a fetus with multiple fractures would guide the management of the remainder of the pregnancy. Some laboratories may be prepared to undertake collagen testing in such situations if the couple chooses to have earlier, although invasive, testing.

Prenatal Ultrasonography for Multifactorial Disorders

A number of isolated abnormalities that may recur in families and that are believed to have multifactorial

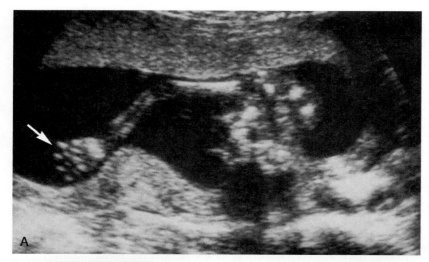

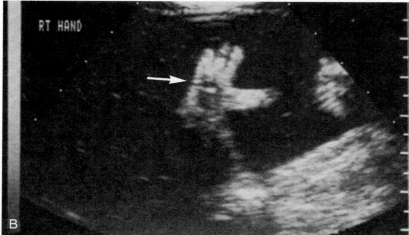

Figure 15-6 ■ Ultrasonograms of hands *(arrows).* **A,** Normal fetus. **B,** Fetus with Holt-Oram syndrome, an autosomal dominant defect with congenital heart defects (often an atrial septal defect) and variable limb abnormalities caused by mutations in the *TBX5* transcription factor gene. Note that there are only three obvious fingers and a thumb. The thumb is abnormal in shape (large and thick) and in position. (Courtesy of A. Toi, Toronto General Hospital, Toronto, Canada.)

Table 15-7

Examples of Defects That Can Be Diagnosed or Ruled Out by Prenatal Diagnostic Ultrasonography

SINGLE-GENE DISORDERS

Holoprosencephaly

Infantile polycystic kidney disease

Meckel-Gruber syndrome (an autosomal recessive disorder with encephalocele, polydactyly, and polycystic kidneys)

Fryns syndrome (an autosomal recessive disorder, generally perinatally lethal, with abnormalities of the face, diaphragm, limbs, genitourinary tract, and central nervous system)

DISORDERS USUALLY THOUGHT OF AS MULTIFACTORIAL

Cleft lip and other facial malformations

Clubfoot

Congenital heart defects

Neural tube defects

ANOMALIES THAT MAY INDICATE A SYNDROME

Abnormal genitalia

Cystic hygroma

Polydactyly

Omphalocele

Radial ray defects

Table 15-8

Prevalence of Chromosome Defects in Fetuses with Selected Isolated and Multiple Sonographically Detected Abnormalities

	Abnormal Karyotype (%)	
Abnormality	Isolated Finding	Multiple Findings
Ventriculomegaly	2	17
Choroid plexus cysts	1	48
Cystic hygroma	52	71
Nuchal edema	19	45
Diaphragmatic hernia	2	49
Heart defects	16	66
Duodenal atresia	38	64
Exomphalos	8	46
Renal abnormalities	3	24

Modified from Snijders RJM, Nicolaides KH: Ultrasound Markers for Fetal Chromosomal Defects. New York, Parthenon, 1996.

Table 15-9

Some Examples of Indications for Fetal Echocardiography*

MATERNAL INDICATIONS (% RISK FOR CONGENITAL HEART DEFECT)

Maternal disease
  Insulin-dependent diabetes mellitus (3%-5%)
  Phenylketonuria (15%)
Teratogen exposure
  Thalidomide (10% if 20-36 days post conception)
  Phenytoin (2%-3%)
  Alcohol (25% with fetal alcohol syndrome)
Maternal congenital heart disease (5%-10% for most lesions)
Abnormal maternal triple screen

FETAL INDICATIONS

Abnormal general fetal ultrasound
Arrhythmia
Chromosome abnormalities
Nuchal thickening
Nonimmune hydrops fetalis

FAMILIAL INDICATIONS

Mendelian syndromes (e.g., tuberous sclerosis, Noonan
  syndrome, velocardiofacial syndrome, Holt-Oram
  syndrome, Williams syndrome)
Paternal congenital heart disease (2%-5%)
Previously affected child (2%-4%, higher for certain lesions)

*This list is not comprehensive, and indications vary between centers.

inheritance can also be identified by ultrasonography (see Table 15-7), including neural tube malformations (see Fig. 15-5). Fetal echocardiography is offered at an increasing number of centers for a detailed assessment of pregnancies at risk for a congenital heart defect (Table 15-9).

Determination of Fetal Sex   Ultrasound examination can be used from 15 weeks of gestation onward to determine fetal sex. This determination may be an important prelude or adjunct in the prenatal diagnosis of certain X-linked recessive disorders (e.g., hemophilia) for those women identified to be at increased risk. A couple may decide not to proceed with invasive testing if a female (and therefore likely unaffected) fetus is identified by ultrasound examination.

The equipment and techniques used by ultrasonographers now allow the detection of many malformations by routine ultrasonography. Once a malformation has been detected or is suspected on routine ultrasound examination, a detailed ultrasound study in three and even four dimensions (three dimensions over time) may be indicated. In addition, a consultation with a clinical genetics unit or perinatal unit should be initiated for counseling and further investigation. The finding of a normal fetus can be cautiously reassuring, whereas the identification of a fetus with an abnormality allows the couple the option of either appropriate pregnancy and delivery management or pregnancy termination.

● LABORATORY STUDIES

Cytogenetics in Prenatal Diagnosis

Either amniocentesis or CVS can provide fetal cells for karyotyping as well as for biochemical or DNA analysis. Preparation and analysis of chromosomes from cultured amniotic fluid cells or cultured chorionic villi require 7 to 10 days, although chorionic villi can also be used for karyotyping after short-term incubation. Although short-term incubation provides a result more quickly, it yields relatively poorer quality preparations in which the banding resolution is inadequate for detailed analysis. Most laboratories use both techniques, but if only one is used, long-term culture of the cells of the mesenchymal core is the technique of choice at present.

Fluorescence in situ hybridization (see Chapters 4 and 5) makes it possible to screen interphase nuclei in fetal cells for the common aneuploidies of chromosomes 13, 18, 21, X, and Y immediately after amniocentesis or CVS. This approach for prenatal cytogenetic assessment requires 1 to 2 days and can be used when rapid aneuploidy testing is indicated.

Chromosome Analysis after Ultrasonography

Because some birth defects detectable by ultrasonography are associated with chromosome abnormalities, karyotyping of amniotic fluid cells, chorionic villus cells, or fetal blood cells obtained by insertion of a needle into an umbilical vessel (**cordocentesis**) may be indicated after ultrasonographic detection of such an abnormality. Chromosome abnormalities are more frequently found when multiple rather than isolated malformations are detected (see Table 15-8). The karyotypes most often seen in fetuses ascertained by abnormal ultrasonographic findings are the common autosomal trisomies (21, 18, and 13), 45,X (Turner syndrome), and unbalanced structural abnormalities. The presence of a cystic hygroma can indicate a 45,X karyotype, but it can also occur in Down syndrome and trisomy 18 as well as in fetuses with normal karyotypes. Thus, complete chromosome analysis is indicated.

Problems in Prenatal Chromosome Analysis

Mosaicism   Mosaicism refers to the presence of two or more cell lines in an individual or tissue sample. When mosaicism is found in cultured fetal cells, there may be problems in interpreting whether the fetus is truly mosaic and in determining the clinical significance of this apparent mosaicism.

Cytogeneticists distinguish three levels of mosaicism in amniotic fluid or CVS cell cultures:

1. **True mosaicism** is detected in multiple colonies from several different primary cultures. Postnatal studies

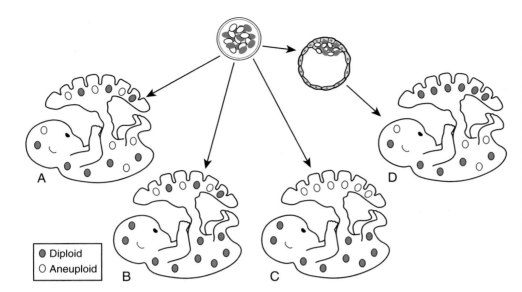

Figure 15-7 ■ The different types of mosaicism that may be detected by prenatal diagnosis. **A,** Generalized mosaicism affecting both the fetus and placenta. **B,** Confined placental mosaicism with normal and abnormal cell lineages present. **C,** Confined placental mosaicism with only an abnormal cell lineage present. **D,** Mosaicism confined to the embryo. (Modified from Kalousek DK: Current topic: confined placental mosaicism and intrauterine fetal development. Placenta 15: 219-230, 1994.)

● Diploid
○ Aneuploid

have confirmed that true mosaicism in culture is associated with a high risk that mosaicism is truly present in the fetus. The probability varies with different situations, however; mosaicism for structural aberrations of chromosomes, for example, is hardly ever confirmed.

2. **Pseudomosaicism,** an unusual karyotype seen in only a single cell, can usually be disregarded.

3. Mosaicism involving several cells or colonies of cells in a single primary culture only is difficult to interpret, but it is generally thought to reflect pseudomosaicism that has arisen in culture.

Maternal cell contamination is a possible explanation of some cases of apparent mosaicism in which both XX and XY cell lines are present. It is more common in long-term CVS cultures than in amniotic fluid cell cultures, as a consequence of the intimate association between the chorionic villi and the maternal tissue (see Fig. 15-2). To minimize the risk of maternal cell contamination, any maternal decidua present in a chorionic villus sample must be carefully dissected and removed, although even the most careful dissection of chorionic villi does not eliminate every cell of maternal origin. When maternal cell contamination is suspected and cannot be disproved (e.g., by DNA genotyping with use of polymorphisms), amniocentesis is recommended to allow a second chromosome analysis.

In CVS studies, discrepancies between the karyotypes found in the cytotrophoblast, villous stroma, and fetus have been reported in about 2% of pregnancies studied at 10 to 11 weeks of gestation. Mosaicism is sometimes present in the placenta but absent in the fetus, a situation termed **confined placental mosaicism** (Fig. 15-7). On occasion, placental mosaicism with a

normal cell line and a trisomic cell line has been reported when a liveborn infant or fetus has nonmosaic trisomy 13 or trisomy 18, the percentage of placental cells with a normal karyotype ranging from 12% to 100%. This finding suggests that when the zygote is trisomic, a normal placental cell lineage established by postzygotic loss of the additional chromosome in a progenitor cell of the cytotrophoblast can improve the probability of intrauterine survival of a trisomic fetus.

Confined placental mosaicism for any chromosome, but particularly for trisomy 15, raises the additional concern that the fetal diploidy may have actually arisen by **trisomy rescue.** This term refers to the loss of an extra chromosome postzygotically, an event that presumably allows fetal viability. If the fetus has retained two copies of chromosome 15 from one parent, however, the result is **uniparental disomy** (see Chapter 5). Because some genes on chromosome 15 are imprinted, uniparental disomy of this chromosome must be excluded because two maternal copies of chromosome 15 cause Prader-Willi syndrome and two paternal copies are associated with Angelman syndrome (see Chapter 5).

Confirmation and interpretation of mosaicism are among the most difficult challenges in genetic counseling for prenatal diagnosis because, at present, clinical outcome information on the numerous possible types and extents of mosaicism is inadequate. Further studies (amniocentesis that follows CVS, or cordocentesis that follows amniocentesis) as well as the medical literature may provide some guidance, but the interpretation sometimes still remains uncertain. Ultrasonographic scanning may provide some reassurance if normal growth is observed and if no congenital anomalies can be demonstrated.

Parents should be counseled in advance of the possibility that mosaicism may be found and that the interpretation of mosaicism may be uncertain. After birth, an effort should be made to verify any abnormal chromosome findings suspected on the basis of prenatal diagnosis. In the case of termination, verification should be sought by analysis of fetal tissues. Confirmation of mosaicism, or lack thereof, may prove helpful with respect to medical management issues as well as for genetic counseling of the specific couple and other family members.

Culture Failure   If couples are to have an opportunity to consider termination of a pregnancy when an abnormality is found in the fetus, they need to be provided with the information at the earliest possible time. Because prenatal diagnosis is always a race against time, the rate of culture failure can be a concern; fortunately, this rate is low. When a CVS culture fails to grow, there is time to repeat the chromosome study with amniocentesis. If an amniotic fluid cell culture fails, either repeated amniocentesis or a cordocentesis can be offered, depending on fetal age.

Unexpected Adverse Findings   On occasion, prenatal chromosome analysis performed primarily to rule out aneuploidy reveals some other unusual chromosome finding, for example, a normal chromosome number but a common variant (such as pericentric inversion of chromosome 9), a rare rearrangement, or a marker chromosome (see Chapter 5). In such a case, because the significance of the finding in the fetus cannot be assessed until the parental karyotypes are known, both parents should be karyotyped to determine whether the finding seen in the fetus is de novo or inherited. Unbalanced or de novo structural rearrangements may cause serious fetal abnormalities. If one parent is found to be a carrier of a structural rearrangement seen in unbalanced form in the fetus, the consequences for the fetus may be serious. On the other hand, if the same finding is seen in a normal parent, it is likely to be a benign change without untoward consequences. Potential exceptions to this guideline include the possibility of uniparental disomy in a region of the genome that contains imprinted genes (see Fig. 5-14). In this situation, an inherited balanced rearrangement may cause serious fetal abnormalities. This possibility can be excluded if there has been a previous transmission of the same balanced rearrangement from a parent of origin of the same sex as the transmitting parent in the current pregnancy.

Biochemical Assays for Metabolic Diseases

More than 100 metabolic disorders can be diagnosed prenatally in chorionic villus tissue or cultured amni-

Table 15-10

Examples of Metabolic Disorders Diagnosed by Enzyme Assay or DNA Analysis in Chorionic Villi or Cultured Amniotic Fluid Cells

AMINO ACID AND ORGANIC ACID DISORDERS

Phenylketonuria
Homocystinuria
Maple syrup urine disease
Methylmalonic acidemia
Propionic acidemia

CARBOHYDRATE DISORDERS

Galactosemia
Glycogen storage diseases, types II, III, IV

CHOLESTEROL AND STEROID METABOLISM DISORDERS

Smith-Lemli-Opitz syndrome
X-linked ichthyosis

LYSOSOMAL DISORDERS

Hurler syndrome
Krabbe disease
Niemann-Pick disease
Tay-Sachs disease

METAL METABOLISM DISORDERS

Menkes syndrome

PEROXISOMAL DISORDERS

Chondrodysplasia punctata
Zellweger syndrome
X-linked adrenoleukodystrophy

PURINE AND PYRIMIDINE DISORDERS

Adenosine deaminase deficiency

MISCELLANEOUS

Oculocerebrorenal syndrome of Lowe

otic fluid cells (Table 15-10), and a few rare conditions can even be identified directly by assay of a substance in amniotic fluid. Most metabolic disorders are rare in the general population but have a high recurrence risk (usually 25% within sibships, because most are autosomal recessive conditions). Because each condition is rare, the experience of the laboratory performing the prenatal diagnostic testing is important; thus, referral to specialized centers is preferable. Whenever possible, biochemical assay on direct chorionic villus tissue—as opposed to cultured tissue—is preferred to avoid misinterpretation of results due to the expansion in culture of the number of contaminating maternal cells. Access to a cultured cell line from a proband in the family is highly advisable so that the laboratory can confirm its ability to detect the biochemical abnormality in the proband before the assay is attempted in CVS or amniotic fluid cells from the pregnancy at risk.

Biochemical tests have one significant advantage over DNA analysis in some cases: whereas DNA analysis by direct detection of a mutation is accurate only for that mutation and not for other alleles at the locus, biochemical testing can detect abnormalities caused by any mutant allele that has a significant effect on the function of the protein. This advantage is particularly significant for disorders characterized by a high degree of allelic heterogeneity or by a high proportion of new mutations.

DNA Analysis

Numerous disorders, many of which were not previously detectable prenatally, can now be diagnosed by DNA analysis. DNA analysis can be performed either by direct detection of the mutation in question or by means of closely linked markers. Any technique used for direct mutation screening (see Chapter 4) can be used for prenatal diagnosis. The number of disorders that can be diagnosed and the precision and efficiency of analysis are increasing rapidly as new approaches are developed, as new mutations are characterized, and as additional genetic diseases are mapped.

When possible, direct methods of detecting a particular mutation are preferred. Because the spectrum of mutations varies from disorder to disorder and often varies between racial and ethnic groups within a particular disorder, the application of DNA analysis to prenatal diagnosis remains highly specialized, except for relatively more frequent diseases such as cystic fibrosis and fragile X syndrome; specific diagnostic laboratories develop particular expertise for the subset of genetic disorders most often seen in their practice or associated with their research. The degree of certainty of the diagnosis approaches 100% when direct detection of a mutation is possible. As noted earlier, however, if the disorder in the patient is due to a mutation different from the one that is being sought, DNA analysis will fail to detect it. Furthermore, prenatal diagnosis by DNA analysis may not be predictive of the exact clinical presentation in an affected pregnancy; for example, in neurofibromatosis type 1, a specific mutation may lead to a severe clinical manifestation in one family member and a mild manifestation in another.

When application of direct methods of DNA diagnosis is impossible or impractical, the indirect approach of genetic linkage analysis can be used. If linked DNA markers are available, the accuracy of diagnosis depends on how closely linked the markers are to the disease gene and on whether appropriate family studies can be performed and are informative (see Chapter 19).

Numerous diseases cannot yet be diagnosed prenatally, but every month additional disorders are added to the list of conditions for which prenatal diagnosis is possible either by biochemical testing or by DNA analysis. As of early 2007, a total of 735 genetic disorders were listed as being diagnosable prenatally in the GeneTests database of genetic testing laboratories. One of the contributions of genetics clinics to medical practice in general is keeping up with the rapid changes and serving as a central source of information about the current status of prenatal testing.

Mitochondrial disorders (see Chapters 7 and 12) that result from mutations in mitochondrial DNA are particularly challenging for prenatal counseling because the mutations are almost always heteroplasmic, and it is difficult to predict the fraction of defective mitochondrial genomes any one fetus will inherit. Although there is uncertainty concerning the degree of heteroplasmy that will be passed on from mother to fetus, DNA analysis of samples from the fetus obtained by CVS or amniocentesis is likely to reflect the overall degree of heteroplasmy in the fetus and therefore should be a reliable indicator of the burden of pathogenic mitochondrial mutations in the fetus.

● EMERGING TECHNOLOGIES FOR PRENATAL DIAGNOSIS

Preimplantation Genetic Diagnosis

Preimplantation genetic diagnosis is the use of molecular or cytogenetic techniques during **in vitro fertilization** to select embryos free of a specific genetic condition for transfer to the uterus. This technology was developed in an effort to offer an alternative option to those couples opposed to pregnancy termination and at significant risk for a specific genetic disorder or aneuploidy in their offspring. Preimplantation genetic diagnosis can be performed by micromanipulation techniques to remove a polar body (see Chapter 2) or by biopsy of a single cell from a six- to eight-cell embryo after in vitro fertilization. Molecular analysis by the polymerase chain reaction has been undertaken for a number of single-gene disorders and appears to give accurate results; chromosome abnormalities have also recently been diagnosed by fluorescence in situ hybridization (see Chapters 4 and 5). Embryos that are found not to carry the genetic abnormality in question after molecular or chromosome analyses can be transferred and allowed to implant, as is routinely done after in vitro fertilization for assisted reproduction. More than 7000 preimplantation genetic diagnoses have been performed worldwide, resulting in more than 1000 healthy liveborns; the few data currently available on this technology suggest that there are no detrimental effects to embryos that have undergone biopsy. Affected embryos are discarded. This practice has raised ethical concerns for those who consider this practice akin to abortion.

Screening for Segmental Duplications or Deletions

The ability of cytogenetic analysis to detect deletions or duplications is limited by the level of resolution of microscopy of banded chromosomes (see Chapter 5). Changes that are below approximately 1 to 2 Mb are usually not visible through the microscope. The technique of comparative genome hybridization onto arrays (see Chapter 4) is moving from the research to the clinical realm and is being applied to evaluations of patients, both in affected individuals and in the prenatal diagnosis setting. Much more needs to be learned about normal variation in copy number polymorphism (see Chapter 9) in order to interpret copy number changes detected in DNA samples from fetuses obtained by CVS or amniocentesis as being either normal variants or pathological changes of clinical significance.

○ PRENATAL PREVENTION AND MANAGEMENT OF GENETIC DISEASE

Disease Prevention Through Elective Pregnancy Termination

In most cases, the findings in prenatal diagnosis are normal, and parents are reassured that their baby will be unaffected by the condition in question. Unfortunately, in a small proportion of cases, the fetus is found to have a serious genetic defect. Because effective prenatal therapy is not available for most disorders, the parents may then choose to terminate the pregnancy. Few issues today are as hotly debated as elective abortion, but despite legal restrictions in some areas, elective abortion is widely used. Among all elective abortions, those performed because of prenatal diagnosis of an abnormality in the fetus account for only a very small proportion. Without a means of legal termination of pregnancy, prenatal diagnosis would not have developed into the accepted medical procedure that it has become.

Some pregnant women who would not consider termination nevertheless request prenatal diagnosis to reduce anxiety or to prepare for the birth of a child with a genetic disorder. The question then is whether the request is justified, because invasive techniques have an associated risk of fetal loss. In practice, the use of prenatal diagnosis by invasive techniques appears to be increasing because the risks are low compared with the couple's a priori risk and because many health care providers believe that parents are entitled to the information. This information may be used for psychological preparation as well as for management of the delivery and of the newborn infant.

At the population level, prenatal diagnosis combined with elective abortion has led to a major decline in the incidence of a few serious disorders, such as β-thalassemia (see Chapter 11) and Tay-Sachs disease (see Chapter 12) in designated population groups. There has also been a decline of nearly 8% in the birth of children with Down syndrome in the United States, primarily to women younger than 35 years, as a result of maternal serum and ultrasound screening followed by CVS or amniocentesis.

The principal advantage of prenatal diagnosis is not to the population but to the immediate family. Parents at risk of having a child with a serious abnormality can undertake pregnancies that they may otherwise not have risked, with the knowledge that they can learn early in a pregnancy whether the fetus has the abnormality. For the population as a whole, there is a theoretical possibility that the frequency of some deleterious genes will increase in the population if couples compensate for the loss of homozygotes by having additional children, who have a two thirds risk of being heterozygotes.

Prenatal Treatment

In a few situations, prenatal diagnosis can be used to identify fetuses at risk for serious birth defects or genetic disorders to provide treatment before the birth of the infant (see Chapter 13). The most successful prenatal treatments have been for metabolic disorders for which maternal medical therapy can be administered. For example, maternal glucocorticoid treatment during pregnancies with fetuses at risk for congenital adrenal hyperplasia is an experimental therapy that can prevent pseudohermaphroditism (see Chapter 6) and improves fetal development. Fetuses affected by vitamin B_{12}–responsive methylmalonic acidemia have been treated successfully by administration of the vitamin during pregnancy. Surgical interventions have also been attempted (see Table 13-2). For example, severe fetal bladder outlet obstruction can be detected by fetal ultrasound examination. If untreated, the consequent reduction in urine production would cause severe oligohydramnios and poor lung development (Potter syndrome). Relief of the bladder obstruction by shunting procedures in utero can prevent irreversible damage to the developing lungs and improve postnatal renal function. Percutaneous introduction of shunts under endoscopic guidance appears to be associated with less morbidity than the use of endoscopy, which in turn generated fewer complications than open hysterotomy. Finally, prenatal bone marrow transplantation has been carried out in a small number of fetuses with severe combined immunodeficiency diagnosed prenatally by direct mutation detection. Bone marrow transplantation from a haploidentical donor (such as a parent) appears to have a greater chance of successful engraftment and more complete immune reconstitution when it is done prenatally rather than postnatally. The procedure is not without its own risks, however, and more experience is required before there is an accurate assessment of benefits and risks.

● GENETIC COUNSELING FOR PRENATAL DIAGNOSIS

The majority of genetic counselors practice in the setting of a prenatal diagnosis program. The complexities posed by the availability of different tests (including the distinction between screening tests and diagnostic tests), the many different and distinctive indications for testing in different families, the subtleties of interpretation of test results, and the personal, ethical, and religious issues that enter into reproductive decision-making all make the provision of prenatal diagnosis services a challenging arena for counselors. The professional staff of the prenatal diagnosis program (physician, nurse, and genetic counselor) must obtain an accurate family history and determine whether other previously unsuspected genetic problems should also be considered on the basis of family history or ethnic background. Ethnic background, even in the absence of a positive family history, may indicate the need for carrier tests in the parents in advance of prenatal diagnostic testing. For example, in a couple referred for any reason, one must discuss carrier testing for autosomal recessive disorders with increased frequency in various ethnic groups. Such disorders include thalassemia in individuals from Mediterranean or Asian background; sickle cell anemia in Africans or African Americans; and Tay-Sachs disease, Canavan disease, cystic fibrosis, familial dysautonomia, Fanconi anemia group C, Gaucher disease, and Niemann-Pick disease types A and B in the fetus of an Ashkenazi Jewish couple.

Parents considering prenatal diagnosis for advanced maternal age, for an abnormal first- or second-trimester screen, or for a specific indication based on family history, carrier testing, or ethnic background need information that will allow them to understand their situation and to give or withhold consent for the procedure. Genetic counseling of candidates for prenatal diagnosis usually deals with the following: the risk that the fetus will be affected; the nature and probable consequences of the specific problem; the risks and limitations of the procedures to be used; the time required before a report can be issued; and the possible need for a repeated procedure in the event of a failed attempt. In addition, the couple must be advised that a result may be difficult to interpret, that further tests and consultation may be required, and that even then the results may not necessarily be definitive.

Although the great majority of prenatal diagnoses end in reassurance, options available to parents in the event of an abnormality—of which termination of pregnancy is only one—should be discussed. *Above all, the parents must understand that in undertaking prenatal diagnosis, they are under no implied obligation to terminate a pregnancy in the event that an abnormality is detected.* The objective of prenatal diagnosis is to determine whether the fetus is affected or unaffected with the disorder in question. Diagnosis of an affected fetus may, at the least, allow the parents to prepare emotionally and medically for the management of a newborn with a disorder.

● GENERAL REFERENCES

Benn PA, Hsu LYF: Prenatal diagnosis of chromosome abnormalities through amniocentesis. In Milunsky A: Genetic Disorders and the Fetus: Diagnosis, Prevention, and Treatment, 5th ed. Baltimore, Johns Hopkins University Press, 2004.

Dimmick JE, Kalousek DK: Developmental Pathology of the Embryo and Fetus. Philadelphia, JB Lippincott, 1992.

Gardner RJM, Sutherland GR: Chromosome Abnormalities and Genetic Counseling, 3rd ed. New York, Oxford University Press, 2003.

● REFERENCES FOR SPECIFIC TOPICS

ACOG Practice Bulletin #77: Screening for fetal chromosomal abnormalities. Obstet Gynecol 109:217-228, 2007.

Eddleman KA, Malone FD, Sullivan L, et al: Pregnancy loss rates after midtrimester amniocentesis. Obstet Gynecol 108:1067-1072, 2006.

Evans MI, Wapner RJ: Invasive prenatal diagnostic procedures 2005. Semin Perinatol 29:215-218, 2005.

Friedman AH, Kleinman CS, Copel JA: Diagnosis of cardiac defects: where we've been, where we are and where we're going. Prenat Diagn 22:280-284, 2002.

Handyside AH, Scriven PN, Ogilvie CM: The future of preimplantation genetic diagnosis. Hum Reprod Suppl 14:249-255, 1998.

Kuliev A, Verlinsky Y: Preimplantation diagnosis: a realistic option for assisted reproduction and genetic practice. Curr Opin Obstet Gynecol 17:179-183, 2005.

Muench MO: In utero transplantation: baby steps towards an effective therapy. Bone Marrow Transplant 35:537-547, 2005.

O'Brien B, Bianchi DW: Fetal therapy for single gene disorders. Clin Obstet Gynecol 48:885-896, 2005.

Orlandi F, Bilardo CM, Campogrande M, et al: Measurement of nasal bone length at 11-14 weeks of pregnancy and its potential role in Down syndrome risk assessment. Ultrasound Obstet Gynecol 22:36-39, 2003.

Reddy UM, Mennutti MT: Incorporating first-trimester Down syndrome studies into prenatal screening. Obstet Gynecol 107:167-173, 2006.

Snijders RJM, Nicolaides KH: Ultrasound Markers for Fetal Chromosomal Defects. New York, Parthenon, 1996.

The Canadian Early and Midtrimester Amniocentesis Trial (CEMAT) Group: Randomised trial to assess safety and fetal outcome of early and midtrimester amniocentesis. Lancet 351: 242-247, 1998.

Wilcox AJ, Lie RT, Solvoll K, et al: Folic acid supplements and risk of facial clefts: national population based case-control study. BMJ 334:464-469, 2007.

● USEFUL WEBSITES

GeneTests: *http://www.genetests.org/* A U.S. government-supported website (copyright, University of Washington) maintained by the University of Washington providing information on testing laboratories as well as educational material on genetic testing, including prenatal diagnosis.

New York Online Access to Health (NOAH). *http://www.noah-health.org/en/search/health.html* A joint effort by the City University of New York, the Metropolitan New York Library Council, the New York Academy of Medicine, and the New York Public Library to provide health information online. Includes information on prenatal diagnosis from the March of Dimes Birth Defects Foundation.

 PROBLEMS

1. Match the term in the top section with the appropriate comment in the bottom section.
   a. Rh immune globulin
   b. 10th week of pregnancy
   c. cordocentesis
   d. mosaicism
   e. 16th week of pregnancy
   f. alpha-fetoprotein in maternal serum
   g. aneuploidy
   h. cystic hygroma
   i. chorionic villi
   j. amniotic fluid

   _____ method of obtaining fetal blood for karyotyping
   _____ usual time at which amniocentesis is performed
   _____ increased level when fetus has neural tube defect
   _____ contains fetal cells viable in culture
   _____ major cytogenetic problem in prenatal diagnosis
   _____ ultrasonographic diagnosis indicates possible Turner syndrome
   _____ risk increases with maternal age
   _____ usual time at which CVS is performed
   _____ derived from extraembryonic tissue
   _____ used to prevent immunization of Rh-negative women

2. A couple has a child with Down syndrome, who has a 21q21q translocation inherited from the mother. Could prenatal diagnosis be helpful in the couple's next pregnancy? Explain.

3. Cultured cells from a chorionic villus sample show two cell lines, 46,XX and 46,XY. Does this necessarily mean the fetus is abnormal? Explain.

4. What two chief types of information about a fetus can be indicated (although not proved) by assay of alpha-fetoprotein, human chorionic gonadotropin, and unconjugated estriol in maternal serum during the second trimester?

5. A couple has had a first-trimester spontaneous abortion in their first pregnancy and requests counseling.
   a. What proportion of all pregnancies abort in the first trimester?
   b. What is the most common genetic abnormality found in such cases?
   c. Assuming that there are no other indications, should this couple be offered prenatal diagnosis for their next pregnancy?

6. A young woman consults a geneticist during her first pregnancy. Her brother was previously diagnosed with Duchenne muscular dystrophy and had since died. He was the only affected person in her family. The woman had been tested biochemically and found to have elevated creatine kinase levels, indicating she is a carrier of the disease.

   Unfortunately, no DNA analysis had been conducted on the woman's brother to determine what type of mutation in the *DMD* gene he had. The woman was investigated by molecular analysis and found to be heterozygous (*A1/A2*) for a microsatellite marker closely linked to the *DMD* gene. No relatives except the parents of the woman were available for analysis.
   a. Can the phase of the mutation in the woman be determined from analysis of the available individuals?
   b. Can this information be used to diagnose her pregnancy?
   c. What other molecular analysis could be performed on the fetus?

7. Discuss the relative advantages and disadvantages of the following diagnostic procedures and cite types of disorders for which they are indicated or not indicated: amniocentesis, CVS, first-semester maternal serum screening.

8. Suppose the frequency of Down syndrome is 1/600 in pregnancies in women younger than 35 years. Consider the following two strategies for prenatal detection of the disorder:
   • All pregnant women younger than 35 years are offered CVS or amniocentesis.
   • All pregnant women undergo a sequential screening strategy, as follows: All participate in first-trimester screening with PAPP-A, hCG, and nuchal translucency. Sensitivity is 84% with a false-positive rate of 5%. Those who score positive are offered CVS, and all use it. Those who score negative are screened during the second trimester with a quadruple maternal serum screening, which has 81% sensitivity and 5% false-positive rate. Those who score positive are offered amniocentesis, and all use it.

   Assuming that a population of 600,000 women younger than 35 years are pregnant:
   a. How many CVS procedures or amniocenteses are done overall given these two strategies?
   b. What fraction of the total expected number of affected fetuses is detected under the two strategies? What fraction is missed?
   c. How many CVS or amniocentesis procedures would need to be done to detect one fetus with Down syndrome under these two strategies?

Chapter 16

Cancer Genetics and Genomics

Cancer is one of the most common and severe diseases seen in clinical medicine. Statistics show that cancer in some form strikes more than one third of the population, accounts for more than 20% of all deaths, and, in developed countries, is responsible for more than 10% of the total cost of medical care. Cancer is invariably fatal if it is not treated. Early diagnosis and early treatment are vital, and identification of persons at increased risk of cancer before its development is an important objective of cancer research.

In this chapter, we describe how molecular genetic studies demonstrate that *cancer is fundamentally a genetic disease.* We describe the kinds of genes that have been implicated in initiating cancer, and the mechanisms by which dysfunction of these genes can result in the disease. Second, we review a number of heritable cancer syndromes and demonstrate how insights gained into their pathogenesis have illuminated the basis of the much more common, sporadic forms of cancer. We also examine some of the special challenges that such heritable syndromes present for medical genetics and genetic counseling. Third, we will show that genetics and genomics have changed both how we think about the causes of cancer and how we diagnose and treat the disease. Genomics—in particular the identification of deletion and duplication of segments of the cancer cell genome and the comprehensive analysis of gene expression and mutation in cancer cells—is truly changing cancer diagnosis and treatment.

Cancer is not a single disease but rather a name used to describe the more virulent forms of **neoplasia,** a disease process characterized by uncontrolled cellular proliferation leading to a mass or tumor (**neoplasm**). For a neoplasm to be a cancer, however, it must also be **malignant,** which means its growth is no longer controlled and the tumor is capable of progression by invading neighboring tissues, spreading (**metastasizing**) to more distant sites, or both. Tumors that do not invade or metastasize are not cancerous but are referred to as **benign** tumors, although their size and location may make them anything but benign to the patient. There are three main forms of cancer: **sarcomas,** in which the tumor has arisen in mesenchymal tissue, such as bone, muscle, or connective tissue, or in nervous system tissue; **carcinomas,** which originate in epithelial tissue, such as the cells lining the intestine, bronchi, or mammary ducts; and **hematopoietic** and **lymphoid** malignant neoplasms, such as leukemia and lymphoma, which spread throughout the bone marrow, lymphatic system, and peripheral blood. Within each of the major groups, tumors are classified by site, tissue type, histological appearance, and degree of malignancy.

● GENETIC BASIS OF CANCER

Neoplasia is an abnormal accumulation of cells that occurs because of an imbalance between cellular proliferation and cellular attrition. Cells proliferate as they pass through the cell cycle and undergo mitosis. Attrition, due to programmed cell death (see Chapter 14), removes cells from a tissue (Fig. 16-1).

The development of cancer (**oncogenesis**) results from mutations in one or more of the vast array of genes that regulate cell growth and programmed cell death. When cancer occurs as part of a **hereditary cancer syndrome,** the initial cancer-causing mutation is inherited through the germline and is therefore already present in every cell of the body. Most cancers, however, are **sporadic** because the mutations occur in a single somatic cell, which then divides and proceeds to develop into the cancer. It is not surprising that somatic muta-

••• The Genetic Basis of Cancer

- Regardless of whether a cancer occurs sporadically in an individual, as a result of **somatic mutation,** or repeatedly in many individuals in a family as a hereditary trait, cancer is a genetic disease.

- Genes in which mutations cause cancer fall into two distinct categories: **oncogenes** and **tumor-suppressor genes** (TSGs). TSGs in turn are either **"gatekeepers"** or **"caretakers"** (Fig. 16-1).

- An **oncogene** is a mutant allele of a **proto-oncogene,** a class of normal cellular protein-coding genes that promote growth and survival of cells. Oncogenes facilitate malignant transformation by stimulating proliferation or inhibiting apoptosis. Oncogenes encode proteins such as:

  - proteins in signaling pathways for cell proliferation
  - transcription factors that control the expression of growth-promoting genes
  - inhibitors of programmed cell death machinery

- **Gatekeeper TSGs** control cell growth. Gatekeeper genes block tumor development by regulating the transition of cells through checkpoints ("gates") in the cell cycle (see Chapter 2) or by promoting programmed cell death and, thereby, controlling cell division and survival. Loss-of-function mutations of gatekeeper genes lead to uncontrolled cell accumulation. Gatekeeper TSGs encode:

  - regulators of various cell-cycle checkpoints
  - mediators of programmed cell death

- **Caretaker TSGs** protect the integrity of the genome. Loss of function of caretaker genes permits mutations to accu-

mulate in oncogenes and gatekeeper genes, which, in concert, go on to initiate and promote cancer. Caretaker TSGs encode:

  - proteins responsible for detecting and repairing mutations
  - proteins involved in normal chromosome disjunction during mitosis
  - components of programmed cell death machinery

- **Tumor initiation.** Different types of genetic alterations are responsible for **initiating cancer.** These include mutations such as:

  - activating or gain-of-function mutations, including gene amplification, point mutations, and promoter mutations, that turn one allele of a proto-oncogene into an oncogene
  - ectopic and heterochronic mutations (see Chapter 11) of proto-oncogenes
  - **chromosome translocations** that cause misexpression of genes or create chimeric genes encoding proteins with novel functional properties
  - loss of function of both alleles, or a dominant negative mutation of one allele, of TSGs.

- **Tumor progression.** Once initiated, a cancer progresses by accumulating additional genetic damage, through mutations or epigenetic silencing, of caretaker genes that encode the machinery that repairs damaged DNA and maintains cytogenetic normality. A further consequence of genetic damage is altered expression of genes that promote vascularization and the spread of the tumor through local invasion and distant metastasis.

tions can cause cancer. Large numbers of cell divisions are required to produce an adult organism of an estimated 10^{14} cells from a single-cell zygote. Given a frequency of 10^{-10} replication errors per base of DNA per cell division, and an estimated 10^{15} cell divisions during

the lifetime of an adult, replication errors alone result in thousands of new DNA mutations in the genome in every cell of the organism. Genome and chromosome mutations add to the mutational burden. The genes mutated in cancer are not inherently more mutable than

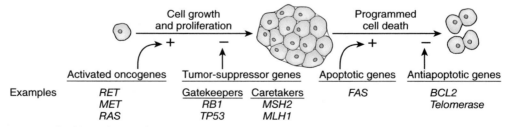

Figure 16-1 ■ General scheme for mechanisms of oncogenesis by proto-oncogene activation, loss of tumor-suppressor gene expression, activation of antiapoptotic genes, or loss of proapoptotic gene expression. The effect of genes that enhance a process is shown as +, whereas the effect of genes that suppress a process is shown as −. Cell division and proliferation are stimulated by the products of proto-oncogenes. Some tumor-suppressor genes directly regulate proto-oncogene function *(gatekeepers);* others act more indirectly by maintaining genome integrity and correcting mutations during DNA replication and cell division *(caretakers).* Activation of an antiapoptotic gene allows excessive accumulation of cells, whereas loss of function of apoptotic genes has the same effect. Activation of oncogenes or antiapoptotic genes is dominant and requires only a single mutant allele. Mutations in tumor-suppressor genes are recessive; when both alleles are mutated or inactivated, cell growth is unregulated or genomic integrity is compromised. Loss of proapoptotic genes may occur through loss of both alleles or through a dominant negative mutation in one allele.

other genes. Many mutations doubtlessly occur in somatic cells and cause one cell among many to lose function or die, but they have no phenotypic effects because the loss of one cell is masked by the vast majority of healthy cells in an organ or tissue. What distinguishes oncogenic mutations is that, by their very nature, they allow even one mutant cell to develop into a life-threatening disease.

The catalogue of genes involved in cancer also includes genes that are transcribed into **noncoding RNAs** from which regulatory **microRNAs (miRNAs)** are generated (see Chapter 3). There are at least 250 miRNAs in the human genome that carry out RNA-mediated inhibition of the expression of their target protein-coding genes, either by inducing the degradation of their targets' mRNAs or by blocking their translation. Approximately 10% of miRNAs have been found to be either greatly overexpressed or down-regulated in various tumors, sometimes strikingly so, and are referred to as **oncomirs**. One example is the 100-fold overexpression of the miRNA miR-21 in **glioblastoma multiforme**, a highly malignant form of brain cancer. Overexpression of some miRNAs can suppress the expression of tumor-suppressor gene targets, whereas loss of function of other miRNAs may allow overexpression of the oncogenes they regulate. Since each miRNA may regulate as many as 200 different gene targets, overexpression or loss of function of miRNAs may have widespread oncogenic effects because many genes will be dysregulated.

Once it is initiated, a cancer progresses by accumulating additional genetic damage through mutations in caretaker genes encoding the cellular machinery that repairs damaged DNA and maintains cytogenetic normality (Fig. 16-2). Damage to these genes produces an ever-widening cascade of mutations in an increasing assortment of the genes that control cellular proliferation and repair DNA damage. In this way, the original clone of neoplastic cells serves as a reservoir of genetically unstable cells, referred to as **cancer stem cells**. These give rise to multiple sublineages of varying degrees of malignancy, each carrying a set of mutations that are different from but overlap with mutations carried in other sublineages. In this sense, cancer is fundamentally a "genetic" disease, and mutations are central to its etiology and progression.

A paradigm for the development of cancer, as illustrated in Figure 16-2, provides a useful conceptual framework for considering the role of genetic changes in cancer, a point we emphasize throughout this chapter. It is a general model that probably applies to many if not most cancers, although it is best elucidated in the case of colon cancer (see later in this chapter).

Cancer in Families

Many forms of cancer have a higher incidence in relatives of patients than in the general population. Most prominent among these familial forms of cancer are the nearly 50 mendelian hereditary cancer syndromes in which the risk of cancer is very high and the approximately 100 additional mendelian disorders listed in *Online Inheritance in Man* that predispose to cancer (Cases 3, 13, 19, and 34). Extensive epidemiological studies

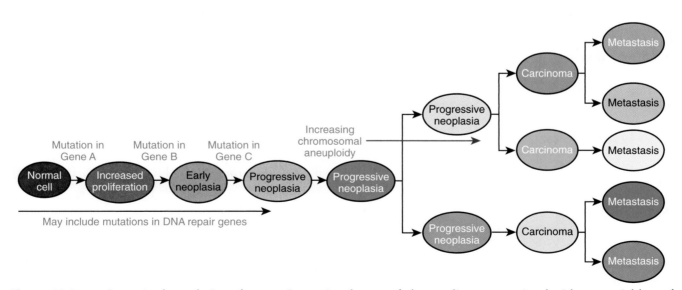

Figure 16-2 ■ Stages in the evolution of cancer. Increasing degrees of abnormality are associated with sequential loss of tumor-suppressor genes from several chromosomes and activation of proto-oncogenes, with or without a concomitant defect in DNA repair. For example, sporadic cancer with DNA repair defects is less common than are cancers without abnormal repair but, when present, may develop along a somewhat different, but parallel, pathway leading to the final common endpoint of malignancy. Multiple lineages carrying somewhat different mutational spectra and epigenetic changes are likely, particularly once metastatic disease appears.

have shown, however, that some families have an above-average risk of cancer even in the absence of an obvious mendelian inheritance pattern. For example, an increased incidence of cancer, in the range of 2- to 3-fold, has been observed in first-degree relatives of probands with most forms of cancer, which suggests that many cancers are complex traits resulting from both genetic and environmental factors (see Chapter 8). Thus, a family history of cancer in multiple first-degree or second-degree relatives of a patient should arouse the physician's suspicion of increased cancer risk in the patient.

Although individuals with a hereditary cancer syndrome represent probably less than 5% of all patients with cancer, identification of a genetic basis for their disease has great importance both for clinical management of these families and for understanding cancer in general. First, the relatives of individuals with strong hereditary predispositions, which are most often due to mutations in a single gene, can be offered testing and counseling to provide appropriate reassurance or more intensive monitoring and therapy, depending on the results of testing. Second, as is the case with many common diseases, understanding the hereditary forms of the disease provides crucial insights into disease mechanisms that go far beyond the rare hereditary forms themselves.

● ONCOGENES

An **oncogene** is a mutant gene whose altered function or expression results in abnormal stimulation of cell division and proliferation. The mutation can be an activating gain-of-function mutation in the coding sequence of the oncogene itself, a mutation in its regulatory elements, or an increase in its genomic copy number, leading to unregulated heterochronic or ectopic function of the oncogene product (see Chapter 11). Oncogenes have a dominant effect at the cellular level; that is, when it is activated or overexpressed, a single mutant allele is sufficient to initiate the change in phenotype of a cell from normal to malignant.

Activated oncogenes encode proteins that act in many steps in the pathway that controls cell growth, including growth factors that stimulate cell division, the receptors and cytoplasmic proteins that transduce these signals, the transcription factors that respond to the transduced signals, and the proteins that counteract programmed cell death (apoptosis) (Fig. 16-3).

Activated Oncogenes in Hereditary Cancer Syndromes

Multiple Endocrine Adenomatosis, Type 2

Multiple endocrine adenomatosis, type 2 (MEN2), in its more common type A variant, is an autosomal domi-

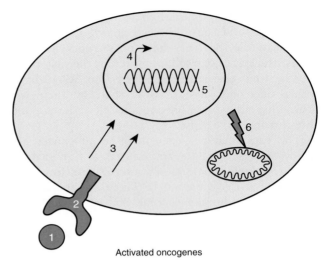

Activated oncogenes

Class	Example	Types of cancer
1. Growth factors	Sis	Glioma
2. Receptor tyrosine kinase	Ret	Multiple endocrine adenomatosis 2
3. Cytoplasmic tyrosine kinase	Abl	Chronic myelogenous leukemia
G protein signaling	K-Ras2	Pancreatic cancer
Phosphoinositide 3-kinase	PTEN	Breast cancer, glioma
4. Transcription factors	Myc	Burkitt lymphoma
5. Telomerase	Telomerase	Many
6. Antiapoptotic proteins	Bcl2	Chronic lymphocytic leukemia

Figure 16-3 ■ Mechanisms of tumorigenesis by oncogenes of various classes. Unregulated growth factor signaling may be due to mutations in genes encoding growth factors themselves (1), their receptors (2), or intracellular signaling pathways (3). Downstream targets of growth factors include transcription factors (4), whose expression may become unregulated. Both telomerase (5) and antiapoptotic proteins that act at the mitochondria (6) may interfere with cell death and lead to tumorigenesis.

nant disorder characterized by a high incidence of medullary carcinoma of the thyroid that is often but not always associated with pheochromocytoma, benign parathyroid adenomas, or both. Patients with the rarer type B variant, termed MEN2B, have, in addition to the tumors seen in patients with MEN2A, thickening of nerves and the development of benign neural tumors, known as **neuromas,** on the mucosal surface of the mouth and lips.

The mutations responsible for MEN2 are in the *RET* gene, which encodes a receptor tyrosine kinase that serves as a receptor for two ligands, glial cell line–derived growth factor and neurturin, and is the same gene implicated in Hirschsprung disease (Case 20) (see Chapter 8). Tyrosine kinase receptors transduce an external signal, such as the binding of the receptor's ligand, by dimerizing and undergoing conformational change. Change in the receptor induced by the ligand activates an intrinsic kinase activity that phosphory-

Table 16-1

Mechanisms of Activation of Proto-oncogenes

Mechanism	Type of Gene Activated	Result
Regulatory mutation	Growth factor genes	Increased expression
Structural mutation	Growth factor receptors, signal-transducing proteins	Allows autonomy of expression
Translocation, retroviral insertion, gene amplification	Transcription factors	Overexpression
Regulatory mutation, translocation, retroviral insertion	Oncomirs	Overexpression, down-regulates tumor-suppressor genes
Deletion, inactivating mutation	Oncomirs	Loss of expression, up-regulates oncogenes

From Miller DM, Blume S, Borst M, et al: Oncogenes, malignant transformation, and modern medicine. Am J Med Sci 300:59-69, 1990; and Esquela A, Slack FJ: Oncomirs—microRNAs with a role in cancer. Nat Rev Cancer 6:259-269, 2006.

lates other cellular proteins, thereby initiating a cascade of changes in protein-protein and DNA-protein interactions and in the enzymatic activity of many proteins. As opposed to the *loss-of-function* mutations in *RET* found in Hirschsprung disease, the *RET* mutations in MEN2A and MEN2B are specific point mutations that *activate* the receptor and cause it to phosphorylate tyrosines even in the absence of binding by ligand. Individuals who inherit an activating mutation in *RET* have an approximately 60% chance of developing symptomatic medullary carcinoma of the thyroid, although more sensitive tests, such as blood tests for thyrocalcitonin or urinary catecholamines synthesized by pheochromocytomas, are abnormal in well above 90% of heterozygotes for MEN2.

Clonality and Tissue Specificity of Multiple Endocrine Adenomatosis Type 2 and Hereditary Papillary Renal Carcinoma

Although we know from the hereditary nature of medullary thyroid carcinoma that mutations in *RET* are the underlying cause of the cancer, not all of the parafollicular cells of the thyroid actually become cancerous, indicating that the oncogenes themselves are not sufficient to cause the disease. Other genome and chromosome mutations are known to occur, such as loss of a portion of chromosome 1p in the medullary thyroid carcinomas in MEN2A. These second events arise at multiple sites in the genomes of individual cells, each of which then divides and develops into a tumor that originates from a single cell and is thus said to be **clonal.**

The *RET* gene is expressed in many tissues of the body and is required for normal embryonic development of autonomic ganglia and kidney. It remains completely unknown why germline activating mutations in this proto-oncogene result in a particular cancer of distinct histological type restricted to specific tissues, whereas other tissues in which the oncogene is expressed do not develop tumors.

Activated Oncogenes in Sporadic Cancer

Well before the discovery of hereditary cancer syndromes due to autosomal dominant inheritance of activated proto-oncogenes, many mutated oncogenes, including *RET* and *MET*, had been identified in sporadic cancers by molecular studies of cell lines derived from these tumors. One of the first activated oncogenes discovered was a mutant *RAS* gene derived from a bladder carcinoma cell line. *RAS* encodes one of a large family of small guanosine triphosphate (GTP)–binding proteins (**G proteins**). G proteins serve as molecular "on-off" switches that activate or inhibit downstream molecules when bound to GTP but then terminate their effect when the bound GTP is cleaved to guanosine diphosphate by an intrinsic GTPase enzymatic activity. Remarkably, the activated oncogene and its normal counterpart proto-oncogene differed at only a single nucleotide. The alteration, a point mutation in a somatic cell, led to synthesis of an abnormal Ras protein that was able to signal continuously, even in the absence of bound GTP. The mutant *RAS* stimulated the growth of the cell line, thus changing it into a tumor. *RAS* point mutations are observed in many tumors, and the *RAS* genes have been shown experimentally to be the mutational target of known carcinogens, a finding that supports a role for mutated *RAS* genes in the development of many cancers. To date, more than 50 human oncogenes (and therefore also their normal proto-oncogenes) have been identified. Only a few of these proto-oncogenes have been found to be inherited in any hereditary cancer syndromes.

Activation of Oncogenes by Chromosome Translocation

Oncogenes are not always the result of a DNA mutation. In some instances, a proto-oncogene is activated by a chromosome mutation, usually through translocation (Table 16-1). More than 40 oncogenic chromosome translocations have been described, primarily in spo-

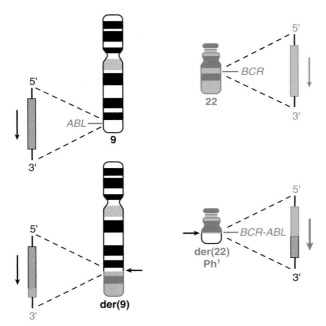

Figure 16-4 ■ The Philadelphia chromosome translocation, t(9;22)(q34;q11). The Philadelphia chromosome (Ph¹) is the derivative chromosome 22, which has exchanged part of its long arm for a segment of material from chromosome 9q that contains the *ABL* oncogene. Formation of the chimeric *BCR-ABL* gene on the Ph¹ chromosome is the critical genetic event in the development of chronic myelogenous leukemia.

radic leukemias and lymphomas but also in a few rare connective tissue sarcomas. In some cases, the translocation breakpoints are within the introns of two genes, thereby fusing two genes into one abnormal gene that encodes a chimeric protein with novel oncogenic properties. The best-known example is the translocation between chromosomes 9 and 22 that is seen in chronic myelogenous leukemia (Fig. 16-4) **(Case 8)**. In others, the translocation activates an oncogene by placing it downstream of a strong, constitutive promoter belonging to another gene. Two well-known

examples are the translocation between chromosomes 8 and 14 in Burkitt lymphoma and the translocation involving chromosome 18 in B-cell lymphoma.

Chronic Myelogenous Leukemia   In chronic myelogenous leukemia, the cytogenetic abnormality seen, the so-called Philadelphia chromosome (Ph¹), is the product of a translocation between chromosomes 9 and 22 **(Case 8)**. The translocation moves the proto-oncogene *ABL*, a tyrosine kinase, from its normal position on chromosome 9q to the "breakpoint cluster region" gene (*BCR*), a gene of unknown function on chromosome 22q. The juxtaposition of *BCR* sequences and *ABL* sequences allows the synthesis of a chimeric protein that is longer than the normal Abl protein and has increased tyrosine kinase activity. The enhanced tyrosine kinase activity of the novel protein encoded by the chimeric gene is the primary event causing the chronic leukemia. A new, highly effective drug therapy for chronic myelogenous leukemia, imatinib, has been developed that is based on inhibition of this tyrosine kinase activity.

Burkitt Lymphoma   Burkitt lymphoma is a B-cell tumor of the jaw that has an unusual geographical distribution; it is the most common tumor of children in equatorial Africa but is rare elsewhere. In most tumors of this type, the *MYC* proto-oncogene is translocated from its normal chromosomal position at 8q24 to a position distal to the immunoglobulin heavy-chain locus at 14q32. Cytogenetically, this mutation is seen as an apparently balanced 8;14 translocation. The translocation presumably brings enhancer or other transcriptional activating sequences, normally associated with the immunoglobulin genes, near to the *MYC* gene. Supporting this hypothesis is the finding that other translocations observed in a smaller proportion of Burkitt lymphoma cases involve translocating immunoglobulin light-chain genes on chromosomes 22 and 2 near to the *MYC* gene (Table 16-2). In either case, these translocations clearly have an important effect on

Table 16-2

Characteristic Chromosome Translocations in Selected Human Malignant Neoplasms

Neoplasm	Chromosome Translocation	Percentage of Cases	Proto-oncogene Affected
Burkitt lymphoma	t(8;14)(q24;q32)	80%	
	t(8;22)(q24;q11)	15%	*MYC*
	t(2;8)(q11;q24)	5%	
Chronic myelogenous leukemia	t(9;22)(q34;q11)	90%-95%	*BCR-ABL*
Acute lymphocytic leukemia	t(9;22)(q34;q11)	10%-15%	*BCR-ABL*
Acute lymphoblastic leukemia	t(1;19)(q23;p13)	3%-6%	*TCF3-PBX1*
Acute promyelocytic leukemia	t(15;17)(q22;q11)	~95%	*RARA-PML*
Chronic lymphocytic leukemia	t(11;14)(q13;q32)	10%-30%	*BCL1*
Follicular lymphoma	t(14;18)(q32;q21)	~100%	*BCL2*

Based on Croce CM: Role of chromosome translocations in human neoplasia. Cell 49:155-156, 1987; Park M, van de Woude GF: Oncogenes: genes associated with neoplastic disease. In Scriver CR, Beaudet AL, Sly WS, Valle D (eds): The Molecular and Metabolic Bases of Inherited Disease, 6th ed. New York, McGraw-Hill, 1989, pp 251-276; Nourse J, Mellentin JD, Galili N, et al: Chromosomal translocation t(1;19) results in synthesis of a homeobox fusion mRNA that codes for a potential chimeric transcription factor. Cell 60:535-545, 1990; and Borrow J, Goddard AD, Sheer D, Solomon E: Molecular analysis of acute promyelocytic leukemia breakpoint cluster region on chromosome 17. Science 249:1577-1580, 1990.

the *MYC* gene, allowing its unregulated expression and resulting in uncontrolled cell growth. The function of the Myc protein is still not entirely known, but it appears to be a transcription factor with powerful effects on the expression of a number of genes involved in cellular proliferation as well as on telomerase expression (see later discussion).

Follicular B-Cell Lymphoma Apoptosis, a major pathway for programmed cell death, is a normal cellular process in which cells are induced to undergo a stereotypic form of suicide characterized by fragmentation of cellular DNA and activation of a family of cysteine proteases, known as caspases, inside cells. Apoptosis plays a critical role in normal development; it is particularly prominent in the development of the immune system, in which the vast majority of developing lymphocytes must be destroyed to protect against cells that might react to one's own antigens. Overexpression of an antiapoptotic protein in lymphocyte lineages could result in vast expansion of lymphocyte populations, thereby contributing to the pathogenesis of lymphoma.

The first apoptotic gene implicated in cancer was identified in sporadic B-cell lymphoma. In nearly all B-cell lymphomas of the follicular type, a gene, *BCL2*, located at 18q21, was found to be activated by a t(14;18) chromosomal translocation that placed the gene under the strong promoter and enhancer of the immunoglobulin heavy-chain gene located at 14q32. The protein encoded by *BCL2* is a mitochondrial inner membrane protein with powerful antiapoptotic effects in B cells. Inappropriate, prolonged expression of this gene, driven by the immunoglobulin promoter, results in a massive expansion of B cells, not because of increased proliferation but because normal apoptosis of these cells is inhibited.

Telomerase as an Oncogene

Another type of oncogene is the gene encoding **telomerase,** a reverse transcriptase that is required to synthesize the hexamer repeat, TTAGGG, as a component of telomeres at the ends of chromosomes. Telomerase is needed because during normal semiconservative replication of DNA (Chapter 2), DNA polymerase, which can only add nucleotides to the 3′ end of DNA, cannot complete the synthesis of a growing strand all the way out to the very 3′ end of the template strand. In human germline cells and embryonic cells, telomeres contain approximately 15 kb of the telomeric repeat. As cells differentiate, telomerase activity declines in all somatic tissues except in the highly proliferative cells of tissues that must undergo self-renewal, such as the bone marrow. As telomerase function is lost, telomeres shorten, with a loss of approximately 35 base pairs of telomeric repeat DNA with each cell division. After hundreds of cell divisions, the chromosome ends will become damaged. DNA damage, in turn, causes cells

to stop dividing and enter G_0 of the cell cycle; the cells will ultimately undergo apoptosis. In contrast, telomerase expression persists in many tumors and permits tumor cells to proliferate indefinitely. In some cases, the appearance of telomerase activity is found to result from chromosome or genome mutations that directly up-regulate the telomerase gene; in others, telomerase may be only one of many genes whose expression is altered by a transforming oncogene, such as *MYC*.

Persistent expression of telomerase has not been shown to be a primary initiating event in any human cancers but is likely to be an important subsequent step that allows the cancer cells to survive despite continuous cell division. Regardless of when telomerase activity re-emerges in cancer, the presence of telomerase activity is now being used as a sensitive diagnostic tool for low levels of cancer in blood samples or in cells obtained by biopsy or needle aspiration of suspected cancerous lesions. Furthermore, given the role of telomerases in enhancing cellular proliferation, inhibition of telomerase is being actively pursued as a new approach to cancer treatment.

● TUMOR-SUPPRESSOR GENES

Whereas the proteins encoded by oncogenes promote cancer, mutations in tumor-suppressor genes (TSGs) contribute to malignancy by a different mechanism, that is, through loss of function of both alleles of the gene. TSGs are highly heterogeneous. Some truly suppress tumors by regulating the cell cycle or causing growth inhibition by cell-cell contact; TSGs of this type are gatekeepers because they regulate cell growth *directly*. Other TSGs, the caretakers, are involved in repairing DNA damage and maintaining genomic integrity. Loss of both alleles of genes that are involved in repairing DNA damage or chromosome breakage leads to cancer *indirectly* by allowing additional secondary mutations to accumulate either in proto-oncogenes or in other TSGs. The products of many TSGs have been isolated and characterized (Table 16-3). Because TSGs and their products are by nature protective against cancer, it is hoped that understanding them will eventually lead to improved methods of anticancer therapy.

The Two-Hit Origin of Cancer

The existence of TSG mutations leading to cancer was originally proposed in the 1960s to explain why certain tumors can occur in both hereditary and sporadic forms. For example, it was suggested that the hereditary form of the childhood cancer **retinoblastoma** might be initiated when a cell in a person heterozygous for a germline mutation in a tumor-suppressor retinoblastoma gene, required to prevent the development of the cancer, undergoes a second, somatic event that inactivates the other allele. As a consequence of this second

Table 16-3

Selected Tumor-Suppressor Genes

Gene	Gene Product and Possible Function	DISORDERS IN WHICH THE GENE IS AFFECTED	
		Familial	Sporadic
Gatekeepers			
RB1	p110 Cell cycle regulation	Retinoblastoma	Retinoblastoma, small cell lung carcinomas, breast cancer
TP53	p53 Cell cycle regulation	Li-Fraumeni syndrome	Lung cancer, breast cancer, many others
DCC	Dcc—receptor Decreases cell survival in the absence of survival signal from its netrin ligands	None known	Colorectal cancer
VHL	Vhl Forms part of a cytoplasmic destruction complex with APC that normally inhibits induction of blood vessel growth when oxygen is present	von Hippel–Lindau syndrome	Clear cell renal carcinoma
Caretakers			
BRCA1, BRCA2	Brca1, Brca2 Chromosome repair in response to double-stranded DNA breaks	Familial breast and ovarian cancer	Breast cancer, ovarian cancer
MLH1, MSH2	Mlh1, Msh2 Repair nucleotide mismatches between strands of DNA	Hereditary nonpolyposis colon cancer	Colorectal cancer

somatic event, the cell loses function of both alleles, giving rise to a tumor. The second hit is most often a somatic mutation, although loss of function without mutation, such as occurs with transcriptional silencing, has also been observed in some cancer cells (see next). In the sporadic form of retinoblastoma, both alleles are also inactivated, but in this case, the inactivation results from two somatic events occurring in the same cell.

The "two-hit" model is now widely accepted as the explanation for many familial cancers besides retinoblastoma, including familial polyposis coli, familial breast cancer, neurofibromatosis type 1 (NF1), hereditary nonpolyposis colon carcinoma, and a rare form of familial cancer known as Li-Fraumeni syndrome. In all of these syndromes, the second hit is often but not always a mutation. Silencing due to **epigenetic** changes such as DNA methylation, associated with a closed chromatin configuration and loss of accessibility of the DNA to transcription factors (see Chapters 3 and 5), is another important, alternative molecular mechanism for loss of function of a TSG. Because an alteration in gene function due to methylation is stably transmitted through mitosis, it behaves like a mutation; because there is no change in the DNA itself, however, the alteration is referred to as an epigenetic rather than a genetic change. Epigenetic silencing of gene expression is a normal phenomenon that explains such widely diverse phenomena as X inactivation (see Chapters 6 and 7), genomic imprinting (see Chapters 5 and 7), and

regulation of a specialized repertoire of gene expression in the development and maintenance of differentiation of specific tissues (see Chapter 14).

Gatekeeper Tumor-Suppressor Genes in Autosomal Dominant Cancer Syndromes

Retinoblastoma

Retinoblastoma, the prototype of diseases caused by mutation in a TSG, is a rare malignant tumor of the retina in infants, with an incidence of about 1 in 20,000 births (Fig. 16-5) (Case 34). Diagnosis of a retinoblastoma must usually be followed by removal of the affected eye, although smaller tumors, diagnosed at an early stage, can be treated by local therapy so that vision can be preserved.

About 40% of cases of retinoblastoma are of the heritable form, in which the child inherits one mutant allele at the retinoblastoma locus (RB1) through the germline. A somatic mutation or other alteration in a single retinal cell leads to loss of function of the remaining normal allele, thus initiating development of a tumor (Fig. 16-6). The disorder is inherited as a dominant trait because the large number of primordial retinoblasts and their rapid rate of proliferation make it very likely that a somatic mutation will occur in one or more of the more than 10^6 retinoblasts. Since the chance of the second hit in the heritable form is so great, the

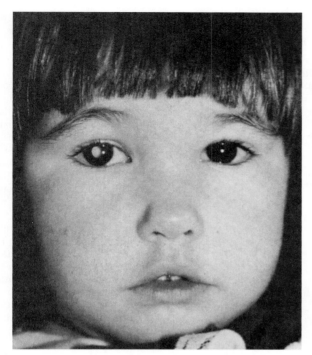

Figure 16-5 ■ Retinoblastoma in a young girl, showing as a white reflex in the affected eye when light reflects directly off the tumor surface. (Photograph courtesy of B. L. Gallie, The Hospital for Sick Children, Toronto.)

hit occurs frequently in more than one cell, and thus heterozygotes for the disorder are often affected with multiple tumors, often affecting both eyes. On the other hand, the occurrence of the second hit is a matter of chance and does not occur 100% of the time; the

penetrance of retinoblastoma, therefore, although high, is not complete.

The other 60% of cases of retinoblastoma are nonheritable (sporadic); in these cases, *both RB1* alleles in a single retinal cell have been inactivated independently. Because two hits in the same cell is a rare event, there is usually only a single clonal tumor and the retinoblastoma is found in one eye only. Although sporadic retinoblastoma usually occurs in one place in one eye only, 15% of patients with unilateral retinoblastoma have the heritable type but by chance develop a tumor in only one eye. Another difference between hereditary and sporadic tumors is that the average age at onset of the sporadic form is in early childhood, later than in infants with the heritable form (see Fig. 16-6).

Loss of Heterozygosity

Geneticists studying DNA polymorphisms in the region close to the *RB1* locus made an unusual but highly significant genetic discovery when they analyzed the alleles seen in tumor tissue from retinoblastoma patients. Individuals with retinoblastoma who were heterozygous at polymorphic loci near *RB1* in normal tissues, such as in their white blood cells, had tumors that contained alleles from only one of their two chromosome 13 homologues, revealing a **loss of heterozygosity** (LOH) in the region of the gene. In familial cases, the retained chromosome 13 markers were the ones inherited from the affected parent, that is, the one with the abnormal *RB1* allele. Thus, LOH represented the second hit of the remaining allele. LOH may occur by interstitial deletion, but there are other mechanisms,

Figure 16-6 ■ Comparison of mendelian and sporadic forms of cancers such as retinoblastoma and familial polyposis of the colon. Mechanisms of somatic mutation are presented in Figure 16-7. See text for discussion.

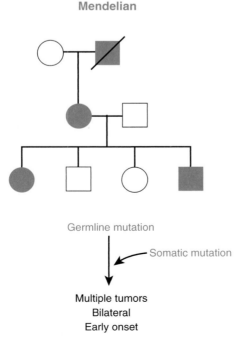

Mendelian

Germline mutation

Somatic mutation

Multiple tumors
Bilateral
Early onset

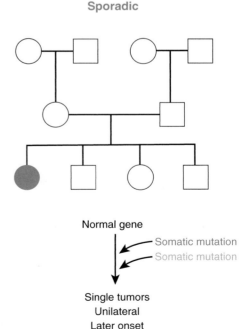

Sporadic

Normal gene

Somatic mutation
Somatic mutation

Single tumors
Unilateral
Later onset

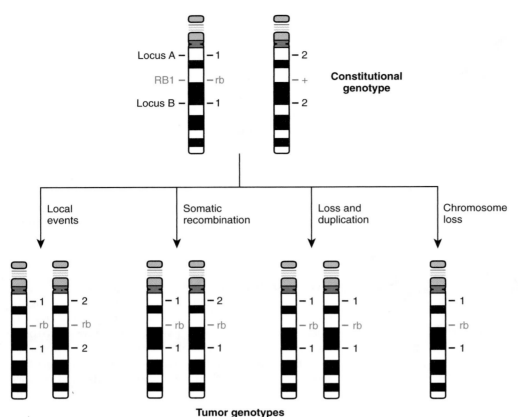

Locus A
RB1
Locus B
Constitutional genotype

Local events

Somatic recombination

Loss and duplication

Chromosome loss

Tumor genotypes

Figure 16-7 ■ Chromosomal mechanisms that could lead to loss of heterozygosity for DNA markers at or near a tumor-suppressor gene in an individual heterozygous for an inherited germline mutation. The figure depicts the events that constitute the "second hit" that leads to retinoblastoma. Local events such as mutation, gene conversion, or transcriptional silencing, however, could cause loss of function of both *RB1* genes without producing loss of heterozygosity. + is the normal allele, *rb* the mutant allele.

such as mitotic recombination or nondisjunction (Fig. 16-7). LOH is the most common mutational mechanism by which the function of the remaining normal *RB1* allele is disrupted in heterozygotes. When LOH is not seen, the second hit is usually a second somatic gene mutation or, occasionally, transcriptional inactivation of a nonmutated allele through methylation. LOH is a feature of a number of other tumors, both heritable and sporadic, and is often considered evidence for the

existence of a TSG, even when that gene is unknown (Table 16-4).

The *RB1* gene maps to chromosome 13, in band 13q14. In a small percentage of patients with retinoblastoma, the first mutation is a cytogenetically detectable deletion or translocation of this portion of chromosome 13. Such chromosomal changes, if they also disrupt genes adjacent to *RB1*, may lead to dysmorphic features in addition to retinoblastoma.

Table 16-4

Examples of Chromosomal Regions That Show Frequent, Repeated LOH in Particular Tumors

Chromosomal Region	Disorder(s)	Associated Tumor-Suppressor Gene
5q	Familial polyposis coli; colorectal carcinoma	*APC*
10q23	Glioblastoma; prostate cancer	*PTEN*
13q	Retinoblastoma; breast carcinoma; osteosarcoma	*RB1*
17p	Colorectal carcinoma; breast carcinoma	*TP53*
18q	Colorectal carcinoma	*DCC*
	Breast carcinoma	
8q	40% of tumors	Unknown
16q	50% of tumors	Unknown
17q	50% of tumors	Unknown (but includes *BRCA1*)
	Small-cell lung carcinoma	
3p	100% of tumors	Unknown
10q	94% of tumors	Unknown
4q, 5q, 13q, and 17p	86% of tumors	Unknown

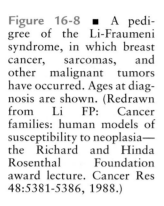

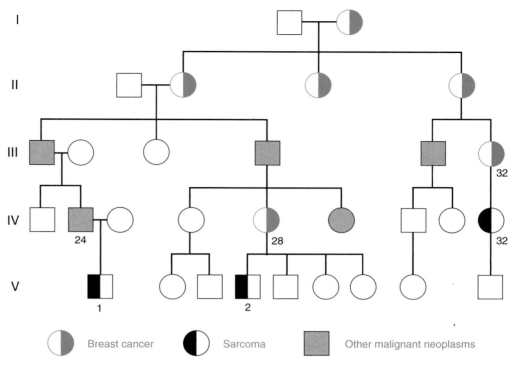

Figure 16-8 ▪ A pedigree of the Li-Fraumeni syndrome, in which breast cancer, sarcomas, and other malignant tumors have occurred. Ages at diagnosis are shown. (Redrawn from Li FP: Cancer families: human models of susceptibility to neoplasia—the Richard and Hinda Rosenthal Foundation award lecture. Cancer Res 48:5381-5386, 1988.)

Breast cancer   Sarcoma   Other malignant neoplasms

Infants with heritable retinoblastoma who survive their childhood cancers have a greatly increased (400-fold) risk for development of other cancers later in adult life. The risk is much higher if the child has received radiotherapy because patients with the heritable form are already carrying a mutation in one *RB1* allele in all the cells of their body and are therefore susceptible to other tumors should the other copy be lost. Mesenchymal tumors that commonly develop in adulthood include osteogenic sarcomas, fibrosarcomas, and melanomas. Although the *RB1* gene is expressed in many tissues, loss of *RB1* initiates tumors only in the retina in childhood and, later in life, in particular tissues of mesenchymal origin. The reason for this tissue specificity is unknown.

The *RB1* gene product, described as p110 Rb1 (a protein 110 kD in size), is a phosphoprotein that is hypophosphorylated and then hyperphosphorylated at different stages of the cell cycle. In its hypophosphorylated state, it blocks cell cycle progression at the boundary between G_1 and S, thereby inhibiting entry into S phase by binding to and inactivating transcription factors that promote DNA synthesis. As p110 Rb1 becomes progressively more phosphorylated, it releases its protein-binding partners, allowing entry of the cell into S phase; it is then progressively dephosphorylated during the course of the cell cycle, allowing it to function again to block entry into S phase of the next cell cycle. Loss of the *RB1* gene deprives cells of an important mitotic checkpoint and allows uncontrolled proliferation. The *RB1* gene is therefore a prototypical gatekeeper TSG. Of note, *RB1* is mutated in a number

of cell lines derived from certain other tumors during their progression (see Table 16-3).

Li-Fraumeni Syndrome

There are rare "cancer families" in which there is a striking history of many different forms of cancer (including several kinds of bone and soft tissue sarcoma, breast cancer, brain tumors, leukemia, and adrenocortical carcinoma), affecting a number of family members at an unusually early age, inherited in an autosomal dominant pattern (Fig. 16-8). This highly variable phenotype is known as the **Li-Fraumeni syndrome** (LFS). Because the TSG *TP53*, encoding the protein p53, is inactivated in the sporadic forms of many of the cancers found in LFS, *TP53* was considered a candidate for the gene defective in LFS. DNA analysis of several families with LFS has now confirmed this hypothesis; affected members in more than 70% of families with LFS carry a mutant form of the *TP53* gene as a germline mutation. As seen also in retinoblastoma, one of the two mutations necessary to inactivate the *TP53* gene is present in the germline in familial LFS, whereas in many sporadic cancers, both mutations are somatic events.

The p53 protein is a DNA-binding protein that appears to be an important component of the cellular response to DNA damage. In addition to being a transcription factor that activates the transcription of genes that stop cell division and allow repair of DNA damage, p53 also appears to be involved in inducing apoptosis in cells that have experienced irreparable DNA damage.

Loss of p53 function, therefore, allows cells with damaged DNA to survive and divide, thereby propagating potentially oncogenic mutations. The *TP53* gene can therefore be considered to also be a gatekeeper TSG.

Neurofibromatosis Type 1

NF1 is a relatively common autosomal dominant disorder that primarily affects the peripheral nervous system and is often characterized by large numbers of benign neurofibromas (Case 29) (see Chapter 7). Certain rare malignant neoplasms, however, are seen with increased frequency in a minority of patients with NF1. These malignant neoplasms include neurofibrosarcoma, astrocytoma, Schwann cell cancers, and childhood chronic myelogenous leukemia, which are extremely rare in patients without NF1. The abnormal cell growth observed in NF1 suggests that the normal gene may function in the regulation of cell division in neural tissue.

The *NF1* gene was mapped to the proximal long arm of chromosome 17 by family linkage studies and was subsequently cloned by application of several of the positional cloning strategies presented in Chapter 10. Inspection of the sequence of the *NF1* gene and its protein product demonstrated significant homology to proteins that activate the GTPase activity of the *RAS* oncogene product (see earlier). This finding strongly suggests that the normal *NF1* product interacts with an unknown member of the *RAS* gene family to regulate proliferative activity in normal cells. The mutant *NF1* gene may fail to regulate growth in the normal cells from which neurofibromas are derived, leading to inappropriate growth and tumor formation.

This model suggests that *NF1* is a TSG. By analogy with other dominantly inherited TSG mutations, loss or inactivation of the remaining normal allele at the *NF1* locus would be required to explain the development of tumors in patients with NF1. In some but not all cases of malignant Schwann cell tumors and juvenile myelogenous leukemia, LOH of the normal *NF1* allele has been demonstrated in the tumor tissues but not in surrounding normal tissues. The finding of LOH for the normal *NF1* gene in some of these tumors does not preclude a role for multiple mutations in other genes leading to unregulated cell division (see Fig. 16-2).

Caretaker Genes in Autosomal Dominant Cancer Syndromes

Familial Breast Cancer due to Mutations in BRCA1 and BRCA2

Breast cancer is common. Population-based epidemiological studies have shown that ~9% of all women in North America and western Europe will develop breast

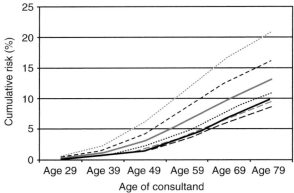

Cumulative risk of developing breast cancer

Age of relative at diagnosis of breast cancer

```
............  20-29      ..........  50-59
- - - -       30-39      - - -       60-69
————          40-49      — — —       70-79
—————         General population
```

Figure 16-9 ■ Breast cancer risks. Cumulative risk, with age, of a female consultand's developing breast cancer when a first-degree relative has breast cancer. The risk for the consultand increases directly with her own age and inversely with the age at which the first-degree relative was first diagnosed with breast cancer. (Modified from Claus EB, Risch N, Thompson WD: Autosomal dominant inheritance of early-onset breast cancer. Implications for risk prediction. Cancer 73:643-651, 1994.)

cancer in their lifetime. Breast cancer has long been recognized to have a strong genetic component; a woman's risk for development of breast cancer is increased up to 3-fold if one first-degree relative is affected and up to 10-fold if more than one first-degree relative is affected. These familial risks are increased even more if the onset of disease in the affected first-degree relative is at 40 years of age or younger (Fig. 16-9). Although as much as 20% of all breast cancer cases may have a significant genetic component as part of a polygenic or multifactorial mode of inheritance (see Chapter 8), only a small proportion of cases appears to be due to a dominantly inherited mendelian predisposition to breast cancer. These families share features characteristic of familial (as opposed to sporadic) cancer: multiple affected individuals in a family, earlier age at onset, frequent bilateral disease, and cancers in other tissues such as ovary and prostate.

Genetic linkage studies in families with early-onset familial breast cancer led to the discovery of mutations in two genes that increase susceptibility to breast cancer, *BRCA1* on chromosome 17q21 and *BRCA2* on chromosome 13q12.3 (Case 5). Together, these two loci account for about one half and one third of autosomal dominant familial breast cancer, respectively, but less than 5% of all breast cancer in the population. Many mutant alleles of both genes have now been catalogued.

Mutations in *BRCA1* and *BRCA2* are also associated with a significant increase in the risk for ovarian cancer in female heterozygotes; mutations in *BRCA2*, but not *BRCA1*, also account for 10% to 20% of all *male* breast cancer, which affects nearly 0.1% of males.

The gene products of *BRCA1* and *BRCA2* are nuclear proteins contained within the same multiprotein complex. This complex has been implicated in the cellular response to double-stranded DNA breaks, such as occurs normally during homologous recombination or abnormally as a result of damage to DNA. As might be expected with any TSG, tumor tissue from heterozygotes for *BRCA1* and *BRCA2* mutations frequently demonstrates LOH with loss of the normal allele.

Penetrance of *BRCA1* and *BRCA2* Mutations Presymptomatic detection of women at risk for development of breast cancer as a result of any of these susceptibility genes is an important aim of current research, both in familial cases and in the larger number of sporadic cases. For the purposes of patient management and counseling, it would obviously be extremely helpful to know the lifetime risk for development of breast cancer in patients carrying particular mutations in the *BRCA1* and *BRCA2* genes, compared with the risk in the general population (Fig. 16-10). Initial studies showed a greater than 80% risk of breast cancer by the age of 70 years in women heterozygous for *BRCA1* or *BRCA2* mutations. These estimates relied on estimates of the risk for development of cancer in female relatives within families ascertained because breast cancer had already occurred many times in family members; that is, the *BRCA1* or *BRCA2* mutation was highly penetrant in the carriers. When similar risk estimates were made from population-based studies, however, in which women carrying *BRCA1* and *BRCA2* mutations were *not* selected because they were members of families in which many cases of breast cancer had already developed, the risk estimates were lower and ranged from 45% to 60% by the age of 70 years. The discrepancy between the penetrance of mutant *BRCA1/2* alleles in families with multiple occurrences of breast cancer and the penetrance seen in women identified by population screening and *not* by family history suggests that other genetic or environmental factors must play a role in the ultimate penetrance of *BRCA1* and *BRCA2* mutations in women heterozygous for these mutations.

Familial Colon Cancer

Familial Polyposis Coli Colorectal cancer, a malignancy of the epithelium of the colon and rectum, is one of the most common forms of cancer. It affects more than 150,000 individuals per year in the United States alone and is responsible for about 15% of all cancer. A small proportion of colon cancer cases are due to the autosomal dominant condition **familial adenomatous**

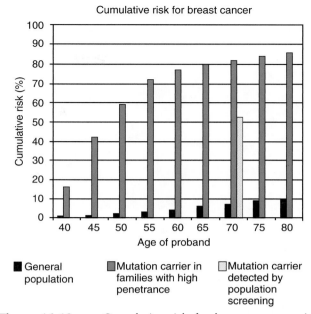

Cumulative risk for breast cancer

Figure 16-10 ■ Cumulative risk for breast cancer, with age, in women carrying a mutation in *BRCA1* or *BRCA2*, calculated by data from families with high penetrance for the mutation (dark blue bars). The risk is compared with the risk for breast cancer in the general population (black bars) as well as the estimated risk (~52%) at the age of 70 years for breast cancer in a mutation carrier for *BRCA1* or *BRCA2* identified through population surveys (light blue bar) rather than in families with high penetrance. See text. (Modified from King MC, Rowell S, Love SM: Inherited breast and ovarian cancer. What are the risks? What are the choices? JAMA 269:1975-1980, 1993; Ford D, Easton DF, Stratton M, et al: Genetic heterogeneity and penetrance analysis of the *BRCA1* and *BRCA2* genes in breast cancer families. The Breast Cancer Linkage Consortium. Am J Hum Genet 62:676-689, 1998; and Brody LC, Biesecker BB: Breast cancer susceptibility genes *BRCA1* and *BRCA2*. Medicine [Baltimore] 77:208-226, 1998.)

polyposis (FAP) (Case 13) and its subvariant, the **Gardner syndrome.** FAP has an incidence of about 1 in 10,000.

In FAP heterozygotes, numerous adenomatous polyps, which themselves are benign growths, develop in the colon during the first two decades of life. In almost all cases, one or more of the polyps becomes malignant. Surgical removal of the colon (colectomy) prevents the development of malignancy. Because this disorder is autosomal dominant, relatives of affected persons must be examined periodically by colonoscopy. The responsible gene, *APC*, was isolated by positional cloning after the disease locus was mapped to chromosome 5q, both by genetic linkage studies in affected families (see Chapter 10) and by demonstration of LOH in colon tumors. Gardner syndrome is also due to mutations in *APC* and is therefore allelic to FAP. Patients with Gardner syndrome have, in addition to the adenomatous polyps with malignant transformation seen in

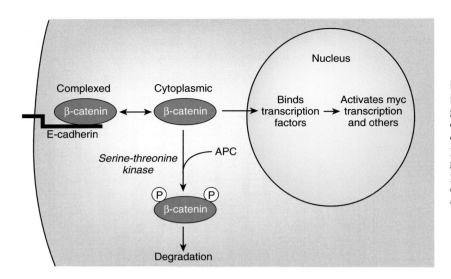

Figure 16-11 ■ Schematic diagram of the interaction between the product of the *APC* gene and β-catenin. β-Catenin forms a complex with the cell adhesion molecule E-cadherin. β-Catenin also exists free in cytoplasm, where it either is targeted by the *APC* gene product for degradation through phosphorylation by a serine-threonine kinase, or enters the nucleus and activates transcription of oncogenic genes, such as *MYC*.

FAP, other anomalies, including osteomas of the jaw and desmoids, which are tumors arising in the muscle of the abdominal wall. Although the FAP phenotype and Gardner phenotype appear to breed true in families, it is unknown presently why some patients with *APC* mutations develop FAP and others develop the Gardner syndrome.

The *APC* gene encodes a cytoplasmic protein that regulates the bifunctional protein known as β-catenin. β-Catenin serves as a link between the cytoplasmic portion of transmembrane cell adhesion molecules (such as the cadherins) and the actin cytoskeleton and is also an activator of transcription (Fig. 16-11). Under normal conditions, when the colonic epithelial layer is intact and no cellular proliferation is required, most β-catenin is present in a large protein complex with E-cadherin. *APC* induces the phosphorylation and subsequent degradation of any unbound β-catenin, thereby keeping free β-catenin levels low in the cell. Loss of *APC* leads to accumulation of free cytoplasmic β-catenin that is translocated into the nucleus, where it activates transcription of cellular proliferation genes, including *MYC*, the same gene that is overexpressed in Burkitt lymphoma. The *APC* gene is therefore a gatekeeper TSG.

Hereditary Nonpolyposis Colon Cancer Approximately 2% to 4% of cases of colon cancer are attributable to a group of familial cancer syndromes known as **hereditary nonpolyposis colon cancer** (HNPCC) (Case 19). HNPCC is characterized by autosomal dominant inheritance of colon cancer occurring during adulthood, but at a relatively young age and without the adenomatous polyps seen with FAP. Male heterozygotes for a mutant HNPCC gene have an approximately 90% lifetime risk for development of cancer of the colon; female heterozygotes have a somewhat smaller risk, approximately 70%, but have an approximately

40% risk for endometrial cancer. There are also additional risks of 10% to 20% for cancer of the biliary or urinary tract and the ovary.

HNPCC is a group of five similar familial cancer syndromes (HNPCC1 through HNPCC5) caused by mutations in one of five distinct DNA repair genes responsible for repairing DNA segments in which correct DNA base pairing (A with T, C with G) has been violated. Although all five of these genes have been implicated in HNPCC in different families, *MLH*, *MSH2*, and *MSH6* are together responsible for the vast majority of HNPCC, whereas the others have been found in only a few very rare patients and are often associated with a lesser degree of mismatch repair deficiency. The HNPCC genes are prototypical caretaker TSGs.

As with other TSGs, the autosomal dominant inheritance pattern of HNPCC comes about through inheritance of one mutant allele followed by mutation or inactivation of the remaining normal allele in a somatic cell. At the cellular level, the most striking phenotype of cells lacking both alleles of one of these genes is an enormous increase in point mutations and in instability of DNA segments containing simple sequence repeats, such as $(A)_n$ or microsatellite polymorphisms, throughout the genome (see Chapter 9). Microsatellite DNA is believed to be particularly vulnerable to mismatch because slippage of the strand being synthesized on the template strand can occur more readily when short tandem DNA repeats are synthesized. Such instability, referred to as the **replication error positive** (or **RER+**) phenotype, occurs at two orders of magnitude higher frequency in cells lacking both copies of a mismatch repair gene. The RER+ phenotype is easily seen in DNA as three, four, or even more alleles of a microsatellite polymorphism in a single individual's tumor DNA (Fig. 16-12). It is estimated that cells lacking both copies of a mismatch repair gene

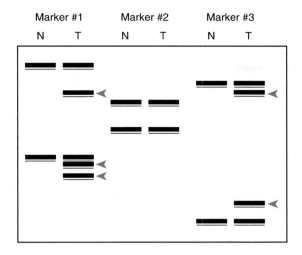

Marker #1   Marker #2   Marker #3
N   T   N   T   N   T

Figure 16-12 ■ Gel electrophoresis of three different microsatellite polymorphic markers in normal (N) and tumor (T) samples from a patient with a mutation in *MSH2* and microsatellite instability. Although marker #2 shows no difference between normal and tumor tissues, genotyping at markers #1 and #3 reveals extra alleles (blue arrows), some smaller, some larger, than the alleles present in normal tissue.

may carry 100,000 mutations within simple repeats throughout the genome. Mutations secondary to the repeat instability occur in many TSGs; two such genes have been isolated and characterized. The first is *APC*, whose normal function and role in FAP were described previously. The second is the gene *TGFBR2* encoding transforming growth factor β receptor II, a serine-threonine kinase that, on binding by ligands such as a transforming growth factor, inhibits intestinal cell division through phosphorylation of downstream signaling molecules. *TGFBR2* has a stretch of 10 adenines encoding three lysines within its coding sequence; deletion of one or more of these adenines in both alleles of the gene occurs with high frequency in RER+ cells and results in frameshift and loss of function of this receptor and, as a consequence, loss of control over growth. Repeat instability can produce many mutations that allow a normal cell to become a fully malignant, metastatic cancer cell.

Caretaker Genes in Autosomal Recessive Chromosome Instability Syndromes

As expected from the important role that DNA replication and repair enzymes play in mutation surveillance and prevention, inherited defects that alter the function of repair enzymes can lead to a dramatic increase in the frequency of mutations of all types, including those that lead to cancer. Autosomal recessive disorders such as **xeroderma pigmentosum** (Case 43), **ataxia-telangiectasia**, **Fanconi anemia**, and **Bloom syndrome** are due to

loss of function of proteins required for normal DNA repair or replication. Thus, the genes that are defective in the chromosome instability syndromes may be viewed as caretaker TSGs. Patients with these conditions have a high frequency of chromosome and gene mutations and, as a result, a markedly increased risk for various types of cancer, particularly leukemia or, in the case of xeroderma pigmentosum, skin cancers in sun-exposed areas. Clinically, radiography must be used with extreme caution if at all in patients with ataxia-telangiectasia, Fanconi anemia, and Bloom syndrome. Furthermore, exposure to sunlight must be avoided in patients with xeroderma pigmentosum.

Although the chromosome instability syndromes are rare autosomal recessive disorders, heterozygotes for these gene defects are much more common and appear to be at an increased risk for malignant neoplasia. For example, Fanconi anemia, in which homozygotes have a number of congenital anomalies in association with bone marrow failure, leukemia, and squamous cell carcinoma of the head and neck, is a chromosome instability syndrome resulting from mutations of at least eight different loci involved in DNA and chromosome repair. One of these Fanconi anemia loci turns out to be the known hereditary cancer gene *BRCA2*. Similarly, female heterozygotes for ataxia-telangiectasia mutations have overall a twofold increased risk of breast cancer compared with controls and a fivefold higher risk for breast cancer before the age of 50 years. Thus, heterozygotes for these chromosome instability syndromes constitute a sizeable pool of individuals at increased risk for cancer.

Loss of Gatekeeper and Caretaker Gene Function in Sporadic Cancer

TP53 and RB1 in Sporadic Cancers

Although Li-Fraumeni syndrome, caused by the inheritance of germline mutations in *TP53*, is a rare familial syndrome, somatic mutation causing a loss of function of both alleles of *TP53* turns out to be one of the most common genetic alterations seen in sporadic cancer (Table 16-3). Mutations of the *TP53* gene, deletion of the segment of chromosome 17p (band p13.1) that includes *TP53*, or both are frequently and repeatedly seen in a wide range of sporadic cancers. These include breast, ovarian, bladder, cervical, esophageal, colorectal, skin, and lung carcinomas; glioblastoma of the brain; osteogenic sarcoma; and hepatocellular carcinoma.

The retinoblastoma gene *RB1* is also frequently mutated in many cancers, including breast cancer. For example, 13q14 LOH observed in human breast cancers is associated with loss of *RB1* mRNA in the tumor tissues. In still other cancers, the *RB1* gene is intact and

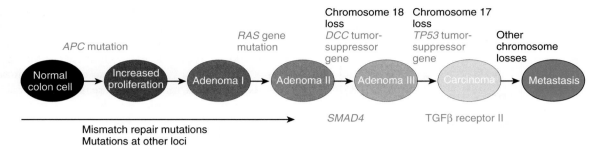

Figure 16-13 ■ Stages in the evolution of colon cancer, serving as a model more generally for cancer evolution (see Fig. 16-2). Increasing degrees of abnormality are associated with sequential loss of tumor-suppressor genes from several chromosomes in addition to activation of the *RAS* proto-oncogene, with or without a concomitant defect in mismatch repair. The order of events is usually but not always as shown here. For example, sporadic cancer with abnormal mismatch repair is less common than are cancers without abnormal repair but, when present, may operate along a somewhat different but parallel pathway leading to malignancy as the final common endpoint. (Modified from Kinzler KW, Vogelstein B: Lessons from hereditary colorectal cancer. Cell 87:159-170, 1996.)

its mRNA appears to be at or near normal levels, and yet the p110 Rb1 protein is deficient. This anomaly has now been explained by the recognition that *RB1* can be down-regulated in association with overexpression of the oncomir *miR-106a*, which targets *RB1* mRNA and blocks its translation. Thus, *miR-106a* might be considered an oncogene that exerts its effect by reducing the expression of the TSG encoding the p110 Rb1 protein.

BRCA1 and BRCA2 in Sporadic Breast and Ovarian Cancer

In familial breast cancer patients carrying *BRCA1* and *BRCA2* mutations, LOH involving the normal allele is often found in the cancer tissues, strongly suggesting that these genes are TSGs. In sporadic breast cancer, however, loss of one allele of *BRCA1* or *BRCA2* is only seen in approximately half of tumors, and even when one allele is mutated, LOH involving the other allele is usually not present. What has been found, however, particularly in more malignant forms of the cancer, is reduced expression of *BRCA1* and *BRCA2*. Reduced expression may be associated with epigenetic changes, such as promoter methylation, or changes in the splicing pattern of the genes. Thus, reduced expression of these TSGs may be an important contributor to the pathogenesis of sporadic breast cancer through a combination of mutation and reduced expression.

A modification of comparative genome hybridization (see Chapter 4) has been used to scan for LOH in breast tumor tissue versus normal tissue in sporadic breast cancer patients. LOH has been found in a number of chromosomal regions, including 1p, 3p, 11p, 13q, 16q, and 17p, which suggests that there may be many genes important for breast tumor progression. Although the gene on chromosome 17p is likely to be *TP53*, the other genes have not been identified.

Hereditary Nonpolyposis Colon Cancer and Familial Adenomatous Polyposis Genes in Sporadic Colon Cancer

In contrast to the low frequency with which *BRCA1* and *BRCA2* are found to be mutated in most sporadic breast cancer, there is ample evidence to support a major involvement of the genes responsible for familial colon cancer, such as *MLH1, MSH2,* and *APC*, in sporadic colon cancer (Fig. 16-13). In nearly 70% of adenomatous polyps in individuals without FAP, the two-hit model for tumorigenesis has been confirmed by finding loss of both copies of *APC* in the adenoma but not in the surrounding normal tissues. In the remaining 30%, in which *APC* is normal, mutations in the gene encoding β-catenin that block its phosphorylation and degradation have been found in nearly half. Similarly, in individuals without an obvious family history for HNPCC, the RER+ phenotype, with associated mutation or transcriptional silencing of both alleles of one or more mismatch repair genes, has been reported in up to 12% of sporadic colon cancer. Activating mutations of one member of the *RAS* gene family (*KRAS*), as well as loss of both copies of *TP53*, are also frequently seen in sporadic colon cancer. Loss of expression of a gene on 18q21 called *DCC* (for *d*eleted in *c*olon *c*arcinoma) is observed in more than 70% of cases of colorectal cancer; this gene encodes a receptor for molecules involved in axonal guidance during normal development of the nervous system; its role in colon cancer is not fully defined. In another 15% of sporadic colon cancers, the *SMAD4* gene, which is involved in signaling downstream from transforming growth factor β receptor II, is mutated.

As important as defects in mismatch repair are in HNPCC and some sporadic colon cancers, most sporadic colon cancer has *no* RER+ phenotype. Instead, these tumors generally have chromosome and genome mutations that reflect defects in either double-stranded break repair or maintenance of the fidelity of how chromosomes segregate during mitosis. Defects in the former generate chromosome translocations, whereas abnormalities in the latter can lead to nondisjunction and aneuploidy. In summary, there are many ways for cell division and growth to become dysregulated, and many more undoubtedly are waiting to be discovered and elucidated.

Issues in Testing for Germline Mutations Causing Hereditary Cancer

BRCA1 and BRCA2 Testing

Identification of a germline mutation in *BRCA1* or *BRCA2* in a patient with breast cancer is of obvious importance for genetic counseling and cancer risk management for the children, siblings, and other relatives of the patient. Testing is important for the patient's own treatment as well. For instance, in addition to removal of the cancer, a woman found to carry a *BRCA1* mutation might also choose to have a prophylactic mastectomy on the unaffected breast or bilateral oophorectomy simultaneously to minimize the number of separate surgeries and anesthesia exposures. However, the percentage of all female breast cancer patients whose disease is caused by a germline mutation in either the *BRCA1* or *BRCA2* gene is small, with estimates that vary between 1% and 3% in populations unselected for family history of breast or ovarian cancer, or age at onset of the disease. Among women with breast cancer who are younger than 50 years, or in women with first- and second-degree relatives with ovarian cancer or breast cancer (particularly if there is the rare male relative with breast cancer), the frequency of finding a germline mutation is much higher, depending on how many and how closely related the family members are. Given the great expense of sequencing these large genes and the uncertainty as to whether all sequence variants in these genes are even pathogenic, it is impractical for all women with breast cancer to undergo gene sequencing to look for *BRCA1* and *BRCA2* mutations.

Genetic counselors and oncologists have worked to develop clinical criteria that will allow them to offer breast cancer patients highly individualized counseling that is specific to each patient's own individual circumstances. Many approaches to individualized counseling are available. One common method uses clinical and genetic variables such as age at onset of disease, family history of breast or ovarian cancer, and penetrance values of different mutant alleles of *BRCA1* and *BRCA2* to calculate the probability that a patient with breast cancer carries a germline mutation in *BRCA1* or *BRCA2* and should therefore be offered *BRCA1* and *BRCA2* sequencing. In addition, expression of the estrogen receptor and the oncogene *HER2* in the biop-

sied malignant tissue, which is already widely used for evaluating prognosis and designing therapy, can also be included in the probability calculation. These markers are useful because the breast cancers in carriers of *BRCA1* mutations (but perhaps not *BRCA2* mutations) are more often found to lack these markers, as compared with sporadic breast cancer. A calculated probability greater than 1 in 10 of carrying a *BRCA1* or *BRCA2* mutation has become widely adopted as an arbitrary threshold for referral for *BRCA1* and *BRCA2* sequencing; for any one patient, however, the decision to undergo testing is a personal one that is made by the patient herself, with guidance and support from her health care provider.

The situation with male breast cancer is quite different. This disease is 100 times less common than female breast cancer, but when it occurs, the frequency of germline mutations in hereditary breast cancer genes, particularly *BRCA2*, is 16%. Thus, all male probands with breast cancer would be candidates for *BRCA1* and *BRCA2* gene sequencing, as would all of their first-degree relatives, if a DNA sample from the proband were no longer available. Finding a mutation in the proband or a first-degree relative would then allow mutation-specific testing in the rest of the family.

HNPCC Germline Mutation Testing

Only 4% of patients with colon cancer, not selected for a family history of cancer, carry a mutation in one of the three mismatch repair genes *MLH1*, *MSH2*, and *MSH6*. Just as with sporadic breast cancer, geneticists need to balance the high cost and low yield of sequencing mismatch repair genes in every patient with colon cancer against the obvious importance of finding such a mutation for the family of a patient. Such clinical factors as an early age at onset (before the age of 50 years), the location of the tumor in more proximal portions of the colon, the presence of a second tumor or history of colorectal cancer, a family history of colorectal or other cancers (particularly endometrial cancer), and cancer in relatives younger than 50 years of age, all boost the probability that a patient with colon cancer is carrying a mutation in a mismatch repair gene. Molecular studies of the tumor tissue, to look for evidence of the RER+ phenotype (as discussed earlier in this chapter) or evidence of absent MLH1, MSH2, or MSH6 protein by antibody staining in the tumor, also increase the probability that an individual patient with colorectal cancer has a mismatch repair mutation. Combining clinical and molecular criteria allows the identification of a small subset (~4%) of all colorectal cancer patients in whom the probability of finding a mismatch repair mutation is 80%. These patients are clearly the most cost-effective group in which sequencing could be recommended. However, as with all such attempts at cost-effectiveness, limiting the number of patients studied to increase the yield of patients with positive sequencing inevitably results in missing a sizeable minority (20%) of patients with germline mismatch repair mutations.

Hereditary Lymphoma with Loss of Expression of Proapoptotic Tumor-Suppressor Genes

Autoimmune Lymphoproliferative Syndrome

Autoimmune lymphoproliferative syndrome is a rare autosomal dominant condition characterized by massive lymphadenopathy and splenomegaly, particularly in childhood, and the development of autoimmune phenomena such as antibody-mediated thrombocytopenia and hemolytic anemia. Although the manifestations of this condition are primarily those of autoimmunity, B-cell and Hodgkin lymphomas have both been described with an increased frequency of 14-fold and 50-fold, respectively.

In autoimmune lymphoproliferative syndrome, the primary abnormality is in the mechanism for lymphocyte apoptosis mediated by the Fas receptor and its ligand, Fas-ligand. Apoptosis is a normal process of cellular suicide in which there is the sudden appearance of openings in mitochondrial membranes that permit the efflux of intramitochondrial proteins and calcium, followed by the activation of intracellular proteases, DNA fragmentation, and cell death. Both Fas-ligand and Fas are homotrimers. Dominant negative mutations (see Chapter 12) in one allele of either of the genes encoding these molecules cause loss of function of the receptor or its ligand, resulting in deficiency of apoptotic signaling and a massive expansion of immature T lymphocytes known as double-negative cells (so called because they lack both the T-helper [T4] and T-suppressor [T8] cell surface markers). Precisely how this defect in apoptosis of T lymphocytes can lead to an increased frequency of various kinds of lymphomas is unknown, but may be due to the markedly increased number of cells that can serve as targets for mutation and therefore malignant transformation.

Cytogenetic Changes in Cancer

Aneuploidy and Aneusomy

As introduced in Chapter 5, cytogenetic changes are hallmarks of cancer, particularly in later and more malignant or invasive stages of tumor development. Such cytogenetic alterations suggest that a critical element of cancer progression includes defects in genes involved in maintaining chromosome stability and integrity and ensuring accurate mitotic segregation.

Initially, most of the cytogenetic studies of tumor progression were carried out in leukemias because the tumor cells were amenable to being cultured and karyotyped by standard methods. For example, when chronic myelogenous leukemia, with a 9;22 Philadelphia chromosome, evolves from the typically indolent chronic phase to a severe life-threatening blast crisis, there may be several additional cytogenetic abnormalities, including numerical or structural changes, such as a second copy of the 9;22 translocation chromosome or an isochromosome for 17q. In advanced stages of other forms of leukemia, other translocations are common.

When the tumor cells can be karyotyped, spectral karyotyping (see Chapters 4 and 5) has also revealed a far greater range of abnormalities than those visible by earlier methods of karyotyping and chromosome identification by banding (Fig. 5-C; see color insert). A vast array of abnormalities is seen in all cancers. Some abnormalities are seen only occasionally in some tumor samples and may be random aberrations, and others are found repeatedly in cancers of the same histological type. Cytogenetic abnormalities found repeatedly in a certain type of cancer are likely to be involved in the initiation or progression of the malignant neoplasm. Still other changes are found only in metastases of a cancer but not in the original primary tumor. A current focus of cancer research is the cytogenetic and molecular definition of these abnormalities, many of which are already known to be related to proto-oncogenes or TSGs and presumably result in enhanced proto-oncogene expression or the loss of TSG alleles.

Gene Amplification

In addition to translocations and other rearrangements, another cytogenetic aberration seen in many cancers is **gene amplification,** a phenomenon in which there are many additional copies of a segment of the genome present in the cell. Gene amplification is common in many cancers, including neuroblastoma, squamous cell carcinoma of the head and neck, colorectal cancer, and malignant glioblastomas of the brain. Amplified segments of DNA are readily detected by comparative genome hybridization and appear as two types of cytogenetic change in routine chromosome analysis: **double minutes** (very small accessory chromosomes) and **homogeneously staining regions** that do not band normally and contain multiple, amplified copies of a particular DNA segment. How and why double minutes and homogeneously staining regions occur are poorly understood, but amplified regions are known to include extra copies of proto-oncogenes, such as the genes encoding Myc, Ras, and epithelial growth factor receptor, which stimulate cell growth or block apoptosis, or both. For example, amplification of the *MYCN* proto-oncogene encoding N-Myc is an important clinical indicator of prognosis in the childhood cancer **neuroblastoma.** *MYCN* is amplified more than 200-fold in 40% of advanced stages of neuroblastoma; despite aggressive treatment, only 30% of patients with advanced disease survive 3 years. In contrast, *MYCN* amplification is found in only 4% of early-stage neuroblastoma, and the 3-year survival is 90%. Amplification of genes encoding the targets of chemotherapeutic agents has also been implicated as a mechanism for the development of drug resistance in patients previously treated with chemotherapy.

● TUMOR PROGRESSION

In familial cancer syndromes, the pattern of inheritance implies that a defect in a single gene, such as an activated proto-oncogene or loss of function of a TSG, inherited in the germline, is capable of initiating the multistep process that leads to cancer. Additional steps occur as the cells evolve into a clinically evident malignant neoplasm (see Fig. 16-2). Sporadic cancers can pose a more difficult problem for dissecting out the steps leading to disease. Although some of the same genes responsible for hereditary cancer syndromes are found to be mutated in sporadic cancers, many other mutations, cytogenetic abnormalities, and epigenetic alterations are already present by the time a cancer is clinically evident. Consequently, it is often difficult to determine the order in which many of the changes occurred and to identify which one actually initiated the malignant process. Whatever the initiating events, however, cancer evolves along multiple lineages as chance mutational and epigenetic events cripple the machinery for maintaining genome integrity, leading to more genetic changes in a vicious circle of more mutations, increasing aneuploidy, and worsening growth control. Such changes do not occur synchronously in every cell in the malignant neoplasm. Rather, different changes occur at random in some of the malignant cells, thereby generating different malignant sublineages. The lineages that experience an enhancement of growth and survival will come to predominate as the cancer evolves and progresses. Furthermore, the surrounding normal tissue probably plays an important role by providing the blood supply that nourishes the tumor, by permitting cancer cells to escape from the tumor and metastasize, and by shielding the tumor from immune attack. Thus, cancer is a complex process, both within the tumor and between the tumor and the normal tissues that surround it.

● APPLYING GENOMICS TO INDIVIDUALIZE CANCER THERAPY

Genomics is already having a major impact on diagnostic precision and optimization of therapy in cancer. In this section, we describe how one such genomic technique, **expression profiling,** is being used to guide diagnosis and treatment.

Gene Expression Profiling and Clustering to Create Signatures

Suppose that one has a number of tissue samples from different cancers and wants to develop a sensitive method to distinguish between these types of tumors in future sets of samples. As described in Chapter 4, comparative hybridization techniques can be used to measure simultaneously the level of mRNA expression of some or all of the approximately 25,000 human genes in any tissue sample, relative to a standard sample. A measurement of mRNA expression in a sample comprises a **gene expression profile** specific to that sample. Figure 16-14 depicts a hypothetical, idealized situation of eight samples, four from each of two types of tumor, A and B, profiled for 100 different genes. The expression profile derived from expression arrays for this simple example is already substantial, consisting of 800 expression values. In a real expression profiling experiment, however, hundreds of samples may be analyzed for the expression for all human genes, which rapidly produces a massive data set of millions of expression values. Organizing the data and analyzing them to extract key information are challenging problems that have inspired the development of sophisticated statistical and bioinformatic tools. Using such tools, one can organize the data to find groups of genes whose expression seems to correlate, that is, move up or down together, between and among the samples. Grouping genes by their patterns of expression across samples is termed **clustering.**

Clusters of gene expression can then be tested to determine if any correlate with particular characteristics of the samples of interest. For example, profiling might indicate that a cluster of genes with a correlated expression profile is found more frequently in samples from tumor A but not from tumor B, whereas another cluster of genes with a correlated expression profile is more frequent in samples derived from tumor B but not from tumor A. Clusters of genes whose expression correlates with each other and with a particular set of samples constitute an **expression signature** characteristic of those samples. In the hypothetical profiles in Figure 16-14, certain genes have a correlated expression that serves as a signature for tumor A; tumor B has a signature derived from the correlated expression of a different subset of these 100 genes.

Application of Gene Signatures

Application of gene expression profiles to characterize tumors can be useful in a number of ways. First, they

EXPRESSION PROFILING

CLUSTERING INTO SIGNATURES

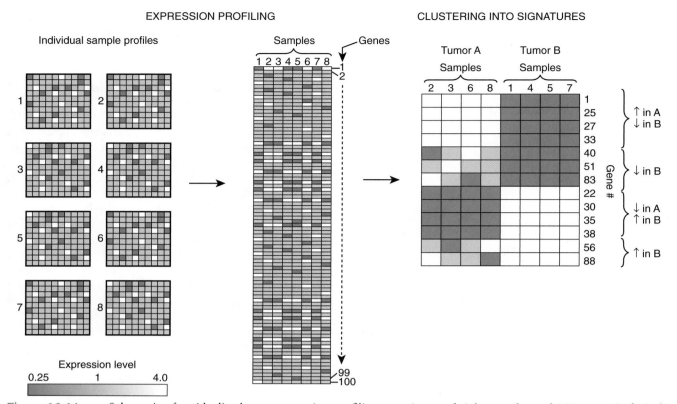

Figure 16-14 ■ Schematic of an idealized gene expression profiling experiment of eight samples and 100 genes. Left: Individual arrays of gene sequences spotted on glass or silicon chips are used for comparative hybridization of eight different samples relative to a common standard. Dark blue indicates decreased expression compared with control, white indicates increased expression, and light blue is unchanged expression. (In this schematic, blue and white represent decreased or increased expression, whereas a real experiment would be quantitative with shades of blue and white.) Center: All 800 expression measurements are organized so that the relative expression for each gene, 1 through 100, is put in order vertically in a column under the number of each sample. Right: Clustering into signatures involves only those 13 genes that showed correlation across subsets of samples. Some genes have reciprocal (high versus low) expression in the two tumors; others show correlated increase or decrease in one tumor and not the other.

increase our ability to discriminate between different tumors in powerful ways that complement the standard criteria applied by pathologists to characterize tumors, such as histological appearance, cytogenetic markers, and expression of specific marker proteins. Once distinguishing signatures for different tumor types (for example, tumor A versus tumor B) are defined with known samples, the expression pattern of *unknown* tumor samples can then be compared with the expression signatures for tumor A and tumor B and classified as A-like, B-like, or neither, depending on how well their expression profiles match the signatures of A and B. Second, different signatures may be found to correlate with clinical outcomes that are known in a set of samples, such as prognosis, response to therapy, or any other outcome of interest. If validated, such signatures could be applied prospectively to help guide therapy in newly diagnosed patients. Finally, for basic research, clustering may reveal previously unsuspected connections of functional importance among genes involved in a disease process.

Gene Expression Profiles in the Management of Cancer Patients

Gene Expression Profiling in Lymphoma Diagnosis

An example of expression profiling to distinguish between similar types of cancers that require different management options is found in the management of **Burkitt lymphoma**. Burkitt lymphoma is a rare but highly aggressive B-cell lymphoma, which we discussed previously in this chapter because of its association with a t(8;14) translocation that dysregulates the *MYC* oncogene. **Diffuse large B-cell lymphoma** is a more common and less aggressive lymphoma. These two lymphomas are distinguished by histological appearance, expression of cell surface proteins, and the t(8;14) translocation, but these parameters can be imperfect discriminators. For example, the t(8;14) translocation is also seen in 5% to 10% of patients with diffuse large B-cell lymphoma. Distinguishing Burkitt lymphoma from diffuse large B-cell lymphoma is important because Burkitt lymphoma requires a harsher chemotherapeutic regimen, including treatment of the cerebrospinal fluid.

In one retrospective study, expression profiling was applied to 35 B-cell lymphoma samples, including 29 that had previously been classified as diffuse B-cell lymphoma and six that could not be classified by a panel of expert pathologists by histological appearance, cell surface protein studies, and cytogenetic analysis. Application of gene expression profiling demonstrated that nine of the 35 patients with diffuse large B-cell lymphoma had a Burkitt lymphoma signature instead,

and were therefore likely to require different treatment. The results of chemotherapy were available in seven of these nine patients with a gene expression signature for Burkitt lymphoma; five received chemotherapy suitable for diffuse large B-cell lymphoma, and none survived more than 2 years. Two received Burkitt lymphoma chemotherapy, and one survived beyond 5 years. Although the numbers are small, this study suggests that application of gene expression signatures may be superior to methods previously employed to distinguish between these two forms of lymphoma, and can contribute to ensuring that patients receive the most appropriate treatment for their lymphoma.

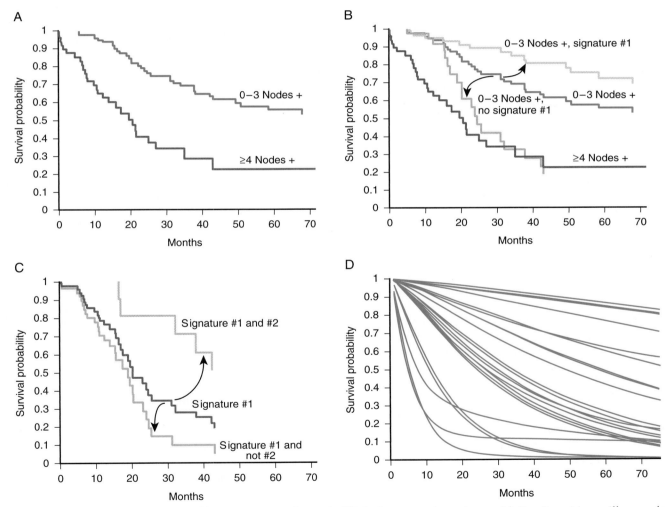

Figure 16-15 ■ Survival curves of breast cancer patients. **A,** Clinical outcome in patients with 0 to 3 positive axillary nodes versus 4 or more positive nodes. **B,** A particular expression profile signature, referred to here as signature #1, was found to correlate well with clinical outcome in that it split the group with 0 to 3+ nodes into two groups, one that had been found to have a better survival and one with worse survival. **C,** Patients with signature #1 could be partitioned as to outcome into those who also had signature #2 and those who did not. **D,** Node status, estrogen receptor status, and multiple gene expression signatures could be combined into a highly personalized profile that correlated well with survival of each individual patient, as represented by her own unique survival curve (in blue). (Modified from Pittman J, Huang H, Dressman H, et al: Integrated modeling of clinical and gene expression information for personalized prediction of disease outcomes. Proc Natl Acad Sci USA 101:8431–8436, 2004.)

Gene Expression Profiling in Breast Cancer Prognosis

Choosing the appropriate therapy for breast cancer is difficult for patients and their physicians because recurrence is common and difficult to predict. Better characterization of each patient's cancer as to recurrence risk and metastatic potential would clearly be beneficial for deciding between more or less aggressive courses of surgery and chemotherapy. Although absence of the estrogen receptor and the presence of metastatic tumor in lymph nodes found during dissection of axillary lymphatics are strong predictors of poorer prognosis and shortened survival, they are still imprecise and uncertain. Expression profiling is opening up a promising new avenue for clinical decision-making in breast cancer treatment.

In a retrospective study of 158 breast cancer patients for whom clinical outcome and survival were already known, patients could, as expected, be readily partitioned into two groups on the basis of their axillary node status, with those with fewer positive nodes having longer survival (Fig. 16-15). Expression profiling was then used to find signatures that correlated best with the known disease outcome. When the gene expression data were analyzed, a particular signature, referred to here as signature #1, was found to correlate well with clinical outcome in that it split the group with 0 to 3+ nodes into two groups, one that had been found to have a better survival and one with worse survival. Signatures themselves could also be combined with each other and the combination analyzed for whether it increased the accuracy with which patients could be divided into those who had had better or worse survival. For example, patients with signature #1 could be partitioned as to outcome into those who also had signature #2 and those who did not. Ultimately, node status, estrogen receptor status, and gene expression signatures could be combined to generate a profile that correlated with survival in each individual patient.

It is hoped that similar studies will allow clinicians to apply such combinations of clinical and gene expression data prospectively in patients newly diagnosed with breast cancer, to provide better estimates of prognosis and to guide the intensity of therapy required. This approach is likely to improve the chances of survival for patients with a predicted poor prognosis by suggesting that the most aggressive radiation and chemotherapy be used. Similarly, finding a signature with a better prognosis may save those patients from the danger of complications from excessively harsh therapeutic modalities.

The fact that the individual prognosis of practically every single patient could be associated with a particular combination of clinical features and expression signatures underscores a crucial point about breast cancer and, in fact, all cancers: each person's cancer is a unique disorder. The heterogeneity among patients who all carry the same cancer diagnosis should not be surprising given what we have learned in this book and this chapter. Every patient is unique in the genetic variants he or she carries, including those variants that will affect how the cancer develops and the body responds to it. Moreover, the clonal evolution of a cancer implies that chance mutational and epigenetic events will likely occur in different and unique combinations in every patient's particular cancer.

Noncoding RNA Expression Profiling

Although most of the evidence to date on expression profiling in cancer has used arrays of protein-coding genes, there is exciting evidence that signatures that rely on *noncoding* RNA expression may be as informative, or even more informative, for classifying different tumor types. With many fewer such genes in the genome, it may be possible to reduce the complexity of the arrays. Furthermore, some highly undifferentiated cancers, which are difficult to classify by expression profiling for protein-coding transcripts, may be classifiable by noncoding RNA expression signatures.

● CANCER AND THE ENVIRONMENT

Throughout this chapter, we have stressed that cancer is a genetic disease, including sporadic cancers that arise from somatic mutations in oncogenes and TSGs. Although the theme of this chapter is that cancer is a genetic disease, there is no contradiction in considering the role of environment in carcinogenesis. By environment, we include exposure to a wide variety of different types of agents—food, natural and artificial radiation, chemicals, and viruses. The risk of cancer shows significant variation among different populations and within the same population in different environments. For example, gastric cancer is almost three times as common among Japanese in Japan as among Japanese living in Hawaii or Los Angeles.

In some cases, environmental agents act as mutagens that cause somatic mutations; the somatic mutations, in turn, are responsible for carcinogenesis. According to some estimates based chiefly on data from the aftermath of the atomic bombings of Hiroshima and Nagasaki, as much as 75% of the risk of cancer may be environmental in origin. In other cases, there appears to be a correlation between certain exposures and risk of cancer, such as the inverse relationship between dietary fiber and colon cancer, without there being a clear mechanistic explanation. The nature of environmental agents that either increase or reduce the risk of cancer, assessment of the additional risk associated with exposure, and ways of protecting the population from such hazards are matters of strong public concern.

Radiation

Ionizing radiation is known to increase the risk of cancer. The data for survivors of the Hiroshima and Nagasaki atomic bombings and other exposed populations show a long latency period, in the 5-year range for leukemia but up to 40 years for some tumors. The risk is dependent on the age at exposure, being greatest for children younger than 10 years and for the elderly. As noted earlier, radiation is much more damaging to persons with inborn defects of DNA repair than to the general population. Everyone is exposed to some degree of ionizing radiation through background radiation (which varies greatly from place to place) and medical exposure. Unfortunately, there are still large areas of uncertainty about the magnitude of the effects of radiation, especially low-level radiation, on cancer risks.

Chemical Carcinogens

Interest in the carcinogenic effect of chemicals dates at least to the 18th century, when the high incidence of scrotal cancer in young chimney sweeps was noticed. Today, there is concern about many possible chemical carcinogens, especially tobacco, components of the diet, industrial carcinogens, and toxic wastes. Documentation of the risk of exposure is often difficult, but the level of concern is such that all clinicians should have a working knowledge of the subject and be able to distinguish between well-established facts and areas of uncertainty and debate.

The precise molecular mechanisms by which most chemical carcinogens cause cancer are still the subject of extensive research. One illustrative example of how a chemical carcinogen may contribute to the development of cancer is that of **hepatocellular carcinoma,** the fifth most common cancer worldwide. In many parts of the world, hepatocellular carcinoma occurs at increased frequency because of ingestion of aflatoxin B1, a potent carcinogen produced by a mold found on peanuts. Aflatoxin has been shown to modify a particular base in the *TP53* TSG, causing a G to T transversion in codon 249, converting an arginine codon to serine in the critically important p53 protein that we discussed earlier in the section on the Li-Fraumeni syndrome. This mutation is found in nearly half of all hepatocellular carcinomas in patients from parts of the world in which there is a high frequency of contamination of foodstuffs by aflatoxin, but it is not found in similar cancers in patients whose exposure to aflatoxin in food is low. The Arg249Ser mutation in p53 enhances hepatocyte growth and interferes with the growth control and apoptosis associated with wild-type p53; LOH of *TP53* in hepatocellular carcinoma is associated with a more malignant appearance of the cancer.

Although aflatoxin B1 alone is capable of causing hepatocellular carcinoma, it also acts synergistically with chronic hepatitis B and C infections.

A more complicated situation occurs with an exposure to complex mixtures of chemicals, such as the many known or suspected carcinogens and mutagens found in cigarette smoke. The epidemiological evidence is overwhelming that cigarette smoke increases the risk for lung cancer and throat cancer as well as other cancers. Cigarette smoke contains polycyclic hydrocarbons that are converted to highly reactive epoxides that cause mutations by directly damaging DNA. The relative importance of these substances and how they might interact in carcinogenesis are still being elucidated.

The case of cigarette smoking also raises another interesting issue. Why do only some cigarette smokers get lung cancer? The case of cancer and cigarette smoking provides an important example of the interaction between environment and genetic factors to either enhance or prevent the carcinogenic effects of chemicals. The enzyme **aryl hydrocarbon hydroxylase** (AHH) is an inducible protein involved in the metabolism of polycyclic hydrocarbons, such as those found in cigarette smoke. AHH converts hydrocarbons into an epoxide form that is more easily excreted by the body but that also happens to be carcinogenic. AHH activity is encoded by members of the *CYP1* family of cytochrome P450 genes (see Chapter 18). One well-studied genetic polymorphism in the *CYP1A1* gene has been associated with susceptibility to lung cancer. The *CYP1A1* gene is inducible by cigarette smoke, but the inducibility is variable in the population because of different alleles at the *CYP1A1* locus. People who carry a "high-inducibility" allele, particularly those who are smokers, appear to be at an increased risk of lung cancer. On the other hand, homozygotes for the recessive "low-inducibility" allele appear to be less likely to develop lung cancer, possibly because their AHH is less effective at converting the hydrocarbons to highly reactive carcinogens. The *CYP1A2* gene is also polymorphic in the population, resulting in variability in the extent of hydrocarbon metabolism in the normal population. A third polymorphic cytochrome P450 gene, *CYP2D6,* has also been associated with an increased susceptibility to lung cancer. A small proportion of people have reduced CYP2D6 activity because they are homozygous for a reduced activity allele at the *CYP2D6* gene. These persons appear to be more resistant to the potential carcinogenic effects of cigarette smoke or occupational lung carcinogens (such as asbestos or polycyclic aromatic hydrocarbons). Normal or ultrafast metabolizers, on the other hand, have a 4-fold greater risk for lung cancer than do slow metabolizers. This risk increases to 18-fold among persons exposed routinely to lung carcinogens. A similar association has been reported for bladder cancer.

Although the precise genetic and biochemical basis for the apparent differences in cancer susceptibility within the normal population remains to be determined, these associations could have significant public health consequences and may point eventually to a way of identifying persons who are genetically at a higher risk for the development of cancer.

● GENERAL REFERENCES

Mitelman F: Catalogue of Chromosome Aberrations in Cancer, 6th ed [on CD-ROM]. New York, John Wiley & Sons, 1998.

Offit K: Clinical Cancer Genetics: Risk Counseling and Management. New York, Wiley-Liss, 1998.

Schneider L: Counseling about Cancer, 2nd ed. New York, Wiley-Liss, 2002.

Vogelstein B, Kinzler KW: The Genetic Basis of Human Cancer, 2nd ed. New York, McGraw-Hill, 2002.

Vogelstein B, Kinzler KW: Cancer genes and the pathways they control. Nat Med 10:789-799, 2004.

Wogan GN, Hecht SS, Felton JS, et al: Environmental and chemical carcinogenesis. Semin Cancer Biol 14:473-486, 2004.

● REFERENCES FOR SPECIFIC TOPICS

Barnetson RA, Tenesa A, Farrington SM, et al: Identification and survival of carriers of mutations in DNA mismatch-repair genes in colon cancer. N Engl J Med 354:2715-2763, 2006.

Chen C-Z: MicroRNAs as oncogenes and tumor suppressors. N Engl J Med 353:1768-1771, 2005.

Dave S, Fu K, Wright GW, et al: Molecular diagnosis of Burkitt's lymphoma. N Engl J Med 354:2431-2442, 2006.

Esquela-Kerscher A, Slack FJ: Oncomirs—microRNAs with a role in cancer. Nat Rev Cancer 6:259-269, 2006.

Esteller M: Cancer epigenetics: DNA methylation and chromatin alterations in human cancer. Adv Exp Med Biol 532:39-49, 2003.

Greenman C, Stephens P, Smith R, et al: Patterns of somatic mutation in human cancer genomes. Nature 446:153-158, 2007.

James PA, Doherty R, Harris M, et al: Optimal selection of individuals for BRCA mutation testing: a comparison of available methods. J Clin Oncol 24:707-715, 2006.

Jones PA, Laird PW: Cancer epigenetics comes of age. Nat Genet 21:163-167, 1999.

Knudson AG: Hereditary cancer: two hits revisited. J Cancer Res Clin Oncol 122:135-140, 1996.

Kops GJP, Weaver BAA, Cleveland DW: On the road to cancer: aneuploidy and the mitotic checkpoint. Nat Rev Cancer 5:773-785, 2005.

Kurzrock R, Kantarjian HM, Druker BJ, Talpaz M: Philadelphia chromosome–positive leukemias: from basic mechanisms to molecular therapeutics. Ann Intern Med 138:819-830, 2003.

Lu J, Getz G, Miska E, et al: MicroRNA expression profiles classify human cancers. Nature 435:834-838, 2005.

Michor F, Iwasa Y, Nowak MA: Dynamics of cancer progression. Nat Rev Cancer 4:197-205, 2004.

Nanda R, Schumm LP, Cummings S, et al: Genetic testing in an ethnically diverse cohort of high-risk women. JAMA 294:1925-1933, 2006.

Parsons DW, Wang T-L, Samuels Y, et al: Colorectal cancer: mutations in a signalling pathway. Nature 436:792, 2005.

Pittman J, Huang E, Dressman H, et al: Integrated modeling of clinical and gene expression information for personalized prediction of disease outcomes. Proc Natl Acad Sci USA 101:8431-8436, 2004.

Shay JW, Wright WE: Telomerase therapeutics for cancer: challenges and new directions. Nat Rev Drug Discov 5:577-584, 2006.

Sjöblom T, Jones S, Wood LD, et al: The Consensus Coding Sequences of Human Breast and Colorectal Cancers. Science 314:268-274, 2006.

Staib F, Hussain SP, Hofseth LJ: TP53 and liver carcinogenesis. Hum Mutat 21:201-216, 2003.

Witt E, Ashworth A: D-Day for BRCA2. Science 297:534, 2002.

PROBLEMS

1. A patient with retinoblastoma has a single tumor in one eye; the other eye is free of tumors. What steps would you take to try to determine whether this is sporadic or heritable retinoblastoma? What genetic counseling would you provide? What information should the parents have before a subsequent pregnancy?

2. Discuss possible reasons why colorectal cancer is an adult cancer, whereas retinoblastoma affects children.

3. Many tumor types are characterized by the presence of an isochromosome for the long arm of chromosome 17. Provide a possible explanation for this finding.

4. Many children with Fanconi anemia have limb defects. If an affected child requires surgery for the abnormal limb, what special considerations arise?

5. Wanda, whose sister has premenopausal bilateral breast cancer, has a greater risk of developing breast cancer herself than does Wilma, whose sister has premenopausal breast cancer in only one breast. Both Wanda and Wilma, however, have a greater risk than does Winnie, who has a completely negative family history. Discuss the role of molecular testing in these women. What would their breast cancer risks be if a pathogenic BRCA1 or BRCA2 mutation were found in the affected relative? What if no mutations were found?

6. Propose a theory for why so few hereditary cancer syndromes, inherited as autosomal dominant diseases, are caused by activated oncogenes, whereas so many are caused by germline mutations in a TSG.

Chapter 17

Personalized Genetic Medicine

More than a century ago, the British physician-scientist Archibald Garrod applied Mendel's laws of heredity to the inheritance of human disease and coined the term **inborn error of metabolism,** thereby creating the field of biochemical genetics. Garrod had more in mind, however, than unusual biochemical changes in patients with autosomal recessive disorders of intermediary metabolism. In a demonstration of prescient scientific and clinical insight, he proposed the much broader concept of **chemical individuality,** in which each of us differs in our health status and susceptibility to various illnesses because of our individual genetic makeup. Indeed, in 1902, he wrote:

> . . . the factors which confer upon us our predis-position and immunities from disease are inher-ent in our very chemical structure, and even in the molecular groupings which went to the making of the chromosomes from which we sprang.

Now, more than a hundred years later in the era of human genomics, we have the means to assess an indi-vidual's genotype at all relevant loci and to characterize the genetic underpinnings of each person's unique "chemical individuality." When the genetic variants rel-evant to maintaining health and preventing or treating illness in each individual are known, and when that knowledge is used in making important clinical deci-sions as a routine part of medical care, we will have entered the era of **personalized genetic medicine,** one of the major goals of the Human Genome Project. However, personalized genetic medicine is only one component of patient-centered medical care in the broadest sense, in which care providers also take each individual's developmental history, environmental exposure, and social experiences into account when providing diagnosis, counseling, preventive interven-tion, management, and therapy.

In the preceding chapter on genetics and cancer, we described powerful new genomic technologies, such as determining which mutations and polymorphisms are present in a tumor and profiling its pattern of RNA expression, that are currently being used for the molec-ular characterization of cancer (see Chapter 16). Such information is proving increasingly helpful for guiding management and therapy for individual cancer patients, as one application of what might be called **genomic medicine.** In this chapter, we explore other applications of genetics and genomics to individualized health care: screening asymptomatic individuals for susceptibility to disease and applying that knowledge to improve health care. First, we describe how the family history can be used to assess risk and to guide preventive and thera-peutic measures in asymptomatic individuals. Next, we discuss population screening and present one of the oldest forms of genetic screening, the detection of abnormalities in newborns at high risk for preventable illness. Finally, we discuss screening of patients for genetic susceptibility based on their genotypes alone and review some of the concepts and methods of genetic epidemiology that are commonly used to evaluate screening for susceptibility genotypes.

FAMILY HISTORY AS PERSONALIZED GENETIC MEDICINE

Physicians have long practiced a form of personalized genetic medicine when they obtain a family history and use it in their clinical decision-making. Family history is clearly of great importance in dealing with single-gene disorders. Applying the known rules of mendelian inheritance allows the geneticist to provide accurate evaluations of risk for disease in relatives of affected individuals (see Chapter 19). Family history is also important when a geneticist assesses the risk for complex

••• Family History in Risk Assessment

High Risk

- Premature disease in a first-degree relative
- Premature disease in a second-degree relative (coronary artery disease only)
- Two affected first-degree relatives
- One first-degree relative with late or unknown disease onset and an affected second-degree relative with premature disease from the same lineage
- Two second-degree maternal or paternal relatives with at least one having premature onset of disease
- Three or more affected maternal or paternal relatives
- Presence of a "moderate-risk" family history on both sides of the pedigree

Moderate Risk

- One first-degree relative with late or unknown onset of disease
- Two second-degree relatives from the same lineage with late or unknown disease onset

Average Risk

- No affected relatives
- Only one affected second-degree relative from one or both sides of the pedigree
- No known family history
- Adopted person with unknown family history

From Scheuner MT, et al: Am J Med Genet 71:315-324, 1997; quoted in Yoon PW, et al: Genet Med 4:304-310, 2002.

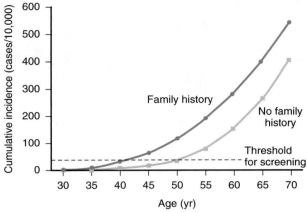

Figure 17-1 ■ Cumulative incidence (per 10,000) of colon cancer versus age in individuals with and without a family history of the disease. (Data from Fuchs CS, Giovannucci EL, Colditz GA, et al: A prospective study of family history and the risk of colorectal cancer. N Engl J Med 331:1669-1674, 1994.)

disorders, as discussed in Chapter 8 and elsewhere in this book. Since a person's genes are shared with his or her relatives, family history provides the clinician with information on the impact that a substantial subset of an individual's genetic makeup might have on one's health, using the medical history of relatives as an indicator of one's own genetic susceptibilities. Furthermore, family members often share environmental factors, such as diet and behavior, and thus relatives provide information about both shared genes and shared environmental factors that may interact to cause most common diseases with complex inheritance. Having a first-degree relative with a common disease of adulthood—such as cardiovascular disease, cancer of the breast, cancer of the colon or prostate, type 2 diabetes, osteoporosis, or asthma—raises an individual's risk for the disease approximately 2-fold to 3-fold relative to the general population, a moderate increase compared with the average population risk (see Box). As discussed in Chapter 8, the more first-degree relatives one has with a complex trait and the earlier in life the disease occurs in a family member, the greater the load of susceptibility genes and environmental exposures likely to be present in the patient's family, leading to a designation of the patient as being at high risk for disease on

the basis of family history. For example, a male with three male first-degree relatives with prostate cancer has an 11-fold greater relative risk for development of the disease than does a man with no family history.

Determining that an individual is at increased risk on the basis of family history can have an impact on individual medical care. For example, two individuals with deep venous thrombosis, one with a family history of unexplained deep venous thrombosis in a relative younger than 50 years and another with no family history of any coagulation disorder, will receive different management with respect to testing for factor V Leiden or prothrombin 20210G>A and anticoagulation therapy (see Chapter 8). Similarly, a family history of colon cancer is sufficient to trigger the initiation of colon cancer screening with more sophisticated screening methods at the age of 40 years, 10 years earlier than for the general population. This is because the cumulative incidence for development of the disease for someone 40 years old with a positive family history equals the risk for someone at the age of 50 years with no family history (Fig. 17-1). The increase in risk is even more pronounced if two or more relatives have had the disease.

Family history is, unfortunately, a relatively underused tool in clinical medicine. In one survey, primary care physicians were found to discuss family history with only half of their new patients and with less than one quarter of their return patients. Only one patient in nine observed by the physicians in that managed care practice was found to have a family tree in the chart. In another survey performed in a managed health care setting, the fact that a patient had one or more first-degree relatives with the disease—and was therefore at increased risk for one of the common adult-onset diseases inherited as a complex trait—was missed in nearly two thirds of patients. It is worth repeating the admonition made by the distinguished pediatrician and geneticist, Barton Childs, quoted in Chapter 1: "to fail to take a good family history is bad medicine."

Of course, with the exception of monozygotic twins, no one shares all his genes with his relatives. Family history is therefore an indirect means of assessing the contribution that an individual's own combination of genetic variants might make to disease. Family history is also an insensitive indicator of susceptibility since it depends on overt disease actually occurring in the relatives of the individual patient. The challenge going forward is to screen populations, independent of family history, for variants relevant to health and disease and to apply this information to make risk assessments that can be used to improve the health care of the individual patient and his or her family. Applying this information requires that we demonstrate that genetic risk factors are valid indicators of actual risk in an individual patient and, if they are valid, how useful such information is in guiding health care.

○ GENETIC SCREENING IN POPULATIONS

Genetic screening is a population-based method for identifying persons with increased susceptibility to or risk for a genetic disease. Screening at the population level is not to be confused with testing for affected persons or carriers within families already identified because of family history. Rather, the objective of population screening is to examine *all* members of a designated population, regardless of family history. Genetic screening is an important public health activity that will become more significant as more and better screening tests become available for determining genetic susceptibilities for disease.

Clinical Validity and Utility

Finding the genetic contributions to health and disease is of obvious importance for research into underlying disease etiology and pathogenesis as well as for identifying potential targets for intervention and therapy. In medical practice, however, whether to screen individuals for increased susceptibilities to illness depends on the **clinical validity** and **clinical utility** of the test. Clinical validity is the extent to which a test result is predictive for disease. The **clinical utility** of a test is the degree to which test results will change what medical care an individual receives and, as a consequence, improve the outcome of care, both medically and economically. Clinical utility can be assessed both for the individual being screened and for the entire population that participates in a screening program.

A genetic **disease association** is the relationship between a susceptibility or protective genotype and a disease phenotype. The susceptibility or protective genotype can be defined as the presence of an allele (in either a heterozygote or a homozygote), the homozygous genotype only, a haplotype containing alleles at neighboring loci, or even combinations of genotypes at multiple unlinked loci. Assuming whatever test being used to detect the genotype gives the correct assignment of the genotype to each person being tested (the **analytic validity** of the test), the clinical validity represents how well the genotype predicts the phenotype, and vice versa. Clinical validity depends on how sensitive and specific the test is for the phenotype, that is, the false-negative and false-positive rates. When faced with an individual patient, however, the practitioner of personalized genetic medicine wants to know more than how sensitive or specific a test is. A third facet of clinical validity is also of concern: to what extent does a particular genotype provide information on whether this patient is at risk for a particular disease, not relative to those without the genotype but in absolute terms? This facet of clinical validity is captured by the **positive predictive value** and **negative predictive value** of the test for that disease. The relationship between some of these factors is best demonstrated by means of a 2×2 table.

Determination of the Predictive Value of a Test

Genotype	DISEASE		
	Affected	Unaffected	Total
Susceptibility genotype present	a*	b	a + b
Susceptibility genotype absent	c	d	c + d
Total	a + c	b + d	a + b + c + d = N

Frequency of the susceptibility genotype = (a + b)/N
Disease prevalence = (a + c)/N (with random sampling or a complete population survey)

Relative Risk Ratio:

$$RRR = \frac{\text{Disease prevalence in carriers of susceptibility genotype}}{\text{Disease prevalence in non-carriers of susceptibility genotype}}$$

$$= \frac{a/(a + b)}{c/(c + d)}$$

Sensitivity: Fraction of individuals with disease who have the susceptibility genotype = a/(a + c)

Specificity: Fraction without disease who do not have the susceptibility genotype = d/(b + d)

Positive predictive value: Proportion of individuals with the susceptibility genotype who have or will develop a particular disease = a/(a + b)

Negative predictive value: Proportion of individuals without the susceptibility genotype who do not have or will not develop a particular disease = d/(c + d)

*The values of a, b, c, and d are derived from a random sample of the population, divided into those with and without the susceptibility genotype, and then examined for the disease (with or without longitudinal follow-up, depending on whether it is a cross-sectional or cohort study) (see later).

Table 17-1

Some Conditions for Which Newborn Screening Has Been Implemented

Condition	Frequency (per 100,000 newborns)*
Congenital hearing loss	200
Sickle cell disease	47
Hypothyroidism	28
Phenylketonuria	3
Congenital adrenal hyperplasia	2
Galactosemia	2
Maple syrup urine disease	≤1
Homocystinuria	≤1
Biotinidase deficiency	≤1

*Approximate values in the United States.

Newborn Screening

The best-known population screening efforts in genetics are the government programs that identify presymptomatic infants with diseases for which early treatment can prevent or at least ameliorate the consequences (Table 17-1). For newborn screening, disease risk is not assessed by determining the genotype directly. Instead, risk is usually measured by detecting abnormally high levels of certain metabolites in the blood of infants who are asymptomatic as newborns but are at greatly increased risk for development of disease later in life. These metabolites are chosen to have high analytic validity for genotypes that have high positive predictive value for serious metabolic disorders later in life. Exceptions to this paradigm of using a biochemical measurement to detect a disease-causing genotype are screening programs for hypothyroidism and abnormalities in hearing, in which the phenotype itself is the target of screening and intervention (see later).

Many of the issues concerning genetic screening in general are highlighted by newborn screening programs. A determination of the appropriateness of newborn screening for any particular condition is based on a standard set of criteria involving analytic validity, clinical validity, and clinical utility (see Box). The clinical validity of test results is obviously important. False-positive results cause unnecessary anxiety to the parents as well as increase the costs because more unaffected infants have to be recalled for retesting. False-negative results vitiate the purpose of having a screening program. The criterion that the public health system infrastructure be capable of handling the care of newborns identified by screening is often underemphasized in discussions of the clinical utility of screening but must also be considered in deciding whether to institute screening for any given condition.

The prototype condition that satisfies all of these criteria is **phenylketonuria** (see Chapter 12). For many

••• General Criteria for an Effective Newborn Screening Program

Analytic Validity

- A rapid and economic laboratory test is available that detects the appropriate metabolite.

Clinical Validity

- The laboratory test is highly sensitive (no false negatives) and reasonably specific (few false positives). Positive predictive value is high.

Clinical Utility

- Treatment is available.
- Early institution of treatment, before symptoms become manifest, reduces or prevents severe illness.
- Routine observation and physical examination will not reveal the disorder in the newborn—a test is required.
- The condition is frequent and serious enough to justify the expense of screening; that is, screening is cost-effective.
- The public health system infrastructure is in place to inform the newborn's parents and physicians of the results of the screening test, to confirm the test results, and to institute effective treatment and counseling.

years, elevated levels of phenylalanine in a spot of blood on filter paper obtained soon after birth has been the mainstay of neonatal screening for phenylketonuria and other forms of hyperphenylalaninemia in all states in the United States, all the provinces of Canada, and nearly all developed countries. A positive screen result, followed by definitive confirmation of the diagnosis, led to the institution of dietary phenylalanine restriction early in infancy, thereby preventing irreversible mental retardation.

Two other conditions that are widely targeted for newborn screening are **congenital deafness** and **congenital hypothyroidism**. Newborn screening for hearing loss is mandated in 37 states in the United States and three provinces in Canada. Approximately half of all congenital deafness is due to single-gene defects (Case 11). Infants found to have hearing impairments by newborn screening receive intervention with sign language and other communication aids early in life, thereby improving their long-term language skills and intellectual abilities beyond that seen if the impairment is discovered later in childhood. Screening for congenital hypothyroidism, a disorder that is genetic only 10% to 15% of the time but is easily treatable, is universal in the United States and Canada and is also routine in many countries. Thyroid hormone replacement therapy started early in infancy completely prevents the severe and irreversible mental retardation caused by congenital hypothyroidism. Thus, both hypothyroidism and

Table 17-2

Disorders Detectable by Tandem Mass Spectrometry

Condition	Substances Present at Increased Levels
Amino acidemias	
Phenylketonuria	Phenylalanine and tyrosine
Maple syrup urine disease	Leucine and isoleucine
Homocystinuria	Methionine
Citrullinemia	Citrulline
Argininosuccinic aciduria	Argininosuccinic acid
Hepatorenal tyrosinemia	Methionine and tyrosine
Organic acidemias	Relevant acylcarnitine metabolites
Propionic acidemia	
Methylmalonic acidemia	
Isovaleric acidemia	
Isolated 3-methylcrotonylglycinemia	
Glutaric acidemia (type I)	
Mitochondrial acetoacetyl-CoA thiolase deficiency	
Hydroxymethylglutaric acidemia	
Multiple CoA carboxylase deficiency	
Fatty acid oxidation disorders	Relevant acylcarnitine metabolites
Short-chain acyl-CoA dehydrogenase deficiency	
Short-chain hydroxy acyl-CoA dehydrogenase deficiency	
Medium-chain acyl-CoA dehydrogenase deficiency	
Very long chain acyl-CoA dehydrogenase deficiency	
Long-chain acyl-CoA dehydrogenase and trifunctional protein deficiency	
Glutaric acidemia type II	
Carnitine palmitoyltransferase II deficiency	

American College of Medical Genetics/American Society of Human Genetics Test and Technology Transfer Committee Working Group: Tandem mass spectrometry in newborn screening. Genet Med 2:267-269, 2000.

deafness easily fulfill the criteria for newborn screening.

A number of other disorders, such as galactosemia, sickle cell disease (Case 37), biotinidase deficiency, and congenital adrenal hyperplasia, are part of neonatal screening programs in many or most states and provinces, but not all. For sickle cell disease, the disorder is more common than phenylketonuria overall in the United States, and identifying asymptomatic newborns with the sickle cell disease genotype means that protective measures can be instituted against the life-threatening bacterial sepsis that can occur before overt manifestations of the disease. For this reason, all but eight states, those with small African American populations, screen newborns routinely for sickle cell disease. Which disorders should be the target of newborn screening varies from state to state and continues to be a matter of debate among government public health agencies.

Tandem Mass Spectroscopy

For many years, most newborn screening was performed by a test specific for each individual condition. For example, phenylketonuria screening was based on a microbial or a chemical assay that tested for elevated phenylalanine. This situation has changed dramatically during the past decade, however, with the application of the technology of **tandem mass spectrometry** (TMS). Not only can a neonatal blood spot be examined accurately and rapidly for an elevation of phenylalanine, with fewer false positives than with the older testing methods, but TMS analysis can simultaneously detect a few dozen other biochemical disorders as well. Some of these were already being screened for by individual tests (Table 17-2). For example, many states were using specific tests for elevated methionine to screen for homocystinuria due to cystathionine β-synthase deficiency (see Chapter 12) or elevated branched-chain amino acids in maple syrup urine disease. A single TMS analysis to measure phenylalanine will also simultaneously detect elevated methionine or branched-chain amino acids. TMS, however, cannot replace the disease-specific testing methods for other disorders currently included in newborn screening, such as galactosemia, biotinidase deficiency, congenital adrenal hyperplasia, and sickle cell disease.

TMS also provides a reliable method for newborn screening for some disorders that fit the criteria for screening but had no reliable newborn screening program in place. For example, **medium-chain acyl-CoA dehydrogenase (MCAD) deficiency** is a disorder of fatty acid oxidation that is usually asymptomatic but manifests clinically when the patient becomes catabolic. Detection of MCAD deficiency at birth can be lifesaving because affected infants and children are at very high risk for life-threatening hypoglycemia in early childhood during the catabolic stress caused by an intercurrent illness, such as a viral infection, and nearly a quarter of children with undiagnosed MCAD deficiency will die with their first episode of hypoglycemia. The metabolic derangement can be successfully managed if it is treated promptly. In MCAD deficiency, alerting parents and physicians to the risk of metabolic compensation is the primary goal of screening since the children are healthy between attacks and do not require daily management other than avoidance of prolonged fasting.

The use of TMS for newborn screening is not without controversy, however. In addition to providing a rapid test for many disorders for which newborn screening either is already being done or can easily be justified, TMS also identifies infants with inborn errors, such as methylmalonic acidemia, that have *not* generally been the targets of newborn screening because of their rarity and difficulty of providing definitive therapy that will prevent the progressive neurological impairment. TMS can also identify abnormal metabolites whose significance for health are uncertain. For example, **short-chain acyl-CoA dehydrogenase (SCAD) deficiency**, another disorder of fatty acid oxidation, is most often asymptomatic, although a few patients may have difficulties with episodic hypoglycemia. Thus, the positive predictive value of a positive TMS screen result for symptomatic SCAD is probably very low. Does the benefit of detecting SCAD deficiency outweigh the negative impact of raising parental concern unnecessarily for most newborns whose test result is positive but who will never be symptomatic? Thus, not every disorder detected by TMS fits the criteria for newborn screening. Some public health experts, therefore, argue that only those metabolites of proven clinical utility should be reported to parents and physicians. Others advocate use of all the information TMS provides and reporting of all abnormal metabolites the TMS screening detects to parents and their physicians, regardless of how well the disorders fit the standard criteria for newborn screening. Patients who show abnormalities of unknown significance can then be carefully observed. For all these reasons, the proper use of TMS for newborn screening remains a subject of debate.

Prenatal Screening

Two tests are commonly used for population screening in fetal life: chromosome analysis for advanced maternal age, and maternal serum alpha-fetoprotein or triple screens for neural tube defects and chromosome aneu-

ploidies. This topic is discussed in the context of prenatal diagnosis in Chapter 15. It has been argued, however, that once the pregnancy has been exposed to the risk of invasive prenatal diagnosis of chromosomal aneuploidy because of advanced maternal age, additional testing should also be offered, such as alpha-fetoprotein levels in amniotic fluid (Chapter 15), genome-wide comparative genome hybridization to find deleterious submicroscopic deletions (Chapters 4 and 5), and mutation screening for cystic fibrosis (see Chapter 12 and Case 10)and other common disorders.

● SCREENING FOR GENETIC SUSCEPTIBILITY TO DISEASE

Genetic Epidemiology

Epidemiological studies of risk factors for disease rely heavily on population studies that measure disease prevalence or incidence and determine whether certain risk factors (genetic, environmental, social, and other) are present in individuals with and without disease. **Genetic epidemiology** is concerned with how genotypes and environmental factors interact to increase or decrease susceptibility to disease. Epidemiological studies generally follow one of three different strategies: the case-control, the cross-sectional, and the cohort design (see Box).

▪▪▪ Strategies Used in Genetic Epidemiology

- **Case-control:** Individuals with and without the disease are selected, and the genotypes and environmental exposures of individuals in the two groups are determined and compared.
- **Cross-sectional:** A random sample of the population is selected and divided into those with and without the disease, and their genotypes and environmental exposures are determined and compared.
- **Cohort:** A sample of the population is selected and observed for some time to ascertain who does or does not develop disease, and their genotypes and environmental exposures are determined and compared. The cohort may be selected at random or may be targeted to individuals who share a genotype or an environmental exposure.

Cohort and cross-sectional studies not only capture information on the relative risk conferred by different genotypes but, if they are random population samples, also provide information on the prevalence of the disease and the frequency of the various genotypes under study. A randomly selected cohort study, in particular, is the most accurate and complete in that phenotypes that take time to appear have a better chance of being detected and scored; they are, however, more expensive and time-consuming. Cross-sectional studies, on the other hand, suffer from underestimation of the frequency of the disease. First, if the disease is rapidly fatal, many of the patients with disease and carrying a risk factor will be missed. Second, if the disease shows age-dependent penetrance, patients carrying a risk factor will actually not be scored as having the disease. Case-control studies, on the other hand, allow researchers to efficiently target individuals, particularly with relatively rare phenotypes that would require very large sample sizes in a cross-sectional or cohort study. However, unless a study is based on complete ascertainment of individuals with a disease, such as in a population register or surveillance program, or uses a random sampling scheme, a case-control study cannot capture information on the population prevalence of the disease.

Susceptibility Testing Based on Genotype

The positive predictive value of a genotype that confers susceptibility to a particular disease depends on the frequency of the genotype in the population, the relative risk for disease conferred by one genotype over another, and the prevalence of the disease. Figure 17-2 provides the positive predictive value for genotype frequencies ranging from 0.5% (rare) to 50% (common), which confer a relative risk that varies from low (2-fold) to high (100-fold), when the prevalence of the disease ranges from relatively rare (0.1%) to more common (5%). As Figure 17-2 shows, the value of the test as a

predictor of disease increases substantially when one is dealing with a common disorder due to a relatively rare susceptibility genotype that confers a high relative risk, compared with the risk for individuals who do not carry the genotype. The converse is also clear: testing for a common genotype that confers a modest relative risk is of limited value as a predictor of disease.

We will illustrate the use of the 2 × 2 table (see earlier in the chapter) in assessing the role of susceptibility genes in a common disorder, **colorectal cancer.** Shown in the following Box are data from a population-based study of colorectal cancer risk conferred by a polymorphic variant in the *APC* gene (see Chapter 16 and Case 13) that changes isoleucine 1307 to lysine (Ile1307Lys). This variant has an allele frequency of about 3.1% among Ashkenazi Jews, which means that approximately 1 in 15 individuals is either a heterozygote or homozygote for the allele. The prevalence of colon cancer in this group of patients is 1%. This variant, common enough to be present in approximately 6% of the Ashkenazi Jewish population and conferring a 2.4-fold increased risk for colon cancer, compared with those without the allele, can be an important risk factor in that nearly 9% of all colon cancer in this population can be attributed to the effect of this allele. However, the small positive predictive value (2%) means that an individual who tests positive for this allele has only a 2% chance of developing colorectal cancer. If this had been a cohort study that allowed complete ascertainment of everyone in whom colorectal cancer was going to develop, the penetrance would, in effect, be only 2%.

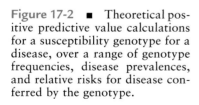

Figure 17-2 ■ Theoretical positive predictive value calculations for a susceptibility genotype for a disease, over a range of genotype frequencies, disease prevalences, and relative risks for disease conferred by the genotype.

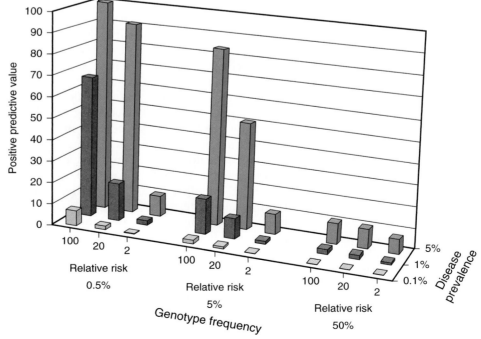

▪▪▪ The Ile1307Lys Allele of the *APC* Gene and Colon Cancer

Genotype	Colon Cancer		
	Affected	Unaffected	Total
Lys1307	7	310	317
Ile1307	38	4142	4180
Total	45	4452	4497

- Relative Risk Ratio = RRR

$$= \frac{\text{Disease prevalence in allele carriers}}{\text{Disease prevalence in non-carriers}}$$

$$= \frac{7/317}{38/4180} = 2.4$$

- Sensitivity: Fraction of individuals with colon cancer who have the allele = 7/45 = 16%
- Specificity: Fraction without colon cancer who do not have the allele = 4142/4452 = 93%
- Positive predictive value: Fraction of individuals with the allele who develop colon cancer = 7/317 = 2%
- Negative predictive value: Fraction of individuals without the allele who do not develop colon cancer = 99%

Data from Woodage T, King SM, Wacholder S, et al. Nat Genet 20:62-65, 1998.

Clinical Utility

In a patient who tests positive for the *APC* Ile1307Lys allele, how does a positive predictive value of 2% translate into medical practice? A complete assessment of the value of testing for genotypes associated with disease does not end with determination of the clinical validity of testing. There is no absolute value of the positive predictive value that determines whether testing is or is not worthwhile. The test must be assessed with regard to clinical utility; that is, do the results of the test influence what care is provided, and more broadly, what are the implications for individual health care and public health if such screening were instituted as part of routine health care?

The clinical utility of a screening test depends on many factors. One critical factor is a public health economic one: can the screening be shown to be **cost-effective**? Is the expense of the testing outweighed by improving health outcomes while reducing health care costs, disability, and loss of earning power? In the example of screening for the *APC* Ile1307Lys allele in Ashkenazi Jews, the utility of certain kinds of testing might indicate the need for a particular regimen of colon cancer surveillance, such as more frequent screening or the use of different approaches to screening. Screening methods (occult stool blood testing versus sigmoidoscopy versus full colonoscopy) differ in expense, sensitivity, specificity, and potential for hazard, and so deciding which regimen to follow has important

implications for the patient's health and health care costs.

Demonstrating that testing improves health care is not always obvious. For example, 1 in 200 to 250 white individuals are homozygous for a Cys282Tyr mutation in the *HFE* gene associated with **hereditary hemochromatosis**, a disorder characterized by iron overload that can silently lead to extensive liver damage and cirrhosis (Case 17). A simple intervention, regular phlebotomy and blood donation to reduce total body iron stores, can prevent hepatic cirrhosis. The susceptibility genotype is common, and 60% to 80% of Cys282Tyr homozygotes show biochemical evidence of increased body iron stores, which suggests that screening to identify asymptomatic individuals who should undergo further testing and, if indicated, the institution of regular phlebotomy, seems a reasonable and cost-effective measure. However, most Cys282Tyr homozygotes remain clinically asymptomatic, leading to the argument that the positive predictive value of *HFE* gene testing for liver disease in hereditary hemochromatosis is too low to justify population screening. Nonetheless, many of these largely asymptomatic patients have signs of silent fibrosis and cirrhosis on liver biopsy, indicating that the Cys282Tyr homozygote may actually be at a higher risk for liver disease than previously thought. Thus, some would argue for population screening to identify individuals in whom regular prophylactic phlebotomy should be instituted. The clinical utility of such population screening remains controversial and will require additional research to determine the natural history of the disease and whether the silent fibrosis and cirrhosis seen on liver biopsy represent the early stages of what will be a progressive illness.

There are other positive and negative outcomes of testing that are psychological in nature and more difficult to assess than the purely economic factors. For example, testing positive for a susceptibility genotype could, on the one hand, empower patients with knowledge of their risks as they make important lifestyle decisions or, on the other hand, cause severe psychological distress or inappropriate fatalism in patients and their relatives who may never develop the disease but test positive for the risk factor. Similarly, patients who test negative could be falsely reassured.

APOE testing in **Alzheimer disease** (AD) (see Chapter 12 and Case 3) provides a clear example of the role of a careful assessment of clinical validity and clinical utility in applying genetic testing to personalized medicine. As discussed in Chapter 8, heterozygotes for the ε4 allele of the *APOE* gene are at a threefold increased risk for development of AD, primarily because the age at onset of AD is shifted 10 to 15 years earlier in them compared with individuals without an *APOE*

Table 17-3

Clinical Validity and Utility of *APOE* Population Screening and Diagnostic Testing for Alzheimer Disease

	Population Screening	Diagnostic Testing
Clinical validity	Asymptomatic individuals aged 65-74 Population prevalence of AD = 3% PPV given ε2/ε4 or ε3/ε4 = 6% PPV given ε4/ε4 = 23%	Individuals aged 65-74 with symptoms of dementia Proportion of dementia patients with AD = ~60% PPV given ε2/ε4 or ε3/ε4 = ~75% PPV given ε4/ε4 = ~98%
Clinical utility	No intervention possible to prevent disease Psychological distress for most people with ε4 alleles who are not likely to develop AD False reassurance for those without ε4 alleles	Increase suspicion that another, potentially treatable cause of dementia may be present Reduce unnecessary testing

Positive predictive value (PPV) calculations are based on a population prevalence of Alzheimer disease (AD) of approximately 3% in individuals aged 65 to 74 years, an allele frequency for the ε4 allele in whites of 10% to 15%, a relative risk of approximately 3 for one ε4 allele, and a relative risk of approximately 20 for two ε4 alleles.

ε4 allele. *APOE* ε4/ε4 homozygotes are at a 20-fold increased risk because their age at onset of AD is shifted by 20 to 30 years. *APOE* testing for the ε4 allele, however, is not recommended in *asymptomatic* individuals but is being used by some practitioners in the evaluation of individuals with symptoms and signs of dementia. An analysis of both the clinical validity and clinical utility of such testing, including calculation of the positive predictive value for asymptomatic and symptomatic individuals, explains why (Table 17-3).

As can be seen from these positive predictive values for asymptomatic people in the age bracket 65 to 74 years, the presence of a single ε4 allele is a very poor predictor of whether AD will develop, despite the 3-fold increased risk for the disease conferred by the ε4 allele compared with those without an ε4 allele. Even with two ε4 alleles, which occurs in approximately 1.5% of the population and is associated with a 20-fold increased risk relative to genotypes without ε4 alleles, there is still less than a 1 in 4 chance of developing AD. In younger asymptomatic individuals, the positive predictive value is smaller still. Thus, in the majority of individuals identified through *APOE* testing as being at increased risk, AD will not develop. Furthermore, knowing that one is at increased risk does not lead to any preventive or therapeutic options and has the potential to cause significant emotional and psychological stress. On the basis of the poor positive predictive value and lack of clinical utility, it should now be clear why *APOE* testing is not recommended in asymptomatic individuals, as discussed in Chapter 8.

On the other hand, individuals who already show signs of dementia are already at a higher prior probability of having AD. *APOE* testing in them may be helpful in deciding whether the disease is indeed AD, or some other form of dementia that would require additional work-up. Of course, with a disorder as devastating and untreatable as AD, it could be argued that even when

APOE testing suggests a high probability of AD, the small chance of a treatable cause for apparent dementia justifies the expense of an additional work-up.

As in all of medicine, balance of the benefits and costs for each component of personalized genetic medicine needs to be clearly demonstrated but also continually reassessed. The need for constant re-evaluation is obvious: imagine how the recommendations for *APOE* testing, despite its low positive predictive value, might change if a low-risk and inexpensive medical intervention is discovered that could prevent the onset of dementia.

Heterozygote Screening

In contrast to screening for genetic disease in newborns or for genetic susceptibility in patients, screening for carriers of mendelian disorders has, as its main purpose, the identification of individuals who are themselves healthy but are at substantial (25%) risk for having children with a severe autosomal recessive or X-linked illness. The principles of heterozygote screening are shown in the accompanying Box.

••• Criteria for Heterozygote Screening Programs

- High frequency of carriers, at least in a specific population
- Availability of an inexpensive and dependable test with very low false-negative and false-positive rates
- Access to genetic counseling for couples identified as heterozygotes
- Availability of prenatal diagnosis
- Acceptance and voluntary participation by the population targeted for screening

To provide a sufficient yield of carriers, current heterozygote screening programs have focused on particular ethnic groups in which the frequency of mutant alleles is high. Heterozygote screening is voluntary and focuses on individuals who identify themselves as being members of a particular high-risk ethnic group. Heterozygote screening has been used extensively for a battery of disorders for which carrier frequency is relatively high: Tay-Sachs disease (Case 38) (the prototype of carrier screening) (see Chapter 12), Gaucher disease, and Canavan disease in the Ashkenazi Jewish population; sickle cell disease (Case 37) in the African American population of North America; and β-thalassemia (Case 39) in high-incidence areas, especially in Cyprus and Sardinia or in extended consanguineous families from Pakistan (see Chapter 11).

The technology for detecting many different mutant alleles in a gene simultaneously in a single procedure (**multiplex testing**) makes it possible to carry out population-based heterozygote screening for cystic fibrosis by examining the *CFTR* gene directly for mutations (see Chapter 12) (Case 10). The most pressing issue for *CFTR* carrier screening by direct detection of mutant alleles is the extreme allelic heterogeneity in many populations and the differences in the mutant alleles present in different ethnic groups. For example, testing with a basic panel of 23 mutations (ΔF508 and the 22 most common other mutations found in non-Hispanic whites) proposed by the American College of Medical Genetics can identify nearly 88% of all mutations and therefore about 80% of the at-risk couples (those in which both partners are heterozygous for a *CFTR* mutation) from this ethnic background. Adding more alleles to the panel only marginally increases the sensitivity of the test in non-Hispanic whites. In other populations, such as Hispanic whites, Asians, and African Americans, the frequency and the distribution of mutant alleles are quite variable. The basic 23-allele panel would detect only 72% of Hispanic carriers, 64% of African American carriers, and 49% of Asian American carriers. Expanded panels that are more ethnic specific are needed for these populations. Thus, for example, many diagnostic laboratories use a panel of mutations in which they test for the ΔF508 mutation plus another four dozen mutant alleles. In contrast, in the Ashkenazi Jewish population, testing for only five mutations detects 94% of carriers, a high sensitivity while testing for fewer mutations.

The impact of carrier screening in lowering the incidence of a genetic disease can be dramatic. Carrier screening for Tay-Sachs disease in the Ashkenazi Jewish population has been carried out since 1969. Screening followed by prenatal diagnosis, when indicated, has already lowered the incidence of Tay-Sachs disease by 65% to 85% in this ethnic group. Prevention of β-thalassemia by carrier detection and prenatal diagnosis has brought about a similar drop in the incidence of the disease in Cyprus and Sardinia. In contrast, attempts to screen for carriers of sickle cell disease in the U.S. African American community have been less effective and have had little impact on the incidence of the disease so far. The success of carrier screening programs for Tay-Sachs disease and β-thalassemia, as well as the relative failure for sickle cell anemia, underscores the importance of community consultation, community education, and the availability of genetic counseling and prenatal diagnosis as critical requirements for an effective program.

GENERAL REFERENCES

Guttmacher AE, Collins FS, Carmona RH: The family history—more important than ever. N Engl J Med 351:2333-2336, 2004.

Snyderman R, Langheier J: Prospective health care: the second transformation of medicine. Genome Biol 7:104, 2006.

REFERENCES FOR SPECIFIC TOPICS

Acheson LS, Wiesner GL, Zyzanski SJ, et al: Family history-taking in community family practice: implications for genetic screening. Genet Med 2:180-185, 2000.

American College of Medical Genetics/American Society of Human Genetics Test and Technology Transfer Committee Working Group: Tandem mass spectrometry in newborn screening. Genet Med 2:267-269, 2000.

Chace DH, Kalas TA, Naylor EW: Use of tandem mass spectrometry for multianalyte screening of dried blood specimens from newborns. Clin Chem 49:1797-1817, 2003.

Feuchtbaum L, Lorey F, Faulkner L, et al: California's experience implementing a pilot newborn supplemental screening program using tandem mass spectrometry. Pediatrics 117:S261-S269, 2006.

Fuchs CS, Giovannucci EL, Colditz GA, et al: A prospective study of family history and the risk of colorectal cancer. N Engl J Med 331:1669-1674, 1994.

Garrod A: The incidence of alkaptonuria: a study in chemical individuality. Lancet 2:1616-1620, 1902.

Khoury MJ, McCabe LL, McCabe ERW: Population screening in the age of genomic medicine. N Engl J Med 348:50-58, 2003.

Marteau TM, Lerman C: Genetic risk and behavior change. Br Med J 322:1056-1059, 2001.

Powell LW, Dixon, JL, Ramm GA, et al: Screening for hemochromatosis in asymptomatic subjects with or without a family history. Arch Intern Med 166:294-301, 2006.

Scheuner MT, Wang SJ, Raffel LJ, et al: Family history: a comprehensive genetic risk assessment method for the chronic conditions of adulthood. Am J Med Genet 71:315-324, 1997.

Schwartz RS: Racial profiling in medical research. N Engl J Med 344:1392-1393, 2001.

Yoon PW, Scheuner MT, Peterson-Oehlke KL, et al: Can family history be used as a tool for public health and preventive medicine? Genet Med 4:304-310, 2002.

USEFUL WEBSITES

Gwinn M, Khoury MJ: Epidemiology. 2001. *http://www.cdc.gov/genomics/training/books/genpractice.htm*

American College of Medical Genetics: Technical Standards and Guidelines for CFTR Mutation Testing, 2006 edition. *http://www.acmg.net/Pages/ACMG_Activities/stds-2002/cf.htm*

PROBLEMS

1. In a population sample of 1,000,000 Europeans, idiopathic cerebral vein thrombosis (iCVT) occurred in 18, consistent with an expected rate of 1 to 2 per 100,000. All the women were tested for factor V Leiden (FVL). Assuming an allele frequency of 2.5% for FVL, how many homozygotes and how many heterozygotes for FVL would you expect in this sample of 1,000,000 people, assuming Hardy-Weinberg equilibrium?

   Among the affected individuals, two were heterozygotes for FVL and one was homozygous for FVL. Set up a 3 × 2 table for the association of the homozygous FVL genotype, the heterozygous FVL genotype, and the wild-type genotype for iCVT.

   What is the relative risk of iCVT in a FVL heterozygote versus the wild-type genotype? What is the risk in a FVL homozygote versus wild-type? What is the sensitivity of testing positive for either one or two FVL alleles for iCVT? Finally, what is the positive predictive value of being homozygous for FVL? heterozygous?

2. In a population sample of 100,000 European women taking oral contraceptives, deep venous thrombosis (DVT) of the lower extremities occurred in 100, consistent with an expected rate of 1 per 1,000. Assuming an allele frequency of 2.5% for factor V Leiden (FVL), how many homozygotes and how many heterozygotes for FVL would you expect in this sample of 100,000 women, assuming Hardy-Weinberg equilibrium?

   Among the affected individuals, 58 were heterozygotes for FVL and 3 were homozygous for FVL. Set up a 3 × 2 table for the association of the homozygous FVL genotype, the heterozygous FVL genotype, and the wild-type genotype for DVT of the lower extremity.

   What is the relative risk of DVT in a FVL heterozygote using oral contraceptives versus women taking oral contraceptives with the wild-type genotype? What is the risk in a FVL homozygote versus wild-type? What is the sensitivity of testing positive for either one or two FVL alleles for DVT while taking oral contraceptives? Finally, what is the positive predictive value for DVT of being homozygous for FVL while taking oral contraceptives? heterozygous?

3. What steps should be taken when a phenylketonuria (PKU) screening test comes back positive? The test is a bacterial inhibition assay on a spot of blood on filter paper (Guthrie test).

4. Newborn screening for sickle cell disease can be performed by hemoglobin electrophoresis, which separates hemoglobin A and S, thereby identifying individuals who are heterozygotes as well as those who are homozygotes for the sickle cell mutation. What potential benefits might accrue from such testing? what harms?

Chapter 18

Pharmacogenetics and Pharmacogenomics

In Chapter 17, we described personalized genetic medicine as the use of an individual patient's genotype to tailor medical care, with the aim of reducing complications and improving outcomes. One area in which personalized genetic medicine is likely soon to become part of routine medical care is drug therapy based on **pharmacogenetics.** Pharmacogenetics is the study of differences in drug response due to allelic variation in genes affecting drug metabolism, efficacy, and toxicity. In one year in the United States alone, more than a billion prescriptions for tens of billions of drug doses are written for more than 10,000 different medications. One frequently cited statistic is that adverse drug reactions occur in more than 2,000,000 patients each year in the United States, resulting in 100,000 excess deaths. The development of a genetic profile with a reasonable positive predictive value for toxicity or an adverse drug reaction is likely to have immediate benefit in allowing physicians to choose a drug or drug dose for which the patient is not at risk for an adverse event, or to decide on a dosage that ensures adequate therapy and minimizes complications. As with all other aspects of personalized medicine, however, the cost-effectiveness of such testing needs to be proved if it is to become part of accepted medical care.

Pharmacogenetics is relevant to individual variation in drug response in two ways. The first is variation in **pharmacokinetics,** that is, the rate at which the body absorbs, transports, metabolizes, or excretes drugs or their metabolites. Examples of pharmacokinetic variation we will discuss in this chapter include polymorphic alleles in the cytochrome P450 system that render codeine ineffective or increase bleeding in warfarin therapy, and the allelic variation in glucuronyltransferase or thiopurine methyltransferase that increases the toxicity of chemotherapeutic agents such as camptothecin (irinotecan) and 6-mercaptopurine. The second is the variation affecting the **pharmacodynamics** of a drug, that is, the genetic causes of variability in the response to the drug due to allelic variation in the drug's downstream targets, such as receptors, enzymes, or metabolic pathways. Examples of pharmacodynamic variation we discuss in this chapter include hemolytic anemia induced by sulfa drugs in individuals deficient in the enzyme glucose-6-phosphate dehydrogenase (Case 16), and difficulties in stabilizing patients receiving a dose of warfarin in optimal therapeutic range due to alleles affecting the level of its target, the vitamin K epoxide receptor complex I. Thus, most broadly, pharmacogenetics encompasses any genetically determined variation in the response to drugs, in terms of both efficacy and toxicity.

● USING RISK INFORMATION TO IMPROVE CARE: PHARMACOGENETICS

Variation in Pharmacokinetic Response

Variation in Phase I Drug Metabolism: Cytochrome P450

The human cytochrome P450 proteins are a large family of 56 different functional enzymes, each encoded by a

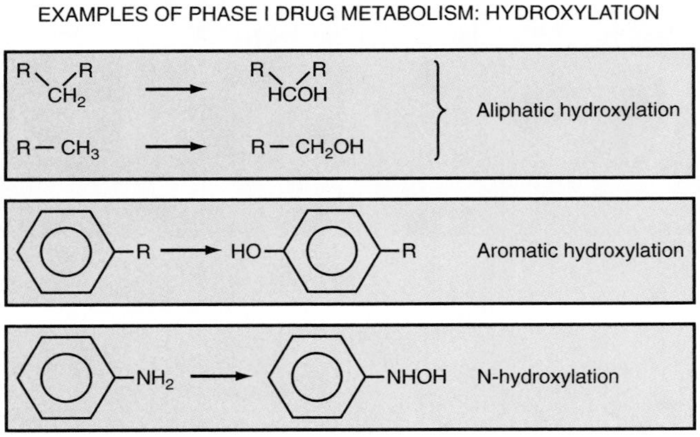

EXAMPLES OF PHASE I DRUG METABOLISM: HYDROXYLATION

Figure 18-1 ■ Typical hydroxylation reactions carried out by cytochrome P450 enzymes in phase I metabolism.

different *CYP* gene. All cytochrome P450 enzymes are heme-containing proteins in the liver; the Fe^{+2} in heme allows them to accept electrons from electron donors, such as NADPH, and use them for catalyzing a number of different reactions, the most common of which is the addition of one of the atoms of oxygen from molecular oxygen (O_2) to a carbon, nitrogen, or sulfur atom. For many drugs, the action of a cytochrome P450 is to add a hydroxyl group to the molecule, a typical step in what is referred to as **phase I** of drug metabolism, defined as the introduction of a more polar group to a compound that allows a side group to be more readily attached (Fig. 18-1). The hydroxyl group attached in phase I provides a site for a sugar or acetyl group to be attached to the drug to detoxify it and make it much easier to excrete in what is referred to as **phase II** of drug metabolism (Fig. 18-2).

The cytochromes P450 are grouped into 20 families according to amino acid sequence homology. Three of these families—*CYP1*, *CYP2*, and *CYP3*—contain enzymes that are promiscuous in the substrates they will act on and that participate in metabolizing a wide array of substances from outside the body (**xenobiotics**), including drugs. Six genes in particular (*CYP1A1*, *CYP1A2*, *CYP2C9*, *CYP2C19*, *CYP2D6*, and *CYP3A4*) are especially important for pharmacogenetics because the six enzymes they encode are responsible for phase I metabolism of more than 90% of all commonly used drugs (Fig. 18-3). *CYP3A4* alone is involved in the metabolism of over 40% of all drugs used in clinical medicine. Furthermore, many of the *CYP* genes are highly polymorphic, with alleles that have real functional consequences for how individuals respond to drug therapy (Table 18-1). *CYP* alleles can result in absent, decreased, or increased enzyme activity, thereby affecting the rate at which many drugs are metabolized. *CYP2D6*, for example, is the primary cytochrome in

phase I metabolism of more than 70 different drugs. There are 26 alleles in the *CYP2D6* gene that affect activity and are classified as reduced, absent, or increased activity alleles (Box). Missense mutations decrease the activity of this cytochrome; alleles with no activity are caused by splicing or frameshift mutations. In contrast, the *CYP2D6*1XN* allele is actually a series of copy number polymorphism alleles in which the *CYP2D* gene is present in three, four, or more copies on one chromosome. Predictably, these copy number polymorphisms produce high levels of the enzyme. There are dozens more alleles that do not affect the function of the protein and are therefore considered to be wild-type. Various combinations of these four classes of alleles produce quantitative differences in metabolizing activity, although some combinations are very rare and not well characterized. Three main phenotypes are generally recognized: **normal** metabolizers, **poor** metabolizers, and **ultrafast** metabolizers (Fig. 18-4).

Poor metabolizers are clearly at risk for accumulation of toxic levels of drugs. Ultrafast metabolizers are at risk for being undertreated with doses inadequate to maintain blood levels in the therapeutic range (see Fig. 18-4).

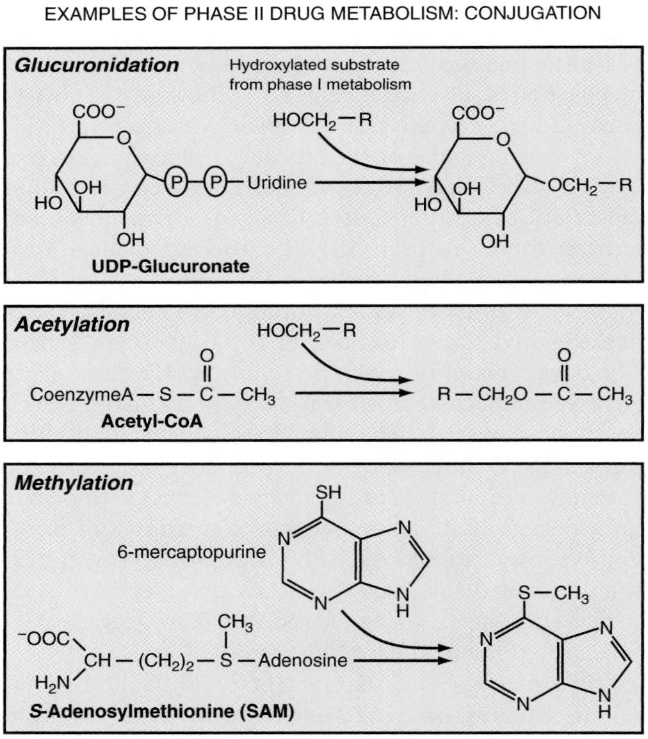

EXAMPLES OF PHASE II DRUG METABOLISM: CONJUGATION

Figure 18-2 ■ Typical phase II conjugation reactions to inactivate drugs and create soluble drug metabolites for excretion.

Metabolizer Phenotypes Arising from Various Combinations of *CYP2D6* Alleles

		Allele on One Chromosome			
		wild-type	*reduced*	*absent*	*increased*
Allele on Other Chromosome	*wild-type*	normal			
	reduced	normal	poor		
	absent	normal	poor	poor	
	increased	ultrafast	—	—	—

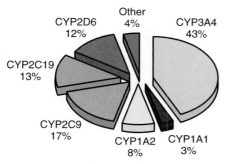

Figure 18-3 ■ Contribution of individual cytochrome P450 enzymes to phase I drug metabolism. (Modified with permission from Guengerich F: Cytochrome P450s and other enzymes in drug metabolism and toxicity. AAPS J 8:E101-E111, 2006.)

Not only are variations in the cytochrome P450 enzymes important in drug detoxification, but they are also involved in activating drugs. For example, codeine is a weak narcotic drug that exerts most of its analgesic effect on conversion to morphine, a bioactive metabolite with a 10-fold higher potency. This conversion is carried out by CYP2D6. Poor metabolizers carrying loss-of-function alleles in *CYP2D6* fail to convert codeine to morphine and thereby receive little therapeutic benefit; in contrast, ultrafast metabolizers can become rapidly intoxicated with low doses of codeine.

The occurrence of poor and ultrafast metabolizers has an additional complication that is important to consider in applying pharmacogenetics to personalized

Table 18-1

Polymorphic Cytochrome P450 Genes Involved in Drug Metabolism

Family	Gene	Alleles of Functional Significance*	Drugs Metabolized (Selected)
CYP1	*CYP1A2*	↑ and ↓ activity alleles	Caffeine Propranolol
CYP2	*CYP2C9*	↑, ↓, and 0 activity alleles	Angiotensin II receptor blockers Nonsteroidal anti-inflammatory drugs Metronidazole Oral hypoglycemics Warfarin
	CYP2C19	↓ and 0 activity alleles	Antiepileptics Antidepressants Antianxiety drugs
	CYP2D6	↑, ↓, and 0 activity alleles	Antiarrhythmics Antidepressants Antipsychotics Beta-adrenergic blockers Narcotic analgesics
CYP3	*CYP3A4*	↑, ↓, and 0 activity alleles	Acetaminophen Antifungals Cocaine Codeine Cyclosporine A Diazepam Erythromycin Cholesterol-lowering statins Taxol Warfarin

*↑, one or more alleles with increased activity; ↓, one or more alleles with reduced activity; 0, one or more alleles with no activity.

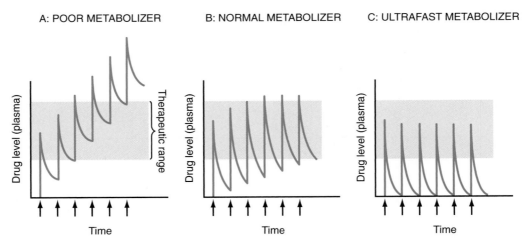

A: POOR METABOLIZER   B: NORMAL METABOLIZER   C: ULTRAFAST METABOLIZER

Figure 18-4 ■ Serum drug levels after repeated doses of a drug *(arrows)* in three individuals with different phenotypic profiles for drug metabolism. **A,** Poor metabolizer accumulates drug to toxic levels. **B,** Normal metabolizer reaches steady-state levels within the therapeutic range. **C,** Ultrafast metabolizer fails to maintain serum levels within the therapeutic range.

genetic medicine. The frequency of many of the alleles in the cytochromes P450 differs among different populations (Table 18-2). For example, a slow metabolizing phenotype for CYP2D6 that is present in 1 in 14 whites is rare in Asia and nearly absent in Native Americans and Pacific Islanders. Similarly, slow metabolizing alleles at *CYP2C19* show striking ethnic variability, with 3% of whites but nearly 16% of Asians having slow metabolism.

Variation in Phase II Metabolism

Glucuronidation Polymorphism and Camptothecin Toxicity Phase I metabolism through the cytochrome P450 enzymes is not the only step in which allelic variation causes individual variability in how drugs are metabolized. Genes encoding phase II metabolism are also functionally polymorphic and provide additional variability among individuals. One important phase II

Table 18-2

Frequency of Poor *CYP2D6* and *CYP2C19* Metabolizers in Various Population Groups

Ethnic Origin of Population	Population Frequency of Poor Metabolizers (%)	
	CYP2D6	*CYP2C19*
Sub-Saharan Africa	3.4	4.0
Amerindian	0	2
Asian	0.5	15.7
White	7.2	2.9
Middle Eastern/North Africa	1.5	2.0
Pacific Islander	0	13.6

Data from Burroughs VJ, Maxey RW, Levy RA: Racial and ethnic differences in response to medicines: towards individualized pharmaceutical treatment. J Natl Med Assoc 94(Suppl):1-26, 2002.

metabolic pathway is glucuronidation by UDP-glycosyl-transferase (see Fig. 18-2), which is part of the normal metabolic pathway for bilirubin excretion into bile. Irinotecan (camptothecin) is a plant alkaloid whose active metabolite (7-ethyl-10-hydroxycamptothecin) has potent antitumor properties because it inhibits the enzyme DNA topoisomerase required for DNA replication. As with most chemotherapeutic agents, there is significant potential for severe toxicity; in the case of camptothecin, treatment is often complicated by bone marrow and gastrointestinal tract toxicity. *UGT1A1* encodes a glucuronate transferase that glucuronidates 7-ethyl-10-hydroxycamptothecin, which is then excreted in the bile. There is a common polymorphism in a variable number tandem repeat A(TA)$_n$TAA in the TATAA box (see Chapter 3) within the *UGT1A1* promoter. The normal allele (*UGT1A1*1*) has six TA repeats, whereas allele 28 (*UGT1A1*28*), a common variant, has seven, which reduces transcription of the gene and the levels of the enzyme. In many populations, rare alleles with 5 copies of the repeat have increased transcription, while others with 8 copies have much reduced transcription. The *UGT1A1*28* allele is frequent in most ethnic groups worldwide (Table 18-3). Case-control studies of patients receiving camptothecin have shown a 3-fold to 5-fold higher relative risk for serious toxicity from typical chemotherapy regimens in individuals homozygous for *UGT1A1*28*. Heterozygotes may also be at increased risk.

N-Acetyltransferase Polymorphism and Tuberculosis Therapy with Isoniazid A second important phase II pathway in drug metabolism is acetylation (see Fig. 18-2). A pharmacokinetic polymorphism in acetylation was first discovered in patients receiving isoniazid therapy for tuberculosis when a high incidence of peripheral neuropathy and bone marrow suppression was observed

Table 18-3

Frequency of *UGT1A1* Genotypes in Various Population Groups

Region/Country	*UGT1A1* Genotype Frequency (%)		
	*1/*1	*1/*28	*28/*28
Sub-Saharan Africa	30	36	34
Southeast Asia	80	19	1
China	78	20	2
Europe	44	47	9
Indian subcontinent	29	49	22
Pacific (Papua New Guinea)	97	3	0
South American Amerindian	33	18	7

Data from Premawardhena A, Fisher CA, Liu YT, et al: The global distribution of length polymorphisms of the promoters of the glucuronosyltransferase 1 gene (UGT1A1): hematologic and evolutionary implications. Blood Cells Mol Dis 31:98-101, 2003; and Adegoke OJ, Shu XO, Gao YT, et al: Genetic polymorphisms in uridine diphospho-glucuronosyltransferase 1A1 (UGT1A1) and risk of breast cancer. Breast Cancer Res Treat 85:239-245, 2004.

in patients who inactivate the drug more slowly than those without adverse reactions. In contrast, rapid acetylators had a higher failure rate with weekly isoniazid therapy for tuberculosis. The slow and rapid inactivation phenotypes are primarily due to allelic differences in an N-acetyltransferase gene, *NAT2*. Three major slow-acetylator alleles have been described along with a large number of rare *NAT2* alleles. Slow acetylators have a substantial decrease in the quantity of N-acetyltransferase in the liver and are homozygous for recessive alleles at this locus. Rapid inactivators are normal homozygotes or heterozygotes and are at increased risk for failure to maintain therapeutic drug levels with a regimen of once a week treatment. The frequency of the slow-acetylator phenotype is markedly different among different population groups (Table 18-4).

In addition to its effect on isoniazid inactivation, the acetylation phenotype affects the disposition of a wide variety of other drugs and xenobiotics. Fast acetylators require larger doses of hydralazine to control hypertension and of dapsone to treat leprosy and other infections. Conversely, slow acetylators are at increased

Table 18- 4

Frequency of Slow-Acetylator Phenotype

Population	Frequency (%)
Sub-Saharan African and African American	51
White	58
Chinese	22
Japanese	10
Inuit	6

Data from Burroughs VJ, Maxey RW, Levy RA: Racial and ethnic differences in response to medicines: towards individualized pharmaceutical treatment. J Natl Med Assoc 94(Suppl):1-26, 2002.

risk for development of a drug-induced systemic lupus erythematosus–like syndrome while receiving hydralazine, and sulfonamide-induced idiosyncratic adverse responses.

Polymorphism in Thiopurine Methyltransferase and 6-Mercaptopurine Efficacy   Another example of the clinical importance of polymorphisms in drug metabolism are the drugs 6-mercaptopurine and 6-thioguanine used in the treatment of childhood leukemias and for immunosuppression (Case 40). These drugs are detoxified by attachment of a methyl group by the enzyme thiopurine methyltransferase encoded by the *TPMT* gene (see Fig. 18-2). Three common missense mutations are known that destabilize the enzyme and cause it to be rapidly degraded. In the aggregate, approximately 10% of whites are heterozygotes and partially deficient; the frequency of heterozygotes in Africa and Asia is approximately half that. Partial deficiency slows metabolism and may either increase drug effectiveness or increase toxicity, depending on the dose used. For example, in a study of more than 800 children treated with a standard dose of 6-mercaptopurine for leukemia, being heterozygous for TPMT deficiency reduced treatment failures from 23% seen in patients with wild-type alleles to 9%, as judged by how many children had minimal residual disease (defined by the ratio of the number of cells with the leukemia-specific gene rearrangement after treatment compared with before treatment, being less than 1 in 10,000).

Cholinesterase Polymorphism and Prolonged Postoperative Paralysis   A final example of a pharmacokinetic polymorphism affecting drug metabolism is variation in serum cholinesterase, leading to prolonged postoperative paralysis after administration of the commonly used paralytic agent succinylcholine during surgery. Succinylcholine is normally hydrolyzed by a serum enzyme, butyrylcholinesterase, a process that reduces the amount of succinylcholine that reaches the motor end plates; this hydrolysis is accounted for when calculating the dose given to the average patient.

The major determinants of cholinesterase activity in the plasma are two codominant alleles of the *BCHE* gene that encodes the butyrylcholinesterase enzyme, known as the usual (*U*) and atypical (*A*) alleles; the atypical allele is the result of a missense mutation (Asp70Gly). Cholinesterase deficiency is usually due to homozygosity for the *A* allele; the enzyme produced by homozygotes is qualitatively altered and has lower activity than the usual type. About 1 in 3300 Europeans is homozygous for an atypical cholinesterase allele; among the Inuits of North America, the frequency of homozygous deficiency is 10-fold higher. Being unable to degrade succinylcholine at the normal rate, homozygotes respond abnormally to its administration with prolonged muscle paralysis (lasting 1 hour to several hours) after surgery and require artificial respiratory support.

Determination of cholinesterase deficiency is not a routine part of preanesthesia evaluation and is performed only if the patient or patient's family gives a history of needing prolonged ventilator support postoperatively. The fact that cholinesterase testing is not routine is a clear example of why genetic testing in personalized medicine depends not only on the clinical validity of the test (i.e., its positive predictive value) but also on the cost and benefits of testing (i.e., clinical utility). It is argued that institution of testing would mean that the expense of testing 3300 individuals routinely to find one at risk outweighs the low cost and minimal potential for serious complication incurred by making the diagnosis after the fact when prolonged apnea occurs and providing the necessary extra ventilator support.

Variation in Pharmacodynamic Response

Glucose-6-Phosphate Dehydrogenase Deficiency and Hemolytic Anemia

Deficiency of glucose-6-phosphate dehydrogenase (G6PD), a ubiquitous X-linked enzyme, is the most common disease-producing enzyme defect of humans, estimated to affect 400 million people worldwide; about 10% of African American males are G6PD deficient and are clinically susceptible to drug-induced hemolysis (Case 16). With more than 400 variants described, G6PD deficiency also appears to be one of the most genetically heterogeneous disorders yet recognized. More than 70 of these variants have been characterized at the molecular level. All but two are point mutations, the exceptions being in-frame deletions of a small number of codons. The high gene frequency of G6PD variants in some populations appears to reflect the fact that G6PD deficiency, like sickle cell hemoglobin and thalassemia, confers some protection against malaria (see Chapter 9). This enzymopathy originally came to attention when the antimalarial drug primaquine was found to induce hemolytic anemia in some African American males, who were subsequently found to have G6PD deficiency.

The mechanism of the drug-induced hemolysis is clear. One of the products of the enzymatic reaction carried out by G6PD, nicotinamide adenine dinucleotide phosphate (NADPH), is the major source of reducing equivalents in the red blood cell. NADPH protects the cell against oxidative damage by regenerating reduced glutathione from its oxidized form. In G6PD deficiency, oxidant drugs such as primaquine deplete the cell of reduced glutathione, and the consequent oxidative damage leads to hemolysis. Additional offending compounds include sulfonamide antibiotics, sulfones such as dapsone, naphthalene (mothballs), and a few others.

Favism, a severe hemolytic anemia that results from ingestion of the broad bean *Vicia faba*, has been known since ancient times in parts of the Mediterranean. Favism is due to extreme G6PD deficiency. The enzyme defect makes the cells vulnerable to oxidants in fava beans. (Pythagoras, the ancient Greek mathematician, warned his followers of the danger of eating these beans.) In areas in which severe deficiency variants like the Mediterranean allele are prevalent, fava beans are a major cause of both neonatal jaundice and congenital nonspherocytic hemolytic anemia.

Malignant Hyperthermia

Malignant hyperthermia is an autosomal dominant condition in which there may be a dramatic adverse response to the administration of many commonly used inhalational anesthetics (e.g., halothane) and depolarizing muscle relaxants such as succinylcholine. Soon after induction of anesthesia, the patients develop life-threatening fever, sustained muscle contraction, and attendant hypercatabolism. The fundamental physiological abnormality in the disease is an elevation of the level of ionized calcium in the sarcoplasm of muscle. This increase leads to muscle rigidity, elevation of body temperature, rapid breakdown of muscle (rhabdomyolysis), and other abnormalities. The condition is an important if not a common cause of death during anesthesia. The incidence is 1 in 50,000 adults undergoing anesthesia but for unknown reasons is 10-fold higher in children.

Malignant hyperthermia is most frequently associated with mutations in a gene called *RYR1*, encoding an intracellular calcium ion channel. However, mutations in *RYR1* account for only about 50% of cases of malignant hyperthermia. At least five other loci have now been identified, one of which is the *CACNL1A3* gene, which encodes the α_1 subunit of a dihydropyridine-sensitive calcium channel. Precisely why the abnormalities in calcium handling in muscle found with *RYR1* or *CACNL1A3* mutations make the muscle sensitive to inhalation anesthetics and muscle relaxants and precipitate malignant hyperthermia is unknown.

The need for special precautions when at-risk persons require anesthesia is obvious. Dantrolene sodium is effective in preventing or reducing the severity of the response if an unsuspected attack occurs, and alternative anesthetics can be given to patients at risk.

Genetic Variation in both Pharmacokinetics and Pharmacodynamics: Warfarin Therapy

The anticoagulant warfarin is an oral medication commonly used for the prevention of thromboembolism. Its mechanism of action is to block the enzyme **vitamin K epoxide reductase complex I** (encoded by the *VKORC1* gene), which serves to reduce vitamin K so that the vitamin can be recycled and used in coagulation factor biosynthesis. Vitamin K is an essential cofactor for the carboxylation of glutamic acid side chains of coagulation factors II, VII, IX, and X, a post-translational modification required for the bioactivity of these clotting factors in the clotting cascade. More than 20,000,000 patients in the United States alone are prescribed warfarin each year. Estimates from different studies indicate that patients receiving warfarin therapy have an annual rate of fatal bleeding of 0.1% to 1% and of serious bleeding of 0.5% to 6.5%. Thus, careful monitoring of anticoagulation status by repeated blood tests is needed to make sure the prolongation of the clotting remains within the therapeutic range needed to prevent thromboembolism.

Establishment of a therapeutic dose of warfarin for a patient is complicated by both genetic and environmental factors. Diet and medications can change how much vitamin K is available, either from food intake or from the supply of vitamin K synthesized by colonic flora. Many medications that interfere with warfarin phase I metabolism can also affect the dose required to remain in the therapeutic range. The risk of bleeding is most pronounced during the first few months of initiation of therapy, when the dose is being adjusted by trial and error according to measurement of the patient's coagulation times. In addition to diet and drug interactions, variability in individual response to warfarin also has a strong genetic basis in polymorphisms both in warfarin metabolism and in its biological target.

Warfarin's most active metabolite undergoes phase I detoxification by CYP2C9. The aggregate frequency of alleles causing deficiency of CYP2C9 is 20% in whites but only 3.5% in African Americans and less than 2% in individuals from Asia. Heterozygotes for deficiency alleles require, on average, a 20% lower dose of warfarin to maintain the same degree of anticoagulation. Using a patient's *CYP2C9* genotype to guide dosage may reduce the time it takes to come to a stable dosing regimen after therapy is initiated.

CYP2C9 variants, however, contribute much less than half of the genetic variability in response to warfarin therapy. Additional variability comes from allelic variants in the target of warfarin, the VKORC1 enzyme. Common alleles at noncoding single nucleotide polymorphisms in the *VKORC1* gene can be used to define two major haplotype families, *A* and *B*, that differ markedly in the dose of warfarin needed to reach and to maintain therapeutic anticoagulation. In one study, homozygous *A/A* individuals required 3.2 mg/day, *B/B* individuals required 6.1 mg/day, and heterozygous *A/B* individuals required intermediate doses of 4.4 mg/day. The mechanism by which these haplotypes confer dif-

ferent sensitivity to warfarin dose is not entirely known, but the *B* haplotype appears to confer a 3-fold increase in mRNA levels for the *VKORC1* gene. Assuming that enzyme levels reflect the levels of mRNA, a 3-fold increase in mRNA translates into a 3-fold increase in the amount of enzyme made, thus requiring a higher dosage of warfarin to achieve the same degree of blockade of vitamin K recycling.

The frequency of the different *VKORC1* haplotypes differs dramatically in different ethnic groups; the more sensitive haplotype, *A*, is present in 33% of whites, 89% of Asians, and 14% of African Americans. The *VKORC1* polymorphism may be responsible for the anecdotal clinical observation that patients of Asian origin are more sensitive to lower doses of warfarin than are individuals of African or European ancestry.

Combining *CYP2C9* and *VKORC1* genotypes explains nearly half of the interindividual difference in warfarin dose required to maintain therapeutic anticoagulation. Homozygotes for *CYP2C9* reduced activity alleles, and *VKORC1 A* alleles require one-fifth to one-sixth the dose of warfarin that a homozygote for normal *CYP2C9* alleles and *VKORC1 B* alleles would need to achieve an appropriate therapeutic response.

Genotypic Risk for Adverse Outcomes After Cardiothoracic Surgery

Nearly 3% of all surgical patients in the United States suffer a perioperative cardiovascular complication, adding $25 billion in costs to the more than $400 billion spent each year on surgical procedures. For example, in coronary artery bypass graft surgery for coronary artery disease, postoperative complications such as prolonged bleeding, myocardial damage, graft failure, and stroke are common complications that are difficult to predict on the basis of clinical characteristics of the patients, such as age, weight, presence of diabetes, or other morbidities. However, by combining information on a patient's genotype at loci involved in postoperative complications with the patient's relevant clinical information, surgeons and anesthesiologists are attempting to bring the methods of personalized medicine to bear on better risk profiling, thereby allowing better selection of patients preoperatively and improved management during and after surgery. Two recent examples demonstrate how such information might be used. Polymorphic alleles at seven loci, including some that encode surface glycoproteins concerned with platelet aggregation and others involved in the coagulation cascade, have been shown to increase the risk of postoperative bleeding. As another example, the risk for stroke in the postoperative period appears to be 3-fold increased in individuals carrying a certain combination of alleles at two loci involved in inflammation, **C-reactive protein** and **interleukin-6**, an increase seen only when both alleles are present. More work will need to be done before a robust profile of polymorphic variants is identified and proved to have sufficient positive predictive value and clinical utility to justify the cost of screening all of the nearly 40,000,000 Americans who undergo some form of surgery each year in the United States.

PHARMACOGENOMICS

Pharmacogenomics, the genomic approach to pharmacogenetics, is concerned with the assessment of common genetic variants in the aggregate for their impact on the outcome of drug therapy. Instead of analyzing individual genes and their variants according to what is known about how they influence pharmacokinetic and pharmacodynamic pathways, sets of alleles at a large number of polymorphic loci (single nucleotide and copy number polymorphisms; see Chapter 9) are being identified that distinguish patients who have responded adversely to what was considered a beneficial drug from those who had no adverse response. Specific knowledge of the metabolism of the drug or how the different alleles might modulate responses to it is not necessary. If this genotypic profile has sufficient positive predictive value, future patients with comparable profiles, who are therefore also at increased risk for an adverse response, could avoid potentially dangerous medications. Meanwhile, the very same drugs could be safely administered to patients without the at-risk profile. Similarly, a genotypic profile can be defined that distinguishes those patients who respond in beneficial ways to a given drug treatment from those who fail to respond. Once again, a genotypic profile with sufficient positive predictive value could be used to predict the probable efficacy of the medication in an individual before the drug is administered, and to identify those patients who should be treated more aggressively and monitored to be sure that the drug achieves therapeutic levels. We expect genomic approaches to pharmacogenetics to become increasingly more important in the delivery of personalized genetic medicine in the years ahead.

ROLE OF ETHNICITY AND RACE IN PERSONALIZED MEDICINE

Racial and ethnic differences in response to drug therapy are a well-known phenomenon. The simplest explanation would be if the differences among various racial groups in the frequencies of alleles of functional consequence for a few major genes involved in pharmacokinetic and pharmacodynamic aspects of drug therapy, were responsible for all of the differences seen in drug response among various groups. The explanation is not that simple, however. Drug response is a complex trait. A drug may have its effect directly or through more active metabolites, each of which may then be metabolized by different pathways and exert its effects on various targets. Thus, variants at more than one locus may interact, synergistically or antagonistically, either to potentiate or to reduce the effectiveness of a drug or to increase its toxic side effects. A comprehensive, pharmacogenomic approach may be necessary before we have testing with truly robust positive predictive values. Furthermore, as with all complex traits, environment is also an important factor. Differences in drug response can be due to differences in diet, concurrent drug therapy, underlying mechanism of disease, lifestyle, or social factors that may also differ between groups.

Given the apparent differences in response to drug therapy among individuals from different ethnic or racial groups, there is currently much debate over whether physicians should be making decisions about the choice of individual drug therapy on the basis of ethnic or racial labels. In one highly publicized example, two studies comparing treatment of white Americans and African Americans for congestive heart failure suggested that African Americans responded less well than did whites to the angiotensin-converting enzyme inhibitor enalapril but more favorably to the combined therapy of a nitrate, isosorbide dinitrate, and an antihypertensive, hydralazine. To what extent can such differences be ascribed to underlying differences between these ethnic groups in the frequency of variant alleles in genes that affect pharmacokinetic and pharmacodynamic aspects of these drugs? Ethnic and racial labels are only approximate surrogates for the real genetic differences underlying differences in response to drug therapy. For example, in one study, individuals from eight geographical areas around the globe were grouped in a blinded manner (without regard to geographical origin) into four populations, according to how many alleles they shared at 39 autosomal and X-linked microsatellite polymorphic loci. When a set of six polymorphic drug metabolizing loci, including four discussed in this chapter (*CYP1A2, CYP2C19, NAT2,* and *CYP2D6*), were analyzed, the frequency of alleles with deficient activity was indeed similar among individuals defined by geographical origin. However, the frequency of alleles with deficient activity was much *more* similar in groups defined by how many alleles they had in common at the microsatellite markers. Thus, labels defined by geographical origin were not as useful as genetic analysis at predicting the underlying differences in frequencies of functional alleles in drug metabolizing genes.

Even if ethnic or racial labels are inadequate for capturing medically relevant genetic variability, some would argue that such categories may still be useful, not so much for what they tell a physician about the genetic make-up of his or her patient, but for what they might tell about other important factors affecting the patient's health, such as social and cultural experiences, including dietary practices, or the effects of discrimination and social alienation. Ultimately, the goal of personalized medicine is to tailor therapy to the individual patient, not by making assumptions about genetic make-up or environmental exposures based on labels defined by physical characteristics, but by using the most accurate predictive testing available, combined with careful attention to the patient—as an individual, as a member of a family, and as a member of society at large—to find the best preventive and therapeutic measures.

● GENERAL REFERENCES

Burroughs VJ, Maxey RW, Levy RA: Racial and ethnic differences in response to medicines: towards individualized pharmaceutical treatment. J Natl Med Assoc 94(Suppl):1-26, 2002.

Need AC, Motulsky AG, Goldstein DB: Priorities and standards in pharmacogenetic research. Nat Genet 37:671-681, 2005.

Sadee W, Dai Z: Pharmacogenetics/genomics and personalized medicine. Hum Mol Genet 14:R207-R214, 2005.

Shastry BS: Pharmacogenetics and the concept of individualized medicine. Pharmacogenomics J 6:16-21, 2006.

Xie HG, Kim RB, Wood AJ, Stein CM: Molecular basis of ethnic differences in drug disposition and response. Annu Rev Pharmacol Toxicol 41:815-850, 2001.

● REFERENCES FOR SPECIFIC TOPICS

American Society of Anesthesiologists Task Force on Preanesthesia Evaluation: Practice advisory for preanesthesia evaluation. Anesthesiology 96:485-496, 2002.

Burchard EG, Ziv E, Coyle N, et al: The importance of race and ethnic background in biomedical research and clinical practice. N Engl J Med 348:1170-1175, 2003.

Cooper RS, Kaufman JS, Ward R: Race and genomics. N Engl J Med 348:1166-1170, 2003.

Exner DV, Dries DL, Domanski MJ, et al: Lesser response to angiotensin-converting-enzyme inhibitor therapy in black as compared with white patients with left ventricular dysfunction. N Engl J Med 344:1351-1357, 2001.

Guengerich FP: Cytochrome P450s and other enzymes in drug metabolism and toxicity. AAPS J 8:E101-E111, 2006.

Haga SB, Burke W: Using pharmacogenetics to improve drug safety and efficacy [commentary]. JAMA 291:2869-2871, 2004.

Marsh S, McLeod HL: Pharmacogenetics of irinotecan toxicity. Pharmacogenomics 5:835-843, 2004.

Podgoreanu MV, Schwinn AD: New paradigms in cardiovascular medicine. Emerging technologies and practices: perioperative genomics. J Am Coll Cardiol 46:1965-1977, 2005.

Rieder MJ, Reiner AP, Gage BF: Effect of *VKORC1* haplotypes on transcriptional regulation and warfarin dose. N Engl J Med 352:2285-2293, 2005.

Voora D, Eby C, Linder W, et al: Prospective dosing of warfarin based on cytochrome P-450 2C9 genotype. Thromb Haemost 93:700-705, 2005.

Wang L, Weinshilboum R: Thiopurine *S*-methyltransferase pharmacogenetics: insights, challenges and future directions. Oncogene 25:1629-1638, 2006.

Wilson JF, Weale ME, Smith AC, et al: Population genetic structure of variable drug response. Nat Genet 29:265-269, 2001.

● USEFUL WEBSITE

Nelson D: Cytochrome P450s in humans. 2003. *http://drnelson.utmem.edu/P450lect.html*

 PROBLEMS

1. Toxic epidermal necrolysis (TEN) and the Stevens-Johnson syndrome (SJS) are two related life-threatening skin reactions that occur in approximately 1 per 100,000 individuals in China, most commonly as a result of exposure to the antiepileptic drug carbamazepine. These conditions carry a significant mortality rate of 30% to 35% (TEN) and 5% to 15% (SJS). It was observed that individuals who suffered this severe allergic reaction carried a particular MHC class 1 allele, *HLA B*1502*, as do 8.6% of the Chinese population. In a retrospective cohort study of 145 patients who received carbamazepine therapy, 44 developed either TEN or SJS. Of these, all 44 carried the *HLA B*1502* allele, whereas only 3 of the patients who received the drug without incident were *HLA B*1502* positive. What is the sensitivity, specificity, and positive predictive value of this allele for TEN or SJS in patients receiving carbamazepine?

2. In 1997, a young female college student died suddenly of cardiac arrhythmia after being startled by a fire alarm in her college dormitory in the middle of the night. She had recently been prescribed an oral antihistamine, terfenadine, for hay fever by a physician at the school. Her parents reported that she would take her medications every morning with breakfast, which consisted of grapefruit juice, toast, and caffeinated coffee. Her only other medication was oral itraconazole, which she was given by a dermatologist in her hometown to treat a stubborn toenail fungus that she considered unsightly. Terfenadine was removed from the U.S. market in 1998.

   Do a literature search on sudden cardiac death associated with terfenadine, relating possibly genetic and environmental factors that might have interacted to cause this young woman's death.

Chapter 19

Genetic Counseling and Risk Assessment

Clinical genetics is concerned with the diagnosis and management of the medical, social, and psychological aspects of hereditary disease. As in all other areas of medicine, it is essential to make a correct diagnosis and to provide appropriate treatment, which must include helping the affected person and family members understand and come to terms with the nature and consequences of the disorder. When a disorder is suspected of being heritable, however, there is an added dimension: the need to inform other family members of their risk and of the means available to them to modify these risks. Just as the unique feature of genetic disease is its tendency to recur within families, the unique aspect of genetic counseling is its focus, not only on the original patient but also on members of the patient's family, both present and future.

Genetic counseling is not limited to the provision of information and calculation of the risk for disease; rather, it is a process of exploration and communication. The ability to define and address the complex psychosocial issues associated with a genetic disorder in a family is central to this practice. Geneticists and genetic counselors can help with prevention and management, be a source of referral to subspecialists, and provide psychologically oriented counseling to help individuals adapt and adjust to the impact and implications of the disorder in the family. Genetic counseling may be most effectively accomplished over time through periodic contact with the family as the medical or social issues become relevant to the lives of those involved (see Box).

THE PROCESS OF GENETIC COUNSELING

Common Indications for Genetic Counseling

Table 19-1 lists some of the most common situations that lead people to pursue genetic counseling. Often, the persons seeking genetic counseling (the **consultands**) are the parents of a child with a potential or known genetic condition, but the consultand may also be an adult who has a disorder of concern or a relative with such a disorder. Genetic counseling is also an integral part of prenatal testing (see Chapter 15) and of genetic testing and screening programs (discussed in Chapter 17).

Established standards of medical care require that providers of genetic services obtain a history that includes family and ethnic information, advise patients of the genetic risks to them and other family members, offer genetic testing or prenatal diagnosis when indicated, and outline the various treatment or management options for reducing the risk of disease. Although genetic counseling case management must be individualized for each patient's needs and situation, a generic approach can be summarized (Table 19-2). In general, patients are *not told* what decisions to make with regard to the various testing and management options but are instead provided with information and support in coming to a decision that seems most appropriate for the patients, the consultands, and their families. This approach to counseling, referred to as **nondirective**

Table 19-1

Common Indications for Genetic Counseling

- Previous child with multiple congenital anomalies, mental retardation, or an isolated birth defect such as neural tube defect or cleft lip and palate
- Family history of a hereditary condition, such as cystic fibrosis, fragile X syndrome, or diabetes
- Prenatal diagnosis for advanced maternal age or other indication
- Consanguinity
- Teratogen exposure, such as to occupational chemicals, medications, alcohol
- Repeated pregnancy loss or infertility
- Newly diagnosed abnormality or genetic condition
- Before undertaking genetic testing and after receiving results, particularly in testing for susceptibility to late-onset disorders, such as cancer or neurological disease
- As follow-up for a positive result of a newborn test, as with PKU; a heterozygote screening test, such as Tay-Sachs; or a positive first- or second-trimester maternal serum screen or abnormal fetal ultrasound examination

counseling, has its origins in the setting of prenatal counseling and is firmly rooted in the guiding principle of respect for an individual couple's right to make reproductive choices free of coercion.

Managing the Risk of Recurrence in Families

Many families seek genetic counseling to ascertain the risk for heritable disease in their children and to learn what options are available to reduce the risk of recurrence of the particular genetic disorder in question. Although prenatal diagnosis is one approach that can often be offered to families, it is by no means a universal solution to the risk of genetic problems in offspring. There are many disorders for which prenatal diagnosis is not feasible, and for many parents, it is not an acceptable option even if it is available. Other measures available for management of recurrence include the following.

- Genetic laboratory tests (karyotyping, biochemical analysis, or DNA analysis) sometimes reassure couples with a family history of a genetic disorder that they themselves are *not* at increased risk of having a child with a specific genetic disease. In other cases, such tests indicate that the couple *is* at increased risk. Genetic counseling is recommended both before and after such testing, to assist consultands in making an informed decision to undergo testing, as well as to understand and to use the information gained through testing.
- If the parents plan to have no more children or no children at all, **contraception or sterilization** may be their choice, and they may need information about the possible procedures or an appropriate referral.
- For parents who want a child or more children, **adoption** is a possibility.

- **Artificial insemination** may be appropriate if the father has a gene for an autosomal dominant or X-linked defect or has a heritable chromosome defect, but it is obviously not indicated if it is the mother who has such a defect. Artificial insemination is also useful if both parents are carriers of an autosomal recessive disorder. In vitro fertilization with a **donated egg** may be appropriate if the mother has an autosomal dominant defect or carries an X-linked disease. In either case, genetic counseling and appropriate genetic tests of the sperm or egg donor should be part of the process.
- In some disorders, DNA analysis of embryos in the preimplantation stage can be carried out by the polymerase chain reaction of a single cell obtained from an early embryo generated by in vitro fertilization (see Chapters 4 and 15). For some parents, a decision not to implant an embryo found to be abnormal would be much more acceptable than abortion at a later stage.

If the parents decide to terminate a pregnancy, provision of relevant information and support is an appropriate part of genetic counseling. Periodic follow-up through additional visits or by telephone is often arranged for a few months or more after a pregnancy termination.

Psychological Aspects

Patients and families dealing with a risk for a genetic disorder or coping with the illness itself are subject to varying degrees of emotional and social stress. Although this is also true of nongenetic disorders, the concern generated by knowledge that the condition might recur, the guilt or censure felt by some individuals, and the need for reproductive decisions can give rise to severe distress. Many persons have the strength to deal personally with such problems; they prefer receiving even bad news to remaining uninformed, and they make their own decisions on the basis of the most complete and accurate information they can obtain. Other

Table 19-2

Genetic Counseling Case Management

- Collection of information
  - Family history (questionnaire)
  - Medical history
  - Tests or additional assessments
- Assessment
  - Physical examination
  - Laboratory and radiological testing
  - Validation or establishment of diagnosis—if possible

- Counseling
  - Nature and consequence of disorder
- Recurrence risk
  - Availability of further or future testing
- Decision-making
  - Referral to other specialists, health agencies, support groups
- Continuing clinical assessment, especially if no diagnosis
- Psychosocial support

••• Genetic Counseling and Risk Assessment

The purpose of genetic counseling is to provide information and support to families at risk for having, or who already have, members with birth defects or genetic disorders. Genetic counseling helps the family or individual:

- to comprehend the medical facts, including the diagnosis, the probable course of the disorder, and the available management;
- to understand the way heredity contributes to the disorder and the risk of recurrence for themselves and other family members;
- to understand the options for dealing with the risk of recurrence;
- to identify those values, beliefs, goals, and relationships affected by the risk for or presence of hereditary disease;
- to choose the course of action that seems most appropriate to them in view of their risk, their family goals, and their ethical and religious standards; and
- to make the best possible adjustment to the disorder or to the risk of recurrence of that disorder, or both, by providing supportive counseling to families and making referrals to appropriate specialists, social services, and family and patient support groups.

persons require much more support and may need referral for psychotherapy. The psychological aspects of genetic counseling are beyond the scope of this book, but several books cited in the General References at the end of this chapter give an introduction to this important field.

Genetic Counseling Providers

Genetic counseling in the past was usually provided by a physician as an integral part of the clinical management of the patient and family; indeed, genetic counseling still remains an important component of medical genetics practice. As the body of genetic knowledge and the extent and sophistication of laboratory diagnosis have expanded, so has the demand for education and counseling to help patients and their families deal with the many complex issues raised by genetic disease. Clinical genetics is particularly time-consuming in comparison with other clinical fields because it requires extensive preparation and follow-up in addition to direct contact with patients. Increasingly, genetic counseling services are being provided by **genetic counselors,** qualified professionals trained in genetics *and* counseling, and **nurse geneticists,** serving as members of a health care team with physicians. Genetic counseling in the United States and Canada is a self-regulating health profession with its own board (the American and Canadian Boards of Genetic Counselors) for accreditation of training programs and certification of practition-

ers. Nurses with genetics expertise are accredited through a separate credentialing commission.

Genetic counselors and nurse geneticists play an essential role in clinical genetics, participating in many aspects of the investigation and management of genetic problems. A genetic counselor is often the first point of contact that a patient makes with clinical genetic services, provides genetic counseling directly to consultands, helps patients and families deal with the many psychological and social issues that arise during genetic counseling, and continues in a supportive role and as a source of information after the clinical investigation and formal counseling have been completed. Counselors are also active in the field of genetic testing; they provide close liaison among the referring physicians, the diagnostic laboratories, and the families themselves. Their special expertise is invaluable to clinical laboratories because explaining and interpreting genetic testing to patients and referring physicians often requires a sophisticated knowledge of genetics and genomics as well as good communication skills.

Referral to family and patient **support groups** is often made by counselors in managing a patient and family with a genetic disorder or birth defect. These organizations, which can be focused either on a single disease or on a group of diseases, can help those concerned to share their experience with others facing the same problem, to learn how to deal with the day-to-day problems caused by the disorder, to hear of new developments in therapy or prevention, and to promote research into the condition. Many support groups have Internet sites and electronic chat rooms through which patients and families give and receive information and advice, ask and answer questions, and obtain much-needed emotional support. Similar disease-specific self-help organizations are active in many nations around the world. In the United States, the Genetic Alliance, a broad coalition of many patient advocacy and family support groups, serves to coordinate the activities of many individual groups.

● DETERMINING RECURRENCE RISKS

The estimation of recurrence risks is a central concern in genetic counseling. Ideally, it is based on knowledge of the genetic nature of the disorder in question and on the pedigree of the particular family being counseled. The family member whose risk of a genetic disorder is to be determined is usually a relative of a proband, such as a sib of an affected child or a living or future child of an affected adult. In some families, especially for some autosomal dominant and X-linked traits, it may also be necessary to estimate the risk for more remote relatives.

When a disorder is known to have single-gene inheritance, the recurrence risk for specific family

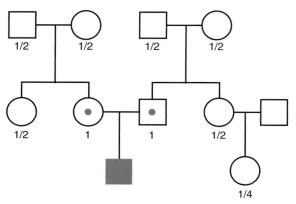

Figure 19-1 ■ Pedigree of a family with an autosomal recessive condition. The probability of being a carrier is shown beneath each individual symbol in the pedigree.

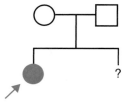

Figure 19-2 ■ Empirical risk estimates in genetic counseling. A family with no other positive family history has one child affected with a disorder known to be multifactorial or chromosomal. What is the recurrence risk? If the child is affected with spina bifida, the empirical risk to a subsequent child is approximately 4% (see Chapter 8). If the child has Down syndrome, the empirical risk of recurrence would be approximately 1% if the karyotype is trisomy 21, but it might be substantially higher if one of the parents is a carrier of a Robertsonian translocation involving chromosome 21 (see Chapter 6).

members can usually be determined from basic mendelian principles (Fig. 19-1; also see Chapter 7). On the other hand, risk calculations may be less than straightforward if there is reduced penetrance or variability of expression, or if disease is frequently the result of new mutation, as in many X-linked and autosomal dominant disorders. Laboratory tests that give equivocal results can add further complications. Under these circumstances, mendelian risk estimates can sometimes be modified by means of applying **conditional probability** to the pedigree (see later), which takes into account information about the family that may increase or decrease the underlying mendelian risk.

In contrast to single-gene disorders, the underlying mechanisms of inheritance for most chromosomal disorders and complex traits are unknown, and estimates of recurrence risk are based on previous experience (Fig. 19-2). This approach to risk assessment is valuable if there are good data on the frequency of recurrence of the disorder in families and if the phenotype is not heterogeneous. However, when a particular phenotype has an undetermined risk or can result from a variety of causes with different frequencies and with widely different risks, estimation of the recurrence risk is hazardous at best. In a later section, the estimation of recurrence risk in some typical clinical situations, both straightforward and more complicated, is considered.

Risk Estimation When Genotypes Are Fully Known by Use of Mendel's Laws

The simplest risk estimates apply to families in which the relevant genotypes of all family members are known or can be inferred. For example, if both members of a couple are known to be heterozygous carriers of an autosomal recessive condition, and one is interested in the chance of the couple's having another affected child, the risk (probability) is one in four with each pregnancy that the child will inherit two mutant alleles and inherit

the disease (Fig 19-3A). Even if the couple were to have six unaffected children subsequent to the affected child (Fig 19-3B), the risk in the eighth, ninth, or tenth pregnancy is still one in four for each pregnancy (assuming there is no misattributed paternity for the first affected child).

Risk Estimation by Use of Conditional Probability When Alternative Genotypes Are Possible

In contrast to the simple case described, situations arise in which the genotypes of the relevant individuals in

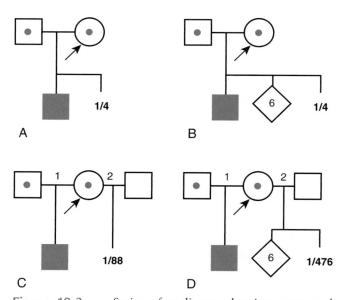

Figure 19-3 ■ Series of pedigrees showing autosomal recessive inheritance with contrasting recurrence risks. **A** and **B**, The genotypes of the parents are known. **C**, The genotype of the consultand's second partner is inferred from the carrier frequency in the population. **D**, The inferred genotype is modified by additional pedigree information. Arrows indicate the consultand. Numbers indicate recurrence risk in the consultand's next pregnancy.

the family are not *definitively* known; the risk of recurrence will be very different, depending on whether or not the consultand is a carrier of an abnormal allele of a disease gene. For example, the chance that a woman who is known from her first marriage to be a carrier of cystic fibrosis (CF) might have an affected child depends on the chance that her husband by her second marriage is a carrier (Fig. 19-3C). The risk of the partner's being a carrier depends on his ethnic background (see Chapter 9). For the general white population, this chance is 1/22. Therefore, the chance that a known carrier and her unrelated partner would have an affected first child is the product of these probabilities, or $1/22 \times 1/4 = 1/88$ (about 1.1%).

Of course, if the husband really were a carrier, the chance that the child of two carriers would be a homozygote or a compound heterozygote for mutant CF alleles is 1/4. If the husband were not a carrier, then the chance of having an affected child is 0. Suppose, however, that one cannot test his carrier status directly. A carrier risk of 1/22 is the best estimate one can make for individuals of his ethnic background and no family history of CF, but in fact, a person either is a carrier or is not. The problem is that we do not know. In this situation, the more opportunities the male in Figure 19-3C (who *may or may not* be a carrier of a mutant gene) has to pass on the mutant gene and fails to do so, the less likely it would be that he is indeed a carrier. Thus, if the couple were to come for counseling already with six children, none of whom is affected (Fig. 19-3D), it would seem reasonable, intuitively, that the husband's chance of being a carrier should be less than the 1/22 risk that the childless male partner in Figure 19-3C was assigned on the basis of the population carrier frequency. In this situation, we apply conditional probability (also known as **Bayesian analysis**, based on Bayes' theorem on probability published in 1763), a method that takes advantage of *phenotypic* information in a pedigree to assess the relative probability of two or more alternative *genotypic* possibilities and to condition the risk on the basis of that information. In Figure 19-3D, the chance that the second husband is a carrier is actually 1/119 and the chance that this couple would have a child with CF is 1/476, not 1/88 as calculated in panel C. Some examples of the use of Bayesian analysis for risk assessment in pedigrees are examined in the following section.

Conditional Probability

To illustrate the value of Bayesian analysis, consider the pedigrees shown in Figure 19-4. In Family A, the mother II-1 is an **obligate carrier** for the X-linked bleeding disorder hemophilia A because her father was affected. Her risk of transmitting the mutant factor VIII (*F8*) allele responsible for hemophilia A is 1/2, and

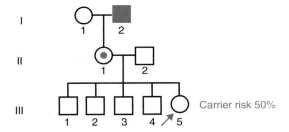

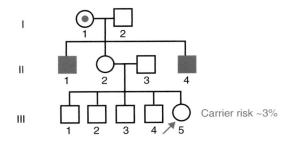

Figure 19-4 ■ Modified risk estimates in genetic counseling. The consultands in the two families are at risk for having a son with hemophilia A. In Family A, the consultand's mother is an obligate heterozygote; in Family B, the consultand's mother may or may not be a carrier. Application of Bayesian analysis reduces the risk of being a carrier to only approximately 3% for the consultand in Family B but not the consultand in Family A. See text for derivation of the modified risk.

the fact that she has already had four unaffected sons does *not* reduce this risk. Thus, the risk that the consultand (III-5) is a carrier of a mutant *F8* allele is 1/2 because she is the daughter of a known carrier.

In Family B, however, the consultand's mother (individual II-2) may or may not be a carrier, depending on whether she has inherited a mutant *F8* allele from her mother, I-1. If III-5 were the only child of her mother, III-5's risk of being a carrier would be 1/2 (her mother's risk of being a carrier) × 1/2 (her risk of inheriting the mutant allele from her mother) = 1/4. Short of testing III-5 directly for the mutant allele, we cannot tell whether she is a carrier. In this case, however, the fact that III-5 has four unaffected brothers is relevant because every time II-2 had a son, the chance that the son would be unaffected is only 1/2 if II-2 *were* a carrier, whereas it is a near certainty (probability = 1) that the son would be unaffected if II-2 were, in fact, *not* a carrier at all. With each son, II-2 has, in effect, tested her carrier status by placing herself at a 50% risk of having an affected son. To have four unaffected sons might suggest that maybe her mother is not a carrier. Bayesian analysis allows one to take this kind

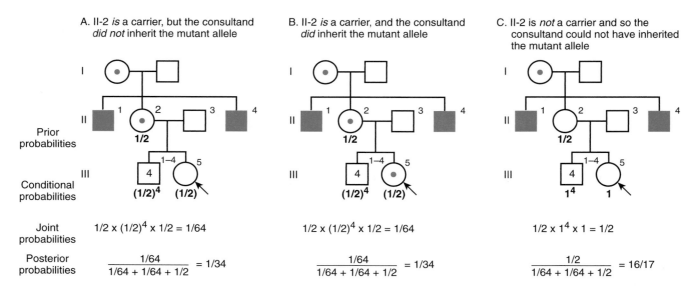

Figure 19-5 ■ Conditional probability used to estimate carrier risk for a consultand in a family with hemophilia in which the prior probability of the carrier state is determined by mendelian inheritance from a known carrier at the top of the pedigree. These risk estimates, based on genetic principles, can be further modified by considering information obtained from family history, carrier detection testing, or molecular genetic methods for direct detection of the mutation in the affected boy, with use of Bayesian calculations. **A** to **C**, The three mutually exclusive situations that could explain the pedigree.

of indirect information into account in calculating whether II-2 is a carrier, thus modifying the consultand's risk of being a carrier and of having an affected child. As we show in the next section, that risk is far lower than 25%.

Identify the Possible Scenarios

To translate this intuition into actual risk calculation, we use a Bayesian probability calculation. First, we list *all* possible alternative genotypes that may be present in the relevant individuals in the pedigree (Fig. 19-5). In this case, there are three scenarios, each reflecting a different combination of alternative genotypes:

- A. II-2 *is* a carrier, but the consultand *is not*.
- B. II-2 and the consultand are *both* carriers.
- C. II-2 is *not* a carrier, which implies that the consultand could not be one either since there is no mutant allele to inherit.

Why do we not consider the possibility that the consultand is a carrier even though II-2 is not? We do not list this scenario because it would require that *two* mutations in the same gene occur independently in the same family, one inherited by the probands and one new mutation in the consultand, a scenario so vanishingly unlikely that it can be dismissed out of hand.

First, we draw the three possible scenarios as pedigrees (see Fig. 19-5) and write down the probability of individual II-2's being a carrier or not. This is referred to as her **prior probability** because it depends simply on her risk of carrying a mutant allele inherited from

her known carrier mother, I-1, and it has not been modified ("conditioned") at all by her own reproductive history.

Next, we write down the probabilities that individuals III-1 through III-4 would be unaffected under each scenario. These probabilities are different, depending on whether II-2 is a carrier or not. If she is a carrier (situations A and B), then the chance that individuals III-1 through III-4 would all be unaffected is the chance that each did not inherit II-2's mutant *F8* allele, which is 1/2 for each of her sons or $(1/2)^4$ for all four. In situation C, however, II-2 is not a carrier, so the chance that her four sons would all be unaffected is 1 since II-2 does not have a mutant *F8* to pass on to any of them. These are called **conditional probabilities** because they are probabilities affected by whether II-2 is a carrier.

Similarly, we write down the probability that the consultand (III-5) is a carrier. In A, she did not inherit the mutant allele from her carrier mother, with probability 1/2. In B, she did inherit the mutant allele (probability = 1/2). In C, her mother is not a carrier, and so III-5 has an approximately 100% chance of not being a carrier. Multiply the prior and conditional probabilities together to form the **joint probabilities** for each situation, A, B, and C.

Finally, we determine what *fraction* of the total joint probability is represented by any scenario of interest—this is called the **posterior probability** of each of the three situations. Since III-5 is the consultand and wants to know her risk of being a carrier, we need the posterior probability of situation B, which is:

$$\frac{1/64}{1/64 + 1/64 + 1/2} = 1/34 = \sim 3\%$$

If we wish to know the chance that II-2 is a carrier, we add the posterior probabilities of the two situations in which she is a carrier, A and B, to get a carrier risk of $1/17 = \sim 6\%$. For every additional child without disease born to II-2 in Family B, the probability that III-5 is a carrier falls, because the joint probability—and therefore the posterior probability—that II-2 is a carrier changes. Similarly, if III-5 also has unaffected sons, her carrier risk could also be modified downward by a Bayesian calculation. However, if II-2 were to have an affected child, then she would have proved herself a carrier, and III-5's risk would become 1/2. Similarly, if III-5 were to have an affected child, then she must be a carrier, and Bayesian analysis would no longer be necessary.

Bayesian analysis may seem like mere statistical maneuvering. However, the analysis allows genetic counselors to quantify what seemed to be intuitively likely from inspection of the pedigree: the fact that the consultand had four unaffected brothers provides support for the hypothesis that her mother is not a carrier. The analysis having been performed, the final risk that III-5 is a carrier can be used in genetic counseling. The risk that her first child will have hemophilia A is $1/34 \times 1/4$, or less than 1%. This risk is appreciably below the prior probability estimated without taking into account the genetic evidence provided by her brothers.

Conditional Probability in X-linked Lethal Disorders

Because any severe X-linked disorder is manifested in the hemizygous male, an isolated case (no family history) of such a disorder may represent either a new gene mutation (in which case the mother is not a carrier) or inheritance of a mutant allele from his unaffected carrier mother (we ignore the small but real chance of mosaicism for the mutation in the mother). Estimation of the recurrence risk depends on knowing the chance that she could be a carrier. Bayesian analysis can be used to estimate carrier risks in X-linked lethal diseases such as Duchenne muscular dystrophy (DMD) and ornithine transcarbamylase deficiency.

Consider the family at risk for DMD shown in Figure 19-6. The consultand, III-2, wants to know her risk of being a carrier. There are three possible scenarios, each with dramatically different risk estimates for the family:

- A. III-1's condition may be the result of a new mutation. In this case, his sister and maternal aunt are not at significant risk of being a carrier.

- B. His mother, II-1, is a carrier, but her condition is the result of a new mutation. In this case, his sister (III-2) has a 1/2 risk of being a carrier but his maternal aunt is not at risk for being a carrier since his grandmother, I-1, is not a carrier.

- C. His mother is a carrier who inherited a mutant allele from her carrier mother (I-1). In this case, all of the female relatives have either a 1/2 or a 1/4 risk of being carriers.

How can we use conditional probability to determine the carrier risks for the female relatives of III-1 in this pedigree? If we proceed as we did previously with the hemophilia family in Figure 19-4, what do we use as the prior probability that individual I-1 is a carrier? We do not have pedigree information, as we did in the hemophilia pedigree, from which to calculate these prior probabilities. We can, however, use some simple assumptions to estimate the prior probability (see Box).

••• Prior Probability that a Female in the Population is a Carrier of an X-Linked Lethal Disorder

Suppose H is the population frequency of female carriers of an X-linked lethal disorder. Assume H is constant from generation to generation.

Suppose the mutation rate at this X-linked locus in any one gamete $= \mu$. Assume μ is the same in males and females. Mutation rate μ is a small number, in the range of 10^{-4} to 10^{-6} (see Chapter 9).

Then, there are three mutually exclusive ways that any female could be a carrier:

1. She inherits a mutant allele from a carrier mother $= 1/2 \times H$.
   or
2. She receives a newly mutant allele on the X she receives from her mother $= \mu$.
   or
3. She receives a newly mutant allele on the X she receives from her father $= \mu$.

The chance a female is a carrier is the sum of the chance that she inherited a preexisting mutation and the chance that she received a new mutation from her mother or from her father.

$$H = (1/2 \times H) + \mu + \mu = H/2 + 2\mu$$

Solving for H, you get the chance that a random female in the population is a carrier of a particular X-linked disorder $= 4\mu$. Note that half of this 4μ, 2μ, is the probability she is a carrier by inheritance, and the other 2μ is the probability that she is a carrier by new mutation.

The chance a random female in the population is *not* a carrier is $1 - 4\mu \approx 1$ (since μ is a very small number).

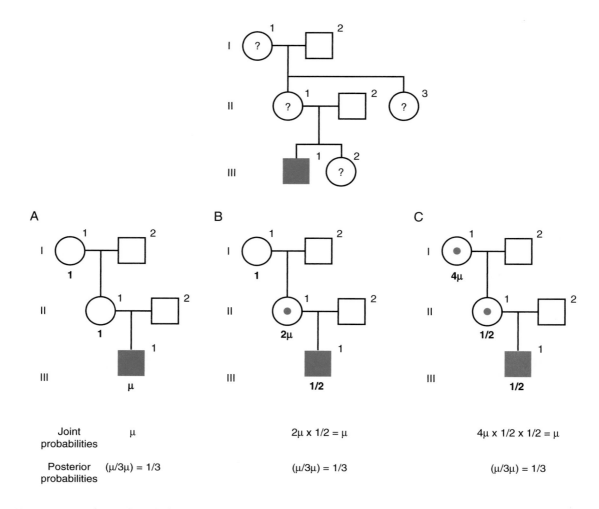

Figure 19-6 ■ Conditional probability used to determine carrier risks for females in a family with an X-linked genetic lethal disorder in which the prior probability of being a carrier has to be calculated by assuming that the carrier frequency is not changing from generation to generation, and that the mutation rates are the same in males and females. **Top,** Pedigree of a family with an X-linked genetic lethal disorder. **Bottom,** The three mutually exclusive situations that could explain the pedigree. **A,** The proband is a new mutation. **B,** The mother of the proband is a new mutation. **C,** The mother of the proband inherited the mutation from her carrier mother, the grandmother of the proband.

Now we can use this value 4μ as the prior probability that a woman is a carrier of an X-linked lethal (see Fig. 19-6). For the purpose of calculating the chance that II-1 is a carrier, we ignore the female relatives II-3 and III-2 because there is nothing about them, such as phenotype, laboratory testing, or reproductive history, that conditions whether II-1 is a carrier.

- In A, III-1 is a new mutation with probability μ. His mother and grandmother are both noncarriers, each of which has a probability of $1 - 4\mu \approx 1$. The joint probability is $\mu \times 1 \times 1 = \mu$.
- In C, individuals I-1 and II-1 are both carriers. As explained in the Box, the chance that I-1 is a carrier has a prior probability of 4μ. For II-1 to be a carrier, she must have inherited the mutant allele from her mother, which has probability 1/2. In addition, the chance that II-1 has passed the mutant allele on to

her affected son is also 1/2. The joint probability is therefore $4\mu \times 1/2 \times 1/2 = \mu$.
- In B, I-1 is designated a noncarrier, and so II-1 must be the product of a maternal or paternal new mutation. The chance that a female will be a carrier by new mutation is $\mu + \mu = 2\mu$ (and *not* 4μ) because we are specifying in scenario B that I-1 is not a carrier. The joint probability is therefore $2\mu \times 1/2 = \mu$.

The posterior probabilities are now easy to calculate as 1/3 each for scenarios A, B, and C. The affected boy has 1/3 chance of being a new mutation (situation A), whereas his mother II-1 is a carrier in both B and C and therefore has a $1/3 + 1/3 = 2/3$ chance of being a carrier. The grandmother, I-1, is a carrier only in C, and so her chance of being a carrier is 1/3.

With these risk figures for the core individuals in the pedigree, we can calculate the carrier risks for the

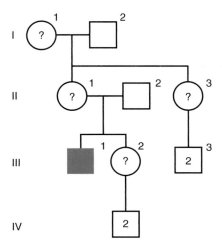

Figure 19-7 ■ The family from Figure 19-6 but now with additional information consisting of unaffected males that must be used to modify the carrier risks for females in the pedigree.

female relatives II-3 and III-2. III-2's risk of being a carrier is $1/2 \times$ [the chance II-1 is a carrier] $= 1/2 \times 2/3 = 1/3$. The risk that II-3 is a carrier is $1/2 \times$ [the chance I-1 is a carrier] $= 1/2 \times 1/3 = 1/6$. In all of these calculations, we are ignoring the small but very real possibility of germline mosaicism (see Chapter 7).

This approach to calculation of conditional probabilities is dependable but can be time-consuming when there are a large number of individuals whose genotypes are in question, because the number of pedigree scenarios increases with every additional individual you add. For example, suppose in the pedigree in Figure 19-6, II-3 and III-2 each had two unaffected sons (Fig. 19-7). There are now additional phenotypic data (unaffected male offspring) that will condition their respective risks for being carriers. The number of situations you have to cover increases from three to seven; situation B in Figure 19-6 splits into B1 and B2, depending on whether or not III-2 inherits the mutant allele from her mother, and situation C breaks into four possibilities (C1 to C4), depending on whether or not II-3 and III-2 inherited the mutant allele from their mothers (Table 19-3).

With this additional information, the chance that III-2 is a carrier is now the posterior risk of situations B2, C3, and C4 = 13/129 = ~10%. With some practice, the tabular approach may allow quicker calculations without drawing out all the pedigrees.

Disorders with Incomplete Penetrance

To estimate the recurrence risk of disorders with incomplete penetrance, the probability that an apparently normal person actually carries the mutant gene in question must be considered. Figure 19-8 shows a pedigree of **split-hand deformity**, an autosomal dominant abnormality with incomplete penetrance discussed in Chapter 7. An estimate of penetrance can be made from a single pedigree if it is large enough, or from a review of published pedigrees; we use 70% in our example. That means that a heterozygote for a mutation that causes split-hand deformity has a 30% chance of *not* showing the phenotype. The pedigree shows several people who must carry the mutant gene but do not express it (i.e., in whom the defect is not penetrant): I-1 or I-2 (assuming no somatic or germline mosaicism) and II-3. The other unaffected family members may or may not carry the mutant gene.

If III-4, the daughter of a known affected heterozygote, is the consultand, she either may have escaped inheriting the mutant allele from her affected mother or did inherit it but is not expressing the phenotype because penetrance is incomplete in this disorder. There are two possibilities (Fig. 19-9). In A, III-4 is not a carrier with prior probability of 1/2. If she does not carry the mutant allele, she will not have the phenotype, so the joint probability for A is 1/2. In B, III-4 is a carrier, also with prior probability 1/2. Here, we must apply the conditional probability that she is a carrier but does not show the phenotype, which has probability of 1 − penetrance = 1 − 0.7 = 0.3, so the joint probability for B is 1/2 × 0.3 = 0.15. The posterior probability

Table 19-3

Conditional Probability Calculation for Fig. 19-7

Situation	FEMALE CARRIER STATUS I-1	II-1	II-3	III-2	Joint Probabilities*
A	No	No	No	No	μ
B1	No	Yes (new mutation)	No	No	$\{2\mu \times {}^1\!/_2\} \times [1] \times [{}^1\!/_2] = \mu/2$
B2	No	Yes (new mutation)	No	Yes	$\{2\mu \times {}^1\!/_2\} \times [1] \times [{}^1\!/_2 \times ({}^1\!/_2)^2] = \mu/8$
C1	Yes	Yes	No	No	$\{4\mu \times {}^1\!/_2 \times {}^1\!/_2\} \times [{}^1\!/_2] \times [{}^1\!/_2] = \mu/4$
C2	Yes	Yes	Yes	No	$\{4\mu \times {}^1\!/_2 \times {}^1\!/_2\} \times [{}^1\!/_2 \times ({}^1\!/_2)^2] \times [{}^1\!/_2] = \mu/16$
C3	Yes	Yes	No	Yes	$\{4\mu \times {}^1\!/_2 \times {}^1\!/_2\} \times [{}^1\!/_2] \times [{}^1\!/_2 \times ({}^1\!/_2)^2] = \mu/16$
C4	Yes	Yes	Yes	Yes	$\{4\mu \times {}^1\!/_2 \times {}^1\!/_2\} \times [{}^1\!/_2 \times ({}^1\!/_2)^2] \times [{}^1\!/_2 \times ({}^1\!/_2)^2] = \mu/64$

*The joint probabilities for the core individuals in the pedigree (I-1, II-1, and III-1 are enclosed in curly brackets { }, and the probabilities for individuals II-3 and III-2 are shown in square brackets [ ]. See Figure 19-7.

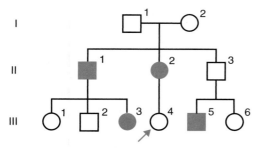

Figure 19-8 ■ Pedigree of family with split-hand deformity and lack of penetrance in some individuals.

that III-4 is a carrier without expressing the phenotype is therefore 3/13 = ~ 23%.

Disorders with Late Age at Onset

Many autosomal dominant conditions characteristically show a late age at onset, beyond the age of reproduction. Thus, it is not uncommon in genetic counseling to ask whether a person of reproductive age who is at risk for a particular autosomal dominant disorder carries the gene. One example of such a disorder is a rare, familial form of **Parkinson disease** (PD) inherited as an autosomal dominant condition.

Consider the dominant PD pedigree in Figure 19-10 in which the consultand, an asymptomatic 35-year-old man, wishes to know his risk for PD. His prior risk of having inherited the *PD* gene from his affected grandmother is 1/4. Considering that perhaps only 5% of persons with this rare form of PD show symptoms at his age, he would not be expected to show signs of the disease even if he had inherited the mutant allele. The more significant aspect of the pedigree,

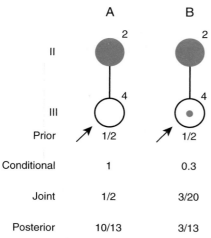

Figure 19-9 ■ Conditional probability calculation for the risk of the carrier state in the consultand in Figure 19-8. There are two possibilities: either she is a carrier (**B**) or she is not (**A**). Her failure to demonstrate the phenotype lowers her carrier risk from the prior probability of 1/2 to 3/13 (23%).

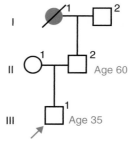

Figure 19-10 ■ Age-modified risks for genetic counseling in dominant Parkinson disease. That the consultand's father is asymptomatic at the age of 60 years reduces the consultand's final risk of carrying the gene to approximately 12.5%. That the consultand himself is asymptomatic reduces the risk only slightly, because most patients carrying the mutant allele for this disorder will be asymptomatic at the age of 35 years.

however, is that the consultand's father (II-2) is also asymptomatic at the age of 60 years, an age by which perhaps two thirds of persons with this form of PD show symptoms and one third do not.

As shown in Figure 19-11, there are three possibilities.

- A. His father did not inherit the mutant allele, so the consultand is not at risk.
- B. His father inherited the mutant allele and is asymptomatic at the age of 60 years, but the consultand did not.
- C. His father inherited the mutant allele and is asymptomatic. The consultand inherited it from his father and is asymptomatic at the age of 35 years.

The father's chance of carrying the mutant allele (situations B and C) is 25%; the consultand's chance of having the mutant allele (situation C only) is 12%. Providing these recurrence risks in genetic counseling requires careful follow-up. If, for example, the consultand or his father were to develop symptoms of PD, the risks change dramatically.

● APPLICATION OF MOLECULAR GENETICS TO DETERMINATION OF RECURRENCE RISKS

Many disease genes can now be detected directly in carriers and affected persons by means of DNA analysis. This represents a major improvement in carrier detection and prenatal diagnosis, in many cases allowing determination of the presence or absence of a particular gene with essentially 100% accuracy.

There are two chief approaches to risk estimation by DNA analysis. The first method is by **direct detection of the mutation** in a patient's or other family member's genomic DNA. Methods such as polymerase chain reaction followed by sequencing or allele-specific

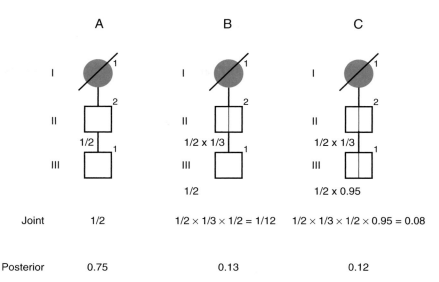

Figure 19-11 ■ Three scenarios pertaining to the Parkinson disease pedigree in Figure 19-10. Individual II-2 is a non-penetrant carrier (vertical line in the symbol) in scenarios B and C. Individual III-1 is a non-penetrant carrier in scenario C.

oligonucleotide (ASO) methods are quick and accurate, and use readily available tissues such as buccal scraping or a blood sample (see Chapter 4). Obviously, direct tests can be used only when the gene or (in the case of ASO) the mutation or mutations responsible for a particular disorder are known. The second is the method of using **flanking markers** that are **closely linked** to the disease locus (see Chapter 10).

Direct Detection of Mutations

Duchenne Muscular Dystrophy

About 60% of patients with DMD have deletions within the gene, and an additional 6% have duplications (see Chapter 12). In the past, Southern blotting with a probe that detects a restriction fragment, formed by the junction of the two segments of DNA on either side of the deletion or duplication ("junctional" fragments), would show fragments that are altered in size compared with the normal fragment and are therefore diagnostic of the deletion or duplication event. Finding the right probe to detect the right junction fragment is not always simple, however. At present, deletions are more frequently detected by a set of polymerase chain reactions designed to amplify the parts of the gene typically deleted in affected patients (see Fig. 12-21). In Figure 19-12A, if the patient with DMD (II-4) had an identifiable deletion, DNA from the fetus (obtained by amniocentesis or chorionic villus sampling, as described in Chapter 15) could be examined directly for the presence or absence of the deletion, and a diagnosis could be made with certainty.

Detecting a duplication by polymerase chain reaction in an affected male is much more difficult; in the absence of a detectable junction fragment, the diagnosis relies on measuring a copy number change of the affected, duplicated segment from 1 to 2 and not on the complete absence of a deleted fragment. A quantitative real-time polymerase chain reaction (qPCR) (see Chapter 4) can be used to measure copy number in DNA and has been applied to this problem with some success.

qPCR is also being used in the more challenging problem of carrier detection in females. A heterozygous female for a dystrophin deletion (III-1 in Fig. 19-12A) has a difference in copy number of the deleted segment of 1:2. Even more difficult is the diagnosis of a carrier of a duplication when there is a copy number ratio of only 3:2 in the carrier versus a normal control DNA segment. Finally, in the absence of a junction fragment, identification of carriers among female family members can still be done indirectly by the use of linked markers (Fig. 19-12B).

In the one third of DMD cases due to point mutations, unless the extensive sequencing work needed to find the pathogenic mutation has been done in the proband, the determination of carrier status may also depend on linked markers.

Cystic Fibrosis

Most mutations in cystic fibrosis (CF) are single-base mutations or deletions or duplications of a small number of nucleotides in the *CFTR* gene (see Chapter 12). Carrier detection and prenatal diagnosis in CF make use of the enormous amount of information that has been accumulated on the types of mutations that cause the disease. More than 1000 different mutations have been described in the *CFTR* gene. Some are rare, occurring in only a few families. Others are much more common, but their frequency can vary enormously in different ethnic groups. As discussed in Chapter 12, about 70% of the CF mutations in individuals of northern European descent are due to the three–base pair deletion that removes the phenylalanine at position 508

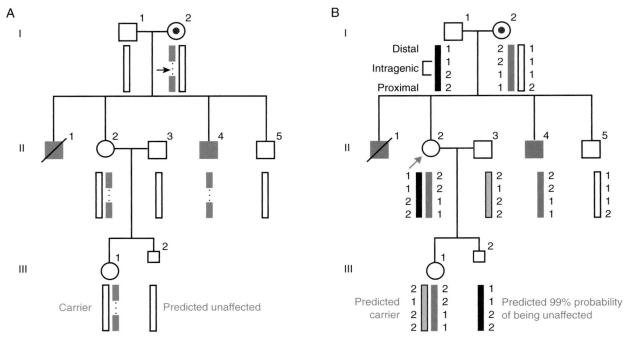

Figure 19-12 ■ Use of direct mutation detection and genetic linkage analysis for genetic counseling in a family with DMD. **A,** The proband has a deletion mutation *(broken blue bar).* Normal *DMD* genes are symbolized by open bars. **B,** The proband's mutation is unknown. Four polymorphic markers were tested, two within the *DMD* gene (intragenic) and one on each side, flanking it. The overall frequency of recombination between the farthest markers is 2%. Haplotypes observed in the family are shown. The haplotype indicated in dark blue contains the mutant *DMD* allele. Predicted genotypes at the *DMD* locus of the consultand's daughter and male fetus are based on the marker haplotypes.

(ΔF508). The ΔF508 mutation is less common or even totally absent in other ethnic groups, in which mutations other than ΔF508 are more frequent. As additional mutations in different patients are identified, laboratories have begun to offer a battery of mutation detection tests in which dozens of the more common mutations in a population can be identified. The polymerase chain reaction and hybridization with oligonucleotides specific for each mutation are used to identify heterozygous carriers and homozygous affected fetuses easily and rapidly. For the minority of families in whom the mutations are unknown, DNA markers very closely linked to the CF locus are available for diagnosis by linkage analysis.

Use of Linked Markers in Molecular Diagnosis

Direct detection of the mutations responsible for genetic disease is not always possible in all cases, for the following reasons.

1. Some diseases, such as Duchenne muscular dystrophy (DMD), neurofibromatosis type 1 (NF1), and osteogenesis imperfecta (OI), have substantial allelic heterogeneity. Extensive sequencing may be necessary to find the mutant alleles responsible in a proband.

2. The problem of allelic heterogeneity is exacerbated when the genes are large with many exons, such as dystrophin in DMD, neurofibromin in NF1, and collagen I in OI. Missense and nonsense mutations in particular are difficult to find without direct sequencing of the gene involved.

3. Time constraints imposed by an ongoing pregnancy may make it difficult to perform the comprehensive sequencing required to find the mutant alleles and to apply that information to a prenatal diagnostic setting.

The linkage approach to mutation detection is *indirect.* One is not detecting the mutant allele itself but is using linked markers that flank the disease locus to track the inheritance of a gene known from the family tree to be harboring a disease-causing mutation. Although indirect, linkage works well if the following requirements can be met:

1. There is close linkage between the mutation and the marker, so that recombination is unlikely.
2. The family is "informative"; that is, crucial family members are available for the study and are heterozygous for the markers.
3. The linkage phase is known or can be reasonably inferred.
4. No recombination has occurred between the markers being followed and the disease gene. If recombination does occur within the disease locus somewhere

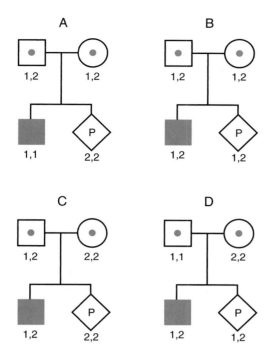

Figure 19-13 ■ Examples of molecular diagnosis in β-thalassemia, with polymorphisms in the β-globin locus, in the second pregnancy (P) of a couple with one affected child. The chance of recombination between the polymorphic marker and the mutation is assumed to be negligible. In Family **A**, phase can be determined from the affected sibling, and a diagnosis that the fetus is unaffected is possible. In Family **B**, phase cannot be determined and no diagnosis is possible because the fetus could be either affected (50% chance) or unaffected (50% chance). In Family **C**, phase cannot be determined completely in both parents, but it is possible to provide a diagnosis that the fetus will be unaffected but could be a carrier of β-thalassemia. In Family **D**, no diagnosis is possible; the family is uninformative.

between the closely linked flanking markers, these markers will alert the diagnostician that a crossover has occurred, and the results may therefore not be reliable.

For a small gene, like β-globin, a linked marker within the gene has a negligible recombination frequency with a mutation anywhere within the gene. However, even with such a tightly linked marker, having an informative family with known linkage phase is critical to indirect molecular diagnosis by linked markers (Fig. 19-13).

The accuracy of diagnosis by genetically linked markers can be increased markedly by use of two informative genetic markers that flank the disease gene. In this instance, the chance of a misdiagnosis is reduced because misdiagnosis will result only if *two* crossovers occur, one on each side of the disease gene. The availability of flanking, tightly linked markers for any disease gene of interest is just one more benefit arising from the Human Genome Project.

Linkage Analysis in Duchenne Muscular Dystrophy

The hypothetical DMD pedigree shown in Figure 19-12B illustrates the use of linked markers to detect a carrier and to diagnose a fetus prenatally. In this family, the maternal grandmother I-2 is clearly a carrier because she has had two affected sons. Her mutation is unknown. She is informative for DNA markers that flank the *DMD* gene and for one of two markers within this large gene. The linkage phase in the maternal grandmother can be inferred from her two living sons, II-4 and II-5, because any phase other than that indicated in Figure 19-12B would require two recombination events (i.e., in the meioses leading to her two living sons). The consultand II-2 has inherited the same maternal haplotype as her affected brother. The markers of her father I-1 are known, and she herself is informative at all four loci. Her linkage phase is known with certainty, and whether she transmits the mutant allele can be determined by following the inheritance of the linked markers. The risk of a recombination occurring in a meiosis in the consultand is about 2%, not negligible with a gene as large as dystrophin. A recombination would be easily detected because the child would inherit a portion of her mother's *DMD* gene (but not necessarily the mutation itself) and a portion of her father's *DMD* gene. Because the consultand's husband's markers are known, it can also be predicted that her daughter III-1 has inherited the mutant *DMD* gene and is a carrier.

● EMPIRICAL RECURRENCE RISKS

Counseling for Complex Disorders

Genetic counselors deal with many conditions that are not single-gene disorders. Instead, counselors may be called on to provide risk estimates for complex trait disorders with a strong genetic component and familial clustering, such as cleft lip and palate, congenital heart disease, meningomyelocele, psychiatric illness, and coronary artery disease (see Chapter 8). In these situations, the risk of recurrence in first-degree relatives of affected individuals may be increased over the background incidence of the disease in the population, but is not at the level expected with autosomal dominant or recessive disorders. In these situations, recurrence risks are estimated empirically by studying as many families with the disorder as possible and observing how frequently the disorder recurs. The observed frequency of a recurrence is taken as an **empirical recurrence risk**.

Genetic counselors must use caution in applying empirical risk figures to a particular family. First, empirical estimates are an average over what is undoubtedly a group of heterogeneous disorders with different mechanisms of inheritance. In any one family, the real recurrence risk may actually be higher or lower than the average. Second, empirical risk estimates use history to make predictions about future occurrences; if the underlying biological causes are changing through time, data from the past may not be accurate for the future. Finally, figures are derived from a particular population, and so the data from one ethnic group, socioeconomic class, or geographical location may not be accurate for an individual from a different background. Nonetheless, such figures are useful when patients ask genetic counselors to give a best estimate for recurrence risk for disorders with complex inheritance.

For example, neural tube defects (myelomeningocele and anencephaly) occur in approximately 0.3% of births in the U.S. white population. If, however, a couple has a child with a neural tube defect, the risk in the next pregnancy is 4% (13 times higher; see Table 8-9). If these risk figures are calculated for different genders, the figures are even more striking: the sister of a girl with a neural tube defect has a 6% chance of also having a neural tube defect. The risks remain elevated compared with the general population risk for more distantly related individuals; a second-degree relative (such as a nephew or niece) of an individual with a neural tube defect is at a 1.7% chance of having a similar birth defect. With folate supplementation before conception and during early pregnancy, however, these recurrence risk figures fall dramatically (see Chapter 8).

Genetic Counseling for Consanguinity

Consanguineous couples sometimes request genetic counseling before they have children because an increased risk of birth defects in their offspring is widely appreciated. In the absence of a family history for a known autosomal recessive condition, we use empirical risk figures for the offspring of consanguineous couples, based on population surveys of birth defects in children born to first-cousin couples compared with nonconsanguineous couples (Table 19-4).

These results provide empirical risk figures in the counseling of first cousins. Although the relative risk of abnormal offspring is higher for related than for unrelated parents, it is still quite low: approximately double in the offspring of first cousins, compared with baseline risk figures for any abnormality of 1.5% to 3% for any child regardless of consanguinity. This increased risk is not exclusively for single-gene autosomal recessive diseases but includes the entire spectrum of single-gene and complex trait disorders. However, any couple, consanguineous or not, who has a child with a birth defect is at greater risk for having another child with a birth defect in a subsequent pregnancy.

Table 19-4

Incidence of Birth Defects in Children Born to Nonconsanguineous and First-Cousin Couples

	Incidence of First Birth Defect in Sibship (per 1000)	Incidence of Recurrence of Any Birth Defect in Subsequent Children in Sibship (per 1000)
First-cousin marriage	36	68
Nonconsanguineous marriage	15	30

Data from Stoltenberg C, Magnus P, Skrondal A, Lie RT: Consanguinity and recurrence risk of birth defects: a population-based study. Am J Med Genet 82:424-428, 1999.

GENERAL REFERENCES

Baker DL, Schuette JL, Uhlmann WR: A Guide to Genetic Counseling. New York, Wiley, 1998.
Harper PS: Practical Genetic Counseling, 6th ed. Oxford, England, Butterworth-Heinemann Medical, 2001.
Kessler S: Genetic Counseling: Psychological Dimensions. London, Academic Press, 1979.
Mahowald MB, Verp MS, Anderson RR: Genetic counseling: clinical and ethical challenges. Annu Rev Genet 32:547-549, 1998.
Weil J: Psychosocial Genetic Counseling. New York Oxford University Press, 2000.
Young ID: Introduction to Risk Calculation in Genetic Counseling, 2nd ed. New York, Oxford University Press, 1999.

REFERENCES FOR SPECIFIC TOPICS

Gardner RJM, Sutherland GR: Chromosome Abnormalities and Genetic Counseling, 3rd ed. New York, Oxford University Press, 2003.
Hodge SE: A simple, unified approach to bayesian risk calculations. J Genet Counsel 7:235-262, 1998.
Stoltenberg C, Magnus P, Skrondal A, Lie RT: Consanguinity and recurrence risk of birth defects: a population-based study. Am J Med Genet 82:424-428, 1999.

USEFUL WEBSITES

Genetic Alliance. *http://www.geneticalliance.org/* An international organization of consumers, professionals, laboratories, hospitals, companies, and not-for-profit foundations dedicated to improving the life of people affected by genetic disease.
GeneClinics. *http://www.geneclinics.org/* A website supported by the Federal government and maintained by the University of Washington and Seattle Children's Hospital, providing information on diagnosis, management, and counseling for specific disorders.
National Society of Genetic Counselors. *http://www.nsgc.org/* The organization in the United States representing the genetic counseling profession. Links to useful websites relevant to genetic counseling.
OMIM: Online Mendelian Inheritance in Man. *http://www.ncbi. nlm.nih.gov/entrez/query.fcgi?db=OMIM* Online database of human genes and genetic diseases maintained by the Johns Hopkins University School of Medicine and supported by the National Library of Medicine, National Institutes of Health.

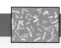

PROBLEMS

1. You are consulted by a couple, Dorothy and David, who tell the following story: Dorothy's maternal grandfather, Bruce, had congenital stationary night blindness, which also affected Bruce's maternal uncle, Arthur; the family history appears to fit an X-linked inheritance pattern. (There is also an autosomal dominant form.) Whether Bruce's mother was affected is unknown. Dorothy and David have three unaffected children: a daughter, Elsie, and two sons, Edward and Eliot. Elsie is planning to have children in the near future. Dorothy wonders whether she should warn Elsie about the risk that she might be a carrier of a serious eye disorder. Sketch the pedigree and answer the following.
   a. What is the chance that Elsie is heterozygous?
   b. An ophthalmologist traces the family history in further detail and finds evidence that in this pedigree, the disorder is not X-linked but autosomal dominant. There is no evidence that Dorothy's mother Cecile was affected. On this basis, what is the chance that Elsie is heterozygous?

2. A deceased boy, Nathan, was the only member of his family with DMD. He is survived by two sisters, Norma (who has a daughter, Olive) and Nancy (who has a daughter, Odette). His mother Molly has two sisters, Maud and Martha. Martha has two unaffected sons and two daughters, Nora and Nellie. Maud has one daughter, Naomi. No carrier tests are available because the mutation in the affected boy remains unknown.
   a. Sketch the pedigree and calculate the posterior risks for all these females, using information provided in this chapter.
   b. In many molecular diagnosis laboratories, prenatal diagnosis by DNA analysis is available only to women with more than a 2% risk that a pregnancy will result in a son with DMD. Which of these women would not qualify?

3. In a village in Wales in 1984, 13 boys were born in succession before a girl was born. What is the probability of 13 successive male births? What is the probability of 13 successive births of a single sex? What is the probability that after 13 male births, the 14th child will be a boy?

4. Let H be the population frequency of carriers of hemophilia A. The incidence of hemophilia A in males (I) equals the chance that a maternal $F8$ gene has a new mutation (μ) from a noncarrier mother *plus* the chance it was inherited as a preexisting mutation from a carrier mother ($1/2 \times H$). Adding these two terms gives $I = \mu + (1/2 \times H)$. H is the chance a carrier inherits the mutation from an affected father ($I \times f$) *plus* the chance of a new paternal mutation (μ) *plus* the chance of a new maternal mutation (μ) *plus* the chance of inheriting it from a carrier mother ($1/2 \times H$). Adding these four terms gives $H = (I \times f) + \mu + \mu + (1/2)H$.
   a. If hemophilia A has a fitness (f) of ~0.70, that is, hemophiliacs have approximately 70% as many offspring as do controls, then what is the incidence of affected males? of carrier females? (Answer in terms of multiples of the mutation rate.) If a woman has a son with an isolated case of hemophilia A, what is the risk that she is a carrier? What is the chance that her next son will be affected?
   b. For DMD, $f = 0$. What is the population frequency of affected males? of carrier females?
   c. Color blindness is thought to have normal fitness ($f = 1$). What is the incidence of carrier females if the frequency of color-blind males is 8%?

5. Ira and Margie each have a sibling affected with CF.
   a. What are their prior risks of being carriers?
   b. What is the risk of their having an affected child in their first pregnancy?
   c. They have had three unaffected children and now wish to know their risk of having an affected child. Using Bayesian analysis to take into consideration that they have already had three unaffected children, calculate the chance that their next child will be affected.

6. A 30-year-old woman with myotonic dystrophy comes in for counseling. Her son, aged 14 years, shows no symptoms, but she wishes to know whether he will be affected with this autosomal dominant condition later in life. Approximately half of individuals carrying the mutant gene are asymptomatic before the age of 14 years. What is the risk that the son will eventually develop myotonic dystrophy? Should you test the child for the expanded repeat in the gene for myotonic dystrophy?

7. A couple arrives in your clinic with their 7-month-old son, who has been moderately developmentally delayed from birth. The couple is contemplating having additional children, and you are asked whether this could be a genetic disorder.
   a. Is this possible, and if so, what pattern or patterns of inheritance would fit this story?
   b. On taking a detailed family history, you learn that both parents' families were originally from the same small village in northern Italy. How might this fact alter your assessment of the case?
   c. You next learn that the mother has two sisters and five brothers. Both sisters have developmentally delayed children. How might this alter your assessment of the case?

8. You are addressing a Neurofibromatosis Association parents' meeting. A severely affected woman, 32 years old, comments that she is not at risk of passing on the disorder because her parents are not affected and her neurofibromatosis, therefore, is due to a new mutation. Comment.

PROBLEMS–cont'd

9. An alternative approach to calculating the carrier risk for III-2 in Figure 19-7 is to break the pedigree apart and do the calculations stepwise, a method referred to as the **dummy consultand method.** Instead of calculating the joint probabilities of all seven scenarios to determine the posterior probability that III-2 is a carrier, one ignores III-2 and her two children for the moment, makes individual II-1 serve as a dummy consultand, and calculates II-1's risk of being a carrier *without using any conditional information provided by III-2.* Then, with the carrier risk for II-1 in hand, determine the prior probability that III-2 is a carrier and then condition that risk by use of the fact she has two unaffected male children. How does the carrier risk for III-2 calculated by the dummy consultand method compare with the risk calculated by the all-encompassing method in Table 19-3? How about the carrier risk for II-1? How does the risk calculated by the dummy consultand method compare with the risk calculated by the complete method in Table 19-3?

Ethical Issues in Medical Genetics

Human genetics has already had a major impact in many areas of medicine. In the future, the knowledge gained from the Human Genome Project will revolutionize clinical medicine as profoundly as did the earlier demonstration that the rules of chemistry are the same whether a reaction takes place in a test tube or in the cells of the body. The challenge confronting us all, both future health professionals and members of society at large, is to make sure that the advances in human genetic knowledge and technology are used responsibly, fairly, and humanely.

Four cardinal principles are frequently considered in any discussion of ethical issues in medicine: **respect for individual autonomy** (safeguarding an individual's rights to control his or her medical care and medical information, free of coercion), **beneficence** (doing good for the patient), **avoidance of maleficence** (*primum non nocere*: "first of all, do no harm"), and **justice** (ensuring that all individuals are treated equally and fairly). Complex ethical issues arise when these principles are perceived to be in conflict with one another. The role of ethicists working at the interface between society and medical genetics is to weigh and balance conflicting demands, each of which has a claim to legitimacy based on one or more of these cardinal principles.

⬤ ETHICAL DILEMMAS ARISING IN MEDICAL GENETICS

In this section, we focus our discussion on some of the ethical dilemmas arising in medical genetics, dilemmas that will only become more difficult and complex as genetics and genomics research expands our knowledge (Table 20-1). The list of issues discussed here is by no means exhaustive, nor are they necessarily independent of one other.

Ethical Dilemmas in Genetic Testing

Prenatal Genetic Testing

Geneticists are frequently asked to help couples use prenatal diagnosis or assisted reproductive technology to avoid having offspring with a serious hereditary disorder. For some hereditary disorders, prenatal diagnosis remains controversial, particularly when the diagnosis leads to a decision to terminate the pregnancy for a disease that, unlike Tay-Sachs disease (Case 38) for example, is not an untreatable, fatal disease of infancy. A debate is ongoing in the community of disabled, mentally retarded, and deaf patients and their families, to name only a few examples, about whether prenatal diagnosis and abortion for these disorders are justified. The ethical dilemma is in attempting to balance respect for the autonomy of parents' reproductive decision-making with an assessment of whether aborting a fetus affected with a disability compatible with life is fair to the fetus or to the broader community of disabled persons or people with hearing impairment.

The dilemma also arises when a couple makes a request for prenatal diagnosis in a pregnancy that is at risk for what most people would not consider a disease or disability. The motivation in seeking prenatal diagnosis might be to avoid recurrence of a disorder associated with a mild or cosmetic defect or for selection of

Table 20-1

Major Ethical and Policy Issues in Medical Genetics

GENETIC TESTING

Prenatal diagnosis, especially for non-disease traits or sex

Testing asymptomatic adults for genotypes that predispose to late-onset disease

Testing asymptomatic children for genotypes that predispose to adult-onset diseases

PRIVACY OF GENETIC INFORMATION

Duty to warn and permission to warn

MISUSE OF GENETIC INFORMATION

Employment discrimination based on an employee's genotype

Discrimination in life and health insurance underwriting based on an employee's genotype

GENETIC SCREENING

Stigmatization

Privacy

Coercion

---

sex. In particular, the issue of sex selection for reasons other than reducing the risk for sex-limited or X-linked disease is a contentious one. Many genetics professionals are concerned that couples are using assisted reproductive technologies, such as in vitro fertilization and blastomere biopsy, or prenatal sex determination and abortion, to balance the sexes of the children in their family or to avoid having children of one or the other sex for social and economic reasons prevalent in their societies.

In the future, particular alleles and genes that contribute to complex traits such as intelligence, personality, stature, and other physical characteristics may possibly be identified. Will such nonmedical criteria be viewed as a justifiable basis for prenatal diagnosis? Some might argue that parents are already expending tremendous effort and resources on improving the *environmental* factors that contribute to healthy, successful children. They might therefore ask why they should not try to improve the *genetic* factors as well. Others consider prenatal selection for particular desirable genes a dehumanizing step that treats children simply as commodities fashioned for their parents' benefit. Once again, the ethical dilemma is in attempting to balance respect for the autonomy of parents' reproductive decision-making with an assessment of whether it is just or beneficial to terminate a pregnancy when a fetus has a strictly cosmetic problem or carries what are perceived to be undesirable alleles or is even of the "wrong" sex. Does a health professional have, on the one hand, a responsibility and, on the other hand, the right to decide for a couple when a disorder is not serious enough to warrant prenatal diagnosis and abortion or assisted reproduction?

There is little consensus among geneticists as to *where* or even *whether* one can draw the line in deciding what constitutes a trait serious enough to warrant prenatal testing.

Genetic Testing for Predisposition to Disease

Another area of medical genetics in which ethical dilemmas frequently arise is genetic testing of asymptomatic individuals for diseases that may have an onset in life later than when the molecular testing is being performed. The ethical principles of respect for individual autonomy and beneficence are central to testing in this context. At one end of the spectrum is testing for late-onset, highly penetrant neurological disorders, such as Huntington disease (see Chapter 12 and Case 22). In such diseases, individuals carrying a mutant allele may be asymptomatic but will almost certainly develop a devastating illness later in life for which there is currently little or no treatment. For these asymptomatic individuals, is knowledge of the test result more beneficial than harmful, or vice versa? There is no simple answer. Studies demonstrate that some individuals at risk for Huntington disease choose not to undergo testing and would rather not know their risk, whereas others choose to undergo testing. Those who choose testing and test positive may have a transient period of depression, with a few suffering severe depression, but many report positive benefits in terms of the help provided in making life decisions about marriage and choice of career. Those who choose testing and are found not to carry the trinucleotide expansion allele report positive benefits of relief but can also experience negative emotional responses due to guilt for no longer being at risk for a disease that either affects or threatens to affect many of their close relatives. In any case, the decision to undergo testing is a highly personal one that must be made only after thorough review of the issues with a genetics professional.

Does the balance for or against testing shift when testing can indicate a predisposition but not a certainty for development later in life of a severe neurological illness for which there is currently little or no treatment, as with *APOE* ε4 allele testing for Alzheimer disease (see Chapter 17 and Case 3)? What if testing indicates a predisposition for a disease for which intervention and early treatment are available? For example, in autosomal dominant hereditary breast cancer, individuals carrying various mutations in *BRCA1* or *BRCA2* have a 50% to 90% chance of developing breast or ovarian cancer (see Chapter 16 and Case 5). Identification of heterozygote carriers would be of benefit because individuals at risk could choose to undergo more frequent surveillance or have preventive surgery, such as mastectomy, oophorectomy, or both, recognizing that these measures can reduce but not completely eliminate the increased risk of cancer. What if surveillance and preventive measures were more definitive, as they are in familial adenomatous polyposis, for which prophylactic colectomy is a proven preventive measure (see Chapter 16 and Case 13)? On being tested for any predisposing gene mutation, individuals incur the risk of serious psychological distress, stigmatization in their social lives, and discrimination in insurance and employment (see later). How are respect for a patient's autonomy, the physician's duty not to cause harm, and the physician's desire to prevent illness to be balanced in these different situations?

Geneticists would all agree that the decision to be tested or not to be tested is not one made in a vacuum. The patient must make an informed decision using all available information concerning the risk for and severity of the disease, the effectiveness of preventive and therapeutic measures, and the potential harm that could arise from testing.

Genetic Testing of Asymptomatic Children

Additional ethical complexity arises when genetic testing involves children because now the basic principles of bioethics need to be considered in the case of both the child and the parents. There are several reasons that parents may wish to have their children tested for a disease predisposition. Testing asymptomatic children for alleles that predispose to disease can be beneficial, even lifesaving, if interventions that decrease morbidity or increase longevity are available. One example is testing the asymptomatic sibling of a child with **medium-chain acyl dehydrogenase deficiency** (see Chapter 17). However, some have argued that even in situations where there are currently no clear medical interventions that might benefit the child, it is the parents' duty to inform and prepare their children for the future possibility of development of a serious illness. The parents may also seek this information for their own family planning or to avoid what some parents consider the corrosive effects of keeping important information about their children from them. Testing children, however, carries the same risks of serious psychological damage, stigmatization, and insurance and employment discrimination as does testing adults (see later). Children's autonomy, their ability to make decisions for themselves about their own genetic constitution, must also now be balanced with the desire of parents to obtain such information.

A different but related issue arises in testing children for the carrier state of a disease that poses no threat to their health but places them at risk for having affected children. Once again, the debate centers on the balance between respect for children's autonomy in regard to their own procreation and the desire on the part of well-meaning parents to educate and prepare children for the difficult decisions and risks that lie ahead once they reach childbearing age.

The preponderance of opinion among bioethicists is that unless there is a clear benefit to the medical care of the child, genetic testing of asymptomatic children for adult-onset disease or for a carrier state should be done only when the child is sufficiently old and mature enough, such as in late adolescence or on reaching adulthood, to decide for himself or herself whether to seek such testing.

Privacy of Genetic Information

Duty to Warn and Permission to Warn

A patient's desire to have his or her medical information kept confidential is one facet of the concept of patient autonomy, in which patients have the right to make their own decisions about how their individual medical information is used and communicated to others. Genetics, however, more than any other branch of medical practice, is concerned with both the patient and the family. A serious ethical and legal dilemma can arise in the practice of genetic medicine when a patient's insistence that his or her medical information be kept strictly private restrains the geneticist from letting other family members know about their risk for a condition, even when such information could be beneficial to them with regard to their own health and the health of their children (see Box). In this situation, is the genetics practitioner strictly obligated to respect the patient's autonomy by keeping information confidential, or is the practitioner obligated to inform other family members (duty to warn)? If so, is informing the patient that he or she should let the relatives know sufficient to discharge the practitioner's duty, or is the practitioner allowed to inform the relatives without authorization, while not being required to do so (permission to warn)?

Guidelines from international health organizations, individual national health policy groups, and professional medical organizations are not unanimous on this issue. Furthermore, in the United States, case law derived from lawsuits in state courts are not consistent with legislative and regulatory mandates, particularly the Privacy Rule of the Health Insurance Portability and Accountability Act (HIPAA).

Judges have ruled in a number of court cases in the United States on whether or not a health care practitioner is permitted or is even required to override a patient's wishes for confidentiality. The precedent-setting case was not one involving genetics. In the 1976 State Supreme Court case in California, *Tarasoff v the Regents of the University of California*, judges ruled that a psychiatrist was liable in the death of a young woman because he failed to take adequate measures to warn her or law enforcement officers that his client had declared an intention to kill her. The judges declared

■■■ Duty to Warn: Patient Autonomy and Privacy Versus Preventing Harm to Others

A woman first presents with an autosomal dominant disorder at the age of 40 years, undergoes testing, and is found to carry a particular mutation in a gene known to be involved in this disorder. She is planning to discuss the results with her teenaged daughter but insists that her younger adult half-siblings (from her father's second marriage after her mother's and father's divorce) not be told that they might be at risk for this disorder and that testing is available. How does a practitioner reconcile the obligation to respect the patient's right to privacy with a desire not to cause her relatives harm by failing to inform them of their risk?

There are many questions to answer in determining whether "a serious threat to another person's health or safety" exists to justify unauthorized disclosure of risk to a relative.

Clinical Questions

- What is the penetrance of the disorder and is it age dependent? How serious is the disorder? Can it be debilitating or life-threatening? How variable is the expressivity? Are there interventions that can reduce the risk of disease or prevent it altogether? Is this a condition that will be identified by routine medical care, once it is symptomatic, in time for institution of preventive or therapeutic measures?
- The risk to half-siblings of the patient is either 50% or negligible, depending on which parent passed the mutant allele to the patient. What does the family history reveal, if anything, about the parent in common between the patient and her half-siblings? Is the patient's mother still alive and available for testing?

Counseling Questions

- Was the patient informed at the time of testing that the results might have implications for other family members? Did she understand in advance that she might be asked to warn her relatives?
- What are the reasons for withholding the information? Are there unresolved issues, such as resentment, feelings of abandonment, or emotional estrangement, that are sources of psychological pain that could be addressed for her own benefit as well as to help the patient clarify her decision-making?
- Are the other family members already aware of the possibility of this hereditary disease and have they made an informed choice not to seek testing themselves? Would the practitioner's warning be seen as an unwarranted intrusion of psychologically damaging information, or would their risk come as a complete surprise?

Legal and Practical Questions

- Does the practitioner have the information and resources required to contact all of the half-siblings without the cooperation of the patient?
- Could the practitioner have reached an understanding, or even a formal agreement, with the patient in advance of testing that she would help in informing her siblings? Would asking for such an agreement be seen as coercive and lead to the patient's depriving herself of the testing she needs for herself and her children?
- What constitutes adequate discharge of the practitioner's duty to warn? Is it sufficient to provide a form letter for the patient to show to relatives that discloses the absolute minimal amount of information needed to inform them of a potential risk?

---

that this situation is no different from one in which physicians have a duty to protect the contacts of a patient with a contagious disease by warning them that the patient has the disease, even against the express wishes of the patient. In the realm of genetics, a duty to warn was mandated in a case in New Jersey, *Safer v Estate of Pack*, in which a panel of three judges concluded that a physician had a duty to warn the daughter of a man with familial adenomatous polyposis of her risk of colon cancer. The judges wrote that "there is no essential difference between the type of genetic threat at issue here and the menace of infection, contagion, or a threat of physical harm." They added that the duty to warn relatives is not automatically fulfilled by telling the patient that the disease is hereditary and that relatives need to be informed.

On the other hand, HIPAA regulations mandate that a patient's authorization is required to release his or her medical information, including the results of genetic testing, and sets criminal and civil penalties for disclosing such information without authorization. There are, however, exceptions under which disclosure without an individual's authorization is permitted for certain "national priority reasons." Among a number of exceptions that involve disclosure for public health and law enforcement reasons, one exception should be highlighted: a serious threat to another person's health or safety. Under the HIPAA, a practitioner can disclose a patient's protected health information to another individual or organization, including the target of the threat, without the patient's authorization only if he or she believes that disclosure can prevent or lessen a serious and imminent threat to a person or the public.

Although the genetics practitioner is most knowledgeable about the clinical aspects of the disease, the relevance of the family history, and the family risk assessment, the many legal and ethical controversies surrounding duty to warn suggest that consultation with legal and bioethics expertise is advisable should a conflict arise over the release of a patient's medical information.

Use of Genetic Information by Employers and Insurers

A third major ethical principle, along with beneficence and respect for autonomy, is justice—the requirement that everyone be able to benefit equally from progress in medical genetics. Justice is a major concern in the area of the use of genetic information in employment and insurance. Is it fair to penalize people who, through no fault of their own, are found to carry a genetic predisposition to disease?

As regards employment, should employers be able to obtain genetic information in making hiring decisions if that information helps them choose dependable and healthy employees with low absenteeism? In particular, some have argued that a small business that funds its employee health care plan itself must have access to such information in making hiring decisions so that it can refuse to hire individuals at risk for development of a serious illness later in life that could bankrupt the entire employee health plan.

In the area of life insurance underwriting, insurers insist that they must have access to all pertinent genetic information about an individual that the individual himself or herself has. Life insurance companies calculate their premiums on the basis of actuarial tables of age-specific survival averaged over the population; premiums will not cover losses if individuals with private knowledge that they are at higher risk for disease conceal this information and buy extra life or long-term disability insurance, a practice referred to as **adverse selection.** If adverse selection were widespread, the premiums for the entire population would have to increase so that in essence, the entire population would be subsidizing the increased coverage for a minority. Adverse selection is likely to be a real phenomenon in some circumstances; in one study of asymptomatic individuals tested for the *APOE* ε4 allele, those who chose to know that they tested positive were found to be nearly six times more likely to purchase extra long-term care insurance than those who did not choose to know their *APOE* genotype. Knowledge that one carried an *APOE* ε4 allele did not, however, affect life, health, or disability insurance purchases. At present, there is little evidence that life insurance companies have actually engaged in discriminatory underwriting practices on the basis of genetic testing. Nevertheless, the fear of such discrimination, and the negative impact discrimination would have on people obtaining clinical testing for their own health benefit as well as on their willingness to participate in genetic research, has led to proposals to ban the use of genetic information in life

underwriting. In the United Kingdom, for example, life insurance companies have voluntarily agreed to an extended moratorium on the use of genetic information in most life underwriting, except when large policies are involved or in the case of Huntington disease, for which disclosure of a positive test result by the patient is required.

The issue of the availability of health insurance for persons carrying alleles for genes that predispose to disease is another vexing problem in societies that lack universal health coverage, such as the United States. Health insurers routinely obtain family history data and smoking history and request blood pressure, serum cholesterol, or urine glucose testing in deciding on availability and setting the premiums for health insurance. Insurers ask why they should be constrained from testing for genes that increase disease risk. Is one's genetic makeup any different from historical and phenotypic data? Many would argue that there is a clear distinction between what are already phenotypic manifestations of a disease, such as hypertension, hypercholesterolemia, and diabetes mellitus, and what are predisposing alleles, such as *BRCA1* mutations (see Chapter 16) and *APOE* ε4 alleles (see Chapters 8 and 17), that may never result in overt disease in the individual who carries them. Some state and federal laws and regulations prohibit discrimination by health insurance companies in providing health insurance based on genetic information. For example, HIPAA regulations specify that genetic susceptibility, without a current diagnosis of illness, cannot be considered a preexisting condition on which coverage can be denied or premiums raised. These regulations provide some protection for the approximately 70% of residents of the United States who are covered either by group health plans offered by large employers or by government-sponsored health plans (Medicare and Medicaid) but not for the approximately 5% to 10% of individuals in the United State who need to buy their own health insurance. Consideration of the impact of genetic testing on the availability of health insurance is, of course, not so serious a problem in societies that provide universal health coverage.

Ethical Dilemmas in Genetic Screening

Although the ultimate objective of genetic screening is to improve the public health, there may also be unintended negative consequences. As with genetic testing, abnormal screening results may lead to stigmatization, adverse psychological consequences, or discrimination in the workplace or the insurance market. Additional, special problems arise from screening programs, however. Because genetic screening is performed on a large number of persons, there is a greater danger than with genetic testing that the screening will not conform to the highest standards of informed consent or may be the result of compulsion, overt or implied, to have the screening done. The right of individuals *not* to know about their deleterious genes may be compromised once a widespread screening program is in operation. Questions arise, such as who has access to samples and data, and how can we make sure that samples, such as DNA, are not used for purposes other than the screening tests for which they were collected and for which consent was given? It is clear that these matters must be considered in the planning of screening programs, which require an ethical review to ensure that concerns are addressed and appropriate safeguards are in place.

⊙ EUGENIC AND DYSGENIC EFFECTS OF MEDICAL GENETICS

The Problem of Eugenics

The term **eugenics,** introduced by Darwin's cousin Francis Galton in 1883, refers to the improvement of a population by selection of only its "best" specimens for breeding. Plant and animal breeders have followed this practice since ancient times. In the late 19th century, Galton and others began to promote the idea of using selective breeding to improve the human species, thereby initiating the so-called eugenics movement, which was widely advocated for the next half-century. The so-called ideal qualities that the eugenics movement sought to promote through the encouragement of certain kinds of human breeding were more often than not defined by social, ethnic, and economic prejudices and fed by anti-immigrant and racist sentiments in society. What we now would consider a lack of education was described then as familial "feeble-mindedness"; what we now would call rural poverty was considered by eugenicists to be hereditary "shiftlessness." The scientific difficulties in determining whether traits or characteristics are heritable and to what extent heredity contributes to a trait were badly underestimated since most human traits, even those with some genetic component, are complex in their inheritance pattern and are influenced strongly by environmental factors. Thus, by the middle of the last century, many scientists began to appreciate the theoretical and ethical difficulties of carrying out eugenics programs. Eugenics is commonly thought to have been largely discredited when it came to be used in Nazi Germany as a justification for mass murder. However, it should be pointed out that in North America and Europe, involuntary sterilization of institutionalized individuals deemed to be mentally incompetent or retarded was carried out under laws passed in the early part of the 20th century in support of eugenics, and was continued for many years after the Nazi regime was destroyed.

Genetic Counseling and Eugenics

Genetic counseling, with the aim of helping patients and their families manage the pain and suffering caused by genetic disease, should not be confounded with the eugenic goal of reducing the incidence of genetic disease or the frequency of alleles considered deleterious in the population. Helping patients and families come to free and informed decisions, particularly concerning reproduction, without coercion, forms the basis for the concept of nondirective counseling (see Chapter 19). Nondirectiveness asserts that individual autonomy and privacy rights are paramount and not to be subordinated to reducing the burden of genetic disease on society or to a theoretical goal of "improving the gene pool," a totalitarian concept that echoes the Nazi doctrine of racial hygiene. Some have argued that true nondirective counseling is a myth, often acclaimed but not easy to accomplish, because of the personal attitudes and values the counselor brings to the counseling session. Nonetheless, despite the difficulties in attaining the ideal of nondirective counseling, the ethical principles of respect for autonomy, beneficence, avoidance of maleficence, and fairness remain at the heart of all genetic counseling practice, particularly in the realm of individual reproductive decision-making.

The Problem of Dysgenics

The opposite of eugenics is **dysgenics,** a deterioration in the health and well-being of a population by practices that allow the accumulation of deleterious alleles. In this regard, the long-term impact of activities in medical genetics that can affect gene frequencies and the incidence of genetic disease may be difficult to predict.

In the case of some single-gene defects, medical treatment can have a dysgenic effect by reducing selection against a particular genotype, thereby allowing the frequency of harmful genes and, consequently, of disease to increase. The effect of relaxed selection is likely to be more striking for autosomal dominant and X-linked disorders than for autosomal recessive disorders, in which the majority of mutant alleles are in silent heterozygous carriers. For example, if successful treatment of Duchenne muscular dystrophy were to be achieved, the incidence of the disease would rise sharply because the *DMD* genes of the affected males would then be transmitted to all their daughters. The effect of this transmission would be to greatly increase the frequency of carriers in the population. In contrast, if all persons affected with cystic fibrosis could survive and reproduce at a normal rate, the incidence of the disease would rise from 1 in 2000 to only about 1 in 1550 over 200 years. Common genetic disorders with complex inheritance, discussed in Chapter 8, could theoretically also become more common if selection is removed, although it is likely that as with autosomal recessive diseases, most of the susceptibility alleles are distributed among unaffected individuals. Consequently, reproduction by affected persons would have little effect on susceptibility allele frequencies.

As prenatal diagnosis (see Chapter 15) becomes widespread, increasing numbers of pregnancies in which the fetus has inherited a genetic defect may be terminated. The effect on the overall incidence of disease is quite variable. In a disorder such as Huntington disease, prenatal diagnosis and pregnancy termination would have a large effect on the incidence of the responsible gene. For most other severe X-linked or autosomal dominant disorders, some reduction might occur, but the disease will continue to recur owing to new mutations. In the case of autosomal recessive conditions, the effect on the frequency of the mutant allele, and consequently of the disease, of aborting all homozygous affected pregnancies would be small because most of these alleles are carried silently by heterozygotes.

One theoretical concern is the extent to which pregnancy termination for genetic reasons is followed by **reproductive compensation,** that is, by the birth of additional, unaffected children, many of whom are carriers of the deleterious gene. Some families with X-linked disorders have chosen to terminate pregnancies in which the fetus was male, but of course, daughters in such families, although unaffected, may be carriers. Thus, reproductive compensation has the potential long-term consequence of increasing the frequency of the genetic disorder that led to the loss of an affected child.

● GENETICS IN MEDICINE

The last half of the 20th century will be remembered as the era that began with the rediscovery of Mendel's laws of inheritance and their application to human biology and medicine, continued with the discovery of the role of DNA in heredity, and culminated in the completion of the Human Genome Project. At the beginning of the 21st century, the human species has, for the first time, a complete representative sequence of its own DNA, a comprehensive inventory of its genes, a vigorous ongoing effort to identify and characterize mutations and polymorphic variants in DNA sequence and copy number, and a rapidly expanding knowledge

base in which various diseases and disease predispositions will be attributable to such variation. With such knowledge comes powerful capabilities as well as great responsibilities. In the end, **genetics in medicine** is about knowledge not for its own sake, but for the sake of improving health, relieving suffering, and enhancing human dignity.

● GENERAL REFERENCES

Beauchamp TL, Childress JF: Principles of Biomedical Ethics, 5th ed. New York, Oxford University Press, 2001.
Kevles D: In the Name of Eugenics: Genetics and the Uses of Human Heredity. Cambridge, Mass, Harvard University Press, 1995.

● REFERENCES FOR SPECIFIC TOPICS

Birn A-E, Molina N: In the name of public health. Am J Public Health 95:1095-1097, 2005.
Godard B, Hurlimann T, Letendre M, et al: Guidelines for disclosing genetic information to family members: from development to use. Fam Cancer 5:103-116, 2006.
Greely HT: Banning genetic discrimination. N Engl J Med 353:865-867, 2005.
Harper PS: Genetic testing, life insurance, and adverse selection. Philos Trans R Soc Lond B Biol Sci 352:1063-1066, 1997.
Lapham EV, Kozma C, Weiss JO: Genetic discrimination: perspectives of consumers. Science 274:621-624, 1996.
Mahowald MB, Verp MS, Anderson RR: Genetic counseling: clinical and ethical challenges. Annu Rev Genet 32:547-549, 1998.
Mayor S: UK insurers postpone using predictive genetic testing until 2011. BMJ 330:617, 2005.
Nowlan W: A rational view of insurance and genetic discrimination. Science 297:195-196, 2002.
Offit K, Groeger E, Turner S: The "duty to warn" a patient's family members about hereditary disease risks. JAMA 292:1469-1473, 2004.
Ossa DF, Towse A: Should genetic information be made available to insurers? Eur J Health Econom 5:116-121, 2004.
Pokorski RJ: Insurance underwriting in the genetic era. Am J Hum Genet 60:205-216, 1997.
Rothenberg KH, Terry SF: Before it's too late—addressing fear of genetic information. Science 297:196-197, 2002.
Sankar P: Genetic privacy. Annu Rev Med 54:393-407, 2003.
Zick CD, Mathews CJ. Roberts JS, et al: Genetic testing for Alzheimer's disease and its impact on insurance purchasing behavior. Health Affairs 24:483-490, 2005.

● USEFUL WEBSITES

Websites of the American Society of Human Genetics, the American College of Medical Genetics, the National Society of Genetic Counselors, and the National Human Genome Research Institute all carry policy statements on various aspects of medical genetics:
http://www.faseb.org/genetics/ashg/ashgmenu.htm
http://www.acmg.net
http://www.nsgc.org/
http://www.nhgri.nih.gov/ELSI/

PROBLEMS

1. A couple with two children is referred for genetic counseling because their younger son, a 12-year-old boy, has a movement disorder for which testing for juvenile Huntington disease (see Case 22) is being considered. What are the ethical considerations for the family in testing?

2. A research project screened more than 40,000 consecutive, unselected births for the number of X chromosomes and the presence of a Y chromosome and correlated the sex chromosome karyotype with the sex assigned by visual inspection in the newborn nursery. The purpose of the project was to observe infants with sex chromosome abnormalities (see Chapter 6) prospectively for developmental difficulties. What are the ethical considerations in carrying out this project?

3. In the case described in the Box in the section on duty to warn, consider what might be your course of action if you were the genetic counselor and the disease in question were the following: hereditary breast and ovarian cancer due to BRCA1 mutations (see Chapter 16 and Case 5); malignant hyperthermia due to RYR1 (ryanodine receptor) mutations (see Chapter 18); early-onset, familial Alzheimer disease due to a PSEN1 (presenilin 1) mutation (see Chapter 12 and Case 3); neurofibromatosis due to NF1 mutations (see Chapter 7 and Case 29); or type 2 diabetes mellitus (see Case 30).

Glossary

Acceptor splice site   The boundary between the 3′ end of an intron and the 5′ end of the following exon. Also called *3′ splice site*.

Acrocentric   A type of chromosome with the centromere near one end. The human acrocentric chromosomes (13, 14, 15, 21, and 22) have satellited short arms that carry genes for ribosomal RNA.

Adverse selection   A term used in the insurance industry to describe the situation in which individuals with private knowledge of having an increased risk for illness, disability, or death buy disproportionately more coverage than those at a lower risk. As a result, insurance premiums, which are based on averaging risk across the population, are inadequate to cover future claims.

Affected pedigree member method   A model-free method of linkage analysis that systematically measures whether relatives affected with a disease share alleles at a locus more frequently than would be predicted by chance alone from their familial relationship. If the relatives are sibs, it is referred to as the *affected sibpair method* of linkage analysis.

Allele   One of the alternative versions of a gene or DNA sequence at a given locus.

Allele-specific oligonucleotide (ASO)   An oligonucleotide probe synthesized to match a particular DNA sequence precisely and allow the discrimination of alleles that differ by only a single base.

Allelic exclusion   In immunogenetics, the observation that only one of the pair of parental alleles for each H chain and L chain of an immunoglobulin molecule is expressed within a single cell.

Allelic heterogeneity   In a population, there may be a number of different mutant alleles at a single locus. In an individual, the same or similar phenotypes may be caused by different mutant alleles rather than by identical alleles at the locus.

Allogenic   In transplantation, denotes individuals (or tissues) that are of the same species but that have different antigens (alternative spelling: allogeneic).

Alpha-fetoprotein (AFP)   A fetal glycoprotein excreted into the amniotic fluid that reaches abnormally high concentration in amniotic fluid (and maternal serum) when the fetus has certain abnormalities, especially an open neural tube defect.

Alu repeat sequence   In the human genome, about 10% of the DNA is made up of a set of about 1,000,000 dispersed, related sequences, each about 300 base pairs long, so named because they are cleaved by the restriction enzyme *Alu*I.

Amniocentesis   A procedure used in prenatal diagnosis to obtain amniotic fluid, which contains cells of fetal origin that can be cultured for analysis. Amniotic fluid is withdrawn from the amniotic sac by syringe after insertion of a hollow needle into the amnion through the abdominal wall and uterine wall.

Amplification   1. In molecular biology, the production of multiple copies of a sequence of DNA. 2. In cytogenetics, amplification refers to the generation of multiple copies of a sequence in the genome that are detectable by comparative genomic hybridization (CGH).

Analytic validity   In reference to a clinical laboratory test, the ability of that test to perform correctly, that is, measure what it is designed to measure.

Aneuploidy   Any chromosome number that is not an exact multiple of the haploid number. The common forms of aneuploidy in humans are *trisomy* (the presence of an extra chromosome) and *monosomy* (the absence of a single chromosome).

Anomalies   Birth defects resulting from malformations, deformations, or disruptions.

Anticipation   The progressively earlier onset and increased severity of certain diseases in successive generations of a family. Anticipation is caused by expansion of the number of unstable repeats within the gene responsible for the disease.

Anticodon   A three-base unit of RNA complementary to a codon in mRNA.

Antisense strand of DNA   The noncoding DNA strand, which is complementary to mRNA and serves as the template for RNA synthesis. Also called the *transcribed strand*.

Apoptosis   Programmed cell death characterized by a stereotypic pattern of mitochondrial breakdown and chromatin degradation.

Array CGH   Comparative genome hybridization performed by hybridizing to a wafer ("chip") made of glass, plastic, or silicon onto which a large number of different nucleic acids have been individually spotted in a matrix pattern. See *microarray*.

Ascertainment   The method of selection of individuals for inclusion in a genetic study.

Ascertainment bias   A difference in the likelihood that affected relatives of affected individuals will be identified, compared with similarly affected relatives of controls. A possible source of error in family studies.

Association   1. In genetic epidemiology, describes the situation in which a particular allele is found either significantly more or significantly less frequently in a group of affected individuals than would be expected from the frequency of the allele in the general population from which the affected individuals were drawn; not to be confused with *linkage*. 2. In dysmorphology, a group of abnormalities of unknown etiology and pathogenesis that is seen together more often than would be expected by chance.

Assortative mating   Selection of a mate with preference for a particular genotype; that is, nonrandom mating. Usually positive (preference for a mate of the same genotype), less frequently negative (preference for a mate of a different genotype).

Assortment   The random distribution of different combinations of the parental chromosomes to the gametes. Nonallelic genes assort independently, unless they are linked.

Autoimmune disorder   A disease characterized by an abnormal immune response apparently directed against antigens of the individual's own tissues; thought to be related to variation in the immune response resulting from polymorphism in immune response genes.

Autologous   Refers to grafts in the same animal from one part to another, or to malignant cells and the cells of the individual in which they have arisen.

Autosome   Any nuclear chromosome other than the sex chromosomes; 22 pairs in the human karyotype. A disease caused by mutation in an autosomal gene or gene pair shows *autosomal inheritance*.

Bacterial artificial chromosomes (BACs)   Vectors capable of carrying 100 to 300 kb of cloned human DNA; propagated in bacteria and used in high-resolution gene mapping and DNA sequencing.

Balanced polymorphism   A polymorphism maintained in the population by heterozygote advantage, allowing an allele, even one that is deleterious in the homozygous state, to persist at a relatively high frequency in the population.

Banding   One of several techniques that stain chromosomes in a characteristic pattern, allowing identification of individual chromosomes and structural abnormalities. See *C bands, G bands, Q bands, R bands* in text.

Barr body   The sex chromatin as seen in female somatic cells, representing an inactive X chromosome.

Base pair (bp)   A pair of complementary nucleotide bases, as in double-stranded DNA. Used as the unit of measurement of the length of a DNA sequence.

Bayesian analysis   A mathematical method widely used in genetic counseling to calculate recurrence risks. The method combines information from several sources (genetics, pedigree information, and test results) to determine the probability that a specific individual might develop or transmit a certain disorder.

Beneficence   The ethical principle of behaving in a way that promotes the well-being of others. See *maleficence*.

Binomial expansion   When there are two alternative classes, one with probability p and the other with probability $1 - p = q$, the frequencies of the possible combinations of p and q in a series of n trials is $(p + q)^n$.

Bioinformatics   Computational analysis and storage of biological and experimental data, widely applied to genomic and proteomic studies.

Birth defect   An abnormality present at birth, not necessarily genetic.

Bivalent   A pair of homologous chromosomes in association, as seen at metaphase of the first meiotic division.

Blastocyst   A stage in early embryogenesis in which the initial ball of cells derived from the fertilized egg (the morula) secrete fluid and form a fluid-filled internal cavity within which is a separate group of cells, the *inner cell mass*.

Blood group   The phenotype produced by genetically determined antigens on a red blood cell. The antigens formed by a set of allelic genes make up a blood group system.

Cap   A modified nucleotide added to the 5′ end of a growing mRNA chain, required for normal processing, stability, and translation of mRNA.

Caretaker genes   Tumor-suppressor genes that are indirectly involved in controlling cellular proliferation by repairing DNA damage and maintaining genomic integrity, thereby protecting proto-oncogenes and gatekeeper tumor-suppressor genes from mutations that could lead to cancer.

Carrier   An individual heterozygous for a particular mutant allele. The term is used for heterozygotes for autosomal recessive alleles, for females heterozygous for X-linked alleles, or, less commonly, for an individual heterozygous for an autosomal dominant allele but not expressing it (e.g., a heterozygote for a Huntington disease allele in the presymptomatic stage).

Case-control study   An epidemiological method in which patients with a disease (the cases) are compared with suitably chosen individuals without the disease (the controls) with respect to the relative frequency of various putative risk factors.

cDNA   See *complementary DNA.*

Cell cycle   The stages between two successive mitotic divisions, described in the text. Consists of the G_1, S, G_2, and M stages.

Centimorgan (cM)   The unit of genetic distance between genes along chromosomes, named for Thomas Hunt Morgan. Two loci are 1 cM apart if recombination is detected between them in 1% of meioses.

Centromere   The primary constriction on the chromosome, a region at which the sister chromatids are held together and at which the kinetochore is formed. Required for normal segregation in mitosis and meiosis.

Centrosomes   A pair of centers that organize the growth of the microtubules of the mitotic spindle; visible at the poles of the dividing cell in late prophase.

CG (or CpG) island   Any region of the genome containing an unusually high concentration of the dinucleotide sequence 5′-CG-3′. Often associated with promoters of genes, in particular housekeeping genes.

CGH   See *comparative genome hybridization.*

Chain termination mutation   A mutation that generates a stop codon, thus preventing further synthesis of the polypeptide chain.

Checkpoint   Positions in the cell cycle, usually at the junction between the G_1 and S or the G_2 and M stages, at which the cell determines whether to proceed to the next stage of the cycle.

Chemical individuality   A term coined by Archibald Garrod to describe the naturally occurring differences in the genetic and biochemical makeup of each individual.

Chiasma   Literally, a cross. The term refers to the crossing of chromatid strands of homologous chromosomes, seen at the diplotene of the first meiotic division. Chiasmata are thought to be evidence of interchange of chromosomal material (crossovers) between members of a chromosome pair.

Chimera   An individual composed of cells derived from two genetically different zygotes. In humans, *blood group chimeras* result from exchange of hematopoietic stem cells by dizygotic twins in utero; *dispermic chimeras,* which are very rare, result from fusion of two zygotes into one individual. Chimerism is also an inevitable result of transplantation.

Chorionic villus sampling (CVS)   A procedure used for prenatal diagnosis at 8 to 10 weeks' gestation. Fetal tissue for analysis is withdrawn from the villous area of the chorion either transcervically or transabdominally, under ultrasonographic guidance.

Chromatids   The two parallel strands of chromatin, connected at the centromere, that constitute a chromosome after DNA synthesis.

Chromatin   The complex of DNA and proteins of which chromosomes are composed. See also *nucleosome.*

Chromosomal satellite   A small mass of chromatin containing genes for ribosomal RNA, at the end of the short arm of each chromatid of an acrocentric chromosome; not to be confused with *satellite DNA.*

Chromosome   One of the threadlike structures in the cell nucleus; consists of chromatin and carries genetic information (DNA).

Chromosome disorder   A clinical condition caused by an abnormal chromosome constitution in which there is duplication, loss, or rearrangement of chromosomal material.

Chromosome mutation   A change in the genetic material at the chromosome level.

Chromosome painting probe   A multilocus probe designed for fluorescence in situ hybridization (FISH) that hybridizes to only one particular chromosome or chromosome arm.

Chromosome segregation   The separation of chromosomes or chromatids in cell division so that each daughter cell gets an equal number of chromosomes.

Chromosome spread   The chromosomes of a dividing cell as seen under the microscope in metaphase or prometaphase.

Cis   Refers to the relationship between two sequences that are on the same chromosome, literally meaning "on the near side of." Contrast with *trans.*

Clinical heterogeneity   The term describing the occurrence of clinically different phenotypes from mutations in the same gene.

Clinical utility   In reference to a clinical laboratory test, the ability of that test to improve the medical care that an individual receives.

Clinical validity   In reference to a clinical laboratory test, the ability of that test to detect the disease that the test was designed to detect.

Clonal evolution   The multistep process of successive genetic changes that occur in a developing tumor cell population.

Clone   1. A cell line derived by mitosis from a single ancestral diploid cell; in embryology, a cell lineage in which the cells have remained geographically close to each other. 2. In molecular biology, a recombinant DNA molecule containing a gene or other DNA sequence of interest. Also, the act of generating such a cell line or clone.

Cloning, molecular   Transfer of a DNA sequence into a single cell of a microorganism, followed by culture of the microorganism to produce large quantities of the DNA sample for analysis.

CNP   See *copy number variant*.

CNV   See *copy number variant*.

Coding strand   In double-stranded DNA, the strand that has the same 5′ to 3′ sense (and sequence, except that in mRNA, U substitutes for T) as mRNA. The coding strand is the strand that is *not* transcribed by RNA polymerase. Also called the *sense strand*.

Codominant   If both alleles of a pair are expressed in the heterozygous state, then the alleles (or the traits determined by them, or both) are codominant.

Codon   A triplet of three bases in a DNA or RNA molecule, specifying a single amino acid.

Coefficient of inbreeding (F)   The probability that an individual homozygous at a locus received both alleles from one ancestor (i.e., the alleles are *identical by descent*).

Cofactor-responsive disease   A genetic disease in which a specific biochemical abnormality affecting a single mutant protein (usually an enzyme) is corrected by the administration of pharmacological amounts of the specific cofactor of the mutant protein (e.g., vitamin B_6-responsive homocystinuria).

Colinearity   The parallel relationship between the base sequence of the DNA of a gene (or the RNA transcribed from it) and the amino acid sequence of the corresponding polypeptide.

Commitment   The transition of an embryonic cell from pluripotency to its particular fate.

Comparative genome hybridization (CGH)   A fluorescence hybridization technique used to compare two different DNA samples with respect to their relative content of a particular DNA segment or segments. CGH can be used with fluorescence in situ hybridization of metaphase chromosomes (FISH) or with hybridization to large numbers of DNA fragments fixed to a solid support (*CGH array*).

Complementarity   The complementary nature of base pairing in DNA.

Complementary DNA (cDNA)   DNA synthesized from a messenger RNA template, through the action of the enzyme reverse transcriptase. See *genomic DNA* for comparison.

Complementation   The ability of cells from patients with two different genetic defects to correct one another, thus demonstrating that the defects are not identical. The complementation may be intergenic or intragenic.

Complex inheritance   A pattern of inheritance that is not mendelian. A trait with complex inheritance usually results from alleles at more than one locus interacting with environmental factors.

Compound (compound heterozygote)   An individual, or a genotype, with two different mutant alleles at the same locus. Not to be confused with *homozygote,* in which the two mutant alleles are identical.

Concordance   Describes a pair of relatives in which (1) both members of the pair have a certain qualitative trait or (2) both members have values of a quantitative trait that are similar in magnitude. See *discordance*.

Conditional probability   1. In Bayesian analysis, this is the chance of an observed outcome given that a consultand has a particular genotype. The product of the prior and conditional probabilities is the joint probability. 2. More generally, a synonym for *Bayesian analysis*.

Confined placental mosaicism   Cytogenetically detectable mosaicism present in the placenta but not present in the fetus, revealed by *chorionic villus sampling* (CVS).

Congenital   Present at birth; not necessarily genetic.

Consanguineous   Related by descent from a common ancestor (the noun is *consanguinity*).

Consensus sequence   In genes or proteins, an idealized sequence in which each base or amino acid residue represents the one most frequently found at that position when many actual sequences are compared; for example, the consensus sequence for splice donor or acceptor sites.

Consultand   In genetic counseling, anyone who consults a genetic counselor for genetic information.

Contiguous gene syndrome   A syndrome resulting from a *microdeletion* of chromosomal DNA extending over two or more contiguous loci. Also called *segmental aneusomy*.

Copy number variant (CNV)   A variation in DNA sequence defined by the presence or absence of a segment of DNA, ranging from 200 bp to 2 Mb. Copy number variants may also have alleles that are tandem duplications of two, three, four, or more copies of a DNA segment. If a variant has an allele frequency >1%, it is referred to as a copy number polymorphism (CNP).

Cordocentesis   A procedure used in prenatal diagnosis to obtain a sample of fetal blood directly from the placenta.

Correlation   A statistical tool applied to a set of paired measurements. A positive correlation exists when the larger the first measurement in the pair is, the larger the second measurement of the pair is. A negative correlation is the opposite, that is, the larger the first measurement, the smaller the second.

Correlation coefficient (r)   A measure of correlation that varies from 1 for perfect positive correlation to −1 for perfect negative correlation; it is 0 when there is no correlation between pairs of measurements.

Coupling   Describes the phase of two alleles at two different but syntenic loci, in which one allele at one of the loci *is* on the same chromosome as the allele at the second locus. See *phase* and *repulsion*.

Crossover, crossing over   The reciprocal exchange of segments between chromatids of homologous chromosomes, a characteristic of prophase of the first meiotic division. See also *recombination*. Unequal crossing over between misaligned chromatids can lead to duplication of the involved segment on one chromatid and deletion on the other, and is a frequent cause of mutation.

Cryptic splice site   A DNA sequence similar to the consensus splice site but not normally used. It is used when the normal splice site is altered by mutation or when a mutation in the cryptic site increases its use by the splicing apparatus. May be in a coding or a noncoding sequence.

Cytogenetics   The study of chromosomes.

Cytotrophoblast   The fetal cells of the chorionic villi that are sampled for karyotyping and DNA analysis.

Daughter chromosomes   The two individual chromosomes formed when a single chromosome composed of paired chromatids separates at the centromere in anaphase of cell division.

Deformation syndrome   A recognizable pattern of dysmorphic features caused by extrinsic factors that affect the fetus in utero.

Degeneracy of the code   The genetic code is described as degenerate because most of the 20 amino acids are specified by more than 1 of the 64 codons.

Degree of relationship   The distance between two individuals in a pedigree. First-degree relatives include parents, siblings, and children. Second-degree relatives are aunts and uncles, nephews and nieces, grandparents and grandchildren.

Deletion   The loss of a sequence of DNA from a chromosome. The deleted DNA may be of any length, from a single base to a large part of a chromosome.

Denaturation (of DNA)   The conversion of DNA from the double-stranded to the single-stranded state, usually accomplished by heating to destroy chemical bonds involved in base pairing.

Deoxyribonucleic acid   See *DNA*.

Determination   During development, the second stage of commitment in which a cell follows its developmental program regardless of whether it is transplanted to a different region of the embryo.

Developmental program   The process by which a cell in an embryo achieves its developmental fate.

Dicentric   A structurally abnormal chromosome with two centromeres.

Dictyotene   The stage of the first meiotic division in which a human oocyte remains from late fetal life until ovulation.

Differentiation   The process whereby a cell acquires a tissue-specific pattern of expression of genes and proteins and a characteristic phenotype.

Diploid   The number of chromosomes in most somatic cells, which is double the number found in the gametes. In humans, the diploid chromosome number is 46.

Discordance   The situation in which (1) one member of the pair has a certain qualitative trait and the other does not or (2) the relatives have values of a quantitative trait that are at opposite ends of the distribution. See *concordance*.

Disomy   See *uniparental disomy*.

Disruption   A birth defect caused by destruction of tissue; may be caused by vascular occlusion, a teratogen, or rupture of the amniotic sac with entrapment.

Dizygotic (DZ) twins   Twins produced by two separate ova, separately fertilized. Also called *fraternal twins*.

DNA (deoxyribonucleic acid)   The molecule that encodes the genes responsible for the structure and function of living organisms and allows the transmission of genetic information from generation to generation.

DNA ligase   An enzyme that can form a phosphodiester bond between the deoxyribose backbones of two strands of DNA. See *ligation*.

DNA methylation   In eukaryotes, the addition of a methyl residue to the 5-position of the pyrimidine ring of a cytosine base in DNA to form 5-methylcytosine.

DNA polymerase   An enzyme that can synthesize a new DNA strand by using a previously synthesized DNA strand as a template.

Domain   A region of the amino acid sequence of a protein that can be equated with a particular function.

Dominant   A trait is dominant if it is phenotypically expressed in heterozygotes. If heterozygotes and homozygotes for the variant allele have the same phenotype, the disorder is a *pure* dominant (rare in human genetics). If homozygotes have a more severe phenotype than do heterozygotes, the disorder is termed *semidominant* or *incompletely dominant*.

Dominant negative   A disease-causing allele, or the effect of such an allele, that disrupts the function of a wild-type allele in the same cell.

Donor splice site   The boundary between the 3′ end of an exon and the 5′ end of the next intron. Also called *5′ splice site*.

Dosage compensation   As a consequence of X inactivation, the amount of product formed by the two copies of an X-linked gene in females is equivalent to the amount formed by the single gene in males. See *X inactivation*.

Double heterozygote   An individual who is heterozygous at each of two different loci. Contrast with *compound heterozygote*.

Double minutes   Very small accessory chromosomes, a form of gene amplification.

Dyschronic expression   Expression of a gene at a time when it is not normally expressed.

Dysmorphism   Morphological developmental abnormalities, as seen in many syndromes of genetic or environmental origin.

Ecogenetic disorder   A disorder resulting from the interaction of a genetic predisposition to a specific disease with an environmental factor.

Ectoderm   One of the three primary *germ layers* of the early embryo. Begins as the layer farthest from the yolk sac and ultimately gives rise to the nervous system, the skin, and neural crest derivatives such as craniofacial structures and melanocytes.

Ectopic expression   Expression of a gene in places where it is not normally expressed.

Embryonic stem cell   A cell derived from the inner cell mass that is self-renewing in culture and, when reintroduced into the inner cell mass of a blastocyst, can repopulate all the tissues of the embryo.

Empirical risk   In human genetics, the probability that a familial trait will occur in a family member, based on observed numbers of affected and unaffected individuals in family studies rather than on knowledge of the causative mechanism.

Endoderm   One of the three primary *germ layers* of the early embryo. Ultimately gives rise to the gut, liver, and portions of the urogenital system.

Enhancer   A DNA sequence that acts in *cis* (i.e., on the same chromosome) to increase transcription of a gene. The enhancer may be upstream or downstream to the gene and may be in the same or the reverse orientation. Contrast with *silencer*.

Enzymopathy   A metabolic disorder resulting from deficiency or abnormality of a specific enzyme.

Epigenetic   The term that refers to any factor that can affect gene function without change in the genotype. Some typical epigenetic factors involve alterations in DNA methylation, chromatin structure, histone modifications, and transcription factor binding that change genome structure and affect gene expression without changing the primary DNA sequence.

Episome   A DNA element that either can exist as an autonomously replicating sequence in the cytoplasm or can integrate into chromosomal DNA. Adeno-associated viral vectors, used in gene therapy, are episomes that exist in the cytoplasm for long periods and can, although rarely, be inserted into the nuclear genome.

Euchromatin   The major component of chromatin. It stains lightly with G banding, decondensing and becoming light-staining during interphase. Contrast with *heterochromatin*.

Eugenics   Increasing the prevalence of desirable traits in a population by decreasing the frequency of deleterious alleles at relevant loci through controlled, selective breeding. The opposite is *dysgenics*.

Eukaryote   A unicellular or multicellular organism in which the cells have a nucleus with a nuclear membrane and other specialized characteristics. See also *prokaryote*.

Euploid   Any chromosome number that is an exact multiple of the number in a haploid gamete (n). Most somatic cells are diploid (2n). Contrast with *aneuploid*.

Exon   A transcribed region of a gene that is present in mature messenger RNA.

Expression profile   A quantitative assessment of the mRNAs present in a cell type, tissue, or tumor. Often used to characterize a cell, tissue, or tumor in comparison to the expression profile of another cell, tissue, or tumor.

Expression vector   A cloning vector engineered to provide for the transcription and translation of a cloned DNA insert so that the host carrying the vector produces the protein encoded by the insert. See *vector.*

Expressivity   The extent to which a genetic defect is expressed. If there is variable expressivity, the trait may vary in expression from mild to severe but is never completely unexpressed in individuals who have the corresponding genotype. Contrast with *penetrance.*

Familial   Any trait that is more common in relatives of an affected individual than in the general population, whether the cause is genetic, environmental, or both.

Fate   The ultimate destination for a cell that has traveled down a developmental pathway. The embryonic *fate map* is a complete description of all the fates of all the different parts of the embryo.

Fetal phase   Stage of intrauterine development from weeks 9 to 40.

Fetoscopy   A technique for direct visualization of the fetus.

FISH   Fluorescence in situ hybridization. See *in situ hybridization.*

Fitness (*f*)   The probability of transmitting one's genes to the next generation compared with the average probability for the population.

Flanking sequence   A region of a gene preceding or following the transcribed region.

Founder effect   A high frequency of a mutant allele in a population founded by a small ancestral group when one or more of the founders was a carrier of the mutant allele.

Fragile site   Nonstaining gap in the chromatin of a metaphase chromosome, such as the fragile site at Xq27 in fragile X syndrome.

Frameshift mutation   A mutation involving a deletion or insertion that is not an exact multiple of three base pairs and thus changes the reading frame of the gene downstream of the mutation.

Gain-of-function mutation   A mutation associated with an increase in one or more of the normal functions of a protein. To be distinguished from *novel property mutation.*

Gamete   A reproductive cell (ovum or sperm) with the haploid chromosome number.

Gatekeeper genes   Tumor-suppressor genes that directly regulate cell proliferation.

Gene   A hereditary unit; in molecular terms, a sequence of chromosomal DNA that is required for the production of a functional product.

Gene dosage   The number of copies of a particular gene in the genome.

Gene-environment interaction   Combined action of alleles at one or more loci with nongenetic factors, such as environmental exposures or random events, in causing a complex disease.

Gene family   A set of genes containing related exons, indicating that the genes have evolved from an ancestral gene by duplication and subsequent divergence.

Gene flow   Gradual diffusion of genes from one population to another across a barrier. The barrier may be physical or cultural and may be breached by migration or mixing.

Gene map   The characteristic arrangement of the genes on the chromosomes.

Gene pool   All the alleles present at a given locus or, more broadly, at all loci in the population.

Gene therapy (gene transfer therapy)   Treatment of a disease by introduction of DNA sequences that will have a therapeutic benefit.

Genetic   Determined by genes; not to be confused with *congenital.*

Genetic code   The 64 triplets of bases that specify the 20 amino acids found in proteins (see Table 3-1).

Genetic complementation   The ability of one mutant allele at a locus to correct for the loss of function associated with another allele at the same or another locus, thus demonstrating that the mutations are not identical. See *complementation.*

Genetic counseling   The provision of information and assistance to affected individuals or family members at risk of a disorder that may be genetic, concerning the consequences of the disorder, the probability of developing or transmitting it, and the ways in which it may be prevented or ameliorated.

Genetic disorder   A defect wholly or partly caused by a gene abnormality.

Genetic drift   Random fluctuation of allele frequencies in small populations.

Genetic epidemiology   A branch of public health research concerned with characterizing and quantifying the influence of genetic variation in the population on the incidence, prevalence, and causation of disease.

Genetic heterogeneity   The production of the same or similar phenotypes by different genetic mechanisms. See *allelic heterogeneity, clinical heterogeneity, locus heterogeneity.*

Genetic lethal   A mutant allele or genetically determined trait that leads to failure to reproduce, although not necessarily to death prior to reproduction.

Genetic load   The sum total of death and disease caused by mutant genes.

Genetic map   The relative positions of the genes on the chromosomes, as shown by linkage analysis. See *physical map* for comparison.

Genetic marker   A locus that has readily classifiable alleles and can be used in genetic studies. It may be a gene or a restriction enzyme site or any characteristic of DNA that allows different versions of a locus (or its product) to be distinguished one from another and followed through families. See *polymorphism.*

Genetic screening   Testing on a population basis to identify individuals at risk of developing or of transmitting a specific disorder.

Genocopy   A genotype that determines a phenotype closely similar to that determined by a different genotype.

Genome   The complete DNA sequence, containing the entire genetic information, of a gamete, an individual, a population, or a species.

Genomic DNA   The chromosomal DNA sequence of a gene or segment of a gene, including the DNA sequence of noncoding as well as coding regions. Also, DNA that has been isolated directly from cells or chromosomes or the cloned copies of all or part of such DNA.

Genomic medicine   The practice of medicine based on large-scale genomic information, such as expression profiling to characterize tumors or to define prognosis in cancer, genotyping of variants in genes involved in drug metabolism or action to determine an individual's correct therapeutic dosage, or analysis of multiple protein biomarkers to monitor therapy or to provide predictive information in presymptomatic individuals.

Genomics   The field of genetics concerned with structural and functional studies of the genome.

Genotype   1. The genetic constitution of an individual, as distinguished from the phenotype. 2. More specifically, the alleles present at one locus.

Germ layer   One of three distinct layers of cells that arise in the inner cell mass, the *ectoderm, mesoderm,* and *endoderm,* each of which develops into a distinctly different tissue in the embryo.

Germline   The cell line from which gametes are derived.

Germline mosaicism   In an individual, the presence of two or more genetically different types of germline cells, resulting from mutation during the proliferation and differentiation of the germline.

Globin switching   Change in expression of the various globin genes during ontogeny.

Haploid   The chromosome number of a normal gamete, with only one member of each chromosome pair. In humans, the haploid number is 23.

Haploinsufficiency   A cause of genetic disease in which the contribution from a normal allele is insufficient to prevent disease because of a loss-of-function mutation at the other allele.

Haplotype   A group of alleles in coupling at closely linked loci, usually inherited as a unit.

HapMap   A set of haplotypes, defined by *tag SNPs,* distributed throughout the genome, used for association studies.

Hardy-Weinberg law   The law that relates allele frequency to genotype frequency, used in population genetics to determine allele frequency and heterozygote frequency when the incidence of a disorder is known.

Hemizygous   A term for the genotype of an individual with only one representative of a chromosome or chromosome segment, rather than the usual two; refers especially to X-linked genes in the male but also applies to genes on any chromosome segment that is deleted on the homologous chromosome.

Heritability (h^2)   The fraction of total phenotypic variance of a quantitative trait that is due to genotypic differences. May be viewed as a statistical estimate of the hereditary contribution to a quantitative trait.

Heterochromatin   Chromatin that stains darkly throughout the cell cycle, even in interphase. Generally thought to be late replicating and genetically inactive. Satellite DNA in regions such as centromeres, acrocentric short arms, and 1qh, 9qh, 16qh, and Yqh constitute *constitutive heterochromatin,* whereas the chromatin of the inactive X chromosome is referred to as *facultative heterochromatin.* Contrast with *euchromatin.*

Heterodisomy   See *uniparental disomy.*

Heterogeneity   See *allelic heterogeneity, clinical heterogeneity, genetic heterogeneity, locus heterogeneity.*

Heteromorphism   A normal morphological or staining variant of a chromosome.

Heteroplasmy   The presence of more than one type of mitochondrial DNA in the mitochondria of a single individual. Contrast with *homoplasmy.*

Heteroploid   Any chromosome number other than the normal.

Heterozygote (heterozygous)   An individual or genotype with two different alleles at a given locus on a pair of homologous chromosomes.

Histocompatibility   A host will accept a particular graft only if it is histocompatible—that is, if the graft contains no antigens that the host lacks.

Histone code   A pattern of histone variants and post-translational modifications that determine specific properties of chromatin associated with epigenetics and differential gene expression.

Histones   Proteins, rich in basic amino acids (lysine or arginine), that are associated with DNA in the chromosomes and are virtually invariant throughout eukaryote evolution.

Holoenzyme   The functional compound formed by the binding of an apoenzyme and its appropriate coenzyme.

Homeobox gene   A gene that contains a conserved 180–base pair sequence termed a *homeobox* in its coding region, encoding a protein motif known as the *homeodomain*. The 60 amino acid residues of the homeodomain are a DNA-binding motif, which is consistent with the role of homeodomain proteins in the transcriptional regulation of genes involved in development.

Homogeneously staining regions (HSRs)   Chromosome regions that stain uniformly and represent amplified copies of a DNA segment.

Homologous chromosomes (homologues)   A pair of chromosomes, one inherited paternally, the other maternally, that pair with each other during meiosis I, undergo crossing over, and separate at anaphase I of meiosis. Homologous chromosomes are generally of similar size and shape when they are viewed under the microscope and contain the same loci, except for the two sex chromosomes in males (X and Y), which are only partially homologous. See *pseudoautosomal region*.

Homologous genes (homologues)   Genes in a single species, or in different species, that have overall similar DNA sequences, that may have related biochemical functions, and that arose from a common ancestral gene. *Orthologous* and *paralogous* genes are types of homologous genes, but their meaning is more restricted.

Homoplasmy   The presence of only one type of mitochondrial DNA in the mitochondria of a single individual. Contrast with *heteroplasmy*.

Homozygote (homozygous)   An individual or genotype with identical alleles at a given locus on a pair of homologous chromosomes.

Host   In molecular genetics, the organism in which a recombinant DNA molecule is isolated and grown; usually *Escherichia coli* or yeast.

Housekeeping genes   Genes expressed in most or all cells because their products provide basic functions.

Housekeeping proteins   Proteins expressed in virtually every cell that have fundamental roles in the maintenance of cell structure and function (versus *specialty proteins*).

Human Genome Project   A major research project, international in scope, that took place in the years 1990-2003 and resulted in the sequencing of a representative human genome and the genomes of many model organisms.

Hybridization   1. In molecular biology, the bonding of two complementary single-stranded nucleic acid molecules according to the rules of base pairing. 2. In somatic cell genetics, fusion of two somatic cells, often from different organisms, to form a hybrid cell containing the genetic information of both parental cell types.

Hydatidiform mole   An abnormality of the placenta in which it grows to resemble a hydatid cyst or bunch of grapes, associated with very abnormal fetal development. In a *complete mole*, the karyotype is 46,XX, representing duplication of the chromosomes of the sperm with no maternal contribution. A *partial mole* is triploid, usually with an extra paternal chromosome set.

Identity by descent   Two individuals in a family who have the same allele or alleles at a locus because they inherited the alleles from a common ancestor. See *coefficient of inbreeding*.

Immunoglobulin gene superfamily   A family of evolutionarily related genes composed of human leukocyte antigen (HLA) class I and class II genes, immunoglobulin genes, T-cell receptor genes, and some other genes encoding cell surface molecules.

Imprinting   The phenomenon of different expression of alleles depending on the parent of origin. See *Prader-Willi syndrome* and *Angelman syndrome* in the text for examples.

In situ hybridization   Mapping a gene or segment of DNA by molecular hybridization to a chromosome spread or cell nucleus on a slide by use of a labeled DNA sequence as a probe corresponding to the gene or DNA segment to be mapped. Usually involves fluorescently labeled probes, in which case it is referred to as fluorescence in situ hybridization (FISH).

Inborn error of metabolism   A genetically determined biochemical disorder in which a specific protein defect produces a metabolic block that may have pathological consequences.

Inbreeding   The mating of closely related individuals. The progeny of close relatives are said to be *inbred*. (Note that some consider the term *inbreeding* to be pejorative when it is applied to human populations.)

Incompletely dominant   A trait that is inherited in a dominant manner but is more severe in a homozygote than in a heterozygote (synonym: semidominant).

Indel   A polymorphism defined by the presence or absence of a segment of DNA, ranging from one base to a few hundred base pairs. Includes simple indels, microsatellites, and minisatellite polymorphisms.

Index case   The family member affected with a genetic disorder who is the first to draw attention to a pedigree. See *proband*.

Induction   The determination of the fate of one region of an embryo by extracellular signals from a second, usually neighboring, region.

In-frame deletion   A deletion that does not destroy the normal reading frame of the gene.

Inner cell mass   A small group of cells within the preimplantation mammalian embryo that will become the primitive ectoderm (or epiblast) after implantation and, ultimately, give rise to the embryo proper and not the placenta.

Insert   In molecular biology, a fragment of foreign DNA cloned into a vector.

Insertion   A chromosomal abnormality in which a DNA segment from one chromosome is inserted into another chromosome.

Intergenic complementation   The ability of cells from patients with similar phenotypes, due to mutations in different genes, to correct one another.

Intergenic DNA   The untranscribed DNA, often of unknown function, that makes up a large proportion of the total DNA in the genome.

Interphase   The stage of the cell cycle between two successive mitoses.

Intervening sequence   See *intron*.

Intron   A segment of a gene that is initially transcribed but then removed from within the primary RNA transcript by splicing together the sequences (exons) on either side of it.

Inversion   A chromosomal rearrangement in which a segment of a chromosome is reversed end to end. If the centromere is included in the inversion, the inversion is *pericentric*; if not, it is *paracentric*.

In vitro fertilization   A reproductive technology in which sperm are allowed to fertilize an egg in tissue culture and the fertilized eggs are then introduced back into the uterus to allow implantation.

Isochromosome   An abnormal chromosome in which one arm is duplicated (forming two arms of equal length, with the same loci in reverse sequence) and the other arm is missing.

Isodisomy   See *uniparental disomy*.

Isolate   A subpopulation in which matings take place exclusively or usually with other members of the same subpopulation.

Isolated case   An individual who is the only member of his or her kindred affected by a genetic disorder, either by chance or by new mutation. See also *sporadic*.

Karyotype   The chromosome constitution of an individual. The term is also used for a photomicrograph of the chromosomes of an individual systematically arranged, and for the process of preparing such a photomicrograph.

kb (kilobase)   A unit of 1000 bases in a DNA or RNA sequence.

Kindred   An extended family.

Kinetochore   A structure at the centromere to which the spindle fibers are attached.

Library   In molecular biology, a collection of recombinant clones that contain a sample of the DNA or RNA (as cDNA) of a tissue.

Ligation   In molecular biology, the process of joining two double-stranded DNA molecules to form a recombinant DNA molecule, by means of phosphodiester bonds, with use of the enzyme DNA ligase.

LINE sequences   A class of repetitive DNA made up of long interspersed nuclear elements, up to 6 kb in length, occurring in several hundred thousand copies in the genome (also called *L1 family*).

Lineage   The progeny of a cell, generally determined by experimentally labeling the cell so that all of its descendants can be identified. See *clone*.

Linkage   Genes on the same chromosome are *linked* if they are transmitted together in meiosis more frequently than chance would allow. Compare with *synteny*.

Linkage analysis   A statistical method in which the genotypes and phenotypes of parents and offspring in families are studied to determine whether two or more loci are assorting independently or exhibiting linkage during meiosis.

Linkage disequilibrium   The occurrence of specific combinations of alleles in coupling phase at two or more linked loci more frequently than expected by chance from the frequency of the alleles in the population.

Linkage disequilibrium block   A set of polymorphic markers whose alleles are in strong linkage disequilibrium with each other. Usually occupies a region of the genome from a few kilobases to a few dozen kilobases in length.

Linkage map   A chromosome map showing the relative positions of genes and other DNA markers on the chromosomes, as determined by linkage analysis.

Locus   The position occupied by a gene on a chromosome. Different forms of the gene (*alleles*) may occupy the locus.

Locus control region (LCR)   A DNA domain, situated outside a cluster of structural genes, responsible for the appropriate expression of the genes within the cluster.

Locus heterogeneity   The production of identical phenotypes by mutations at two or more different loci.

LOD score   A statistical method that tests genetic marker data in families to determine whether two loci are linked. The lod score is the *log*arithm of the *od*ds in favor of linkage. By convention, a LOD score of 3 (odds of 1000 : 1 in favor) is accepted as proof of linkage and a LOD score of −2 (100 : 1 against) as proof that the loci are unlinked.

L1 family   See *LINE sequences.*

Loops   Arrangement of chromatin, packaged as solenoids, attached to the chromosome scaffold. Thought to be a structural or functional unit of chromosomes.

Loss-of-function mutation   A mutation associated with a reduction or a complete loss of one or more of the normal functions of a protein.

Loss of heterozygosity (LOH)   Loss of a normal allele from a region of one chromosome of a pair, allowing a defective allele on the homologous chromosome to be clinically manifest. A feature of many cases of retinoblastoma, breast cancer, and other tumors due to mutation in a tumor-suppressor gene.

Lyonization   Term used for the phenomenon of X inactivation, which was first described by the geneticist Mary Lyon. See *X inactivation.*

Major histocompatibility complex (MHC)   The complex locus on chromosome 6p that includes the highly polymorphic human leukocyte antigen (HLA) genes.

Maleficence   Behavior that harms others. Avoidance of maleficence is one of the cardinal principles of ethics. See *beneficence.*

Male-to-male transmission   A pattern of inheritance of a trait from a father to all of his sons and none of his daughters (also referred to as *holandric* inheritance).

Malformation syndrome   A recognizable pattern of dysmorphic features having a single cause, either genetic or environmental.

Manifesting heterozygote   A female heterozygous for an X-linked disorder in whom, because of nonrandom X inactivation, the trait is expressed clinically, although not usually to the same degree of severity as in hemizygous affected males.

Maternal inheritance   The transmission of genetic information only through the mother.

Maternal serum screening   Laboratory test that relies on measurement of the levels of particular substances, such as alpha-fetoprotein, human chorionic gonadotropin, and unconjugated estriol, in a pregnant woman's blood, to screen for fetuses affected with certain trisomies or with neural tube defects.

Mb (megabase)   A unit of 1,000,000 bases or base pairs in genomic DNA.

Meiosis   The type of cell division occurring in the germ cells, by which gametes containing the haploid chromosome number are produced from diploid cells. Two meiotic divisions occur: meiosis I and meiosis II. Reduction in chromosome number takes place during meiosis I.

Mendelian   Patterns of inheritance that follow the classic laws of Mendel: autosomal dominant, autosomal recessive, and X-linked. See *single-gene disorder.*

Mesoderm   The middle *germ layer* in the early embryo; the source of cells that go on to make bones, muscles, connective tissue, heart, hematopoietic system, kidney, and other organs.

Messenger RNA (mRNA)   An RNA, transcribed from the DNA of a gene, that directs the sequence of amino acids of the encoded polypeptide.

Metacentric   A type of chromosome with a central centromere and arms of apparently equal length.

Metaphase   The stage of mitosis or meiosis in which the chromosomes have reached their maximal condensation and are lined up on the equatorial plane of the cell, attached to the spindle fibers. This is the stage at which chromosomes are most easily examined.

Metastasis   Spread of malignant cells to other sites in the body.

Methemoglobin   The oxidized form of hemoglobin, containing iron in the ferric rather than the ferrous state, that is incapable of binding oxygen.

MicroRNA   A particular class of noncoding RNAs that are processed into short interfering RNAs (siRNA), double stranded RNAs approximately 22 nucleotides in length, that affect mRNA stability or translation. siRNAs are involved in gene regulation in development and differentiation.

Microarray   Miniaturized wafer ("chip") made of glass, plastic, or silicon onto which a large number of different nucleic acids have been individually spotted. See also *CGH, expression profile.*

Microdeletion   A chromosomal deletion that is too small to be seen under the microscope. See also *contiguous gene syndrome.*

Microsatellite marker   See *short tandem repeat polymorphism (STRP).*

Minisatellite   See *VNTR.*

Missense mutation   A mutation that changes a codon specific for one amino acid to specify another amino acid.

Mitochondrial bottleneck   A step in oogenesis in which only a small sample of the total number of mitochondria in an oocyte precursor is passed on to daughter cells, thereby allowing significant variation in the proportions of mutant and wild-type mitochondria inherited by the daughter cells.

Mitochondrial DNA (mtDNA)   The DNA in the circular chromosome of the mitochondria. Mitochondrial DNA is present in many copies per cell, is maternally inherited, and evolves 5 to 10 times as rapidly as genomic DNA.

Mitochondrial inheritance   The inheritance of a trait encoded in the mitochondrial genome. Because the mitochondrial genome is maternally inherited, with only very rare exceptions, inheritance of the mitochondrial genome occurs almost always through the female line.

Mitosis   The process of ordinary cell division, resulting in the formation of two cells genetically identical to the parent cell.

Model-based linkage analysis   Linkage analysis that relies on assuming a particular mode of inheritance to infer when crossovers have occurred between two loci. Also referred to as *parametric linkage analysis.*

Model-free linkage analysis   Linkage analysis that makes no assumptions as to the mode of inheritance. This form of analysis relies on determining whether the extent of allele sharing at any loci among related individuals who either do or do not share a disease or trait deviates significantly from what would be expected by chance alone. See *affected pedigree member method.* Also referred to as *nonparametric linkage analysis.*

Modifier gene   A gene that alters the phenotype associated with mutations in a nonallelic gene.

Monosomy   A chromosome constitution in which one member of a chromosome pair is missing, as in 45,X Turner syndrome.

Monozygotic (MZ) twins   Twins derived from a single zygote and thus genetically identical. Also termed *identical twins.*

Morphogen   A substance produced during development in a localized region of the organism that diffuses out to form a concentration gradient and directs cells into two or more specific developmental pathways, depending on its concentration.

Morphogenesis   The process whereby changes in cell shape, adhesion, movement, and number lead to three-dimensional structure.

Mosaic   An individual or tissue with at least two cell lines differing in genotype or karyotype, derived from a single zygote; not to be confused with *chimera.*

Mosaic development   Embryological development in which different regions of the embryo develop independently from surrounding regions. See *regulative development.*

Multifactorial inheritance   The type of non-mendelian inheritance shown by traits that are determined by a combination of multiple factors, genetic and environmental. Also termed *complex inheritance.*

Multiplex   A pedigree in which there is more than one case of a particular disorder.

Multiplex testing   A laboratory method that allows many different tests to be performed simultaneously on the same sample.

Mutagen   An agent that increases the spontaneous mutation rate by causing changes in DNA.

Mutant   A gene that has been altered by mutation; also used to refer to a nonhuman organism carrying a mutant gene.

Mutation   Any permanent heritable change in the sequence of genomic DNA.

Mutation rate (μ)   The frequency of mutation at a given locus, expressed as mutations per locus per gamete (or per generation, which is the same).

Negative predictive value   With respect to a clinical test for a disease, the extent to which testing negative indicates that one does not have or will not develop the disease.

Neoplasia   An abnormal growth produced by imbalance between normal cellular proliferation and normal cellular attrition. May be benign or malignant (cancer).

Noncoding strand   See *antisense strand of DNA.*

Nondisjunction   The failure of two members of a chromosome pair to disjoin during meiosis I, or of two chromatids of a chromosome to disjoin during meiosis II or mitosis, so that both pass to one daughter cell and the other daughter cell receives neither.

Nonsense mutation   A single-base substitution in DNA resulting in a chain-termination codon.

Northern blotting A technique analogous to Southern blotting, for detection of RNA molecules by hybridization to a complementary DNA probe.

Novel property mutation A mutation that confers a new property on the protein.

Nuchal translucency An ultrasonographic finding of an echo-free space between the skin line and the soft tissue overlying the cervical spine in the subcutaneous tissue of the fetal neck. Increased nuchal translucency occurs in fetal aneuploidy.

Nucleic acid hybridization See *hybridization*.

Nucleosome The primary structural unit of chromatin, consisting of 146 base pairs of DNA wrapped twice around a core of eight histone molecules.

Nucleotide A molecule composed of a nitrogenous base, a 5-carbon sugar, and a phosphate group. A nucleic acid is a polymer of many nucleotides.

Null allele An allele that results either in the total absence of the gene product or in the total loss of function of the product.

Obligate heterozygote An individual who may be clinically unaffected but on the basis of pedigree analysis must carry a specific mutant allele.

Odds A ratio of probabilities or risks. Often calculated as a ratio of the probability of an event's occurring versus the probability of the event's not occurring, as one way to assess the relative chance of the event. Odds can vary in value from 0 to infinity.

Odds ratio A comparison of the odds that individuals who share a particular factor (e.g., a genotype, an environmental exposure, or a drug) will have a disease or trait versus the odds for individuals who lack the factor.

	Affected	Unaffected	Total
Factor present	a	b	a + b
Factor absent	c	d	c + d
Total	a + c	b + d	a + b + c + d

Among individuals in whom the factor is present, the *odds* of being affected = (a/b). Among individuals in whom the factor is absent, the *odds* of being affected = (c/d), and the odds ratio = (a/b)/(c/d) = ad/bc. [Strictly speaking, this definition of odds ratio is a **disease** odds ratio. A more traditional odds ratio used in epidemiology is an **exposure** odds ratio, which is a comparison of the odds that individuals affected with a particular disease were exposed to a particular factor = (a/c) versus the odds that unaffected individuals were exposed = (b/d), giving an odds ratio of (a/c)/(b/d). Note that both formulations result in the same ratio = ad/bc. Using a disease odds ratio formulation makes it easier to show arithmetically that a disease odds ratio approximates the relative risk ratio when the disease is rare (c << d and a << b)]. See *relative risk*.

Oligonucleotide A short DNA molecule (usually 8 to 50 base pairs), synthesized for use as a probe or for use in the polymerase chain reaction.

Oncogene A dominantly acting gene responsible for tumor development. Mutation, overexpression, or amplification of oncogenes in somatic cells may lead to neoplastic transformation. Contrast with *proto-oncogene* and with *tumor-suppressor gene*.

Ontogeny The developmental history of an organism.

Open reading frame The interval between the start and stop codons of a nucleotide sequence that encodes a protein.

Orthologous Refers to genes in different species that are similar in DNA sequence and also encode proteins that have the same function—at least at the biochemical level—in each species. Orthologous genes originate from the same gene in a common ancestor. Contrast with *paralogous* and *homologous*.

P 1. In cytogenetics, the short arm of a chromosome (from the French *petit*). 2. In population genetics, the frequency of the more common allele of a pair. 3. In biochemistry, abbreviation of *protein* (e.g., p53 is a 53-kD protein).

PACs (P1 artificial chromosomes) Vectors capable of cloning DNA inserts 100 to 300 kb in size, used in high-resolution mapping and gene sequencing.

Painting probe See *chromosome painting probe*.

Paired domain A DNA-binding motif found in the members of a large class of developmentally important mammalian transcription factors encoded by *PAX* genes. Named originally for the *Drosophila* paired gene in which it was first described.

Palindrome In molecular biology, a nucleotide sequence in which the 5′ to 3′ sequence of one strand of a segment of DNA is the same as that of its complementary strand. The sites of restriction enzymes are usually palindromes.

Paralogous Refers to two or more genes in a single species that are similar in DNA sequence and are likely to encode proteins with similar and perhaps overlapping but not identical functions. Paralogous genes are likely to have originated from a common ancestral gene. Example, α- and β-globin genes.

Parental transmission bias A phenomenon seen with the inheritance of unstable repeat expansion mutations in which expansions of the repeat occur preferentially when the mutation is transmitted by one parent versus the other.

PCR   See *polymerase chain reaction.*

Pedigree   In medical genetics, a family history of a hereditary condition, or a diagram of a family history indicating the family members, their relationship to the proband, and their status with respect to a particular hereditary condition.

Penetrance   The fraction of individuals with a genotype known to cause a disease who have any signs or symptoms of the disease. Contrast with *expressivity.*

Pharmacodynamics   The effects of a drug or its metabolites on physiological function and metabolic pathways.

Pharmacogenetics   The area of biochemical genetics concerned with the impact of genetic variation on drug response and metabolism.

Pharmacogenomics   The application of genomic information or methods to pharmacogenetic problems.

Pharmacokinetics   The rate at which the body absorbs, transports, metabolizes, or excretes a drug or its metabolites.

Phase   In an individual heterozygous at two syntenic loci, the designation of which allele at the first locus is on the same chromosome as which allele at the second locus. See *coupling* and *repulsion.*

Phenocopy   A mimic of a phenotype that is usually determined by a specific genotype, produced instead by the interaction of some environmental factor with a normal genotype.

Phenotype   The observed biochemical, physiological, and morphological characteristics of an individual, as determined by his or her genotype and the environment in which it is expressed. Also, in a more limited sense, the abnormalities resulting from a particular mutant gene.

Philadelphia chromosome (Ph¹)   The structurally abnormal chromosome 22 that typically occurs in a proportion of the bone marrow cells in most patients with chronic myelogenous leukemia. The abnormality is a reciprocal translocation between the distal portion of 22q and the distal portion of 9q.

Physical map   A map showing the order of genes and markers along a chromosome and their distances apart in units such as cytogenetic bands or base pairs. Physical mapping is performed by techniques such as radiation hybrid mapping, fluorescence in situ hybridization (FISH), and nucleotide sequencing, not by data from linkage analysis. See *genetic map* for comparison.

Plasmids   Independently replicating, extrachromosomal circular DNA molecules, used in molecular biology as vectors for cloned segments of DNA.

Pleiotropy   Multiple phenotypic effects of a single allele or pair of alleles. The term is used particularly when the effects are not obviously related.

Pluripotent   Describes an embryonic cell that is capable of giving rise to different types of differentiated tissues or structures, depending on its location and environmental influences.

Point mutation   A single nucleotide base pair change in DNA.

Polyadenylation site   In the synthesis of mature mRNA, a site at which a sequence of 20 to 200 adenosine residues (the polyA tail) is added to the 3′ end of an RNA transcript, aiding its transport out of the nucleus and, usually, its stability.

Polygenic   Inheritance determined by many genes at different loci, with small additive effects; not to be confused with *complex (multifactorial) inheritance,* in which environmental as well as genetic factors may be involved.

Polymerase chain reaction (PCR)   The molecular genetic technique by which a short DNA or RNA sequence is amplified enormously by means of two flanking oligonucleotide primers used in repeated cycles of primer extension and DNA synthesis with DNA polymerase.

Polymorphism   The occurrence together in a population of two or more alternative genotypes, each at a frequency greater than that which could be maintained by recurrent mutation alone. A locus is arbitrarily considered to be polymorphic if the rarer allele has a frequency of .01, so that the heterozygote frequency is at least .02. Any allele rarer than this is a *rare variant.*

Polyploid   Any multiple of the basic haploid chromosome number other than the diploid number; thus, 3n, 4n, and so forth.

Positional cloning   The molecular cloning of a gene on the basis of knowledge of its map position, without prior knowledge of the gene product.

Positive predictive value   With respect to a clinical test for a disease, the extent to which testing positive indicates that one has or will develop the disease.

Preimplantation diagnosis   A type of prenatal diagnosis in which a cell is removed from a multicell embryo generated by in vitro fertilization and tested for the presence of a disease-causing mutation.

Premutation   In unstable repeat disorders (e.g., fragile X syndrome), a moderate expansion of the number of repeats that is at increased risk of undergoing further expansion during meiosis and causing the full disorder in the offspring. Premutations can be asymptomatic, as in Huntington disease, or they may be associated with a distinct syndrome, such as the *fragile X–associated tremor/ataxia syn-*

drome in individuals with triplet repeat expansions in the premutation range in their *FMR1* gene.

Primary constriction   See *centromere*.

Primary structure   The amino acid sequence of a polypeptide.

Primary transcript   The initial, unprocessed RNA transcript of a gene that is co-linear with the genomic DNA, containing introns as well as exons.

Primer   A short oligonucleotide designed to hybridize to a single-stranded DNA template and provide a free DNA end to which DNA polymerase can add bases and synthesize DNA complementary to the template.

Proband   The affected family member through whom the family is ascertained. Also called the *propositus* or *index case*.

Probe   In molecular genetics, a labeled DNA or RNA sequence used to detect the presence of a complementary sequence by molecular hybridization; or a reagent capable of recognizing a desired clone in a mixture of many DNA or RNA sequences. Also, the process of using such a molecule.

Prokaryote   A simple unicellular organism, such as a bacterium, lacking a separate nucleus. See *eukaryote*.

Promoter   A DNA sequence, located in the 5′ end of a gene, at which transcription is initiated.

Prophase   The first stage of cell division, during which the chromosomes become visible as discrete structures and subsequently thicken and shorten. Prophase of the first meiotic division is further characterized by pairing (synapsis) of homologous chromosomes.

Propositus   See *proband*.

Proteome   The collection of all proteins present in a cell, tissue, or organism at a particular time. Contrast with *transcriptome*, the collection of all RNA transcripts, and *genome*, the collection of all DNA sequences.

Proteomics   A field of biochemistry encompassing the comprehensive analysis and cataloguing of the structure and function of all the proteins present in a given cell or tissue (see *proteome*). Parallels *genomics*, a similarly comprehensive approach to the analysis of DNA sequence and mRNA expression.

Proto-oncogene   A normal gene involved in some aspect of cell division or proliferation that may become activated by mutation or other mechanism to become an oncogene.

Pseudoautosomal region   Segment of the X and Y chromosome, located at the most distal portion of their respective p and q arms, at which crossing over occurs during male meiosis. Traits due to alleles at

pseudoautosomal loci will appear to be inherited as autosomal traits despite the physical location of these loci on the sex chromosomes.

Pseudodeficiency allele   A clinically benign allele that has a reduction in functional activity detected by in vitro assays but that has sufficient activity in vivo to prevent haploinsufficiency.

Pseudogene   1. An inactive gene within a gene family, derived by mutation of an ancestral active gene and frequently located within the same region of the chromosome as its functional counterpart (*nonprocessed pseudogene*). 2. A DNA copy of an mRNA, created by retrotransposition and inserted randomly in the genome (*processed pseudogene*). Processed pseudogenes are probably never functional.

Pseudomosaicism   The occurrence of a single cytogenetically abnormal cell in a cytogenetic analysis of a chorionic villus sampling or amniocentesis specimen. Generally considered artifactual and of no clinical significance.

q   1. In cytogenetics, the long arm of a chromosome. 2. In population genetics, the frequency of the less common allele of a pair.

Qualitative trait   A trait that an individual either has or does not have. Contrast with *quantitative trait*.

Quantitative trait   A measurable quantity that differs among different individuals, often following a normal distribution in the population. Contrast with *qualitative trait*.

Random mating   Selection of a mate without regard to the genotype of the mate. In a randomly mating population, the frequencies of the various matings between individuals with particular genotypes are determined solely by the frequencies of the alleles concerned.

Reading frame   One of the three possible ways of reading a nucleotide sequence as a series of triplets. An *open reading frame* contains no termination codons and thus is potentially translatable into protein.

Rearrangement   Chromosome breakage followed by reconstitution in an abnormal combination. If *unbalanced*, the rearrangement can produce an abnormal phenotype.

Recessive   A trait that is expressed only in homozygotes, compound heterozygotes, or hemizygotes.

Reciprocal translocation   See *translocation*.

Recombinant   An individual who has a new combination of alleles not found in either parent.

Recombinant chromosome   A chromosome that results from exchange of reciprocal segments by crossing over between a homologous pair of parental chromosomes during meiosis.

Recombinant DNA technology Methods by which a DNA molecule is constructed in vitro from segments from more than one parental DNA molecule.

Recombination The formation of new combinations of alleles in coupling by crossing over between their loci.

Recombination fraction (θ) The fraction of offspring of a parent heterozygous at two loci who have inherited a chromosome carrying a recombination between the loci.

Recurrence risk The probability that a genetic disorder present in one or more members of a family will recur in another member of the same or a subsequent generation.

Reduction division The first meiotic division, so called because at this stage the chromosome number per cell is reduced from diploid to haploid.

Redundancy The situation in which genes (often paralogous) have overlapping functions.

Regulative development A developmental stage during which removal or destruction of a particular region of the embryo is compensated for by other embryonic regions, thereby allowing normal development.

Regulatory gene A gene that codes for an RNA or protein molecule that regulates the expression of other genes.

Regulatory region of a gene A DNA segment, such as a promoter, enhancer, or locus control region, within or near a gene that regulates the expression of the gene.

Relative risk A comparison of the *risk* for a disease or trait in individuals who share a particular factor (such as genotype, an environmental exposure, or a drug) versus the *risk* among individuals who lack the factor.

	Affected	Unaffected	Total
Factor present	a	b	a + b
Factor absent	c	d	c + d
Total	a + c	b + d	a + b + c + d

The *risk* of being affected in individuals who have the factor = (a/a + b), the *risk* of being affected when the factor is absent = (c/c + d), and the relative risk ratio = (a/a + b)/(c/c + d) = a(c + d)/c(a + b). Note that relative risk ratio ≈ ad/bc, the odds ratio, when the disease is relatively rare (c < < d and a < < b). See *odds ratio*.

Relative risk ratio (λ_r) In complex disorders, the risk that a disease will occur in a relative of an affected person compared with the risk for disease in any random person in the general population.

Repetitive DNA (repeats) DNA sequences that are present in multiple copies in the genome.

Replication error positive A phenotype of cancer cells in which loss of function of mismatch repair genes causes errors such as slipped mispairing to go unrepaired when microsatellite sequences are replicated. These errors lead to tissue mosaicism so that the cancer appears to contain more than two alleles at many short tandem repeat polymorphic loci.

Replicative segregation Random distribution of mitochondria into daughter cells.

Repulsion Describes the phase of two alleles at two different but syntenic loci, in which one allele at one of the loci is *not* on the same chromosome as the allele at the second locus. See *phase* and *coupling*.

Restriction endonuclease (restriction enzyme) An enzyme, derived from bacteria, that can recognize a specific sequence of DNA and cleave the DNA molecule within the recognition site or at some nearby site.

Restriction fragment length polymorphism (RFLP) A polymorphic difference in DNA sequence between individuals that can be recognized by restriction endonucleases. See *polymorphism*.

Restriction map A linear array of sites on DNA cleaved by various restriction endonucleases.

Restriction site A short sequence in DNA that can be recognized and cut by a specific restriction endonuclease.

Retrovirus A virus, with an RNA genome, that propagates by conversion of the RNA into DNA by the enzyme reverse transcriptase.

Reverse transcriptase An enzyme, RNA-dependent DNA polymerase, that catalyzes the synthesis of DNA on an RNA template.

RFLP See *restriction fragment length polymorphism*.

Ribonucleic acid See *RNA*.

Ribosome A cytoplasmic organelle composed of ribosomal RNA and protein, on which polypeptides are synthesized from messenger RNA.

Ring chromosome A structurally abnormal chromosome in which the telomere of each chromosome arm has been deleted and the broken arms have reunited in ring formation.

Risk The probability of an event's occurring. Often calculated as the number of times the event occurs divided by the total number of opportunities there were for the event to occur. As with all probabilities, risk varies from 0 to 1.

RNA (ribonucleic acid)   A nucleic acid formed on a DNA template, containing ribose instead of deoxyribose. *Messenger RNA (mRNA)* is the template on which polypeptides are synthesized. *Transfer RNA (tRNA)*, in cooperation with the ribosomes, brings activated amino acids into position along the mRNA template. *Ribosomal RNA (rRNA)*, a component of the ribosomes, functions as a nonspecific site of polypeptide synthesis.

RNA polymerase   An enzyme that synthesizes RNA on a DNA template.

RNAi   RNA interference. A system for regulating gene expression in which short RNA segments, approximately 22 bases in length, form double-stranded structures with an mRNA and either target it for destruction or block its translation. (See *microRNA*.) Scientists have taken advantage of this normal, endogenous system of gene regulation to design new and powerful technologies for gene silencing by use of exogenously supplied RNAi sequences.

Robertsonian translocation   A translocation between two acrocentric chromosomes by fusion at or near the centromere, with loss of the short arms.

Sanger sequencing   Currently, the method most widely used to determine the nucleotide sequence of a DNA molecule. The DNA whose sequence is to be determined is used as a template for a polymerase that extends a complementary primer in the presence of four different dideoxynucleotides ("chain-terminating" nucleotides) corresponding to the four bases, ACGT, found in DNA. The length of each of the different strands produced corresponds to which dideoxynucleotide was incorporated and terminated the extension reaction for that strand. The particular dideoxynucleotide incorporated is determined by the rules of DNA base-pairing by the base that was present at that site in the template.

Satellite DNA   DNA containing many tandem repeats of a short basic repeating unit; not to be confused with *chromosomal satellite*, the chromatin at the distal end of the short arms of the acrocentric chromosomes.

Scaffold   The nonhistone structure observed when histones are experimentally removed from chromosomes. Believed to represent a structural component of the nucleus and of chromosomes.

Segmental aneusomy   Loss of a small segment from one chromosome of a pair, resulting in hemizygosity for genes in that segment on the homologous chromosome. See also *contiguous gene syndrome*.

Segmental duplication   See *segmental aneusomy*.

Segregation   In genetics, the disjunction of homologous chromosomes at meiosis.

Segregation analysis   A statistical method that assesses the phenotypes of individuals in families to determine the most likely mode of inheritance of a disease or trait.

Selection   In population genetics, the operation of forces that determine the relative fitness of a genotype in the population, thus affecting the frequency of the gene concerned.

Sense strand   See *coding strand*.

Sensitivity   In diagnostic tests, the frequency with which the test result is positive when the disorder is present.

Sequence   1. In genomics and molecular genetics, the order of nucleotides in a segment of DNA or RNA. 2. In clinical genetics, a recognizable pattern of dysmorphic features due to a number of different causes; to be distinguished from *malformation syndrome*.

Sex chromatin   See *Barr body*.

Sex chromosomes   The X and Y chromosomes.

Sex-influenced   A trait that is not X-linked in its pattern of inheritance but is expressed differently, either in degree or in frequency, in males and females.

Sex-limited   A trait that is expressed in only one sex, although the gene that determines the trait is not X-linked.

Sex-linked   Old term for *X-linked*, now little used because formally it fails to distinguish between X and Y linkage.

Short tandem repeat polymorphism (STRP)   A polymorphic locus consisting of a variable number of tandemly repeated binucleotide, trinucleotide, or tetranucleotide units such as $(TG)_n$, $(CAA)_n$, or $(GATA)_n$; different numbers of units constitute the different alleles. Also termed a *microsatellite marker*.

Sib, sibling   A brother or sister.

Sibpair analysis   A form of model-free linkage analysis in which pairs of siblings either concordant or discordant for a phenotype or trait are analyzed at loci throughout the genome to determine whether there are any loci at which they share alleles significantly more or less than the expected average of 50%.

Sibship   All the sibs in a family.

Silencer   A DNA sequence that acts in *cis* (i.e., on the same chromosome) to decrease transcription of a nearby gene. The silencer may be upstream or downstream to the gene and may be in the same or the reverse orientation (contrast with *enhancer*).

Silent allele   A mutant gene that has no detectable phenotypic effect.

Single-copy DNA   The type of DNA that makes up most of the genome.

Single-gene disorder   A disorder due to one or a pair of mutant alleles at a single locus.

Single nucleotide polymorphism (SNP)   A polymorphism in DNA sequence consisting of variation in a single base.

Sister chromatid exchange   The exchange of segments of DNA between sister chromatids, either in the four-strand stage of meiosis or in mitosis. Occurs with particularly high frequency in patients with Bloom syndrome.

SKY   See *spectral karyotyping.*

Slipped mispairing   A mutational mechanism that occurs during DNA replication of sequences with repeats of one or more nucleotides, in which a repeat on one strand mispairs with a similar repeat on the complementary strand, generating a deletion or expansion of the number of repeats.

SNP   See *single nucleotide polymorphism.*

Solenoid   A fiber composed of compacted strings of nucleosomes, forming the fundamental unit of chromatin organization.

Somatic mutation   A mutation occurring in a somatic cell rather than in the germline.

Somatic rearrangement   Rearrangement of DNA sequences in the chromosomes of lymphocyte precursor cells, thus generating antibody and T-cell receptor diversity.

Southern blotting   A technique, devised by the British biochemist Ed Southern, for preparation of a filter to which DNA has been transferred, following restriction enzyme digestion and gel electrophoresis to separate the DNA molecules by size. Specific DNA molecules can then be detected on the filter by their hybridization to labeled probes.

Specialty proteins   Proteins, expressed in only one or a limited number of cell types, that have unique functions contributing to the individuality of the cells in which they are expressed. Contrast with *housekeeping proteins.*

Specification   The first stage of commitment in which a cell will follow its developmental program if it is explanted but can still be reprogrammed to a different fate if it is transplanted to a different part of the embryo.

Specificity   In diagnostic tests, the frequency with which a test result is negative when the disease is absent.

Spectral karyotyping (SKY)   A procedure that uses the fluorescence in situ hybridization (FISH) technique to stain each of the 24 human chromosomes distinctively.

Splicing   The splicing out of introns and splicing together of exons in the generation of mature mRNA from the primary transcript.

Sporadic   In medical genetics, a disease that is not the result of inheritance of a disease-causing allele from a parent. Often the result of a new germline or somatic mutation.

Stem cell   A type of cell capable both of self-renewal and of proliferation and differentiation.

Stop codon   See *termination codon.*

Stratification   The situation in which a population contains a number of subgroups whose members have not freely and randomly mated with the members of other subgroups.

Structural gene   A gene coding for any RNA or protein product.

Structural protein   A protein that serves a structural role in the body, such as collagen.

Submetacentric   A type of chromosome with arms of different lengths.

Synapsis   Close pairing of homologous chromosomes in prophase of the first meiotic division.

Syndrome   A characteristic pattern of anomalies, presumed to be causally related.

Synpolydactyly   A birth defect of the hands and feet characterized by extra digits and the fusion of adjoining digits.

Synteny   The physical presence together on the same chromosome of two or more gene loci, whether or not they are close enough together for linkage to be demonstrated.

Tag SNPs   A select, minimal subset of all the SNPs in a genomic region, chosen because they are in linkage disequilibrium with one another in the population. Tag SNPs are useful because they form a minimum set of SNPs whose alleles constitute haplotypes capable of representing all the common haplotypes in that region. See *HapMap.*

Tandem repeats   Two or more copies of the same (or similar) DNA sequence arranged in a direct head-to-tail succession along a chromosome.

TATA box   A consensus sequence in the promoter region of many genes that is located about 25 base pairs upstream from the start site of transcription and that determines the start site.

T-cell antigen receptor (TCR)   Genetically coded receptor on the surface of T lymphocytes that specifically recognizes antigen molecules.

Telomerase   A ribonucleoprotein reverse transcriptase that uses its own RNA template to add species-specific hexamers (such as TTAGGG in humans) to telomeres.

Telomere   The end of each chromosome arm. Human telomeres end with tandem copies of the sequence $(TTAGGG)_n$, which is required for the proper replication of chromosome ends.

Telophase   The stage of cell division that begins when the daughter chromosomes reach the poles of the dividing cell and that lasts until the two daughter cells take on the appearance of interphase cells.

Teratogen   An agent that produces congenital malformations or increases their incidence.

Termination codon   One of the three codons (UAG, UAA, and UGA) that terminate synthesis of a polypeptide. Also called a *stop codon*. (See Table 3-1.)

Tertiary structure   Three-dimensional configuration.

Trans   Refers to the relationship between two sequences located across from each other on the two homologous chromosomes, or to interactions between a protein and a chromosome locus. Literally means "across from." Contrast with *cis*.

Transcription   The synthesis of a single-stranded RNA molecule from a DNA template in the cell nucleus, catalyzed by RNA polymerase.

Transcription factor   One of a large class of proteins that regulate transcription by forming large complexes with other transcription factors and RNA polymerase; these complexes then bind to regulatory regions of genes either to promote or to inhibit transcription.

Transfer RNA (tRNA)   See *RNA*.

Transformation   An in vitro phenomenon in which certain cell lines, such as cancer cells, are able to grow indefinitely in culture. More generally, the process in vivo by which a normal cell in a tissue becomes a cancerous cell.

Transition mutation   Substitution of one purine for another purine or one pyrimidine for another pyrimidine.

Translation   The synthesis of a polypeptide from its mRNA template.

Translocation   The transfer of a segment of one chromosome to another chromosome. If two nonhomologous chromosomes exchange pieces, the translocation is *reciprocal*. See also *Robertsonian translocation*.

Transversion   A mutation caused by substitution of a purine for a pyrimidine or vice versa.

Triploid   A cell with three copies of each chromosome, or an individual made up of such cells.

Trisomy   The state of having three representatives of a given chromosome instead of the usual pair, as in trisomy 21 (Down syndrome).

tRNA   Transfer RNA; see *RNA*.

Tumor-suppressor gene   A normal gene involved in the regulation of cell proliferation, in which recessive mutations can lead to tumor development, as in the retinoblastoma gene or the p53 gene. Contrast with *oncogene*.

Two-hit model   The hypothesis that some forms of cancer can be initiated when both alleles of a tumor-suppressor gene become inactivated in the same cell.

Ultrasonography   A technique in which high-frequency sound waves are used to examine internal body structures; useful in prenatal diagnosis.

Uniparental disomy   The presence in the karyotype of two copies of a specific chromosome, both inherited from one parent, with no representative of that chromosome from the other parent. If both homologues of the parental pair are present, the situation is *heterodisomy*; if one parental homologue is present in duplicate, the situation is *isodisomy*. See *Prader-Willi syndrome* and *Angelman syndrome* in the text.

Unstable repeat expansion disorders   Diseases that occur when a gene contains tandemly repeating units of a few nucleotides and the number of such units increases beyond a threshold and interferes with the expression or function of that gene. Most commonly, the nucleotide unit involved in the expansion contains three nucleotides (*triplet repeat expansion*), as with CAG in Huntington disease or CGG in fragile X syndrome.

Vector   In molecular genetics, the DNA molecule into which a gene or DNA fragment has been cloned, capable of replicating in a specific host and thereby replicating the cloned DNA segment as well. Vectors include plasmids, bacteriophage lambda, cosmids, both bacterial and yeast artificial chromosomes, and viruses.

VNTR (variable number of tandem repeats)   A type of DNA polymorphism created by a tandem arrangement of multiple copies of short DNA sequences. Highly polymorphic, used in linkage studies and in DNA "fingerprinting" for paternity testing and forensic medicine.

Western blotting   A technique analogous to Southern blotting, used for the detection of proteins, usually by immunological methods.

Wild-type   A term used to indicate the normal allele (often symbolized as +) or the normal phenotype.

X;autosome translocation   Reciprocal translocation between an X chromosome and an autosome.

X inactivation   Inactivation of genes on one X chromosome in somatic cells of female mammals, occurring early in embryonic life, at about the time of implantation. See *lyonization.*

X linkage   The distinctive inheritance pattern of alleles at loci on the X chromosome that do not undergo recombination (crossing over) during male meiosis.

Y linkage   Genes on the Y chromosome, or traits determined by such genes, are Y-linked.

Zinc finger proteins   One class of transcription factor proteins containing loop-shaped tandem repeating segments that bind zinc atoms.

Zygosity   The number of zygotes from which a multiple birth is derived. For example, twins may be either monozygotic (MZ) or dizygotic (DZ). To determine whether a certain pair of twins is MZ or DZ is to determine their zygosity.

Zygote   A fertilized ovum.

Answers to Problems

Chapter 2   The Human Genome and the Chromosomal Basis of Heredity

1. (a) *A* and *a*.   (b) i. At meiosis I. ii. At meiosis II.
2. Meiotic nondisjunction.
3. $(1/2)^{23} \times (1/2)^{23}$; you would be female.
4. (a) 23; 46.   (b) 23; 23.
   (c) At fertilization; at S phase of the next cell cycle.
5. Chromosome 1, ~9 genes/Mb; chromosome 13, ~3-4 genes/Mb; chromosome 18, ~4 genes/Mb; chromosome 19, ~19 genes/Mb; chromosome 21, ~5 genes/Mb; chromosome 22, ~10 genes/Mb. Because of the higher density of genes, one would expect that a chromosome abnormality of chromosome 19 would have a greater impact on phenotype than an abnormality of chromosome 18. Similarly, chromosome 22 defects are expected to be more deleterious than those of chromosome 21.

Chapter 3   The Human Genome: Gene Structure and Function

1. There are several possible sequences because of the degeneracy of the genetic code. One possible sequence of the double-stranded DNA is
   5′ AAA AGA CAT CAT TAT CTA 3′
   3′ TTT TCT GTA GTA ATA GAT 5′
   RNA polymerase "reads" the bottom (3′ to 5′) strand. The sequence of the resulting mRNA would be 5′ AAA AGA CAU CAU UAU CUA 3′.
      The mutants represent the following kinds of mutations:
   Mutant 1: single nucleotide substitution in fifth codon; for example, UAU → UGU.
   Mutant 2: frameshift mutation, deletion in first nucleotide of third codon.
   Mutant 3: frameshift mutation, insertion of G between first and second codons.
   Mutant 4: in-frame deletion of three codons (nine nucleotides), beginning at the third base.
2. The sequence of the human haploid genome consists of nearly 3 billion nucleotides, organized into 24 types of human chromosome. Chromosomes contain chromatin, consisting of nucleosomes. Chromosomes contain G bands that contain several thousand kilobase pairs of DNA (or several million base pairs) and hundreds of genes, each containing (usually) both introns and exons. The exons are a series of codons, each of which is three base pairs in length. Each gene contains a promoter at its 5′ end that directs transcription of the gene under appropriate conditions.

3. A mutation in a promoter could interfere with or eliminate transcription of the gene. Mutation of the initiator codon would prevent normal translation. Mutations at splice sites can interfere with the normal process of RNA splicing, leading to abnormal mRNAs. A 1 bp deletion in the coding sequence would lead to a frameshift mutation, thus changing the frame in which the genetic code is read; this would alter the encoded amino acids and change the sequence of the protein. (See examples in Chapter 11.) A mutation in the stop codon would allow translation to continue beyond its normal stopping point, thus adding new, incorrect amino acids to the end of the encoded protein.

4. Mutations in introns can influence RNA splicing, thus leading to an abnormally spliced mRNA (see Chapter 11). *Alu* or L1 sequences can be involved in abnormal recombination events between different copies of the repeat, thus deleting or rearranging genes. L1 repeats can also actively transpose around the genome, potentially inserting into a functional gene and disrupting its normal function. Locus control regions influence the proper expression of genes in time and space; deletion of a locus control region can thus disrupt normal expression of a gene (see Chapter 11). Pseudogenes are, generally, nonfunctional copies of genes; thus, in most instances, mutations in a pseudogene would not be expected to contribute to disease.

5. RNA splicing generates a mature RNA from the primary RNA transcript by combining segments of exonic RNA and eliminating RNA from introns. RNA splicing is a critical step in normal gene expression in all tissues of the body and operates at the level of RNA. Thus, the genomic DNA is unchanged. In contrast, in somatic rearrangement, segments of genomic DNA are rearranged to eliminate certain sequences and generate mature genes during lymphocyte precursor cell development, as part of the normal process of generating immunoglobulin and T-cell receptor diversity. Somatic rearrangement is a

highly specialized process, specific only to these genes and specific cell types.

Chapter 4 Tools of Human Molecular Genetics

1. (a) Southern blot or polymerase chain reaction (PCR) of DNA obtained from chorionic villus sampling or amniotic fluid cell sample. In either case, Southern blot or PCR of another locus must be done simultaneously to make sure that failure to obtain a hybridization signal (Southern blot) or an amplified product (PCR) was caused by the deletion and not by technical difficulties with the DNA sample or the procedure used.
   (b) Northern blot or quantitative PCR.
   (c) Many laboratories would simply amplify the segment and sequence it. An alternative is allele-specific oligonucleotide analysis of a PCR product that spans the segment of DNA containing the base change; or, if the base change creates or destroys a restriction enzyme recognition site, you can use restriction digestion of the PCR product that spans the segment containing the mutation to determine whether the mutation is present.

2. The chief advantage of PCR is that much less DNA is required for an analysis than that required in Southern blotting. In addition, PCR is much faster and less expensive. A potential disadvantage is that PCR can "see" only relatively short stretches of genomic DNA (in each assay), whereas Southern blotting can "examine" an entire gene. PCR is also much more sensitive to contamination by extraneous DNA. In comparison with biochemical assays, PCR has the same advantage of speed. However, biochemical testing is a functional assay that can detect a range of mutations at a locus (including any unknown mutation that interferes with enzyme activity). PCR is best suited to examination of specific, known mutations.

3. All except red blood cells. However, even samples of red blood cells or serum may contain enough DNA from contaminating white blood cells that testing could be done by PCR because PCR is so sensitive.

4. Establishes the gene responsible for a given disorder; may demonstrate allelic and locus heterogeneity; provides immediate tools for diagnosis and genetic counseling; provides opportunity to determine the molecular basis of a disorder, through extensive laboratory research; could be used to design gene replacement therapy; may highlight a physiological pathway that could be manipulated with medication or diet and thereby ameliorate or prevent the condition.

5. (a) A C to T transition converting an arginine codon to a stop codon, resulting in premature termination.

(b) Oligonucleotides 2, 3, and 4 would be usable. Oligonucleotide 1 is specific for the mutant sequence, but the mismatch with the normal sequence would occur at the next to last base. It would be difficult to establish hybridization conditions such that this oligonucleotide would hybridize stably to the mutant but not the normal sequence. Oligonucleotide 2 is specific for the normal sequence. By placement of the base that is mutated in the center, it is easy to design conditions such that this oligonucleotide will form a stable duplex with the normal sequence but not the mutant. Oligonucleotide 3 is specific for the mutant sequence and would be an excellent discriminator between normal and mutant sequences. Oligonucleotide 4 is specific for the mutant sequence but would hybridize to the strand complementary to the one shown here and would serve to discriminate between normal and mutant. Oligonucleotide 5 is too short for there to be conditions that would allow discrimination between normal and mutant sequences.

Chapter 5 Principles of Clinical Cytogenetics

1. (a) Forty-six chromosomes, male; one of the chromosome 18's has a shorter long arm than is normal.
   (b) To determine whether the abnormality is de novo or inherited from a balanced carrier parent.
   (c) Forty-six chromosomes, male, only one normal 7 and one normal 18, plus a reciprocal translocation between chromosomes 7 and 18. This is a balanced karyotype. For meiotic pairing and segregation, see text, particularly Figure 5-12.
   (d) The del(18q) chromosome is the der(18) translocation chromosome, 18pter → 18q12::7q35 → 7qter. The boy's karyotype is unbalanced; he is monosomic for the distal long arm of 18 and trisomic for the distal long arm of 7. Given the number of genes on chromosomes 7 and 18 (see Fig. 2-8), one would predict that the boy is monosomic for about 100 genes on chromosome 18 and trisomic for about 100 genes on chromosome 7.

2. (a) About 95%.
   (b) No increased risk, but prenatal diagnosis may be offered.

3. Postzygotic nondisjunction, in an early mitotic division. Although the clinical course cannot be predicted with complete accuracy, it is likely that she will be somewhat less severely affected than would a nonmosaic trisomy 21 child.

4. (a) Abnormal phenotype, unless the marker is exceptionally small and restricted only to the centromeric sequences themselves. Gametes may be normal or abnormal; prenatal diagnosis indicated.

(b) Abnormal phenotype (trisomy 13; see Chapter 6); will not reproduce.

(c) Abnormal phenotype in proband and approximately 50% of offspring.

(d) Normal phenotype, but risk for unbalanced offspring (see text).

(e) Normal phenotype, but risk for unbalanced offspring, depending on the size of the inverted segment (see text).

5. (a) Not indicated.

(b) Fetal karyotyping indicated; at risk for trisomy 21, in particular.

(c) Karyotype indicated for child to determine whether it is trisomy 21 or translocation Down syndrome. If it is translocation, parental karyotypes are indicated.

(d) Not indicated, unless other clinical findings might suggest a contiguous gene syndrome (see Chapter 6).

(e) Karyotype indicated for the boys to rule out deletion or other chromosomal abnormality. If clinical findings indicate possibility of fragile X mental retardation, a specific DNA diagnostic test would be indicated.

6. (a) Paracentric inversion of the X chromosome, between bands Xq21 and Xq26, determined by karyotyping.

(b) Terminal deletion of 1p in a female, determined by karyotyping.

(c) Female with deletion within band q11.2 of chromosome 15, determined by in situ hybridization with probes for the *SNRPN* gene and D15S10 locus.

(d) Female with interstitial deletion of chromosome 15, between bands q11 and q13, determined by karyotyping. In situ hybridization analysis confirmed deletion of sequences within 15q11.2, with use of probes for the *SNRPN* gene and D15S10 locus.

(e) Female with deletion of sequences in band 1q36.3, determined by array CGH with the three BAC probes indicated.

(f) Male with duplicated sequences within Xq28, determined by in situ hybridization with a probe for the *MECP2* gene.

(g) Male with an extra marker chromosome, determined by karyotyping. Marker was identified as an r(8) chromosome by in situ hybridization with a probe for D8Z1 at the centromere.

(h) Female with Down syndrome, with a 13q;21q Robertsonian translocation in addition to two normal chromosome 21's, determined by karyotyping.

(i) Presumably normal male carrier of a 13q;21q Robertsonian translocation, in addition to a single normal chromosome 21 (and a single normal chromosome 13), as determined by karyotyping.

7. For Figure 5-5: *top*, 46,XX arr cgh 1-22(#BACs) × 2,X(#BACs) × 2,Y(#BACs)0; *bottom*, 47,XY, + 18 arr cgh 18(BAC names) × 3.

For Figure 5-9: **A,** arr cgh 12p(BAC name ← BAC name) × 3; **B,** arr cgh 1p36.2(BAC names) × 1; **C,** arr cgh 7q22(BAC names) × 1.

Chapter 6   Clinical Cytogenetics: Disorders of the Autosomes and the Sex Chromosomes

1. Theoretically, X and XX gametes in equal proportions; expected XX, XY, XXX, and XXY offspring (25% each). In actuality, XXX women have virtually all chromosomally normal offspring, XX and XY, implying that XX gametes are at a significant disadvantage or are lost.

2. (a) To determine whether presence of an X-linked recessive disorder in the girl is due to a chromosome defect (such as an X;autosome translocation or 45,X Turner syndrome), to the presence of a condition (such as androgen insensitivity) allowing a female phenotype in an XY person, or to homozygosity or nonrandom X inactivation in a 46,XX individual. See text.

(b) The break probably disrupts one copy of the hemophilia A (*F8*) gene; the normal X, as is usual with this type of translocation, is preferentially inactivated in most or all cells. See Figure 6-16.

3. No. XYY can result only from meiosis II nondisjunction in the male, whereas XXY can result from nondisjunction at meiosis I in the male or at either division in the female.

4. Translocation of Y chromosome material containing the sex-determining region (and the *SRY* gene) to the X chromosome or to an autosome.

5. 46,XY; androgen insensitivity (testicular feminization); the mother or child may be the result of a de novo mutation, but if the mother is heterozygous, the usual X-linked risks apply.

6. 46,XX; autosomal recessive; prenatal diagnosis possible; need for clinical attention in neonatal period to determine sex and to forestall salt-losing crises.

7. (a) None; the short arms of all acrocentric chromosomes are believed to be identical and contain multiple copies of rRNA genes.

(b) None if the deletion involves only heterochromatin (Yq12). A more proximal deletion might delete genes important in spermatogenesis (see Fig. 6-10).

(c) Cri du chat syndrome, severity depending on the amount of DNA deleted (see Fig. 6-7B).

(d) Some features of Turner syndrome, but with normal stature; the Xq⁻ chromosome is preferentially inactivated in all cells (provided that the X inactivation center is not deleted), thus reducing the potential severity of such a deletion.

Different parts of the genome contain different density of genes. Thus, deletion of the same amount of DNA on different chromosomes might delete a vastly different number of genes, thus leading to different phenotypic expectations (see Fig. 2-8).

8. Question for discussion. See text for possible explanations.

9. (a) A 1% risk is often quoted, but the risk is probably not greater than the population age-related risk.

   (b) Age-related risk is greater than 1%.

   (c) No increased risk if the niece with Down syndrome has trisomy 21; but if the niece carries a Robertsonian translocation, the consultand may be a carrier and at high risk.

   (d) 10% to 15%; see text.

   (e) Only a few percent; see text. The woman's age-related risk may be relevant.

10. 46,XX,rob(21;21)(q10;q10) or 46,XX,der(21;21)(q10;q10). (There is no need to add +21 to the karyotype, since the 46 designates that she must have a normal 21 in addition to the translocation.)

Chapter 7   Patterns of Single-Gene Inheritance

1. (b) Autosomal recessive; 1/4.

   (c) Calvin and Cathy are obligatory heterozygotes. Given that Calvin and Cathy are first cousins, it is also very likely that they inherited their mutant allele through Betty and Barbara from the same grandparent. Thus, Betty and Barbara are very likely to be carriers, but it is not obligatory. It is theoretically possible that Cathy inherited her CF allele from Bob and that Calvin inherited his from his father, Barbara's husband. DNA-based carrier testing will answer the question definitively.

2. (a) Heterozygous at each of two loci; for example, *A/a B/b*.

(b) The parents (Gilbert and Gisele, Horace and Hedy) are all homozygous for the *same* recessive allele for congenital deafness.

3. Variable expressivity—d; uniparental disomy—i; consanguinity—j; inbreeding—c; X-linked dominant inheritance—g; new mutation—e; allelic heterogeneity—h; locus heterogeneity—a; homozygosity for an autosomal dominant trait—b; pleiotropy—f.

4. (b) They are homozygous.

   (c) 100%; virtually zero if Elise's partner is unaffected.

   (d) 50%; virtually zero if Enid's partner is unaffected.

5. All are possible except (c), which is unlikely if the parents are completely unaffected.

6. (a) New mutation.   (b) Mutation rate.

   (c) Mutation rate.   (d) 50%.

7. The consultand and her partner are first cousins once removed. The simplest way to calculate coefficient of inbreeding, F, in simple pedigrees like this is the path method, in which one determines all the paths by which an allele from a common ancestor can be transmitted to the individual whose coefficient of inbreeding one is seeking to calculate.

   Form all the paths connecting all the pertinent individuals in this pedigree (see figure below). Each path that gives a closed loop is a consanguineous path. There are two closed loops: A-D-H-K-L-I-E-A and B-D-H-K-L-I-E-B. To calculate F, count all the "nodes" (the dots representing each of the individuals) in each of the closed loops, counting each node only once. Call that n. The coefficient of inbreeding due to that loop is then given by $(1/2)^{n-1}$. So, in this example, the loop A-D-H-K-L-I-E-A contains 7 unique nodes, n = 7. Add all the coefficients for each loop together to find F. For the pedigree, then:

   $(1/2)^{n-1} = (1/2)^6 = 1/64$ for loop A-D-H-K-L-I-E-A
   $(1/2)^{n-1} = (1/2)^6 = 1/64$ for loop B-D-H-K-L-I-E-B
   and F = 1/32

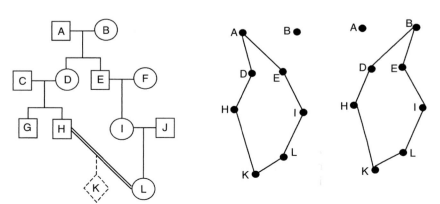

Figure for answering question 7, Chapter 7.

8. AD is most likely. Vertical transmission, including male to male, from generation to generation, males and females affected.

AR and XR are possible but unlikely. AR would require that both of the spouses of the two affected individuals in generations I and II be carriers, which is unlikely unless the pedigree comes from a genetic isolate (so-called pseudodominant inheritance of a recessive disorder due to high frequency of carriers in the population). XR would require that the same two women be carriers and, in addition, that there be something unusual in the X inactivation pattern for the female in generation III to be affected while neither of the females in generation II (who are both obligatory carriers) is affected.

Mitochondrial and XD inheritance are incompatible. There is male-to-male transmission, which eliminates both of these modes of inheritance. In addition, there are female offspring of affected males who are not affected.

Chapter 8   Genetics of Common Disorders with Complex Inheritance

1. (a) Autosomal dominant with reduced penetrance. If it were truly multifactorial, the risk for more distantly related relatives would drop by more than 50%.
   (b) In dominant disease, you would expect no increase in risk after an affected person has had two affected children. In multifactorial inheritance, the risk after two affected children would be greater than after only one affected child because, with two affected, there is a greater likelihood that the parents are carrying a significant load of predisposing alleles at multiple loci; see text.
2. Male-to-male transmission can disprove X-linkage; other criteria of multifactorial inheritance can be examined, as in the text.
3. For autosomal recessive but not for multifactorial inheritance, there is very little chance that a parent will be affected unless the families come from an inbred population where "pseudodominant" inheritance may occur; for other criteria, see text.

Chapter 9   Genetic Variation in Individuals and Populations: Mutation and Polymorphism

1. Assuming 20 years is one generation, 41 mutations/9 million alleles/2 generations = ~2.3×10^{-6} mutations/generation at the aniridia locus. The estimate is based on assumptions that ascertained cases result from new mutation, that the disease is fully penetrant, that all new mutants are liveborn (and ascertained), and that there is only a single locus at which mutations can lead to aniridia. If there are multiple loci, the estimated rate is too

high. If some mutations are not ascertained (because of lack of penetrance or death in utero), the estimated rate might be too low.

2. Chances are greater that the mother is a heterozygote by virtue of her having received a new mutation in the X chromosome she received from her father. As you will see in Chapter 19, if male and female mutation rates are equal in an X-linked genetic lethal condition, you would expect two thirds of the mothers of an isolated affected male to be carriers. However, if point mutations are much more likely in the male germline, she will have a >90% chance of being a carrier.

3. One way of determining this is to reverse the question and ask instead what proportion of individuals would be *homozygous*. Then the proportion who are heterozygous is 1 minus the proportion who are homozygous. For each allele, the frequency of homozygotes would be 0.20×0.20, or 0.04. Thus, 5×0.04, or 20%, of individuals would be homozygous for allele 1 *or* allele 2 *or* . . . allele 5. Therefore, 80% of individuals would be heterozygous at this locus.

4. Yes; greater during subsequent pregnancies; disease can be prevented by use of antibodies to Rh D (RhoGAM) to clear the maternal circulation of Rh-positive blood cells before they can elicit a primary immune response; if the man is also Rh-negative, the child would have to be Rh-negative, and no hemolytic disease would occur.

5. $q = 0.26$, $p = 0.74$, $p^2 = 0.55$, $2pq = 0.38$, $q^2 = 0.07$
   Frequency of $Rh-/-$ genotype in mother = 7%. Frequency of $Rh+/+$ in father = 55%. Frequency of $Rh+/-$ in father = 38%.
   First pregnancy:
   All matings of $Rh-/-$ mother $\times$ $Rh +/+$ father will sensitize = $0.07 \times 0.55 = 3.8\%$.
   Expect half of matings of $Rh-/-$ mother by $Rh+/-$ father will sensitize = $0.07 \times 0.38 \times 1/2 = 1.3\%$.
   Total at risk for sensitization = 5.1%.

   Second pregnancy:
   All second pregnancies of sensitized $Rh-/-$ mother $\times$ $Rh+/+$ father are at risk for Rh incompatibility = 3.8%.
   Expect half of the pregnancies of sensitized $Rh-/-$ mother by $Rh+/-$ father will be at risk for Rh incompatibility = $1.3\% \times 1/2 = 0.65\%$.
   Total at risk for incompatibility = 4.45%.

6. (a) a, 0.1; A, 0.9.   (b) Same.   (c) $(0.18)^2$.
7. (a) 0.02.
   (b) $(0.04)^2$ or about 1 in 600 (homozygotes do not reproduce).   (c) 0.0004.   (d) 1/4.
8. Only (d) is in equilibrium. Selection for or against particular genotypes; nonrandom mating; recent migration.

9. (a) Abby has a 2/3 chance of being a carrier. Andrew has about a 1/150 chance of being a carrier. Therefore, their risk of having an affected child is $2/3 \times 1/150 \times 1/4$, or 1/900.

(b) $2/3 \times 1/4 \times 1/4 = 1/24$.

(c) $2/3 \times 1/22 \times 1/4 = 1/132$; $2/3 \times 1/4 \times 1/4 = 1/24$.

10. (a) Facioscapulohumeral muscular dystrophy: $q = 1/50,000$, $2pq = 1/25,000$. Friedreich ataxia: $q = 1/158$, $2pq = 1/79$. Duchenne muscular dystrophy is X-linked recessive and occurs mostly in males, so we will ignore any of the rare females affected. If it occurs in the population at a frequency of 1 in 25,000, then, assuming half of the population is male, the frequency in males must be 1 in 12,500, so $q = 1/12,500$, $2pq = 1/6,250$.

(b) The autosomal dominant and X-linked disorders would increase rapidly, within one generation, to reach a new balance. The autosomal recessive disorders would increase also, but only very slowly, because the majority of the mutant alleles are not subject to selection.

11. Approximately 1/26 and 1/316.

Chapter 10   Human Gene Mapping and Disease Gene Identification

1. The HD and MNSs loci map far enough apart on chromosome 4 to be unlinked, even though they are syntenic.

2. The LOD scores indicate that this polymorphism is closely linked to the polycystic kidney disease gene. The peak LOD score, 25.85, occurs at 5 cM. The odds in favor of linkage at this distance compared with no linkage at all are $10^{25.85}:1$ (i.e., almost $10^{26}:1$). The data in the second study indicate that there is *no* linkage between the disease gene and the polymorphism in this family. Thus, there is genetic heterogeneity in this disorder, and linkage information can therefore be used for diagnosis only if there is previous evidence that the disease in that particular family is linked to the polymorphism.

3. Every parent who passed on the cataract was also informative at the γ-crystallin locus, that is, was heterozygous for the polymorphic alleles at this locus. The phase is known by inspecting the pedigree in individuals IV-7 and IV-8 since these two individuals received both the cataract allele and the A allele at the γ-crystallin locus from their father (but note, we do not know what the phase was in the father simply by inspection). We do not know the phase in individuals IV-3 or IV-4 because we do not know if they inherited the cataract mutation along with the A or the B allele at the γ-crystallin locus from their mother. Phase is also known in individuals V-1, V-2, V-6, and V-7. The cataract seems to co-segregate with the "A" haplotype. There

are no crossovers. A complete LOD score analysis should be performed. In addition, one might examine the γ-crystallin gene itself for mutations in affected persons since it would be a reasonable candidate for being the gene in which mutations could cause cataracts.

4. (a) The phase in the mother is probably B/WAS, according to the genotype of the affected boy. This phase can be determined with only 95% certainty because there is a 5% chance that a crossover occurred in the meiosis leading to the affected boy. On the basis of this information, there is a $(0.95 \times 0.95) + (0.05 \times 0.05) = 0.9045$ chance that the fetus (who is male) will be *unaffected*.

(b) This surprising result (assuming paternity is as stated) indicates that the mother has inherited the A allele (and the WAS allele) from her mother and her phase is A/WAS, not B/WAS. Thus, there must have been a crossover in the meiosis leading to the affected boy. To confirm this, one should examine polymorphisms on either side of this one on the X chromosome to make sure that the segregation patterns are consistent with a crossover. On the basis of this new information, there is now a 95% chance that the fetus in the current pregnancy is *affected*.

5. Discovery of the gene has made specific, accurate diagnosis by DNA testing, including prenatal diagnosis, and carrier detection possible for most families. Knowledge of the allelic variation that causes Duchenne and Becker dystrophy allows better prognosis for management and counseling. Continued research on which proteins interact with dystrophin has revealed a whole new set of muscle proteins whose members have been shown to carry mutations in other forms of muscular dystrophies (particularly of the limb-girdle type) that were of unknown etiology before the discovery of their interaction with dystrophin (see Chapter 12). Discovery of the gene has also led to increasing efforts at gene replacement as a treatment. Unfortunately, no successful therapy has yet emerged. The NOD2 variants are less likely to provide substantial diagnostic help since having the predisposing gene variant is not necessary or sufficient for development of Crohn disease. For example, a patient in whom you suspect Crohn disease might very well have the disorder without carrying the NOD2 variant. The impact of knowing about NOD2 is likely to be in the area of expanding our knowledge of the pathogenesis and suggesting novel therapies for this disorder.

6. The risk estimates are just that, estimates, that are based on measures that have uncertainty. It is important also to keep in mind that there may be substantial differences in which genes contribute the most to AMD in different ethnic groups and in different environments, and so one should not assume one

can generalize findings that are for the most part obtained from white populations to the entire world.

Chapter 11   Principles of Molecular Disease: Lessons from the Hemoglobinopathies

1. The pedigree should contain the following information: Hydrops fetalis is due to a total absence of α chains. The parents each must have the genotype αα/– –. The α– genotype is common in some populations, including Melanesians. Parents with this genotype cannot transmit a – –/– – genotype to their offspring.

2. Except in isolated populations, patients with β-thalassemia will often be genetic compounds because there are usually many alleles present in a population in which β-thalassemia is common. In isolated populations, the chance that a patient is a true homozygote of a single allele is greater than it would be in a population in which thalassemia is rare. In the latter group, more "private mutations" might be expected (ones found solely or almost solely in a single pedigree). A patient is more likely to have identical alleles if he or she belongs to a geographical isolate with a high frequency of a single allele or a few alleles, or if his or her parents are consanguineous. See text in Chapter 7.

3. Three bands on the RNA blot could indicate, among other possibilities, that (a) one allele is producing two mRNAs, one normal in size and the other abnormal, and the other allele is producing one mRNA of abnormal size; (b) both alleles are making a normal-sized transcript and an abnormal transcript, but the aberrant ones are of different sizes; or (c) one allele is producing three mRNAs of different size, and the other allele is making no transcripts.

    Scenario (c) is highly improbable, if possible at all. Two mRNAs from a single allele could result from a splicing defect that allows the normal mRNA to be made, but at reduced efficiency, while leading to the synthesis of another transcript of abnormal size, which results from either the incorporation of intron sequences in the mRNA or the loss of exon sequences from the mRNA. In this case, the other abnormal band comes from the other allele. A larger band from the other allele could result from a splicing defect or an insertion, whereas a smaller band could be due to a splicing defect or a deletion. Hb E is caused by an allele from which both a normal and a shortened transcript are made (see Fig. 11-12); the normal mRNA makes up 40% of the total β-globin mRNA, producing only a mild anemia.

4. These two mutations affect different globin chains. The expected offspring are 1/4 normal, 1/4 Hb M Saskatoon heterozygotes with methemoglobine-

mia, 1/4 Hb M Boston heterozygotes with methemoglobinemia, and 1/4 double heterozygotes with four hemoglobin types: normal, both types of Hb M, and a type with abnormalities in both chains. In the double heterozygotes, the clinical consequences are unknown—probably more severe methemoglobinemia.

5. $2/3 \times 2/3 \times 1/4 = 1/9$.

6. 1/4.

7. 8, 1, 2, 7, 10, 4, 9, 5, 6, and 3.

8. Exceptions to this rule can arise, for example, from splice site mutations that lead to the mis-splicing of an exon. The exon may be excluded from the mRNA, generating an in-frame deletion of the protein sequence or causing a change in the reading frame, leading to the inclusion of different amino acids in the protein sequence.

9. About two thirds of the couples to whom such infants were born did not know about thalassemia or the prevention programs. About 20% refused abortion, and false paternity was identified in 13% of cases.

Chapter 12   The Molecular, Biochemical, and Cellular Basis of Genetic Disease

1. Three types of mutations could explain a mutant protein that is 50 kilodaltons larger than the normal polypeptide:

    A mutation in the normal stop codon that allows translation to continue.

    A splice mutation that results in the inclusion of intron sequences in the coding region. The intron sequences would have to be free of stop codons for sufficient length to allow the extra 50 kilodaltons of translation.

    An insertion, with an open reading frame, into the coding sequence.

    For any of these, approximately 500 extra residues would be added to the protein, if the average molecular weight of an amino acid is about 100. Five hundred amino acids would be encoded by 1500 nucleotides.

2. A nucleotide substitution that changes one amino acid residue to another should be termed a *putative pathogenic mutation*, and possibly a *polymorphism*, unless (a) it has been demonstrated, through a functional assay of the protein, that the change impairs the function to a degree consistent with the phenotype of the patient or (b) instead of or in addition to a functional assay, it can be demonstrated that the nucleotide change is found *only* on mutant chromosomes, which can be identified by haplotype analysis in the population of patients and their parents and *not* on normal chromosomes in this population.

The fact that the nucleotide change is only rarely observed in the normal population and found with significantly higher frequency in a mutant population is strong supportive evidence but not proof that the substitution is a pathogenic mutation.

3. If Johnny has CF, the chances are about 0.85×0.85, or 70%, that he has a previously described mutation that could be readily identified by DNA analysis. His parents are from northern Europe; therefore, the probability that he is homozygous for the ΔF508 mutation is 0.7×0.7, or 50%, because about 70% of CF carriers in northern Europe have this mutation. If he does not have the ΔF508 mutation, he could certainly still have CF, because about 30% of the alleles (in the northern European population, at least) are not ΔF508. Steps to DNA diagnosis for CF include the following: (a) look directly for the ΔF508 mutation; if it is not present, (b) look for other mutations common in the specific population; (c) then look directly for other mutations based on probabilities suggested by the haplotype data; (d) if all efforts to identify a mutation fail (or if time does not allow), perform linkage analysis with polymorphic DNA markers closely linked to CF.

4. James may have a new mutation on the X chromosome because Joe inherited the same X chromosome from his mother, and the deletion was present in neither Joe nor his mother. If this is the case, there is no risk of recurrence. Alternatively, the mother may be a mosaic, and the mosaicism includes her germline. In this case, there is a definite risk that the mutant X could be inherited by another son or passed to a carrier daughter. About 5% to 15% of cases of this type appear to be due to maternal germline mosaicism. Thus, the risk is half of this figure for her male offspring because the chance that a son will inherit the mutant X is $1/2 \times 5\%$ to $15\% = 2.5\%$ to 7.5%.

5. For DMD, as a classic X-linked recessive disease that is lethal in males, one third of cases are predicted to be new mutations. The large size of the gene is likely to account for the high mutation rate at this locus (i.e., it is a large target for mutation). The ethnic origin of the patient will have no effect on either of these phenomena.

6. The limited number of amino acids that have been observed to substitute for glycine in collagen mutants reflects the nature of the genetic code. Single nucleotide substitutions at the three positions of the glycine codons allow only a limited number of missense mutations. See Table 3-1.

7. Two bands of G6PD on electrophoresis of a red cell lysate (see Chapter 18) indicate that the woman has a different *G6PD* allele on each X chromosome and that each allele is being expressed in her red cell population. However, no single cell expresses both alleles, because of X inactivation. Males have only a single X chromosome and thus express only one *G6PD* allele. A female with two bands could have two normal alleles with different electrophoretic mobility, one normal allele and one mutant allele with different electrophoretic mobility, or two mutant alleles with different electrophoretic mobility. Because the two common deficiency alleles (A^- and B^-) migrate to the same position as the common normal-activity alleles (A and B), the woman is unlikely to have a common deficiency allele at both loci. Apart from that, one cannot say much about the possible pathological significance of the two bands without measuring the enzymatic activity. If one of the alleles has low activity, she would be at risk for hemolysis to the extent that the high-activity allele is inactivated as a result of X inactivation.

8. The box in Chapter 12 entitled "Enzyme Deficiencies and Disease" lists the possible causes of loss of multiple enzyme activities: they may share a cofactor whose synthesis or transport is defective; they may share a subunit encoded by the mutant gene; they may be processed by a common enzyme whose activity is critical to their becoming active; or they may normally be located in the same organelle, and a defect in the organelle's biological processes can affect all four enzymes. For example, they may not be imported normally into the organelle and may be degraded in the cytoplasm. Almost all enzymopathies are recessive (see text), and most genes are autosomal.

9. Haploinsufficiency. Thus, in some situations, the contributions of both alleles are required to provide a sufficient amount of protein to prevent disease. An example of haploinsufficiency is provided by heterozygous carriers of LDL receptor deficiency.

10. This situation is well illustrated by diseases due to mutations in mtDNA or in the nuclear genome that impair the function of the oxidative phosphorylation complex. Nearly all cells have mitochondria, and therefore oxidative phosphorylation occurs in nearly all cells, yet the phenotypes associated with defects in oxidative phosphorylation damage only a subset of organs, particularly the neuromuscular system with its high energy requirements.

11. One example is phenylketonuria, in which mental retardation is the only significant pathological effect of deficiency of phenylalanine hydroxylase, which is found not in the brain but solely in the liver and kidneys, organs that are unaffected by this biochemical defect. Hypercholesterolemia due to deficiency of the LDL receptor is another example. Although the LDL receptor is found in many cell types, the hepatic deficiency of it is

primarily responsible for the increase in LDL cholesterol levels in blood.

12. There are two defining characteristics of these alleles: the hex A activity that they encode is sufficiently reduced to allow their detection in screening assays (when the other allele is a common Tay-Sachs mutation with virtually no activity); and their hex A activity is nevertheless adequate to prevent the accumulation of the natural substrate (GM$_2$ ganglioside). There are probably only a few substitutions in the hex A protein that would reduce activity to only a modest degree (i.e., without crippling the protein more substantially). Thus, the region of residues 247 to 249 appears to be relatively tolerant of substitutions, at least of Trp for Arg. Substitutions that more dramatically alter the charge or bulk of the residues at these positions may well be disease-causing alleles.

13. A gain-of-function mutation leads to an abnormal increase in the activities performed by the wild-type protein. Consequently, the overall integrity of the protein and each of its functional domains must remain intact despite the gain-of-function mutation. In addition, of course, the mutation must confer the gain of function. Consequently, the mutation must do nothing to disturb the normal properties of the protein and must enhance at least one of them, if not more, to confer the gain of function. Mutations other than missense mutations (e.g., deletions, insertions, premature stops) are almost uniformly highly disruptive to protein structure.

14. As discussed in Chapter 9, the presence of three common alleles for Tay-Sachs disease in the Ashkenazi population seems likely to be due either to a heterozygote advantage or to genetic drift (one form of which is the founder effect). The high frequency of these alleles might also be due to gene flow, although the population of origin of the three common mutations is not apparent, making this explanation seem less likely (in contrast, say, to the evidence indicating that the most common PKU alleles in many populations around the world are of Celtic origin).

15. The two forms of myotonic dystrophy are characterized by an expansion of a CUG trinucleotide in the RNA, which is thought to lead to an RNA-mediated pathogenesis. According to this model, the greatly enhanced number of CUG repeats bind an abnormally large fraction of RNA-binding proteins, including, for example, regulators of splicing, thereby depleting the cell of these critical proteins. One approach to therapy might be to prevent this binding. This might be achieved by introducing, perhaps by gene transfer (see Chapter 13), a viral vector that expresses a GAC trinucleotide repeat, which would bind to the CUG repeat sequences in the RNA and block the binding of the RNA-binding proteins to the expanded CUG repeats. Expression of too large a number of GAC repeat–containing molecules might itself have undesirable side effects, however, including binding to CUG codons that encode leucine, blocking their translation.

Chapter 13   The Treatment of Genetic Disease

1. Unresponsive patients may have mutations that drastically impair the synthesis of a functional gene product. Responsive patients may have mutations in the regulatory region of the gene. The effects of these mutations may be counteracted by the administration of IFN-γ. These mutations could be in the DNA-binding site that responds to the interferon stimulus or in some other regulatory element that participates in the response to IFN-γ. Alternatively, responsive patients may produce a defective cytochrome b polypeptide that retains a small degree of residual function. The production of more of this mutant protein, in response to IFN-γ, increases the oxidase activity slightly but significantly.

2. An enzyme that is normally intracellular can function extracellularly if the substrate is in equilibrium between the intracellular and extracellular fluids and if the product is either nonessential inside the cell or in a similar equilibrium state. Thus, enzymes with substrates and products that do not fit these criteria would not be suitable for this strategy. This approach may not work for phenylalanine hydroxylase because of its need for tetrahydrobiopterin. However, if tetrahydrobiopterin could diffuse freely across the polyethylene glycol layer around the enzyme, the administration of tetrahydrobiopterin orally may suffice. This strategy would not work for storage diseases because the substrate of the enzyme is trapped inside the lysosome. In Lesch-Nyhan syndrome, the most important pathological process is in the brain, and the enzyme in the extracellular fluid would not be able to cross the blood-brain barrier. Tay-Sachs disease could not be treated in this way because of the nondiffusibility of the substrate from the lysosome.

3. Rhonda's mutations prevent the production of any LDL receptor. Thus, the combination of a bile acid–binding resin and a drug (e.g., lovastatin) to inhibit cholesterol synthesis would have no effect in increasing the synthesis of LDL receptors. The boy must have one or two mutant alleles that produce a receptor with some residual function, and the increased expression of these mutant receptors on the surface of the hepatocyte reduces the plasma LDL-bound cholesterol.

4. Unresponsive patients probably have alleles that do not make any protein, that decrease its cellular abundance in some other way (e.g., make an unstable protein), or that disrupt the conformation of the protein so extensively that its pyridoxal-phosphate binding site has no affinity for the cofactor, even at high concentrations. The answer to the second part of this question is less straightforward. The answer given here is based on the generalization that most patients with a rare autosomal recessive disease are likely to have two different alleles, which assumes that there is no mutational hotspot in the gene and that the patients are not descended from a "founder" and are not members of an ethnic group in whom the disease has a high frequency. In this context, Tom is likely to have two alleles that are responsive; first cousins with the same recessive disease are likely to share only one allele, so that Allan is likely to have one responsive allele that he shares with Tom and another allele that is either unresponsive or that responds more poorly to the cofactor than Tom's other allele.

5. (a) You need both a promoter that will allow the synthesis of sufficient levels of the mRNA in the target tissue of choice and the phenylalanine hydroxylase cDNA. In reality, you also need a vector to deliver the "gene" into the cell, but this aspect of the problem has not been dealt with much in the text.
(b) A phenylalanine hydroxylase "gene" will probably be effective in any tissue that has a good blood supply for the delivery of phenylalanine and an adequate source of the cofactor of the enzyme, tetrahydrobiopterin. The promoter would have to be capable of driving transcription in the target tissue chosen for the treatment.
(c) Any mutation that severely reduces the abundance of the protein in the cell but has no effect on transcription. This group includes those mutations that impair translation or that render the protein highly unstable. The thalassemias include examples of all these types.
(d) Liver cells are capable of making tetrahydrobiopterin, whereas other cells may not be. The target cell for the gene transfer should thus be capable of making this cofactor; otherwise, the enzyme will not function unless the cofactor is administered in large amounts.
(e) Human phenylalanine hydroxylase probably exists as a homodimer or homotrimer. In patients whose alleles produce a mutant polypeptide (versus none at all), these alleles may manifest a dominant negative effect on the product of the transferred gene. This effect could be overcome by making a gene construct that produces more of the normal phenylalanine hydroxylase protein (thus diluting out the effect of the mutant polypeptide) or by transferring the gene into a cell type that does not normally express phenylalanine hydroxylase and that would therefore not be subject to the dominant negative effect.

6. One must consider the kinds of mutations that decrease the abundance of a protein but that are associated with residual function. One class of such mutations are those that decrease the abundance of the mRNA but do not alter the protein sequence (i.e., each protein molecule produced has normal activity, but there are fewer molecules). Mutations of this type might include enhancer or promoter mutations, splice mutations, or others that destabilize the mRNA. In this case, one could consider strategies to increase expression from the normal allele and perhaps also the mutant allele, as is done with hereditary angioedema, in which danazol administration increases the expression of the product from both the wild-type and mutant alleles. A second class of such mutations are those within the coding sequence that destabilize the protein but still allow some residual function. Here, a strategy to increase the stability or the function of the mutant protein should be considered. For example, if the affected protein has a cofactor, one could administer increased amounts of the cofactor, provided such an approach would not have unacceptable side effects.

7. Gentamicin can facilitate the skipping of a premature stop codon, allowing the translational apparatus to misincorporate an amino acid that has a codon comparable to that of the mutant termination codon. Although this treatment might allow the synthesis of a protein of normal size, the amino acid that is substituted in place of the premature stop codon may not necessarily allow normal folding, processing, or function of the mutant protein, unless it is the amino acid that is normally located in that position.

Chapter 14   Developmental Genetics and Birth Defects

1. Before determination, an embryo can lose one or more cells, and the remaining cells can undergo specification and ultimately develop into a complete embryo. Once cells are determined, however, mosaic development takes place—an embryonic tissue will follow its developmental program regardless of what happens elsewhere in the embryo. Regulative development means that an embryonic cell can be removed by blastomere biopsy for the purpose of preimplantation diagnosis without harming the rest of the embryo.

2. a–3, b–2, c–4, d–1.

3. a–4, b–3, c–5, d–2, e–1.

4. Mature T or B cells that have somatically rearranged their T-cell receptor or immunoglobulin loci would not be appropriate. This change is not epigenetic; it is a permanent alteration of the DNA sequence itself. Animals derived from a single nucleus from a mature T or B cell are incapable of mounting an appropriately broad immune response.

5. Consider issues of regulation versus simple capacity to carry out a biochemical reaction. Also, consider dominant negative effects of transcription factors, taking into account the frequent binary nature of such factors (DNA-binding and activation domains).

Chapter 15   Prenatal Diagnosis

1. c, e, f, i and j, d, h, g, b, i (and, in part, j), and a.

2. No, the child can have only Down syndrome or monosomy 21, which is almost always lethal. Thus, they should receive counseling and consider other alternatives for having children.

3. No, not necessarily; the problem could be maternal cell contamination.

4. The level of maternal serum alpha-fetoprotein (MSAFP) is typically elevated when the fetus has an open neural tube defect. The levels of MSAFP and unconjugated estriol are usually reduced and the human chorionic gonadotropin is usually elevated when the fetus has Down syndrome.

5. (a) About 15% (see Table 5-5).
   (b) At least 50% are chromosomally abnormal.
   (c) No, prenatal diagnosis or karyotyping of the parents would be indicated only after three such abortions (although some practitioners suggest offering testing after only two), provided there are no other indications, such as advanced maternal age.

6. (a) Yes. The phase can be determined from analysis of her father, who has to have transmitted a normal X chromosome to his daughter, the consultand.
   (b) Yes. A male fetus who receives her father's allele linked to *DMD* will be unaffected. If a male fetus receives her mother's allele linked to *DMD*, it will be affected. This, of course, assumes no recombination in the transmitted chromosome.
   (c) Deletion analysis looking for one of the common deletion mutations.

7. Question for discussion. Consider issues of sensitivity and specificity of each of the different forms of testing, the psychosocial issues of prenatal diagnosis and termination at different stages of pregnancy, and risk of complications of the two invasive methods.

8. 600,000 women, 1000 pregnancies affected.
   Assume everyone is willing to participate in the sequential screening. Of 1000 true positives, first-trimester screening picks up 840 high-risk "posi-

tives" (84%) who undergo CVS; 160 are low risk, and they get a second-trimester screen. Of these 160, 130 (81%) are positive and undergo amniocentesis and are found to have an affected fetus; 30 affected pregnancies are missed.

Of the 599,000 unaffected false positives in the first-trimester screen, 29,950 positives need CVS. The remaining 569,050 are low risk and get a second-trimester screen. You get 28,452 positives in the second-trimester screen who undergo amniocentesis; the remaining 540,598 unaffected pregnancies are reassured.

In summary, with sequential screening, you will detect 970 of the 1000 (97%) and will miss 30 (3%). You will do 970 invasive tests in affected pregnancies while also doing $29,950 + 28,452 = 58,402$ invasive tests in unaffected pregnancies.

You will do 62 invasive tests to detect each affected pregnancy.

This compares to the situation if you just offered invasive testing to everyone. Depending on the uptake, you will miss some fraction of affecteds. If uptake were 97% (very, very unlikely for an invasive test), you would end up doing 582,000 invasive tests to find 970 affected pregnancies. You would miss the same 30 affected pregnancies as with the sequential testing but would have to do a 10 times greater number of invasive tests to achieve the same detection rate.

Chapter 16   Cancer Genetics and Genomics

1. Family history, careful examination of both parents' retinas, cytogenetic analysis if the tumor is associated with other malformations, mutation identification. Advise the parents of the risk, but point out that a future child could be examined immediately after birth and at short intervals for some time to make sure that if tumors develop, they are detected and treated early. The parents should be informed of the risk of disease in subsequent pregnancies, the availability of prenatal diagnosis, and the impact of the disease should it recur.

2. Colorectal cancer seems to require a number of sequential mutations in several genes, a process that may take longer than one (in hereditary) or two (in sporadic) mutations in the retinoblastoma gene. Age dependence may also reflect the number, timing, and rate of cell divisions in colon cells and in retinoblasts.

3. A cell line with i(17q) is monosomic for 17p and trisomic for 17q. Thus, formation of the isochromosome leads to loss of heterozygosity for genes on 17p. This may be particularly important if one or more tumor-suppressor genes (such as *TP53*) are present on 17p. In addition, a number of proto-

oncogenes map to 17q. It is possible that increasing their dosage may confer a growth advantage on cells containing the i(17q).

4. The chief concern is the need to reduce radiation exposure to the lowest possible level because of the risk of cancer in children with this genetic defect.

5. Although most (>95%) breast cancer appears to follow multifactorial inheritance, there are two known genes (*BRCA1* and *BRCA2*) and at least one other suspected locus (*BRCA3*) in which mutations cause autosomal dominant premenopausal breast cancer that may be bilateral. The empirical risk figures are consistent with an overall multifactorial model with admixture of dominant forms of the disease with somewhat reduced lifetime penetrance. Direct mutation detection could be performed if desired by the probands in Wanda's and Wilma's families, and if a mutation were found in *BRCA1* or *BRCA2*, a direct test for cancer risk could be offered to their relatives.

6. It is likely that many activated oncogenes, if inherited in the germline, would disrupt normal development and be incompatible with survival. There are a few rare exceptions, such as activating *RET* mutations in MEN2 and activating *MET* mutations in hereditary papillary kidney cancer. These activated oncogenes must have tissue-specific oncogenic effects. Although it is not known why such specific types of cancers occur in individuals who inherit germline mutations in these oncogenes, one plausible theory is that other genes expressed in most of the tissues of the body counteract the effect of these activating mutations, thereby allowing normal development and suppressing oncogenic effects in most of the tissues in heterozygotes.

Chapter 17   Personalized Genetic Medicine

1.

IDIOPATHIC CEREBRAL VEIN THROMBOSIS (ICVT) AND FACTOR V LEIDEN (FVL)

Genotype	iCVT Affected	iCVT Unaffected	Total
Homozygous FVL	1	624	625
Heterozygous FVL	2	48,748	48,750
Wild-type	15	950,610	950,625
Total	18	999,982	1,000,000

You would expect 625 FVL homozygotes and 48,750 heterozygotes.

Relative risk for iCVT in FVL homozygotes = $(1/625)/(15/950,625) = \sim101$.

Relative risk for iCVT in FVL heterozygotes = $(2/48,750)/(15/950,625) = \sim3$.

Sensitivity of testing positive for either one or two FVL alleles = 3/18 = 17%.

Positive predictive value for homozygotes = 1/625 = 0.16%.

Positive predictive value for heterozygotes = 2/48,748 = 0.004%.

Although the relative risks are elevated with FVL, particularly when the individual is homozygous for the allele, the disorder itself is very rare and thus the PPV is low.

2.

DEEP VENOUS THROMBOSIS (DVT) IN THE LEGS, ORAL CONTRACEPTIVE (OC) USE, AND FACTOR V LEIDEN (FVL)

Genotype	DVT Affected	DVT Unaffected	Total
Homozygous FVL	3	59	62
Heterozygous FVL	58	4,825	4,875
Wild-type	39	95,025	95,063
Total	100	99,000	100,000

You would expect ~62 FVL homozygotes and 4,875 heterozygotes.

Relative risk for DVT in FVL homozygotes taking OC = ~118.

Relative risk for DVT in FVL heterozygotes taking OC = ~30.

Sensitivity of testing positive for either one or two FVL alleles = 62%.

Positive predictive value for homozygotes = 3/62 = ~5%.

Positive predictive value for heterozygotes = 58/4,875 = 1.2%.

Note that DVT is more common than the example of idiopathic cerebral vein thrombosis given in Question 1, whereas the relative risks for homozygotes are of similar magnitude (101 versus 118); thus, the PPV of testing homozygous is accordingly much higher but still only 5%.

3. You should first explain to the parents that the test is a routine one performed on all newborns and that the results, as in many screening tests, are often falsely positive. The parents should also be told that the test result may be a true positive, and if it is, a more accurate and definitive test needs to be done before we will know what the child's condition really is and what treatment will be required. The child should be brought in as soon as possible for examination and the appropriate samples obtained to confirm the elevated phenylalanine level, to determine if the child has classic or variant PKU or hyperphenylalaninemia, and to test for abnormalities in tetrabiopterin metabolism. Once a diagnosis is made, dietary phenylalanine restriction is instituted to bring blood phenylalanine levels down below the range considered toxic (>300 μmol/L). The child must then be

observed for dietary adjustments to be made to keep the blood phenylalanine levels under control.

4. Questions to consider in formulating your response are as follows:

Consider benefits of preventing disease by knowing a newborn's genotype at the β-globin locus. Can knowing the genotype help prevent pneumococcal sepsis? other complications of sickle cell anemia?

Compare and contrast how sickle cell screening was introduced versus Tay-Sachs carrier screening with respect to community involvement and leadership. Consider the historical context in which screening was undertaken and the extent to which the African American community was involved in planning and implementing testing.

Distinguish between *SS* homozygotes and *AS* heterozygotes. What harm might accrue from the identification of *SS* and *AS* individuals? What does identification of a newborn with *SS* or *AS* tell you about the genotypes of the parents and genetic risks for future offspring to the parents?

Chapter 18   Pharmacogenetics and Pharmacogenomics

1.

CARBAMAZEPINE-INDUCED TEN OR SJS

HLA B*1502 allele present	TEN or SJS		
	Affected	*Unaffected*	*Total*
+	44	3	47
−	0	98	98
Total	44	101	145

Sensitivity = 44/44 = 100%.
Specificity = 98/101 = 97%.
Positive predictive value = 44/47 = 94%.

2. Terfenadine blocks the HERG cardiac-specific potassium channel encoded by *KCNH2*.

Various alleles in the coding portion of *KCNH2* are associated with prolongation of the QT interval on electrocardiography, which is associated with sudden death.

Terfenadine is metabolized by the cytochrome P450 enzyme CYP3A4, which has numerous alleles associated with reduced metabolism.

Itraconazole is an antifungal that blocks CYP3A4 cytochrome and increases serum levels of drugs metabolized by this cytochrome.

Grapefruit juice contains a series of naturally occurring compounds, furanocoumarins, that interfere with CYP3A4 metabolism of numerous drugs, including terfenadine.

Caffeine is unlikely to be involved in that caffeine has very little effect on CYP3A4, which has only a minor role in caffeine metabolism. Most caffeine is metabolized by CYP1A2.

Chapter 19   Genetic Counseling and Risk Assessment

1. (a) Prior risk, 1/4; posterior risk (two normal brothers), 1/10.

(b) Zero, unless the autosomal dominant form can show nonpenetrance, in which case there is a very small probability that Cecile, Dorothy, and Elsie would all be nonpenetrant carriers. Without knowing the penetrance, we cannot calculate the exact risk that Elsie is heterozygous.

2. (a) Restrict your attention and conditional probability calculations to those women for whom we have conditional probability information that could alter their carrier risk. These individuals are Lucy, who has an affected grandson and two unaffected grandsons; her daughter Molly, who has an affected son; and Martha, who has two unaffected sons. Maud does not contribute any additional information because she has no sons. Write down an abbreviated pedigree (see illustration) and calculate all the possible prior probabilities.

In A, Nathan is a new mutation with probability μ.

In B, Molly is the new mutation—but because Lucy is *not* a carrier, Molly can only carry a new mutation and did not inherit the mutation; her prior probability is 2μ (*not* 4μ) because the new mutation could have occurred on either her paternal or her maternal X chromosome.

In C, Lucy is a carrier. As shown earlier in this chapter in the Box describing the calculation for the probability that any female is a carrier of an X-linked lethal disorder, Lucy's prior probability = 4μ. Molly inherits the mutant gene, but Martha does not, so the probability her two sons would be unaffected is essentially 1.

In D, Lucy is a carrier, as is Molly, but so is Martha, and yet she did not pass the mutant gene to her two sons.

(We do not consider all the other combinations of carrier states because they are so unlikely, they can be ignored. For example, the possibility that Lucy is a mutation carrier, but Molly does not inherit a mutation from Lucy, and then Nathan is *another* new mutation is vanishingly small because the joint probability of such an event would require *two* new mutations and would contain μ^2 terms in the joint probability that are too small to contribute to the posterior probability.)

The conditional probabilities can then be calculated from these various joint probabilities.

For Molly, she is a carrier in situations B, C, and D, so her probability of being a carrier is 13/21.

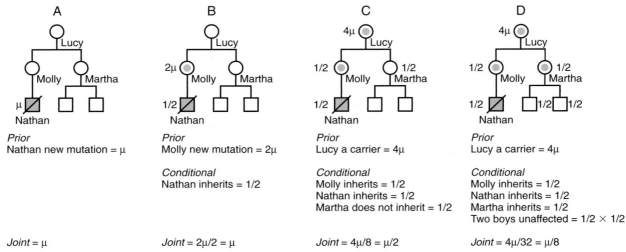

Figure for question 2, Chapter 19.

Similarly, Molly's mother Lucy, 5/21; Norma and Nancy, 13/42; Olive and Odette, 13/84; Martha, 1/21; Nora and Nellie, 1/42; Maud, 5/42; Naomi, 5/84.

(b) To have a 2% risk of having an affected son, a woman must have an 8% chance of being a carrier; thus, Martha, Nora, and Nellie would not be obvious candidates for prenatal diagnosis by DNA analysis because their carrier risk is less than 8%.

3. $(1/2)^{13}$ for 13 successive male births.
$(1/2)^{13} \times 2$ for 13 consecutive births of the same sex. (The 2 arises because this is the chance of 13 consecutive male births *or* 13 consecutive female births, before any children are born.)
1/2. The probability of a boy is 1/2 for each pregnancy, regardless of how many previous boys were born (assuming there is straightforward chromosome segregation, no abnormality in sexual development that would alter the underlying 50% to 50% segregation of the X and Y chromosomes during spermatogenesis, and no sex-specific lethal gene carried by a parent).

4. (a) Use the first equation, $I = \mu + 1/2H$, to solve for H and substitute it for H in the second equation, $H = 2\mu + 1/2H + If$. Solve for I, $I = 3\mu/(1-f)$. Substituting 0.7 for f gives:
the incidence of affected males $I = 10\mu$
the incidence of carrier females $H = 18\mu$

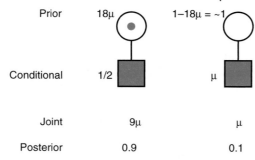

Chance next son will be affected is $1/2 \times 0.9 = 0.45$.
(b) Substitute $f = 0$ into the equations and you get $I = 3\mu$ and $H = 4\mu$.
(c) 0.147.

5. (a) The prior risk that either Ira or Margie is a cystic fibrosis carrier is 2/3; therefore, the probability that both are carriers is $2/3 \times 2/3 = 4/9$.
(b) Their risk of having an affected child in any pregnancy is $1/4 \times 4/9 = 1/9$.
(c) Bayesian analysis is carried out.

	Both Carriers	Not Both Carriers
Prior	4/9	5/9
Conditional (3 normal children)	$(3/4)^3$	1
Joint	$4/9 \times (3/4)^3 = 3/16$ = .19	5/9 = .56
Posterior	.19/(.19 + .56) = 1/4	.56/.75 = ~3/4

Thus, the chance that Ira's and Margie's next child will be affected is $1/4 \times 1/4 = 1/16$.

6. The child's prior probability of carrying a mutant myotonic dystrophy gene is 1/2. If it is assumed that he has a 1/2 chance of being asymptomatic even if he carries the mutant gene, then his chance of carrying it and showing no symptoms is 1/3. Testing is a complex issue. Many would think that testing an asymptomatic child for an incurable illness with adult onset is improper because the child should be allowed to make that decision for himself or herself (see Chapter 20).

7. (a) Yes; autosomal recessive, autosomal dominant (new mutation), X-linked recessive, and multifactorial inheritance and a chromosome disorder all need to be considered, as would nongenetic factors such as prenatal teratogen exposure and intrauterine infection. A careful physical examination and labo-

ratory testing are required for a proper assessment of risks for this couple.

(b) This increases suspicion that the disorder is autosomal recessive, but the possibility of consanguinity does not prove autosomal recessive inheritance, and all other causes must still be investigated thoroughly.

(c) This fact certainly supports the likelihood that the problem has a genetic explanation. The pedigree pattern would be consistent with autosomal recessive inheritance only if the sister's husband were carrying the same defect (possible if he is from the same village, for example). An X-linked recessive pattern (particularly if the affected children are all boys) or a chromosome defect (such as the mothers of the affected children having balanced translocations with unbalanced karyotypes in the affected children) ought to be considered. The mother and her son should receive a genetic evaluation appropriate to the clinical findings, such as karyotype and fragile X analysis.

8. The woman needs genetic counseling. She has a 1/2 risk of passing the mutant *NF1* gene to her offspring. The fact that she carries a new mutation only reduces the recurrence risk elsewhere in the family.

9. Make II-1 the dummy consultand. With use of all information in the pedigree except III-2 and her two unaffected children, the risk that II-1 is a carrier is covered in situations B, C1, and C2 in Table 19-3, giving a posterior probability of 13/21.

STEP ONE OF DUMMY CONSULTAND METHOD

| Situation | Female Carrier Status | | II-3 | Joint Probabilities |
	I-1	II-1		
A	No	No	No	$\{1 \times 1 \times \mu\} = \mu$
B	No	Yes (new mutation)	No	$\{1 \times 2\mu \times {}^1/_2\} = \mu$
C1	Yes	Yes	No	$\{4\mu \times {}^1/_2 \times {}^1/_2\} \times [{}^1/_2] = \mu/2$
C2	Yes	Yes	Yes	$\{4\mu \times {}^1/_2 \times {}^1/_2\} \times [{}^1/_2 \times ({}^1/_2)^2] = \mu/8$

One can then use this calculation as a starting point to determine that the prior probability that III-2 is a carrier, ignoring her two unaffected sons, is $^1/_2$ the probability her mother, II-1, is a carrier $= {}^1/_2 \times 13/21 = 13/42$; the prior probability that she is not a carrier is $1 - (13/42) = 29/42$ (see Table 19-3). Then we use another round of conditional probability to see what effect the two unaffected sons of III-2 have, to determine the posterior risk that III-2 is a carrier.

STEP TWO OF DUMMY CONSULTAND METHOD

Situation	Female Carrier Status III-2	Joint Probabilities
A	No	29/42
B	Yes	$13/42 \times ({}^1/_2)^2$

The posterior probability that III-2 is a carrier, given her two unaffected sons, is 13/129, the same as when we used the approach in Table 19-3. So far, so good.

Some consider the dummy consultand method to be faster than the all-encompassing approach, but it is also easy to misapply, resulting in miscalculation. However, note that the dummy consultand method, as outlined here, gives the correct result only for the consultand III-2 herself and not necessarily for other females in the pedigree. For example, the 13/21 (62%) carrier risk for individual II-1, calculated in the first step of the two-step dummy consultand method without use of the information for individual III-2, is actually incorrect. The correct result for II-1 is the posterior probability of all the situations except A in Table 19-3, which equals 65/129 (50%). (We thank Susan Hodge from Columbia University for pointing out this problem with the dummy consultand method.)

Chapter 20   Ethical Issues in Medical Genetics

1. The first consideration is testing the boy for an incurable disease. Because the boy has symptoms and the family is seeking a diagnosis, this is *not* the same situation as if an asymptomatic child is being considered for myotonic dystrophy testing. However, because Huntington disease in a child is overwhelmingly the result of an expansion of an enlarged triplet repeat in one of the parents, usually the father, finding a markedly enlarged expansion in the child will automatically raise the possibility that one of the parents, probably the father, is a carrier of a repeat that is enlarged enough to cause adult-onset Huntington disease. Thus, by testing the child, one might inadvertently discover something about a parent's risk. Testing should therefore be carried out with informed consent from the parents. Other issues: If one of the parents carries the *HD* gene, what do you do about testing the asymptomatic older sib? Neither parent is currently symptomatic; what if neither parent carries an expanded *HD* allele, but the symptomatic child does carry an expanded allele?

2. To justify screening, one must show that the good that comes from screening, the beneficence of the testing, outweighs the harm. Consider the issue of

autonomy because implicit in the act of informing families that their child has a chromosomal abnormality is the fact that the child cannot decide whether she or he wants such testing later in life. One might argue that because abnormalities in learning and behavior occur in some individuals with sex chromosome anomalies, informing the parents and providing educational and psychological intervention before major problems arise might be beneficial. There is also, however, the concern about "the self-fulfilling prophecy," that telling parents there might be a problem increases the risk that there will be a problem by altering parental attitudes toward the child. There is a large amount of literature on this subject that is worth investigating and reading. See, for instance:

Bender BG, Harmon RJ, Linden MG, Robinson A: Psychosocial adaptation of 39 adolescents with sex chromosome abnormalities. Pediatrics 96(pt 1):302-308, 1995.

Puck MH: Some considerations bearing on the doctrine of self-fulfilling prophecy in sex chromosome aneuploidy. Am J Med Genet 9:129-137, 1981.

Robinson A, Bender BG, Borelli JB, et al: Sex chromosomal aneuploidy: prospective and longitudinal studies. Birth Defects Orig Artic Ser 22:23-71, 1986.

3. You must consider the extent to which withholding information constitutes "a serious threat to another person's health or safety." In these different disorders, consider how serious the threat is and whether there is any effective intervention if the relative were informed of his or her risk.

Index

Note: Page numbers followed by b indicate boxed material; those followed by f indicate figures; those followed by t indicate tables.

A

ABO blood groups, 187t, 187–188
Abortion(s)
  elective, for disease prevention, 457
  spontaneous, chromosome abnormalities in, incidence of, 76–77
N-Acetyltransferase polymorphism, isoniazid therapy and, 500–501, 501t
Achondroplasia, 128, 128f, 232–233
  cell-to-cell signaling and, 436
  etiology and incidence of, 232
  germline mosaicism and, 137
  inheritance risk for, 233
  management of, 232–233
  mutation in, 183
    rate of, 180, 181, 181t
  pathogenesis of, 232
  phenotype and natural history of, 232
Acrocentric chromosomes, 62
Active chromatin hub, 328
Acute intermittent porphyria, 359f, 359–360
Acute lymphoblastic leukemia, chromosome translocation in, 466t
Acute lymphocytic leukemia, chromosome translocation in, 466t
Acute myelocytic leukemia, chromosome translocation in, 466t
Adenine, 7, 7f
Adeno-associated viruses, as gene therapy vectors, 413, 414
Adenosine deaminase deficiency
  severe combined immunodeficiency due to, gene therapy for, 416
  treatment of, 402–403, 403f
Adenoviruses, as gene therapy vectors, 413, 414
Adjacent-1 segregation, 75
Adjacent-2 segregation, 75
Adrenal hyperplasia, congenital, 110–111, 111f
  HLA alleles and, 191, 191t
  major histocompatibility complex in, 189
  newborn screening for, 488
Affected pedigree member method, 222–223
Affected sibpair method, 222–223
Aflatoxin, hepatocellular carcinoma and, 483
AFP. See Alpha-fetoprotein.
Age at onset, 120–121
  late, conditional probability in disorders with, 516, 517f
Age-related macular degeneration, 234–235
  etiology and incidence of, 234
  inheritance risk for, 235
  management of, 235
  pathogenesis of, 234

Age-related macular degeneration (Continued)
  phenotype and natural history of, 234–235
  positional cloning of, by genome-wide association, 228–229
Albright hereditary osteodystrophy, genomic imprinting and, 137–138, 138f, 138t
Alleles, 2, 7. See also specific alleles.
  codominant, 119
  dominant negative, 375
  heterogeneity of, phenotype variation and, 347t, 347–348
  at loci on different chromosomes, independent assortment of, 207–209, 209f
  at loci on same chromosome, independent assortment of, 209, 210f
  mutant (variant), 116
  segregation of, 20b
  sharing of, among relatives, 153–154, 154f, 154t
  wild-type (common), 116
Allele-specific oligonucleotide probes, 49–50, 51f, 53b
Allelic exclusion, 38
Allelic heterogeneity, 122
Alpha₁-antitrypsin deficiency, 347, 358f, 358–359, 359f
  as ecogenetic disease, 358–359
  population differences in incidence, gene frequency, and heterozygote frequency for, 201t
  treatment of, 402
Alpha-fetoprotein
  in amniotic fluid, 445, 446t
  in maternal serum, 445
    Down syndrome and, 448f, 448–450
    neural tube defects and, 447–448, 448f, 448t
  prenatal, neural tube defects and, 168
  prenatal measurement of, 445–446, 446t
Alpha-globin/beta-globin deficiency, 312–313
Alpha-globin genes, deletions of, 333, 334f, 335, 335t
Alpha-satellite DNA, 13
  and FISH, 63f, 64, 85f
Alpha-thalassemia, 324, 333–336
  deletions of α-globin genes and, 333, 334f, 335, 335t
  forms of, 334–335, 335f
  myelodysplasia associated with, 336
Alternate segregation, 75
Alu family, 13
Alzheimer disease, 236–237, 377–381
  environmental factors in, 164–166, 165t
  etiology and incidence of, 236

Alzheimer disease (Continued)
  genetics of, 164–166, 165t, 377–381
  genetics of
    amyloid precursor gene and, 377–378, 378t, 379f, 380f
    APOE gene and, 165t, 165–166, 379–381, 380t
    presenilin 1 and 2 genes and, 378–379
    susceptibility to, 379–381, 380t
  inheritance risk for, 237
  management of, 237
  pathogenesis of, 236, 377
  phenotype and natural history of, 236–237
  susceptibility testing for, 492–493
Aminoacidopathies, 348–351
  hyperphenylalaninemias as, 348–351, 349f
Amniocentesis, 443, 444–446, 446f, 446t
Amnion disruption, 420, 421f
Amniotic fluid
  alfa-fetoprotein in, 445, 446t
  interphase cells of, fluorescence in situ hybridization of, 87f
ß-Amyloid peptide, in Alzheimer's disease, 377
  amyloid precursor protein and, 377–378, 378t, 379f, 380f
Amyoplasia, 421f
Analogous structures, 423–424
Analytic validity, 487
Anaphase
  of meiosis, 19
  of mitosis, 15
Ancestry informative markers, 216
Androgen insensitivity syndrome, 111–112, 112f
  incidence of, 105t
Anemia. See also Sickle cell disease.
  Fanconi, caretaker genes in, 475
  hemolytic, 329, 330–332
    glucose-6-phosphate dehydrogenase deficiency and, 502
Anencephaly, genetic and environmental factors in, 166–168, 167f
Aneuploidy, 65, 67f, 67–68, 68f, 86f, 87f, 175. See also specific disorders.
  in cancer, 478
  prenatal screening for, 448–450
Aneusomy
  in cancer, 478
  segmental, 144
Angelman syndrome, 96t
  genomic imprinting and, 78–79, 80f, 80t, 137
Aniridia, mutation rate in, 181t
Ankylosing spondylitis, HLA alleles and, 190–191, 191t
Anterior-posterior axis, 432

Anticipation, 139, 140, 388
Anticodons, 32
Antisense DNA, 31
α_1-Antitrypsin deficiency, 347, 358f, 358–359, 359f
   as ecogenetic disease, 358–359
   population differences in incidence, gene frequency, and heterozygote frequency for, 201t
   treatment of, 402
APC gene, 258–259, 473–474, 475, 476
Apert syndrome, mutation in, 183
APOE gene, in Alzheimer's disease, 165t, 165–166, 379–381, 380t
Apoprotein B-100, familial hypercholesterolemia and, 361t
Apoptosis, 14, 427, 439
   in follicular B-cell lymphoma, 467
ARH adaptor protein, familial hypercholesterolemia and, 361t
Array comparative genome hybridization, 56, 186
Arthritis, rheumatoid
   HLA alleles and, 191t
   juvenile, HLA alleles and, 191t
Arthrogryposes, 420, 421f
Artificial chromosomes, 414
Artificial insemination, to avoid genetic disease recurrence, 508
Aryl hydrocarbon hydroxylase, 483
Ascertainment, 156
   population-based, 156
   volunteer-based, 156
Ascertainment bias, in case-control studies, 153
Assisted reproductive technologies. See also specific techniques.
   increased risk with, of Beckwith-Wiedemann syndrome, 239
Association analysis, 207, 223–226
   linkage analysis compared with, 226b
   strengths and weaknesses of, 224–225
Assortative mating, Hardy-Weinberg law and, 196
Ataxia
   fragile X-associated tremor/ataxia syndrome and, 142
      pathogenesis of, 389
   Friedreich, 140t, 143–144, 387, 387f
      pathogenesis of, 389
   spinocerebellar, slipped mispairing mechanism in, 388, 388f
Ataxia-telangiectasia, caretaker genes in, 475
Atherosclerosis
   genetic and environmental factors in, 172, 172f
   plaques in, pathogenesis of, in familial hypercholesterolemia, 364
ATRX gene, 110, 335–336
ATR-X syndrome, 334
Autism, relative risk ratio for, 153t
Autoimmune disorders, 190
Autoimmune lymphoproliferative syndrome, 478
Autonomy, respect for, 523
Autosomal disorders, 89–98. See also specific disorders.
   deletion syndromes as, 95
   dominant, 126–129, 127f
      cancer syndromes as
         caretaker tumor-suppressor genes in, 472–475

Autosomal disorders (Continued)
   dominant
      gatekeeper tumor-suppressor genes in, 468–472
      fitness in, 129
      incompletely dominant, 128, 128f
      new mutations in, 128–129
      sex-limited phenotype in, 129, 129f, 130f
   genomic, 95–98, 96t, 97f, 98f
   recessive, 123–126
      carrier frequency and, 123–124
      chromosome instability syndromes as, caretaker tumor-suppressor genes in, 475
      consanguinity and, 124f, 124–125, 125f, 125t
      gene frequency and, 123–124
      Hardy-Weinberg law in, 194
      inbreeding and, 125–126
      new mutations in, 126
      positional cloning by model-based linkage mapping, 226–227
      rare, in genetic isolates, 126
      sex-influenced, 123
Autosomal inheritance, 122–129
   dominant, 126–129, 127f, 130b
   recessive, 122–126, 123f
Autosomally transmitted deletions in mtDNA, 386
Autosomes, 6, 118
Avoidance of maleficence, 523
Axis specification, 432–433
Azoospermia, 96t
Azoospermia factor, 100–101

B
Bacterial artificial chromosome libraries, 48
Bacterial artificial chromosome vectors, 45
Bayesian analysis, 511
B-cell lymphoma(s)
   diffuse, diagnosis of, gene expression profiling in, 480–481
   follicular, chromosome translocation in, 466t, 467
BCR-ABL oncogene, 248–249, 466
Becker muscular dystrophy, 368–372
   clinical phenotype of, 368, 369f
   inheritance of, 368
Beckwith-Wiedemann syndrome, 79, 238–241
   etiology and incidence of, 238
   increased risk of, with assisted reproductive technologies, 239
   management of, 239
   pathogenesis of, 238–239
   phenotype and natural history of, 239
   recurrence risk for, 239
Beneficence, 523
Benign tumors, 461
Berg, Paul, 25
Beta-globin gene. See ß-Globin gene expression.
Beta-globin Glu6Val mutation, 308–309
Beta-globulin mRNA, capping and tailing defects of, 340
Beta-thalassemia, 324, 333, 336f, 336–340
   complex, 337
   simple, 337
      molecular basis of, 337, 337t, 338f, 340
   variant hemoglobins with thalassemia phenotypes and, 340
Beta-thalassemia homozygotes, 347

Bias
   ascertainment, in case-control studies, 153
   in case-control studies, 153
   recall, in case-control studies, 153
Biochemical assays, prenatal, for metabolic disease, 455t, 455–456
Biochemical genetics, 323
Biotinidase deficiency, newborn screening for, 488
Bipolar disorder
   genetic and environmental factors in, 171t, 171–172
   relative risk ratio for, 153t
Blastocyst(s), 428
   definition of, 426
Blood group antigens, 187–188
   ABO system and, 187t, 187–188
   hemolytic disease of the newborn and, 188
   Rh system and, 188
Bloom syndrome, caretaker genes in, 475
Bone marrow, for cytogenetic analysis, 60
Bone marrow transplantation, HLA alleles and, 192
Branchio-oto-renal dysplasia syndrome, 422
BRCA1 gene, 29f
BRCA1/BRCA2 genes, 468t, 472–473, 475–477
   mutations of
      germline mutation testing for, 477
      mutations of, 242–243, 472f, 472–473, 473f
      penetrance of, 473, 473f
BRCA2 gene, 468t, 475
Break, symbol for, 66t
Break and join, symbol for, 66t
Breast cancer
   diagnosis of, 481f, 482
   familial
      caretaker genes in, 472f, 472–473, 473f
      due to BRCA1/BRCA2 mutations, 472f, 472–473, 473f
      germline mutation testing for, 477
   hereditary, 242–243
      etiology and incidence of, 242
      inheritance risk for, 243
      management of, 243
      pathogenesis of, 242
      phenotype and natural history of, 242
   loss of gatekeeper and caretaker function in, 476
   loss of heterozygosity in, 470t
Burkitt lymphoma(s)
   chromosome translocation in, 466t, 466–467
   diagnosis of, gene expression profiling in, 480–481

C
C banding, 62
CACNL1A3 gene, 502
Camptomelic dysplasia, 110
Camptothecin toxicity, glucuronidation polymorphism and, 500, 501t
Cancer, 461–484. See also specific types and sites.
   cytogenetic analysis in, 82–83
   cytogenetics of, 5, 82–83
   environment and, 482–484
      chemical carcinogens in, 483–484
      radiation and, 483

Cancer (Continued)
  in families, 463–464
  genetic basis of, 461–464, 462b, 462f,
      463f
  initiation of, 462b
  oncogenes and, 464f, 464–467
    activated
      in hereditary cancer syndromes,
          464–465
      in sporadic cancer, 465–467
    sporadic, 461–462
  stages in evolution of, 463, 463f
  treatment of, gene expression profiling
      and clustering for individualization
      of, 479–482, 480f
  tumor progression in, 462b, 479
  tumor-suppressor genes and. See
      Tumor-suppressor genes.
  two-hit origin of, 467–468
Cancer stem cells, 463
Carcinomas, 461
CARD15 gene, cloning of, 227–228
Cardiac ion channel gene mutations,
    282–284
Cardiothoracic surgery, genotypic risk for
    adverse outcomes after, 503–504
Carriers, 116
  frequency of, 123–124
Cartilage hair hypoplasia, 385
Case-control studies, of familial
    aggregation, 153
Cat-eye syndrome, 96t, 98
CCR5 gene, HIV resistance and, 192
cDNA
  definition of, 42
  libraries of, 46, 46f
Celiac disease, HLA alleles and, 191t
Cell cycle, 13–14, 14f
Cell death, programmed, 439
Cell division, 13–20. See also Meiosis;
    Mitosis.
  cell cycle and, 13–14, 14f
  human karyotype and, 15–16, 16f–18f
Cell migration, 438–439, 439f, 440f
Cell shape and function, 437–438, 438f
Cell-to-cell signaling, morphogens and,
    435–437, 437f
Centimorgans, 212–213
Centromere(s), 13, 14, 14f
  position of, 61–62
Centrosomes, 14–15
Cerebral vein thrombosis, disease
    association of, 224
CFTR gene, 122, 123–124, 252–253, 365,
    366f, 494
  cloning of, 227, 227b
  genetic and environmental modifiers and,
      159
  mutations in, 365–366
Chain termination mutations, 179
Charcot-Marie-Tooth disease, 96t, 97
  type 1A, 244–245, 325
    etiology and incidence of, 244
    inheritance risk for, 245
    management of, 245
    pathogenesis of, 244
    phenotype and natural history of,
        244–245
CHARGE syndrome, 246–247
  etiology and incidence of, 246
  inheritance risk for, 247
  management of, 247
  pathogenesis of, 246
  phenotype and natural history of, 247
CHD7 gene, 246–247

Checkpoints, 14
Chemical carcinogens, 483–484
Chemical individuality, 186–187, 485
Chiasmata, 18
Childs, Barton, 487
Chimera, 433
  definition of, 426
Cholesterol, uptake of, by LDL receptor,
    361–362, 363f
Cholinesterase polymorphism, prolonged
    postoperative paralysis and, 501–502
Chondroplasia, 325
Chorion, definition of, 426
Chorion frondosum, 447
Chorion levae, 447
Chorionic villus sampling, 443, 444–445,
    446–447, 447f
Choroid plexus cysts, prevalence of, 452t
Choroideremia, founder effect and, 202,
    202f
Chromatids, sister, 14, 14f
Chromatin, 8
Chromosome(s), 5. See also Chromosome
    abnormalities.
  acrocentric, 62
  arms of, 16
  artificial, 414
  daughter, 15, 15f
  deletions of, 70–71, 87f, 88f
    interstitial, 70
  derivative, 66t
  dicentric, 66t, 72
  duplications of, 71
    fragile site, 66t
  fluorescence in situ hybridization to, 55,
      62f, 63–64, 85f–88f
  fragile sites on, 62–63
  homologous, 6
    random assortment of, 20b
  identification of, methods for, 60–63
    C banding as, 62
    fragile sites and, 62–63
    high-resolution banding as, 62, 63f
    Q banding as, 60–61
    R banding as, 61f, 61–62, 62d
  insertions of, 66t, 75
  inversions of, 66t, 72f, 72–74, 73f
    paracentric, 72–73
    pericentric, 73, 73f
  karyotype and, 15–16, 16f–18f
  marker, 66t, 71
  in meiosis, cytogenetic studies of,
      81–82
  metacentric, 62
  mitochondrial, 10
  mutations of, 175
    frequency of, 176t
    frequency of disease due to, 152t
    origin of, 176
  nonrecombinant, 209
  number of
    abnormalities of, 65, 67–68
      aneuploidy as, 67f, 67–68, 68f
      tetraploidy as, 65, 67
    reduction of, 20b
  organization of, 8–10, 9f, 11f
  pseudodicentric, 72
  recombinant, 209, 210f
  ring, 66t, 71
  sex. See Sex chromosomes; X
      chromosome; Y chromosome.
  structurally abnormal, extra, 71
  submetacentric, 62
  supernumerary, 71
  telocentric, 62

Chromosome(s) (Continued)
  translocations of, 74f, 74–75
    in cancer, 462b
    oncogene activation by, 465t, 465–467,
        466f, 466t
Chromosome abnormalities, 2, 65, 65t,
    66t, 67–77
  abbreviations for, 66t
  of chromosome number, 65, 67–68
    aneuploidy as, 67f, 67–68, 68f
    tetraploidy as, 65, 67
  of chromosome structure, 68–75, 69f
    balanced rearrangements as, 68, 72–75
      inversions as, 66t, 72f, 72–74, 73f
      translocations as, 74f, 74–75
    unbalanced rearrangements as, 68–72,
        70f, 87f
      deletions as, 70–71, 87f, 88f
      dicentric chromosomes as, 72
      duplications as, 71
      isochromosomes as, 71–72
      marker and ring chromosomes as, 71
  family history of, chromosome analysis
      in, 60
  incidence of, 76t, 76–77, 77t
    in live births, 76
    in spontaneous abortions, 76–77
  mosaicism as, 75–76
Chromosome analysis
  applications of, 5–6
  cytogenetic. See Cytogenetics.
Chromosome instability syndromes, 82,
    82f
Chromosome "painting" probes, 55, 63f
Chromosome segregation, 14
Chromosome spread, 15, 16f
Chronic lymphoblastic leukemia,
    chromosome translocation in, 466t
Chronic myelogenous leukemia, 248–249
  chromosome translocation in, 466, 466t
  etiology and incidence of, 248
  inheritance risk for, 249
  management of, 249
  pathogenesis of, 248
  phenotype and natural history of,
      248–249
Chronic progressive external
    ophthalmoplegia, 384t, 385
Cigarette smoking, carcinogenesis and,
    483
Cleft lip/palate, 168–169, 169t
  nonsyndromic, 168, 169
  syndromic, 168–169, 169t
Clinical heterogeneity, 122
Clinical utility, 487
Clinical validity, 487
Clones, 41
  definition of, 42
  libraries of, 45–47
    complementary DNA libraries as, 46,
        46f
    genomic, 45f, 45–46
    library screening by nucleic acid
        hybridization as, 47, 47f
    screening of, 47, 47f
  oligonucleotide, 47
Cloning
  molecular, 41, 43f
  positional, 208
    of autosomal recessive disorder, by
        model-based linkage mapping,
        226–227
    of complex disease
      by genome-wide association,
          228–229

Cloning *(Continued)*
  positional, by model-free linkage mapping, 227–228
  reproductive, 406–407
  therapeutic, 406
Clustering, to create signatures, 479
Codominant alleles, 119
Codons, 31–32, 32t
  repeat expansion of, diseases due to, 389–390
  stop (nonsense), 32
Coefficient of correlation, 157
Coefficient of inbreeding, 124, 125t
Cofactors
  impaired binding of, 356, 356f
  metabolism of, abnormalities of, 356–357
Colitis, ulcerative, positional cloning of, by model-free linkage mapping, 227–228
Collagen
  molecular abnormalities of, in osteogenesis imperfecta, 375, 376f
  structural genes and, in osteogenesis imperfecta, 372–373, 372f–374f, 373t, 375–377
  type I, diminished production of, in osteogenesis imperfecta, 375
  types II, III, and IV, in osteogenesis imperfecta, 375
Colon cancer. *See also* Colorectal carcinoma; Familial polyposis coli; Hereditary nonpolyposis colorectal cancer.
  sporadic, loss of gatekeeper and caretaker function in, 476f, 476–477
Color blindness, red-green, Hardy-Weinberg law in, 194–195, 195t
Colorectal carcinoma, loss of heterozygosity in, 470t
Common alleles, 116
Comparative genome hybridization, 55–56, 56f, 64f, 64–65
  array, 56
  cytogenetics, 64f, 64–65
Complement factor H variants, 234–235
Complementary DNA
  definition of, 42
  libraries of, 46, 46f
Complementation analysis, 355
Complex inheritance. *See* Multifactorial disorders; Multifactorial inheritance.
Complex traits, gene mapping of, model-free linkage analysis for, 222–223
  of qualitative traits, 222–223
  of quantitative traits, 223
Compound heterozygotes, 116, 332
  in phenylketonuria, 350
Concordance, 152
  in dizygotic vs. monozygotic twins, 155, 155t
  in monozygotic twins, 155
  among relatives, 153–154, 154f, 154t
  studies of, limitations of, 158–159
  in twins reared apart, 155
Conditional probability, 511f, 511–512
  in disorders with incomplete penetrance, 515–516, 516f
  in disorders with late age at onset, 516, 517f
  in X-linked lethal disorders, 514f, 514–515, 515f, 515t
Confined placental mosaicism, 81, 454, 454f

Conformational diseases, 358
Congenital adrenal hyperplasia, 110–111, 111f
  HLA alleles and, 191, 191t
  major histocompatibility complex in, 189
  newborn screening for, 488
Congenital anomalies
  deformations as, 420, 421f
  disruptions as, 420, 421f
  malformations as, 420, 420f
  multifactorial, 166t, 166–170
  public health impact of, 419
Congenital bilateral absence of the vas deferens, 365
Congenital disorders, 120
Congenital heart disease
  genetic and environmental factors in, 169–170, 170f, 170t
  protection against, by PCSK9 protease sequence variants, 363–364, 364t
Congenital hypothyroidism, treatment of, 398
Congenital myotonic dystrophy, 139, 140t
Conjoined twins, 432
Conotruncal anomaly face, 97–98
Consanguinity, 118, 124f, 124–125
  Hardy-Weinberg law and, 196–197
  measurement of, 124–125, 125f, 125t
  recurrence risk and, genetic counseling for, 520
Constitutive heterochromatin, 62
Consultands, 116, 117f, 120
Contiguous gene syndromes, 96, 144, 180
Contraception, to avoid genetic disease recurrence, 508
Controls, unrelated family member, 154
Convergent evolution, 424
Copy number polymorphisms, 65, 186
Corneal stem cells, 407
Coronary artery disease, genetic and environmental factors in, 172, 172f
Correlation
  coefficient of, 157
  negative, 157
  positive, 157
  of quantitative traits, 157t, 157–158
Counseling. *See* Genetic counseling.
Coupling, 211
CpG islands, 35
Cranial-caudal axis, 432
Craniosynostoses
  cell-to-cell signaling and, 436
  mutation in, 183
C-reactive protein, 503–504
CREB binding protein, 442
Cri du chat syndrome, 95, 96f
Crick, Francis, 7
Critical interval, 223
Crohn disease, 250–251
  etiology and incidence of, 250
  inheritance risk for, 251
  management of, 251
  pathogenesis of, 250
  phenotype and natural history of, 251
  positional cloning of, by model-free linkage mapping, 227–228
  relative risk ratio for, 153t
Crossing over, 17, 20b
  unequal, 179, 180f
Crouzon syndrome, mutation in, 183
Cryptic splice sites, 338
Cutaneous xanthomas, in familial hypercholesterolemia, 128, 128f
CYP2C9 genotype, 503

Cystathionine synthase deficiency, 356, 356f
Cystic fibrosis, 79, 81, 122, 123–124, 252–253, 347, 364–367
  CFTR gene and protein and, 365, 366f
  direct determination of mutation in, 517–518
  etiology and incidence of, 252
  genetic analysis of families of patients and, 367
  genetic and environmental modifiers in, 159
  genetics of, 365–367
    CFTR in populations and, 367
    epithelial sodium channel gene *SCNN1* mutations and, 366
    genotype-phenotype correlations and, 366–367
    mutations in CFTR polypeptide and, 365–366
  genotype-phenotype correlations in, 366–367
  inheritance risk for, 253
  linkage disequilibrium in, 227
  management of, 253
  natural history of, 252–253
  pathogenesis of, 252
  pathophysiology of, 365
  phenotypes of, 252–253, 365
  population differences in incidence, gene frequency, and heterozygote frequency for, 201t
  population screening for, 367
  positional cloning by model-based linkage mapping, 226–227
  prenatal diagnosis of, 367
  treatment of, 367
Cystic hygroma, prevalence of, 452t
Cytochrome P450, variation in pharmacokinetic response and, 497–500, 498f–500f, 499t
Cytogenetics, 5, 59–83
  in cancer, 5, 82–83
  chromosome abnormalities and, 65, 65t, 66t, 67–77. *See also* Chromosome abnormalities.
  chromosome identification methods in, 60–63
    C banding as, 62
    fragile sites and, 62–63
    high-resolution banding as, 62, 63f
    Q banding as, 60–61
    R banding as, 61f, 61–62, 62d
  comparative genome hybridization in, 55–56, 56f, 64f, 64–65
  fluorescence in situ hybridization in, 55, 62f, 63–64
  indications for, 60
  in mendelian disorders, 82, 82f
  molecular, 63
  parent-of-origin effects and, 77–81
    confined placental mosaicism and, 81
    genomic imprinting and, 77–81, 78f, 79f
    hydatidiform mole and ovarian teratoma cytogenetics and, 81
  in prenatal diagnosis, 453–455
    problems in, 453–455
    after ultrasonography, 453
  studies of chromosomes in meiosis and, 81–82
Cytokinesis, 15
Cytosine, 7, 7f

D

Daughter chromosomes, 15, 15f
DCC gene, 468t
Deafness. *See* Hearing loss.
Deep vein thrombosis (DVT), 160–162, 161f
Deficiency, of chromosome segments, pericentric inversions leading to, 73
Deformations, 420, 421f
Degenerate genetic code, 32
Deletion(s), 70–71, 87f, 88f, 177b
  centromere, 66t
  chromosomal, 70–71, 87f, 88f
    interstitial, 70
  of DNA sequences, 179–180
  prenatal screening for, 457
  small, 179, 181b
Deletion syndromes, 95
Denys-Drash syndrome, 110
Deoxyribonucleic acid. *See* DNA.
Depletion, for metabolic abnormality treatment, 399
Derivative chromosomes, 66t
Determination, 427, 429–432
  definition of, 426
Development
  mosaic, 430, 432
  regulative, 430
    twinning and, 430–431, 431f, 432f, 433
Developmental biology, 419–442
  axis specification and pattern formation and, 432–434
    HOX gene system and, 433–434, 434f
  cellular and molecular mechanisms in, 434–439
    cell migration and, 438–439, 439f, 440f
    cell shape and organization and, 437–438, 438f
    gene regulation by transcription factors and, 435, 435f, 436f
    morphogens and cell-to-cell signaling and, 435–437, 437f
    programmed cell death and, 439
  clinical dysmorphology and, 419–422
    genetic and environmental causes of malformations and, 421f, 421–422
    malformation, deformations, and disruptions and, 420f, 420–421, 421f
    pleiotropy and, 422, 423, 424f
  core concepts in, 426–427
  developmental processes and, 424–426
    environmental factors and, 425–426
    probability and, 425
  embryological development and, 426–429
    cellular processes during, 427, 428f
    germ cells and, 428
    human, 427–428, 429f, 430f
    stem cells and, 428–429, 431f
  evolution and, 422–424, 425f
  fate, specification, and determination and, 429–432
    mosaic development and, 432
    regulative and mosaic development and, 430
    regulative development and twinning and, 430–431, 431f, 432f, 433
  interaction of developmental mechanisms in embryogenesis and, 440–442
  limb as model of organogenesis and, 440–442, 441f

Developmental biology *(Continued)*
  public health impact of birth defects and, 419
  terminology in, 426–427
Developmental disorders, chromosome analysis in, 60
Diabetes mellitus
  type 1 (insulin dependent; IDDM), 278–279
    etiology and incidence of, 278
    genetic and environmental factors in, 163–164
    HLA alleles and, 191t
    inheritance risk for, 279
    management of, 279
    MHC association in, 163–164
    pathogenesis of, 278–279
    phenotype and natural history of, 279
    relative risk ratio for, 153t
  type 2 (non-insulin dependent; NIDDM), 163, 294–295
    etiology and incidence of, 294
    HLA alleles and, 191t
    inheritance risk for, 295
    management of, 295
    pathogenesis of, 294–295
    phenotype and natural history of, 295
Diakinesis, 18
Diaphragmatic hernia, prevalence of, 452t
Dicentric chromosomes, 66t, 72
Dichorionic twins, 430
  definition of, 426
Dietary restriction, for metabolic abnormality treatment, 396, 398
Differentiation, 427
  definition of, 426
DiGeorge syndrome, 96t, 97–98, 170, 170f
  fluorescence in situ hybridization of, 87f
  programmed cell death in, 439
  schizophrenia and, 171
Diploid cells, 13
Diplotene, 18
Direct determination of mutations, 516–518
Discordance, for disorders, 152
Disease associations, 223–226
  genome-wide association and haplotype map and, 225–226
Disease concordance. *See* Concordance.
Disease-containing haplotype, 215f, 216
Disease states, molecular phenotypes characterizing, 57
Disomy, uniparental, 78
Disruptions, 420, 421f
Diversion, for metabolic abnormality treatment, 398f, 398–399, 399f
Dizygotic twins, 153–154
  twin studies of genetic environmental factors in disease and, 154–156
DMD gene, 256–257, 368–369, 370f, 371
  molecular analysis and, 371, 371f
  post-translational modification of dystrophin complex and, 371
DMPK gene, 143, 144
DNA
  allele-specific oligonucleotide probes and, 49–50, 51f, 53b
  antisense (noncoding), 31
  bases of, 7, 7f, 8f
  in chromatin, 8–10
  cloning and. *See* Clones; Cloning.
  comparative genome hybridization and, 55–56, 56f

DNA *(Continued)*
  complementary
    definition of, 42
    libraries of, 46, 46f
  damage to, gene mutations and, 177
  deletions of sequences of, 179–180
  human karyotype and, 16–17
  informational relationships among RNA and proteins and, 27–28
  insertion of sequences of, 179–180
  mitochondrial. *See* mtDNA.
  naked, 414
  origins of replication of, 14
  packaged in liposomes, 414
  polymerase chain reaction and, 50–52, 52f
  polymorphisms in
    insertion-deletion, 184–186
      copy number polymorphisms and, 186
      microsatellites and, 185, 185f
      minisatellites and, 185f, 185–186, 186f
    single nucleotide, 184
  pseudogenes and, 30
  recombinant, 4, 43
  repetitive, 10, 12–13
    disease and, 13
  sense (coding), 31
  single-copy (unique), 10, 12
  Southern blotting and, 48, 49f, 50f
  structure of, 7–8, 7f–9f
  synthesis of
    in cell-cycle phases, 13–14, 14f
    in meiosis, 16
  transfer into cells, nonviral vectors for, 414
  vectors and, 43–45
    definition of, 42
    expression vectors as, 46
    plasmids as, 44–45
DNA analysis, prenatal, 456
DNA fingerprinting, 186
DNA hypomethylation, 404–405
DNA libraries, 45–47
  cDNA, 46, 46f
  definition of, 42
  genomic, 45f, 45–46
  screening of, 47, 47f
DNA ligase, 43
DNA mismatch repair genes, 270–271
DNA repair, gene mutations and, 177
DNA replication errors, gene mutations and, 176–177
DNA sequence(s), individual, molecular genetic tools for analysis of, 41–48, 43f
  genome database resources as, 47–48
  libraries as, 45–47
    complementary DNA libraries as, 46, 46f
    genomic, 45f, 45–46
    screening of, 47, 47f
  molecular cloning as, 41
  restriction enzymes as, 41, 43, 44f
  vectors as, 43–45
    plasmids as, 44–45
DNA sequence analysis, 53–55, 54f
Dominant disorders
  autosomal. *See* Autosomal disorders, dominant.
  selection in, 197–198, 198t
Dominant inheritance, 118, 119
  autosomal, 126–129, 127f, 130b

Dominant inheritance (Continued)
  of X-linked disorders, 131, 133f,
    133–135
    characteristics of, 133b
    with male lethality, 134f, 134–135
Dominant negative alleles, 375
Donated eggs, to avoid genetic disease
  recurrence, 508
Double helix, of DNA, 8, 8f, 9f
Double minutes, 478
Down, Langdon, 89
Down syndrome, 67, 67f, 81, 89–94, 90f,
    325
  chromosomes in, 91–93
  etiology of, 93
  mosaic, 92–93
  partial trisomy 21 in, 93
  phenotype in, 90, 91f
  prenatal and postnatal survival in, 90–91
  21q21q translocation in, 92
  recurrence risk of, 93–94
  risk of, 93
  Robertsonian translocation in, 91–92, 92f
DQB1 gene, diabetes mellitus and, type 1,
    164
Drug metabolism
  normal, poor, and ultrafast, 498, 500f
  phase I of, 498, 498f
    variation in, 497–500, 498f–500f, 499t
  phase II of, 498, 498f
    variation in, 500–502
Duchenne muscular dystrophy, 256–257,
    367–372
  clinical phenotype of, 368, 368f
  direct determination of mutation in, 517,
    518f
  DMD gene and its product and,
    368–369, 370f, 371
    molecular analysis and, 371, 371f
    post-translational modification of
      dystrophin complex and, 371
  etiology and incidence of, 256
  fitness in, 135
  gene therapy for, 416t
  germline mosaicism and, 137
  inheritance of, 368, 369t
    risk for, 257
  linkage analysis in, 519
  management of, 257
  maternal mosaicism and, 372
  mutation rate in, 180–181, 181t
  pathogenesis of, 256
  phenotype and natural history of,
    256–257
    in females, 256–257
    in males, 256
  prenatal diagnosis and carrier detection
    for, 371–372
  therapy for, 372
  X inactivation and, 130, 131f
Duodenal atresia, prevalence of, 452t
Duplications
  of chromosome segments, pericentric
    inversions leading to, 73
  of chromosomes, 71
    fragile site, 66t
  prenatal screening for, 457
Duty to warn, 525–527, 526b
Dynamic mutations, 180, 387
Dyschondrosteosis, 135, 135f
Dysgenics, 528–529
Dysmorphology, clinical, 419–422
Dystrophia myotonica. See Myotonic
  dystrophy.

E
Echocardiography, fetal, 453, 453t
Ecogenetics, 358–359
Ectoderm, 426–427
  definition of, 426
Edema, angioneurotic, hereditary,
    treatment of, 404
Eggs, 22
  donated, to avoid genetic disease
    recurrence, 508
Ellis-van Creveld syndrome, 201, 202f
Embryo, definition of, 426
Embryogenesis
  definition of, 426
  human, 427–428, 429f, 430f
  interaction of developmental mechanisms
    in, 440–442
Embryology, of reproductive system,
    99–100, 100f
Embryonic stem cell(s), definition of, 426
Embryonic stem cell technology, 433,
    433f
Empirically derived risk figures, 151–152
Employers, use of genetic information by,
    527
Encephalomyopathy, gastrointestinal,
    mitochondrial, 386
Endocardial cushions, 439
Endoderm, 427
  definition of, 426
Endonucleases, restriction, 41, 43, 44f
  definition of, 42
Enhancers, 28, 35
Environmental factors
  in Alzheimer disease, 164–166, 165t
  in anencephaly, 166–168, 167f
  in atherosclerosis, 172, 172f
  in bipolar disorder, 171t, 171–172
  in cancer, 482–484
    chemical carcinogens and, 483–484
    radiation and, 483
  causes of malformations and, 421f,
    421–422
  in congenital heart disease, 169–170,
    170f, 170t
  in coronary artery disease, 172, 172f
  in cystic fibrosis, 159
  in development, 425–426
  gene-environment interactions and, 151
  in Hirschsprung disease, 162–163, 163f
  in mental illness, 170–171, 171t
  in multifactorial disorders. See
    Multifactorial disorders.
  in neural tube defects, 166–168, 167f
  in schizophrenia, 170–171, 171t
  in single-gene disorders, 159–160
  in spina bifida, 166–168, 167f
  twin studies of, 154–156
  in type 1 diabetes mellitus, 163–164
Enzyme(s)
  diseases involving, 348–360, 357b,
    357f
    acute intermittent porphyria as, 359f,
      359–360
    altered protein function due to
      abnormal post-translational
      modification and, 355–356
    aminoacidopathies as, 348–351
    α₁-antitrypsin deficiency as, 358f,
      358–359, 359f
    loss of protein function due to
      impaired binding or metabolism of
      cofactors and, 356–357
    lysosomal storage diseases as, 351–355

Enzyme(s) (Continued)
  inhibition of, for metabolic abnormality
    treatment, 399
Enzyme replacement therapy, 403–404
  for lysosomal storage diseases, 352
Enzymopathies, 399
Epigenetic(s), 77
Epigenetic changes, 429, 468
Epilepsy, myoclonic, with ragged-red fibers,
    290–291
  etiology and incidence of, 290
  inheritance risk for, 291
  management of, 291
  pathogenesis of, 290–291
  phenotype and natural history of, 291
Episomes, 410
Estriol, unconjugated, in prenatal
    screening, 449, 449t
Ethical issues, 523–529
  dysgenics as, 528–529
  eugenics as, 528
  in gene therapy, 415
  in genetic screening, 527–528
  in genetic testing, 523–525
    of asymptomatic children, 525
    for predisposition to disease,
      524–525
    prenatal, 523–524
    principles of, 523
  privacy of genetic information as,
    525–527
    duty to warn and permission to warn
      and, 525–527, 526b
    employers' and insurers' use of genetic
      information and, 527
Ethnicity
  differences in frequency of genetic
    diseases and, 199–204, 201t
    genetic drift and, 200–202
    heterozygote advantage and, 202–204
  in personalized medicine, 504–505
Eugenics, 528
Eukaryotes, 26–27
Euploidy, 65
Evolution
  convergent, 424
  development and, 422–424, 425f
Exomphalos, prevalence of, 452t
Exons, 28
Expansion, 139
Expression profiling, for cancer therapy
    individualization, 479–482, 480f
Expression signatures, 85f, 479
  application of, 479–480
Expression vectors, 46
Expressivity, 119–120, 119f–121f
  variable, 119
Extra structurally abnormal chromosomes,
    71

F
Factor V Leiden
  testing for, consensus recommendations
    for, 162b
  venous thrombosis and, 160–162, 161f
Familial adenomatous polyposis, 258–259
  caretaker genes in, 473–474
  etiology and incidence of, 258
  inheritance risk for, 259
  management of, 259
  pathogenesis of, 258
  phenotype and natural history of,
    258–259

Familial aggregation
  of disease, 152
    measurement of, 152–153, 153t
  of quantitative traits, 157f, 157–158
  studies of, limitations of, 158–159
Familial hypercholesterolemia, 126–128,
    128f, 260–261, 360–364, 361f,
    361t
  atherosclerotic plaque pathogenesis in,
    364
  coronary artery disease and, 172
  etiology and incidence of, 260
  inheritance risk for, 261
  LDL receptor mutations and, 360–362
    cholesterol uptake and, 361–362, 363f
    classes of, 362, 364f
    genetics of, 360–361, 362f
  management of, 261, 398–399, 399f
  pathogenesis of, 260
  PCSK9 protease and, 362–364
  phenotype and natural history of,
    260–261
  population differences in incidence, gene
    frequency, and heterozygote
    frequency for, 201t
Familial polyposis coli
  caretaker genes in, 473–474, 474f
  loss of heterozygosity in, 470t
Family history
  of chromosomal abnormalities,
    chromosome analysis in, 60
  as personalized genetic medicine,
    146–147, 485–487, 486b, 486f
  positive, 153
Fanconi anemia, caretaker genes in, 475
Fate, 429–432
  definition of, 426
FBN1 gene, 286–287
Female pseudohermaphroditism, 110–111,
    111f
Fertility disorders, chromosome analysis in,
    60
Fertilization, 22
  in vitro, preimplantation genetic
    diagnosis and, 430–431, 432f, 433,
    456, 508
Fetal alcohol syndrome, 426
Fetal cells, for cytogenetic analysis, 60
Fetal hemoglobin, hereditary persistence of,
    337
Fetal phase, of development, 428
Fetal retinoid syndrome, 425–426
Fetus
  definition of, 426
  prenatal diagnosis and. See Prenatal
    diagnosis.
  prenatal treatment and, 457–458
  sex determination of, 453
F8/F9 genes, 268–269
FGFR3 gene, 232–233
Fibroblasts, for cytogenetic analysis, 60
First degree relatives, 116, 117f
FISH, 62f, 63–64, 85f–88f
Fitness, 118, 197
  in autosomal dominant inheritance, 129
Fluorescence in situ hybridization, 55, 62f,
    63–64, 85f–88f
Fluorescence-tagged nucleotides, digital
    image capture of, 55–57
  comparative genome hybridization as,
    55–56, 56f
  fluorescent in situ hybridization to
    chromosomes as, 55
  RNA expression arrays as, 56–57

FMR1 gene, 144, 262–263
FMRP protein, 388
Folic acid, in maternal diet, neural tube
    defects and, 168
Formin gene, 425
Founder effect, 199, 201–202, 202f
FOXL2 gene, 110
Fragile sites, 62–63
  chromosome duplications and, 66t
  in fragile X syndrome, 142f
Fragile X syndrome, 62–63, 133, 142,
    142f, 143f, 262–263, 387, 387f
  etiology and incidence of, 262
  inheritance risk for, 263
  management of, 263
  mutation in, 180
  pathogenesis of, 262, 388
  phenotype and natural history of,
    262–263
  severe, 139, 140t
Fragile X–associated tremor/ataxia
    syndrome, 142
  pathogenesis of, 389
Frameshift mutations, 180
Frasier syndrome, 110
FRDA gene, 144
Friedreich ataxia, 140t, 143–144, 387,
    387f
  pathogenesis of, 389
Functional pathways, 57
FV gene, 316–317

G
G banding, 60
G_0 phase, of cell cycle, 14
G_1 phase, of cell cycle, 13–14, 14f
G_2 phase, of cell cycle, 14, 14f
G proteins, 465
Gain, of symbol for, 66t
Gains of glycosylation, 325
Galactosemia
  newborn screening for, 488
  treatment of, 395
Galton, Francis, 528
Gametes, 13
Gametogenesis, 20–22, 21f, 22f
Gangliosidosis, GM_2. See Tay-Sachs
    disease.
Gardner syndrome, caretaker genes in,
    473–474
Garrod, Archibald, 485
Gastrointestinal encephalomyopathy,
    mitochondrial, 386
Gastrulation, definition of, 426
Gaucher disease, treatment of, 403–404,
    404f
Gaussian distribution, 156, 156f
G-banding, 16, 16f
Gene(s), 5. See also specific genes.
  in development, 424–425
  essential, insertional inactivation of, 415
  frequency of, 123–124
  microRNA, 30
  modifier, 151
    phenotype variation and, 348
  molecular definition of, 28
  nuclear, modification of mtDNA disease
    phenotypes by, 386–387
  organization and structure of, 28–30,
    29f
  promoter region of, 28
  RNA, noncoding, 30
  signatures of, 479–480

Gene(s) (Continued)
  single-gene inheritance and. See Single-
    gene inheritance.
  structure of, 28
  transcription of, 30–31
  variation in, 116
  Y-linked, in spermatogenesis, 100–101
Gene amplification, in cancer, 478–479
Gene analysis, applications of, 5–6
Gene dosage, hemoglobinopathies and,
    329
Gene-environment interactions, 151
Gene expression, 30–36, 31f. See also
    specific genes.
  of dominant mutant gene product,
    reducing, 405
  ectopic, mutations associated with, 325
  of ß-globin gene, 33, 33f, 34f, 35–36
  heterochronic, mutations associated with,
    325
  initiation of transcription and, 35
  from locus not affected by disease,
    increasing, 404–405, 406f
  modulation of, therapeutic, 404–405
  pleiotropic, 116
  polyadenylation and, 36
  post-translational processing and, 33
  profiling, for cancer therapy
    individualization, 479–482, 480f
  regulation of, defect in, 359f, 359–360
  RNA splicing and, 35–36
    alternative, 36
  transcription and, 30–31
    initiation of, 35
  of mitochondrial genome, 33
  translation and genetic code and, 31–32,
    32t
  variation in
    gene regulation and, 36–38
    medically relevant, 38
  of X-linked genes, X inactivation and,
    130, 131f
Gene families, 28–30
Gene flow, 199, 200f
  Hardy-Weinberg law and, 199, 200f
Gene-gene interactions, 151
Gene identification, 226–229
  positional cloning of autosomal recessive
    disorder by model-based linkage
    mapping and, 226–227
  positional cloning of complex disease and
    by genome-wide association, 228–229
  by model-free linkage mapping,
    227–228
Gene mapping, 5, 207–229
  of complex traits, 222–226
    disease association approach for,
    222–225
      genome-wide association and
        haplotype map and, 225–226
      strengths and weaknesses of,
        224–225
    model-free linkage analysis for,
      222–223
      of qualitative traits, 222–223
      of quantitative traits, 223
  contribution to medical genetics, 208b
  gene identification and, 226–229
    positional cloning of autosomal
      recessive disorder by model-based
      linkage mapping and, 226–227
    positional cloning of complex disease
      by genome-wide association and,
      228–229

Gene mapping *(Continued)*
  gene identification and
    positional cloning of complex disorder by model-free linkage mapping and, 227–228
  haplotype map and, 216–217, 217f, 218f
  independent assortment and homologous recombination in meiosis and, 208f, 208–209
    of alleles at loci on different chromosomes, 208–209, 209f
    on same chromosome, with crossover in every meiosis, 209, 210f
  by linkage analysis, 217–222
    determining whether two loci are linked and, 217–220
    phase in, 220–222
  linkage equilibrium and disequilibrium and, 213–216, 214f–216f
  recombination frequency and, 209, 211–213
    genetic maps and physical maps and, 212–213, 213f
    heterozygosity and phase effects on detection of recombination events and, 211f, 211–212, 212f
    linkage and recombination frequency and, 212
    recombination frequency as measure of distance between two loci and, 209, 211, 211f
Gene mutations. *See* Mutation(s).
Gene pools, 192
Gene regulation, by transcription factors, 435, 435f, 436f
Gene superfamilies, 30
Gene therapy, 410–416
  diseases amenable to, 415–416
  essential requirements of, 411b
  ethical considerations in, 415
  future for, 416, 416t
  gene transfer strategies for, 411, 413f
  general considerations for, 410–411, 412f
  risks of, 414–415
  target cells for, 411, 413
  vectors for
    nonviral, 414
    viral, 413–414
Genetic code, 27, 32
  degenerate, 32
Genetic complementation, 355
Genetic counseling, 507–509, 509b
  for complex disorders, 519–520
  for consanguinity, 520, 520t
  duty to warn and, 526b
  of families with multifactorial traits, 173b
  indications for, 507–508, 508t
  for prenatal diagnosis, 458
  providers for, 509
  psychological aspects of, 508–509
  risk of recurrence and, 508
  for unbalanced karyotypes, 65b
Genetic counselors, 509
Genetic disorders. *See also* Chromosome abnormalities; Multifactorial disorders; Single-gene disorders; *specific disorders.*
  classification of, 2
Genetic diversity, human, 183–184
  genetic polymorphism concept and, 183–184
Genetic drift
  founder effect and, 199, 201–202, 202f
  heterozygote advantage versus, 203–204

Genetic drift *(Continued)*
  in small populations, Hardy-Weinberg law and, 196–197
Genetic epidemiology, 159, 490b, 490–491
Genetic heterogeneity, 122
  treatment and, 396
Genetic isolates, rare recessive disorders in, 126
Genetic lethals, 129, 198
Genetic markers, 208
Genetic polymorphism. *See* Polymorphisms; Population genetics.
Genetic redundancy, 347
Genetic screening, 487–490
  clinical validity and utility of, 487
  ethical dilemmas in, 527–528
  for genetic susceptibility to disease, 490–494
    based on genotype, 491f, 491–492
    clinical utility of, 492–493
    genetic epidemiology and, 490b, 490–491
    heterozygote screening as, 493b, 493–494
  of libraries of clones, 47, 47f
    by nucleic acid hybridization, 47, 47f
  of newborns, 488t, 488–490
    for phenylketonuria, 349, 488
    tandem mass spectroscopy for, 489t, 489–490
  population, for cystic fibrosis, 367
  prenatal, 490
    for aneuploidies, 448–450, 449f, 450f, 450t
    for aneuploidy, 448–450
    for deletions, 457
    for Down syndrome, 448–450, 449f, 449t, 450t
    for duplications, 457
    human chorionic gonadotropin in, 449, 449t
    inhibin A in, 449, 449t
    for neural tube defects, 447–448, 448f, 448t
    pregnancy-associated plasma protein A in, 449, 449t
    ultrasonography for, 449, 449f
    unconjugated estriol in, 449, 449t
Genetic testing
  of asymptomatic children, 525
  ethical issues in, 523–525
  for predisposition to disease, 524–525
  prenatal, 523–524
Genetics
  applications of, 1–2
  biochemical, 323
  future directions for, 2–3
  as medical specialty, 1–2
  in other medical specialties, 2
Genetics in medicine, 529
Genocopies, 152
Genome(s)
  changes in activity of, 36–38
    allelic exclusion and, 38
    immunoglobulin and T-cell receptor diversity, 36–38, 37f
  haplotype map of, 216–217, 217f, 218f
  human. *See* Human genome.
  mitochondrial, interaction with nuclear genome, 385–386
  mutations of, frequency of disease due to, 152t

Genome(s) *(Continued)*
  nuclear
    interaction with mitochondrial genome, 385–386
    transcription of, 27, 30–31
    somatic, modification of, by transplantation. *See* Transplantation.
Genome database resources, 47–48
Genome hybridization, comparative, 55–56, 56f
Genome mutations, 175
  frequency of, 176t
  origin of, 176
Genome scans, 223
Genomic arrays, 66t
Genomic disorders, 96t, 97
Genomic imprinting, 38, 77–81, 78f, 79f
  Angelman syndrome as example of, 78–79, 80f, 80t
  Prader-Willi syndrome as example of, 78–79, 80f, 80t, 88f
  unusual inheritance patterns due to, 137–139, 138f, 138t, 319f
Genomic libraries, 45f, 45–46
Genotype
  correlation with phenotype, 121–122, 347
  definition of, 116
  phenotype related to, 347–348
  susceptibility testing based on, 491f, 491–492
Germ cells, transmission of genetic information by, 428
Germ layers, 428
  definition of, 426–427
Germline, 6
Germline mosaicism, 136–137, 137f
Giemsa banding, 60
Gilbert, Walter, 53
GJB2 gene, 254–255
Glioblastoma, loss of heterozygosity in, 470t
Glioblastoma multiforme, 463
ß-Globin gene expression, 33, 33f, 34f, 35–36
  developmental regulation of, 327–329, 329f
  initiation of transcription and, 35
  polyadenylation and, 36
  RNA splicing and, 35–36
α-Globin genes, deletions of, 333, 334f, 335, 335t
Globin genes, developmental expression of, 327
ß-Globin Glu6Val mutation, 308–309
Globin switching, 327, 328f
α-Globin/ß-globin deficiency, 312–313
Globoid cell leukodystrophy, treatment of, 408, 409
ß-Globulin mRNA, capping and tailing defects of, 340
Glucose-6-phosphate dehydrogenase deficiency, 264–265
  etiology and incidence of, 264
  hemolytic anemia and, 502
  management of, 265
  pathogenesis of, 264
  phenotype and natural history of, 264–265
Glucuronidation, polymorphism in, camptothecin toxicity and, 500, 501t
Glycosylation
  gains of, 325, 355–356
  loss of, 355–356

GNAS gene, 138t, 138–139
Gonad(s), embryology of, 99–100, 100f
Gonadal development, disorders of, 109t, 109–112, 110t
Gonadal dysgenesis, 109–110
G6PD gene, 264–265
Graves disease, HLA alleles and, 191t
Greig cephalopolysyndactyly, 420, 420f, 441
Growth, 427
Growth disorders, chromosome analysis in, 60
Guanine, 7, 7f
Gyrate atrophy, 202

H
Haploid cells, 13
Haploinsufficiency, 70
Haplotype(s), 116, 190, 190f
Haplotype maps (HapMaps), 216–217, 217f, 218f
    genome-wide, association analysis with, 225–226
Hardy, Geoffrey, 193
Hardy-Weinberg law, 193b, 193–199
    in autosomal recessive disease, 194
    factors disturbing, 195–199
        exception to large population with random mating as, 195–197
        exceptions to constant allele frequencies as, 196–199
    in X-linked disease, 194–195, 195t
Hb C, 330t, 332
Hb E, 330t, 340
Hb Hammersmith, 330t, 332
Hb Hyde Park, 330t, 333
Hb Kempsey, 325, 330t, 333, 347
Hb S, 329, 330t
    molecular pathology of, 331
    origins of, 331–332, 332f
HD gene, 276–277
Health Insurance Portability and Accountability Act, 525, 526
Hearing loss, 384t
    congenital, newborn screening for, 488
    inheritance risk for, 255
    nonsyndromic, 254–255
        etiology and incidence of, 254
        management of, 254–255
        pathogenesis of, 254
        phenotype and natural history of, 254
Heart disease
    congenital
        genetic and environmental factors in, 169–170, 170f, 170t
        protection against, by PCSK9 protease sequence variants, 363–364, 364t
    prevalence of, 452t
Hedgehog protein, 436
Hematopoietic malignant neoplasms, 461
Hematopoietic stem cells, 407
    from bone marrow, transplantation of, 407f, 407–408, 408f
    from placental cord blood, transplantation of, 408–409, 409f
Hemizygosity, 116
    X-linked inheritance and, 130
Hemochromatosis, 123
    hereditary, 266–267
        etiology and incidence of, 266
        inheritance risk for, 267
        management of, 266–267
        pathogenesis of, 266
        susceptibility testing for, 492

Hemochromatosis *(Continued)*
    HLA alleles and, 191, 191t
    major histocompatibility complex in, 189
    treatment of, 399
Hemoglobin
    developmental expression of globin genes and globin switching and, 327, 328f
    developmental regulation of ß-globin gene expression and, 327–329, 329f
    fetal, hereditary persistence of, 337
    gene dosage, ontogeny, and clinical disease and, 329
    Hb C, 330t, 332
    Hb E, 330t, 340
    Hb Hammersmith, 330t, 332
    Hb Hyde Park, 330t, 333
    Hb Kempsey, 325, 330t, 333, 347
    human hemoglobin genes and, 327, 328f
    monomers of, 332
    with novel physical properties, 330–332
    sickle cell, 329, 330t
        molecular pathology of, 331
        origins of, 331–332, 332f
    structure and function of, 326f, 326–327
    tetramers of, 332
    unstable, 332
Hemoglobinopathy, 329–342
    gene dosage, ontogeny, and clinical disease and, 329
    hemoglobin structural variants and, 329–333, 330t
        with altered oxygen transport, 332–333
        in hemolytic anemias, 330–332
        with thalassemia phenotypes. *See* Thalassemia.
    heterozygote advantage versus, 203–204
    thalassemia as. *See* Thalassemia.
Hemolytic anemias, 329, 330–332
    glucose-6-phosphate dehydrogenase deficiency and, 502
Hemolytic disease of the newborn, 188
Hemophilia, 268–269
    etiology and incidence of, 268
    fitness in, 135
    inheritance risk for, 269
    management of, 269
    pathogenesis of, 268
    phenotype and natural history of, 268–269
Hemophilia A, 131–132
    germline mosaicism and, 137
    mutation rate in, 181t
Hemophilia B
    gene therapy for, 416t
    germline mosaicism and, 137
    mutation in, 183
    mutation rate in, 181t
Hepatocellular carcinoma, aflatoxin and, 483
Hereditary angioneurotic edema, treatment of, 404
Hereditary cancer syndromes, 461, 463–464. *See also specific syndromes.*
    activated oncogenes in, 464–465
Hereditary hemochromatosis, 266–267
    etiology and incidence of, 266
    inheritance risk for, 267
    management of, 266–267
    pathogenesis of, 266
    susceptibility testing for, 492

Hereditary nonpolyposis colorectal cancer, 270–271
    caretaker genes in, 474–475, 475f
    etiology and incidence of, 270
    germline mutation testing for, 477–478
    inheritance risk for, 271
    management of, 271
    pathogenesis of, 270
    phenotype and natural history of, 270–271
Hereditary persistence of fetal hemoglobin, 337
Heritability, 158
    estimating from twin studies, 158
    studies of, 158–159
Hermaphroditism, 109
Hernia, diaphragmatic, prevalence of, 452t
Heterochromatin, constitutive, 62
Heterodisomy, 78
Heterogeneity
    allelic, 122
    clinical (phenotypic), 122
    locus, 122
Heteromorphisms, 61
Heteroplasmy, 381
    mitochondrial, 145–146
Heteroploidy, 65
Heterozygosity, 116
    loss of, 469–471, 470f, 470t
    recombination event detection and, 211f, 211–212, 212f
Heterozygote(s), 116
    compound, 116, 332
    manifesting, 130, 132–133
Heterozygote advantage, 199, 202–204
    drift versus, 203–204
    hemoglobinopathies and, 203–204
    malaria and, 203–204
Heterozygote screening, 493b, 493–494
Hex A pseudodeficiency alleles, 353
HEXA gene, 310–311
HFE gene, 123, 266
Highly discordant sibpair method, 223
High-resolution banding, 62, 63f
HIPAA, 525, 526
Hirschsprung disease, 122, 272–273, 438
    etiology and incidence of, 272
    genetic and environmental factors in, 162–163, 163f
    inheritance risk for, 273
    management of, 272–273
    pathogenesis of, 272
    phenotype and natural history of, 272
Histone code, 9–10, 77
HIV, resistance to, genetic factors in, 192–193, 193t
HLA, 189–192, 190f
    disease association and, 190–191, 191t
    tissue transplantation and, 191–192
HLA-DR3 gene, diabetes mellitus and, type 1, 164
Holoprosencephaly, 274–275, 436–437, 437f
    etiology and incidence of, 274
    inheritance risk for, 275
    management of, 274
    pathogenesis of, 274
    phenotype and natural history of, 274
Homeobox gene
    pattern formation and, 433–434, 434f
    synpolydactyly and, 435, 436f
Homocystinuria, 356, 356f
    newborn screening for, 488
    treatment of, 401, 401f

Homologous chromosomes, 6
  random assortment of, 20b
Homologous recombination, independent
    assortment and, 208f, 208–209
  of alleles at loci on different
      chromosomes, 208–209, 209f
  on same chromosome, with crossover in
      every meiosis, 209, 210f
Homologous structures, 423, 425f
Homologously staining regions, 478
Homologues, 6
  random assortment of, 20b
Homoplasmy, mitochondrial, 145
Homozygosity, 116
Host, definition of, 42
"Hotspots," for mutation, 178–179
Housekeeping proteins, 345–347
HOX gene
  pattern formation and, 433–434, 434f
  synpolydactyly and, 435, 436f
Human chorionic gonadotropin, in prenatal
    screening, 449, 449t
Human Gene Mutation database, 355–356
Human genome, 5, 6f, 6–13, 25–38
  chromosomes of. See Chromosome(s).
  DNA structure and, 7–8, 7f–9f
  gene expression and, 30–36, 31f, 33f,
      34f
    variations in, relevance to medicine, 38
  gene mapping and. See Gene mapping.
  gene organization and structure and,
      28–30, 29f
  gene regulation and changes in activity
      of, 36–38
  information content of, 25–26, 26f, 27f
  in meiosis, 20b
  organization of, 10, 12f, 12–13
  variation in, 116
Human Genome Project, 1, 25, 28
  comparative genome hybridization and,
      64f, 64–65
  DNA sequencing in, 54–55
  genome database resources and, 47–48
Human immunodeficiency virus, resistance
    to, genetic factors in, 192–193, 193t
Human leukocyte antigen, 189–192, 190f
  disease association and, 190–191, 191t
  tissue transplantation and, 191–192
Hunter syndrome, 133, 354t, 354–355
Huntington disease, 140t, 140–141, 141f,
    276–277, 387, 387f
  etiology and incidence of, 276
  inheritance risk for, 277
  management of, 277
  mutation in, 180
  pathogenesis of, 276, 389–390
  phenotype and natural history of,
      276–277
  slipped mispairing mechanism in, 388,
      388f
Hurler syndrome, 354f, 354t, 354–355
Hybridization, definition of, 42
Hybridization arrays, 66t
Hydatidiform moles
  complete, 81
  cytogenetics of, 81
  partial, 67, 81
Hydrops fetalis, 333
Hypercholesterolemia, familial. See
    Familial hypercholesterolemia.
Hyperlipoproteinemia, 360. See also
    Familial hypercholesterolemia.
Hyperornithinemia, with gyrate atrophy,
    202

Hyperphenylalaninemia, 348–351, 349f
  locus heterogeneity of, 348, 348t
  nonphenylketonuria, 350
  phenylalanine hydroxylase gene and,
      molecular defects in, 350f, 350–351
  phenylketonuria as, 349–350
    variant, 350
  tetrahydropterin metabolism defects in,
      351
Hypophosphatemic rickets, X-linked
    (vitamin D–resistant), 133–134
Hypothyroidism
  congenital, treatment of, 398
  newborn screening for, 488

I
I-cell disease, 355–356
Identity by descent, 124–125, 125f
Idiopathic cerebral vein thrombosis, 160
Iduronate sulfatase deficiency, 133
Immunodeficiency, severe combined, 403,
    410
  due to adenosine deaminase deficiency,
      gene therapy for, 416
  X-linked, gene therapy for, 415–416
Immunoglobulins, somatic rearrangement
    of, 36–38, 37f
Imprinting centers, 77
In situ hybridization, 66t
In vitro fertilization, preimplantation
    genetic diagnosis and, 430–431, 432f,
    433, 456, 508
Inborn errors of metabolism, vitamin-
    responsive, treatment of, 400–401,
    401f, 401t
Inbreeding, 125–126
  coefficient of, 124
  Hardy-Weinberg law and, 196–197
Incompletely dominant disease, 119
Independent assortment, homologous
    recombination and, in meiosis, 208f,
    208–209
  of alleles at loci on different
      chromosomes, 208–209, 209f
  on same chromosome, with crossover in
      every meiosis, 209, 210f
Index case, 116, 117f
Individual autonomy, respect for, 523
Infertility, chromosomally abnormal sperm
    in, 82
Inflammatory bowel disease, positional
    cloning of, by model-free linkage
    mapping, 227–228
Informative meioses, 212
Inhibin A, in prenatal screening, 449,
    449t
Inhibition, for metabolic abnormality
    treatment, 399
Inner cell mass, 428
  of blastocyst, 426
Insert(s), definition of, 42
Insertion(s), 177b
  of DNA sequences, 179–180
  small, 179, 181b
Insertion-deletion genetic polymorphism,
    184–186
  copy number polymorphisms and, 186
  microsatellites and, 185, 185f
  minisatellites and, 185f, 185–186, 186f
Insurers, use of genetic information by, 527
Interleukin-6, 503–504
Interphase, 10, 13
  fluorescence in situ hybridization in, 87f

Intrauterine growth restriction, 280–281
  etiology and incidence of, 280
  inheritance risk for, 281
  management of, 280–281
  pathogenesis of, 280
  phenotype and natural history of,
      280
Intron(s), 28
Intron mutations, 338
Isochromosomes, 66t, 71–72
Isodisomy, 78
Isolate(s), 196
Isolated cases, 118
Isoniazid therapy, N-acetyltransferase
    polymorphism and, 500–501, 501t

J
Joint probability, 512
Juvenile rheumatoid arthritis, HLA alleles
    and, 191t

K
Karyotype(s), 5
  human, 15–16, 16f–18f
    unbalanced, in liveborns, counseling
        guidelines for, 65b
Karyotype analysis, 59–60
Kearns-Sayre syndrome, 383, 384t
Kindreds, 116, 117f
Klinefelter syndrome, 81, 106f, 106–107
  follow-up observations in, 106t
  incidence of, 105t
Krabbe disease, treatment of, 408, 409

L
LCGR gene, 129, 129f, 130f
LD blocks, 216–217
LDL receptor, mutations in, familial
    hypercholesterolemia due to, 260–261,
    360–362, 361t, 362f
Leber congenital amaurosis, gene therapy
    for, 416t
Leber hereditary optic neuropathy, 146,
    147f, 384t
Leigh syndrome, 384t
Lentiviruses, as gene therapy vectors, 414
Leptotene, 17
Leukemia. See also specific types of
    leukemia.
  chromosome translocation in, 466t
Library screening, 47, 47f
Li-Fraumeni syndrome, gatekeeper
    tumor-suppressor genes in, 471f,
    471–472
Ligands, 436
Ligation, definition of, 42
Limb, as model of organogenesis, 440–442,
    441f
Limb buds, 441
LINE family, 13
LINE sequences, 180
Linkage, recombination frequency and, 212
Linkage analysis, 207, 217–222
  association analysis compared with, 226b
  determining whether two loci are linked
      and, 217–220
  in Duchenne muscular dystrophy, 519
  gene identification and, 226–229
    positional cloning of autosomal
        recessive disorder by model-based
        linkage mapping and, 226–227

Linkage analysis (*Continued*)
  gene identification and,
    positional cloning of complex disease
        and
      by genome-wide association,
          228–229
      by model-free linkage mapping,
          227–228
  model-based (parametric), for mapping
      mendelian traits, 217–220
  model-free (nonparametric), for mapping
      complex traits, 222–223
    of qualitative traits, 222–223
    of quantitative traits, 223
  phase in, 220–222
    phase-known and phase-unknown
        pedigrees and, 220f, 220–221, 221t
Linkage disequilibrium, 190, 213–216,
    214f–216f
  in cystic fibrosis, 227
  LD blocks and, 216–217
  measure of, 216
Linkage equilibrium, 213–216, 214f–216f
Linked markers, in molecular diagnosis,
    518–519, 519f
Liposomes, DNA packaged in, 414
Lissencephaly, 438
Live births
  chromosome abnormalities in, incidence
      of, 76
  in Down syndrome, 90–91
  unbalanced karyotypes in, counseling
      guidelines for, 65b
Liver transplantation, modification of
    somatic genome by, 409
Locus(i)
  distance between, recombination
      frequency as measure of, 209, 211,
      211f
  heterogeneity of, phenotype variation
      and, 348, 348t
  independent assortment and homologous
      recombination and, 208f, 208–209
    of alleles at loci on different
        chromosomes, 208–209, 209f
    of alleles at loci on same chromosome,
        with crossover in every meiosis,
        209, 210f
  map distances between, 212–213, 213f
  mutant, increasing gene expression from,
      404, 405t
  not affected by disease, increasing gene
      expression from, 404–405, 406f
  tightly linked, 212
  unlinked, 212
  wild-type, increasing gene expression
      from, 404, 405t
Locus control regions, 28, 35, 327–329, 329f
Locus heterogeneity, 122
LOD score method, 212, 218–223
  combining LOD score information across
      families and, 220, 220t
  nonparametric, 223
  parametric, 219
Long interspersed nuclear element family, 13
Long interspersed nuclear element
    sequences, 180
Long QT syndrome, 282–285
  etiology and incidence of, 282
  inheritance risk for, 283
  management of, 283
  pathogenesis of, 282
  phenotype and natural history of,
      282–283

Loops, of solenoids, 10
Loss of, symbol for, 66t
Loss-of-function mutations, 118–119
Loss of heterozygosity, 469–471, 470f,
    470t
Lowe syndrome, 421–422
LUC7L gene, 334–335, 335f
Lymphoblastoid cell lines, for cytogenetic
    analysis, 60
Lymphoid malignant neoplasms, 461
Lymphoma(s)
  B-cell
    diffuse, diagnosis of, gene expression
        profiling in, 480–481
    follicular, chromosome translocation
        in, 466t, 467
  Burkitt
    chromosome translocation in, 466t,
        466–467
    diagnosis of, gene expression profiling
        in, 480–481
  diagnosis of, gene expression profiling in,
      480–481
  hereditary, with loss of expression of
      proapototic tumor-suppressor genes,
      478
Lysosomal storage diseases, 351–355
  Tay-Sachs disease as. *See* Tay-Sachs
      disease.
  treatment of, 407–409
    hematopoietic stem transplantation for,
        407f, 407–408, 408f
    placental cord blood cell
        transplantation for, 408–409,
        409f

M
Macular degeneration, age-related,
    234–235
  etiology and incidence of, 234
  inheritance risk for, 235
  management of, 235
  pathogenesis of, 234
  phenotype and natural history of,
      234–235
  positional cloning of, by genome-wide
      association, 228–229
Major histocompatibility complex, 188f,
    188–192, 189, 189f
  class I, 189
  class II, 189
  diabetes mellitus and, type 1, 163–164
Malaria, heterozygote advantage versus,
    203–204
Male pseudohermaphroditism, 111–112,
    112f
Maleficence, avoidance of, 523
Male-limited precocious puberty, 129,
    129f, 130f
Male-to-male transmission, 133
Malformations, 420, 420f
  genetic and environmental causes of,
      421f, 421–422
Malignant hyperthermia, 502
Malignant tumors, 461. *See also* Cancer;
    specific malignant tumors.
Manic-depressive disorder, relative risk
    ratio for, 153t
Manifesting heterozygotes, 130, 132–133
Mannose-binding lectin, cystic fibrosis and,
    159
Map distance, 212–213, 213f
  sex differences in, 213

Maple syrup urine disease, newborn
    screening for, 488
Marfan syndrome, 286–287
  etiology and incidence of, 286
  inheritance risk for, 287
  management of, 287
  pathogenesis of, 286
  phenotype and natural history of,
      286
Marker chromosomes, 66t, 71
Maternal age, advanced, cytogenetic studies
    and, 60
Maternal inheritance, of mtDNA diseases,
    381
Maternal origin, 66t
Mating, assortative, Hardy-Weinberg law
    and, 196
MBL2 gene, genetic and environmental
    modifiers and, 159–160
McKusick, Victor A., 115
Mean, 156, 156f
Meconium ileus, 365
MECP2 gene, 134–135, 304–305
Medium-chain acyl-CoA dehydrogenase
    deficiency, 489–490
Medulloblastoma, spectral karyotyping
    analysis of, 86f
Meiosis, 16–20, 18f
  biological significance of, 22–23
  cytokinesis and, 19–20, 20f
  first division of (meiosis I), 17–19
    anaphase of, 19
    metaphase of, 18–19
    prophase of, 17–18
    telophase of, 19
  human, cytogenetic analysis in,
      81–82
  human genome in, 20b
  independent assortment and homologous
      recombination in, 208f, 208–209
    of alleles at loci on different
        chromosomes, 208–209, 209f
    on same chromosome, with crossover
        in every meiosis, 209, 210f
  informative, 212
  second division of (meiosis II), 20
Meiotic crossover, 17, 20b
MELAS, 384t, 385
MEN
  type 2A, 122, 183
  type 2B, 122, 183
Mendel, Gregor, 115
Mendelian disorders, cytogenetics in, 82,
    82f
Mendelian inheritance. *See* Single-gene
    inheritance.
Mendelian Inheritance in Man (McKusick),
    115, 323
Mendelian susceptibility to mycobacterial
    disease, 325, 355
Mental illness, genetic and environmental
    factors in, 170–171, 171t
Mental retardation, X-linked, 105
6-Mercaptopurine, efficacy of,
    polymorphism in, 501
MERRF, 145, 290–291, 384t
  etiology and incidence of, 290
  inheritance risk for, 291
  management of, 291
  pathogenesis of, 290–291
  phenotype and natural history of,
      291
Mesoderm, 426–427
  definition of, 427

Mesonephric ducts, development of, 100
Messenger RNA. *See* mRNA.
MET oncogene, 465
Metabolic abnormalities
    inborn errors of metabolism as, vitamin-responsive, treatment of, 400–401, 401f, 401t
    prenatal diagnosis of, biochemical assays for, 455t, 455–456
    treatment of, 396, 398t, 398–399
        depletion as, 399
        dietary restriction as, 396, 398
        diversion as, 398f, 398–399, 399f
        inhibition as, 399
        replacement as, 398
Metacentric chromosomes, 62
Metaphase, 59
    of meiosis, 18–19
    of mitosis, 15
Metastasis, 461
Methemoglobins, 333
Methionine synthase, loss of activity of, 357
Methylation, 179
5-Methylcytosine, 77
MHC. *See* Major histocompatibility complex.
Micro RNAs, 463
Microarray(s), definition of, 42
Microarray technology, 55, 85f
MicroRNA genes, 30
Microsatellites, 185, 185f
Migration, 427
Miller-Dieker syndrome, 288–289, 438
    etiology and incidence of, 288
    inheritance risk for, 288–289
    management of, 288
    pathogenesis of, 288
    phenotype and natural history of, 288
Minisatellites, 185f, 185–186, 186f
miRNAs, 463
Missense mutations, 179
Mitochondrial chromosomes, 10
Mitochondrial disorders, prenatal diagnosis of, 456
Mitochondrial DNA. *See* mtDNA.
Mitochondrial gastrointestinal encephalomyopathy, 386
Mitochondrial genetic bottlenecks, 146, 382–383
Mitochondrial genome, 145–146
    homoplasmy and heteroplasmy and, 145–146
    mutations in, maternal inheritance of disorders caused by, 146, 147f
    replicative segregation and, 145
    transcription of, 33
Mitochondrial inheritance, 144–146
    characteristics of, 146b
    homoplasmy and heteroplasmy and, 145
    maternal inheritance of mtDNA and, 146, 147f
    mitochondrial genome and, 145–146
    replicative segregation and, 145
Mitosis, 14–15, 15f
    biological significance of, 22–23
    phases of, 14–15
Mitotic spindle, 14
MLH gene, 474
MLH1 gene, 270–271, 476
MLH1/MLH2 genes, 468t
Model-free linkage analysis, 222–223

Modifier genes, 151
    phenotype variation and, 348
Molecular cloning, 41, 43f
Molecular cytogenetics, 63
Molecular genetic tools, 41–57
    for analysis of individual DNA and RNA sequences, 41–48, 43f
        genome database resources as, 47–48
        libraries as, 45–47
            complementary DNA libraries as, 46, 46f
            genomic, 45f, 45–46
            screening of, 47, 47f
        molecular cloning as, 41
        restriction enzymes as, 41, 43, 44f
        vectors as, 43–45
            expression vectors as, 46
            plasmids as, 44–45
    DNA sequence analysis as, 53–55, 54f
    for nucleic acid analysis, 48–50
        allele-specific oligonucleotide probes as, 49–50, 51f, 53b
        Northern (RNA) blotting as, 50
        Southern blotting as, 48, 49f, 50f
    polymerase chain reaction as, 50–52, 52f
        quantitative, 52, 53f
    using digital image capture of fluorescence-tagged nucleotides, 55–57
        comparative genome hybridization as, 55–56, 56f
        fluorescence in situ hybridization to chromosomes as, 55
        RNA expression arrays as, 56–57
    Western blot analysis of proteins as, 57, 57f
Molecular medicine, 399–416, 400f. *See also* Treatment, molecular.
Molecular phenotypes, 57
Mongolism, 90. *See also* Down syndrome.
Monoamniotic twins, 430
    definition of, 427
Monochorionic twins, 430
    definition of, 427
Monomers, of hemoglobin, 332
Monosomy, 67
Monosomy 11q, partial, fluorescence in situ hybridization of, 87f
Monozygotic twins, 153, 426
    definition of, 427
    twin studies of genetic environmental factors in disease and, 154–156
Morphogen(s), 429
    cell-to-cell signaling and, 435–437, 437f
    definition of, 427
Morphogenesis, 426, 427–428
    definition of, 427
Morula, 426
    definition of, 427
Mosaic(s), definition of, 427
Mosaic development, 430, 432
    definition of, 427
Mosaicism, 75–76, 135–137, 136f
    confined to embryo, 454f
    in Down syndrome, 92–93
    generalized, affecting fetus and placenta, 454f
    germline, 136–137, 137f
    involving several cells or colonies of cells, 454
    placental, confined, 81, 454, 454f
    prenatal cytogenetic diagnosis of, 453–455, 454f
    pseudo-, 454

Mosaicism *(Continued)*
    somatic, 136
    true, 453–454
mRNA, 27, 27f
    ß-globulin, capping and tailing defects of, 340
    nonfunctional, 338, 340
    nonsense-mediated decay of, 179
    reading frame of, 32
    synthesis of, 28
    translation and, 30
    translation of, 31–32
MSH2 gene, 474, 476
MSH6 gene, 474
mtDNA
    deletions in, autosomally transmitted, 386
    diseases of, 381–387
        genetics of, 381, 382f
        mtDNA mutations and, 381–383, 383f, 384t
        phenotypes of, 383, 385–387
            interactions between mitochondrial and nuclear genomes and, 385–386
            modification by nuclear gene, 386–387
            mutations in tRNA and rRNA genes of mitochondrial genome and, 385, 386f
            oxidative phosphorylation and, 383, 385
            unexplained and unexpected, 385
    maternal inheritance of, 146, 147f
mtDNA depletion syndrome, 386
Mucopolysaccharidoses, 354f, 354t, 354–355
Multifactorial disorders, 151–173, 152t. *See also specific disorders.*
    congenital, 166t, 166–170
    examples of, with known genetic and environmental factors, 160–173
    genetic and environmental modifiers of, 159–160
    limitations of studies of, 158–159
    positional cloning of
        by genome-wide association, 228–229
        by model-free linkage mapping, 227–228
    prenatal diagnosis of, ultrasonography for, 451, 453
    qualitative traits of, genetic analysis of, 152–153
        of concordance and discordance, 152
        of familial aggregation, measurement of, 152–153, 153t
    quantitative traits of, genetic analysis of, 156–158
        of familial aggregation, 157f, 157–158
        heritability and, 158
        normal distribution and, 156, 156f
        normal range and, 156–157
    recurrence risk for, genetic counseling for, 519–520
    relative contributions of genes and environment to
        of concordance and allele sharing among relatives, 153–154, 154f, 154t
        determining, 153–156
        twin studies for, 154–156
        unrelated family member controls for, 154
    treatment of, 393–394, 394t

Multifactorial inheritance, 2, 124. *See also* Multifactorial disorders; *specific disorders.*
  characteristics of, 159b
  frequency of disease due to, 152t
  genetic counseling and, 173b
Multigenic effects, 151
Multiple endocrine adenomatosis, type 2, 464–465
  clonality and tissue specificity of, 465
Multiple endocrine neoplasia
  type 2A, 122, 183
  type 2B, 122, 183
Multiple sclerosis
  case-control studies of, 153
  HLA alleles and, 191t
  relative risk ratio for, 153t
Multiplex testing, 494
Multipotent cells, definition of, 427
Muscular dystrophy
  Becker, 368–372
    clinical phenotype of, 368, 369f
    inheritance of, 368
  Duchenne, 256–257
    fitness in, 135
    germline mosaicism and, 137
    X inactivation and, 130, 131f
  oculopharyngeal, 139
Mutagens, 176
Mutant alleles, 116
Mutant gene products, dominant, reducing expression of, 405
Mutant locus(i), increasing gene expression from, 404, 405t
Mutation(s), 175–177. *See also specific mutations.*
  cancer and, 462–463
  chromosome, 175
    frequency of, 176t
    origin of, 176
  definition of, 116
  deletions as, 177b
  direct determination of, 516–518
  dynamic, 180, 387
  fitness and, 118
    in autosomal dominant inheritance, 129
  frameshift, 180
  frequency of, 176t
  gene, 175–176
    frequency of, 176t
    origin of, 176–177, 177f
  genome, 175
    frequency of, 176t
    origin of, 176
  insertional metaplasia causing malignant neoplasia and, 414–415
  insertions as, 177b
  intron, 338
  missense, 179
  molecular analysis of, 53b
  new
    in autosomal disorders, 126
    in autosomal dominant inheritance, 128–129
    in X-linked disorders, 135
  nomenclature for, 180, 181b
  nonsense (chain termination), 179
  origin of, 176–177, 177f
  point (nucleotide substitutions), 177b
    chain termination mutations as, 178
    "hotspots" of mutation and, 178–179
    missense mutations as, 178
    RNA processing mutations as, 178

Mutation(s) *(Continued)*
  protein function and, 323–325, 324f
    gain-of-function, 324–325
    loss-of-function, 323–324
    mutations associated with heterochronic or ectopic gene expression and, 325
    novel property mutations and, 325
  rates of
    in humans, estimates of, 180–182, 181t
    sex differences in, 182f, 182–183
  RNA processing, 179
  selection and, Hardy-Weinberg law and, 197–199
  selectively neutral, 183
  somatic, 176
  splice junction, 338
  synonymous, 338
MYCN gene, 478–479
Mycobacterial infection, mendelian susceptibility to, 325, 355
Myelodysplasia, associated with α-thalassemia, 336
Myoclonic epilepsy with ragged-red fibers, 290–291
  etiology and incidence of, 290
  inheritance risk for, 291
  management of, 291
  pathogenesis of, 290–291
  phenotype and natural history of, 291
Myotonic dystrophy, 140t, 143, 143f
  congenital, 139, 140t
  pathogenesis of, 389
  population differences in incidence, gene frequency, and heterozygote frequency for, 201t
  unstable repeat expansions and trinucleotide sequence in, 387, 387f, 388

N
Naked DNA, 414
Narcolepsy, HLA alleles and, 191t
NARP syndrome, 384t
Negative correlation, 157
Negative predictive value, 487
Neonates. *See* Newborns.
Neoplasia, 461. *See also* Cancer; *specific neoplasias.*
  chromosome analysis in, 60
  malignant, insertional metaplasia causing, 414–415
Neoplasm(s), 461. *See also* Cancer; *specific neoplasias.*
Neural tube defects
  folic acid and, 168
  prenatal screening for, 447–448, 448f, 448t
  prevention of, 168, 448
Neuroblastoma, 478–479
Neurocristopathy, 272–273
  etiology and incidence of, 272
  inheritance risk for, 273
  management of, 272–273
  pathogenesis of, 272
  phenotype and natural history of, 272
Neurodegenerative diseases, 377–390
  Alzheimer disease as. *See* Alzheimer disease.
  due to expansion of unstable repeat sequences, 387f, 387–390, 388f
  pathogenesis of, 388–390
  of mtDNA. *See* mtDNA, diseases of.

Neurofibromatosis, 96t
  segmental, 136
  type 1, 292–293
    etiology and incidence of, 292
    gatekeeper tumor-suppressor genes in, 472
    inheritance risk for, 293
    management of, 293
    mutation rate in, 180–181, 181t
    pathogenesis of, 292
    penetrance and expressivity and, 119f, 119–120, 120f
    phenotype and natural history of, 292–293
    somatic mosaicism and, 136
Neuromas, in multiple endocrine adenomatosis, type 2, 464
Nevoid basal cell carcinoma syndrome, 442
Newborns
  death of, chromosome analysis in, 60
  hemolytic disease of, 188
  screening of, 488t, 488–490
    for phenylketonuria, 349, 488
    tandem mass spectroscopy for, 489t, 489–490
NF1 gene, 120, 120f, 292–293
NOD2 gene, 250–251
  cloning of, 227–228
Noncoding RNA(s), 463
  expression profiling of, 482
Noncoding RNA genes, 30
Nondisjunction, 67–68, 68f
Nonparametric linkage analysis, 222–223
Nonparametric LOD score, 223
Nonprocessed pseudogenes, 30
Nonrecombinant chromosomes, 209
Nonsense codons, 32
Nonsense-mediated mRNA decay, 179, 340
Nonsense mutations, 179
Nonsyndromic cleft lip/palate, 168, 169
Normal distribution, 156, 156f
Normal range, 156–157
Northern blotting, 50
  definition of, 42
Novel property mutations, 325
Nuchal edema, prevalence of, 452t
Nuchal translucency, 449, 449f
Nuclear transplantation, modification of somatic genome by, 406–407
Nucleic acid hybridization probes, library screening by, 47, 47f
Nucleic acids, molecular genetic tools for analysis of, 48–50
  allele-specific oligonucleotide probes as, 49–50, 51f, 53b
  Northern (RNA) blotting as, 50
  Southern blotting as, 48, 49f, 50f
Nucleosomes, 9
Nucleotide substitutions, 177b
  chain termination mutations as, 178
  "hotspots" of mutation and, 178–179
  missense mutations as, 178
  RNA processing mutations as, 178
Nurse geneticists, 509

O
Oculopharyngeal muscular dystrophy, 139
Odds ratio, 224
Oligonucleotide(s) (oligonucleotide clones), 47
  definition of, 42
  microarray of, 85f

Oligonucleotide probes, allele-specific, 49–50, 51f, 53b
Oncogenes, 325, 462b, 464f, 464–467
    activated
        activation by chromosome translocation, 465t, 465–467, 466f, 466t
        in hereditary cancer syndromes, 464–465
        in sporadic cancer, 465–467
        telomerase as, 467
Oncogenesis, 461
Oncomirs, 463
Ontogeny, hemoglobinopathies and, 329
Oocytes, primary, 21–22
Oogenesis, 21–22, 22f
Optic neuropathy, hereditary, Leber, 146, 147f, 384t
Organ transplantation, HLA alleles and, 191–192
Organogenesis, 426, 428
    definition of, 427
    limb as model of, 440–442, 441f
Origins, of DNA replication, 14
Ornithine transcarbamylase deficiency, 296–297
    etiology and incidence of, 296
    inheritance risk for, 297
    management of, 297
    pathogenesis of, 296
    phenotype and natural history of, 296–297
Osteogenesis imperfecta, 136
    clinical management of, 376
    collagen structural genes in, 372–373, 372f–374f, 373t, 375–377
    genetics of, 375–376
    germline mosaicism and, 137, 137f
    molecular abnormalities of collagen in, 375, 376f
    novel forms of, 375
    prenatal diagnosis of, 376
Osteosarcoma(s), loss of heterozygosity in, 470t
OTC gene, 296–297
Ovarian cancer
    hereditary, 242–243
        etiology and incidence of, 242
        inheritance risk for, 243
        management of, 243
        pathogenesis of, 242
        phenotype and natural history of, 242
    loss of gatekeeper and caretaker function in, 476
Ovarian failure, premature, 110, 142
Ovarian teratomas, cytogenetics of, 81
Ovum(a), 22
    donated, to avoid genetic disease recurrence, 508
Oxygen transport, altered, hemoglobin variants with, 329

P
p arm, of chromosomes, 16
Pachytene, 18, 19f
Palindromes, 43
Pallister-Hall syndrome, 441
Pallister-Killian syndrome, 71
Paracentric chromosome inversions, 72–73
Paralysis, postoperative, cholinesterase polymorphism and, 501–502
Paramesonephric ducts, development of, 100
Parental transmission bias, 139

Parent-of-origin effects, 77–81
    confined placental mosaicism and, 81
    genomic imprinting and, 77–81, 78f, 79f
    hydatidiform mole and ovarian teratoma cytogenetics and, 81
Parkinson disease, 383
Paternal origin, 66t
Pattern formation, 433–434, 434f
PCR. See Polymerase chain reaction.
PCSK9 protease
    familial hypercholesterolemia and, 361t, 362–364
    protection against congenital heart disease by, 363–364, 364t
Pearson syndrome, 384t
Pedigrees, 116, 117f, 118
    medical history and, 146–147
    patterns of, 119–121
        age at onset as, 120–121
        penetrance and expressivity as, 119–120, 119f–121f
        phase determination from, 221–222
        phase-known, 221
        phase-known and phase-unknown, linkage analysis and, 220f, 220–221, 221t
        unusual inheritance patterns due to genomic imprinting and, 137–139, 138f, 138t, 319f
Penetrance, 119–120, 119f–121f
    incomplete, conditional probability in disorders with, 515–516, 516f
    reduced, 119
Pericentric chromosome inversions, 73, 73f
Permission to warn, 525–527
Personalized genetic medicine, 485–494
    ethnicity and race in, 504–505
    family history as, 485–487, 486f
    genetic screening and, 487–490
        clinical validity and utility of, 487
        of newborns, 488t, 488–490
        prenatal, 490
    screening for genetic susceptibility to disease and, 490–494
        based on genotype, 491f, 491–492
        clinical utility of, 492–493
        genetic epidemiology and, 490b, 490–491
        heterozygote screening as, 493b, 493–494
Pfeiffer syndrome, mutation in, 183
Pharmacodynamics, 497
    variation in both pharmacokinetic and pharmacodynamic response and, 502–503
    variation in pharmacodynamic response and, 502
        glucose-6-phosphate dehydrogenase deficiency and hemolytic anemia and, 502
        malignant hyperthermia and, 502
Pharmacogenetics, 497–504
    genotypic risk for adverse outcomes after cardiothoracic surgery and, 503–504
    variation in both pharmacokinetic and pharmacodynamic response and, 502–503
    variation in pharmacodynamic response and, 502
        glucose-6-phosphate dehydrogenase deficiency and hemolytic anemia and, 502
        malignant hyperthermia and, 502

Pharmacogenetics (Continued)
    variation in pharmacokinetic response and, 497–502
        cytochrome P450 and, 497–500, 498f–500f, 499t
        in phase II metabolism, 500–502
Pharmacogenomics, 504
Pharmacokinetics, 497
    variation in both pharmacokinetic and pharmacodynamic response and, 502–503
    variation in pharmacokinetic response and, 497–502
        cytochrome P450 and, 497–500, 498f–500f, 499t
        in phase II metabolism, 500–502
Phase, recombination event detection and, 211f, 211–212, 212f
Phase-known pedigrees, 221
Phenocopies, 152, 356–357
Phenotypes, 2. See also specific disorders.
    clinical, therapy directed at, 396
    definition of, 116
    genotype correlation with, 121–122
    genotype related to, 347–348
    molecular, 57
    replication error positive, 474–475
    sex-limited, in autosomal dominant disease, 129, 129f, 130f
Phenotypic heterogeneity, 122
Phenotypic threshold effect, 385
Phenotypic variance, 156, 156f
Phenylalanine hydroxylase gene, molecular defects in, in hyperphenylalaninemias, 350f, 350–351
Phenylketonuria, 324, 346–347
    classic, 349
    compound heterozygotes in, 350
    Hardy-Weinberg law in, 194
    maternal, 351
    mutation causing, 197
    newborn screening for, 349, 488
    population differences in incidence, gene frequency, and heterozygote frequency for, 201t
    tetrahydropterin metabolism defects in, 351
    variant, 350
Philadelphia chromosome, 466
Phosphorylation, oxidative, mtDNA diseases and, 383, 385
PKD1/PKD2 genes, 298–299
PKU. See Phenylketonuria.
Placental artery thrombosis, 161
Placental cord blood cell transplantation, for lysosomal storage diseases, 408–409, 409f
Placental mosaicism, confined, 81
Plasmids, as vectors, 44–45
Pleiotropic gene expression, 116
Pleiotropy, 422, 423f, 424f
PMP22 gene, 244–245
Point mutations, 177b
    chain termination mutations as, 178
    "hotspots" of mutation and, 178–179
    missense mutations as, 178
    RNA processing mutations as, 178
Polyadenylation, 36
Polycystic kidney disease, 437–438
    autosomal dominant, 298–299
        etiology and incidence of, 298
        inheritance risk for, 299
        management of, 298–299

Polycystic kidney disease *(Continued)*
    autosomal dominant
        pathogenesis of, 298
        phenotype and natural history of, 298
    type 1, mutation rate in, 181t
Polydactyly, 420, 420f
Polygenic effects, 151
Polyglutamine disorders, 140–142
    Huntington disease as, 140t, 140–141,
        141f
    spinobulbar muscular atrophy as, 142
Polymerase chain reaction, 41, 50–52, 52f
    definition of, 42
    quantitative, 52, 53f
        definition of, 42
    reverse transcriptase, 51–52
Polymorphisms, 116, 183–184
    N-acetyltransferase, isoniazid therapy
        and, 500–501, 501t
    cholinesterase, prolonged postoperative
        paralysis and, 501–502
    in DNA
        insertion-deletion, 184–186
            copy number polymorphisms and,
                186
            microsatellites and, 185, 185f
            minisatellites and, 185f, 185–186,
                186f
        single nucleotide, 184
    in glucuronidation, camptothecin toxicity
        and, 500, 501t
    in populations. *See* Population genetics.
    in proteins, inherited variation and,
        186–192
        blood groups and, 187–188
        major histocompatibility complex and,
            188f, 188–192, 189f
    in thiopurine methyltransferase and 6-
        mercaptopurine efficacy, 501
Population genetics, 192–199
    of *CFTR* gene, 367
    ethnic differences in genetic disease
        frequency and, 199–204, 201t
        genetic drift and, 200–202
            founder effect and, 201–202, 202f
        heterozygote advantage and, 101–104
        Hardy-Weinberg law and, 193–194,
            194t
            in autosomal recessive disease, 194
            factors disturbing Hardy-Weinberg
                equilibrium and, 195–199
            in X-linked disease, 194–195, 195t
        HIV resistance and, 192–193, 193t
    of Tay-Sachs disease, 353, 353f
Population stratification, 225
    genome-wide association and haplotype
        map and, 225–226
Positional cloning, 208
    of autosomal recessive disorder, by model-
        based linkage mapping, 226–227
    of complex disease
        by genome-wide association, 228–229
        by model-free linkage mapping,
            227–228
Positive correlation, 157
Positive family history, 153
Positive predictive value, 487
Posterior probability, 512–513
Postoperative paralysis, prolonged,
        cholinesterase polymorphism and,
        501–502
Prader-Willi syndrome, 96t, 300–301
    etiology and incidence of, 300
    genomic imprinting and, 137

Prader-Willi syndrome *(Continued)*
    genomic imprinting in, 78–79, 80f, 80t,
        88f
    inheritance risk for, 301
    management of, 301
    pathogenesis of, 300
    phenotype and natural history of,
        300–301
Predictive value, positive and negative, 487
Predisposition, to genetic disease, genetic
    testing for, 524–525
Pregnancy
    termination of, for disease prevention, 457
    in woman of advanced age, chromosome
        analysis in, 60
Pregnancy-associated plasma protein A, in
    prenatal screening, 449, 449t
Preimplantation diagnosis, 430–431, 432f,
    433, 456, 508
Premature ovarian failure, 110, 142
Premutations, 141
Prenatal diagnosis, 5, 443–458
    biochemical assays for, 455t, 455–456
    of cystic fibrosis, 367
    cytogenetics for, 453–456
    DNA analysis for, 456
    genetic counseling and, 458. *See also*
        Genetic counseling.
    methods of, 444–453, 445t
        invasive, 445–447
            indications for, 443–444, 444b,
                445t
        noninvasive, 447–453
    of multifactorial disorders, by
        ultrasonography, 451, 453
    of neural tube defects, 168
    preimplantation genetic diagnosis as,
        430–431, 432f, 433, 456, 508
    prevention and management of genetic
        disease and, 457–458
    risks of, 446
    screening tests for
        for aneuploidies, 448–450, 449f, 450f,
            450t
        for neural tube defects, 447–448, 448f,
            448t
        for segmental duplications or deletions,
            457
    of single-gene disorders, by
        ultrasonography, 451
    by ultrasonography, 450, 451f, 452f, 452t
Prenatal treatment, 457–458
Presenilin 1 and 2 genes, in Alzheimer
    disease, 378–379
Prevention, of genetic disease, 457
Primary chorionic villi, 446
Primary constriction, 16
Primary oocytes, 21–22
Primary spermatocytes, 21
Primers, for polymerase chain reaction,
    definition of, 42
Prior probability, 512, 513b
Privacy, of genetic information, 525–527
    duty to warn and permission to warn
        and, 525–527, 526b
    employers' and insurers' use of
        information and, 527
Probability
    conditional, 511f, 511–512
    in development, 425
    joint, 512
    posterior, 512–513
    prior, 512, 513b
Probands, 116, 117f

Probes
    chromosome "painting," 55
    definition of, 42
    nucleic acid hybridization, library
        screening by, 47, 47f
PROC gene, 316–317
Processed pseudogenes, 30
Progenitor cells, definition of, 427
Programmed cell death, 439
Proliferation, 427
Prometaphase, of mitosis, 15
Prometaphase banding, 62, 63f
Promoter regions, 28
Pronuclei, 22
Prophase
    of meiosis I, 17–18
    of mitosis, 14–15
Propositus, 116, 117f
Prostate cancer, loss of heterozygosity in,
    470t
Protein(s)
    augmentation of, 402
    biologically normal, mutations disrupting
        formation of, 325, 326t
    C-reactive, 503–504
    function of. *See* Protein function.
    G proteins as, 465
    housekeeping, 345–347
    informational relationships among DNA
        and RNA and, 27–28
    mutant, small molecule therapy to
        enhance function of, 400–402
    polymorphisms in, inherited variation
        and, 186–192
        blood groups and, 187–188
        major histocompatibility complex and,
            188f, 188–192, 189f
    post-translational processing of, 33
    receptor, defects in, 360–364
        hypercholesterolemia and, 360–364,
            361f, 361t
    specialty, 345–347
    structural, disorders of, 367–377
        in collagen structural genes, 372–373,
            372f–374f, 373t, 375–377
        dystrophin disorders as, 367–372
    Western blot analysis of, 57, 57f
Protein function
    altered
        due to abnormal post-translational
            modification, 355–356
        gains of glycosylation and, 355–356
        loss of glycosylation and, 355
    loss of
        due to abnormalities in cofactor
            metabolism, 356–357
        due to impaired binding or metabolism
            of cofactors, 356–357
    mutations and, 323–325, 324f
        gain-of-function, 324–325
        loss-of-function, 323–324
        mutations associated with
            heterochronic or ectopic gene
            expression and, 325
        novel property, 325
Protein scaffold, 10
Protein-DNA conjugates, 414
Proteome, 25
Prothrombin gene, 161
Proto-oncogenes, 462b
Pseudoautosomal inheritance, 135, 135f
Pseudoautosomal loci, 118
Pseudoautosomal region, of sex
    chromosomes, 99

Pseudodicentric chromosomes, 72
Pseudogenes, 30
    nonprocessed, 30
    processed, 30
Pseudohermaphroditism
    female, 110–111, 111f
    male, 111–112, 112f
Pseudohypoparathyroidism
    genomic imprinting and, 137–138, 138t
    type 1a, genomic imprinting and,
        137–138, 138f, 138t
    type 1b, genomic imprinting and, 138t,
        139, 139f
Pseudomosaicism, 75–76
Pseudopseudohypoparathyroidism, genomic
    imprinting and, 138
Psoriasis vulgaris, HLA alleles and, 191t
Pure dominant disease, 119
Purines, 7, 7f
Pyrimidines, 7, 7f

Q
q arm, of chromosomes, 16
Q banding, 60–61
21q21q translocation, in Down syndrome,
    92
Quadrivalent formations, 74f, 75
Quadruple screen, 449–450
Qualitative traits, in multifactorial
        disorders, genetic analysis of, 152–153
    of concordance and discordance, 152
    of familial aggregation, measurement of,
        152–153, 153t
Quantitative phenotype, 156, 156f
Quantitative polymerase chain reaction, 52,
    53f
    definition of, 42
Quantitative traits, of multifactorial
        inheritance, genetic analysis of,
        156–158
    of familial aggregation, 157f, 157–158
    heritability and, 158
    normal distribution and, 156, 156f
    normal range and, 156–157

R
R banding, 61f, 61–62, 62d
Race, in personalized medicine, 504–505
Radiation, cancer associated with, 483
Random assortment, of homologues, 20b
Range, normal, 156–157
Rare variants, 183
RAS oncogene, 465
RAS proto-oncogene, 476f
RB1 gene, 302–303, 468t, 468–471,
    475–476
Reading frame, 32
Recall bias, in case-control studies, 153
Receptor proteins, defects in, 360–364
Recessive disorders
    autosomal. See Autosomal disorders,
        recessive.
    selection in, 197
    X-linked, 198–199
Recessive inheritance, 118–119
    autosomal. See Autosomal inheritance,
        recessive.
    of X-linked disorders, 131–133, 132b, 132f
        in homozygous affected females, 132
        manifesting heterozygotes and
            unbalanced inactivation for X-
            linked disease and, 132–133

Reciprocal translocation, 66t, 74–75
Recombinant chromosomes, 209, 210f
Recombinant DNA, 4, 43
Recombination, 17
    deletions or duplications due to,
        179–180, 180f
    HapMap and, 217, 218f
    homologous, independent assortment
        and, 208f, 208–209
    of alleles at loci on different
        chromosomes, 208–209, 209f
    on same chromosome, with crossover
        in every meiosis, 209, 210f
Recombination frequency, 209, 211–213
    genetic maps and physical maps and,
        212–213, 213f
    heterozygosity and phase effects on
        detection of recombination events
        and, 211f, 211–212, 212f
    linkage and recombination frequency
        and, 212
    recombination frequency as measure of
        distance between two loci and, 209,
        211, 211f
Recurrence
    determining risk of, 509–516, 510f
        molecular genetics applied to, 516–519
            direct detection of mutations by,
                517–518
            linked markers in, 518–519, 519f
        when alternative genotypes are
            possible, 510–516
        when genotypes are fully known, 510,
            510f
    empirical risk of, 519–520
        of complex disorders, 519–520
        consanguinity and, 520, 520t
    managing risk of, 508
Red-green color blindness, Hardy-Weinberg
    law in, 194–195, 195t
Reduced penetrance, 119
5α-Reductase, 111
Reduction division, 16
Regulative development, 426, 430
    definition of, 427
    twinning and, 430–431, 431f, 432f, 433
Regulatory elements, 28
Reiter syndrome, HLA alleles and, 191t
Relative risk, 152, 224
Relative risk ratio, 152–153, 153t
Relatives, 116, 118. See also Familial
        entries; Family history; Pedigrees.
    allele sharing among, 153–154, 154f,
        154t
    concordance among, 153–154, 154f, 154t
Renal abnormalities, prevalence of, 452t
Renal aplasia, 425
Renal carcinoma, papillary, hereditary,
        clonality and tissue specificity of, 465
Repeat expansions, unstable, diseases due
        to expansion of, 387f, 387–388, 388f
    pathogenesis of, 388–390
Repetitive DNA, 10, 12–13
    disease and, 13
Replacement, for metabolic abnormality
        treatment, 398
Replication error positive phenotype,
    474–475
Replicative segregation, 146, 381
Reproductive cloning, 406–407
Reproductive compensation, 529
Reproductive system, embryology of,
    99–100, 100f
Repulsion, 211

RER+ phenotype, 474–475
Residual function, 347
Respect for individual autonomy, 523
Restriction endonucleases, 41, 43, 44f
    definition of, 42
Restriction enzymes, 41, 43, 44f
RET gene, 162–163, 163f, 464, 465
Retinitis pigmentosa, 122
    digenic, 160, 160f
    heterozygosity and phase in, 211–212, 212f
Retinoblastoma(s), 302–303, 324, 467–468
    etiology and incidence of, 302
    gatekeeper tumor-suppressor genes in,
        468–469, 469f
    inheritance risk for, 303
    loss of heterozygosity in, 469–471, 470f,
        470t
    management of, 302–303, 395
    mutation rate in, 181t
    pathogenesis of, 302
    phenotype and natural history of, 302
Retrotransposition, 30
Retroviruses, as gene therapy vectors,
    413–414
Rett syndrome, 134f, 134–135, 304–305
    etiology and incidence of, 304
    inheritance risk for, 305
    management of, 304–305
    pathogenesis of, 304
    phenotype and natural history of, 304
Reverse transcriptase, 46, 46f
Reverse transcriptase PCR, 51–52
Rh system, 188
Rheumatoid arthritis
    HLA alleles and, 191t
    juvenile, HLA alleles and, 191t
Ribonucleic acid. See RNA.
Ribosomal RNA, 27, 27f
Ribosomes, 27, 27f
Ring chromosomes, 66t, 71
Risk assessment, 509b
Risk figures, empirically derived, 151–152
Risk ratio, in relatives, 224
RNA, 27
    informational relationships among DNA
        and proteins and, 27–28
    messenger. See mRNA.
    noncoding, 30
        expression profiling of, 482
    Northern blotting and, 42, 50
    ribosomal, 27, 27f
    splicing of, 35–36
        alternative, 36
        medical significance of, 36
    structure of, 27, 27f
    synthesis of, 27
    transcription and, 30–31
    transfer, 27, 27f
RNA expression arrays, 56–57
    clinical applications of, 57
RNA interference, 405
RNA processing mutations, 179
RNA sequences, individual, molecular
        genetic tools for analysis of, 41–48, 43f
    genome database resources as, 47–48
    libraries as, 45–47
        complementary DNA libraries as, 46,
            46f
        genomic, 45f, 45–46
        screening of, 47, 47f
    molecular cloning as, 41
    restriction enzymes as, 41, 43, 44f
    vectors as, 43–45
        plasmids as, 44–45

RNA splicing, 30
  mutations of, in ß-thalassemias, 337–338, 339f
RNA viruses, as gene therapy vectors, 413–414
Robertsonian translocation, 66t, 72, 75
  in Down syndrome, 91–92, 92f
Robin sequence, 422, 424f
rRNA, 27, 27f
RT-PCR, 51–52
Rubenstein-Taybi syndrome, 422, 423f, 442
RYR1 gene, 502

S
S phase, of cell cycle, 14, 14f
Safer v Estate of Pack, 526
Sanger, Fred, 53
Sanger sequencing, 53–55, 54f
Sarcoma(s), 461
α-Satellite DNA, 12
  and heteromorphisms, 61
  and FISH, 63f, 64, 85f
Satellites, 62
Scaffold, protein, 10
Scheie syndrome, 354t, 354–355
Schizoaffective disorder, 172
Schizophrenia
  genetic and environmental factors in, 170–171, 171t
  relative risk ratio for, 153t
  velocardiofacial syndrome and, 171
SCNN1 gene, mutations in, 366
Second degree relatives, 116, 117f
Secondary spermatocytes, 21
Secondary villi, 446
Segmental aneusomy, 87f, 88f, 96, 96t, 144
Segmental duplications, 13
  prenatal screening for, 457
Segmental neurofibromatosis, 136
Segregation, replicative, 145, 381
Selection
  in dominant disorders, 197–198, 198t
  Hardy-Weinberg law and, 197–199
  in recessive disease, 197
    X-linked, 198–199
Semidominant disease, 119
Sense, DNS, 31
Sequences, definition of, 422
Severe combined immunodeficiency, 403, 410
  due to adenosine deaminase deficiency, gene therapy for, 416
  X-linked, gene therapy for, 415–416
Sex
  autosomal recessive disorders influenced by, 123
  determination of
    chromosomal basis of, 98–99
    fetal, 453
Sex chromosomes, 6, 98–109. *See also* X chromosome; Y chromosome.
  cytogenetic abnormalities of, 105t, 105–109, 106t
  pseudoautosomal region of, 99
  sex determination and, 98–99
Sex differences
  in map distances, 213
  in mutation rates, 182f, 182–183
Sex reversal, 306–307
  etiology and incidence of, 306
  inheritance risk for, 307
  management of, 307
  pathogenesis of, 306

Sex reversal *(Continued)*
  phenotype and natural history of, 306–307
Sex-limited phenotypes, in autosomal dominant disease, 129, 129f, 130f
Sex-reversed 46,XY females, 110
Sexual development, disorders of, 109t, 109–112, 110t
Short-chain acyl-CoA dehydrogenase deficiency, 490
SHOX gene, 135
Sibs, 116, 117f
Sibship, 116, 117f
Sickle cell disease, 122, 308–309, 323, 325, 330–331, 488
  clinical features of, 330–331
  etiology and incidence of, 308
  inheritance risk for, 309
  management of, 309
  molecular pathology of, 331
  origins of Hb S mutation and, 331–332, 332f
  pathogenesis of, 308
  phenotype and natural history of, 308
  population differences in incidence, gene frequency, and heterozygote frequency for, 201t
  sickling and its consequences and, 331, 331f
Sickle cell trait, 330
Significance, of disease associations, 224
Silencers, 28
Single-copy DNA, 10, 12
Single-gene disorders, 2, 116
  genetic and environmental modifiers of, 159–160
  prenatal diagnosis of, ultrasonography for, 451
  treatment of, 394f, 394–395, 395t
Single-gene inheritance, 115–147. *See also* Single-gene disorders.
  autosomal, 118
  conditions mimicking, 144
  dominant, 118, 119
  family history as personalized medicine and, 146–147
  genotype and, 116
    phenotype correlated with, 121–122
  mendelian, autosomal patterns of. *See* Autosomal *entries.*
  mosaicism and. *See* Mosaicism.
  mutations in mitochondrial genome and, disorders caused by maternal inheritance of, 144–147
  pedigrees and, 116, 117f, 118
    factors affecting, 119–121
      age at onset as, 120–121
      penetrance and expressivity as, 119–120, 119f–121f
      imprinting in, 137–139
      unusual inheritance patterns due to, 137–139, 138f, 138t, 139f
  phenotype and, 116
    genotype correlated with, 121–122
  pseudoautosomal, 135, 135f
  recessive, 118–119
  unstable repeat patterns and, 139–144, 140t
    fragile X syndrome and, 142, 142f, 143f
    Friedreich ataxia and, 140t, 143–144
    myotonic dystrophy and, 143, 143f
    polyglutamine disorders and, 140–142

Single-gene inheritance *(Continued)*
  unstable repeat patterns and, similarities and differences among disorders with, 144
  variation in genes and, 116
  X-linked. *See* X-linked inheritance.
Single-gene mutations, frequency of disease due to, 152t
Single nucleotide genetic polymorphisms, 184
  tag, genome-wide association and haplotype map and, 225
Sister chromatid(s), 14, 14f
Sister chromatid exchange, 82, 82f
Skewed inactivation, 133
Slipped mispairing, 139
Small-cell lung carcinoma, loss of heterozygosity in, 470t
Smith-Lemli-Opitz syndrome, 421–422
Smith-Magenis syndrome, 96t, 97
Smoking, carcinogenesis and, 483
Smooth chorion, 447
SNPs. *See* Single nucleotide polymorphisms.
Solenoids, 10
Somatic cells, 6, 6f
Somatic mosaicism, 136
Somatic mutations, 176
Somatic rearrangement, 36–38, 37f
Sonic hedgehog mutation, 274–275
Soto syndrome, 96t
Southern blot, 48, 49f, 50f
  definition of, 42
SOX9 gene, 110
Specialty proteins, 345–347
Specification, 429–432
  definition of, 427
Spectral karyotyping, 55, 85f
Sperm, 21
  chromosomally abnormal, in infertility, 82
  fluorescence in situ hybridization of, 86f
Spermatids, 21
Spermatocytes
  primary, 21
  secondary, 21
Spermatogenesis, 21, 21f
  Y-linked genes in, 100–101
Spermatogonia, 21
Spina bifida, genetic and environmental factors in, 166–168, 167f
Spinobulbar muscular atrophy, 142
Spinocerebellar ataxias, slipped mispairing mechanism in, 388, 388f
Spinocerebellar atrophies, 387
Splice junction mutations, 338
Split-hand deformity, penetrance and expressivity and, 120, 121f
Spontaneous abortions, chromosome abnormalities in, incidence of, 76–77
Sporadic cancer, 461–462
  activated oncogenes in, 465–467
    activation by chromosome translocation and, 465t, 465–467, 466f, 466t
    telomerase as oncogene and, 467
  loss of gatekeeper and caretaker gene function in, 475–477
Sporadic cases, 118
SRY gene, 100, 101f, 306–307
Standard deviation, 156, 156f
Stem cell(s)
  definition of, 427
  maintenance of regenerative capacity in tissues by, 428–429, 431f

Stem cell transplantation,
　　of bone marrow cells, 407f, 407–408,
　　　　408f
　　for lysosomal storage diseases, 407–409
　　modification of somatic genome by, 406,
　　　　407–409
　　in nonstorage diseases, 407
　　of placental cord blood cells, 408–409,
　　　　409f
Sterilization, to avoid recurrence, 508
Stickler syndrome, 422
Stillbirth, chromosome analysis in, 60
Stop codons, 32
　　mutant, small molecule therapy to allow
　　　　skipping over, 402
Stratification, Hardy-Weinberg law and,
　　　195–196
Submetacentric chromosomes, 62
Supernumerary chromosomes, 71
Susceptibility testing, 490–494
　　based on genotype, 491f, 491–492
　　clinical utility of, 492–493
　　genetic epidemiology and, 490b,
　　　　490–491
　　heterozygote screening as, 493b,
　　　　493–494
Synapsis, 18
Synaptonemal complex, 18, 19f
Syndactyly, 420, 420f
Syndrome, definition of, 422
Syndromic cleft lip/palate, 168–169, 169t
Synonymous mutations, 338
Synpolydactyly, 435, 436f

T
Tandem mass spectroscopy, 489t, 489–490
Tarasoff v the Regents of the University of
　　　California, 525–526
Target cells, for gene therapy, 411, 413
TATA box, 35
Tau protein, in Alzheimer disease, 377
Tay-Sachs disease, 126, 310–311, 347,
　　　352f, 352–353, 353t
　　etiology and incidence of, 310
　　hex A pseudodeficiency alleles and, 353
　　inbreeding and, 196
　　inheritance risk for, 311
　　management of, 310–311
　　pathogenesis of, 310
　　phenotype and natural history of, 310
　　population differences in incidence, gene
　　　　frequency, and heterozygote
　　　　frequency for, 201t
　　population genetics of, 353, 353f
T-cells, somatic rearrangement of
　　　immunoglobulins and, 36–38, 37f
Telocentric chromosomes, 62
Telomerase, 14, 467
Telomere(s), 14, 14f, 66t
Telophase, of mitosis, 15
Teratoma(s), ovarian, cytogenetics of, 81
Terminal, 66t, 70, 88f
Tertiary villi, 447
Testicular feminization, 111–112, 112f
　　incidence of, 105t
Testis-determining gene, 100, 101f
Tetrads, 18
Tetrahydropterin, metabolism of, defects
　　　in, in hyperphenylalaninemias, 351
Tetramers, of hemoglobin, 332
Tetraploidy, 65, 67
　　c, 65, 67
TGFBR2 gene, 475

Thalassemia, 312–313, 329, 333–342
　　complex, 337, 340–341, 341f
　　etiology and incidence of, 312
　　inheritance risk for, 313
　　management of, 313
　　pathogenesis of, 312
　　phenotype and natural history of,
　　　　312–313
　　public health approaches to preventing,
　　　　341–342
　　α-thalassemia as, 324, 333–336
　　　　deletions of α-globin genes and, 333,
　　　　　　334f, 335, 335t
　　　　forms of, 334–335, 335f
　　　　myelodysplasia associated with,
　　　　　　336
　　ß-thalassemia as, 324, 333, 336f,
　　　　336–340
　　　　complex, 337
　　　　simple, 337
　　　　　　molecular basis of, 337, 337t, 338f,
　　　　　　　　340
　　　　variant hemoglobins with thalassemia
　　　　　　phenotypes and, 340
ß-Thalassemia homozygotes, 347
Thalassemia minor, 336–337
Thalidomide syndrome, 426
Therapeutic cloning, 406
Therapy. See Treatment; specific diseases
　　and treatments.
Thiopurine S-methyltransferase
　　deficiency of, 314–315
　　　　etiology and incidence of, 314
　　　　inheritance risk for, 314
　　　　management of, 314
　　　　phenotype and natural history of, 314
　　efficacy of, polymorphism in, 501
Third degree relatives, 116, 117f
Thrombophilia, 316–317
　　etiology and incidence of, 316
　　inheritance risk for, 317
　　management of, 317
　　pathogenesis of, 316
　　phenotype and natural history of,
　　　　316–317
Thymine, 7, 7f
Thyroiditis, subacute, HLA alleles and, 191t
Tightly linked loci, 212
Tobacco use, carcinogenesis and, 483
Totipotent cells, definition of, 427
TP53 gene, 468t, 475, 483
TPMT gene, 314–315
Transcription
　　enhancers and, 35
　　initiation of, 35
　　of mitochondrial genome, 33
　　of nuclear genome, 27, 30–31
Transcription factors, 30, 35
　　gene regulation by, 435, 435f, 436f
Transcriptional regulatory molecules, 435
Transfer RNA, 27, 27f
Transforming growth factor ß, cystic
　　　fibrosis and, 159
Transitions, 179
Translation, 27, 27f
　　genetic code and, 31–32, 32t
　　post-translational processing of proteins
　　　　and, 33
Translocation, 66t
　　reciprocal, 66t, 74–75
　　Robertsonian, 66t, 72, 75
Transplantation, modification of somatic
　　　genome by, 405–410
　　liver transplantation for, 409

Transplantation (Continued)
　　nuclear transplantation for, 406–407
　　problems and future of, 410
　　stem cell transplantation for, 406,
　　　　407–409
Transport defects, 364–367. See also Cystic
　　　fibrosis.
Transversions, 179
Treatment, 393–416. See also specific
　　　diseases and treatments.
　　current state of, 393–395
　　　　for genetically complex diseases,
　　　　　　393–394, 394t
　　　　for single-gene diseases, 394f,
　　　　　　394–395, 395t
　　directed at clinical phenotype, 396
　　genetic heterogeneity and, 396
　　long-term assessment of, need for,
　　　　395–396
　　of metabolic abnormalities, 396, 398t,
　　　　398–399
　　　　depletion as, 399
　　　　dietary restriction as, 396, 398
　　　　diversion as, 398f, 398–399, 399f
　　　　inhibition as, 399
　　　　replacement as, 398
　　molecular, 399–416, 400f
　　　　gene therapy as. See Gene therapy.
　　　　at level of protein, 399–404
　　　　　　enzyme replacement therapy as,
　　　　　　　　402–404
　　　　　　protein augmentation as, 402
　　　　　　small molecule therapy treatment and
　　　　　　　　prevention of enhanced mutant
　　　　　　　　protein function as, 400–402
　　　　to modulate gene expression,
　　　　　　404–405
　　　　transplantation as, 405–410
　　　　　　liver, 409
　　　　　　nuclear, 406–407
　　　　　　problems and future of, 410
　　　　　　stem cell, 407–409
　　prenatal, 457–458
Trinucleotide repeat disorders, 183. See
　　　also Unstable repeat expansions.
Triple screen, 449–450
Trisomy, 67
Trisomy 3p, partial, fluorescence in situ
　　　hybridization of, 87f
Trisomy 13, 89, 94–95, 95f
Trisomy 16, 81
Trisomy 18, 64f, 67, 89, 94, 94f
Trisomy 21. See Down syndrome.
　　prenatal diagnosis of, 443–444,
　　　　445t
　　prenatal screening for, 448–450, 449f,
　　　　449t, 450t
Trisomy rescue, 454
Trisomy X, 107–108
　　follow-up observations in, 106t
　　incidence of, 105t
tRNA, 27, 27f
　　in mitochondrial disorders, 384f, 385
　　in mitochondrial genome, 382f, 386f
Tumor initiation, 462b
Tumor-suppressor genes, 462b, 467–479,
　　　468t
　　caretaker, 462b, 462f, 468t
　　in autosomal dominant cancer
　　　　syndromes, 472–475
　　in autosomal recessive chromosome
　　　　instability syndromes, 475
　　loss of, in sporadic cancer, 475–477
　　cytogenetic changes and, 478–479

Tumor-suppressor genes (Continued)
gatekeeper, 462b, 462f, 468t
in autosomal dominant cancer
syndromes, 468–472
loss of, in sporadic cancer, 475–477
proapoptotic, hereditary lymphoma with
loss of expression of, 478
testing for germline mutations causing
hereditary cancer and, 477–478
two-hit origin of cancer and, 467–468
Turner syndrome, 67, 81, 108f, 108–109,
318–319
etiology and incidence of, 105t, 318
follow-up observations in, 106t
inheritance risk for, 319
management of, 318–319
pathogenesis of, 318
phenotype and natural history of, 318
Twin(s)
conjoined, 432
dichorionic, 430
definition of, 426
dizygotic, 153–154
twin studies of genetic environmental
factors in disease and, 154–156
monoamniotic, 430
definition of, 427
monochorionic, 430
definition of, 427
monozygotic, 153, 426
definition of, 427
twin studies of genetic environmental
factors in disease and, 154–156
regulative development and, 430–431,
431f, 432f, 433
Twin studies
estimating heritability from, 158
of genetic environmental factors in
disease, 154–156
limitations of, 155–156
Two-hit origin, of cancer, 467–468
Tyrosinemia, type I, founder effect and,
201

U
Ulcerative colitis, positional cloning of, by
model-free linkage mapping, 227–228
Ultrasonography
prenatal diagnosis using, 450–453, 451f,
452f, 452t
chromosome analysis after, 453
for multifactorial disorders, 451, 453
for neural tube defects, 168
for single-gene disorders, 451
prenatal screening using, 449, 449f
Unbalanced inactivation, 133
Unconjugated estriol, in prenatal screening,
449, 449t
Unequal crossing over, 179, 180f
Uniparental disomy, 78
Unique DNA, 10, 12
Unlinked loci, 212
Unrelated family member controls, 154
Unstable repeat expansions, 139–144,
140t
fragile X syndrome as, 142, 142f, 143f
Friedreich ataxia as, 140t, 143–144
myotonic dystrophy as, 143, 143f

Unstable repeat expansions (Continued)
polyglutamine disorders and, 140–142
Huntington disease as, 140t, 140–141,
141f
spinobulbar muscular atrophy as, 142
similarities and differences among
disorders and, 144
Urea cycle disorders, treatment of, 398, 398f
Uveitis, anterior, acute, HLA alleles and,
191t

V
Validity
analytic, 487
clinical, 487
Variable expressivity, 119
Variable number tandem repeats (VNTRs),
185f, 185–186, 186f
Variance, 156, 156f
Variant(s), 65
rare, 183
Variant alleles, 116
Vas deferens
congenital absence of, 347
congenital bilateral absence of, 365
Vectors, 43–45
definition of, 42
expression, 46
for gene therapy
adverse response to, 414
nonviral, 414
viral, 413–414
plasmids as, 44–45
Velocardiofacial syndrome, 96t, 97–98,
170, 170f
fluorescence in situ hybridization of, 87f
programmed cell death in, 439
schizophrenia and, 171
Venous thrombosis, 160–162, 161f
Ventriculomegaly, prevalence of, 452t
VHL gene, 468t
Viral vectors, 413–414
Vitamin D–resistant rickets,
hypophosphatemic, 133–134
VKORC1 gene, 503

W
Waardenburg syndrome, 438, 440f
Warfarin therapy, genetic variation in
pharmacokinetics and
pharmacodynamics and, 502–503
Watson, James, 7
Webbing, of digits, 435, 436f
Weinberg, Wilhelm, 193
Western blot, definition of, 42
Western blot analysis, 57, 57f
Wild-type alleles, 116
Wild-type locus(i), increasing gene
expression from, 404, 405t
Williams syndrome, 96t
WT1 gene, 110

X
X chromosome, 7, 101–105
inactivation of, 101–105, 102f, 102t,
103b, 103f, 130, 131f

X chromosome (Continued)
inactivation of
nonrandom, 104f, 104–105
X inactivation center and XIST gene
and, 103–104
X inactivation, 101–105, 102f, 102t, 103b,
103f, 130, 131f
nonrandom, 104f, 104–105
skewed, 133
unbalanced, 132–133
X inactivation center and XIST gene and,
103–104
X inactivation center, 103–104
Xanthoma(s), cutaneous, in familial
hypercholesterolemia, 128, 128f
Xeroderma pigmentosum, 320–321
caretaker genes in, 475
etiology and incidence of, 320
inheritance risk for, 321
management of, 321
pathogenesis of, 320
phenotype and natural history of,
320–321
XIST gene, 103–104
X-linked disorders. See also specific
disorders.
dominant inheritance of, 131, 133f,
133–135
characteristics of, 133b
with male lethality, 134f, 134–135
Hardy-Weinberg law in, 194–195,
195t
lethal, conditional probability in, 514f,
514–515, 515f, 515t
new mutation in, 135
recessive, mutation and selection balance
in, 198–199
recessive inheritance of, 131–133, 132b,
132f
X-linked inheritance, 118, 129–135
X inactivation and, 130, 131f
X-linked mental retardation, 105
X-linked rickets (vitamin D–resistant),
hypophosphatemic, 133–134
XX males, 100, 101f
incidence of, 105t
XY females, 100, 101f
incidence of, 105t
47,XXX syndrome, 107–108
47,XYY syndrome, 107–108
follow-up observations in, 106t
incidence of, 105t

Y
Y chromosome, 7, 99f, 99–100
embryology of reproductive system and,
99–100, 100f
spermatogenesis and, 100–101
testis-determining gene and, 100,
101f

Z
α-ZF deletion, 334–335, 335f
Zone of polarizing activity, 436, 437f
Zygote, 13, 22
definition of, 427
Zygotene, 17–18, 19f